Clinical Obstetrics

Clinical Obstetrics

Edited by

Carl J. Pauerstein, M.D.

Professor and Chairman of Obstetrics and Gynecology
The University of Texas Health Science Center at San Antonio

Churchill Livingstone
New York, Edinburgh, London, Melbourne

Library of Congress Cataloging in Publication Data:

Clinical obstetrics.

(A Wiley medical publication)
Includes bibliographies and index.
1. Obstetrics. I. Pauerstein, Carl J., 1932–
II. Series. [DNLM: 1. Obstetrics. 2. Perinatology.
3. Pregnancy Complications. WQ 100 C6412]
RG524.C574 1987 618.2 86-19052
ISBN 0-471-89586-5

CONTRIBUTORS

Richard A. Becker, M.D.
Clinical Associate Professor
Department of Medicine
The University of Texas Health Science Center at San Antonio
San Antonio, Texas

Thomas J. Benedetti, M.D.
Associate Professor
Director, Division of Perinatal Medicine
Department of Obstetrics and Gynecology
University of Washington
Seattle, Washington

Michael D. Berkus, M.D.
Clinical Assistant Professor
Department of Obstetrics and Gynecology
The University of Texas Health Science Center at San Antonio
San Antonio, Texas

Jorge D. Blanco, M.D.*
Associate Professor
Department of Obstetrics and Gynecology
The University of Texas Health Science Center at San Antonio
San Antonio, Texas

Yves W. Brans, M.D.
Associate Professor
Departments of Pediatrics and Obstetrics and Gynecology
The University of Texas Health Science Center at San Antonio
San Antonio, Texas

* Present address: Memorial Medical Center, Savannah, Georgia.

Robert K. Creasy, M.D.
Emma Sue Hightower Professor and Chairman
Department of Obstetrics, Gynecology and Reproductive Sciences
The University of Texas Health Science Center at Houston
Chief of Obstetrics and Gynecology
Herman Hospital
Houston, Texas

John M. Davison, M.D.
Scientific Staff and Consultant Obstetrician and Gynaecologist
Medical Research Council Human Reproduction Group
Princess Mary Maternity Hospital
Newcastle upon Tyne, England

Jeffrey M. Dicke, M.D.
Assistant Professor
Department of Obstetrics and Gynecology
The University of Texas Health Science Center at San Antonio
San Antonio, Texas

Raymond A. Dombroski, M.D.
Assistant Professor
Department of Obstetrics and Gynecology
The University of Texas Health Science Center at San Antonio
San Antonio, Texas

Patrick Duff, M. D.
Assistant Director
Division of Maternal–Fetal Medicine
Department of Obstetrics and Gynecology
Madigan Army Medical Center
Tacoma, Washington

Dale R. Dunnihoo, M.D., Ph.D.
Director
Department of Obstetrics and Gynecology
E.A. Conway Memorial Hospital
Monroe, Louisiana
Professor
Louisiana State University School of Medicine
Shreveport, Louisiana

Robert D. Eden, M.D.
Assistant Professor
Department of Obstetrics and Gynecology
Division of Maternal–Fetal Medicine
University of Illinois College of Medicine
Chicago, Illinois

Sergio E. Fabro, M.D., Ph.D.
Director
Department of Obstetrics and Gynecology
Columbia Hospital for Women
Professor
Georgetown University School of Medicine
Washington, DC

Brent E. Finley, M.D.
Assistant Professor
Department of Obstetrics and Gynecology
University of Kansas Medical Center
Kansas City, Kansas

John I. Fishburne, M.D.
Professor and Chairman
Department of Obstetrics and Gynecology
The University of Oklahoma
Oklahoma City Campus—Health Sciences Center
Oklahoma City, Oklahoma

Jack FitzSimmons, M.D.
Assistant Professor
Department of Obstetrics and Gynecology
University of Wisconsin Medical School
Madison General Hospital
Madison, Wisconsin

Barbara Freeman, J.D.
Attorney-at-Law
Chicago, Illinois

Steven G. Gabbe, M.D.
Professor
Departments of Obstetrics and Gynecology and Pediatrics
University of Pennsylvania School of Medicine
Director of Jerrold R. Golding Division of Fetal Medicine
Hospital of the University of Pennsylvania
Philadelphia, Pennsylvania

C. E. Gibbs, M.D.
Professor
Department of Obstetrics and Gynecology
The University of Texas Health Science Center at San Antonio
San Antonio, Texas

Ronald S. Gibbs, M.D.
Professor
Director, Division of Obstetrics
Department of Obstetrics and Gynecology
The University of Texas Health Science Center at San Antonio
San Antonio, Texas

Martin L. Gimovsky, M.D.
Director, Maternal–Fetal Medicine
White Memorial Medical Center
Assistant Professor
Department of Obstetrics and Gynecology
University of Southern California
School of Medicine
Los Angeles, California

Guy M. Harbert, Jr., M.D.
Maime A. Jessup Professor
Director, Division of Maternal and Fetal Medicine
Department of Obstetrics and Gynecology
University of Virginia School of Medicine
Charlottesville, Virginia

C. R. Harmon, M.D.
Assistant Professor
Director, Fetal Assessment Unit
Department of Obstetrics, Gynecology and Reproductive Sciences
The University of Manitoba
Winnipeg, Manitoba, Canada

Dennis Horan, J.D.
Attorney-at-Law
Chicago, Illinois

Robert W. Huff, M.D.
Professor and Deputy Chairman
Department of Obstetrics and Gynecology
The University of Texas Health Science Center at San Antonio
San Antonio, Texas

S. Jason Kapnick, M.D.
Instructor in Gynecology
Harvard Medical School
Fellow in Gynecologic Oncology
Brigham and Women's Hospital
Boston, Massachusetts

E. Michael Kelly, J.D.
Attorney-at-Law
Chicago, Illinois

Nancy Wolfert Kirshenbaum, M.D.
Instructor in Obstetrics and Gynecology
Fellow, Division of Maternal–Fetal Medicine
New York University School of Medicine
New York, New York

Robert C. Knapp, M.D.
William H. Baker Professor of Gynecology
Harvard Medical School
Chief of Gynecology and Gynecologic Oncology
Brigham and Women's Hospital and Dana Farber Cancer Institute
Boston, Massachusetts

Mark B. Landon, M.D.
Fellow in Maternal–Fetal Medicine
Jerrold R. Golding Division of Fetal Medicine
Hospital of the University of Pennsylvania
Philadelphia, Pennsylvania

Oded Langer, M.D.
Assistant Professor
Department of Obstetrics and Gynecology
Albert Einstein College of Medicine of Yeshiva University
Belfer Educational Center
Bronx, New York

Leonard Laufe, M.D.
Professor
Department of Obstetrics and Gynecology
The University of Texas Health Science Center at San Antonio
San Antonio, Texas

Marshall D. Lindheimer, M.D.
Professor
Departments of Obstetrics–Gynecology and Medicine
The University of Chicago
Chicago, Illinois

Ian MacGillivray, M.D.
Emeritus Professor
Department of Obstetrics and Gynecology
University of Aberdeen
Scotland

Frank A. Manning, M.D.
Professor and Head
Department of Obstetrics, Gynecology and Reproductive Sciences
The University of Manitoba
Women's Hospital
Winnipeg, Manitoba, Canada

Irwin R. Merkatz, M.D.
Professor and Chairman
Department of Obstetrics and Gynecology
Albert Einstein College of Medicine of Yeshiva University
Belfer Educational Center
Bronx, New York

Warren N. Otterson, M.D.
Professor and Vice-Chairman
Department of Obstetrics and Gynecology
Louisiana State University School of Medicine
Shreveport, Louisiana

Stephen F. Pariser, M.D.
Clinical Assistant Professor
Department of Obstetrics and Gynecology
The Ohio State University
Columbus, Ohio

Tim H. Parmley, M.D.
Associate Professor
Division of Maternal–Fetal Medicine
Department of Gynecology and Obstetrics
The Johns Hopkins Hospital
Baltimore, Maryland

Robert M. Patterson, M.D.
Assistant Professor
Department of Obstetrics and Gynecology
The University of Texas Health Science Center at San Antonio
San Antonio, Texas

Carl J. Pauerstein, M.D.
Professor and Chairman
Department of Obstetrics and Gynecology
The University of Texas Health Science Center at San Antonio
San Antonio, Texas

Richard H. Paul, M.D.
Professor
Director, Division of Maternal–Fetal Medicine
Department of Obstetrics and Gynecology
University of Southern California
School of Medicine
Los Angeles, California

Edward J. Quilligan, M.D.
Professor and Chairman
Department of Obstetrics and Gynecology
University of California–Davis
Sacramento, California

I. Jon Russell, M.D., Ph.D.
Assistant Professor
Department of Medicine
The University of Texas Health Science Center at San Antonio
San Antonio, Texas

Rudy E. Sabbagha, M.D.
Professor
Department of Obstetrics and Gynecology
Northwestern University Medical School
Director, Diagnostic Ultrasound Center
Northwestern Memorial Hospital
Chicago, Illinois

Barry S. Schifrin, M.D.
Director of Maternal–Fetal Medicine
Medical Center of Tarzana
Tarzana, California

John W. Seeds, M.D.
Assistant Professor
Division of Maternal and Fetal Medicine
Department of Obstetrics and Gynecology
The School of Medicine
The University of North Carolina at Chapel Hill
Chapel Hill, North Carolina

Joe Leigh Simpson, M.D.
Professor and Chairman
Department of Obstetrics and Gynecology
University of Tennessee, Memphis
The Health Science Center
Memphis, Tennessee

Norman Talal, M.D.
Professor
Head, Division of Clinical Immunology
Departments of Medicine and Microbiology
The University of Texas Health Science Center at San Antonio
San Antonio, Texas

Darl E. Vander Ploeg, M.D.
Professor and Head
Division of Dermatology
Department of Medicine
The University of Texas Health Science Center at San Antonio
San Antonio, Texas

Bruce K. Young, M.D.
Professor
Director, Division of Maternal–Fetal Medicine
Department of Obstetrics and Gynecology
New York University School of Medicine
Chief, Obstetrical Service
Bellevue Hospital Center
New York, New York

Frederick P. Zuspan, M.D.
Richard L. Meiling Professor and Chairman
Department of Obstetrics and Gynecology
The Ohio State University
College of Medicine
Columbus, Ohio

To Marie Louise of the Irish eyes

PREFACE

This book arose out of the belief that none of the existing textbooks of obstetrics is a completely satisfactory guide to clinical practice. The text is intended to provide comprehensive coverage of the current practice of obstetrics. It will be useful to medical students, but it is designed to be most valuable to house officers and physicians actively engaged in obstetrical practice.

My colleagues and I concluded that a textbook of clinical obstetrics is approached best from the perspective of the clinician consulted by a pregnant woman because of a given problem or set of problems. Therefore, problems commonly encountered in practice are reviewed in depth. Areas of consensus and controversy are identified. Where consensus exists, it is stated. Where controversy rules, the conflicting views are presented, and the author's opinion as to the best managment is given without equivocation.

To achieve an authoritative text, it seemed advisable to ask acknowledged experts to write about their areas of special interest. Their contributions offer comprehensive, practical, and authoritative information about the clinical management of obstetrical problems.

In keeping with the clinical emphasis, certain chapters usually not found in textbooks of obstetrics were added. Among these additions are chapters dealing with induction and stimulation of labor, malignancy in pregnancy, management of shoulder dystocia, invasive cardiovascular monitoring, and medical–legal considerations.

Another goal was to make the book easily readable. To this end, I thoroughly edited each chapter, not to alter the information that the authors intended to convey, but rather to achieve uniformity of style.

The material is presented in 50 chapters, organized in six sections. Chapters 1 through 10 deal with aspects of normal pregnancy, labor and delivery, the puerperium, and the newborn infant. Chapters 11 through 14 deal with antepartum and intraparatum evaluation of the fetus. Individual chapters discuss clinical teratology, prenatal diagnosis of genetic problems, ultrasonography, and electronic and biophysical fetal monitoring. Chapters 15 through 26 are concerned with problems specific to pregnancy and labor, such as induction of labor, management of abnormal presentation, premature labor, postdate pregnancy, and abnormal labor. Chapters 27 through 42 discuss maternal illnesses in pregnancy, varying from vulvovaginitis to malignancy. Wherever applicable, the effects of the maternal condition on the pregnancy and the effects of pregnancy on the mother's condition are discussed fully. Chapters 43 through 49 are devoted to various aspects of operative obstetrics, including management of shoulder dystocia, invasive cardiovascular monitoring of acutely ill obstetrical patients, use of forceps and vacuum extractor, and management of puerperal hemorrhage. These chapters discuss operative techniques such as cesarean section, cesarean hysterectomy, and hypogastric artery ligation in detail, with step-by-step descriptions of the operative techniques. The final chapter, devoted to a discussion of medical–legal considerations, is written by members of a prominent law firm that specializes in defending physicians and hospitals in malpractice litigation.

Illustrations have been used liberally throughout the book to enhance the clarity of exposition. Drawings have been used to particular advantage in the descriptions of techniques and operative procedures.

I am most grateful to the contributors for their willingness to add this task to their already busy lives. I thank Ms. Cleteann Luce, my Administrative Assistant, for her untiring efforts in handling a multitude of details, communications, and other critical tasks during the entire preparation of the manuscript. My thanks also are due to Ms. Gretta Small, Editor in the Department of Obstetrics and Gynecology at The University of Texas Health Science Center in San Antonio, for her skills in editing and word processing, for her patience, and for her cheerful participation in preparing the manuscript. Ms. Herlinda Carreon, my Administrative Secretary, handled many onerous small chores during the review of galley and page proofs. I am indebted to Dr. Ronald S. Gibbs and Dr. Robert W. Huff of this Department of Obstetrics and Gynecology for their advice, support, and friendship. Special thanks are due Master John Stronge and Past Masters Kieran O'Driscoll, Declan Meagher, and Dermot MacDonald of the National Maternity Hospital in Dublin, Ireland, for allowing me to partake of their experience, knowledge, and gracious hospitality. I am grateful to Mr. Ray Moloney for encouraging me to undertake this effort. Finally, I thank Ms. Linda Turner, Ms. Elaine Kiang and Mr. Sidney Landau of John Wiley & Sons for their support of the project.

CARL J. PAUERSTEIN

San Antonio, Texas
December 1986

CONTENTS

PART I NORMAL OBSTETRICS

PART II ABNORMAL OBSTETRICS

SECTION A ANTEPARTUM AND INTRAPARTUM EVALUATION OF THE FETUS

SECTION C. MATERNAL PROBLEMS IN PREGNANCY

PART I

NORMAL OBSTETRICS

1

OBSTETRICS—AN OVERVIEW

Perhaps in very earliest times human babies were born with only their mothers in attendance, but the oldest traditions and records attest to society's interest in and assistance with birth. In some societies husbands attended, but in others they were excluded. Egyptian papyri 3500 years old give illustrated instructions for assistants during pregnancy and delivery. The Old Testament records activities of Hebrew midwives and ancient Hindu literature gives explicit instructions for diagnosis and treatment of various obstetrical phenomena.

Assistants at birth in Greece had to be mothers who were past the age of childbirth.[5] They were considered members of the healing profession and also cared for various gynecological problems. Roman practices were similar. Throughout the Middle ages, women giving birth were cared for by community women recognized for their interest and skills. The English name for these individuals is "midwife" with many local and ethnic terms. "Midwife" means "the woman (wife) with (mid)."

European physicians (always male) began to play a consultant's role in the delivery process during the 16th century. The Chamberlen family, through three generations in France, developed and kept secret the obstetrical forceps as a means of dealing with difficult deliveries. William Harvey, in England in the 17th century, published a book with a chapter entitled "De Partu," based on his observations as a consultant to the midwives of his day. Graham[5] calls this the first work on midwifery in English and William Harvey the "Father of British Midwifery." In the United States, the medical profession early on accepted the responsibility and role of the birth attendant, although midwives were commonly used in rural areas and urban ghettos.

The term *obstetrics* comes from a similar Latin word meaning midwife. Owsei Temkin, in *Williams Obstetrics*,[9] gives an interesting discussion of the possible origins of the term.

Both obstetrics and midwifery may be defined as that body of knowledge dealing with human reproduction.

Modern obstetrics as a branch of medicine considers preconceptional issues and deals with pregnancy from conception to the onset of labor (antepartum), during labor and delivery (intrapartum), and for an extended period afterward (postpartum). Obstetrics also has accepted research and clinical challenges related to family planning and population.

PURPOSES OF OBSTETRICAL CARE

The purposes of obstetrical care are to assure that:

- Each woman is in the best possible physiologic and psychological health at the time of conception.
- The gestation progresses with normal fetal growth and development and with good maternal health.
- Labor and delivery occur under the circum-

stances best suited for the conditions present at the time.
- Each newborn is "well born" in terms of its health and environment.
- Each mother recovers from the experience without sequelae.

The goal of obstetrical care often is expressed as "a healthy mother with a healthy baby." The American College of Obstetricians and Gynecologists has stated, "Excellence in maternal health care is the foundation for the physical, intellectual, social, and economic success of any society. It is the basic determinant of the health of future generations"[2]

DEMOGRAPHIC AND VITAL DATA

The number and health status of human births have great implication for all facets of local and national life. As a result, many data are defined and collected rather precisely by agencies of government, private business, and scientific organizations.

Live Birth and Stillbirth

All jurisdictions in the United States require the certification of a birth, living or dead, which results from pregnancy of 20 weeks' duration or longer. These Life Birth Certificates (Fig. 1-1) and Fetal Death (Stillbirth) Certificates (Fig. 1-2) may be signed by anyone who witnesses the birth and is willing to certify to it. Each certificate contains demographic and clinical information about the parents as well as the newborn or fetus. Most states issue annual reports based on the data from these certificates and cooperate with the National Center for Health Statistics in compilation of nationwide data sets.

Abortion

A termination of pregnancy prior to the 20th week of gestation is defined as an *abortion* (spontaneous or induced), and the product of conception is called an *abortus*. Certification is not necessary for these terminations in most jurisdictions, although some states may have a reporting system for induced abortions.

Birth Rate

For the past several years, between 3.4 and 3.8 million births have been certified in the United States. This represents a birth rate (number of births/100,000 population) of around 16 and a fertility rate (number of births/1000 women 15–44 years of age) of about 65. As recently as 1957, 4.3 million births were reported in the United States (birth rate of 25) with a correspondingly high fertility rate. The estimate for 1983 (Ref. 8, p. 2) is 3.6 million births with a birth rate of 15.5. These U.S. data are compared with estimates of other nations in Table 1-1.

Health Status Data

Various data sets are useful for evaluation of the health status of populations and of health care delivery systems.

Birth Weight. The weight at birth reflects duration of gestation and intrauterine growth, both of which are influenced by nutrition, complications of pregnancy, and the general health of women in the reproductive age. Limits of "normal" are 2500 g (5½ lb) and 4500 g (9 lb 15 oz). Abnormalities of birth weight are associated with increased likelihood of newborn death and long-term disability. Jurisdictions and population groups in the United States report rates of low-birth-weight infants (LBWI) ranging from 3.5 to 16/100 live births. The low-birth-weight rate sharply influences the outcome rates.

Neonatal Mortality. Neonatal mortality means the death within the first 28 days of life of an infant born alive. The rate is calculated per 1000 live births. The reported range in the United States is 6–15/1000, depending on population and institution.

Weight-Specific Neonatal Mortality. This term means the death of a live born infant within certain birth weight groupings. The rate is calculated per 1000 live born infants in that weight range. The weight-specific mortality at 1000–1250 g birth weight may be 450/1000 live births, whereas, between 2500 and 3000 g, it might be 4/1000 live births. The weight-specific neonatal mortality is often used to appraise the quality of care during birth and in the first few days of the newborn's life. It also is helpful in comparing data from one nation or city to another. The United States, for example, ranks tenth or eleventh among developed nations in overall neonatal mortality, but second in weight-specific neonatal mortality[6]—probably a

Form Approved
OMB No. 68R 1900

TYPE OR PRINT IN PERMANENT INK
FOR INSTRUCTIONS SEE HANDBOOK

U.S. STANDARD

CERTIFICATE OF LIVE BIRTH

LOCAL FILE NUMBER | BIRTH NUMBER

CHILD

CHILD—NAME FIRST MIDDLE LAST 1.	SEX 2.	DATE OF BIRTH *(Mo., Day, Yr.)* 3a.	HOUR 3b. M
HOSPITAL—NAME *(If not in hospital, give street and number)* 4a.	CITY, TOWN OR LOCATION OF BIRTH 4b.	COUNTY OF BIRTH 4c.	

CERTIFIER

I certify that the stated information concerning this child is true to the best of my knowledge and belief. 5a. *(Signature)* ▶	DATE SIGNED *(Mo., Day, Yr.)* 5b.	NAME AND TITLE OF ATTENDANT AT BIRTH IF OTHER THAN CERTIFIER *(Type or print)* 5c.
CERTIFIER—NAME AND TITLE *(Type or print)* 5d.	MAILING ADDRESS *(Street or R.F.D. No., City or Town, State, Zip)* 5e.	
REGISTRAR 6a. *(Signature)* ▶	DATE RECEIVED BY REGISTRAR *(Month, Day, Year)* 6b.	

MOTHER

MOTHER—MAIDEN NAME FIRST MIDDLE LAST 7a.			AGE *(At time of this birth)* 7b.	STATE OF BIRTH *(If not in U.S.A., name country)* 7c.
RESIDENCE—STATE 8a.	COUNTY 8b.	CITY, TOWN OR LOCATION 8c.	STREET AND NUMBER OF RESIDENCE 8d.	INSIDE CITY LIMITS *(Specify yes or no)* 8e.
MOTHER'S MAILING ADDRESS—*If same as above, enter Zip Code only* 9.				

FATHER

FATHER—NAME FIRST MIDDLE LAST 10a.	AGE *(At time of this birth)* 10b.	STATE OF BIRTH *(If not in U.S.A., name country)* 10c.
I certify that the personal information provided on this certificate is correct to the best of my knowledge and belief. 11a. *(Signature of Parent or other Informant)* ▶	RELATION TO CHILD 11b.	

INFORMATION FOR MEDICAL AND HEALTH USE ONLY

RACE—MOTHER (e.g., White, Black, American Indian, etc.) *(Specify)* 12.	RACE—FATHER (e.g., White, Black, American Indian, etc.) *(Specify)* 13.	BIRTH WEIGHT 14.	THIS BIRTH—Single, twin, triplet, etc. *(Specify)* 15a.	IF NOT SINGLE BIRTH—Born first, second, third, etc. *(Specify)* 15b.	IS MOTHER MARRIED? *(Specify yes or no)* 16.

PREGNANCY HISTORY (Complete each section)

LIVE BIRTHS *(Do not include this Child)*		OTHER TERMINATIONS *(Spontaneous and Induced)*	
17a. Now living Number ____ None ☐	17b. Now dead Number ____ None ☐	17d. Before 20 weeks Number ____ None ☐	17e. After 20 weeks Number ____ None ☐
DATE OF LAST LIVE BIRTH *(Month, Year)* 17c.		DATE OF LAST OTHER TERMINATION *(as indicated in d or e above)* *(Month, Year)* 17f.	

DEATH UNDER ONE YEAR OF AGE
Enter State File Number of death certificate for this child

MULTIPLE BIRTHS
Enter State File Number for mate(s)

LIVE BIRTH(S)

FETAL DEATH(S)

EDUCATION—MOTHER *(Specify only highest grade completed)*		EDUCATION—FATHER *(Specify only highest grade completed)*		
Elementary or Secondary (0-12) 18.	College (1-4 or 5+)	Elementary or Secondary (0-12) 19.	College (1-4 or 5+)	
DATE LAST NORMAL MENSES BEGAN *(Month, Day, Year)* 20.	MONTH OF PREGNANCY PRENATAL CARE BEGAN First, second, etc. *(Specify)* 21a.	PRENATAL VISITS Total number *(If none, so state)* 21b.	APGAR SCORE 1 min. 22a.	5 min. 22b.

COMPLICATIONS OF PREGNANCY *(Describe or write "none")*
23.

CONCURRENT ILLNESSES OR CONDITIONS AFFECTING THE PREGNANCY *(Describe or write "none")*
24.

COMPLICATIONS OF LABOR AND/OR DELIVERY *(Describe or write "none")* 25.	CONGENITAL MALFORMATIONS OR ANOMALIES OF CHILD *(Describe or write "none")* 26.

DEPARTMENT OF HEALTH, EDUCATION, AND WELFARE—PUBLIC HEALTH SERVICE—NATIONAL CENTER FOR HEALTH STATISTICS
1978 REVISION

Figure 1-1. Example of U.S. Standard Certificate of Live Birth.

Form Approved
OMB No. 68R 1901

U. S. STANDARD

REPORT OF FETAL DEATH

STATE FILE NUMBER

TYPE OR PRINT IN PERMANENT INK
SEE HANDBOOK FOR INSTRUCTIONS

HOSPITAL—NAME *(If not in ho~~ital, give street and number)* 1a. | CITY, TOWN OR LOCATION OF DELIVERY 1b. | COUNTY OF DELIVERY 1c.

DATE OF DELIVERY *(Month, Day, Year)* 2a. | HOUR OF DELIVERY 2b. M | SEX OF FETUS 3. | WEIGHT OF FETUS 4.

MOTHER

MOTHER—MAIDEN NAME FIRST MIDDLE LAST 5a. | AGE *(At time of this delivery)* 5b. | RESIDENCE—STATE 6a. | COUNTY 6b.

CITY, TOWN OR LOCATION 6c. | STREET AND NUMBER 6d. | INSIDE CITY LIMITS *(Specify yes or no)* 6e.

RACE—(e.g., White, Black, American Indian, etc.) *(Specify)* 7. | EDUCATION *(Specify only highest grade completed)* (Elementary or Secondary (0-12) | College (1-4 or 5+) 8. | DATE LAST NORMAL MENSES BEGAN *(Month, Day, Year)* 9. | IS MOTHER MARRIED? *(Specify yes or no)* 10.

PREGNANCY HISTORY *(Complete each section)*

LIVE BIRTHS: 11a. Now living Number___ None ☐ | 11b. Now dead Number___ None ☐

OTHER TERMINATIONS *(Spontaneous and Induced)*: 11d. Before 20 weeks Number___ None ☐ | 11e. After 20 weeks Number___ *(Do not include this fetus)* None ☐

DATE OF LAST LIVE BIRTH *(Month, Year)* 11c. | DATE OF LAST OTHER TERMINATION *(as indicated in d or e above)* *(Month, Year)* 11f.

MONTH OF PREGNANCY PRENATAL CARE BEGAN First, second, etc. *(Specify)* 12a. | PRENATAL VISITS—Total number *(If none, so state)* 12b. | THIS BIRTH—Single, twin, triplet, etc. *(Specify)* 13a. | IF NOT SINGLE BIRTH—Born first, second, third, etc. *(Specify)* 13b.

FATHER

FATHER—NAME FIRST MIDDLE LAST 14a. | AGE *(At time of this delivery)* 14b. | RACE—(e.g., White, Black, American Indian, etc.) *(Specify)* 14c. | EDUCATION *(Specify only highest grade completed)* Elementary or Secondary (0-12) | College (1-4 or 5+) 14d.

CAUSE OF FETAL DEATH

15. **PART I** Fetal or maternal condition directly causing fetal death. IMMEDIATE CAUSE *[ENTER ONLY ONE CAUSE PER LINE FOR (a), (b), AND (c).]* (a) | Specify Fetal or Maternal

Fetal and/or maternal conditions, if any giving rise to the immediate cause (a), stating the underlying cause last. DUE TO, OR AS A CONSEQUENCE OF: (b) | Specify Fetal or Maternal

DUE TO, OR AS A CONSEQUENCE OF: (c) | Specify Fetal or Maternal

PART II OTHER SIGNIFICANT CONDITIONS OF FETUS OR MOTHER: Conditions contributing to fetal death but not related to cause given in (a) | FETUS DIED BEFORE LABOR, DURING LABOR OR DELIVERY, UNKNOWN *(Specify)* 16. | PHYSICIAN'S ESTIMATE OF GESTATION 17. Weeks | AUTOPSY *(Specify yes or no)* 18.

MULTIPLE BIRTHS Enter State File Number for mate(s)

LIVE BIRTH(S)

COMPLICATIONS OF PREGNANCY *(Describe or write "none")* 19. | COMPLICATIONS OF LABOR AND/OR DELIVERY *(Describe or write "none")* 20.

CONCURRENT ILLNESSES OR CONDITIONS AFFECTING THE PREGNANCY *(Describe or write "none")* 21. | CONGENITAL MALFORMATIONS OR ANOMALIES OF FETUS *(Describe or write "none")* 22.

FETAL DEATH(S)

NAME OF PHYSICIAN OR ATTENDANT *(Type or print)* 23. | NAME OF PERSON COMPLETING REPORT *(Type or print)* TITLE 24.

DEPARTMENT OF HEALTH, EDUCATION, AND WELFARE—PUBLIC HEALTH SERVICE—NATIONAL CENTER FOR HEALTH STATISTICS
1978 REVISION

Figure 1-2. Example of death certificate that must be filed when a stillborn infant is delivered.

TABLE 1-1. WORLD POPULATION ESTIMATES—1983

Country	Number of Births	Population (millions)	Birth Rate (per 100,000)	Years to Double Population at Current Rate
Egypt	1.9 million	45.9	43	22
Israel	98 thousand	4.1	24	41
India	25.0 million	730.0	36	33
Mexico	2.4 million	75.7	32	27
United Kingdom	730 thousand	56.0	13	533
United States	3.8 million	234.0	15	95

Source: Ob-Gyn News, April 1–14, 1984.

more discriminant measurement of the medical care received.

Postneonatal Mortality. Postneonatal mortality indicates the death of an infant after the first 28 days, but within the first year after birth. This rate is calculated per 1000 live births and ranges from 5 to 10/1000 in the United States. Postneonatal mortality may reflect the quality of immunization, sanitation, and water supply, but also may contain deaths from neonatal causes postponed as a result of technological support systems.

Infant Mortality. This term designates the death of a live born infant prior to the first anniversary of birth (the sum of neonatal and postneonatal mortality). The rate is calculated per 1000 live births. Infant mortality is commonly used in evaluating societal development and general health status of population groups. In 1983, the infant mortality in the United States was 10.9 (Ref. 8, p. 5).

Fetal Death. Fetal death indicates the death of a fetus prior to birth (stillbirth). Most jurisdictions require the pregnancy to have completed 20 weeks' duration and the fetus to have attained a certain length or weight (25 cm crown heel, 500 g). The rate is calculated per 1000 live births.

Perinatal Mortality. This term means fetal deaths plus neonatal deaths. The rate is calculated per 1000 *total births*. The Perinatal Mortality rate is used as an index of the quality of obstetrical and newborn care. Fetal deaths and neonatal deaths often contribute equally to the perinatal mortality. Rates of 12–14/1000 total births are now being reported from some hospitals and jurisdictions.

Maternal Mortality. Maternal mortality means the death of a pregnant woman or of a woman who was pregnant within 42 days* before death. The causes of maternal death usually are classified as follows:

Direct Obstetrical. This indicates death due to an obstetrical disorder. The "big three" are hemorrhage (postpartum atony, ectopic pregnancy, abruptio placentae), pregnancy-induced hypertension (cerebral hemorrhage, cardiac failure), and infection (puerperal sepsis). Abortion-related deaths have decreased from 89 in 1972 to 16 in 1980.[1] Direct causes make up 60–65% of the maternal deaths in most studies.

Indirect Obstetrical. This indicates death resulting from previously existing disease or from a nonobstetrical disorder that developed during pregnancy, labor, or the puerperium, where the disease or disorder was aggravated by the physiologic effects of pregnancy. Common causes include pulmonary vascular embolus, cardiac disease, anesthesia complications, and cerebral hemorrhage due to vascular malformation.

Unrelated (Nonobstetric). These are deaths from disorders incidental to and not aggravated by pregnancy. Suicide, homicide, accidents, and carcinoma are the leading causes in this group.

The *Maternal Mortality Rate* is calculated by adding direct and indirect causes per 100,000 live births. The reported rate in recent years in the United States has been 8–10, but many maternal deaths are not identified.[4]

Maternal mortality rates have been used as an indicator of the quality of nutrition, sanita-

*Some jurisdictions and professional groups use periods of 90–180 days.

tion, water supply, and health services. In the United States, studies of individual maternal deaths often have great instructional value and have called attention to previously unrecognized syndromes such as septic shock and sepsis from IUD complications.

Maternal mortality rates increase after age 30, becoming, at 40, 5–6 times that of women aged 20–25.[4,11] These increases are associated more with indirect causes, such as cardiovascular and renal disease, than with direct events.[4,11]

Maternal, infant, and perinatal mortality rates in the United States differ among racial and age groups. For example, United States maternal mortality rates for whites have been one-fourth to one-half that of other races. Infant mortality shows a similar difference (Table 1-2). These differences are believed to be related to socioeconomic status as well as to access to health care and offer a continuing challenge to society and to the health care system of the United States.

PATTERNS AND TRENDS IN THE DELIVERY OF OBSTETRICAL SERVICES

Medical care is provided to pregnant women in the United States in a variety of styles. In 1940, slightly more than 50% of American births occurred in hospitals, but by 1960 hospital births exceeded 95%, where it has remained since. Out-of-hospital births in 1980 were 35,548, or slightly less than 1% of the total.[7] These births occurred in a variety of facilities, such as birthing centers, patients' homes, and homes of midwives. The states of Texas, California, Oregon, and Washington contributed about 75% of these nonhospital births.

Physicians attend the births of over 97% of infants born in the United States. ln 1980, midwives attended 62,669 births or 1.7% of the total. Of these, about 83% were in a hospital.[7]

TABLE 1-2. MORTALITY PER 100,000 LIVE BIRTHS—UNITED STATES, 1950–1980

	Maternal*		Infant†	
	Nonwhite	White	Nonwhite	White
1950	220	61	45	28
1960	98	26	41	22
1970	56	14	30	17
1980	26	8	21	11

* Wallace, H. M., Gold, E. M. and Oglesby, A. C.: *Maternal and Child Health Practices: Problems, Resources, and Methods of Delivery*, 2nd Edition. New York, Wiley, 1982. Copyright © 1982 by John Wiley & Sons, Inc. Reprinted by permission of John Wiley & Sons, Inc.

† Monthly vital statistics report: Advance report of final natality statistics, 1980. *USDHHS* **31**:8, p. 17, 1982.

Mortality and morbidity associated with human births have markedly decreased in the last four decades. This improvement has occurred for many reasons, including better understanding of the physiology and pathophysiology of reproduction, maternal nutrition, hospitalization for birth, better-trained attendants, blood transfusions, antibiotics, anesthesia, fetal monitoring and intrauterine fetal diagnosis. Especially noteworthy has been the development of Maternal and Fetal Medicine and of Neonatology as medical specialties and the establishment of maternal and neonatal special-care units.

Many obstetrical patients require few if any of the new and expensive technologies, but if outcome is to be optimal, these advances must be accessible to all. Each patient's needs must be accurately perceived and the type and complexity of care must be appropriate to meet those needs. To this end, a geographic *regional approach* has been initiated in several states or portions of states.[10] In this system, institutions and physicians with various skill levels are identified and referral/consultation mechanisms are developed among them. For instance, one or two hospitals with a highly expert staff and elaborate equipment might be a regional "level 3" institution serving 5–25 other hospitals that give safe and skillful care to patients with less complex problems. Success of this system depends on early and accurate diagnosis and risk assessment, a willingness to transfer and accept patients, a prompt and well-trained transport system, good communication between providers and patients, and assurance of access to various levels of care. The rapidly growing cost of care and the increasing complexity of the applied technology contribute to the development of such systems.

Another factor modifying traditional obstetrical services has been the demand for a "family oriented" birth experience that allows more active participation by a parturient and her family. To accomplish this, hospitals are providing "home-like" birthing rooms and free-standing birthing centers are appearing in many localities. Nonhospital birthing centers vary widely in quality and safety. Many are not subject to licensing or other third party review.

An additional significant influence is personal injury litigation (malpractice, etc.) brought by patients and families against physicians and hospitals. Not only have suits against

TABLE 1-3. PROFESSIONAL LIABILITY INSURANCE, ANNUAL PREMIUM—1983, $1M/1M COVERAGE, OB/GYN, SELECTED STATES

State	Premium
Arkansas	$6,900
California	$25,300
Illinois	$32,500
New York	$51,700
South Carolina	$8,900

obstetrical providers increased in numbers, but awards have become much larger than heretofore. The contribution of litigation to the cost of obstetrical care is significant (Table 1-3). Liability insurance premiums are very high in some states and unnecessary diagnostic and therapeutic measures may be performed for "defensive" purposes (see Chapter 50).

One specific change in care is particularly noteworthy—that of delivery by cesarean section. As late as 1960 most hospitals in the United States reported that about 3–4% of births were by the abdominal route, but by 1978 this figure was approaching 25% in some institutions and exceeded 15% nationwide.[3] Factors influencing the cesarean delivery include the enhanced safety of major surgery (anesthesia, technical skills) and concern with long-term outcome of the newborn. Especially important in the latter category are professional liability litigation, electronic and biochemical fetal monitoring and intensive care nurseries. Concern about the newborn is now the motivation for most cesarean sections, whereas this was not true before 1960. Recently, this practice has come under review. Issues of personal and economic costs have been raised and the results in terms of the newborn have been questioned. The interest in "family centered," "natural" childbirth is also contrary to the rising cesarean section rate.

Other issues important to the rapidly changing patterns and styles of care include methods of funding, environmental and dietary influences on the developing fetus, intrauterine diagnosis and therapy, and career orientation of many women in the reproductive age.

REFERENCES

1. Abortion surveillance: Annual Summary 1979–1980, Centers for Disease Control. Atlanta, GA, USHHS, Public Health Service, May 1983.
2. American College of Obstetricians and Gynecologists: Maternal health policy. Statement of policy as issued by the Executive Board of The American College of Obstetricians and Gynecologists, Chicago, IL, 1977.
3. Cesarean childbirth: Report of a consensus, development conference. NIH, Bethesda, MD, U.S. Department of Health and Human Services, Public Health Service, Sept. 22–24, 180, NIH Publication No. 82-2067, Oct. 1981.
4. Gibbs, C. E. and Locke, W. E.: Maternal deaths in Texas, 1969 to 1973. *Am. J. Obstet. Gynecol.* **126**:687–692, 1976.
5. Graham, H.: *Eternal Eve: The History of Gynaecology and Obstetrics.* Garden City, NY, Doubleday, 1951, p. 38.
6. Lee, K. S., Paneth, N., Gartner, L. M. and Pearlman, M.: The very low-birth-weight rate: Principal predictor of neonatal mortality in industrialized populations. *J. Pediatr.* **97**:759–764, 1980.
7. Monthly Vital Statistics Report: Advance report of final natality statistics, 1980. United States Department of Health and Human Services, **31**:8, p. 17, 1982.
8. Monthly Vital Statistics Report: Annual summary of births, deaths, marriages, and divorces: United States, 1983, United States Department of Health and Human Services, **32**:13, 1984.
9. Pritchard, J. A. and MacDonald, P. C.: *Williams Obstetrics,* 16th Edition. Norwalk, CT, Appleton-Century-Crofts, 1980, p. 1.
10. Toward improving the outcome of pregnancy: Recommendations for the regional development of maternal and perinatal health services. Committee on Perinatal Health, The National Foundation–March of Dimes, White Plains, NY, 1977.
11. Wallace, H. M., Gold, E. M. and Oglesby, A. C.: *Maternal and Child Health Practices: Problems, Resources, and Methods of Delivery,* 2nd Edition. New York, John Wiley & Sons, 1982, p. 87.

2

FETAL AND PLACENTAL DEVELOPMENT: OVULATION, FERTILIZATION, AND DEVELOPMENT OF THE BLASTOCYST

Successful sexual reproduction is a continuum arbitrarily assigned a beginning and ending. Each member of a species begins with fertilization—the successful merging of two different pools of genetic information to form a new individual.

The uniqueness of this individual is suggested by the following calculations: In a species with 23 pairs of chromosomes, there are 2^{23} potential chromosome distributions for any given gamete. As the probability of any two events is the product of the two individual probabilities, 2^{46} is the number of potential chromosome distributions in the zygote. The number of potential gene distributions is, of course, larger yet. This figure must be multiplied by the probabilitics of mutational events, the variation produced by crossing over during meiosis, and the variation produced by the delicate interplay between genetic, epigenetic, and environmental factors that alter development at every stage of the process.[59] The range of possible results becomes inconceivably large. Consequently, variability is one of the most fundamental attributes of development subsequent to sexual reproduction. All standard descriptions like the one that follows are thus inherently misleading.

When ovulation occurs, the egg that escapes from the follicle is a secondary oocyte in the process of a second meiotic division which has proceeded only to the point of metaphase.[3] After mitotic development in the embryonic gonad, the oogonium is encapsulated in primitive granulosa in a primordial follicle and is halted in the dictyotene stage of the first meiotic prophase (Fig. 2-1). This is a primary oocyte (Fig. 2-2). The relationship between the oocyte and the follicle is poorly understood but is known to be complex and changing.[6,7] Initially, the follicle inhibits further development of the oocyte and, with variable effectiveness, maintains it until future ovulation. The follicular apparatus also controls the resumption of meiosis I in the primary oocyte when follicular maturation begins (Fig. 2-3). The follicle further regulates the progression to metaphase of meiosis II and probably regulates other more subtle aspects of oocyte maturation in preparation for ovulation. For example, during the immediate preovulatory period, the follicular cells send messages into the oocytes that alter protein synthesis. Cells fertilized before they have had time to translate these messages are not viable.[44] The ovulated oocyte is approximately 150–200 microns in diameter.[31] The whole is encased in a glycoprotein membrane, the zona pellucida, produced by the follicle cells. The zona pellucida and the oocyte are enclosed in a collection of granulosa cells, the cumulus oophorus (Fig. 2-4). As the oocyte in its cumulus coating is extruded from the follicle through an avascular portion of the follicular wall, it is swept off of the ovarian surface by mobile fimbria which aid the cilia of the tubal epithelium, transporting it into the ampullary portion of the fallopian tube. [12] It is probably fertilizable for less than 24 hours at this site.

Spermatozoa initially proliferate beginning

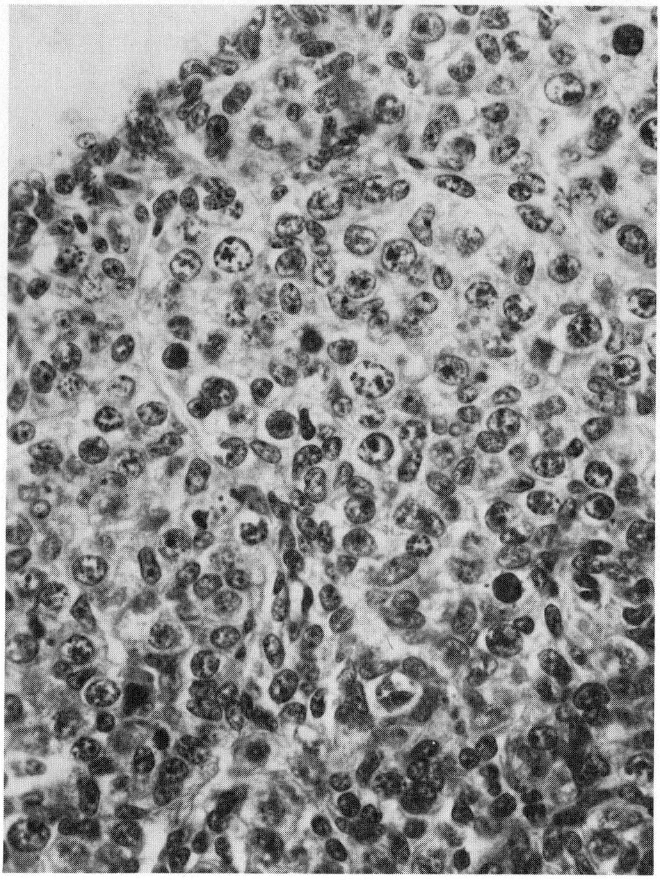

Figure 2-1. In this embryonic ovary, large germ cells are seen in a matrix of smaller cells which will invest the germ cells in follicles and then differentiate into granulosa cells. Some of the cellular matrix will become the ovarian theca.

at puberty and, after several divisions, are termed primary spermatocytes. Meiosis and spermiogenesis result in the development of four spermatids. Several weeks are required for a complete cycle in a healthy male. The spermatozoon that achieves fertilization has been highly selected. Of the several hundred million sperm deposited in the vagina, only a few million reach the uterine lumen and only a few thousand reach the tubal ostia. A few hundred reach the ampulla. There is evidence that they may do this in as short a period of time as 5 minutes.[57]

Healthy sperm are motile and sperm motility is demonstrably important, but this rapid transit time implies active transport by the genital tract. Sperm motility may be particularly involved in transit through the cervical mucus and penetration of the corona radiata. During the course of transit through the genital canal, the sperm become capacitated.[27] Vaginal sperm are not capable of fertilizing the oocyte. Although capacitation (the acquisition by the sperm of the ability to fertilize) is not fully understood, it is known to involve the acrosome reaction. This consists of the development of perforations in the acrosomal membrane which covers the tip of the sperm head. These perforations have been demonstrated ultrastructurally. The perforations allow the release of an enzyme, hyaluronidase, which digests the corona radiata and the zona pellucida and allows the sperm to penetrate both. It has been suggested that the reason many sperm are required for normal fertility, although only one fertilizes the oocyte, is that many are required to digest the corona allowing one to enter.

When the first sperm penetrates the zona pellucida, it contacts the surface of the oocyte, the vitelline membrane. The cell membrane of the sperm fuses with the vitelline membrane and the sperm enters the oocyte. The fusion of sperm and vitelline membrane initiates a change in the vitelline membrane which generally makes it impenetrable to subsequent sperm, although errors occur. The clinical phenomena of triploidy or of hydatidiform moles may be the results of such errors.[26,36,61] The

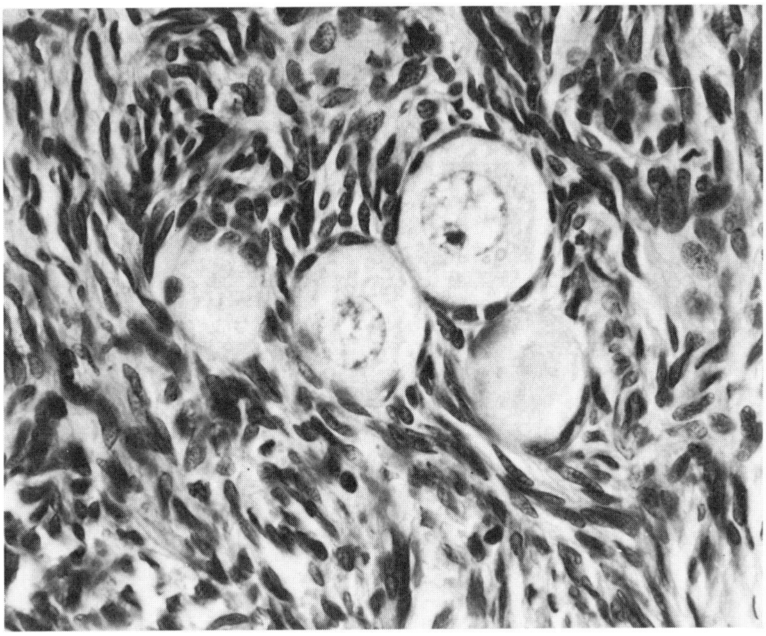

Figure 2-2. This primite oocyte is encapsulated by a single flattened layer of primitive granulosa, forming a primordial follicle. Several adjacent follicles are seen sectioned in varying diameters.

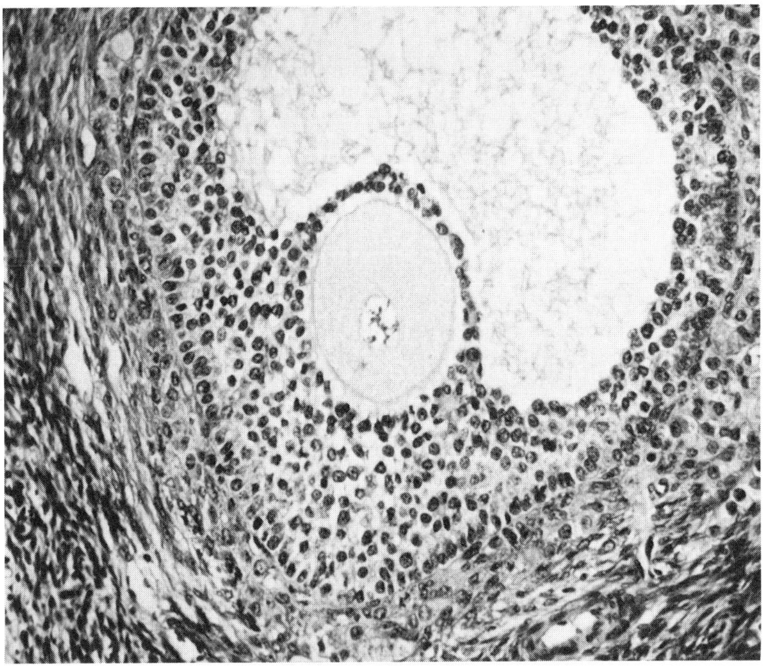

Figure 2-3. This developing preovulatory follicle is surrounded by an outer layer of normal ovarian stroma, the theca externa, and an inner layer of ovarian stroma, the theca interna, which consists of cuboidal cells. Granulosa cells have proliferated to form a thick epithelium lining the follicular cyst. The antral cavity has developed eccentrically, leaving the secondary oocyte embedded in a cumulus oophorous.

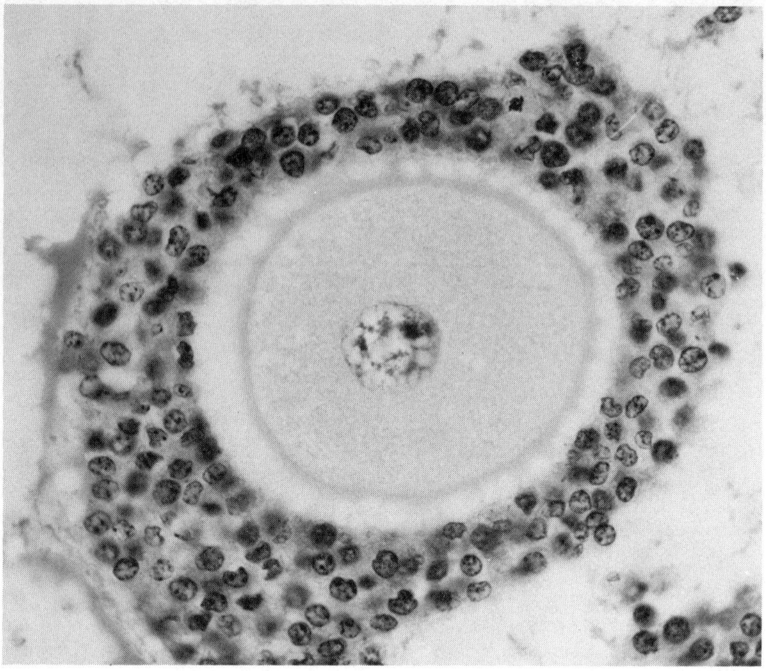

Figure 2-4. The secondary oocyte seen here has a well developed zona pellucida and string-like cytoplasmic extensions of the granulosa cells are attached to it. The separation of zona pellucida and granulosa cells is artifactual, but the "strings" are not.

membrane change is termed the zona reaction. It consists of the dissolution of previously observable granules, lying immediately beneath the oocyte cell surface. Subsequently, the vitelline membrane which has previously been applied to the zona pellucida retracts.

Penetration of the oocyte by sperm also initiates completion of the second meiotic division. When fusion of the vitelline membrane and the plasma membrane of the sperm occurs, the second meiosis resumes and is completed and the second polar body is extruded. Reconstitution of the now haploid female pronucleus is accomplished. The haploid chromosomal contribution of the male is similarly reconstituted in a pronucleus and the two pronuclei approach each other. When the male and female pronuclei come into contact, the nuclear envelopes fuse and disappear. The two haploid chromosomal complements are then intermingled on a metaphase spindle, which is formed with the aid of the centriole contributed by the male. Immediately upon formation of the metaphase spindle, the first cleavage division begins. Therefore, the one-cell stage embryo is extremely transitory. A new individual has begun. The significance and the uniqueness of this biologic phenomenon are so profound that, historically, they have inspired mysticism. Greater understanding only increases the wonder.

With the achievement of syngamy, the ovum (one-cell stage, Streeter's Horizon I) begins to divide, resulting in two daughter cells or blastomeres (Streeter's Horizon II—segmenting ovum). This division and all subsequent ones until the loss of the zona pellucida on approximately day 5 are achieved by decreasing cell size and without increase in mass of the total conceptus which remains approximately 200 microns in diameter.[31]

Hertig's descriptions of preimplantation human conceptuses suggest that, after the first cleavage division, subsequent divisions occur at approximately 12-hour intervals in an asynchronous manner. The result is an increasing number of smaller and smaller cells encased in a zona pellucida approximately 200 microns in diameter. This structure has the appearance of a mulberry and is termed a morula. Hertig described a morula of 12 cells that he thought was approximately 72 hours postfertilization. This example was of particular interest because it demonstrated what may be the earliest differentiation in the morula. Of the 12 cells, Hertig noticed that one was larger than all the rest and situated centrally.

This observation raises the more general question of what differentiation may take place in the preimplantation conceptus. Little is known, but based on other systems, cleavage divisions are not random but are oriented with respect to up and down, right and left.[58] The position of any given cell with respect to the whole determines its fate. This principle extends back to the ovum where the organization of the cytoplasm may determine up and down, right and left. In some lower species, polarity is determined by the site of sperm penetration where the zona reaction is initiated. Hertig also noticed that the second polar body was directly opposite the first within the zona and wondered if this was significant. In any case, potential differentiation is very plastic. Cells can be moved experimentally from one site to another, thereby altering their fate. This is even more true of nuclei, which remain undifferentiated much longer in development than do whole cells. Irreversibility in the process of differentiation is achieved at different times in different tissues.

In a 58-cell morula believed to be about 96 hours old, Hertig described the next recognizable stage in development, the development of a fluid-filled space within the morula, converting it into a blastocyst (Streeter's Horizon III). The fluid-filled space develops eccentrically in the morula so that it is largely enclosed by a single layer of cells, except at one pole, where this layer is thickened by all other cells collected into a single mass. The cells of the blastocyst wall are destined by their position to be the future trophoblast. The cells in the single mass will become the embryo. In Hertig's 58-cell examples, 53 cells were found in the cyst wall and five in the inner cell mass.

About this time or hours before, during the fourth day postovulation, the conceptus reaches the uterine cavity. Prior to this time, it has been nurtured in the fallopian tube. Appropriate tubal function involves provision of the correct environment for fertilization and cleavage and correct timing of its entry into the endometrial cavity.[12] During the fifth day, several critical steps occur. The blastocyst becomes fully developed. In a 107-cell example described by Hertig, there were eight cells in the inner cell mass. The zona is largely lost, although remnants of it are present. In addition, the cells on the ventral surface of the inner cell mass form a distinct one-cell layer, the first germ layer, the endoderm. The blastocyst is now ready to implant on the sixth postovulatory day.

On the sixth day, the blastocyst floats freely in the endometrial cavity. The inner cell mass displays the differentiation implied by the development of the endoderm. The trophoblast also displays differentiation. Mitoses are prominent in the trophoblast but many of the cells are flattened in apparent response to distension of the cyst from within. Ideally, implantation occurs in the midportion of the anterior or posterior uterine wall. The blastocyst invades the endometrium to the appropriate depth and is so positioned that the implanting pole of the blastocyst contains the inner cell mass (Fig. 2-5). Variation in any of these mechanisms may be responsible for abnormalities to be discussed below.

GROWTH, DEVELOPMENT, AND AGING

With implantation (Streeter's Horizon IV) or perhaps shortly before, when the zona is lost, growth begins. Growth is a complex phenomenon that may be expressed at many levels but is easily expressed in terms of cell size and number.[75] Most tissues initially grow by simple cell division, a proliferative phase. The cells remain small with minimal cytoplasm that ultrastructurally contains a few mitochondria and little reticulum, that is, they are undifferentiated. Although larger than most cells, germ cells are useful examples of the general phenomena. First identified in the wall of the yolk sac at the end of the third week of development, they migrate during the fourth, fifth, and sixth weeks into the medial portion of the urogenital ridge via the hindgut mesentery (Fig. 2-6).[77] Here they divide mitotically at a rate that is maximal between the eighth and 20th week of development (Fig. 2-1).[2] Mitotic division drops off rapidly after 20 weeks and is completed by birth. About 60,000 oogonia are present in the gonad at 8 weeks. The number increases to approximately 7 million by 20 weeks of fetal age. It is characteristic of the proliferative phase of growth that it has a specific developmental time course. After it is over, there is little additional proliferation. The time course is specific for a given tissue. Under some circumstances in some tissues, such as the liver, proliferation can be

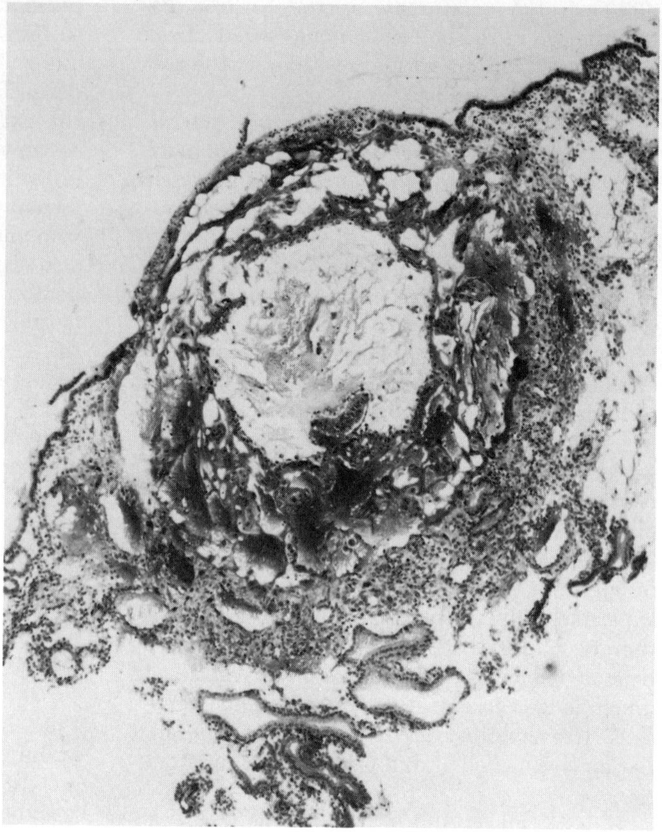

Figure 2-5. The implantation is so oriented that the embryonic pole is the deepest. A bilaminar disc consisting of an ectoderm and an endoderm is suspended beneath a tiny amniotic sac. The whole is suspended from the chorionic membrane by a small amount of extraembryonic mesoderm. The chorionic membrane contains a very thin layer of extraembryonic mesoderm, an equally thin layer of cytotrophoblast and a well-developed syncytium containing intercommunicating lacunae that are filled with maternal blood.

reinitiated. It also persists in some tissues at a maintenance level, such as epithelia, but it does not normally contribute to further growth.

The second phase of growth, which overlaps the first, is cell enlargement or hypertrophy. This consists of multiple changes in the cell and is limited if nutritional deprivation occurs, but, as a developmental process, it is the result of cell differentiation.[75] Ultrastructurally, this is manifested by development of large amounts of cytoplasmic organelles designed to perform biologic work. Differentiation is relative. An example is the smooth muscle cell of the myometrium. It is differentiated with respect to the embryonic muscle cell, but it differentiates additionally in response to the hormonal stimulation of pregnancy. Another fundamental attribute of cell differentiation is that, with rare exceptions, differentiated cells do not reenter mitotic cycles. They acquire mortality and have fairly specific limited life spans after which they die.[72] The time course of this life span is tissue specific, years in the case of neurons and 120 days in the case of red blood cells.

The germ cells illustrate the phenomenon of differentiation-associated growth. At about 15 weeks, while mitosis is still occurring, some of the oogonia begin to differentiate (Fig. 2-1). They enlarge and enter meiotic prophase. Their 46 chromosomes are first condensed (leptotene stage) and become arranged as 23 pairs of homologous chromosomes (zygotene stage). As each chromosome splits, the pairs become tetrads. An important source of genetic variation results. By a mechanism known as crossing over, the arm of one member of the pair exchanges genetic material with an arm of the other member, resulting in new chromosomes that are unlike either of the original pair (diplotene stage). The cell then enters a resting phase (dictyotene stage) preceding the metaphase of the first meiotic division. It is encapsulated in this state by the primitive granulosa. The germ cell is now termed a primary oocyte and the

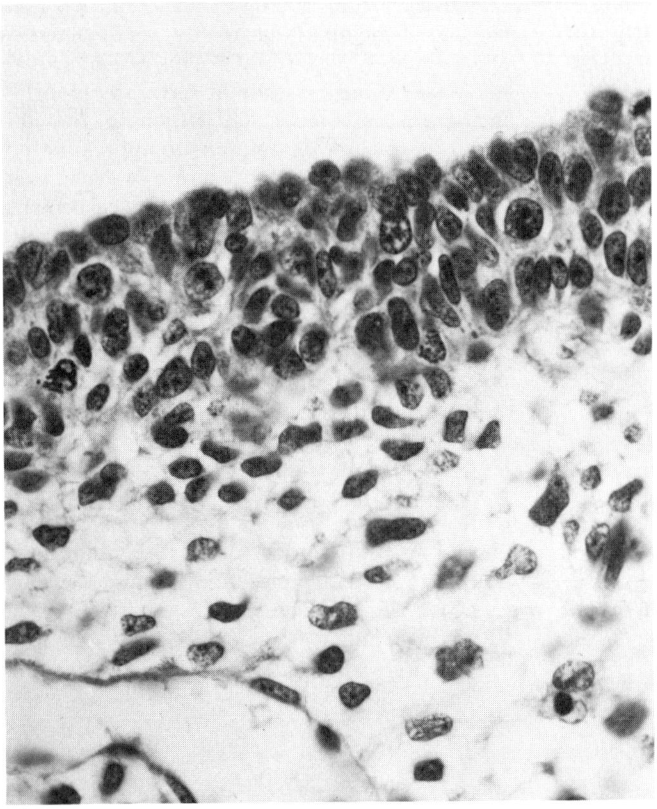

Figure 2-6. This view of the medial surface of the urogenital ridge during the fifth week of development shows large germ cells embedded in the proliferating surface epithelium. Both germ cells and epithelial cells proliferate at this site.

capsule of granulosa cells that contains it constitutes the primordial follicle. The cells of the primordial follicle secrete a glycoprotein membrane which coats the oocyte, called the zona pellucida. The zona pellucida is penetrated by cytoplasmic processes of the granulosa cell which make contact with the oocyte within and make possible the control of further development. Gonadotrophins are also important in maintaining the continued good health of the oocyte.

The primary oocyte is partially differentiated at this point. It has an elaborate set of cytoplasmic organelles and is much larger than the oogonia (Figs. 2-1–2-4, 2-6). It also illustrates the other facet of differentiation described above. It has a defined life span. Germ cells that are not encapsulated die promptly. Those that are encapsulated die more slowly, but just as surely, beginning at 15 weeks. Germ cell death begins when meiosis (differentiation) begins. Only 1–2 million oocytes survive until birth and only 3–4 hundred thousand are present at menarche.[9] On the average, the last of these die by the time the woman reaches age 50.

In the 2–3 weeks immediately preceding ovulation with follicular maturation, the primary oocyte undergoes additional differentiation. Just prior to ovulation, it completes the first meiotic division and extrudes the polar body. Thus, a secondary oocyte is ovulated.[3] This cell with its additional differentiation has a very short, predetermined life span. Only fertilization allows the secondary oocyte to escape mortality. The unequal nature of the first meiotic division resulting in the majority of the cytoplasm remaining with the secondary oocyte is significant. As mentioned above, the detailed organization of the constituents of this cytoplasm probably controls differentiation.[58,59]

Thus, germ cells illustrate both the proliferative phase of growth and the hypertrophic phase associated with cell differentiation. They also illustrate the principal biologic result of growth and development, which is programmed cell death.

An embryo begins as a population of undifferentiated cells, all of which subsequently divide. Development is associated with the conversion of some portion of this population to differentiated end stage cells that do not further divide, but enlarge, age, and die (Figs. 2-7–2-9). These processes occur according to very different schedules in different tissues of the same organism. The final adult size of any tissue or organ is determined by this process. Early differentiation of its entire cell population precludes unlimited growth. The time course of differentiation may also presage the early demise of this tissue or organ, as exemplified by the germ cells.

In gross terms, the growth of the human embryo consists of the accumulation of mass from that of a drop of water approximately 200 microns in diameter to the mass of a full-term infant.[22,55] Although this latter figure has a wide range, 3465 g was selected as "perfect" size by this author approximately 18 years ago. From fertilization until implantation, little increase in mass occurs, but from day 6 postovulation until the end of the first lunar month, mass increases approximately 8000 times.[55] This rate of growth decreases rapidly so that, at term, the monthly increase is only about 30%. In length, the conceptus goes from 200 microns to approximately a 50 cm infant at birth. The rate of growth decreases from the initial astronomical one to about 6.5% per month at term.[60] Whether or not there is a limitation on growth just preterm, based on decreasing placental capacity, is debatable, but, in general, prenatal growth curves are continuous with those that occur in the postnatal period, birth appearing as only an incidental event.

Growth does not occur uniformly. In general, it occurs first in that portion of the conceptus that is to give rise to the head region of the embryo. This is immediately behind the prochordal plate. It spreads posteriorly, anteriorly, and laterally with differentiation and development following the same general pattern.[35] The future head and neck region are 45% of the total

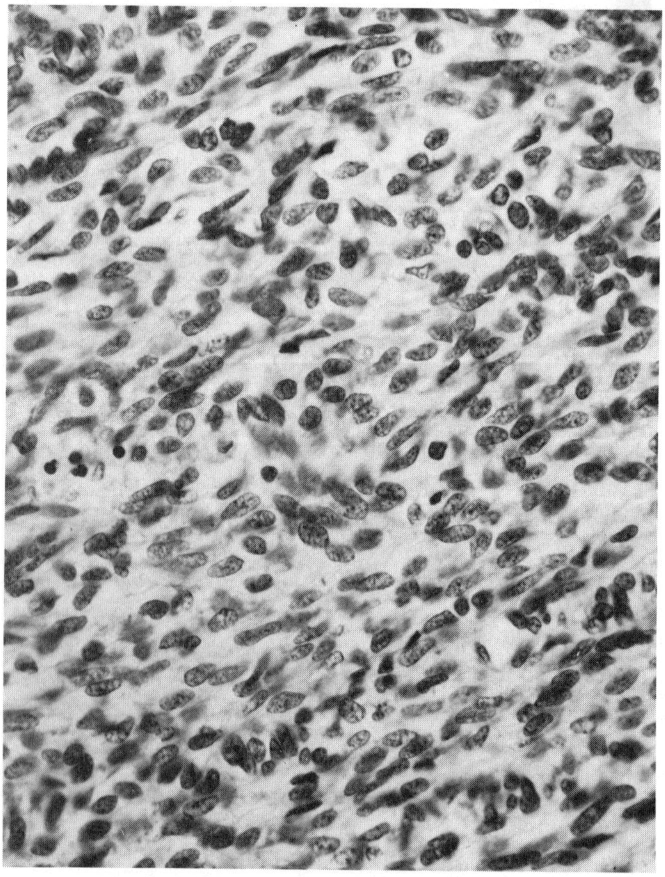

Figure 2-7. The cervical stroma of a 20-week embryo consists largely of undifferentiated cells with little cytoplasm.

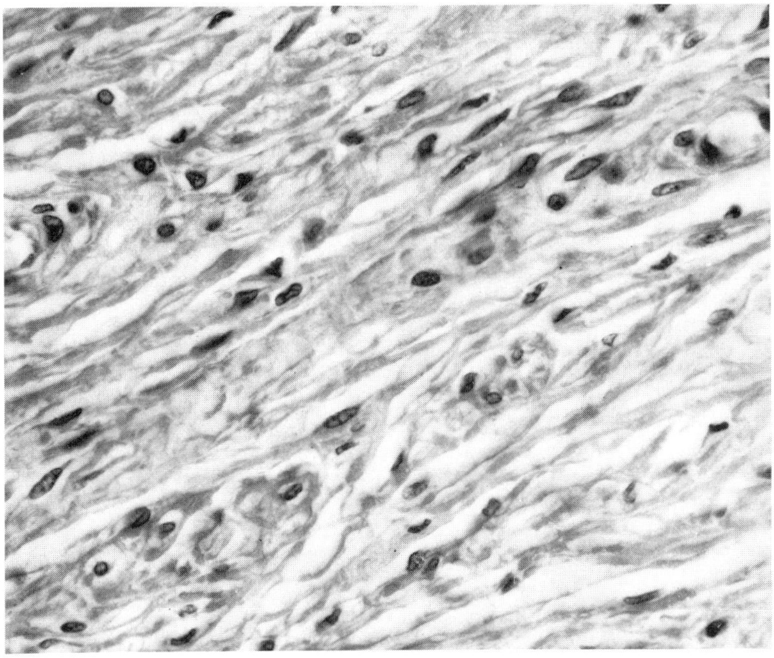

Figure 2-8. At term the cells of the cervical stroma have large amounts of differentiated cytoplasm, but most of the tissue is still cellular.

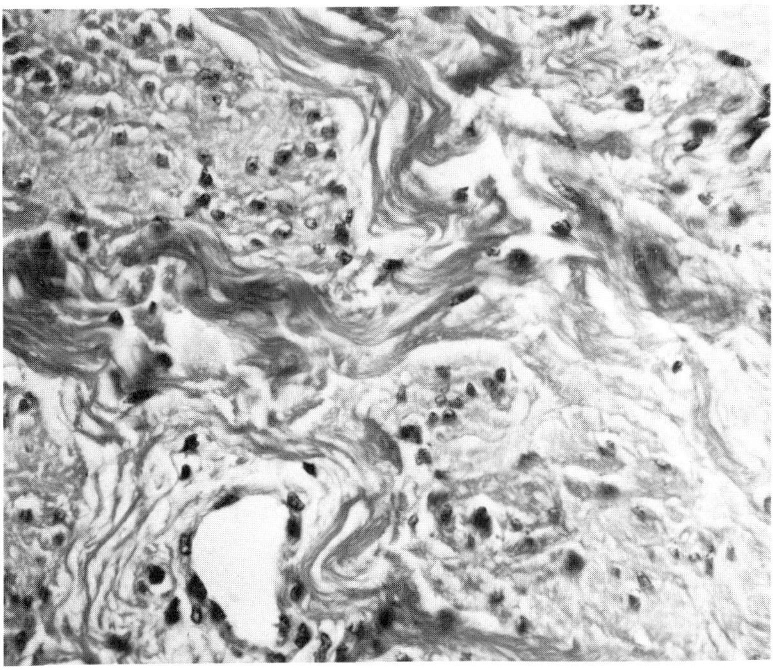

Figure 2-9. In a 25-year-old woman, the cervical stroma contains much acellular collagen and other structural proteins. An older woman may possess tissues that are even less cellular.

volume of the embryo at 1 lunar month, and the lower extremities are only 2%. At term, the head and neck are only 30% of the total volume of the embryo and the lower extremities are 15%.[55,60]

Specific organ systems tend to appear, grow rapidly, and then slow their rate of growth as other systems catch up. The central nervous system is one of the first to grow rapidly, next the viscera, and last the musculoskeletal system. Genital organs do not exhibit maximal growth until puberty and the lymph organs not until late childhood.[55] An even more dramatic example of differential growth is seen by comparing the placenta and embryo. Initially, most of the conceptus is placenta, but at term the placental weight is often less than one-fifth the fetal weight.[75]

Specific tissues also grow nonuniformly.[55] Nervous tissue constitutes 21% of total body weight at 6 lunar months and 15% at birth. Viscera and muscle stay the same at 16% and 25%, respectively. The skeleton decreases from 22% to 18%. The skin is 4% of body weight at 6 lunar months and the same at birth. The subcutaneous support of the skin is only a trace at 6 lunar months and 12% at birth.

Biochemical changes also accompany development.[55] The most fundamental change is in water content, which is 96% at 3 lunar months and less than 73% at birth. Fat weight is 0.1 g at 3 lunar months, 6–7 g at 6 lunar months, and 380 g at birth. Protein weight at 3 lunar months is 1.5 g and at birth is 120 g. The biochemical changes parallel the development of differentiated tissues.

IMPLANTATION AND PLACENTAL DEVELOPMENT

The first fetal tissue to go through a cycle of growth and development is the trophoblast. As we have seen, growth and differentiation begin in the trophoblast before implantation. With implantation, the process is accelerated.[29,30] As the flattened trophoblastic cells of the blastocyst come into contact with the endometrium, they become cuboidal and are now designated the cytotrophoblast. The cytotrophoblast acts as a proliferating or germinal layer to produce a much more differentiated tissue, the multinucleated syncytiotrophoblast, which lies between the cytotrophoblast and the maternal tissues. As the blastocyst sinks into the endometrium, the syncytiotrophoblast extends all around its circumference so that the blastocyst becomes entirely surrounded by a syncytium supported by an underlying layer of cytotrophoblast, one cell thick. Although it is the syncytiotrophoblast that carries the blastocyst into the endometrium by directly invading the maternal tissues, the process is aided by the fact that the blastocyst collapses shortly after implantation and does not redistend until it is almost completely contained within the endometrium.

The syncytiotrophoblast is a remarkable tissue. It numbers among its abilities the capacity to avoid immune rejection by the maternal organism utilizing mechanisms that are still problematic. It is the source of a host of hormone products, including hCG, which is produced as soon as implantation occurs and in smaller quantities even before implantation, as well as progesterone. Chorionic progesterone takes over support of the pregnancy from the corpus luteum in the eighth gestational week.[8] Within the syncytiotrophoblast, multiple vacuoles develop and coalesce to form an intracellular labyrinth that extends entirely around the blastocyst and throughout the syncytiotrophoblastic layer (Fig. 2-5). The syncytiotrophoblast then invades maternal vascular channels and endometrial glands, so that the contents of the glands and capillaries escape into the labyrinth of lacunar spaces to circulate passively around the blastocyst. The labyrinth is therefore the precursor to the intervillous space. The blastocyst is completely buried in the endometrium by the 12th day.

During implantation, changes also take place inside the blastocyst. The cytotrophoblast not only gives rise to the overlying syncytium but also to a loose connective tissue, the extraembryonic mesoderm which lines the inner wall of the blastocyst and separates the inner cell mass from it (Fig. 2-10). As early as the eighth day, a cystic space develops in the extraembryonic mesoderm which connects the inner cell mass to the cytotrophoblastic wall of the blastocyst.[29,30] This is the amniotic cavity. The extraembryonic mesoderm lining the blastocyst begins to fill in the center except for a central space beneath the inner cell mass.[32] This space is soon lined by endoderm which has extended beyond the edges of the inner cell mass to produce what is now the yolk sac. Secondarily, coalescing spaces develop in the extraembryonic mesoderm to produce an extraembryonic coelom. This space

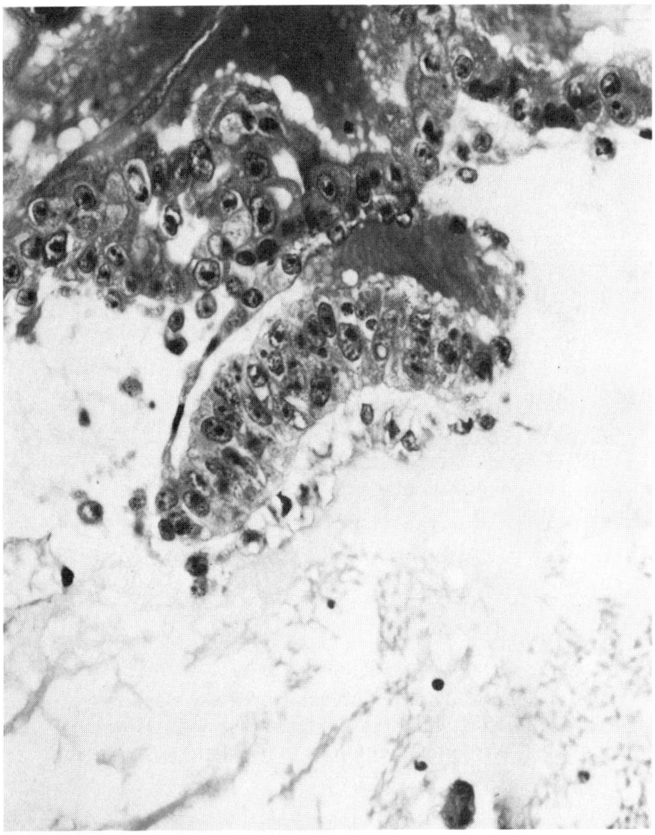

Figure 2-10. Above and to the left, maternal blood circulates through the lacunar spaces of the syncytium. The thin strip-like syncytial cells are supported by a single layer of cuboidal cells, the cytotrophoblast. Below and within the blastocystic cavity, a bilaminar embryonic disc lies in the floor of an early amniotic sac. The disc contains a formative cell layer and an endodermal cell layer. The amniotic sac is roofed over by a one-cell layered amnion; the whole embryonic structure is suspended from the chorionic membrane by a few cells of extraembryonic mesoderm.

splits the mesoderm so that one layer invests the yolk sac (Fig. 2-10), the inner cell mass, and the amniotic sac and connects through a connecting stalk or body stalk with the mesoderm layer that lines the inner surface of the cytotrophoblast. Meanwhile, the inner cell mass has become a bilaminar disc lying between the amniotic sac and the yolk sac. It forms the floor of the amniotic sac and the roof of the yolk sac. The nonendodermal cells of the inner cell mass form the superior layer of the bilaminar disc. They become columnar and arrange themselves so that their long axis is perpendicular to the endodermal layer beneath them. This is the formative layer. lt gives rise to both ectoderm and mesoderm.

The bilaminar disc is slightly oval. Near one pole the cells of the endoderm become somewhat more columnar than their fellows and attach themselves to the overlying ectoderm This spot of attachment of the two layers is the prochordal plate It is the site of the future mouth and provides cephalad to caudad and right to left orientation to the bilaminar embryonic disc. This polarity occurs by the end of the second week. Before proceeding with embryonic development, we will turn attention to the placenta. This distinction is artificial because the placenta is only an exteriorized embryonic organ.

PLACENTA

The placenta develops from the chorionic membrane which consists of the trophoblastic epithelium and its supporting stroma of extraembryonic mesoderm.[24] Beginning earlier, but becoming prominent in the third week of development, the cytotrophoblast begins to proliferate to produce radial columns that project outward from the blastocyst wall (Fig. 2-11). They extend through the syncytial labyrinth until they reach the maternal tissue and then

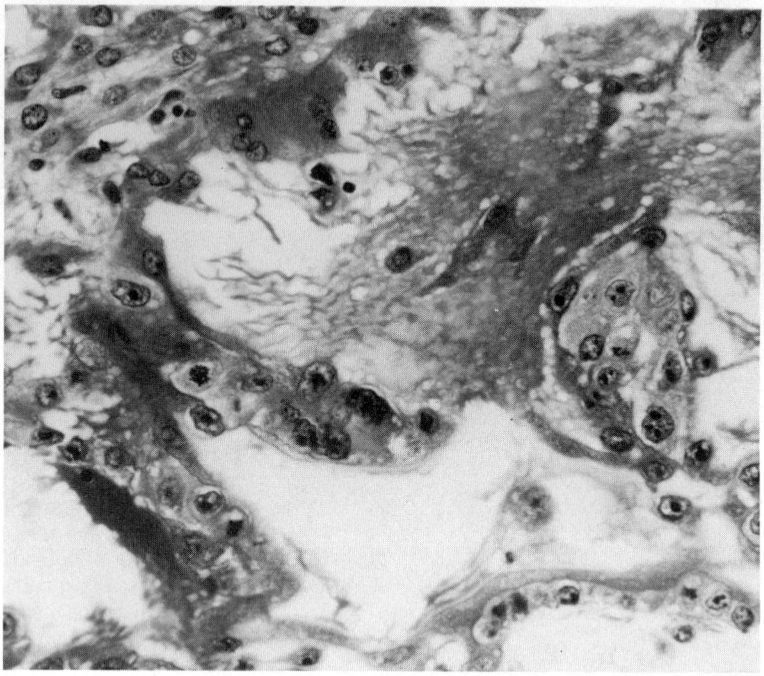

Figure 2-11. To the lower right, a one-cell layer of cytotrophoblast supports the syncytium which, as a labyrinth, extends to the upper left where maternal tissue is seen. However, masses of proliferating cytotrophoblast are forming columns that extend through the labyrinth almost to the maternal tissues.

spread between the syncytium and the maternal tissue entirely around the conceptus (Fig. 2-12). Thus, a single shell, the cytotrophoblastic shell, is formed. Via the cytotrophoblastic cell columns, the cytotrophoblastic shell is continuous with the undifferentiated cytotrophoblast of the chorionic membrane. It encloses the preexisting mass of syncytiotrophoblastic tissue (Fig. 2-13). Maternal glands and blood vessels continue to open into this labyrinth through the cytotrophoblastic shell. Although it is conventional to refer to the shell as a cytotrophoblast, it is significantly differentiated.[39,76] Many of the cells composing it are those termed "intermediate trophoblast" and are the source of human placental lactogen (hPL). The only truly undifferentiated cytotrophoblastic cells are those that remain basal along the chorionic membrane. Isolated cells penetrate the maternal tissues beyond the trophoblastic shell. They invade the muscular and elastic walls of the spiral arterioles supplying the implantation site (Fig. 2-14).[50] They may penetrate within the walls of these vessels, fairly deeply into the myometrium. This invasion has the effect of destroying the capacity of the spiral arterioles to respond to catecholamines during maternal "fight or flight" reactions.[21] Additionally, trophoblastic cells invade both decidua and myometrium in a nonspecific pattern that has been termed syncytial endometritis or myometritis. Maturing into mononuclear or multinuclear intermediate trophoblast, these cells produce hPL.[39] When this process is exaggerated, it may be responsible for the "placental site tumor."[38]

As described above, the blastocyst is probably completely buried in the endometrium and surrounded by syncytium by the 12th postovulatory day. Subsequent growth results in its reemergence above the endometrial surface. When this occurs, the reemerging surface of the chorionic membrane is denied a vascular supply, atrophies, and becomes the decidua capsularis. Only that portion of the chorion remaining in contact with the endometrium continues to grow to become the definitive placenta. The cytotrophoblastic shell expands laterally and extends deeper into maternal tissues so that the contained space enlarges. This space is filled by developing placental cotyledons.

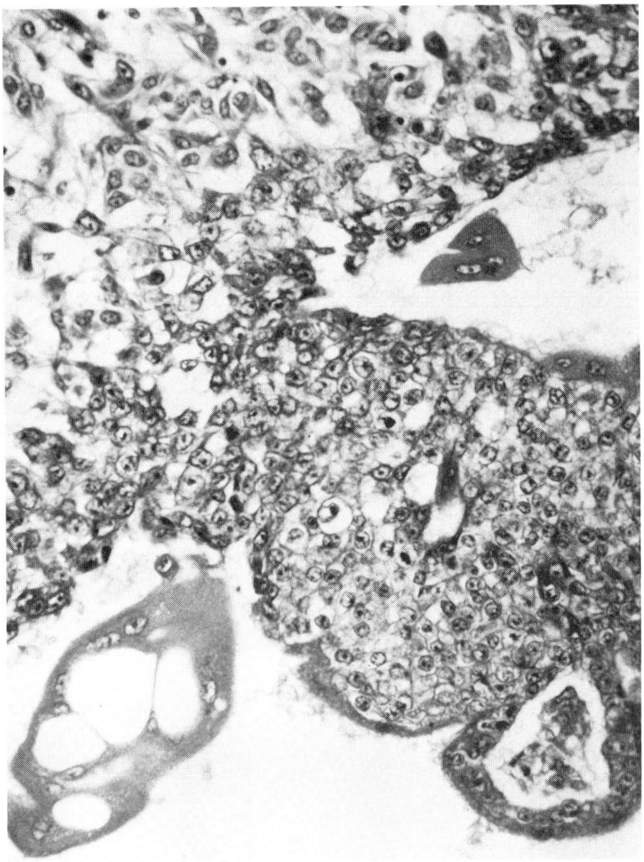

Figure 2-12. The cytotrophoblastic column coming from the lower right has reached the maternal tissue in the upper left. It has begun to spread out laterally and has turned the syncytiotrophoblast back into the intervillous space. There is no clear-cut demarcation between maternal and trophoblastic tissue.

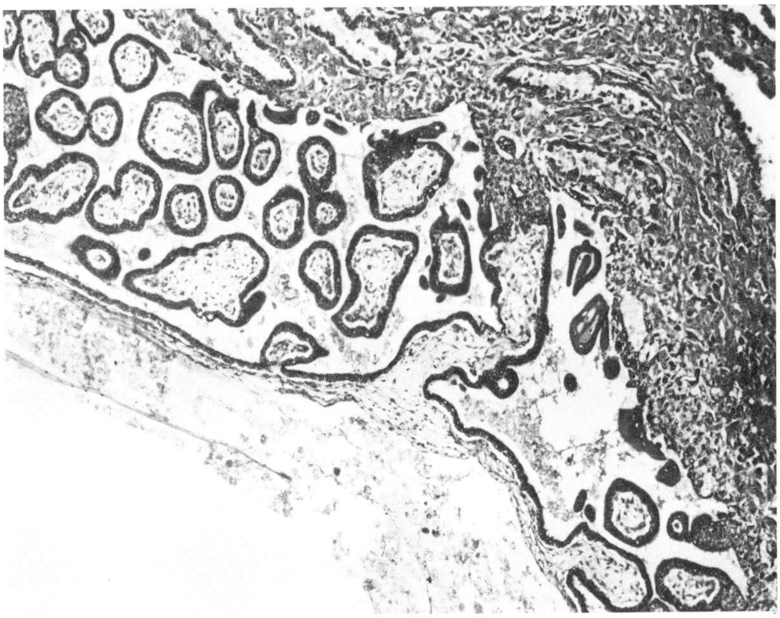

Figure 2-13. The extraembryonic mesoderm has extended up into the base of the cytotrophoblastic cell columns, producing anchoring villi. The cotyledons will develop in the intervillous space between the chorionic membrane and the basal plate, that is, the combination of maternal and fetal tissues.

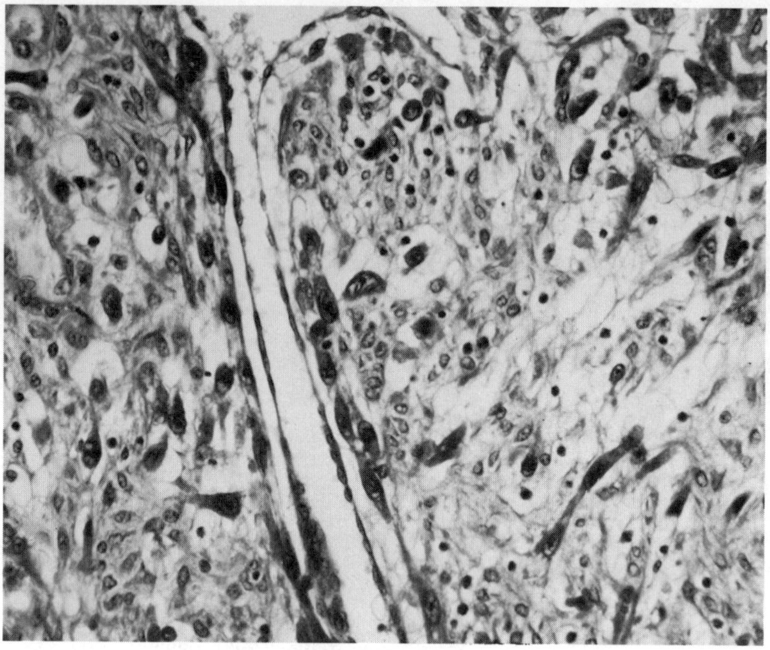

Figure 2-14. The intervillous space is above. This maternal vessel has had almost its entire endothelium stripped off by trophoblast invading from the implantation above. Trophoblastic cells also infiltrate the surrounding decidua.

If implantation is sufficiently superficial or is located in a particularly confined site, such as the cornua, attachment may take place on the opposing wall, as well as on the primary one. Under such circumstances, an accessory placental lobe or a succenturiate lobe may develop. Such abnormal implantations are also frequently associated with malorientation of the implanting blastocyst, such that the inner cell mass is not in the implanting pole, therefore velamentous insertion of the umbilical cord or body stalk is common in this circumstance. In experimental systems, implantation in which the inner cell mass is directly opposite the implanting pole of the blastocyst results in splitting of the inner cell mass and monozygotic twinning with which velamentous insertion of the umbilical cord is also highly associated.[33]

If the blastocyst is implanted at the proper depth, it remains spherical when it begins to reemerge above the surface of the endometrium, but if implantation has been too deep and has spread laterally beneath the endometrial surface, an hourglass configuration results. Depending on how arced its development is, it may lead to placenta marginata or circumvallata.[65] It is not known what regulates the depth of implantation. Presumably the regulatory mechanisms reside at least partially in the decidua because defects in this tissue are the universal finding when placenta accreta is observed.

Placental cotyledons begin as proliferations of cytotrophoblast extending from the chorionic membrane into the intervillous space. Covered by syncytiotrophoblast and supported internally by extraembryonic mesoderm from the chorionic membrane, these trunci chorii grow toward the maternal surface of the intervillous space, the basal plate.[24] As they do so, they divide many times, producing finer and finer terminal villi which extend laterally and vertically to fill the intervillous space. The first branching villi appear in the middle of the third week of development (Streeter's Horizon VII). True cotyledons begin to develop in the seventh week at the same time that spiral arterioles are tapped. The cotyledons develop tropically so that they become oriented to the sites at which maternal spiral arterioles enter the intervillous space through the cytotrophoblastic shell.[17] This results in proliferation of villi around the orifices of maternal vessels such that maternal blood enters the center of a cotyledon and diffuses laterally through it.

During the third week of development, angioblastic activity begins in the villi and body stalk (Fig. 2-15).[25] By the end of the fourth week of embryonic life, there is a fetal circulation and nucleated red blood cells can be seen in the capillaries within the stroma of the villi (Fig. 2-16).

As the placenta matures, it goes through a sequence of phenomena which results in increased surface area for exchange.[62] The first is a dramatic increase in the number of terminal villi in the intervillous space. The second is the modification of the terminal villi. During the first trimester, they possess well-defined cytotrophoblastic and syncytiotrophoblastic epithelial layers. Few capillaries are present in a large amount of stroma. During the second trimester, the capillaries proliferate and become copious, but both the trophoblast and the stroma are still prominent. During the third trimester, the terminal villi are converted to structures that contain a high proportion of capillaries to stroma (Fig. 2-17). The cytotrophoblast is scanty and the syncytium is so thin that electron microscopy is required to confirm its presence at specialized sites of exchange termed epithelial plates.[42,76]

Consistent with this differentiation, placental growth has almost ceased by term. Initially growing faster than the fetus, it slows after 20 weeks.[29] The observable progression from a population of undifferentiated proliferating cells to a population largely composed of differentiated nonproliferating cells is the principal theoretical reason for wondering if the placenta ages. Growth, development, and aging are empirically related as discussed above.[47,71,72] The placenta is demonstrably not senescent at term, although the putative role of placental senescence in some prolonged pregnancies remains a question.[16] However, senescence is not the issue, as a tissue may be quite mature while still far from senescent.

Syncytial knots, collections of degenerating trophoblastic nuclei, increase as the placenta

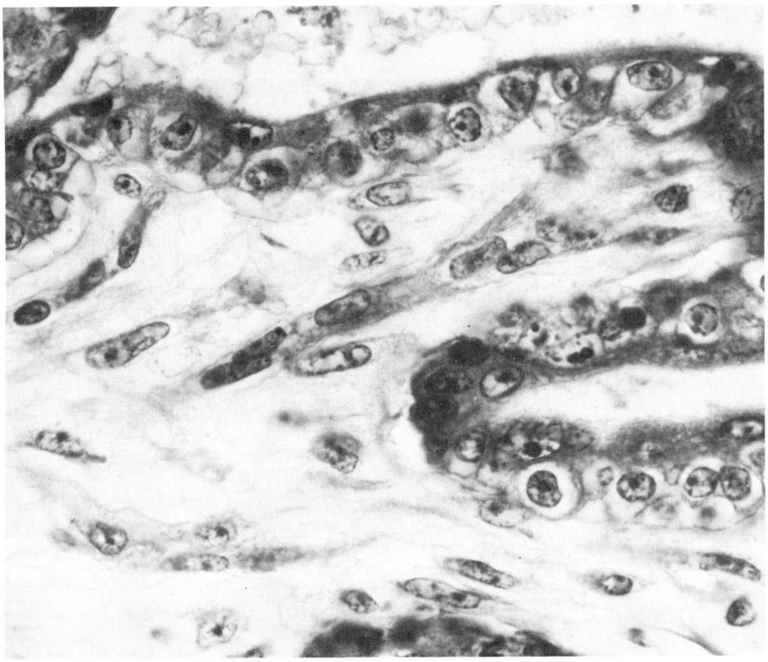

Figure 2-15. In the mesoderm of this anchoring villus, elongated angioblasts have arranged themselves in a linear aggregation that will soon develop a lumen and become a capillary.

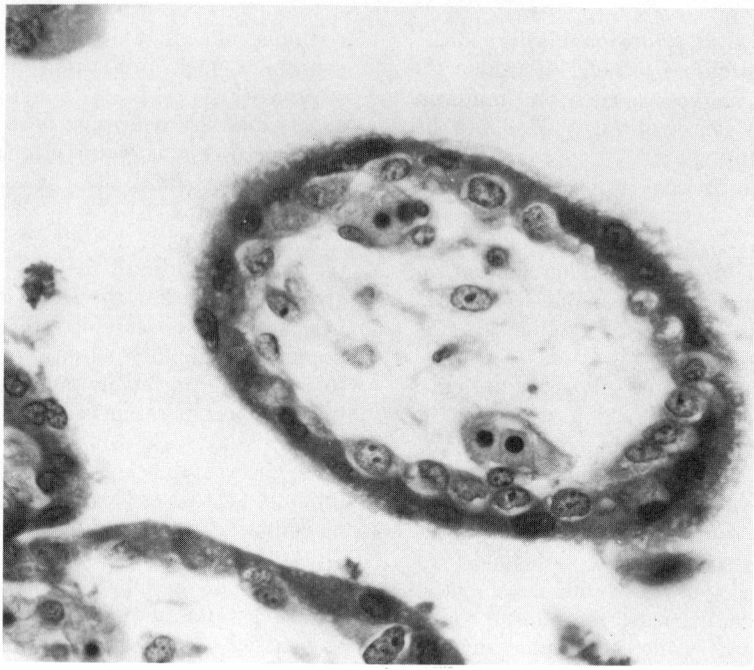

Figure 2-16. Nucleated fetal red cells occupy the two capillaries in the stromal core of his villus. The trophoblastic epithelium is clearly two cell layers with well-developed cytotrophoblast.

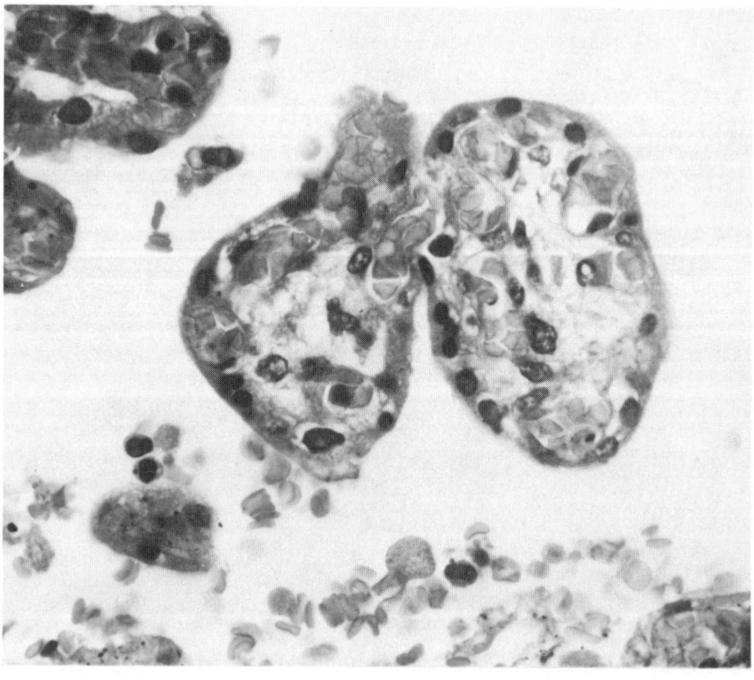

Figure 2-17. Only a one-cell-layered epithelium surrounds the mesodermal core of these term villi which contain capillaries filled with non-nucleated red cells. The gaps in the syncytium are only apparent.

approaches term. They are reminiscent of nuclear pyknosis occurring in mature stratified squamous epithelia and may represent only maturation. Intervillous thrombi which are the results of leaks in the fetal vascular system also increase as term approaches and passes. Their presence certainly suggests loss of integrity of the fetal vascular channels. Whether or not this is related to placental aging is not clear.

If the placenta does not represent a model for aging, it does represent a model for the control of growth and development. The placenta associated with anencephalics demonstrates histologic immaturity at term in that there is persistence of a proliferating cytotrophoblastic cell population (Fig. 2-18). In contrast, corticosteroids not only can induce differentiation in the fetal lung but can induce premature maturation in the rodent placenta.[5,74] Furthermore, corticosteroids given to pregnant monkeys result in smaller final size of some fetal organs.[4] All these observations are consistent with the view that the rate at which the proliferative phase of growth is converted to the cell hypertrophy phase and secondarily halted is at least partially under hormonal control.[59] Differentiation sets limits to growth and starts the clock that measures aging. The placenta may not get old, but its aging clock certainly appears to have been started.[10,14,40]

DEVELOPMENT OF THE MESODERM

At the end of the second week of embryonic life, the embryonic disc is bilaminar with the formative cell layer and the endoderm attached at the prochordal plate. The formative cells begin to proliferate rapidly in the posterior portion of the disc and move toward the midline of the disc where they produce a linear elevation, the primitive streak.[45,64,66] They then migrate down into the space between the formative layer and the endoderm. This migration converts the primitive streak into a linear depression, the primitive groove. The new tissue that arises be-

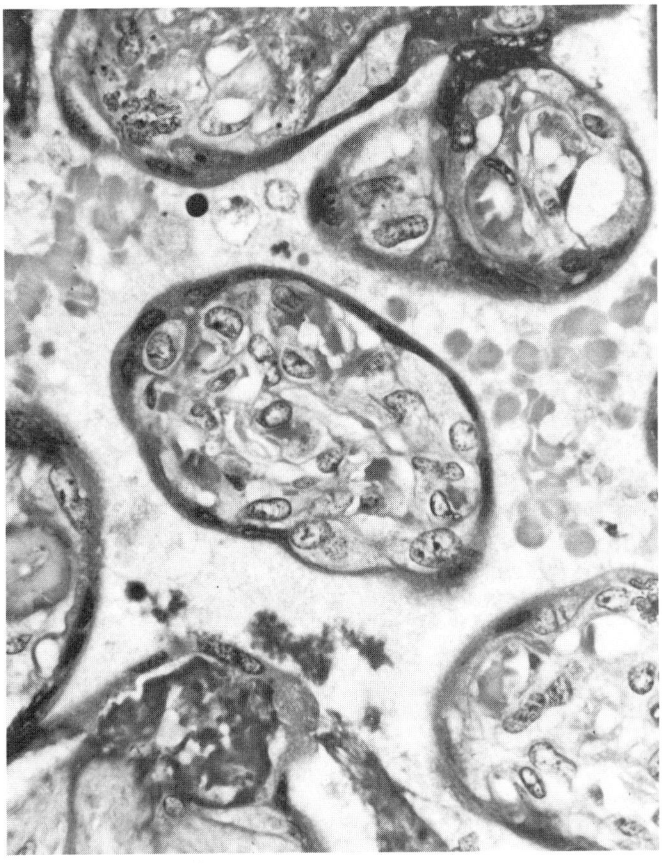

Figure 2-18. A large number of prominent cytotrophoblastic cells are present in the terminal villi of this placenta associated with an anencephalic fetus.

tween the two original layers is the mesoderm. The cells at the apex of the groove, the cephalic end, first form a bulge, designated Hensen's node, and then extend as a solid midline cord forward into the space between the formative layer and the endoderm, until they reach the posterior edge of the prochordal plate. This is the notochord. As the disc grows, the primitive groove is displaced posteriorly and the notochord lengthens. Just posterior to the primitive groove, the endoderm and the formative cell layer form another attachment similar to the prochordal plate. This cloacal plate will become the site of the anal and urogenital orifices.

The cells dropping into the space between the two layers from the edges of the primitive groove extend forward, laterally and posteriorly, to fill the space between the formative cell layer, now termed ectoderm, and the endoderm. This new mesodermal layer is continuous with the extraembryonic mesoderm at the lateral edges of the embryonic disc. It separates ectoderm and endoderm everywhere except at the prochordal and cloacal plates.

The intraembryonic mesoderm becomes organized into bilateral columns of tissue that are parallel to the notochord (Figs. 2-19, 2-20). The para-axial mesoderm, the most medial of the columns, runs from the prochordal plate, caudad to the cloacal plate. Subsequently, the para-axial mesoderm becomes segmented into approximately 42 pairs of somites (Fig. 2-20). These give rise to portions of the subcutaneous tissue, the axial skeleton, and musculature and impart to the body between the head and the pelvis the segmental nature of its organization. They probably are not the determinants of this segmental structure, but only its first recognizable results. The intermediate mesoderm just lateral to the para-axial mesoderm has a similar distribution. The most lateral portion of the mesoderm is referred to as lateral plate mesoderm and it extends around the cephalic end of the prochordal plate and the caudad end of the cloacal plate. The para-axial mesoderm will give rise to the somatic musculature and to the skeleton as well as the dermis. The lateral plate mesoderm gives rise to the visceral musculature and some of the branchial arch mesoderm.

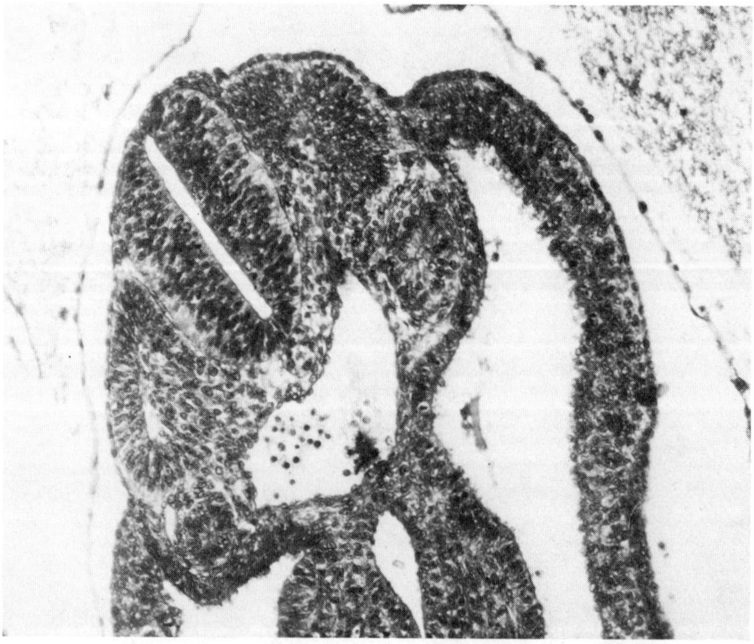

Figure 2-19. This section of an embryo in the somite stage of development reveals most peripherally an amnion. A single-cell layer of ectoderm surrounds the tubular embryo. To the upper left in the embryo is the neural tube, underlain in succession by the notochord, the dorsal aorta, and the endoderm of the gut. Laterally are seen the paired intraembryonic coeloms.

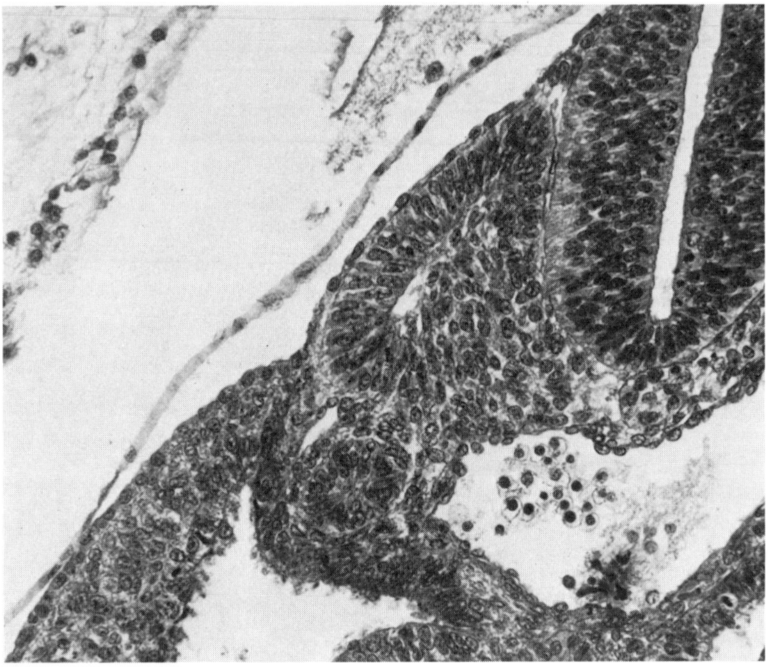

Figure 2-20. The neural canal occupies the upper right hand corner of the picture. In the angle between it and the overlying ectoderm, there is a small nest of neural crest cells. Beneath the neural canal is the notochord. Immediately lateral to it is a developing somite and in the lower left is the intraembryonic coelom, splitting the lateral plate mesoderm. Between the coelom and the somite, intermediate mesoderm contains an early nephrocele.

During the latter part of the third week, coalescing cavities form in the lateral plate mesoderm and produce a continuous horseshoe-shaped space, the intraembryonic coelom (Figs. 2-19, 2-20). lt extends in the lateral plate mesoderm from the posterior lateral edge of the embryonic disc around the cephalic end of the prochordal plate to join a similar cavity on the other side. The intraembryonic coelom communicates with the extraembryonic coelom through the posterolateral wall of the embryonic disc. The portion of the intraembryonic coelom anterior to the prochordal plate becomes the pericardial sac. The portions lateral to this structure become the pleural sacs and the most caudal portions of the intraembryonic coelom become the right and left sides of the peritoneal cavity. Although the functions of the various spaces involved in early development, that is, the yolk sac, the amniotic sac, and the intra and extraembryonic coeloms, are not clearly known, adult physiology and comparative studies suggest that circulatory functions are prominent among them. They share many biologic characteristics with blood vessels and lymphatics.

The subsequent development of the mesoderm is complex. Significant milestones include the following.[45,64,66] Differentiation of most muscle groups is complete by the end of the seventh week of development with the intrinsic muscles of the eye and the perineal muscles following in a few days. Primary ossification centers appear in the neurocranium, ribs, and lung bones in the latter part of the first trimester. Ossification centers in the vertebrae, hips, and digits follow. Calcification is not really established until the second trimester. Bone marrow function begins in the humerus at the end of the seventh week of development.

DEVELOPMENT OF THE NEURAL ECTODERM

When, during the third week of development, the notochord forms, it induces in the overlying ectoderm a linear thickening which becomes the

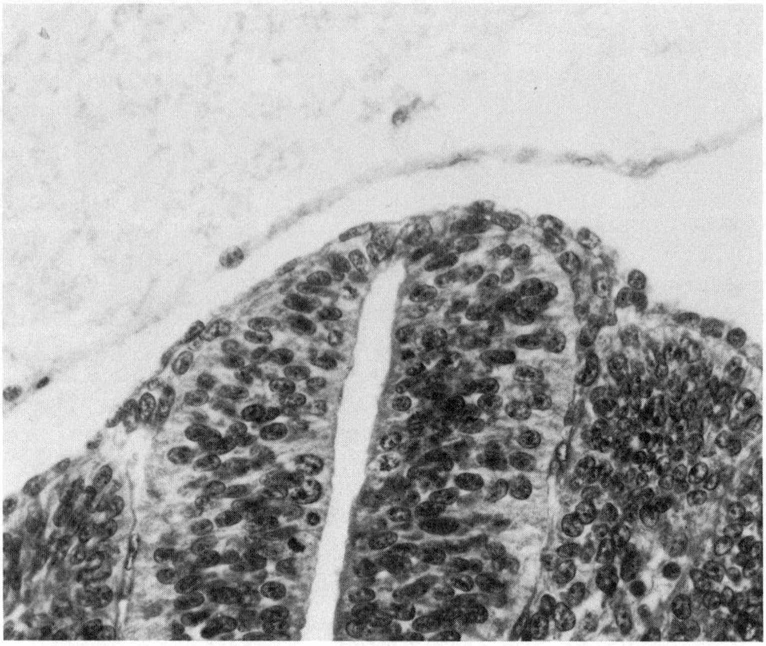

Figure 2-21. The amniotic membrane surrounds the embryo which is covered by a one-cell-layered ectoderm. The neural canal occupies the center of the embryo and in the angle between it and the ectoderm, a nest of fewer than 10 neural crest cells is seen bilaterally.

neuroectoderm.[25] This results in a thickened plate, the neural plate, extending from the caudal edge of the prochordal plate to Hensen's node. The neural plate folds from side to side, producing a neural groove. The cells at the edge of the neural plate where it joins the ectoderm become a specified population, neural crest cells (Fig. 2-21).

During the fourth week of development, the lateral folds of the neural plate fuse over the central neural groove at the level of the future neck, forming a neural canal (Figs. 2-19–2-21). The neural canal then closes over sequentially cephalad to caudad. The anterior end, the anterior neuropore, becomes completely closed late in week 4 (Streeter's Horizon XII) and the posterior end, the posterior neuropore, is closed early in week 5. During week 4, the neural tube grows in length and two ventral flexures develop in it. The most caudad, the cervical flexure, develops at the junction of the future spinal cord and brain stem. The most cephalic, the mesencephalic flexure, develops at the level of the future midbrain. The portion of the brain between these two is the rhombencephalon. Its contained neural canal expands to become the fourth ventricle. The portion of the neural tube anterior to the mesencephalic flexure becomes dilated to form the third ventricle. Between the third and fourth ventricle, the neural canal remains small as the aqueduct of Sylvius. The portion of the neural tube anterior to the mesencephalic flexure is termed the forebrain. During week 4, the optic vesicles develop from it. They will extend to the overlying ectoderm and result in development of the eye.

In the neural canal, tissue proliferation is confined to the ependymal or pericanalicular layer of cells (Fig. 2-22). Once formed, the cells migrate out into the mantle layer of the neural tube. Their cell processes extend further out into the marginal layer. Because the ventral portion of the neural tube grows more rapidly than does the dorsal portion, the floor bulges into the lumen of the neural canal, resulting in a lateral groove which runs from the mesencephalic flexure to the caudal end of the neural tube (Fig. 2-23). Dorsal to this sulcus limitans, most cells become sensory, and ventral to it, they become motor. That portion of the forebrain which is to give rise to the cerebral hemisphere is largely dorsal, thus sensory, in this

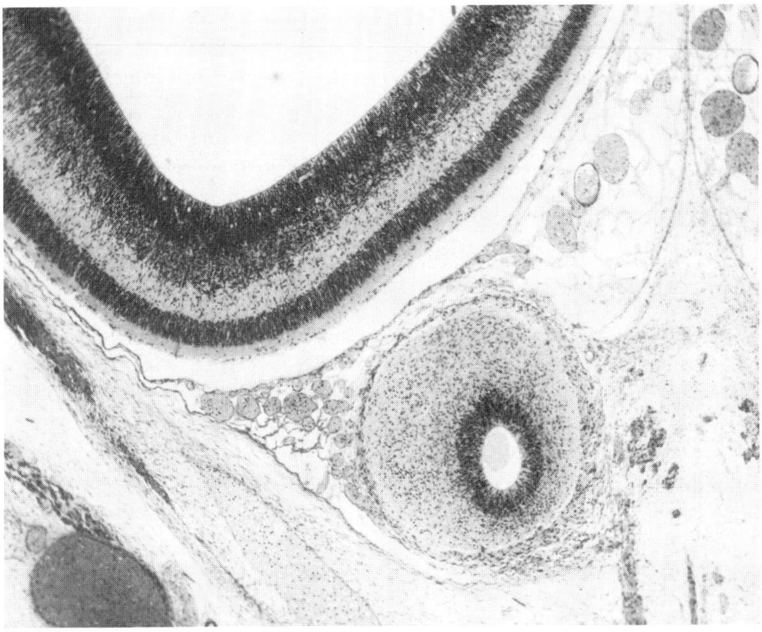

Figure 2-22. This section illustrates a portion of the wall of the developing cerebral hemisphere and the underlying olfactory bulb. The latter has the primitive organization of the early central nervous system with proliferation around the central canal and subsequent cell migration into the mantle layer. Cell processes without nuclei occupy the peripheral marginal layer. The cerebral cortex, however, already has a much more complicated structure derived from the more primitive one.

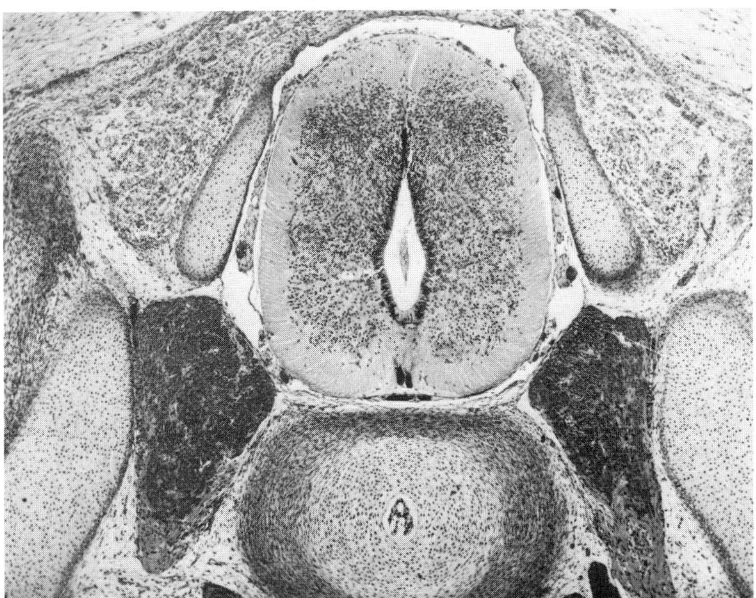

Figure 2-23. Remnants of the notochord occupy the center of the vertebral body immediately beneath this section of the developing spinal cord. Beneath and lateral to the vertebral body are sympathetic ganglia. In the angle between the vertebral body and the central nervous system are the dorsal root ganglia. The spinal cord has the original three-layered organization of the central nervous system but is divided by the sulcus limitans into dorsal and ventral components.

sense.[25,45,64,66] The lens and otic primordia develop from the surface ectoderm during the fourth week. By the end of the fourth week, the latter has sunk beneath the surface ectoderm and has become the otocyst.

During the fifth week, the brain grows rapidly. The prosencephalon or forebrain is divided into a caudal diencephalon and a cephalic telencephalon. The telencephalon is the terminal end of the forebrain, plus two lateral outpouchings. These outpouchings are the eventual cerebral hemispheres and their cavities will be the lateral ventricles. The cerebral hemispheres arise in the fifth week and grow dorsally and caudally to cover the diencephalon by the end of week 6. During week 5, the primordia of the cerebral cortex, corpus striatum, and internal capsule form. Layers of the cerbral cortex are established by the end of the sixth lunar month.

Also during week 5 the diencephalon begins to develop into the pineal, epithalamus, thalamus, hypothalamus, and posterior pituitary, as well as to contribute with the cerebral hemisphere to the choroid plexus. The mesencephalon at the same time is becoming organized into the superior and inferior colliculi and the cerebral peduncles.

During the fifth week, the hindbrain is folded dorsally as the pontine flexure develops, resulting in division of the hindbrain into an anterior metencephalon and a caudal myelencephalon becomes the medulla oblongata.

When the neural tube closes, it entraps some mesoderm which develops a capillary vasculature and expands into the ventricles as the choroid plexus (Fig. 2-24). The mesoderm containing capillaries is invested by a layer of ependyma (Fig. 2-25).

The population of cells previously identified as neural crest gives rise to a variety of tissues, including the spinal root ganglia, the peripheral ganglia of the autonomic nervous system, the adrenal medulla, melanocytes in the skin, and portions of the mesenchymal tissue of the branchial arches (Fig 2-23).[25,35] Neural crest cells migrate to the appropriate site and then differentiate. By the end of week 4, sensory ganglia of the cranial nerves and some dorsal root ganglia

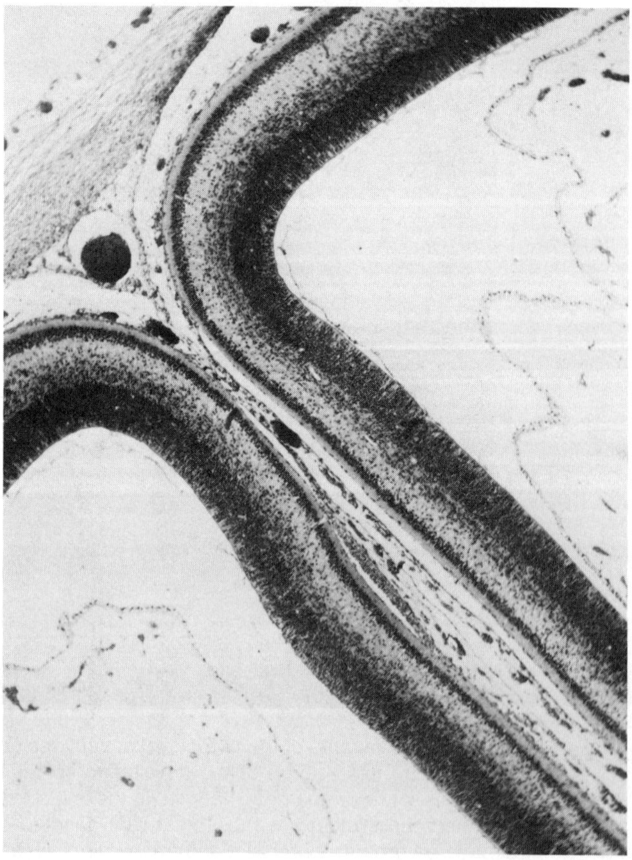

Figure 2-24. Bulging cerebral hemispheres are divided by vascular mesoderm.

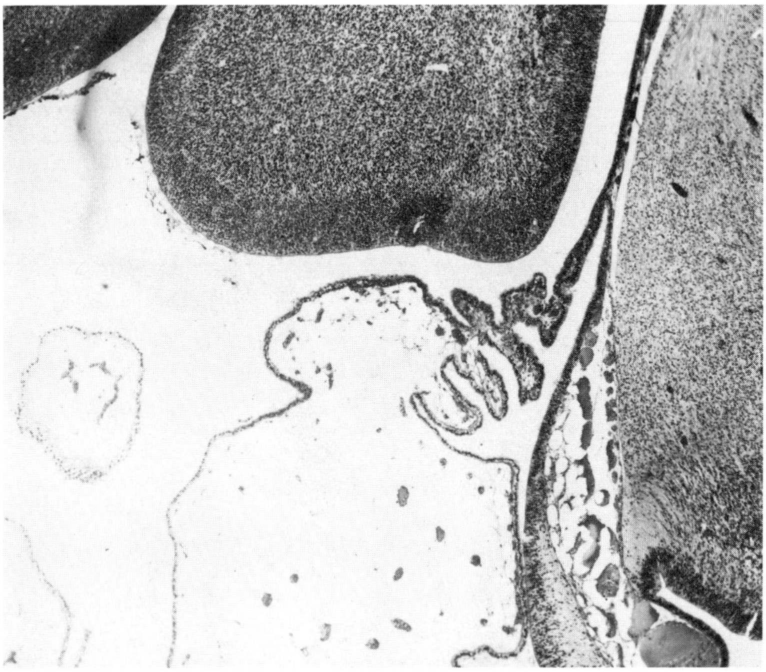

Figure 2-25. Vascular mesoderm invested by neural ependyma forms fronds, the choroid plexus, which extend into the ventricles.

are forming. The sympathetic ganglia and adrenal medulla begin to develop in week 5. Neural crest cells migrate into the skin and become melanocytes late in the first trimester. In the face and pharyngeal region, neural crest cells extensively contribute to soft tissues, sensory receptors, and endocrine and neuroendocrine type cells.

The development of the central nervous system illustrates a fundamental principle in fetal growth and development which is that growth tends to start cephalically and spreads first caudally in the midline and then laterally.[58] It must be noted, however, in this context that the cephalic pole of the trilaminar disc is immediately caudad to the prochordal plate.[35] This region will be the head of the eventual body and gradients of growth and development extend from it in all directions.

FOLDING OF THE TRILAMINAR DISC

The growth and development of the central nervous system just described constitutes the most dramatic expression of the relative increase in growth rates in the head region and central axis of the trilaminar disc during the fourth week of development. This results in bulging of the disc upward into the amniotic sac so that the edges become folded under the bulging disc.[45] The consequence is that the most anterior portion of the trilaminar disc folds down over the front of the embryo. The mesoderm anterior to the intraembryonic coelom is at the level of the future upper abdomen and becomes the septum transversus or future diaphragm. The anterior or transverse part of the intraembryonic coelom becomes the pericardial sac with the heart developing in its floor. The prochordal plate becomes the mouth and the top of the neural tube is the brain.

Posteriorly, the posterior end of the embryo folds at the level of the future sacrum. The cloacal plate is folded forward to become the site of the anus and urogenital orifices and the mesoderm posterior to the cloacal plate contributes to the lower anterior abdominal wall. The lateral edges of the embryo come together in the midline. Cephalic to the level of the septum transversus, the lateral intraembryonic coelom remains separate as the pleural cavities, but caudal to this level, the mesodermal l- which separate the cavities disappear

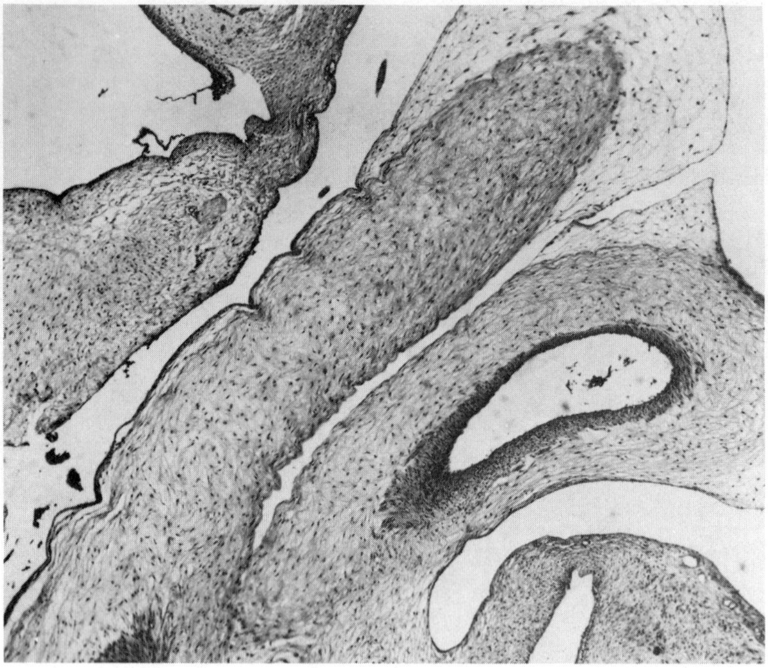

Figure 2-26. The coelomic cavity lies to the upper right. At the top left and lower right edges of the photograph are seen the edges of the anterior abdominal wall. The large vessel containing body stalk (umbilical cord) runs between them to the lower left corner of the photograph. The coelomic cavity extends beyond the abdominal wall into the body stalk.

and left sides join in a common peritoneal cavity. The posterior folding also results in the rotation of the body stalk from the dorsal and posterior aspect of the trilaminar disc to the lower anterior abdominal wall of the tubular embryo (Fig. 2-26).

DEVELOPMENT OF EXTERNAL BODY FORM

When the embryo has achieved a tubular form, due to this folding, it is ready to be transformed into something recognizable as body-like. After the folding movements have produced the basic orientation, development of limbs and a face is next. Limb buds first develop near the end of the fourth week, the arm buds preceding the leg buds by a few days.[13] These consist of subectodermal condensations of mesoderm. They elongate and assume a paddle shape at their extremities. The paddle then differentiates digits fac[illegible]umes the form of a hand or a foot. Ini-[illegible]hs are oriented so that flexor sur-[illegible]ard the body, but the arms rotate laterally and the legs rotate medially to produce the adult orientation.

The development of the head and face is complex.[13,35] When the folding at the anterior end of the trilaminar disc described above has occurred, the result is that a diverticulum of endoderm, the foregut, extends forward from the orifice of the yolk sac to the prochordal plate. It is surrounded by mesoderm at all sites, except at the prochordal plate. This mesoderm is further surrounded by ectoderm as soon as the neural tube closes. During the latter part of the fourth week, linear ridges of subectodermal mesoderm develop and extend around the future face and neck region from dorsally to ventrally. These are the branchial arches (Fig. 2-27). Four are well defined and the fifth and sixth less well developed. Linear grooves separate them. Internally, the foregut endoderm balloons out to form pharyngeal pouches which fuse with the ectoderm in the base of each of the grooves, forming branchial membranes. The first and second branchial arches contain cartilages that may be of neural crest origin. The most dorsal part of the first and second arch will form the ex-

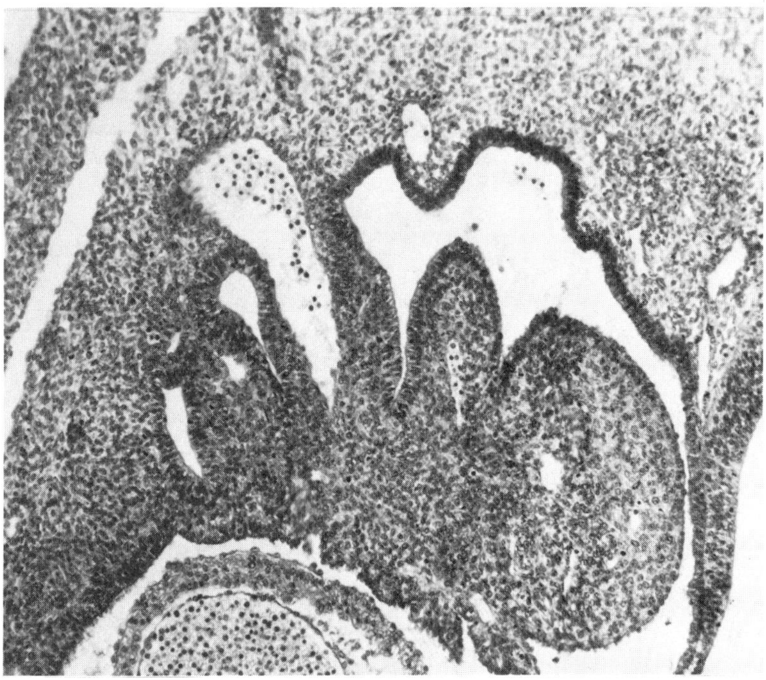

Figure 2-27. This section through the oropharynx demonstrates the linear divisions produced by the branchial arches. At least three pharyngeal pouches have been cut across. The heart lies below.

ternal ear. The branchial membrane in the groove between these two arches forms the tympanum and the associated pharyngeal pouch will form the middle ear chamber and the eustachian tube (Fig. 2-28). The cartilages of the first and second arch give rise to the bones of the middle ear. The ventral part of the first arch divides into two processes which project forward above and below the prochordal plate, now known as the buccopharyngeal membrane. The process below, the mandibular process, will give rise to the lower jaw and much of the tongue (Fig. 2-29). The upper process, the maxillary process, will fuse above the buccopharyngeal membrane with a mass of mesoderm that has developed just above the future mouth, the frontonasal elevation. This results in the formation of the upper jaw. The buccopharyngeal membrane breaks down, resulting in a mouth on about the 24th day.

At the site of the future nares, at the end of the fourth week, surface ectodermal thickenings or nasal placodes develop just lateral to the future nasal elevation. The most anterior extension of the foregut lies close behind this site within the body of the embryo. Thus, converting these sites to nasal passages requires only that the mesoderm around the nasal placodes grow up around them, forming a nose and converting them into pits, and that the tissue between the placode and the foregut disappear, establishing continuity (Fig. 2-30). Ectodermal cells in the roof of this nasal passage differentiate into olfactory cells and send fibers to the olfactory bulb of the forebrain.

Also during the fourth week, induced by the development of optic vesicles from the forebrain, the surface ectoderm at the site of the future eyes thickens, forming lens placodes. These, in turn, invaginate to form lens vesicles. The lens vesicles separate from the surface ectoderm and become the lens of the future eye. The cornea then develops from the surface ectoderm and underlying mesoderm (Fig. 2-31).

While facial development is occurring, the second branchial arch has been expanding over the third, fourth, and fifth branchial arches to fuse with the expanding sixth arch. This covers the other arches and gives the neck its sm
contour.

The hyoid bone is derived fr

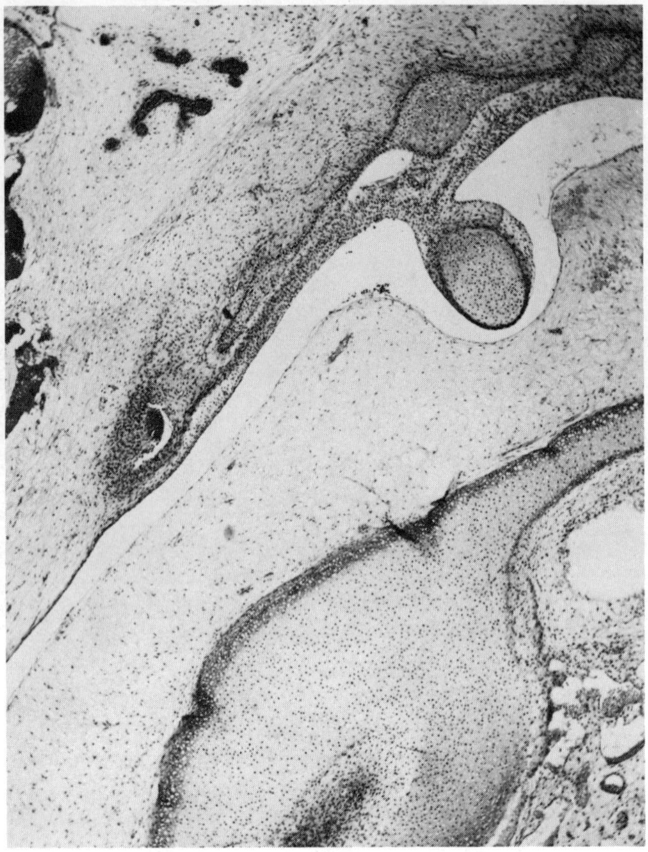

Figure 2-28. The first pharyngeal pouch or eustachian tube extends from the lower left to upper right where middle ear ossicles can be seen to be forming.

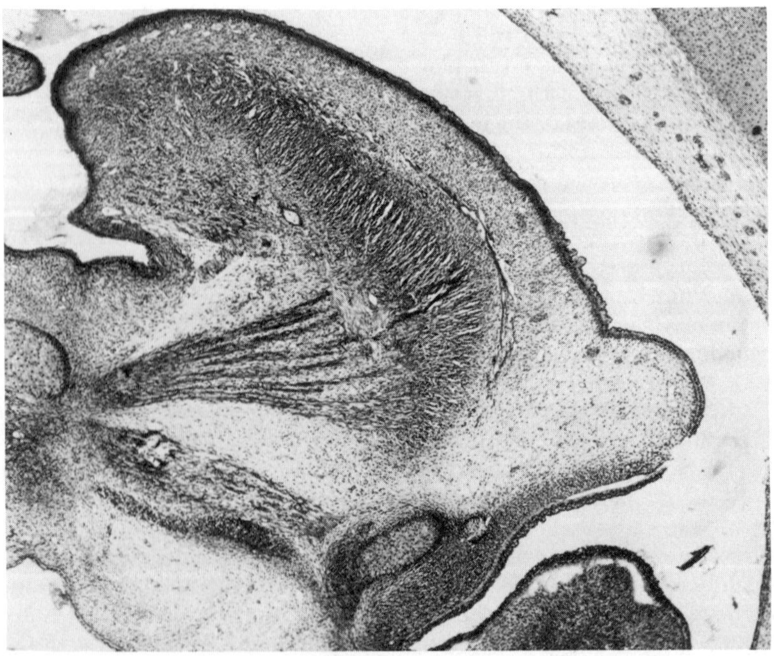

The primitive tongue lies in the floor of the future oral cavity. Muscle strips ifferentiate within it.

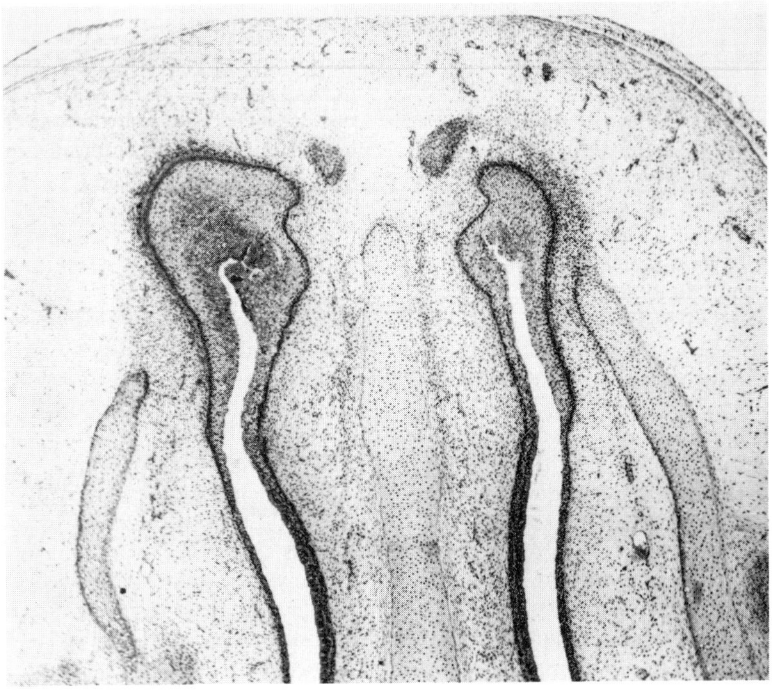

Figure 2-30. This section through the tip of the nose enters the nares from above. The epithelium of the anterior portion of the nares is derived from the surface ectoderm, but that of the posterior nares comes from the foregut.

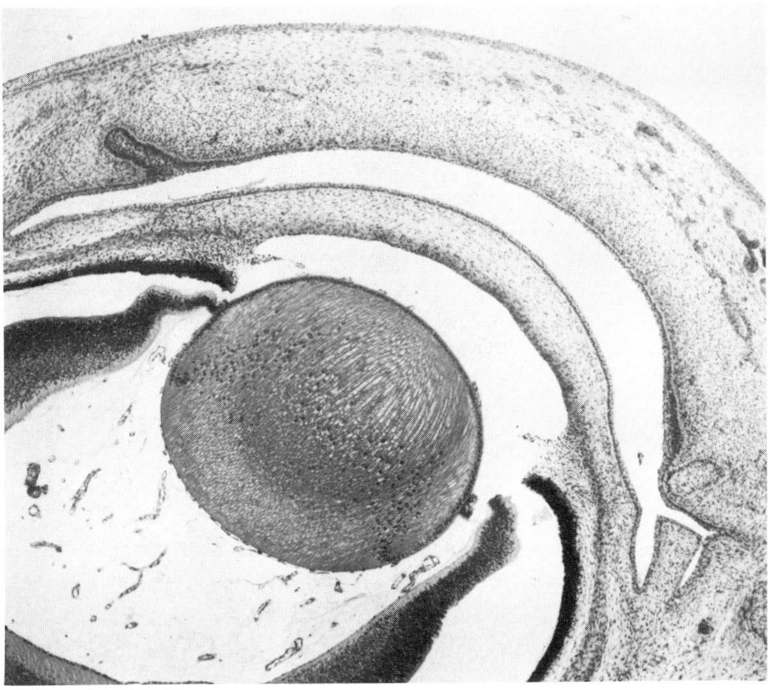

Figure 2-31. The lids are not yet open in this early eye. The cornea can be seen to be composed of an ectodermal epithelium supported by mesoderm. The lens is ectodermal as is the retina to the lower left.

branchial arch. The second pharyngeal pouch, that is, the one between the second and third branchial arches, gives rise to the palatine fossa and the palatine tonsil. The dorsal part of the third pharyngeal pouch gives rise to the inferior parathyroid glands and the ventral part of this pouch gives rise to the thymus. The dorsal part of the fourth pharyngeal pouch gives rise to the superior parathyroid gland and the ventral part to the ultimobranchial body or the thyrocalcitonin-producing cells of the thyroid gland. All these pouch structures reach their eventual normal site by a combination of differential growth and cell migration.

At the other end of the embryo, the external genitalia begin in the fifth week of development as a subectodermal mound of mesoderm, the genital tubercle, immediately cranial to the cloacal membrane.[13] This will become the clitoris in the female and the penis in the male (Fig. 2-32). Subsequently, subectodermal ridges of mesoderm run from this tubercle dorsally around the cloacal membrane. These are the urogenital folds. They will be the labia minora in the female. Anterior to the genital tubercle, a more generalized mesodermal collection develops which extends posteriorly as paired ridges, lateral to the urogenital fold. This is the pubic mound and the labioscrotal folds. In the female, the pubic mound will become the mons pubis and the folds, the labia majora. After week 6, the cloacal membrane has been divided into a posterior or dorsal anal membrane and an anterior or ventral urogenital membrane. These membranes subsequently disappear.[64] Subsequent female development consists of little more than growth of these structures, but male development is more complex. In the male, during the ninth week, the urogenital folds fuse in the midline from posteriorly to anteriorly enclosing the urogenital sinus and forming the penile urethra. Final closure is achieved in week 10. The labial scrotal folds also become approximated to form the scrotum and the testes descend over the course of several days at about 28 weeks.

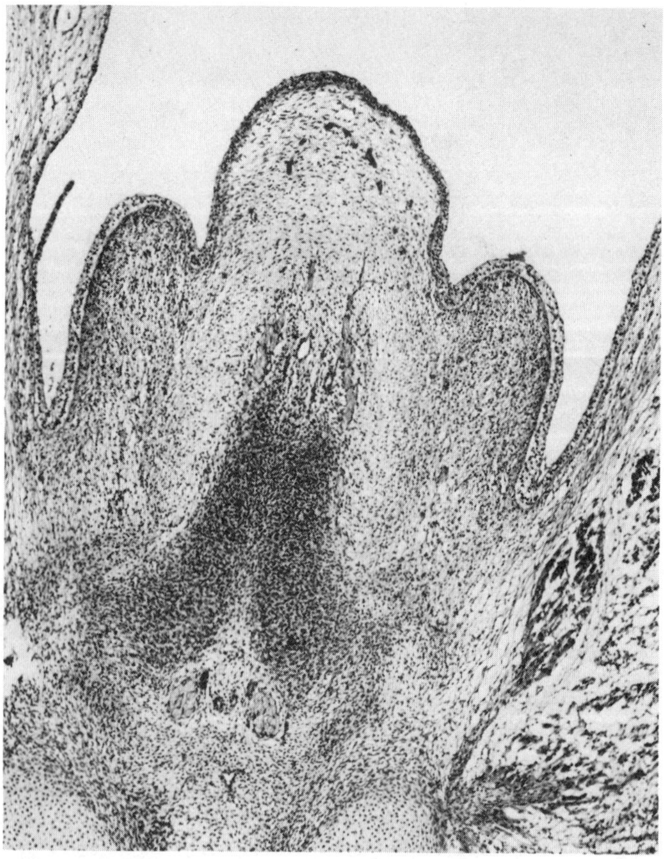

Figure 2-32. Labio-scrotal folds flank the genital tubercle between the thighs. The primordia of the cavernosa of the clitoris are forming. The symphysis pubis is developing at the lower left.

THE ENDODERM

The gastrointestinal tract, the lungs, and portions of the urogenital system have their origin in the very early events that produce the endoderm.[29-32] The endoderm is the first of the definitive germ cell layers to become apparent. The first derivative of the endoderm is the yolk sac (Fig. 2-33). This cavity develops a posterior diverticulum, the allantois, which extends into the body stalk. When folding takes place during week 4, the endodermal roof of the yolk sac is converted into an anterior diverticulum that extends forward to the prochordal plate, the foregut; a central portion that continues to communicate with the yolk sac, the midgut; and a posterior diverticulum that is continuous past the cloacal plate into the allantois, the hindgut. As the body stalk is rotated forward, so is the allantois which then runs from the cloacal plate through the ventral body wall to the body stalk.

The endoderm is now a tube invested with mesoderm at all sites except at the buccopharyngeal and cloacal membranes. The buccopharyngeal membrane ruptures at about 24 days, but the cloacal one disappears only during the seventh week, after it has been divided into anal and urogenital membranes.

The foregut gives rise to the pharynx, the lower respiratory tract, the esophagus which reaches its approximate relative length by week 7, and the stomach which develops as a dilatation of which subsequent rotation and differential growth produce the adult orientation. Glandular epithelium in the stomach may begin to function in the sixth lunar month. The duodenum is formed from both foregut and midgut with the junction of the two in the center of the C-loop.

With the future mouth, just anterior to the most cephalic extension of the endoderm, ectodermal cells form a diverticulum in the midline which separates from the oropharyngeal cavity and becomes the anterior pituitary (Fig. 2-34).[25]

The thyroid gland develops from endodermal cells in the floor of the foregut.[25] Beginning about day 24, at a site corresponding to the base of the future tongue, these cells form a down-

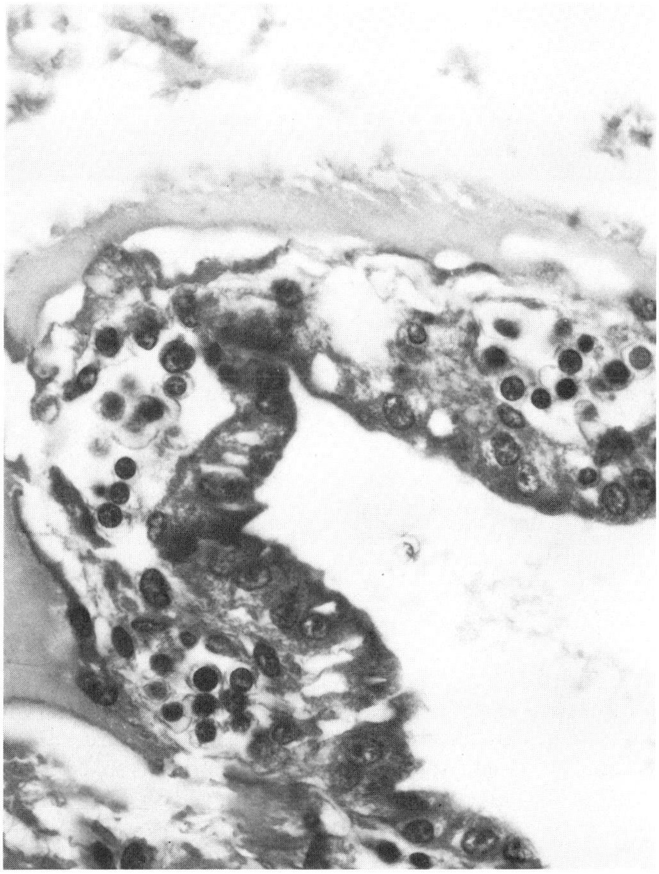

Figure 2-33. Endoderm forms a dense layer of cuboidal cells that is invested by extraembryonic mesoderm containing capillaries. Nucleated red cells are budding off from the wall of these capillaries. These are the blood islands in the wall of the yolk sac.

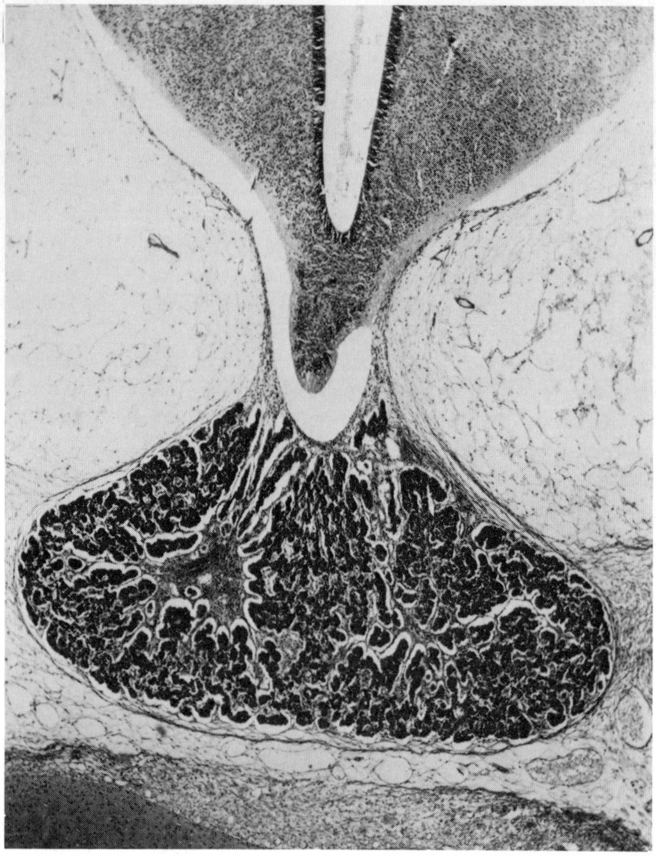

Figure 2-34. The anterior pituitary is developing beneath an extension of the midbrain which will become the posterior pituitary. The bony floor of the sella is developing.

growing diverticulum that by differential growth is displaced to the base of the neck. Differentiation and colloid formation occur by the 11th week (Fig. 2-35).

The pulmonary system has its onset in a ventral groove that develops in the anterior wall of the foregut on day 26.[13,25] This groove enlarges to become a vertical diverticulum which divides caudally into two lung buds by day 28. These two buds become the lungs and the fused portion of the diverticulum becomes the trachea. During week 5, the smaller left lung bud divides into two tubes and the right lung bud into three tubes (Fig. 2-36). The right main stem bronchus is more vertical than the left even at this stage. By week 9, growth and development have occurred to the point that the lobules are present. By week 10, the lungs have an adult form and by week 24, they will support life. Alveoli continue to form, however, until approximately 8 years of age.

Endodermal cells from the caudal foregut form the hepatic diverticulum (Fig. 2-37). They extend into the septum transversus, where they produce cords of liver parenchyma, growing between umbilical and vitelline veins, thus producing sinusoids between liver cords. The Kupffer cells of the liver and the hemopoietic portions are mesodermal. Hemopoiesis begins in the liver in the sixth week (Fig. 2-38). By 9 weeks, the weight of the liver is 10% of the total weight of the fetus. A second division of the hepatic diverticulum becomes the gallbladder and the cystic duct. During the 13th–16th weeks, bile is excreted.

The pancreas forms from two buds (Fig. 2-39). The dorsal one arises directly from the duodenum. The ventral one is carried to the region as the duodenum rotates. The ventral bud then fuses with the dorsal bud (Fig. 2-40). The exocrine pancreatic glands develop from the ventral and dorsal buds. Proteolytic enzymes are produced in the sixth lunar month. The islets of Langerhans arise from cells that subsequently bud off from the developing tubules of the exocrine gland. This occurs during the fourth lunar month. Insulin secretion begins about 20 weeks. The spleen develops from a

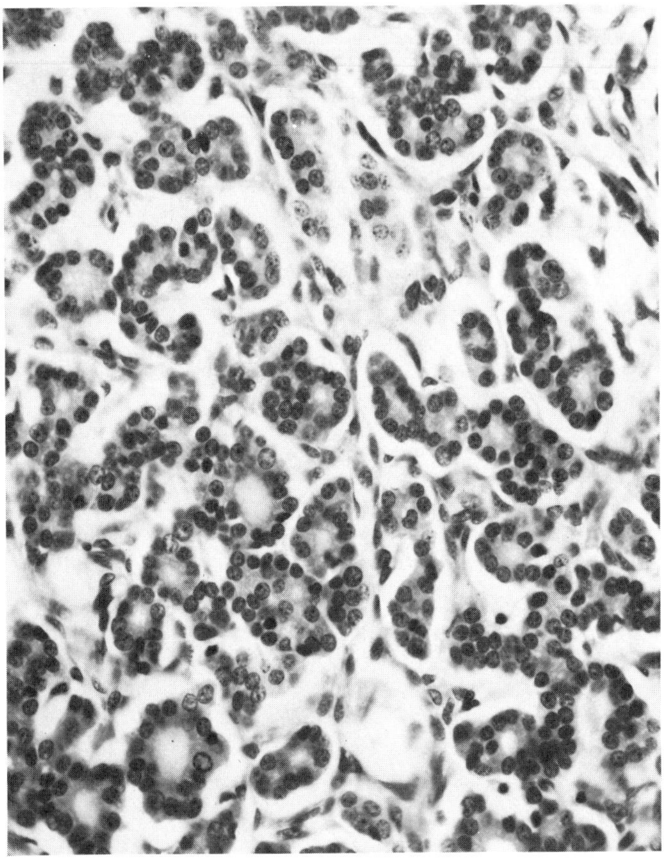

Figure 2-35. Colloid is present in the acini of the larger of these thyroid follicles. Some portions of the gland are not as well differentiated.

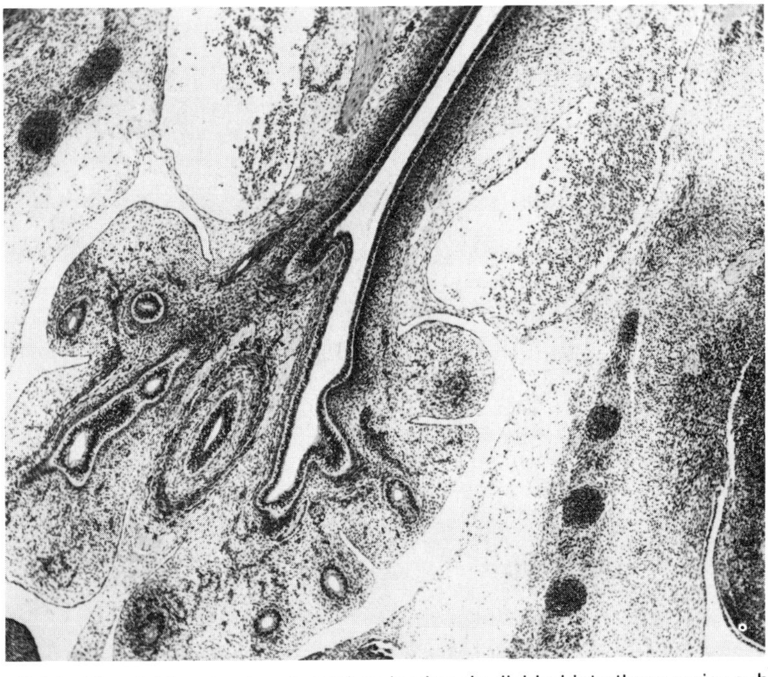

Figure 2-36. The right main stem bronchus is already divided into three major subdivisions serving three lobes as opposed to the left which possesses only two.

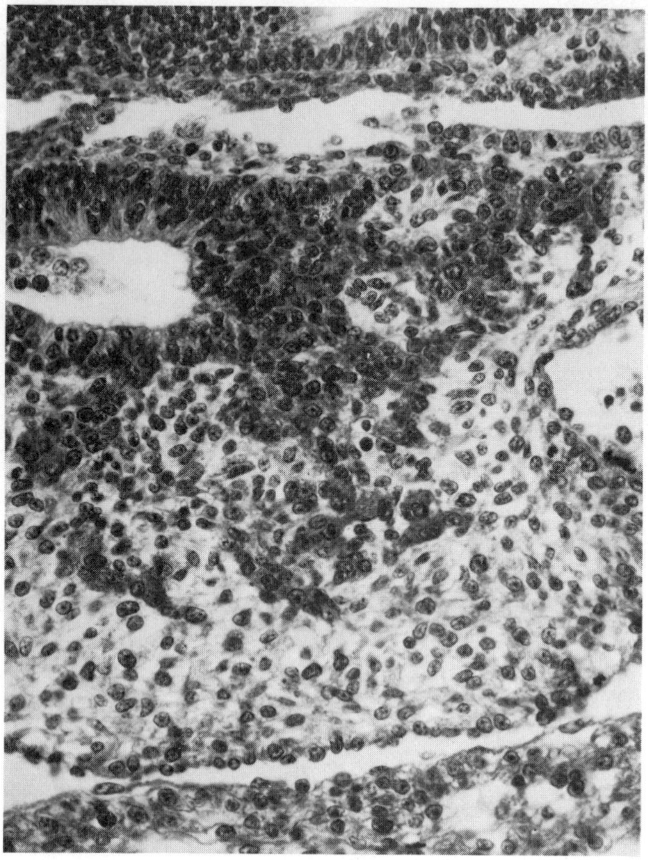

Figure 2-37. Primitive liver cells are arising in the wall of the foregut and migrating into the septum transversus. An attempt at cord-like arrangement is beginning.

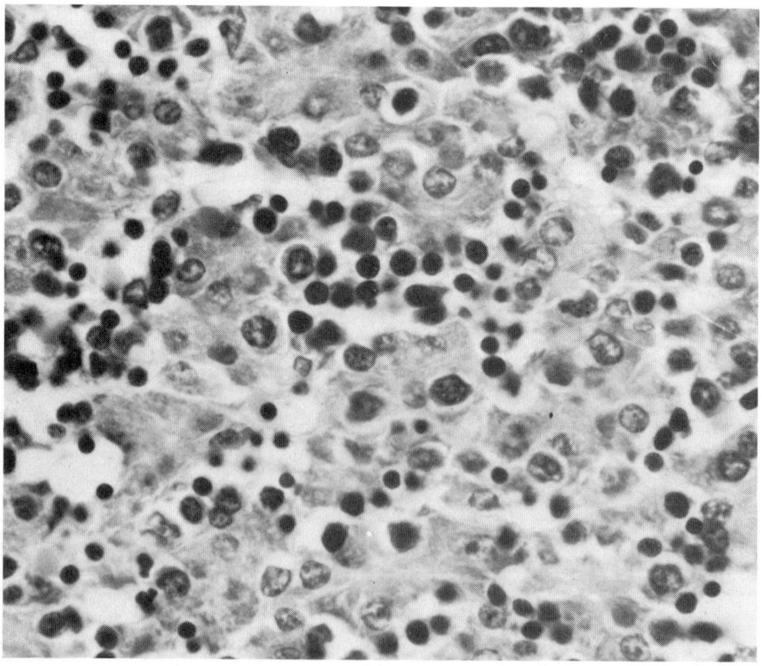

Figure 2-38. Hemopoiesis is occurring in the endothelial walls of the vascular channels between the cords of liver cells. Nucleated erythroblasts are the predominant cell type.

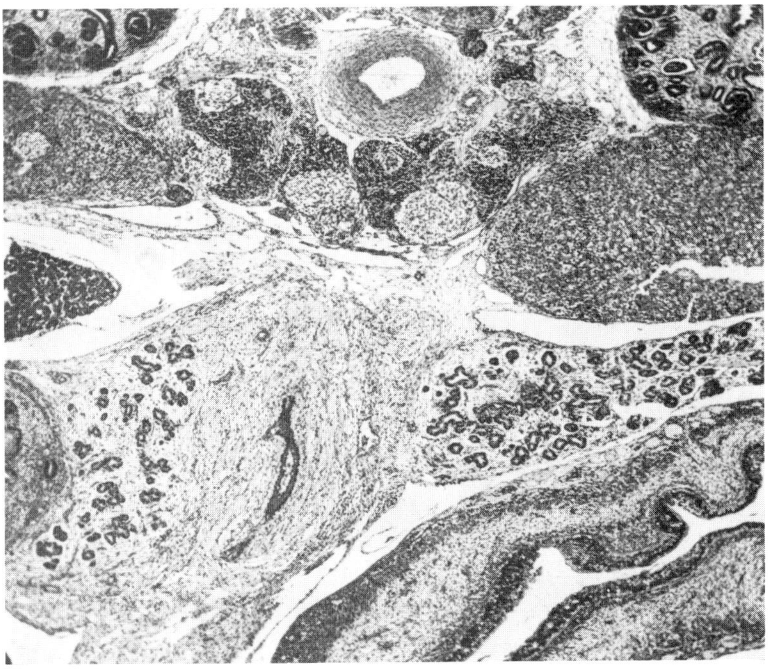

Figure 2-39. The two buds of the pancreas are seen. The dorsal one on the left is closely associated with the duodenum. The ventral one will be rotated into place. The stomach is below. The kidneys are in the upper corners of the photograph.

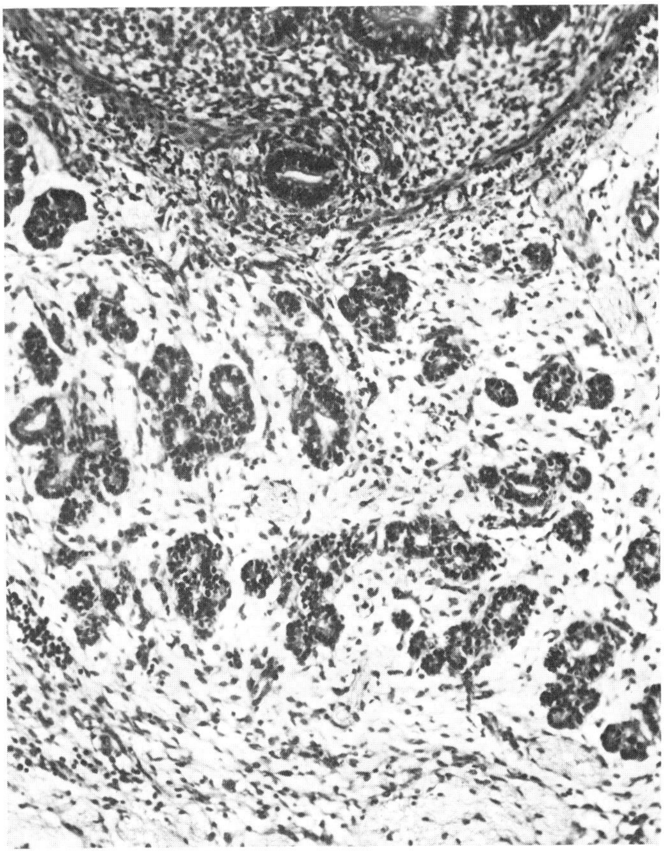

Figure 2-40. The dorsal bud of the pancreas is seen here to be arising within the wall of the duodenum.

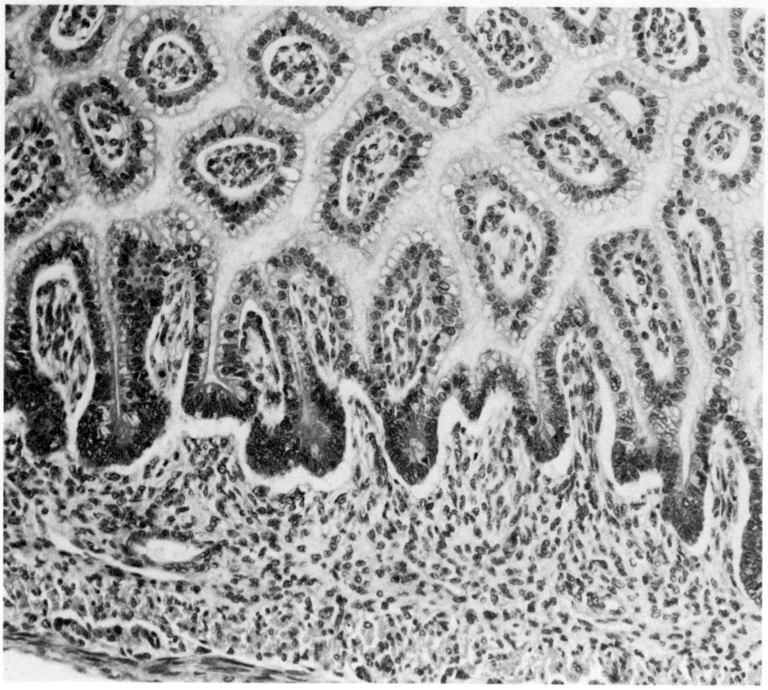

Figure 2-41. The villous form of the small bowel is apparent in the early second trimester.

mesodermal primordium in the dorsal mesogastrium of the foregut.

The midgut gives rise to the small intestine from the point of entrance of the common bile duct to the ileocecal valve (Fig. 2-41). From it also develop the appendix and colon to the midportion of the transverse colon. During the fifth week, the cecal diverticulum appears. Differential growth subsequently divides it into a cecum and appendix.

As the embryo grows, the yolk sac aperture becomes relatively smaller and the midgut becomes more of a tube. It is only loosely suspended from the posterior wall of the coelom by its mesentery and, as it lengthens, it herniates into the umbilical cord. During the 10th week, the midgut herniation returns to the abdominal cavity. This phenomenon is believed to be due simply to physical factors of size related to mesonephric development. During the second month, the mesonephric kidneys are maximal in size and extend from the septum transversus to the pelvis. Around the 10th week, they begin to degenerate and the metanephros becomes functional.[67,68]

The hindgut gives rise to the gastrointestinal tract from the middle of the transverse colon to the anus (Fig. 2-42). A more caudal extension, the tailgut, soon disappears. The ventral extension, the allantois, is separated from the hindgut by the urorectal septum. This structure arises in the fourth week in the angle between the hindgut and allantois. It consists of a mass of growing mesoderm that pushes into the angle and, by growing to the cloacal membrane, separates the allantois, now the urogenital sinus, from the hindgut, now the rectum and anus. This is achieved by the end of the sixth week. The dorsal portion of the cloacal membrane is now the anal membrane and the urogenital membrane is the ventral portion. The urogenital sinus will become the urachus, bladder, urethra, and vestibule in the female and the urachus, bladder, and a portion of the urethra in the male. The mesonephric (Wolffian) ducts empty into the urogenital sinus at about the level where the future urethra will join the vestibule in the fifth week (Fig. 2-43). Both portions of the cloacal membrane disappear in the seventh week.[64]

UROGENITAL SYSTEM

During the fourth week, the first nephric structures develop in the intermediate mesoderm,

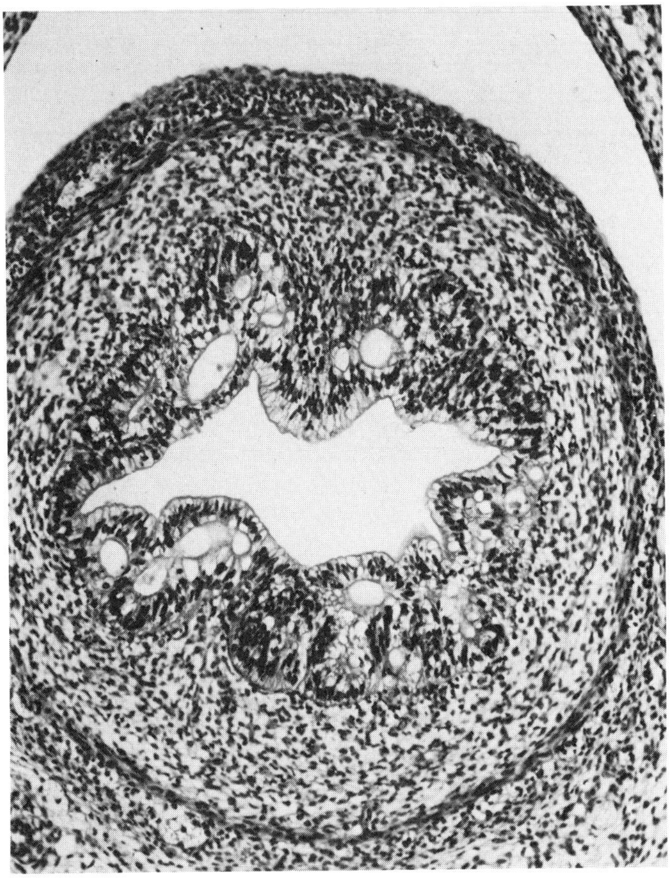

Figure 2-42. The muscular wall of the large bowel and its less complex lining make it distinguishable from the small bowel in the early second trimester. The coelomic cavity is above.

immediately lateral to the somites and in the posterior wall of the intraembryonic coelom.[67,68] Occurring at the level of the first somite, these consist of nephroceles, in essence cystic spaces in the intermediate mesoderm (Figs. 2-19, 2-20). They lack capillary glomeruli and may or may not communicate with the coelom by peritoneal funnels. As development proceeds, these structures occur sequentially and then degenerate in a cephalad to caudad manner in the intermediate mesoderm. At about the level of the ninth somite on the dorsolateral wall of the nephroceles, a nephric cord appears from which subsequently develops the nephric duct (Wolffian duct). This structure becomes continuous and, as subsequent nephric segments develop, it moves caudalward, reaching and entering the cloaca early in the fifth week of development (Figs. 2-43, 2-44). By the time the sequential process reaches the level of the future abdominal cavity, the nephroceles are well developed and contain glomeruli supplied by capillaries (Fig. 2-45). These more fully developed structures in the midportion of the column of intermediate mesoderm result in a bulge of this mesoderm into the adjacent coelomic cavity. Termed the urogenital ridges, these bilateral vertical ridges lie in the angle between the mesentery of the midgut and hindgut and the posterior wall of the coelom. They fill most of the coelomic or peritoneal cavity prior to 10 weeks of development and are believed responsible for the herniation of the midgut. The gonads will develop on their medial surface and the paramesonephric (Müllerian) ducts on their lateral one.

When the nephric or Wolffian duct enters the cloaca, it does so at about the level where the future urethra will enter the vestibule in the female. During the fifth week, the nephric or Wolffian duct gives off a diverticulum, the ureteric bud just above where it enters the cloaca. This diverticulum, the future ureter, grows dorsolaterally into the most caudal portion of the column of intermediate mesoderm. Here it bifurcates. With subsequent bifurcation and growth, it will induce development of the definitive kidney (Figs. 2-46, 2-47). Those glomeruli

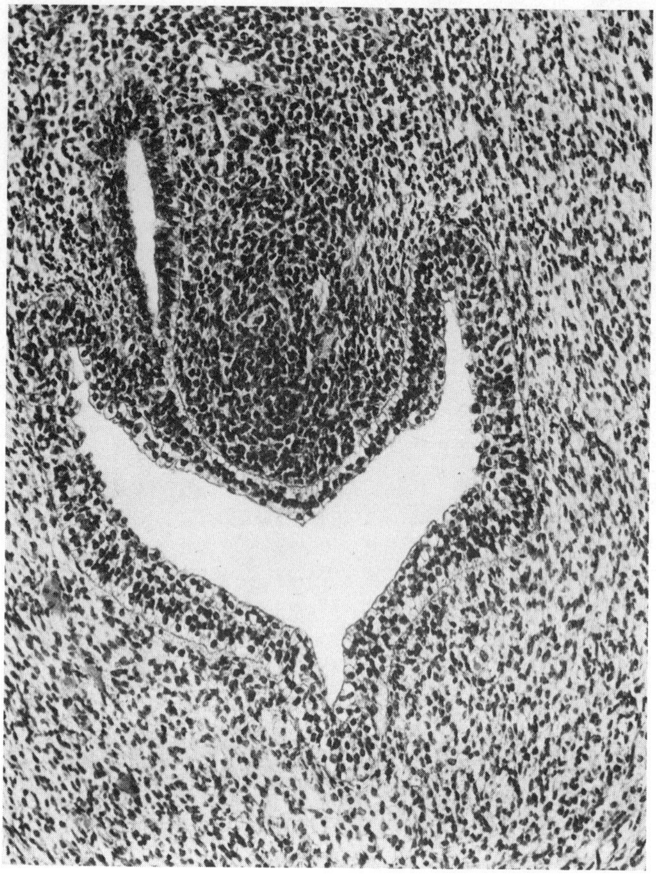

Figure 2-43. The urogenital sinus lies below. In the upper left the Wolffian duct enters the sinus. The other Wolffian duct is out of the plane of the picture. The epithelium of the posterior wall of the urogenital sinus is more consistent with that of the Wolffian duct than with that of the anterior wall of the urogenital sinus.

in the urogenital ridge which are connected to the Wolffian duct then degenerate.

With subsequent growth, the urogenital sinus expands. Consequently, it takes up and includes more and more of the Wolffian duct until it has taken up the duct back to the point where the ureteric bud develops. The sinus continues to expand, however, and now includes portions of the ureter as well. The result is that the ureter and Wolffian duct come to have separate orifices into the urogenital sinus. The ureter enters at the sites that will, with subsequent development, become the corners of the base of the trigone of the bladder. The Wolffian ducts enter at sites just below and lateral to where the urethra will enter the vestibule. Because the Wolffian duct is a mesodermal structure, the further implication of this developmental step is that the epithelium of the trigone, the posterior wall of the urethra, and the posterior wall of the urogenital sinus or vestibule between the orifices of the two Wolffian ducts are mesodermal epithelium or behave as one (Figs. 2-43, 2-44). This is particularly relevant to genital tract development because it means that the portion of the wall of the urogenital sinus which lies between the orifices of the two Wolffian ducts and which will give rise to the hymenal membrane and the lower vagina is at least partially Wolffian.[15]

This comes about in the following way: On the lateral surface of the urogenital ridges, late in the fifth week of embryonic life, the coelomic epithelium thickens to form the Müllerian placodes.[23,43] This is the site of the future fimbria of the tube. During the sixth week, the Müllerian placode forms multiple frond-like evaginations that coalesce into a single tube and migrate in the urogenital ridge down the lateral border of the preexisting Wolffian duct (Fig. 2-48). As they reach the pelvis, they move anteriorly over the Wolffian duct to fuse in the midline. The fused tip of the Müllerian duct then abuts upon the posterior wall of the urogenital sinus between the orifices of the two Wolffian ducts (Fig. 2-49). This site is mesodermal and lies immediately below the urethral orifice. When abutment

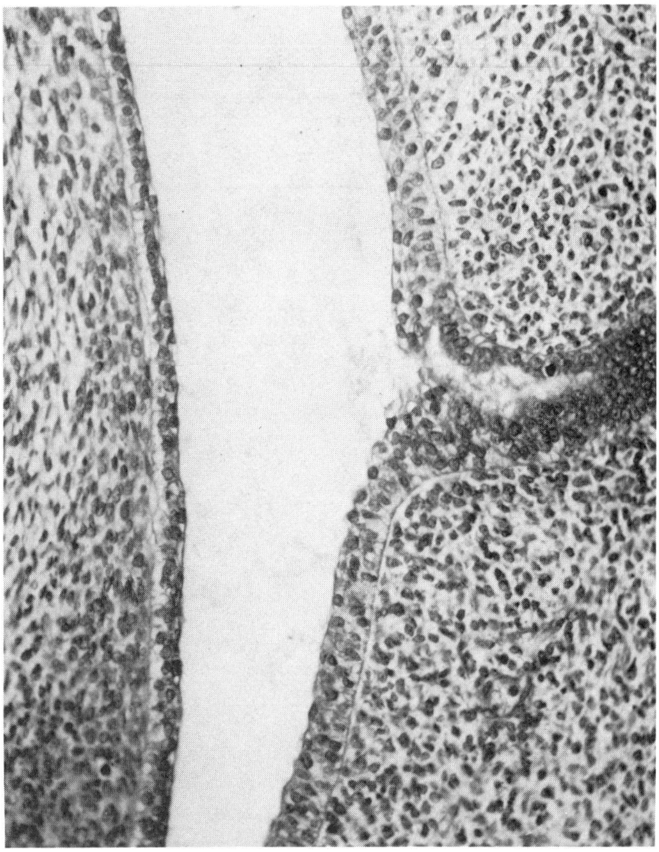

Figure 2-44. The nephric or Wolffian ducts enter the posterior wall of the urogenital sinus. Note that the epithelium surrounding this orifice is dissimilar from that of the opposite wall of the sinus.

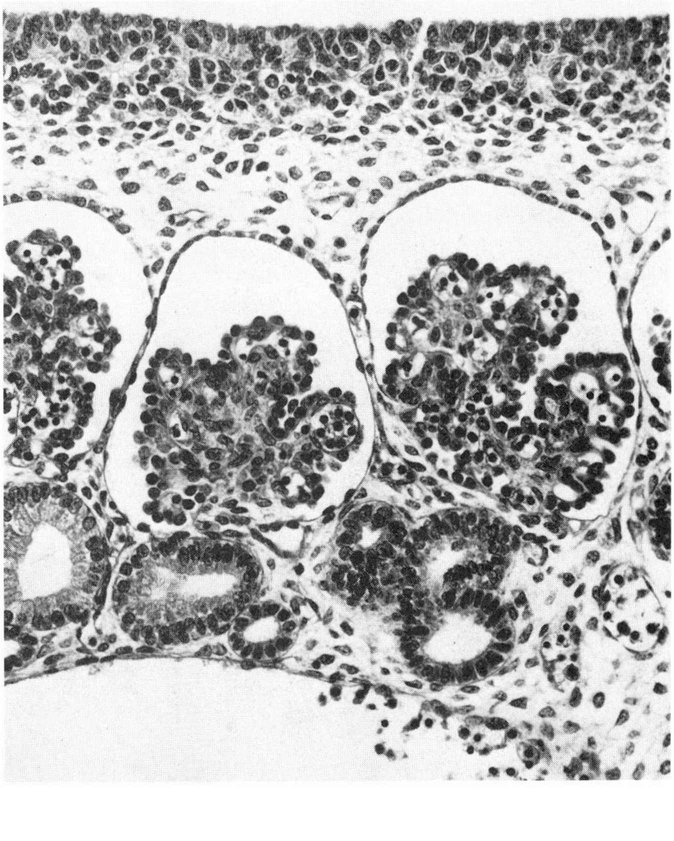

Figure 2-45. This section illustrates three of the sequential glomeruli that develop in the urogenital ridge. The surface is the medial surface and an indifferent gonad is developing there. Below the glomeruli are the nephric tubules and segments of the nephric duct may be seen.

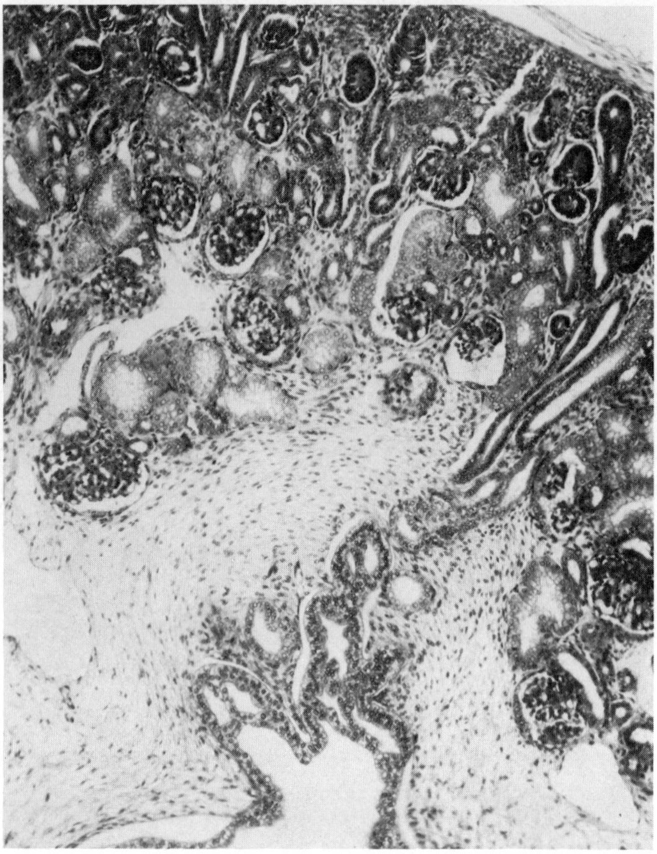

Figure 2-46. The ureteric bud has extended into the lowermost portion of the intermediate mesoderm and there has expanded into the renal pelvis which is below in the photograph. The renal cortex is developing in the mesoderm beyond it.

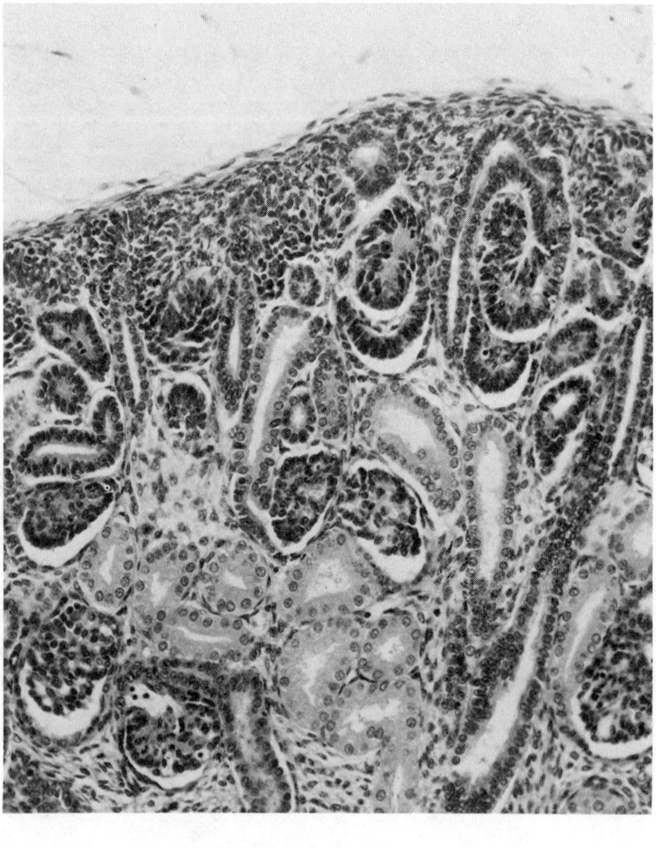

Figure 2-47. The renal cortex develops sequentially. The most peripheral glomeruli differentiate only after the more central ones so that the outer surface is more immature than the medulla.

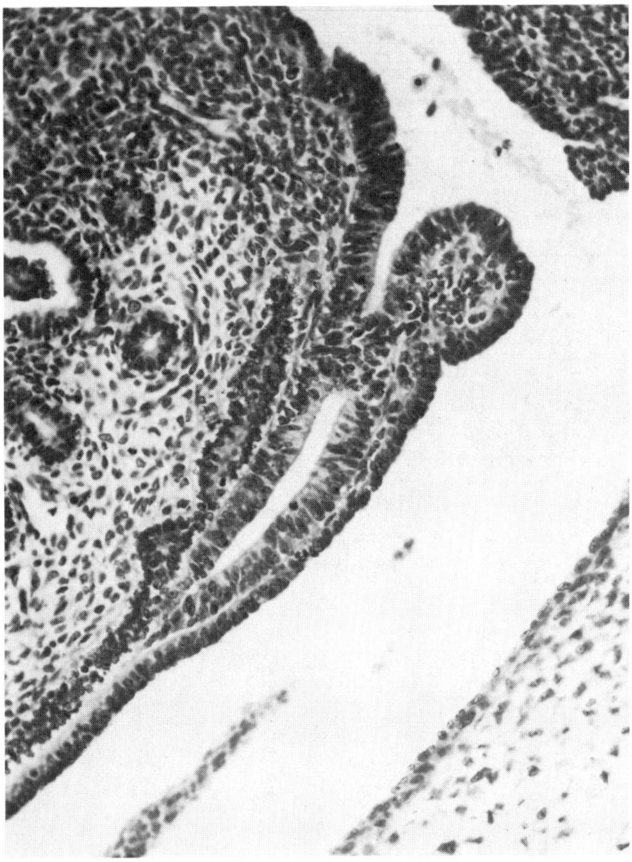

Figure 2-48. The Müllerian duct extends as an evagination from the coelom into the space between the Wolffian duct and the coelomic epithelium. It will remain closely applied to the surface of the Wolffian duct as it migrates into the pelvis.

occurs, the mesodermal epithelium begins to produce a cord of squamous epithelium, the vaginal plate (Fig. 2-50). This will become the lower vagina. In contrast, the upper vagina is derived from the Müllerian duct.[9,54] As differential growth occurs, the vaginal plate fills the elongating space between the tip of the Müllerian duct and the posterior wall of the urogenital sinus or future vestibule. In contrast to previous thought, the vaginal plate is continuously patent with the Müllerian duct all the way into the coelomic cavity as early as the first part of the second trimester.[63] Apparently, during normal development, the hymenal membrane is never intact. However, remnants of a transverse septum between the Müllerian duct portion of the vagina and the urogenital sinus portion of the vagina are visible in second-trimester embryos.

If this transverse septum does not break down, one of the major anomalies may occur. The vaginal plate is from the outset a squamous epithelium. Clinical observation suggests that the conversion of the Müllerian duct columnar epithelium, to the squamous epithelium of the upper vagina depends on vaginal patency. If the transverse septum remains intact, the Müllerian duct epithelium is not converted to a squamous one, but remains columnar. Under normal circumstances, conversion occurs beginning caudad and proceeding cephalad.[15,54] In the past, this has been interpreted to mean that the squamous epithelium migrated from the urogenital sinus, but more recent experimental work suggests that the squamous epithelium of the upper vagina develops de novo from Müllerian duct columnar epithelium if patency exists.

Subsequently, the upper vagina is functionally isolated from the rest of the upper genital tract by development of the cervix. As the vagina lengthens and enlarges, the stroma around the eventual endocervical canal begins to differentiate and to become more functionally rigid. This portion of the Müllerian duct becomes the cervix. As the vagina enlarges and swells around the lower portion of this segment, the vaginal fornices are formed. Presumably, because of the

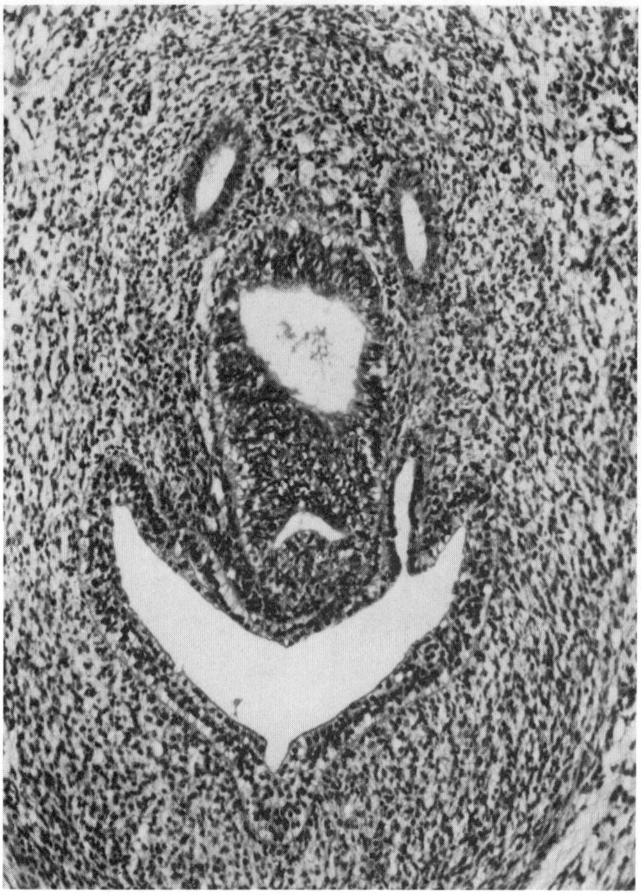

Figure 2-49. The tip of the fused Müllerian ducts has now reached the posterior wall of the urogenital sinus where it lies between the orifice of the two Wolffian ducts. One of the Wolffian ducts is slightly out of the plane of the section.

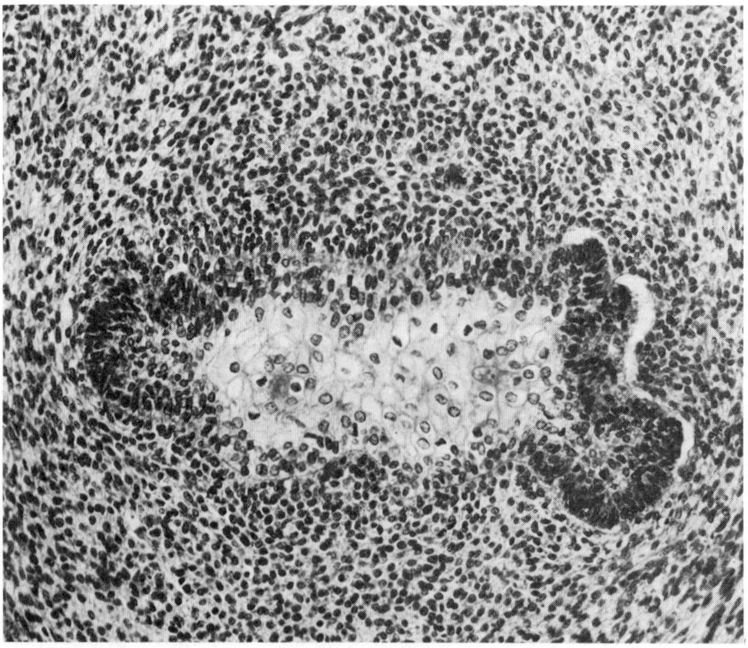

Figure 2-50. This cross section of the vaginal plate just below the tip of the Müllerian duct demonstrates squamous maturation. Cavitation will soon follow.

functional obstruction that results from cervical development, which is as effective an obstruction as if patency did not exist, conversion of the mucus-secreting columnar epithelium of the Müllerian duct to squamous epithelium is stopped. A junction of squamous and columnar epithelium is formed at the anatomic external os of the cervix. This conversion is re-initiated in later life by any eversion of the endocervical epithelium into the vaginal environment. The wall of the rest of the genital canal differentiates later in development, usually after the 20th week.[46,49] This circumstance is revealed in the location of Wolffian duct remnants in the adult genital canal. Because the cervical stroma develops very early when the Wolffian duct and Müllerian duct are still very close to each other, Wolffian duct remnants in the adult cervix are no more than about 5 mm from the endocervical surface and are deeply embedded in the cervical wall. Later, by the time that the vaginal, uterine, and tubal walls differentiate, the Müllerian and Wolffian ducts have become more widely separated. Wolffian duct remnants thus lie outside the walls of these portions of the adult genital canal (Fig. 2-51).

The myometrium, endometrial stroma, and epithelium become fully differentiated between 20 weeks and term, but responsiveness to sex steroids is very variable. A few female infants bleed because maternal hormones have decidualized their endometrium and withdrawal produces slough, but, in general, the infant's endometrium is not fully responsive. Teratologic studies with diethylstilbestrol suggest, however, that the vaginal plate epithelium is sensitive to estrogen as early as 10 weeks because DES seems to inhibit its development.[54] DES also prevents the conversion of the Müllerian duct epithelium to a squamous one and disorganizes the stromal maturation that forms the walls of the cervix, myometrium, and tubes.[37] As described above, the germ cells migrate from the yolk sac via the hindgut mesentery into the medial wall of the urogenital ridge primarily during the fifth week of embryonic life. Assuming that the embryo is a normal genetic male, the Y chromosome either carries or controls the expression of the genes that result in the production of the HY antigen in embryonic tissue.[28] In the presence of this antigen, the arrival of the germ cells results in the devel-

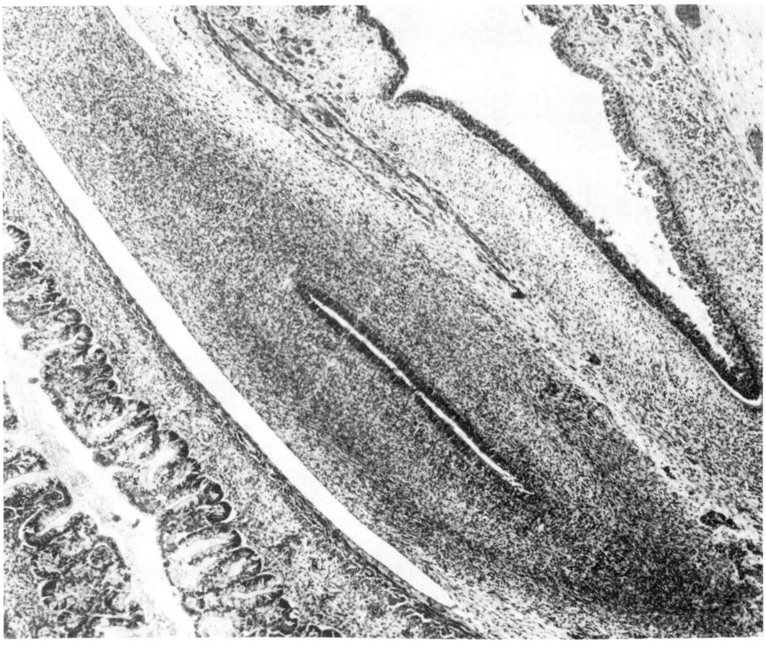

Figure 2-51. This uterus shows no differentiation of myometrium or endometrium. Only the epithelium is clearly delineated. The urogenital sinus (bladder) lies above and the hindgut (colon) lies below.

opment of a testis. The epithelial cells on the surface of the gonad proliferate and produce radial cords, so-called sex cords, that extend from the coelomic surface to the center of the urogenital ridge, the medulla of the future gonad (Fig. 2-52). The germ cells become embedded in the sex cords. Those that do not become embedded die. These sex cords soon separate from the surface and differentiate into the testicular tubules (Fig. 2-53). The epithelial cells of the cords become the Sertoli cells. Although the germ cells in the male remain largely undifferentiated and perhaps, therefore, are less fragile than the same cells in the ovary, their continued good health depends upon their maintenance within a healthy tubule with healthy Sertoli cells. The testicular tubules connect through the rete with the epididymis and vas deferens. These structures derive from the mesonephric tubules and duct. The interstitial or Leydig cells develop in the stromal tissue of the testis (Fig. 2-54). These testosterone producers develop sufficiently early that they exhibit significant response to the chorionic gonadotrophin produced by the placenta in the first trimester. Experimental studies suggest that the testosterone surge which accompanies the hCG peak may be critically important in effecting the simultaneously occurring development of the male central nervous system.[34] Various aspects of sexual behavior can be modified in animals by preventing this androgen peak. The cyclicity of the central nervous system which underlies the female reproductive cycle seems to be inherent in development unless it is inhibited by this large dose of androgen early in male embryogenesis.

If the embryo is female, an ovary develops when the germ cells reach the gonadal ridge. True sex cords do not develop in the ovary, but gonadal development seems to be a few days behind that seen in the male (Fig. 2-1). Portions of the adult rete ovarii also seem to originate in the coelomic epithelial in some cases. Mention has already been made of the necessity that the early differentiating germ cells be incorporated into primordial follicles by cells of the coelomic epithelium. The formation of these follicles and the secretion of the zona pellucida by the primitive granulosa postpones the inevitable demise for a small portion of the millions of germ cells that are initially present in the embryonic ovary (Figs. 2-1–2-4). The ovarian stroma differentiates into cells resembling rather plump fibroblasts, the theca (Fig. 2-2). When, in conjunction with the follicle, these cells become further differen-

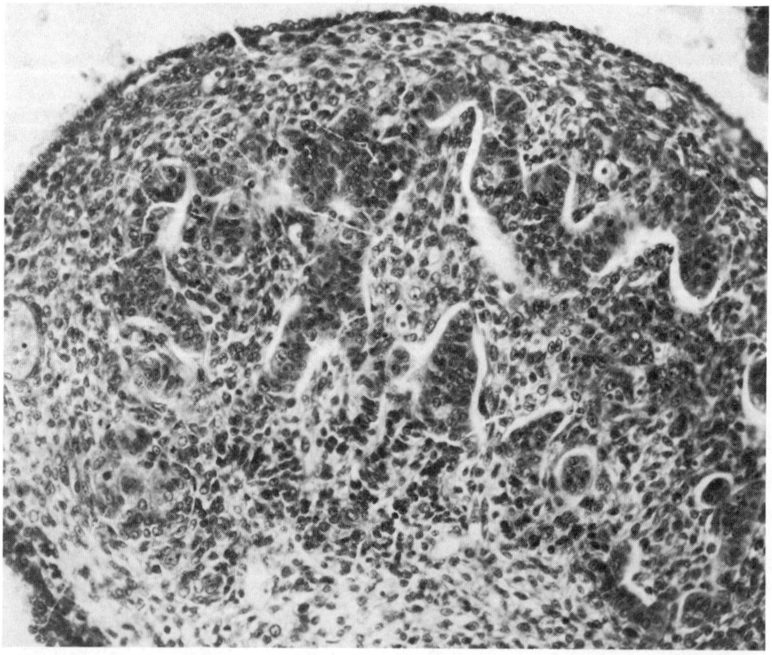

Figure 2-52. Radial cords of epithelium are developing within the stroma of this gonad. No Leydig cells are apparent.

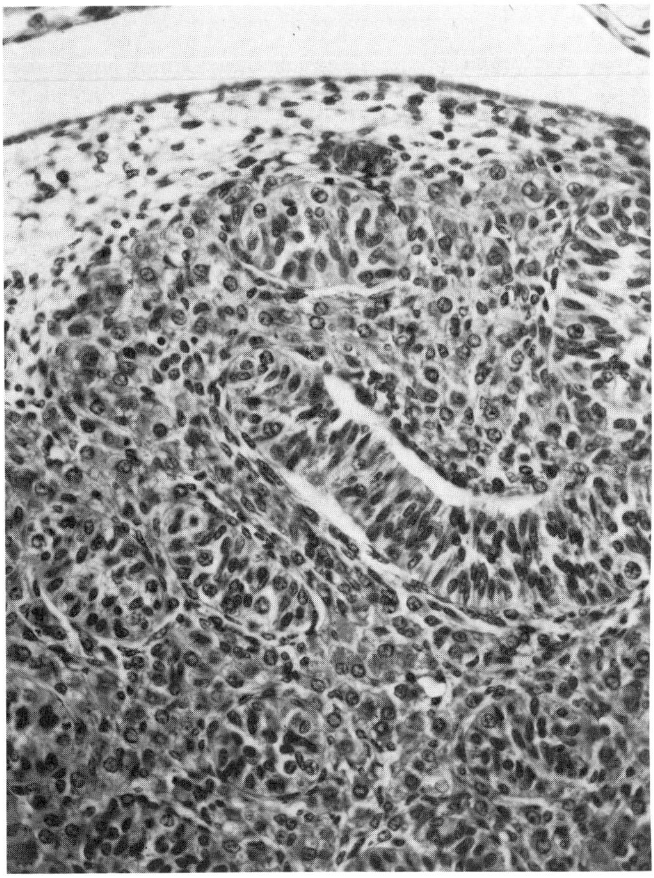

Figure 2-53. Epithelial cords are becoming clear-cut tubules, but no lumina are apparent. Large germ cells can be seen in the primitive tubules. Leydig cell development is suggested and the tunica albuginea is forming.

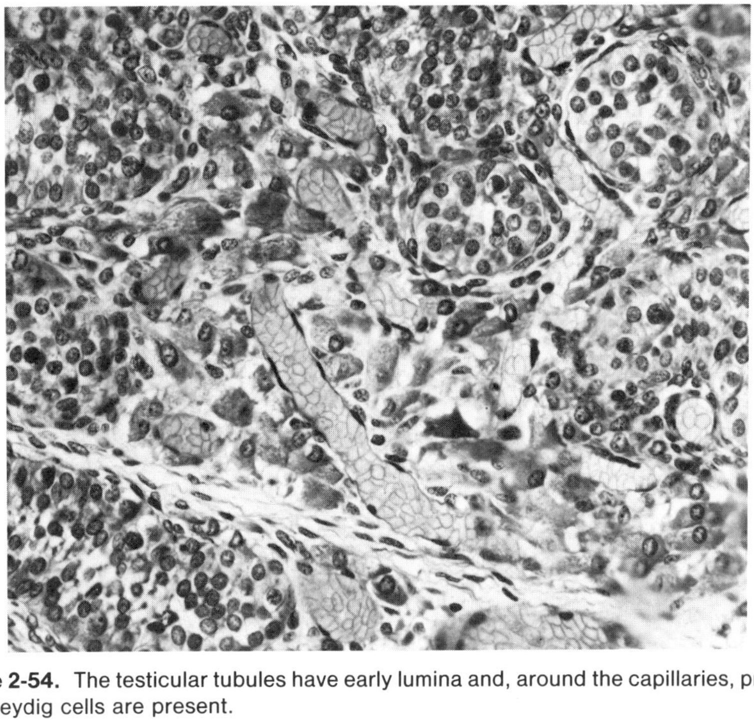

Figure 2-54. The testicular tubules have early lumina and, around the capillaries, prominent Leydig cells are present.

tiated into polyhedral hormone producers, they are capable of producing estrogen. In the absence of follicles or infiltration with neoplastic cells, ovarian theca usually produces only androgens (Fig. 2-3).

CARDIOVASCULAR

The cardiovascular system is the first physiologic system to function in the embryo. Consistent with what has been suggested above about the interrelationship of growth, development, and aging, this early onset of function may be associated with the fact that almost 70% of the North American population dies of cardiovascular disease.

On about day 15, angiogenesis begins in the extraembryonic mesoderm in the wall of the yolk sac, the body stalk, and the chorion (Fig. 2-15). The first sign is the aggregation of mesodermal cells in linear groups that soon develop lumina converting them into vascular channels. Some of the mesodermal cells differentiate into endothelial cells lining the channels and some into blood cell precursors. When significant amounts of blood formation are taking place, primarily in the yolk sac at first, these collections are known as blood islands (Fig. 2-55). Blood vessels develop in the embryo about 2 days after they occur in the extraembryonic mesoderm.[25] In the middle of the third week, paired linear aggregates of mesodermal cells collect in the lateral plate mesoderm that forms the floor of that portion of the intraembryonic coelom that is anterior to the prochordal plate. These heart tubes develop lumina and establish continuous connections with all other developing vessels throughout the embryo and the extraembryonic mesoderm. When the trilaminar disc is folded, the lateral folding brings the heart tubes together and they fuse into a single structure, the future heart. As the head fold develops, the heart is rotated down to a site just above the septum transversus or future diaphragm. Myogenic contractions of the heart tubes begin as early as day 22. It is believed that directional flow exists by the end of the fourth

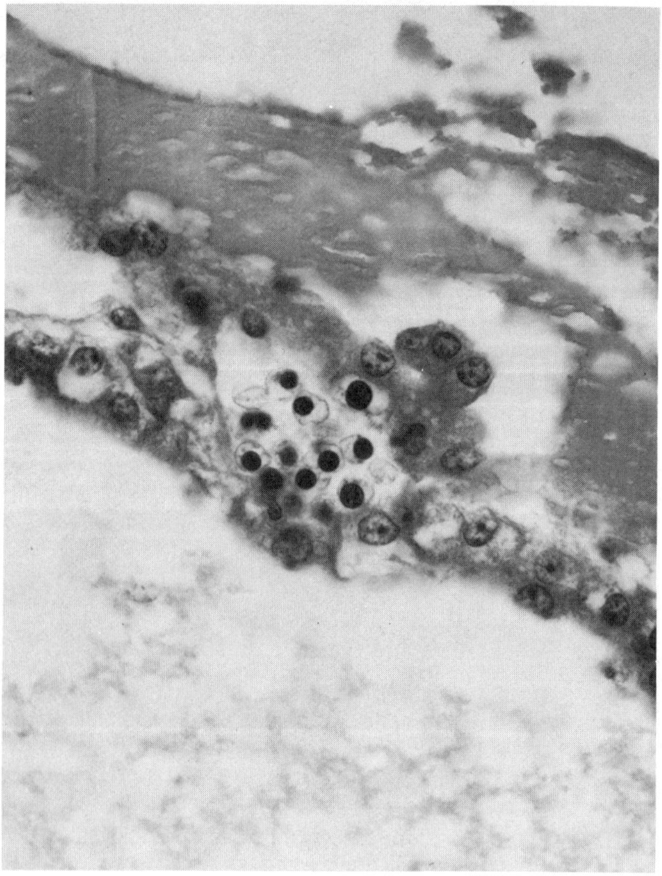

Figure 2-55. The endodermal cell layer of this yolk sac wall is at the bottom. The overlying mesoderm contains a capillary. Multiple nucleated erythroblasts are budding off the endothelium of this capillary.

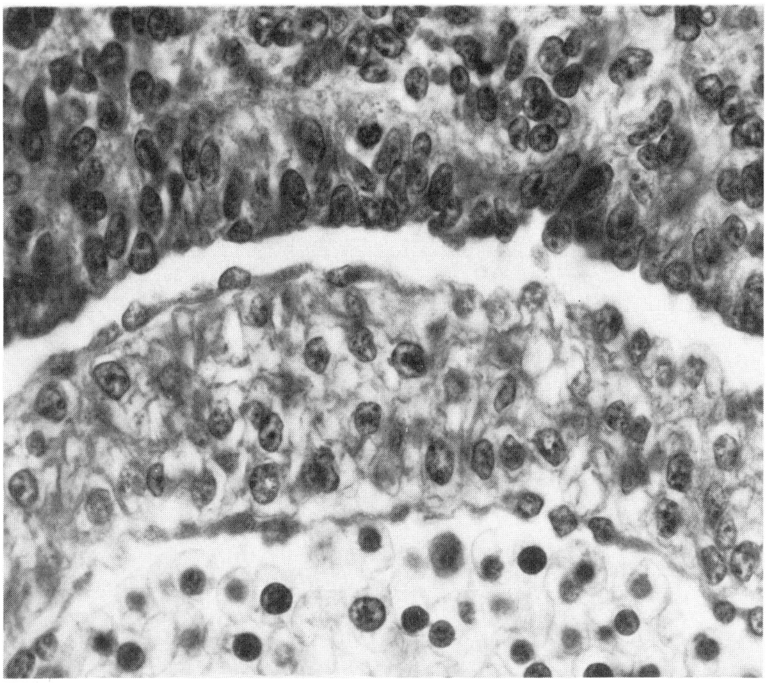

Figure 2-56. Nucleated red cells fill the ventricle in this developing heart. The three-layered construction of the heart wall is apparent. The endocardial layer, a single-cell layer, is derived from the heart tubes. A multiple-cell layer, the future myocardium, separates the endocardium from the single-cell-layered pericardium.

week of embryonic life. As the heart enlarges, it bulges into the adjacent intraembryonic coelom, now the pericardial sac. The mesoderm around the heart tube differentiates into both the muscular myocardium and the visceral pericardium. The endocardium of the mature heart is derived from the mesodermal cells that have formed the heart tubes (Fig. 2-56).

Speculatively, the blood islands, which develop in the yolk sac at 15 days, the fetal liver after 6 weeks, and the bone marrow after the first trimester, give rise to all the blood cells but the lineage of the red cell is best defined (Fig. 2-38). Yolk sac blood islands produce largely primitive erythroblasts that are nucleated and contain hemoglobin E. As erythropoiesis moves to the liver between the sixth and eighth weeks, definitive erythroblasts that are somewhat smaller and that contain hemoglobin F become prominent. Nucleated red blood cells are largely gone by the 10th week. Hepatic erythropoiesis is maximal at about 30 weeks and is almost gone in the normal newborn. Erythropoiesis begins in the bone marrow early in the second trimester and occurs in the sternum by the end of the sixth month. After it is established, hemoglobin A begins to appear. The correlation of anatomic site, cell type, and hemoglobin type presented here is not absolute.[25] The early development of blood and circulation is paralleled by prominent iron transport by the placenta starting early in development.[19]

INTEGUMENTARY SYSTEM

The skin is composed of an epithelium of ectodermal origin and a dermis of mesodermal origin. The dermis is derived partially from the somites of the para-axial mesoderm and partially from the lateral plate mesoderm. In the head and neck region, a remarkable amount of the dermis and other connective tissue structures are derived from the neural crest.[35] The epithelium or epidermis begins as a one-cell layer of ectoderm which, with closure of the neural tube, completely surrounds the embryo by the end of week 4 (Figs. 2-20, 2-21).[25,45] This one-cell layer proliferates as a germinal layer and produces a more superficial cell layer, the periderm. The cells of the periderm are polyhedral and possess ultrastructural features that suggest that they are capable of transport (Fig. 2-57). During the third lunar month of gestation, the skin achieves three more milestones in its development. The epithelium produces intermediate type cells and therefore begins to resemble a stratified squamous epithelium. It is also invaded by melanocytes from the neural crest. Both the dermis and the epidermis begin to arrange themselves in the genetically determined pattern of ridges produced by the dermal papillae. Although present throughout the skin, the ridges are most prominent over the palmar surfaces of the hands and soles of the feet. They provide the basis for fingerprinting. These structures are generally complete by the fifth lunar month of gestation.

The epidermis subsequently develops a complex set of appendages and a fully cornified surface. Although the antecedents of this development occur early in the second trimester, it is not completed until approximately the 28th week of gestational age.[49] Beginning first over the eyebrows and lips, the cells of the germinal layer proliferate and produce keratinoblasts which, as they rise through the overlying squamous epithelium, differentiate into fully flattened anucleated squames containing only keratin. The surface of the cell is coated with lipid. These cells form the impervious stratum corneum of the mature skin. Simultaneously, the cells of the germinal layers produce buds that project down into the dermis. These become club-shaped. When the bulbous end is secondarily invaded by a dermal papillus, they become hair follicles (Fig. 2-58). Sebaceous glands develop from the basal germinal cells along the side of the hair follicles or, in some cases such as in the labia minora, directly from the surface epithelium. Eccrine sweat glands are also the result of down growth from the basal germinal layer of the epidermis. They are seen in the palms and soles as early as the first part of the second trimester. Nails develop as thickenings of the epidermis, beginning in the early second trimester. After the development of the stratum corneum begins around the eyebrows, development proceeds in a cephalad to caudad manner. It moves back over the scalp and down the trunk and out the extremities. As it occurs somewhat prematurely in the hands and feet, the last portions of skin to be keratinized are the wrists and ankles. Complete keratinization is achieved by about 28 weeks. The stratum corneum imparts opacity to the fetal skin so that

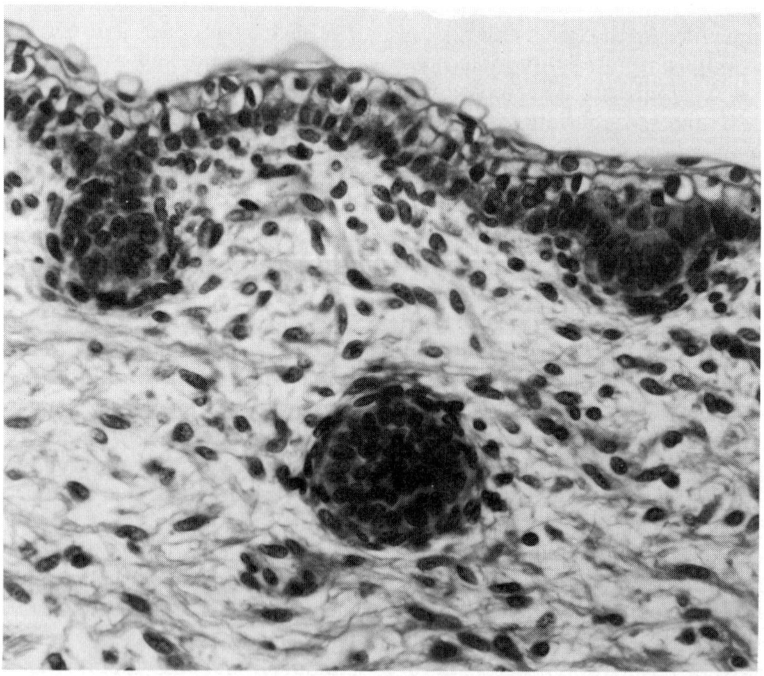

Figure 2-57. The epithelium is approximately three cell layers thick. A basal cell layer and a layer of intermediate cells are surmounted by balloon-like periderm cells. The basal cell layer is beginning to form the buds which will give rise to the appendages.

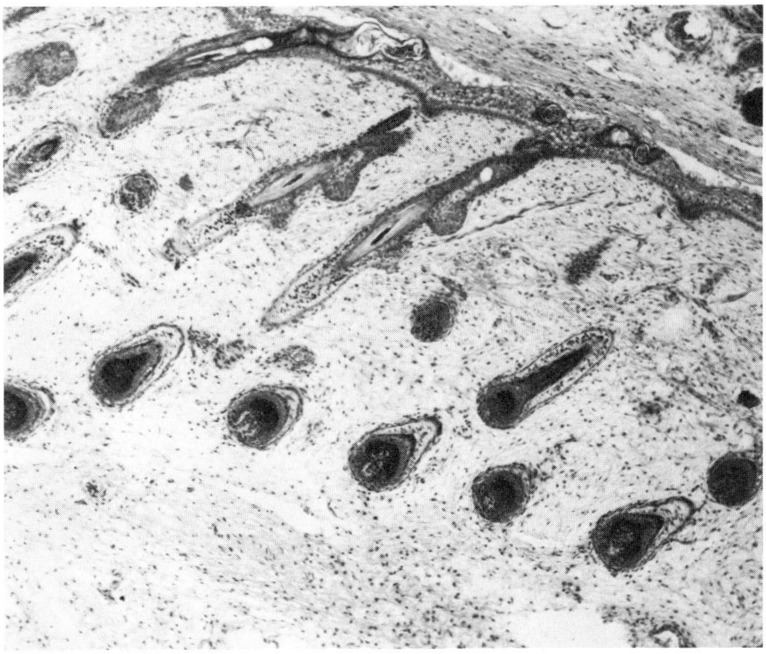

Figure 2-58. This skin from the scalp of the second-trimester fetus has hair follicles with associated sebaceous glands.

the degree to which it has developed can be ascertained simply by inspecting the prematurely born infant. If the stratum corneum is present, the subcutaneous vasculature is not visible. Prior to development of the stratum corneum, the fetal skin is freely permeable to water and probably to many other substances. The stratum corneum renders the skin relatively impermeable, a fact that probably has physiologic consequence.[47]

Additional skin appendages of particular importance in reproduction are the apocrine sweat glands, the most notable of which are the breasts.[1] Mammals evolved approximately 100 million years ago as the dinosaurs were dying. In addition to being capable of controlling their temperatures, mammals possess modified skin appendages which nourish the young. The initial development of the mammae takes place in so-called milk lines (Fig. 2-59). These paired structures run from the posterior surface of the shoulders through the axilla onto the ventral surfaces of the chest. They extend down across the abdomen into the groin and minimally out over the posterior buttocks. Mammae may be found in this distribution in any of several different species of mammals. Subsequent mammary development is rudimentary along most of the milk line, but over this distribution, extramammary breast disease may occasionally be seen in adults. Examples are extramammary nipples, aberrant breast tissue, extramammary Paget's disease, or apocrine gland infections or tumors. By the end of week 5, the milk line consists of a thickening along its entire course, produced by bud-like proliferations of the basal germinal cells of the epidermis. By the end of week 6, most of the budding has disappeared, although the apocrine sweat glands in the axilla and labia majora are developed from it. However, over the anterior chest, development proceeds more definitively. The subepithelial bud enlarges and projects further into the dermis (Fig. 2-60). At about 12 weeks of embryonic life, roughly 20 sprouts develop from this bud. These will be the lactiferous ducts. Secondary sprouts that will become breast tissue develop a few weeks later. Differentiation of breast secretory epithelium and myoepithelial cells occurs in the second trimester from an undifferentiated epithelial cell. Some neonatal breasts are sufficiently responsive to maternal hormones that they produce small quantities of secretion at term. The epithelial development of the breast is probably controlled by the preceding development of the associated mesoderm. The adipose

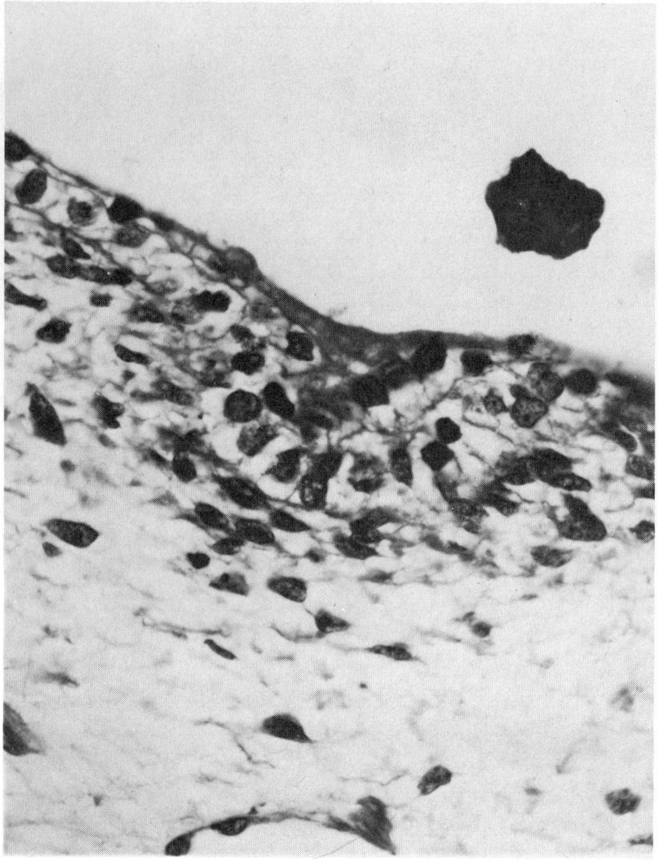

Figure 2-59. This invagination and thickening of the surface epithelium is the earliest sign of future breast development.

tissue in the breast is among the first of the mesodermal tissues to develop. For unknown reasons, most supernumerary nipples in women are caudal, but a few are located superior to the breast. In some Asian populations, most accessory nipples are superior to the breast. Polymastia without nipples is seen on occasion. In the vulva, swelling of accessory breast tissue may complicate pregnancy.

AMNIOTIC FLUID

The amniotic cavity develops as a fluid collection in the body stalk immediately above the inner cell mass during the eighth postovulatory day.[30] It seems to be a transudate at this time, and subsequently. Studies of its constituents suggest that it is in rough equilibrium with the fetal serum, reflecting changes in that fluid. Although fetal urination and swallowing probably play a role in its production and removal, its volume during the first half of pregnancy is directly related to fetal volume and surface area, suggesting that it in some way reflects fetal size.[41,53,70] The ready permeability of the unkeratinized fetal skin and the copious capillary vasculature of the fetal dermis make it likely that the fetal skin is a significant site of exchange and perhaps the most significant early in pregnancy. That this might be so is further suggested by the fact that when the skin keratinizes fully and becomes impermeable late in the second trimester, the character of the amniotic fluid begins to change.[20,47,56] Its volume decreases slightly from a maximum of approximately 1000 cc.[18,53] It becomes more and more hypotonic and is no longer in equilibrium with fetal serum. This is particularly true for large molecules such as bilirubin and alpha-feto-protein that are not excreted by the fetal kidney. In the third trimester, the principal known sources of exchange between the fetus and the amniotic fluid are the 400–500 cc of urine produced per day by the fetal kidney and the similar amount swallowed.[51,52] Exchange exists via the fetal lung as well.[11] When significant variation exists in either the rate of urine production or of swal-

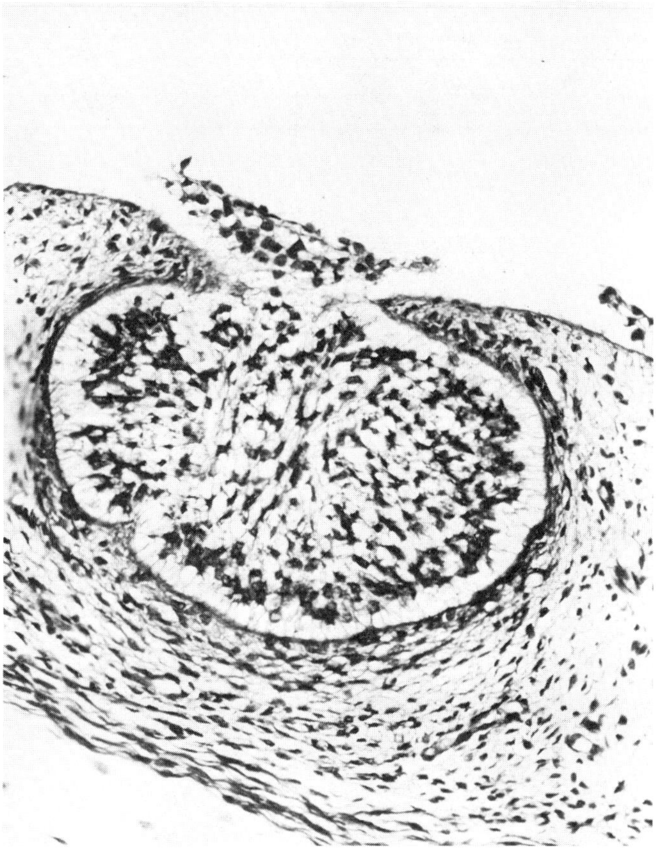

Figure 2-60. A well-developed subepithelial bud has been formed by invaginating epithelium. This is the future breast.

lowing, oligohydramnios or polyhydramnios may develop. Again, it may not be merely coincidental that these entities tend to develop in the early third or late second trimester as the fetal skin becomes impermeable.

ADRENAL

The adrenal cortex, a mesodermal derivative, develops from cells of the coelomic epithelium during the fifth week.[25,45,66] They begin in the area between the root of the hindgut mesentery and the developing gonadal ridge. They then migrate to their final site just above the kidney. The migration occurs in two waves. The primary wave produces the large fetal zone of the cortex, whereas the secondary wave produces the smaller definitive cortex (Fig 2-61). The adrenal cortex develops autonomously until the fifth month of gestation, after which ACTH from the fetal pituitary is required for further development. In the presence of ACTH, the cells of the initial migration form a large fetal zone which will regress after birth, leaving only the definitive cortex. The development of the fetal zone is associated with the production of steroid hormone precursors that are converted to estriol by the placenta. The fetal zone may also be related to the development of other maturational changes such as skin desquamation, muscle catabolism, and surfactant production in the lung.[48] In some species, development of the fetal zone of the adrenal cortex appears to be clearly linked with the initiation of labor, but in primates the relationship is more complex. As noted above, developmental failure may occur in anencephalics in which the fetal zone of the adrenal is poorly developed.

CONCLUSION

The fetal development described in this chapter is complex, but there are some unifying principles: (1) Although the precise combinations of genetic and environmental influences that result in the development of any given individual

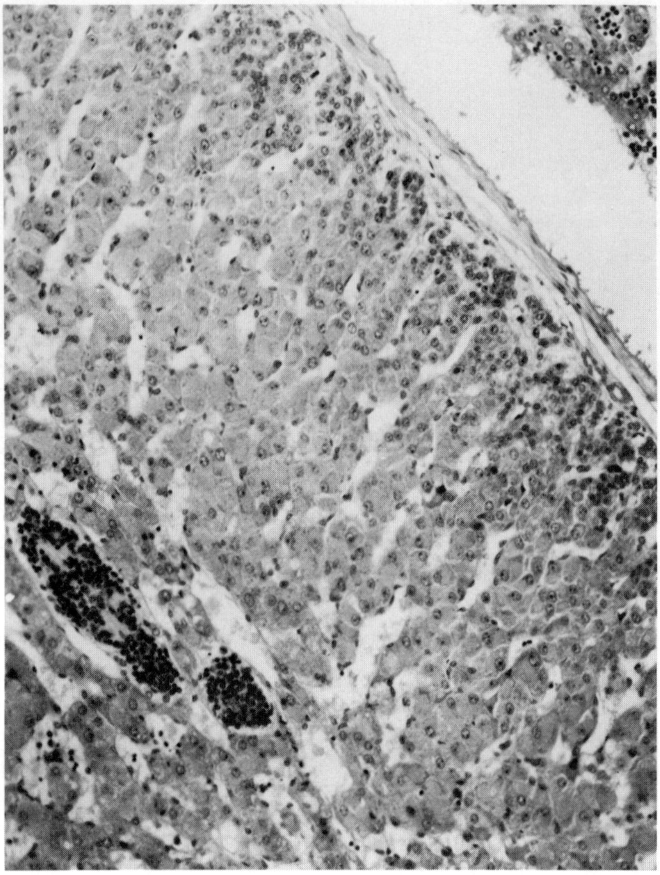

Figure 2-61. The future adrenal medulla is represented by two islands of dark cells to the lower left and the future adrenal cortex is represented by the thin layers of dark cells on the outer edge of the gland. All else is the fetal zone of the adrenal cortex.

are unique to that individual, development, in general, occurs in a predictable sequence that follows a fairly narrow time-course in all individuals of a given species. (2) This developmental sequence is based upon a more fundamental sequence of growth and development that consists first of growth by proliferation and then of growth by differentiation and cell hypertrophy. (3) Although cell hypertrophy and differentiation culminate in mature function, they also presage mortality in most cases. (4) The cycle of growth, maturation, and aging occurs on a different time table among different cell populations in the same organism.

REFERENCES

1. Anderson, R. R.: Embryonic and fetal development of the mammary apparatus. In: *Lactation*, Vol. 4. B. L. Larson (Ed.). New York, Academic Press, 1978, pp. 367–370.
2. Baker, T. G.: A quantitative and cytological study of germ cells in human ovaries. *Proc. R. Soc. Lond. (Biol.)* **158:**417-433, 1963.
3. Baker, T. G.: Oogenesis and ovulation. In: *Reproduction in Mammals: I. Germ Cells and Fertilization.* C. R. Austin and R. V. Short (Eds.). Cambridge, Cambridge Unversity Press, 1978, pp. 14–45.
4. Beck, J. C. and Johnson, J. W. C.: Maternal administration of glucocorticoids. *Clin. Obstet. Gynecol.* **23:**93–113, 1980.
5. Blackburn, W. R., Kaplan, H. S., and McKay, D. G.: Morphologic changes in the developing rat placenta following prednisolone administration. *Am. J. Obstet. Gynecol.* **92:**234–246, 1965.
6. Channing, C. P., Anderson, L. D., Hoover, D. J., Kolena, J., Osteen, K.G., Pomerantz, S. H., and Tanabe, K.: The role of non-steroidal regulators in control of oocyte and follicular maturation. *Rec. Prog. Horm. Res.* **38:**331–407, 1982.
7. Channing, C. P. and Pomerantz, S. H.: Studies on an oocyte maturation inhibitor partially purified from porcine and human follicular fluids. In: *Intragonadal Regulation of Reproduction.* P. Franchimont and C.P. Channing (Eds.). New York, Academic Press, 1981, pp. 81–96.

8. Csapo, A. I., Pulkkinen, M. O., and Wiest, W. O.: Effects of lutectomy and progesterone replacement therapy in early pregnant patients. *Am. J. Obstet. Gynecol.* **115**:759–765, 1973.
9. Cunha, G. R.: The dual origin of vaginal epithelium. *Am. J. Anat.* **143**:387–392, 1975.
10. Diamant, S., Kissilveitz, R., and Diamant, Y.: Lipid peroxidation system in human placental tissue: General properties and the influence of gestational age. *Biol. Reprod.* **23**:776–781, 1980.
11. Duenholter, J. H. and Pritchard, J. A.: Fetal respiration: Quantitative measurements of amniotic fluid inspired near term by human and rhesus fetuses. *Am. J. Obstet. Gynecol.* **125**:306–309, 1976.
12. Eddy, C. A. and Pauerstein, C. J.: Anatomy and physiology of the fallopian tube. *Clin. Obstet. Gynecol.* **23**:1177–1193, 1980.
13. England, M. A.: *Color Atlas of Life Before Birth.* Chicago, Year Book Medical Publishers, 1983.
14. Flexner, L. B., Cowie, D. B., Hellman, L. M., Wilde, W. S., and Vosburgh, G. J.: The permeability of the human placenta to sodium in normal and abnormal pregnancies and the supply of sodium to the human fetus as determined with radioactive sodium. *Am. J. Obstet. Gynecol.* **55**:469–480, 1948.
15. Forsberg, J. G.: Cervicovaginal epithelium: Its origin and development. *Am. J. Obstet. Gynecol.* **115**:1025–1043, 1973.
16. Fox, H.: The placenta as a model for organ ageing. In: *Placenta, A Neglected Experimental Animal.* P. Beaconsfield and C. Fillee (Eds.). New York, Pergamon Press, 1979, pp. 351–385.
17. Freese, U.: Vascular relations of placenta exchange areas in primates and man. In: *Respiratory Gas Exchange and Blood Flow in the Placenta.* L. D. Longo and H. Bartels (Eds.). National Institutes of Health, Department of Health, Education and Welfare Publication, NIH# 73361, 1972, pp. 31–53.
18. Fuchs, F.: Volume of amniotic fluid at various stages of pregnancy. *Clin. Obstet. Gynecol.* **9**:449–460, 1966.
19. Galbraith, G. M. P., Galbraith, R. M., and Faulk, W. P.: Immunological studies of transferrin and transferrin receptors of human placental trophoblast. *Placenta* **1**:33–46, 1980.
20. Gillibrand, P. N.: Changes in amniotic fluid volume with advancing pregnancy. *J. Obstet. Gynaecol. Br. Commonw.* **76**:527–529, 1969.
21. Greiss, F.: Uterine and placental blood flow. In:. *Gynecology and Obstetrics*, Vol. 3, Chap. 62. J. J. Sciarra (Ed.). Hagerstown, MD, Harper & Row, 1982, pp. 1–19.
22. Gruenwald, P.: Growth of the human foetus. In: *Advances in Reproductive Physiology.* A. McLaren (Ed.). New York, Academic Press, 1967, pp. 279–309.
23. Gruenwald, P.: The relation of growing Müllerian duct to the Wolffian duct and its importance for the genesis of malformations. *Anat. Rec.* **81**:1–19, 1941.
24. Hamilton, W. J. and Boyd, J. D.: Development of the human placenta. In: *Scientific Foundations of Obstetrics and Gynecology.* E. E. Philip, J. Barnes, and M. Newton (Eds.). Philadelphia, F. A. Davis Co., 1970, pp. 185–254.
25. Hamilton, W. J. and Mosman, H. W.: *Human Embryology*, 4th Edition. Baltimore, Williams & Wilkins, 1972.
26. Harris, M. J., Poland, B. J., and Dill, F. J.: Triploidy in 40 human spontaneous abortuses: Assessment of phenotype in embryos. *Obstet. Gynecol.* **57**:600–606, 1981.
27. Hartmann, J. F. and Gwatkin, R. B. L.: Alteration of sites on the mammalian sperm surface following capacitation. *Nature* **234**:479–481, 1971.
28. Haseltine, F. P.: Defects in H-Y antigen expression and related gonadal failure. *Semin. Reprod. Endocrinol.* **1**:113–119, 1983.
29. Hertig, A. T. and Rock, J.: On the development of the early human ovum with special reference to the trophoblast of the pre-villous stage: A description of 7 normal and 5 pathological human ova. *Am. J. Obstet. Gynecol.* **47**:149–184, 1944.
30. Hertig, A. T. and Rock, J.: Two human ova in the previllous stage, having a developmental age of about 7 and 9 days respectively. *Contrib. Embryol.* **31**:65–84, 1945.
31. Hertig, A., Rock, J., Adams, E. C., and Mulligan, W. J.: On the preimplantation stages of the human ovum: A description of four normal and four abnormal specimens ranging from the second to the fifth day of development. *Contrib. Embryol.* **35**:201–220, 1954.
32. Heuser, C., Hertig, A. T., and Rock, J.: Two human embryos showing early stages of the definitive yolk sac. *Contrib. Embryol.* **31**:85–99, 1945.
33. Hsu, Y. C.: Monozygotic twin formation in mouse embryos in vitro. *Science* **209**:605–606, 1980.
34. Hutchinson, J. B. (Ed.): *Biological Determinants of Sexual Behavior.* New York, John Wiley & Sons, 1978.
35. Johnston, M. C.: Embryology of the pharyngeal and facial areas. In: *Development of Upper Respiratory Anatomy and Function.* U.S. Government Printing Office #617-046-00033-1, 1976.
36. Kajii, T. and Ohama, K.: Androgenetic origin of hydatidiform mole. *Nature* **268**:633–634, 1977.
37. Kaufman, R. H., Adam, E., Binder, G. L., and Gerthoffer, E..: Upper genital tract changes and pregnancy outcome in offspring exposed in utero to diethylstilbestrol. *Am. J. Obstet. Gynecol.* **137**:299–308, 1980.
38. Kurman, R. J., Scully, R. E., and Norris, H. J.: Trophoblastic pseudotumor of the uterus. An exaggerated form of syncytial endometritis simulating a malignant tumor. *Cancer* **38**:1214–1226, 1976.

39. Kurman, R. J., Young, R. H., Norris, H. J., Main, C. S., Lawrence, W. D., and Scully, R. E.: Immuno-cytochemical localization of placental lactogen and chorionic gonadotrophin in the normal placenta and trophoblastic tumors, with emphasis on intermediate trophoblast and the placenta site trophoblastic tumor. *Int. J. Gynecol. Pathol.* **3**:101–121, 1984.
40. Kusamran, T., Drake, R., Wunderlich, S. M., Lau, A., Balinga, B. S., and Munro, H. N.: Control of RNA content of developing human placenta. *Placenta* **1**:157–167, 1980.
41. Lind, T., Kendall, A., and Hytten, F. E.: The role of the fetus in the formation of amniotic fluid. *Br. J. Obstet. Gynaecol.* **79**:289–298, 1972.
42. Ludwig, K. S.: The morphologic structure of the placenta in relation to its exchange function. In: *Respiratory Gas Exchange and Blood Flow in the Placenta.* L.D. Longo and H. Bartels (Eds.). National Institutes of Health, Department of Health, Education and Welfare, NIH 73-361, 1972, pp. 13–22.
43. Marshall, F. F. and Beisel, D. S.: The association of uterine and renal anomalies. *Obstet. Gynecol.* **51**:559–562, 1978.
44. Moor, R. M., Osborn, J. C., and Crosby, I. M.: Cell interactions and oocyte regulation in mammals. In: *Follicular Maturation and Ovulation.* R. Rolland, E. V. Van Hall, S. G. Hillier, K. P. McNatty, and J. Schoemaker (Eds.). Princeton, Excerpta Medica, 1982, pp. 249–264.
45. Moore, K. L.: *The Developing Human.* Philadelphia, W.B. Saunders Co., 1973.
46. O'Rahilly, R.: The embryology and anatomy of the uterus. In: *The Uterus.* H. J. Norris and A. T. Hertig (Eds.). Baltimore, Williams & Wilkins, 1973, pp. 17–39.
47. Parmley, T. H., Gupta, P. K., and Walker, M. A.: "Aging" pigments in term human placenta. *Am. J. Obstet. Gynecol.* **139**:760–766, 1981.
48. Parmley, T. H. and Miller, E.: Fetal maturity and amniotic fluid analysis. *Am. J. Obstet. Gynecol.* **105**:354–362, 1969.
49. Parmley, T. H. and Seeds, A. E.: Fetal skin permeability to isotopic water (THO) in early pregnancy. *Am. J. Obstet. Gynecol.* **108**:128–131, 1970.
50. Pijnenborg, R., Dixon, G., Robertson, W. B., and Brosens, I.: Trophoblastic invasion of human decidua from 8 to 18 weeks of pregnancy. *Placenta* **1**:3–19, 1980.
51. Pritchard, J. A.: Deglutition by normal and anencephalic fetuses. *Obstet. Gynecol.* **25**:289–297, 1965.
52. Pritchard, J. A.: Fetal swallowing and amniotic fluid volume.*Obstet. Gynecol.* **28**:606–610, 1966.
53. Queenan, J. T., Thompson, W., Whitfield, C. R., and Shah, S. I.: Amniotic fluid volumes in normal pregnancy. *Am. J. Obstet. Gynecol.* **114**:34–38, 1972.
54. Robboy, S. J., Taguchi, O., and Cunha, G. R.: Normal development of the human female reproductive tract and alterations resulting from experimental exposure to diethylstilbestrol. *Hum. Pathol.* **13**:190–197, 1982.
55. Scammon, R. E.: Developmental anatomy. In: *Morris' Human Anatomy.* J. P. Schaeffer (Ed.). Philadelphia, Blakiston Co., 1942, pp. 9–52.
56. Seeds, A. E.: Current concepts of amniotic fluid dynamics. *Am. J. Obstet. Gynecol.* **138**:575–586, 1980.
57. Settlage, D. S. F., Motoshima, M., and Tredway, D. R.: Sperm transport from the external cervical os to the fallopian tubes in women: A time and quantitation study. *Fertil. Steril.* **24**:655–661, 1973.
58. Slack, J. M. W.: *From Egg to Embryo.* Melbourne, Australia, Cambridge University Press, 1983.
59. Stewart, A. D. and Hunt, D. M.: *The Genetic Basis of Development.* New York, John Wiley & Sons, 1982.
60. Streeter, G. L.: Weight, sitting height, head size, foot length, and menstrual age of the human embryo. *Contrib. Embryol.* **11**:143–170, 1920.
61. Surti, U., Szulman, A. E., and O'Brien, S.: Dispermic origin and clinical outcome of three complete hydatidiform moles with 46, XY karyotype. *Am. J. Obstet. Gynecol.* **144**:84–87, 1982.
62. Teasdale, F.: Gestational changes in the functional structure of the human placenta in relation to fetal growth: A morphometric study. *Am. J. Obstet. Gynecol.* **137**:560–568, 1980.
63. Terruhn, V.: A study of impression moulds of the genital tract of female fetuses. *Arch. Gynecol.* **229**:207–217, 1980.
64. Thomas, J. B.: *Introduction to Human Embryology.* Philadelphia, Lea and Febiger, 1968.
65. Torpin, R.: *The Human Placenta.* Springfield, IL, Charles C Thomas, 1969.
66. Tuchmann-Duplessis, H., Auroux, M., and Haegel, P.: *Illustrated Human Embryology.* New York, Springer-Verlag, 1975.
67. Torrey, T. W.: The early development of the human nephros. *Contrib. Embryol.* **35**:175–197, 1954.
68. Torrey, T. W.: Morphogenesis of the vertebrate kidney. In:. *Organogenesis.* R. L. DeHaan and H. Ursprung (Eds.). New York, Holt, Rinehart and Winston, 1965, pp. 559–579.
69. Valdes-Dapena, M. A.: The development of the uterus in late fetal life, infancy, and childhood. In: *The Uterus.* H. Norris and A. Hertig (Eds.). Baltimore, Williams & Wilkins, 1973, pp. 40–67.
70. Vanotterlo, L. C., Waldimiroff, J. W., and Wallenburg, H. C. S.: Relationship between fetal urine production and amniotic fluid volume in normal pregnancy and pregnancy complicated by diabetes. *Br. J. Obstet. Gynaecol.* **84**:205–209, 1977.
71. Vincent, R. A., Huang, P. C., and Parmley, T. H.: Proliferative capacity of cell cultures derived from the human placenta. *In Vitro* **12**:649–653, 1976.

72. Walton, J.: The role of limited cell replicative capacity in pathologic age change. A review. *Mech. Aging Dev.* **19**:217–244, 1982.
73. Weinberg, P. C., Cameron, I. L., Parmley, T. H., Jter, J. R., and Pauerstein, C. J.: Gestational age and placental cellular replication.*Obstet. Gynecol.* **36:** 692–696, 1970.
74. Wellmann, C. F. and Volk, B. W.: Fine structural changes in the rabbit placenta induced by cortisone. *Arch. Pathol.* **94**:147–157, 1972.
75. Winnick, M., Coscia, A., and Noble, A.: Cellular growth in human placenta. I. Normal placental growth. *Pediatrics* **39**:248–251, 1967.
76. Wislocki, G. B. and Dempsey, D. W.: Electron microscopy of the human placenta. *Anat. Rec.* **123**:133–167, 1955.
77. Witschi, E.: Migration of the germ cells of human embryos from the yolk sac to the primitive gonadal folds. *Contrib. Embryol.* **32**:67–80, 1948.

3

PHYSIOLOGY OF THE PREGNANT WOMAN

Pregnancy is a wondrous thing! The idea of a newly conceived individual receiving nurture from the mother as it grows and develops, to be finally born into independent existence intrigues everyone. Among the remarkable phenomena of pregnancy are the maternal physiologic adaptations. Changes in the mother's appearance as pregnancy progresses are usually obvious to even the casual observer. Less obvious, but more fascinating, are the multitude of adjustments in function and composition of tissues and organs which are interactive and interdependent.

Maternal physiologic adaptations in pregnancy are designed to meet the needs of the developing embryo and fetus. However, many of these changes occur in advance of any manifest needs of the growing conceptus, under the influence of the hormones of the placenta. Later in pregnancy, additional physiologic changes occur in the mother, secondary to the increasing metabolic needs and physical bulk of the conceptual mass.

ENDOCRINOLOGIC CHANGES

Changes in the endocrine system make a good starting point in a discussion of maternal physiologic changes in pregnancy, because many of the other changes are related to those in the endocrine system.

The Placenta

Changes in the endocrine system in pregnancy begin with, and often occur in consequence of, the endocrinology of the placenta.

Protein Hormones. The placenta produces steroid and protein hormones. The first placental hormone to be isolated was human chorionic gonadotropin (hCG), a glycoprotein composed of α and β subunits. The α subunit of hCG is identical to that of follicle stimulating hormone (FSH), luteinizing hormone (LH), and thyroid stimulating hormone (TSH). The β subunit has some structural and immunologic properties in common with LH, but β-hCG contains a unique 30 amino acid terminal peptide sequence. The concentration of hCG in maternal blood rises rapidly in pregnancy to reach peak levels at about day 60. hCG production then decreases steadily until about 18 weeks, when a plateau is reached that continues to term (see Chapter 5).

Although we can efficiently measure the biologic and immunologic presence of hCG, we know very little about the control of the synthesis of hCG, nor do we fully understand its role in pregnancy. We do know that hCG rescues the corpus luteum and supports the corpus luteum until the placenta becomes the major steroid hormone producer in the pregnant woman.

A second protein hormone, human placental lactogen (hPL), sometimes designated human chorionic somatomammotropin (hCS), is synthesized by the trophoblast.[16] hPL can be measured in the serum at the eighth week of pregnancy. Unlike hCG, the serum concentration of hPL rises throughout pregnancy. Production may exceed 2 g/day at term. hPL stimulates the development of the breasts and acts in concert with steroid hormones to prepare the breasts for lactation. In addition to acting on the breasts, hPL also acts as a regulator of metabolism. Its effects are similar to the anabolic effects of human growth hormone, to which it is structurally related. Metabolic effects of hPL include protein sparing and nitrogen retention, lipolysis resulting in elevated levels of free fatty acids in maternal blood, and increased peripheral resistance to insulin.[28,29]

Steroid Hormones

Estrogen. The estrogens circulating in pregnant women are produced by the placenta and fetus acting in synergism. Because of this obligatory synergism, serial determinations of specific estrogen levels can be useful indicators of changes in the condition of the fetus. The placenta is unable to initiate estrogen synthesis from acetate and therefore must have access to cholesterol. Although the fetus can utilize acetate as a precursor, most of the steroid hormone synthesis in the fetal adrenal starts with cholesterol, which is found in fetal blood combined with proteins. Fetal low density lipoproteins (LDL) provide three-quarters of the cholesterol utilized for fetal steroidogenesis. Cholesterol synthesis from fetal acetate and transferred cholesterol from the mother together account for about one-quarter of the fetal cholesterol pool.[41]

The major estrogen synthesized during pregnancy is estriol, which is largely derived from the precursor dehydroepiandrosterone sulfate (DHEAS) secreted by the fetal adrenal. DHEAS is subsequently hydroxylated in the fetal liver to 16α-hydroxydehydroepiandrosterone sulfate (16α OHDHEAS). The placenta cannot accomplish this hydroxylation because it lacks an efficient 16 hydroxylase system. However, the placenta is rich in sulfatase and removes the sulfate to form 16α-hydroxyepiandrosterone (16α-OHDHEA). Free 16α-hydroxyepiandrosterone is then converted to 16α-hydroxyandrostenedione (16α-OHDHA) which is aromatized to 16α-hydroxyestrone. The latter compound is converted to estriol via a 17 reductase. Less than 10% of the 16α-OHDHEAS that converts to estriol is derived from the mother.

Estrone and estradiol together make up only about 10% of total estrogen production in pregnancy. Estradiol and estrone are largely derived from maternal and fetal DHEAS. A placental sulfatase hydrolyzes DHEAS to free DHEA, which is converted to androstenedione by placental Δ^5-Δ^4 isomerase and 3β-dehydrogenase. Androstenedione is then aromatized to estrone. Estrone is converted to 17β-estradiol by a 17β-hydroxyoxidoreductase.

A fourth estrogen, estetrol, which is 15α-hydroxylated estriol, is also found in the fetal and maternal circulations. Estetrol is formed almost exclusively by the fetal liver, mainly from fetal precursors. Estetrol thus has the potential to be a sensitive index of fetal well-being. However, supportive clinical data are lacking.

Progesterone. The normal life span of the corpus luteum is about 12 days. Should conception occur, the life of the corpus luteum is extended, perhaps for the duration of the pregnancy. The corpus luteum produces most of the progesterone measured early in pregnancy. Chorionic gonadotropin secreted by the syncytiotrophoblast supports the corpus luteum, which produces the progesterone that is critical to the maintenance of pregnancy during the five weeks immediately following fertilization, that is, for seven weeks from the last menstrual period (LMP). After the seventh week (counting from the LMP), the progesterone required for pregnancy maintenance is produced by the placenta.

The fetus is not essential for progesterone synthesis. Demise of the intrauterine fetus does not significantly lower maternal blood levels of progesterone. Rather, the placenta synthesizes progesterone from cholesterol carried to it in the maternal blood in the form of lipoproteins. Maternal cholesterol provides about 90% of the substrate for progesterone synthesis in pregnancy. Presumably the low-density lipoproteins are bound by receptors on the cell membrane of the trophoblast cells, from which they can be incorporated into the cells for use as a substrate. Cholesterol then undergoes a series of reactions which form pregnenolone, which, in turn, is converted to progesterone.

In addition to the circulating hormonal products of the placenta, changes in the maternal endocrine organs are also noted in pregnancy.

The Pituitary Gland

The pituitary gland enlarges significantly in pregnancy. Putative evidence suggests that this enlargement is due to the effects of estrogen on pituitary cells. Much of the enlargement is due to hyperplastic and hypertrophic growth of the lactotrophs. A decrease in the number of somatotrophs has been described, but this may be relative rather than absolute.[14,40] The morphologic changes in the pituitary are accompanied by functional changes. Levels of pituitary LH are diminished in early pregnancy and fall progressively, so that LH is undetectable near term.[8] Several investigators have reported similar findings concerning FSH. Release of LH and FSH in response to stimulation with gonadotropin releasing hormone (GnRH) is markedly diminished in pregnancy. The mechanisms underlying the diminished response to GnRH have not been defined.

Prolactin. In 1971, prolactin (PRL) was isolated from the human pituitary and a radioimmunoassay for human prolactin was developed. The increase in number and size of the lactotrophs in pregnancy is accompanied by an increase of 10-fold or more in serum PRL concentrations which begins before the eighth week of pregnancy[10,45] and continues to term. Most of the circulating PRL is secreted by the mother's pituitary gland. In spite of the elevated PRL levels, the normal diurnal variation is observed. Responses to sulpiride are unchanged,[17] and responses to thyrotropin releasing hormone (TRH) stimulation are either normal or increased during pregnancy. The major physiologic roles of PRL are classically considered to be priming the breasts for lactation and the initiation and maintenance of lactation in the puerperium. However, some authorities suggest that, in humans, the major physiologic function of PRL is its impact on maternal metabolism which is designed to provide substrates to the fetus.

Growth Hormone. During pregnancy, human growth hormone (hGH) levels are not much different from those in the nonpregnant woman.[50,56] However, the secretion of hGH in response to L-arginine infusion or insulin-induced hypoglycemia is blunted in pregnancy. The response patterns are somewhat different for each of these stimuli. Normal or increased response to arginine occurs during the first trimester; the response is either normal or blunted in the second trimester and clearly blunted during the third trimester and in the puerperium.[51,-54,55] hGH secretion in response to insulin-induced hypoglycemia is diminished from the second trimester through the puerperium. The reasons for the changes in response to challenges are not completely clear, but the placental steroid and protein hormones may be involved.

Adrenocorticotropic Hormone (ACTH). Available studies are in disagreement concerning the concentrations of ACTH during pregnancy. At this writing it is unclear as to whether ACTH rises, falls, or remains the same in pregnancy.

Thyroid Stimulating Hormone (TSH). Blood concentrations of TSH are either unchanged or rise slightly. The release of TSH in response to thyrotropin releasing hormone (TRH) is unchanged by pregnancy.

The Thyroid Gland

Iodide is produced from dietary iodine in the intestine, from which it is absorbed into the bloodstream. The iodide is then concentrated within the thyroid gland under the influence of TSH. Stored iodide is oxidized to iodine, which iodinates the tyrosyl group of thyroglobulin (TG). This results in the formation of monoiodothyronine (MIT) and diiodothyronine (DIT). These molecules combine to form triiodothyronine (T_3) and thyroxine (T_4). The latter compounds are stored in the thyroid gland bound to thyroglobulin (TG). Prior to release into the circulation, they are freed from TG by proteases under the influence of TSH. They are bound in the bloodstream to thyroxin binding globulin (TBG), to thyroxine binding prealbumin (TBPA), and to albumin.

During pregnancy, TBG is increased, due to increased hepatic synthesis. The ability of TBG to bind thyroxine increases markedly in pregnancy, starting in the first trimester. Because TBG has a very high affinity for thyroxines, it accounts for most of the serum binding of the latter. Along with the doubling of TBG concentrations in pregnancy,[39] the capacity of TBG to bind thyroxine doubles.[46] The percentage of thyroxine bound to the second significant carrier, TBPA, diminishes during pregnancy. Thus, total T_3 and T_4 concentrations rise during pregnancy, which increases the serum protein-bound iodine (PBI). Circulating unbound (free) T_3 and T_4 levels are minimally altered by gestation. Because only free T_3 and T_4 are physiologically active, the elevated PBI does not reflect hyperthyroidism. Similarly, the apparent increased functional iodine uptake by the thyroid is relative rather than absolute and actually reflects the decrease in the total iodine pool. This decrease in the iodine pool is secondary to increased renal excretion of iodine. Thyroid function does not change in pregnancy. The basal metabolic rate (BMR), when corrected for the increased surface area of mother and fetus, remains unchanged, as does T_4 metabolism. (See also Chapter 36.)

The Adrenal Gland

The anatomy and function of the adrenal gland do not change significantly in pregnancy. The adrenal is divided into three histologic zones: the outer zona glomerulosa, which synthesizes the mineralocorticoids, aldosterone and corticosterone; the middle zona fasciculata, which produces corticoids; and the inner zona reticularis, which produces corticoids and androgens. ACTH stimulates the production of corticoids and androgens by driving the conversion of cholesterol to pregnenolone.

Cortisol. During pregnancy, transcortin, the cortisol-binding protein, increases in concentration due to estrogen-driven hepatic synthesis. Cortisol that is bound to transcortin has no biologic activity. Some cortisol is bound to albumin, and about 7–8% circulates as free, biologically active cortisol. Free cortisol is progressively increased in pregnancy. At term, the amount of free cortisol is 2.5 times that found in nonpregnant women.[37] In spite of the increase in free cortisol, pregnant women do not manifest symptoms of hypercortisolism, with the possible exceptions of some alteration in glucose tolerance, aminoaciduria (which may be explained by other mechanisms), and striae gravidarum.

11-Deoxycorticosterone (DOC). DOC levels are elevated from the late second trimester to term. In the third trimester some of the DOC found in the mother arises from 21 hydroxylation or progesterone.

Aldosterone. Aldosterone levels are elevated in pregnancy. Presumably the increase in progesterone, which antagonizes aldosterone influence at the renal tubule, causes a compensatory rise in plasma renin activity. At the same time, under the influence of estrogen, hepatic synthesis of angiotensinogen (renin substrate) increases. These changes result in increased production of angiotensin II. Angiotensin II, in turn, stimulates the zona glomerulosa, increasing aldosterone synthesis. In the last trimester of pregnancy, this results in a sixfold increase in blood levels of aldosterone over nonpregnant levels.

Testosterone. Testosterone production does not increase during pregnancy. Although plasma levels of testosterone are elevated during pregnancy, the increase is secondary to a fivefold increase in sex hormone binding globulin (SHBG). Levels of free testosterone are either unaltered or slightly lower when compared to the nonpregnant state. Thus, there is no change in the biologic impact of testosterone.

Androstenedione. Androstenedione is poorly bound to SHBG. Therefore, the slight increase in androstenedione synthesis during pregnancy results in higher plasma levels of free androstenedione. However, no androgenic effects result from this phenomenon, because the conversion of androstenedione to estrogen is increased 10-fold in pregnancy.[9]

Dehydroepiandrosterone. Dehydroepiandrosterone (DHEA) and its sulfated form (DHEAS) arise mainly from the adrenal, with some ovarian production of DHEA. The concentration of DHEA in the blood of pregnant women is either unchanged or somewhat lower than in nonpregnant women. Although the production rate of DHEA doubles in pregnancy, so does its clearance rate.[20] In addition, plasma binding of DHEA is increased in pregnancy. DHEA is converted to estrone and estradiol by the placenta.

The production rate of DHEAS is increased during pregnancy to double the prepregnant levels at term. However, the metabolic clearance rate increases about eightfold at the same time.[1,11] Thus, plasma levels are about half as high as those in nonpregnant women. DHEAS is cleared through three pathways in pregnancy, each accounting for about one-third of the total clearance. One is conversion to E_1 and E_2. About half of maternal E_1 and E_2 are derived from maternal DHEAS. The second is conversion to 16α-OHDHEAS and thence to estriol. About 10% of estriol at term is derived from maternal DHEAS. The third pathway is by metabolism into steroid by-products.[32]

The Ovaries

The corpus luteum functions well only in early pregnancy. Progesterone and 17-dehydroxy-progesterone (17 OHP) rise steadily for the first month of pregnancy. After the fifth week of pregnancy (seventh week after the last normal menstrual period), production of these steroids by the corpus luteum nearly ceases, as evidenced by the observation that progesterone levels do not drop significantly if the corpus luteum is removed and the fact that blood levels of 17 OHP, which is not synthesized by the placenta, decline. The corpus luteum also secretes relaxin, which is detectable soon after implantation occurs. Relaxin is secreted for the entire duration of pregnancy. The function of relaxin in human pregnancy is unknown. Removal of the corpus luteum with resultant loss of relaxin has no obvious effect on pregnancy.

HEMATOLOGIC CHANGES

Changes in the hematologic system are among the most dramatic of the physiologic adaptations to pregnancy. Of these changes, none are more striking or significant than the changes in blood volume. Healthy primigravidas increase their plasma volume from a mean of about 2600 ml in the prepregnant state to about 3800 ml at 34 weeks. Plasma volume then either remains constant to term or may decline by about 200 ml.

Changes in red cell volume are less well defined because of large individual variations and because of differences from study to study. Other factors, such as body mass, diet, iron supplementation, and size of the conceptus, also obfuscate interpretation. A fair approximation seems to be that the red cell mass increases linearly from the first trimester to term, at which time a total of 200–400 ml has been gained.

Thus, if one assumes an average prepregnant red cell volume of 1400 ml, along with a plasma volume of 2600 ml, an approximation of the changes in normal pregnancy can be reconstructed as in Table 3-1.

If pregnancy is to be successful, the pregnant woman must produce this large increase in plasma volume.[20] High risk pregnancies are frequently associated with failure to expand plasma volume. Several studies have demonstrated a relationship between decreased plasma volume, or hemoconcentration, and entities such as pregnancy-induced hypertension and intrauterine growth retardation. Measurement of plasma volume expansion may provide the single best index of progression of the pregnancy.[15] Indeed, fetal growth and health correlate more closely with maternal plasma volume expansion than with maternal red cell mass.[31]

A low hematocrit in pregnancy may signify a disproportionate rise in plasma volume, rather than a true deficiency in erythropoiesis. The erythrocyte count normally falls to about 3.7 million/mm^3 at about 30 weeks, from average prepregnant values of about 4.5 million/mm^3. The hematocrit and hemoglobin concentration fall in similar fashion. The hematocrit drops from an average of about 40% to about 34% near term. Hemoglobin concentration reaches its lowest value of about 11.5 g/dl at 25 weeks, then increases as term approaches to a mean of about 12.6 g/dl. The fall in hemoglobin seems to be a harbinger of normal fetal growth, so that birth weights are negatively correlated with hemoglobin concentration at any given time in pregnancy.[30] Additional evidence that the apparent anemia of pregnancy is physiologic rather than pathologic is the fact that the arterial–venous (A-V) oxygen difference is lower in pregnant

TABLE 3-1. PLASMA VOLUME, RED CELL VOLUME, TOTAL BLOOD VOLUME, AND HEMATOCRIT IN PREGNANCY

		Weeks of Pregnancy			
	Nonpregnant	**20**	**30**	**34**	**40**
Plasma volume ml	2600	3150	3750	3830	3600
Red cell volume ml	1400	1450	1550	1600	1650
Total blood volume ml	4000	4600	5200	5430	5250
"Body hematocrit" %	35.0	31.5	29.8	29.5	31.5
Venous hematocrit* %	39.8	35.8	34.0	33.5	35.8

* Assuming a hematocrit ratio of 0.88.

Source: Hytten, F. E. and Leitch, I.: The volume and composition of the blood. In: *The Physiology of Human Pregnancy*, 2nd Edition. Oxford, Blackwell Scientific Publications, 1971, p. 26.

than in nonpregnant women. Since oxygen consumption rises somewhat in pregnancy, it is clear that the rise in total hemoglobin is more than adequate for the needs of pregnancy.

Serum iron concentrations are lower in late pregnancy than they are in nonpregnant women. This fact, considered in concert with the fall in hemoglobin and hematocrit noted above, suggests to some observers that anemia does exist in pregnancy because of iron deficiency, rather than as the physiologic consequence of hemodilution. However, others argue that serum iron concentrations do not correlate with hemoglobin concentrations in pregnancy and, furthermore, that total serum iron is probably increased, because of the increased plasma volume in pregnancy (Ref. 25, p. 38).

In any individual pregnant woman, hemoglobin concentration does not indicate health or deficiency. For example, although most women with hemoglobin concentrations of less than 11 g/dl in late pregnancy are likely to be iron-deficient, some gravidas conduct normal activities and are completely asymptomatic with hemoglobin concentrations of less than 9 g/dl. The question for the obstetrician is whether or not to recommend prophylactic supplemental iron to pregnant patients who demonstrate no current evidence of iron deficiency. Our answer is "yes," based upon the following reasoning: Most women begin pregnancy with a total body iron content of about 2.5 g. During pregnancy, the mother needs sufficient iron to satisfy the manufacture of about 200–400 ml of added erythrocytes (say 400 mg of iron), 300 mg for transfer to the conceptual mass, and 200 mg which is excreted. Thus, a significant proportion of the total iron stores is utilized during pregnancy. Although iron reserves are probably restored between pregnancies, it is also likely that most pregnant women cannot provide the 6–7 mg of iron needed per day in the last half of pregnancy from their diet plus their iron stores.[42] Thus, it seems reasonable to prescribe supplemental iron. The supplement is likely to be utilized. Iron is absorbed from the intestine more efficiently in pregnant than in nonpregnant women. In addition to increased absorption, the concentration of transferrin, the β-globulin responsible for binding of iron in plasma, is increased in pregnancy from about 3 to 5–6 mg/liter. This increase occurs even in the presence of normal hemoglobin and serum iron concentrations and is only slightly decreased when exogenous iron is given.[12,36]

The mean corpuscular hemoglobin (MCH), mean corpuscular hemoglobin concentration (MCHC), and mean corpuscular volume (MCV) do not change significantly in pregnancy. The osmotic fragility of the erythrocytes increases in pregnancy but declines toward normal late in the third trimester.

A marked leukocytosis occurs in pregnancy. The mean leukocyte count rises from about 7200 per mm^3 in nonpregnant women to a mean of about 10,000 (range 5000–16,600) per mm^3 in late pregnancy.[25]

Serum Electrolytes

The concentrations of most serum electrolytes fall in pregnancy. The falls are not dramatic and the mean values are within the range for the nonpregnant (Table 3-2). An exception to this generalization is bicarbonate, which falls more dramatically due to the compensated respiratory alkalosis of pregnancy.

Proteins

Serum total protein concentration falls during the third trimester, to reach a level at midpregnancy which is about 10 g/liter lower than the prepregnant value. Most of the fall in total proteins is due to a fall in serum albumin concentrations. In contrast, serum α- and α_2-globulins

TABLE 3-2. CHANGES IN SERUM CONCENTRATIONS OF ELECTROLYTES DURING PREGNANCY

	Na*	K	Ca	Mg
Nonpregnant	138.7 ± 0.8	4.3 ± 0.1	5.0	1.6
Pregnant				
20 weeks	136.4 ± 0.4	4.0 ± 0.1	4.9 ± 0.3	1.5 ± 0.3
32 weeks	137.3 ± 0.9	4.1 ± 0.2	4.6 ± 0.2	1.5 ± 0.2
40 weeks	136.7 ± 1.3	4.2 ± 0.2	4.6 ± 0.3	1.5 ± 0.2

* All concentrations in mEq/liter.

Source: Modified from Hytten, F. E. and Lind, T.: *Diagnostic Indices in Pregnancy.* Basel, Switzerland, Ciba-Geigy Ltd., 1973, p. 40.

each increase about 1 g/liter during pregnancy. β-Globulin concentrations rise by about 3 g/liter. There is a small fall in γ-globulin concentration, specifically in the γG fraction. Fibrinogen values are increased in pregnancy by 100–200 mg/dl to levels of 300–400 mg/dl. The significance of the lower concentrations of protein during pregnancy is unknown, particularly because the total body quantities are increased.

Alpha-fetoprotein, an α_1-gycoprotein made in the fetus, can be measured in the maternal blood in pregnancy. Other new glycoproteins also appear in maternal blood during pregnancy.

The elevation of plasma fibrinogen and globulin levels in pregnancy causes erythrocytes to sediment more quickly in pregnant women. Thus, the erythrocyte sedimentation rate is not a useful diagnostic procedure in pregnant women.

Enzymes

The concentrations of many enzymes do not change in pregnancy (Table 3-3). Some of those that do change are noteworthy. Serum alkaline phosphatase increases in pregnancy because of placental synthesis. Thus, this enzyme is not useful in the evaluation of hepatic disease during pregnancy. The increase in alkaline phosphatase in pregnancy is due to a heat-stable fraction synthesized by the placenta. Because this fraction accounts for up to 67% of total serum alkaline phosphatase activity in the third trimester, it has been suggested to be an index of placental function. The drop in creatinine kinase during the first half of pregnancy could mask the elevated creatinine kinase found in carriers of X-linked Duchenne muscular dystrophy. Finally, the 30% depression of serum pseudocholinesterase activity found in late pregnancy may diminish the ability of pregnant women to hydrolyze succinylcholine. Thus, the paralysis induced by this agent could be prolonged in late pregnancy (Ref. 25, pp. 43–45).

TABLE 3-3. CHANGES IN SERUM ENZYME CONCENTRATIONS IN PREGNANCY

Enzyme	Change
Acid phosphatase	↔
Alkaline phosphatase	↑
α-Amylase	↔
Ceruloplasmin	↑
Creatine kinase	↓
Cystein aminopeptidase	↑
Diamine oxidase	↑
Hydroxybutyrate dehydrogenase	↔
Isocitrate dehydrogenase	↔
Lactate dehydrogenase	↔
Leucine aminopeptidase	↔
Lipase	↓
Monoamine oxidase	↔
Pseudocholinesterase	↓
SGOT	↔
SGPT	↔

Source: Constructed from data in Hytten, F. E. and Lind, T.: *Diagnostic Indices in Pregnancy*. Basel, Switzerland, Ciba-Geigy Ltd., 1973, pp. 43–46.

Lipids

Lipids circulate in the form of lipoproteins. The α-lipoproteins are designated high-density lipoproteins, and the β-lipoproteins are designated low-density lipoproteins. The increase in β-lipoproteins is disproportionately greater than the increase in α-lipoproteins. The elevation in cholesterol and phospholipid levels is mainly in the low-density fraction, whereas the increase in triglycerides occurs in both high- and low-density fractions.

The concentration of free (nonesterified) fatty acids increases during pregnancy. Palmitic and stearic acid levels rise disproportionately to oleic, linoleic, and arachidonic acids.

CHANGES IN METABOLIC FUNCTION

Body Water

In addition to water contained in the intravascular compartment in the plasma, other extracellular water is found in cerebrospinal fluid, lymph, various body secretions, and as the interstitial fluid. The remainder of the body water is intracellular.

The average weight gain during pregnancy is about 12 kg in women whose diets are not restricted. Of this, about 3.4 kg is accounted for by the baby, 0.65 kg by the placenta, and 0.8 kg by the amniotic fluid. An additional 2.6 kg are due to increases in the weight of the reproductive organs and in blood volume (Table 3-4). This leaves about 3.4 kg unaccounted for. The unaccounted-for weight is partly due to the accumulation of fat mass and mostly due to the accumulation of extra body water. Body water increases steadily during pregnancy. This is true in women who have no generalized edema and is

TABLE 3-4. ANALYSIS OF WEIGHT GAIN

Tissues and Fluids Accounted for and Total Weight Gained	Increase in Weight up to: 10 wk	20 wk	30 wk	40 wk
	g	g	g	g
Fetus	5	300	1500	3400
Placenta	20	170	430	650
Amniotic fluid	30	350	750	800
Uterus	140	320	600	970
Mammary gland	45	180	360	405
Blood	100	600	1300	1250
Extracellular extravascular fluid				
(1) No edema or leg edema	0	30	80	1680
(2) Generalized edema	0	500	1526	4897
Total				
(1) No edema or leg edema	340	1950	5020	9155
(2) Generalized edema	340	2420	6466	12372
Total weight gained				
(1) No edema or leg edema	650	4000	8500	12500
(2) Generalized edema	650	4500	10000	14500
Weight not accounted for				
(1) No edema or leg edema	310	2050	3480	3345
(2) Generalized edema	310	2080	3534	2128

Source: Hytten, F. E. and Leitch, I.: Changes in the maternal body. In: *The Physiology of Human Pregnancy,* 2nd Edition. Oxford, Blackwell Scientific Publications, 1971, p. 356.

exaggerated in those who display clinical signs of edema.[26]

About 2.5 liters of extracellular water is added during pregnancy. Most of it is stored in the ground substance of connective tissue, under the influence of estrogen. Although the ground substance therefore contains extra water during pregnancy, many pregnant women do not demonstrate generalized edema. A significant number do develop edema of the legs, but leg edema accounts for relatively little of the excess water. Leg edema is due to the effect of gravity and is enhanced by the increased venous pressure in the lower extremities. It tends to decrease after elevation of the legs. About 15% of pregnant women have leg edema and an additional 25% display dependent edema. Thirty percent of clinically normal women have some edema. The incidence of edema is doubled in women with elevated blood pressure and increases to 85% in women with hypertension and proteinuria. Edematous women have bigger infants than nonedematous women do, and a lower incidence of babies weighing less than 2500 g. The infants born of edematous mothers are not edematous. The difference in weight is due to a more rapid fetal growth rate in the fetuses of edematous women. The difference in weight persists after correction for maternal height and weight, parity, length of gestation, and preeclampsia. Although the cause of generalized edema is unknown, the presence of edema, even generalized, in otherwise normal women does not compromise pregnancy outcome.[38]

Changes in Metabolism

Carbohydrate Metabolism. Maternal glucose metabolism is altered in pregnancy. Glucose is the major source of energy for the fetus, but changes in fat and protein metabolism also influence carbohydrate metabolism.

Pregnancy may be considered a state of balance among diabetogenic factors, such as the placental hormones, and the increased metabolic needs of the fetus and the mother. Human placental lactogen (hPL) promotes lipolysis so that the concentration of free fatty acids in maternal plasma rises. hPL concentrations rise when maternal blood glucose concentrations drop. The resulting rise in free fatty acids spares glucose for fetal metabolic needs. hPL also increases peripheral tissue resistance to the action of insulin, thereby making maternal carbohydrate metabolism less efficient. hPL inhibits maternal gluconeogenesis, which elevates plasma protein levels. Since hPL also increases circulating insulin levels, protein synthesis is enhanced. Thus, maternal amino acids are made available to the fetus.

The effects of estrogen and progesterone on carbohydrate metabolism have not been clearly defined. In animals, both estrogen and progesterone cause increased insulin secretion in response to a given load of glucose. Estrogen also decreases the hypoglycemic response elicited by injected insulin. However, data for human pregnancy are nonextant.

Lipid Metabolism. Plasma lipid concentrations are elevated in pregnancy particularly after the 20th week. These increases are related to the increased utilization of fat to supply maternal energy needs, while sparing glucose for the fetus.

Protein Metabolism. Protein is utilized for fetal growth and for the growth of the organs that increase in mass during pregnancy. The concentrations of the amino acids in maternal serum, with the exception of glutamic acid and histidine, are lowered in pregnancy.

CHANGES IN ORGANS AND SYSTEMS

Pregnancy is accompanied by profound structural and functional changes in many tissues, organs, and organ systems. The most obvious change is the change in contour due to the enlarging uterus. The abdominal bulge tends to be greater in multiparous women than in primigravidas. The enlarging uterus causes many patients to change their gait to a broader base, and to lean backward to maintain balance. The loosening of the ligaments along with the postural change results in an increased lumbar lordosis. Thus, low back pain is a common complaint in advanced pregnancy.

The Skin

Increased pigmentation, especially of the areolae, abdominal midline (linea nigra), axillae, and perineum, is very common in pregnancy. Chloasma gravidarum (the mask of pregnancy) is less common. Facial hyperpigmentation occurs in 50–70% of pregnant women, usually starting during the second half of pregnancy. The hyperpigmentation is usually symmetrically distributed on the forehead, cheeks, and nose, and less often in perioral and mental areas. Chloasma is more common in dark-haired, brown-eyed women and is progressive during pregnancy. Unless the hyperpigmentation is deep, complete disappearance or significant regression occurs after delivery.[57]

Although melanocyte stimulating hormone (MSH) is not increased in pregnancy, progesterone and estrogen are melanogenic stimulants and probably cause the hyperpigmentation.

Striae gravidarum are seen in about 90% of pregnant women. The striae begin as pink or violaceous streaks, usually during the 2nd half of pregnancy, and tend to occur in areas of maximum stretch, such as the abdomen, breasts, and thighs. They are probably caused by a combination of increased hormonal activity and distention. During pregnancy, the content of collagen and nonsulfated mucopolysaccharides in the dermis increases. The mucopolysaccharides bind more water, so that interfibrous cohesive forces are decreased. The distention produced by the enlarging uterus and breast tissue may cause the collagen fibers to become frayed and oriented along the lines of stress, producing the striae. The increased edema and subcutaneous fat of pregnancy probably add to the stress forces.

The Breasts

Many women note enlargement of the breasts and a sensation of heaviness as early signs of pregnancy. Throughout pregnancy, changes occur in the areolae, the nipples, and the breast. The nipples enlarge in diameter in most pregnant women. Along with the enlargement, the nipple becomes more mobile, so that it can be forced outward by the grip of the nursing infant's gums at the base of the nipple. The areolae increase in diameter by about 50%. Among primigravidas, this increase is more marked in younger women, but there is no relationship to age among multiparas.[21] During first pregnancies, the areolae become more darkly pigmented, and the tubules of Montgomery become more prominent.

The breast enlarges rapidly during the first two months of pregnancy, due largely to vascular engorgement. After this time, progressive breast enlargement continues at a slower rate throughout pregnancy. This enlargement is due to increase in the mass of the glandular tissue, probably under the influence of hPL acting in concert with the steroid hormones. Enlargement of the breasts is quite variable among pregnant women. In primigravidas especially, the increases in breast mass are age-related. Women under age 20 note much greater increases than do women over 30. Genetic differences also influence the amount of enlargement of the breasts.[24] Efficiency of lactation is directly correlated with incremental enlargement of the breasts.

The Fallopian Tubes and Ovaries

The fallopian tubes do not exhibit marked changes during pregnancy. The major change in the ovaries is the persistence of the corpus luteum of pregnancy. The corpus luteum at term is considerably smaller than that seen at 8–12 weeks of gestation. Another change that is often observed is the presence of decidual tissue on the surface of both ovaries.

The Uterus

The uterus grows in pregnancy in humans as it does in all animals[22] (Table 3-5). The uterus must grow in order to accommodate the growing conceptual mass without increasing intrauterine pressure. In the first three months of pregnancy, the uterus doubles its weight. During this trimester, mitotic proliferation of myocytes, largely due to estrogen stimulation, accounts for a major proportion of total uterine growth. The nonpregnant uterus of a nulliparous woman weighs about 40 g, and that of a parous woman about 70 g. In contrast, the pregnant uterus at term weighs about 1200 g. After the first trimester, most further growth is due to hypertrophy of myocytes. Individual myocytes measure an average of 2.5–5 x 50–90 μm in the nonpregnant uterus, and 5–10 x 500–800 μm in the pregnant uterus at term.[43]

During the first trimester, the uterus grows more rapidly than does the conceptual mass. After the first trimester, the conceptus grows faster than the uterus and the conceptual mass expands to fill the entire uterine cavity. The *decidua capsularis*, a layer of decidua that covers the implantation site shortly after implantation and isolates the developing conceptus from the general uterine cavity (Fig. 3-1), then fuses with the *decidua vera* (the decidua that lines the general uterine cavity) so that the uterine cavity is obliterated. Soon after the decidua capsularis fuses with the decidua vera, the former disappears. As the conceptual mass continues to expand, pressure is exerted upon the uterine isthmus. (The uterine isthmus is that portion of the uterine muscular wall that is limited superiorly by the lowest portion of the uterine cavity and inferiorly by the fibrous tissue of the cervix.) During the third month of pregnancy, the isthmic segment elongates before the products of conception have filled the available space in the corpus. This elongation is accompanied by a thickening of the wall of the lower uterine segment and corpus. The incorporation of the isthmic segment into the general uterine cavity coincides with the filling of the uterine cavity by the conceptus. Isthmic incorporation is not secondary to distention but is an adjustment of the musculature of the lower pole of the uterus to the growth of the conceptus. The incorporation of the isthmus into the uterine cavity is accompanied by thinning of its musculature. The process stops at the junction of the isthmus with the cervix. After incorporation has been completed, the junction of the corpus with the isthmic segment cannot be identified by gross or microscopic examination of the uterine wall[5] (Fig. 3-2).

The uterus converts from the pyriform configuration of the nonpregnant state to a more spherical contour as midpregnancy is reached. After the 20th week of pregnancy, the uterus begins to elongate and assumes a cylindroid shape. As elongation of the uterus begins, the transverse diameter of the fundus also begins to increase. The increase in width of the uterus

TABLE 3-5. INCREASE IN WEIGHT OF THE UTERUS

	Weeks of Pregnancy				
	0	10	20	30	40
	g	g	g	g	g
Gross weight	50	200	400	700	1100
Contained blood (8%)	4	16	32	56	88
Blood-free uterus	46	184	368	644	1012
Rounded increase above nonpregnant weight of blood-free uterus		140	320	600	970

Source: Hytten, F. E. and Leitch, I.: Changes in the maternal body. In: *The Physiology of Human Pregnancy*, 2nd Edition. Oxford, Blackwell Scientific Publications, 1971, p. 334.

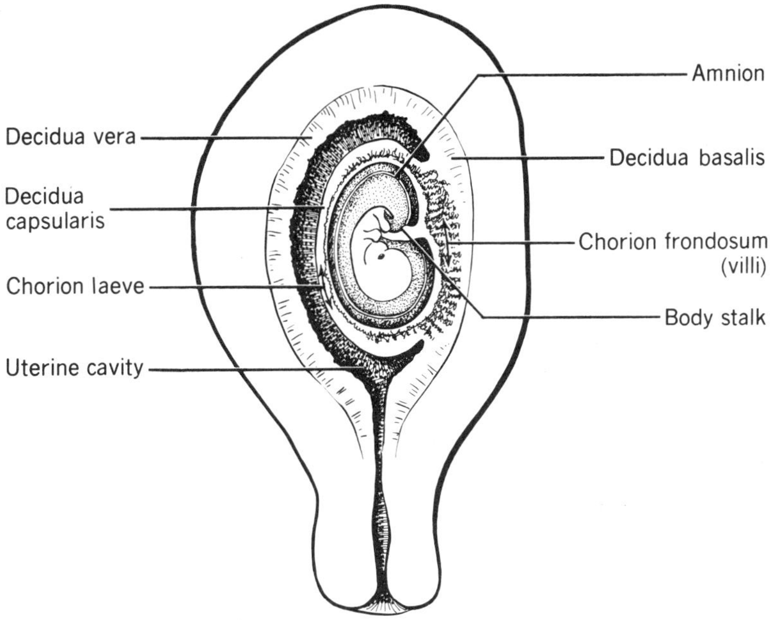

Figure 3-1. During the first trimester of pregnancy, the decidua capsularis isolates the conceptual mass from the remainder of the uterine cavity.

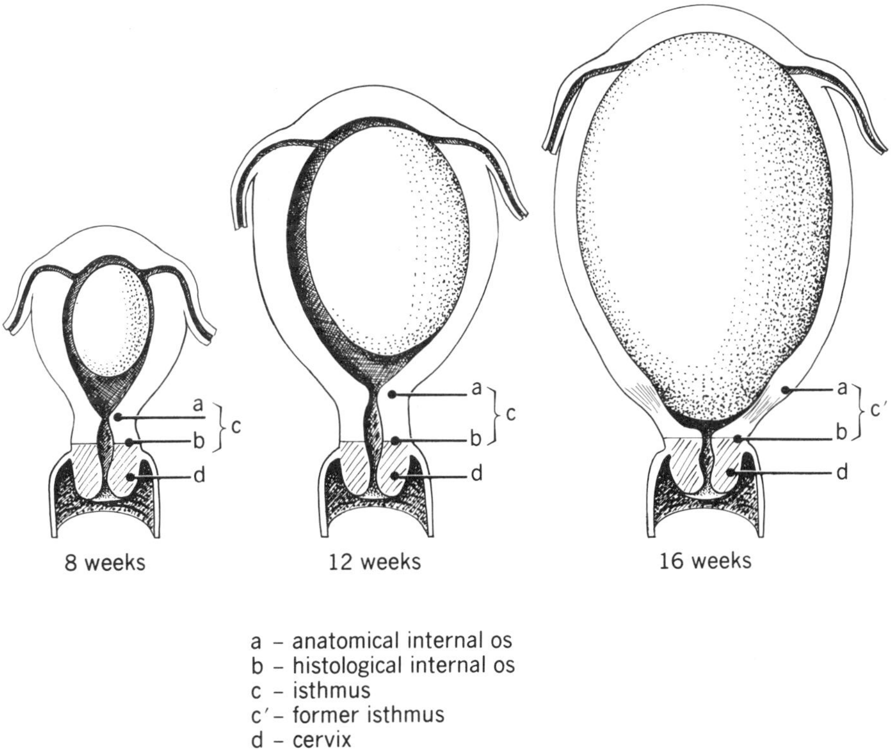

Figure 3-2. During early pregnancy, the cervix does not change significantly, but the corpus grows rapidly. The isthmus elongates during the third month of pregnancy. Later the isthmus is incorporated into the lower uterine segment.

continues to term, but the rate of increase diminishes during the last month of pregnancy. After 20 weeks of pregnancy, uterine *accommodation* to fetal growth occurs largely by hypertrophy of the myofibrils, rather than by replication.[13]

The muscle bundles of the human uterus are arranged in helical configurations. The left and right spirals, which presumably originate in the unfused Müllerian ducts, meet in the midline of the fused uterus simplex. The population density of myofibrils is highest in the corpus and least in the isthmus. These architectural arrangements account for the salient features of uterine behavior during normal labor. The preponderant concentration of contractile elements in the corpus allows for the phenomenon designated *fundal dominance*. In normal labor, the contractile forces exerted by the fundus are much stronger than those generated by the midportion of the uterus, which, in turn, contracts more strongly than the lower uterine segment.[44] Because of the helical arrangement of the muscle bundles, the fibers in the upper and midcorpus pull longitudinally toward the top of the uterus, exerting upward and outward traction on the musculature of the lower uterine segment, which is predominantly arranged in horizontally oriented circular muscle bundles. During labor, total uterine length decreases. The upper uterine segment thickens and the lower uterine segment thins.

The Cervix

The cervix becomes softer in pregnancy due to a loosening of the connective tissue, especially the collagen fibrils' association with each other. As part of the connective tissue reaction, the stroma becomes looser and more edematous. Increased vascularity of the cervix contributes to the softening and also causes the cervix to appear cyanotic. All of these changes increase as pregnancy progresses.

The epithelium of the ectocervix may demonstrate more proliferative activity in the basal layer and persistence of large nuclei into the midzone. These changes would be interpreted as dysplasia in nonpregnant women. The endocervical glands proliferate markedly and produce thick, tenacious mucus.

The Vulva and Vagina

Vulvar vascularization increases in pregnancy. In some women, usually multiparas, vulvar varices are noted in pregnancy. Edema of the vulva is also common and can be severe. The vagina shares in the general connective tissue loosening of pregnancy; it becomes more pliable and is edematous. The mucosa thickens, the underlying smooth muscle hypertrophies, and vascularization increases. The vagina, like the cervix, is cyanotic during pregnancy.

The Cardiovascular System

The Heart. "The heart is often displaced upward and to the left as pregnancy progresses, so that during the last few months of gestation the apex impulse may be in the fourth left interspace and the left border of dullness at or outside the midclavicular line."[18] As a result of this displacement, the heart also may appear to be enlarged in its transverse diameter by as much as 3.6 cm. Thus, it is very difficult to establish the presence of mild cardiac enlargement in the pregnant woman.

The clinical picture is further confused by changes in the heart sounds and by the appearance of innocent murmurs. The first heart sound becomes louder in early pregnancy and reaches peak volume in the second trimester. The increased intensity is accompanied by splitting of the mitral and tricuspid components of the first heart sound, due to early mitral valve closure. A large percentage of pregnant women develop a third heart sound which reaches peak intensity at about 30 weeks, and which disappears or diminishes markedly during the first week of the puerperium. Systolic murmurs are noted in about 95% and diastolic murmurs in about 20% of normal pregnant women at some time during gestation.[4]

Blood Pressure. During most of pregnancy, the systolic blood pressure is slightly below prepregnant levels. The diastolic pressure is significantly below levels in nonpregnant women until the last trimester, when it begins to rise toward prepregnant levels.

Cardiac Output. Cardiac output increases early in the first trimester. By the 10th week of pregnancy, cardiac output has increased from the nonpregnant value of 4.5 liters/min to 6 liters/min. Cardiac output increases by an additional 10% during the second trimester. The increase in cardiac output persists until the end of pregnancy. The major antecedent of the increased cardiac output is decreased peripheral resistance. In addition to a diminution of peripheral resistance in the systemic circulation, the uteroplacental circulation also provides a low-resistance shunt. The increase in heart rate, which averages 15 beats per minute, accounts for some of the increase in cardiac output, but the major contribution is made by increased stroke volume. Cardiac output increases by about 30%, whereas heart rate increases by only 20%. The required increase in stroke volume is about 64–71ml.[23]

Oxygen consumption does not rise in proportion to the rise in cardiac output. Therefore, relatively less oxygen is extracted from arterial blood, so that the A-V oxygen difference decreases by about 30% in the first trimester, then steadily rises during pregnancy, to reach prepregnancy levels at term.

The Respiratory System

The earliest change in respiratory function is hyperventilation. Progesterone increases the sensitivity of the hypothalamic respiratory center to the partial pressure of CO_2 in plasma. Pregnant women also demonstrate greatly increased hyperventilatory response to increases in alveolar CO_2 tension. The hyperventilation washes CO_2 out of the lungs so that the alveolar concentration of CO_2 is decreased. The decrease in the partial pressure of CO_2 in the alveoli is accompanied by an increase in plasma pH. The consequent respiratory alkalosis requires that plasma bicarbonate be lowered in order to maintain normal pH Decreased plasma bicarbonate concentrations are compensated for by increased renal retention of hydrogen ion.[35]

In addition to the observed hyperventilation, more than 60% of pregnant women complain of dyspnea, which often begins in the first trimester. In spite of much speculation and some investigation, the cause of dyspnea remains enigmatic. It is clear that pregnancy does not impair pulmonary function. Pulmonary function is described in terms of lung volumes and lung capacities. The *tidal volume* (TV) is the volume of air moved in or out with each respiration. After inspiration, the lungs passively return to their original volume, which is the lung volume at rest in the absence of contraction of the respiratory muscles, and is designated the *functional residual volume* (FRV). When the volume of air that can be inspired with a maximum of effort, called the *inspiratory capacity* (IC), is added to the FRV, the *total lung capacity* (TLC) is reached. In contrast, the volume moved out of the lungs by forced expiration from a position of rest is called the *expiratory reserve volume* (ERV), which, when subtracted from the FRV, leaves the *residual volume*

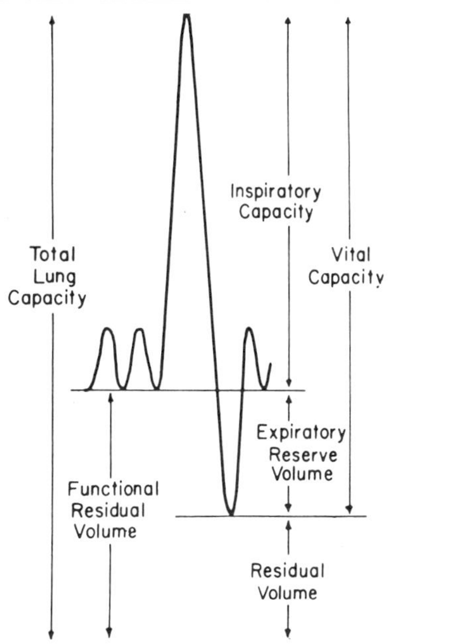

Figure 3-3. See text for explanation. (Reprinted from Prowse, C. M. And Gaensler, E. A.: Respiratory and acid–base changes during pregnancy. *Anesthesiology* **26**:351–392, 1965, by permission of *Anesthesiology* and Lippincott/Harper & Row.)

(RV). The *vital capacity* (VC) is the sum of the inspiratory capacity and the expiratory reserve volume (Fig. 3-3). The *minute volume*, a measure of ventilation, is calculated by multiplying the respiratory rate and the tidal volume. The *ventilatory equivalent* (VE) for oxygen is the number of liters of air moved for every 100 ml of oxygen used by the body.

In pregnancy, the subcostal angle widens, the transverse diameter of the chest increases, and the excursions of the diaphragm increase. These changes allow for normal pulmonary function, in spite of the enlarged abdomen. Although the respiratory rate remains unchanged, the tidal volume increases by about 40%. Therefore, the minute volume increases significantly. Because this increase is accomplished by deeper rather than faster breathing, alveolar ventilation, which is the tidal volume less the volume of anatomic dead space, increases even more than total ventilation. Although vital capacity is essentially unchanged in pregnancy, the lung contains less end expiratory volume, so that the expiratory reserve volume is decreased. However, the inspiratory capacity is increased, so that vital capacity is unchanged. Total lung volume and residual volume are, of course, decreased. The timed vital capacity is not significantly altered by pregnancy, nor is the maximum breathing capacity.

The Urinary Tract

Pregnancy brings about anatomic and functional changes in the urinary tract. The urinary tract dilates during pregnancy in about 90% of women. For reasons yet unknown, primigravidas are particularly likely to display dilation of the urinary tract, and the dilation is more marked in them than it is in multiparous women. The ureter begins to dilate late in the first trimester, which suggests that the dilation is secondary to decreased smooth muscle tone under the influence of progesterone. As pregnancy progresses, the right ureter becomes more dilated than the left. We now believe that ureteral dilation of pregnancy is secondary to mechanical obstruction rather than to progesterone. The left side is less affected than the right side because of regional anatomic relationships. Neither ureteral contractility nor ureteral tone are diminished in pregnancy.[2,19,47-49] The chronic partial obstruction results in increased dead space in the urinary tract. The only putative physiotropic consequence of the increased dead space is that stasis of urine makes pregnant women more vulnerable to urinary tract infections.

In contrast to the anatomic changes, the physiologic changes have profound impact on fluid and electrolyte balance. As noted above, the average woman gains roughly 12 kg of weight. About 60% of this, or 6–8 kg, is fluid, of which about 4 kg is extracellular fluid. To keep the sodium concentration in the region of 142 mEq/liter requires the retention of about 800 mEq (about 20 g) of sodium. Therefore, normal pregnant women are in positive sodium balance of about 0.5 g/week in early pregnancy and about 1 g/week in later pregnancy.

Sodium balance and, in consequence, the size of the extracellular space are basically regulated in the kidney. In pregnancy, factors that favor both sodium gain and sodium loss are either activated or initiated. Increased secretion of aldosterone enhances sodium reabsorption, but progesterone, which is also increased, antagonizes the action of aldosterone at the renal tubule. Water retention is induced in the distal tubule under the influence of the pituitary antidiuretic hormone (ADH). In addition to regulation of sodium and water excretion in the kidney by these two mechanisms (GFR and aldosterone), a *third factor* that influences sodium retention in the proximal tubule has been identified.

Glomerular Filtration Rate (GFR). Blood flow to the kidneys increases early in pregnancy and remains elevated to term. Thus, an increased volume of plasma is presented to the glomerulus per unit time. At the glomerulus, an essentially protein-free plasma ultrafiltrate is formed. The rate at which this protein-free filtrate is formed is called the glomerular filtration rate (GFR). Since blood flow to the kidneys designated in terms of renal plasma flow (RPF) increases about 25–30% in pregnancy, whereas GFR increases about 50%, a greater proportion of the renal plasma flow is filtered, so that the filtration fraction (GFR/RPF) is increased. In consequence, renal excretion of amino acids, glucose, proteins, electrolytes, and vitamins is increased in pregnancy.

The urinary excretion of substances is the result of glomerular filtration and tubular processing, by either reabsorption or secretion. Urea and creatinine, for example, are excreted only by glomerular filtration. Thus, plasma concentrations of these substances are significantly diminished during pregnancy. Uric acid is freely filtered at the glomerulus, but a portion of the filtered uric acid is reabsorbed in the proximal tubule. In early pregnancy, the serum concentration of uric acid is decreased by 25%. Uric acid clearance may decrease in the last trimester due to an increase in tubular reabsorption.[6]

Tubular reabsorption can occur either passively or actively, depending upon the concentration gradient of the substance under consideration. Active reabsorption transport systems depend upon either the duration of exposure of the solute in the ultrafiltrate to the resorbing membrane, or upon active transport mechanisms that are saturated when the solute reaches a certain concentration in the ultrafiltrate. The maximum rate of resorption of a solute by the tubules is designated the transport maximum (Tm). In pregnancy, tubular resorption cannot always accommodate to the increased GFR, so that many solutes are excreted in the urine. This glomerulo-tubular imbalance leads to glycosuria, aminoaciduria, and increased urinary excretion of other nutrients and vitamins in pregnancy.

Since the filtration fraction reflects the proportion of plasma traversing the glomerulus that is filtered off as pre-urine, more sodium is presented to the tubules. This requires adjustments in tubular reabsorption, to avoid sodium depletion. For example, a GFR of 120 ml/min with a serum sodium of 145 mEq/liter would mean that 25,056 mEq sodium was filtered each 24 hours (120 x 0.145 x 1440 minutes). If 98% were resorbed, 501 mEq would be excreted in 24 hours (29 g). If 99% were resorbed, 250 mEq would be excreted (14.6 g). Because the changes in GFR from 120 to 180 ml/min mean a filtered load difference of 24,200–36,300 mEq/24 hours, some tubular adjustments must take place.

Aldosterone. The juxtoglomerular apparatus of the kidney senses pressure differences between the renal artery and the surrounding renal parenchyma. When renal artery pressure is high, the apparatus acts to decrease renal blood flow. When arterial pressure is low, renal blood flow is increased, except that the apparatus loses function if the pressure drops much below 60 mmHg. Any decrease in renal blood flow, whether due to a drop in systemic perfusion pressure or to renal artery obstruction, activates the juxtoglomerular apparatus. However, the definitive stimulus that activates the juxtoglomerular cells is sodium. The cells produce renin, which acts on an α_2-globulin to form the decapeptide *angiotensin I*, which is subsequently converted to an octapeptide, *angiotensin II*. Angiotensin II, besides being the most potent natural pressor substance known in the body, also stimulates the zona glomerulosa of the adrenal gland which, in turn, secretes *aldosterone*. As noted above, aldosterone then acts on the proximal renal tubule to increase sodium retention. The mechanism of this action appears to be a classic target organ hormone reaction. The aldosterone binds to specific proteins on the renal tubule cells, enters the nuclei, and directs synthesis of a specific protein which increases sodium reabsorption and decreases potassium reabsorption.

In normal pregnancy, or during salt depletion in the nonpregnant state, angiotensin II does not elicit its pressor response but does elicit the aldosterone response. Plasma renin, angiotensin, and aldosterone are all increased in normal pregnancy. The highest plasma renin concentrations are noted in the first trimester, after which they decline. Plasma angiotensin II levels are elevated throughout pregnancy.[53] Although some investigators suggest that these increases reflect a relative sodium deficit during pregnancy, this contention has not been proved. Although all components of the renin–angiotensin–aldosterone system are elevated in pregnancy, the normal pregnant patient responds appropriately to sodium loading or restriction. Normal pregnant women are resistant to the pressor effects of angiotensin, so that the isopressor dose is 2.5 times that of nonpregnant women.

The Third Factor. The putative third factor is a humoral factor produced by volume expansion. Under steady-state conditions, a constant fraction of filtered sodium is reabsorbed in the proximal tubule despite fluctuations in GFR. The third factor resets this balance. Although the third factor always decreases fractional sodium reabsorption, total reabsorption may increase, decrease, or remain constant, depending on fluctuations in GFR. The third factor inhibits reabsorptive capacity of the tubal epithelium so that tubular reabsorption of sodium in the proximal tubule is decreased. Sodium excretion is increased by the third factor even if the GFR is reduced. Contraction of the effective circulatory blood volume causes third factor activity to disappear and sodium is again resorbed in the proximal tubule due to the absence of the third factor.

Antidiuretic Hormone (ADH). The role of ADH in pregnancy is not well defined. Women are less sensitive to ADH during pregnancy. In late pregnancy, the retention of water exceeds the retention of salt, that is, increase in total body water exceeds the increase in the total exchangeable sodium.

Antidiuretic hormone is made in the supraoptic nuclei of the hypothalamus and stored in the hypophysis. Its release and synthesis are under the control of three kinds of receptors:

1. Osmoreceptors that monitor plasma osmolality.
2. Volume receptors that monitor the volume of blood and other extracellular space. The volume receptors are located in the aorta, the atrium, and the kidney. The renal pathway involves the renin–angiotensin system and angiotensin-mediated release of ADH.
3. The neural receptors in the midbrain are activated by drugs, fever, stress, and systemic illness. Thirst activates receptors close to the supraoptic nuclei.

Loss of sodium and water, with a resultant contracture of the extracellular space, signals ADH release. ADH then causes water retention, and the serum sodium falls. Extracellular fluid shifts into the cells, the glomerular filtration rate falls, and the urea nitrogen rises.

Under some conditions, a dilutional hyponatremia may occur, with an inappropriate ADH response. These syndromes are characterized by hyponatremia, urinary sodium loss, normal or expanded extracellular volume, and a urine that is hyperosmolal to plasma. Central neural receptors apparently drive the ADH secretion in these conditions. They may be ameliorated by fluid restriction.

Other Electrolytes. Potassium passes readily through the glomerulus and is then completely resorbed from the lumen of the proximal tubule. All of the potassium found in the urine is secreted into the lumen of the distal convoluted tubule and collecting duct under the influence of aldosterone. Excretion of potassium decreases in pregnancy. Although serum concentrations of potassium are not increased in pregnancy, potassium balance is positive during pregnancy.

Serum calcium and phosphate concentrations fall in pregnancy. Urinary excretion of calcium is increased, so that the diet should include 2 g of calcium per day to assure that maternal calcium is not depleted.

Renal acid–base balance must be adjusted to compensate for the respiratory alkalosis which occurs because of the lowering of Pco_2 secondary to hyperventilation. This compensation is accomplished by renal retention of hydrogen ions and reduction of serum bicarbonate levels.

Glucose excretion increases in a significant percentage of, but not in all, pregnant women. At least two mechanisms underlie the glycosuria. The first is the increased filtered load of glucose which is a function of the increased GFR. In addition, it seems likely that in some women the TMG for glucose is decreased in pregnancy, so that the capacity of the proximal tubules to resorb glucose is diminished as compared to the nonpregnant state.[7] The practical consequence of the glycosuria of pregnancy is that pregnant diabetics cannot be monitored satisfactorily by following urinary glucose concentrations.

The Gastrointestinal System

Pregnancy presents a series of gastrointestinal symptoms, sometimes paradoxical. During the first trimester, nausea and vomiting are so common that they are considered as physiologic symptoms of pregnancy. When these symptoms abate, a majority of pregnant women note increased appetite. (See Chapter 5.)

In addition, some pregnant women scrupulously avoid certain foods, either to minimize pyrosis or because of inexplicable aversions. At the same time, a craving for certain foods may be noted which, in the extreme, is manifested as *pica*—a craving for strange or unnatural foods such as clay, chalk, and laundry starch.

The cause of the nausea and vomiting of pregnancy is not known. Many observers suggest that it is related to endocrinologic changes, particularly the increased levels of estrogen or hCG. It seems likely that the pathologic vomiting of pregnancy, designated "hyperemesis gravidarum," is secondary to psychodynamic factors. (See Chapter 5.) The other common complaint of pregnant women, heartburn, is probably due to reflux of gastric acids into the lower esophagus due to relaxation of the lower esophageal sphincter. Although earlier reports suggested that pregnant women experiencing heartburn, indigestion, bloating, and belching often had hiatus hernias, most women with these symptoms do not have hiatus hernias, and some women with hiatus hernias are asymptomatic. In any case, the incidence of hiatus hernia is increased in pregnancy.[34,52]

Muscle tone in the gastrointestinal tract is lower in pregnancy. The consequent relaxation of the cardiac sphincter and stomach, coupled with the increased mass of the intra-abdominal contents, may account for the reflux of gastric contents into the esophagus. The acidity of the gastric secretions probably diminishes during the first six months of pregnancy, to return to prepregnant values in the last trimester. Although direct evidence for this statement is not absolute, available studies support this contention, as does the observation that peptic ulcers are rarely encountered in pregnant women.

The motility of the stomach is also diminished in pregnancy. Emptying of the stomach after a solid meal is slower in pregnant than in nonpregnant women. Motility of the small intestine is decreased in pregnancy. Thus, the contents are moved from the duodenum to the cecum at a more leisurely pace. The relative prolongation of the exposure of foodstuffs to the intestinal mucosa may facilitate absorption of nutrients from the lumen. The motility of the colon is diminished in pregnancy. Thus, water absorption is increased, which contributes to the constipation noted in pregnancy.

The gallbladder is often enlarged during

pregnancy due to relative atony of the walls. The gallbladder also empties more slowly. Little firm information is available concerning changes in liver function in pregnancy. (See Chapter 35.) Changes in various enzymes are summarized in Table 3-3.

REFERENCES

1. Belisle, S., Osathanondh, R., and Tulchinsky, D.: The effect of constant infusion of unlabelled dehydroepiandrosterone sulfate on maternal plasma androgens and estrogens. *J. Clin. Endocrinol. Metab.* **45**:544–550, 1977.
2. Bellina, J. H., Dougherty, C. M., and Mickal, A.: Pyeloureteral dilation and pregnancy. *Am. J. Obstet. Gynecol.* **108**:356–363, 1970.
3. Boonshaft, B., O'Connell, J. M. B., Hayes, J. M., and Schreiner, G. E.: Serum renin activity during normal pregnancy: Effect of alternations of posture and sodium intake. *J. Clin. Endocrinol. Metab.* **28**:1641–1644, 1968.
4. Cutforth, R. and MacDonald, C. B.: Heart sounds and murmurs in pregnancy. *Am. Heart J.* **71**:741–747, 1966.
5. Danforth, D. N.: The fibrous nature of the human cervix, and its relation to the isthmic segment in gravid and nongravid uteri. *Am. J. Obstet. Gynecol.* **53**:541–557, 1947.
6. Davison, J. M. and Dunlop, W.: Renal hemodynamics and tubular function in normal human pregnancy. *Kidney Int.* **18**:152, 1980.
7. Davison, J. M. and Hytten, F. E.: The effect of pregnancy on the renal handling of glucose. *J. Obstet. Gynaecol. Br. Commonw.* **82**:374, 1975.
8. de la Lastra, M. and Llados, C.: Luteinizing hormone content of the pituitary gland in pregnant and nonpregnant women. *J. Clin. Endocrinol. Metab.* **44**:921–923, 1977.
9. Edman, C. D., MacDonald, P. C., and Gant, N. F.: Placental clearance of maternal plasma androstenedione through estradiol formation (PC-AE2). Scientific Abstracts, The 26th Annual Meeting of The Society for Gynecologic Investigation, San Diego, 1979, p. 67 (Abstract 110).
10. Friesen, H. G., Fournier, P., and Desjardins, P.: Pituitary prolactin in pregnancy and normal and abnormal lactation. *Clin. Obstet. Gynecol.* **16**:25–45, 1973.
11. Gant, N. F., Hutchinson, H. T., Siiteri, P. K., and MacDonald, P. C.: Study of the metabolic clearance rate of dehydroisoandrosterone sulfate in pregnancy. *Am. J. Obstet. Gynecol.* **111**:555–563, 1971.
12. Gerritsen, T. and Walker, A. R. P.: The effect of habitually high iron intake on certain blood values in pregnant Bantu women. *J. Clin. Invest.* **33**:23–26, 1954.
13. Gillespie, C. E.: Principles of uterine growth in pregnancy. *Am. J. Obstet. Gynecol.* **59**:949–959, 1950.
14. Goluboff, L. G. and Ezrin, C.: Effect of pregnancy on the somatotroph and the prolactin cell of the human adenohypophysis. *J. Clin. Endocrinol. Metab.* **29**:1533–1538, 1969.
15. Goodlin, R. C.: Heading off plasma volume problems of pregnancy. *Contemp. OB/GYN* **20**:165–180, 1982.
16. Grumbach, M. M. and Kaplan, S. L.: On the placental origin and purification of chorionic "growth hormone–prolactin" and its immunoassay in pregnancy. *Trans. N.Y. Acad. Sci.* **27**:167–188, 1964.
17. Guitelman, A., Aparicio, N. J., Mancini, A., and Debeljuk, L.: Release of prolactin during pregnancy: Effect of sulpiride. *Fertil. Steril.* **30**:42–44, 1978.
18. Hamilton, B. E. and Thompson, K. J.: The circulation in normal pregnant women. In: *The Heart in Pregnancy and the Child-Bearing Age*, Book II, *Physiology of the Circulation in Normal Pregnancy and in Pregnant Women with Heart Disease.* Boston, Little, Brown and Company, 1941, pp. 127–171.
19. Harrow, B. R., Sloane, J. A., and Salhanick, L.: Etiology of the hydronephrosis of pregnancy. *Surg. Gynecol. Obstet.* **119**:1042, 1964.
20. Hytten, F. E.: Metabolic adaptations of pregnancy. In: *Prevention of Handicaps Through Antenatal Care.* A. C. Turnbull and F. Woodford (Eds.). New York, Associated Scientific Publishers, 1976, pp. 35–39.
21. Hytten, F. E. and Baird, D.: The development of the nipple in pregnancy. *Lancet* **i**:1201–1204, 1958.
22. Hytten, F. E. and Cheyne, G. A.: The size and composition of the human pregnant uterus. *J. Obstet. Gynaecol. Br. Commonw.* **76**:400–403, 1969.
23. Hytten, F. E. and Leitch, I.: Cardiovascular dynamics. In: *The Physiology of Human Pregnancy*, 2nd edition. Oxford, Blackwell Scientific Publications, 1971, pp. 69–110.
24. Hytten, F. E. and Leitch, I.: Preparations for breast feeding. In: *The Physiology of Human Pregnancy*, 2nd edition. Oxford, Blackwell Scientific Publications, 1971, pp. 234–241.
25. Hytten, F. E. and Lind, T.: *Diagnostic Indices in Pregnancy.* Summit, NJ, Pharmaceuticals Division, Ciba-Geigy Corp, 1973.
26. Hytten, F. E. and Thomson, A. M.: Weight gain in pregnancy. In: *Hypertension in Pregnancy.* M. D. Lindheimer, A. I. Katz, and F. P. Zuspan (Eds.). New York, John Wiley & Sons, 1976, pp. 179–187.
27. Ivy, A.C.: The functional anatomy of labor, with special reference to the human being. *Am. J. Obstet. Gynecol.* **44**:952–972, 1942.
28. Josimovich, J. B. and Mintz, D. H.: Biological and immunochemical studies on human placental lactogen. *Ann. N.Y. Acad. Sci.* **148**:488–500, 1968.
29. Kalkhoff, R. K., Richardson, B. L., and Beck, P.:

Effects of steroids and human placental lactogen on carbohydrate tolerance. *Clin. Res.* **15**:413, 1967.

30. Koller, O.: The clinical significance of hemodilution during pregnancy. *Obstet. Gynecol. Surv.* **37**:649–652, 1982.
31. Letsky, E.: The haematological system. In: *Clinical Physiology in Obstetrics.* F. E. Hytten and G. Chamberlain (Eds.). Oxford, Blackwell Scientific Publications, 1980, pp. 43–78.
32. Madden, J. D., Siiteri, P. K., MacDonald, P. C., and Gant, N. F.: The pattern and rates of metabolism of maternal plasma dehydroisoandrosterone sulfate in human pregnancy. *Am. J. Obstet. Gynecol.* **125**:915–920, 1976.
33. Mitchell, G. W., Jr., McRipley, R. J., Selvaraj, R. J., and Sbarra, A. J.: The role of the phagocyte in host–parasite interactions. *Am. J. Obstet. Gynecol.* **6**:687–695, 1966.
34. Mixon, W. T. and Woloshin, H. J.: Hiatus hernia in pregnancy. *Obstet. Gynecol.* **8**:249, 1956.
35. Moore, L. A., Jahnigen, D., Rounds, S. S., Reeves, J. T., and Grover, R. F.: Maternal hyperventilation helps preserve arterial oxygenation during high-altitude pregnancy. *J. Appl. Physiol.* **52**:690–694, 1982.
36. Morgan, E. H.: Plasma-iron and haemoglobin levels in pregnancy. *Lancet* **i**:9–12, 1961.
37. O'Connell, M. and Welsh, G. W., III: Unbound plasma cortisol in pregnant and Enovid-E treated women as determined by ultrafiltration. *J. Clin. Endocrinol. Metab.* **29**:563–568, 1969.
38. Oedema in Pregnancy, editorial. *Lancet* **ii**:197–198, 1967.
39. Parslow, M. E., Oddie, T. H., and Fisher, D. A.: Evaluation of serum triiodothyronine and adjusted triiodothyronine (free triiodothyronine index) in pregnancy. *Clin. Chem.* **23**:490–492, 1977.
40. Pasteels, J. L., Gausset, P., Danguy, A., Ectors, F., Nicoll, C. S., and Varavidhi, P.: Morphology of the lactotropes and somatotropes of man and Rhesus monkeys. *J. Clin. Endocrinol. Metab.* **34**:959–967, 1972.
41. Pitkin, R. M., Connor, W. E., and Lin, D. S.: Cholesterol metabolism and placental transfer in the pregnant rhesus monkey. *J. Clin. Invest.* **51**:2584–2592, 1972.
42. Pritchard, J. A. and Scott, D. E.: Iron demands during pregnancy. In: *Iron Deficiency.* L. Hallberg, H.-G. Harwerth, and A. Vanotti (Eds.). London, Colloquia Geigy, Academic Press, 1970, pp. 173–182.
43. Reynolds, S. R. M.: *Physiology of the Uterus.* New York, Hafner Publishing Company, 1965.
44. Reynolds, S. R. M., Harris, J. S., and Kaiser, I. H.: *Clinical Measurement of Uterine Forces in Pregnancy and Labor*, Chapter VIII. Springfield, IL, Charles C Thomas, 1954, pp. 164–180.
45. Rigg, L. A., Lein, A., and Yen, S. S. C.: Pattern of increase in circulating prolactin levels during human gestation. *Am. J. Obstet. Gynecol.* **129**:454–456, 1977.
46. Robin, N. L., Refetoff, S., Fang, V., and Selenkow, H. A.: Parameters of thyroid function in maternal and cord serum at term pregnancy. *J. Clin. Endocrinol. Metab.* **29**:1276–1280, 1969.
47. Rubi, R. A. and Sala, N. L.: Ureteral function in pregnant women. III. Effect of different positions and of fetal delivery upon ureteral tonus. *Am. J. Obstet. Gynecol.* **101**:230, 1968.
48. Sala, N. L., Rubi, R. A.: Ureteral function in pregnant women. *Am. J. Obstet. Gynecol.* **92**:918, 1965.
49. Sala, N. L. and Rubi, R. A.: Ureteral function in pregnant women. II. Ureteral contractility during normal pregnancy. *Am. J. Obstet. Gynecol.* **99**:228, 1967.
50. Samaan, N. A., Bradbury, J. T., and Goplerud, C. P.: Serial hormonal studies in normal and abnormal pregnancy. *Am. J. Obstet. Gynecol.* **104**:781–794, 1969.
51. Samaan, N. A., Goplerud, C. P., and Bradbury, J. T.: Effect of arginine infusion on plasma levels of growth hormone, insulin and glucose during pregnancy and the puerperium. *Am. J. Obstet. Gynecol.* **107**:1002–1007, 1970.
52. Sutherland, C. G., Atkinson, J. C., Brogdon, B. G., Crow, N.E., and Brown, W. E.: Esophageal hiatus hernia in pregnancy. *Obstet. Gynecol.* **8**:261, 1956.
53. Symonds, E. M.: The renin-angiotensin system and sodium excretion during gestation. In: *Hypertension in Pregnancy.* M. D. Lindheimer, A. I. Katz, and F. P. Zuspan (Eds.). New York, John Wiley & Sons, 1976, pp. 271–279.
54. Tyson, J. E., Rabinowitz, D., and Merimee, T. J.: Plasma insulin and hGH responses to arginine in pregnancy. *Clin. Res.* **16**:526, 1968.
55. Tyson, J. E., Rabinowitz, D. , Merimee, T. J., and Friesen, H.: Response of plasma insulin and human growth hormone to arginine in pregnant and postpartum females. *Am. J. Obstet. Gynecol.* **103**:313–319, 1969.
56. Varma, S. K., Sonksen, P. H., Varma, K., Soeldner, J. S., Selenkow, H. A., and Emerson, K.: Measurement of human growth hormone in pregnancy and correlation with human placental lactogen. *J. Clin. Endocrinol. Metab.* **32**:328–332, 1971.
57. Wade, T. R., Wade, S. L. and Jones, H. E.: Skin changes and diseases associated with pregnancy. *Obstet. Gynecol.* **52**:233–242, 1978.

4

IMMUNOLOGIC ASPECTS OF PREGNANCY

Pregnancy is of interest to immunologists because it is the classical exception to a fundamental immunologic rule. The rule states that the immune system recognizes unique cell surface molecules (antigens), is immunologically tolerant of self, and rejects all that is foreign. This mechanism allows the individual to ward off infecting organisms and has given rise to the notion that the immune system exists for host defense. On the other hand, this self/nonself discrimination is the bane of transplant surgeons who must poison the immune system with cytotoxic drugs to prevent rejection of implanted allogenic kidney, heart, liver, or bone marrow cells. Despite this cardinal principle, females of every mammalian species have, for thousands of years, nurtured within their bodies offspring that are foreign, since half of their cell surface antigens are genetically derived from the father.

A complex network of immunologic changes occurs early in pregnancy to attenuate the mother's immune response and to protect the developing fetus from immunologic injury. These changes are more easily measured than explained, so it is not yet possible to diagram, from beginning to end, the sequence of interactive immunologic events. Table 4-1 offers a classification of immunologic phenomena with no attempt to identify major or minor roles in the overall process.

The immunomodulation of pregnancy is not without risk. During pregnancy, the woman's immune system appears to be less effective in screening for all nonself-antigens. As a result, pregnant women are more susceptible to infectious organisms and to progressive growth of neoplastically transformed cells.

This chapter reviews the functions of the normal immune system in the nonpregnant state and examines some of the changes that occur during pregnancy.

CELLULAR IMMUNITY

Development of Immune Cells

Immunopotent leukocytes originate from the embryonic stem cells which progressively move from the embryo to the yolk sac, then to the fetal liver, and ultimately to the bone marrow, where they reside in the adult (Fig. 4-1). As they differentiate, first in the liver and then in the bone marrow, immature lymphocytes can be identified as T cells by the presence of unique cell surface T cell antigens, and as B cells by detectable surface immunoglobulins of the IgM class.

T cells migrate from the bone marrow to the thymus, where new surface markers appear as the cells mature in the thymic microenvironment. There is selection within the thymus in favor of cells that react against foreign but not against self-antigens. Several phenotypically and functionally distinct T cell subsets migrate

TABLE 4-1. MECHANISMS OF MATERNAL–FETAL ALLOGRAFT TOLERANCE

1. Separation of maternal and fetal circulations
   a. Selective transfer of IgG but not IgM and IgA antibodies
   b. Virtual exclusion of immune cell transfer
2. Afferent blockade of immune system
   a. Impairment of lymph drainage from placenta
   b. Avoidance of lymph vessels by invading trophoblast
3. Immunologic barrier at maternal–fetal interface
   a. Alloantigens poorly expressed by trophoblast
   b. Blocking antibody on trophoblast modulates antigen expression
4. Masking of surface alloantigens
   a. Local synthesis of sialomucin coat
   b. Maternal transferrin and blocking antibodies
5. Pinocytosis and digestion of maternal antibodies
6. Synthesis by trophoblast of suppressor factors
   a. Estrogen
   b. Progesterone
   c. Human chorionic gonadotropin
7. Fetal suppressor mechanisms
   a. Alpha-fetoprotein
   b. Suppressor cells
   c. Natural killer cells
8. Maternal suppressor mechanisms
   a. Corticosteroids
   b. Alpha-2-macroglobulin
   c. Blocking antibodies
   d. Suppressor cells

Source: Adapted from Beer, A. E. and Billingham, R. E.: Mechanisms of nonrejection of foeto-placental allografts. *Folia Biol.* **26**:225–243, 1980, Academia Publishing House of the Czechoslovak Academy of Sciences.

from the thymus to the spleen and lymph nodes, where they occupy the medullary and parafollicular regions.

Mature T lymphocytes can be separated into several subpopulations defined by the presence of distinct antigens on their membrane surfaces. Those antigens can be detected by monoclonal antibodies produced by hybridomas. Each hybridoma is capable of synthesizing large quantities of immunoglobulin specific for a single T cell surface antigen. Such antibodies are now commercially available from two sources that use different nomenclature but detect comparable subpopulations of T cells (see legend Fig. 4-1).

The phenotypically different subpopulations of T cells have different functions. Helper T cells, which are recognized by OKT4 or Leu 3a antibodies, proliferate in response to mitogen or antigen. They produce interleukins (also called T cell growth factors), interact with other T cells to promote T effector functions, and promote B lymphocyte differentiation into antibody-producing plasma cells. Suppressor T lymphocytes, identified by monoclonal OKT8 or Leu 2a antibodies, inhibit those functions.

The interactive effects of helper and suppressor T cells illustrate a natural mechanism by which positive and negative signals regulate the immune response to antigens. Immune cells capable of reacting against self-antigens are, in normal individuals, prevented from doing so by antigen-specific suppressor cells and by other mechanisms. When these regulatory mechanisms fail, the result can be an autoimmune disease[49] or decreased resistance to infection.[27]

Mammalian B cells remain within the bone marrow throughout their maturation. Pre-B lymphocytes begin immunoglobulin production at about 10 weeks of gestation with antigen-specific IgM, which is inserted into the cell surface membrane.[83] At that point, B cells are very susceptible to immunosuppression. Exposure to self-antigens at this critical stage renders potentially immunopotent cells specifically tolerant to those antigens. Foreign-antigen-specific B cells mature further by developing surface IgD. Upon activation by antigen, the surface IgD is lost and terminal differentiation to antibody-secreting plasma cells can occur. A single clone of B cells is capable of producing IgM, IgG, or IgA antibody, with each antibody class having the same antigenic specificity. Most B cells exhibit other surface molecules such as receptors for the third component of complement (C3R), receptors for the constant portion of immunoglobulin (Fc), and small molecular weight protein products (Ia or DR) of immune response genes. All these surface proteins are involved in the interactions of B cells with other components of the immune system.

Peripheral blood monocytes and the mononuclear phagocytic cells of the reticuloendothelial system develop from a marrow cell line different from that giving rise to lymphocytes. Mature monocytes exhibit surface histocompatibility antigens (HLA A,B,C, DR, in addition to FcR and C3Rs.

Normal Cellular Immune Mechanisms

Monocytes are crucial to nearly all functions of lymphocytes (Fig. 4-2) because they process antigen for specific lymphocyte activation and release a soluble factor (interleukin-1) that

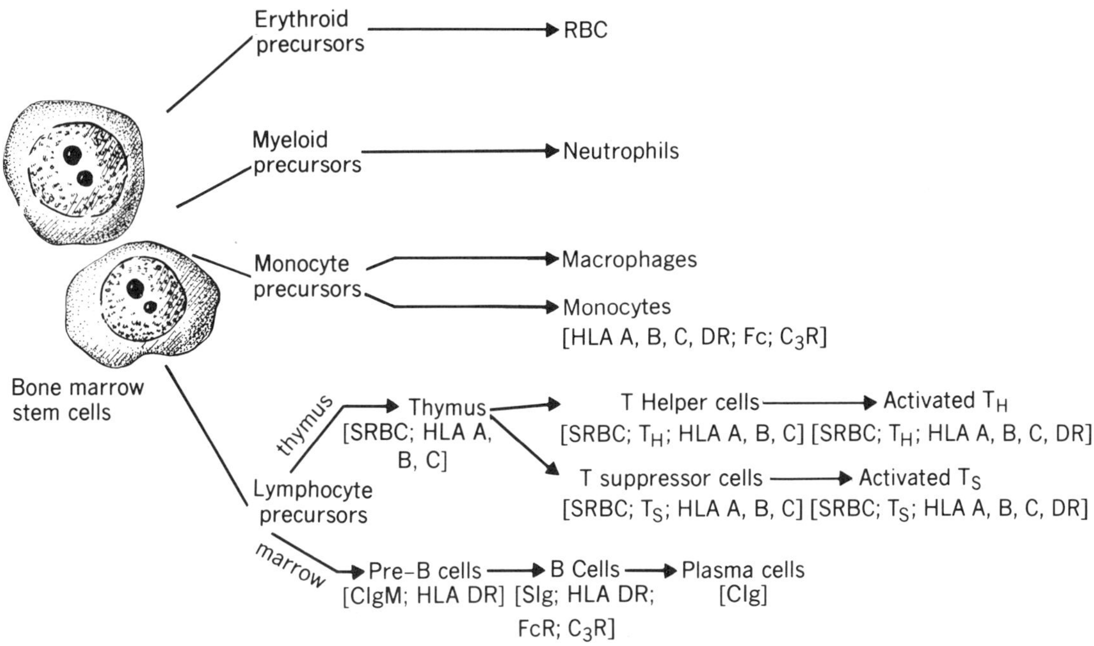

Figure 4-1. Schematic representation of leukocyte ontogeny showing characteristic cell surface markers. SRBC—Receptor for sheep red blood cell surface antigen; HLS A,B,C,DR—human leukocyte antigens A,B,C, and DR; T_H—helper T cell antigen, recognized by OKT_4 or Leu 3_a monoclonal antisera; T_S—suppressor T cell antigen, recognized by OKT_8 or Leu 2 monoclonal antisera; CIgM—cytoplasmic IgM; SIg—surface immunoglobulin; FcR—receptor for constant region of immunoglobulin molecules; C_3R—receptor for third component of complement; Clq—cytoplasmic immunoglobulin of one or more classes.

stimulates T cell proliferation. After phagocytosing antigen, monocytes degrade it into fragments. Some fragments become closely associated with Ia (DR) antigens on the monocyte surface.[98] That complex of self with foreign antigens then initiates the entire cascade of interacting cells and soluble factors that constitutes the immune response.[54]

Activation of T effector cells results in cell-mediated immunity (CMI) against foreign antigens through two major mechanisms. First, activated T lymphocytes produce a myriad of soluble factors such as interleukins, lymphotoxins, vasodilators, mitogens, and interferons which amplify the local immune response and recruit other cell types. Second, a cytotoxic T cell is generated that is capable of killing target cells on contact.

CMI is exemplified by delayed-type hypersensitivity reactions and by the destruction of virus-infected cells that express viral neoantigens on their surfaces. CMI can be measured in vitro by the mixed-lymphocyte reaction (MLR), which closely parallels the immunologic confrontation predicted to occur between maternal and fetal tissues during pregnancy. To demonstrate this phenomenon in the laboratory, mononuclear leukocytes from a donor are inactivated with mitomycin-C or by irradiation to prevent them from proliferating. The treated cells are then cultured together with untreated mononuclear cells from an unrelated (allogenic) donor. Cells from the second donor respond to the "foreign" HLA antigens on the surface of the first donor's cells by proliferating, demonstrated by the incorporation of radioactive thymidine into newly synthesized DNA. The cytotoxic cells generated as a result of that proliferation then progressively lyse the target leukocytes.

Fetal lymphocytes do not develop cytotoxic or natural killer cell activity until late in pregnancy or even a few days postpartum.[83] The absence of those cyto-destructive cells prevents anti-maternal allograft reactivity and tends to decrease the inflammatory potential at the

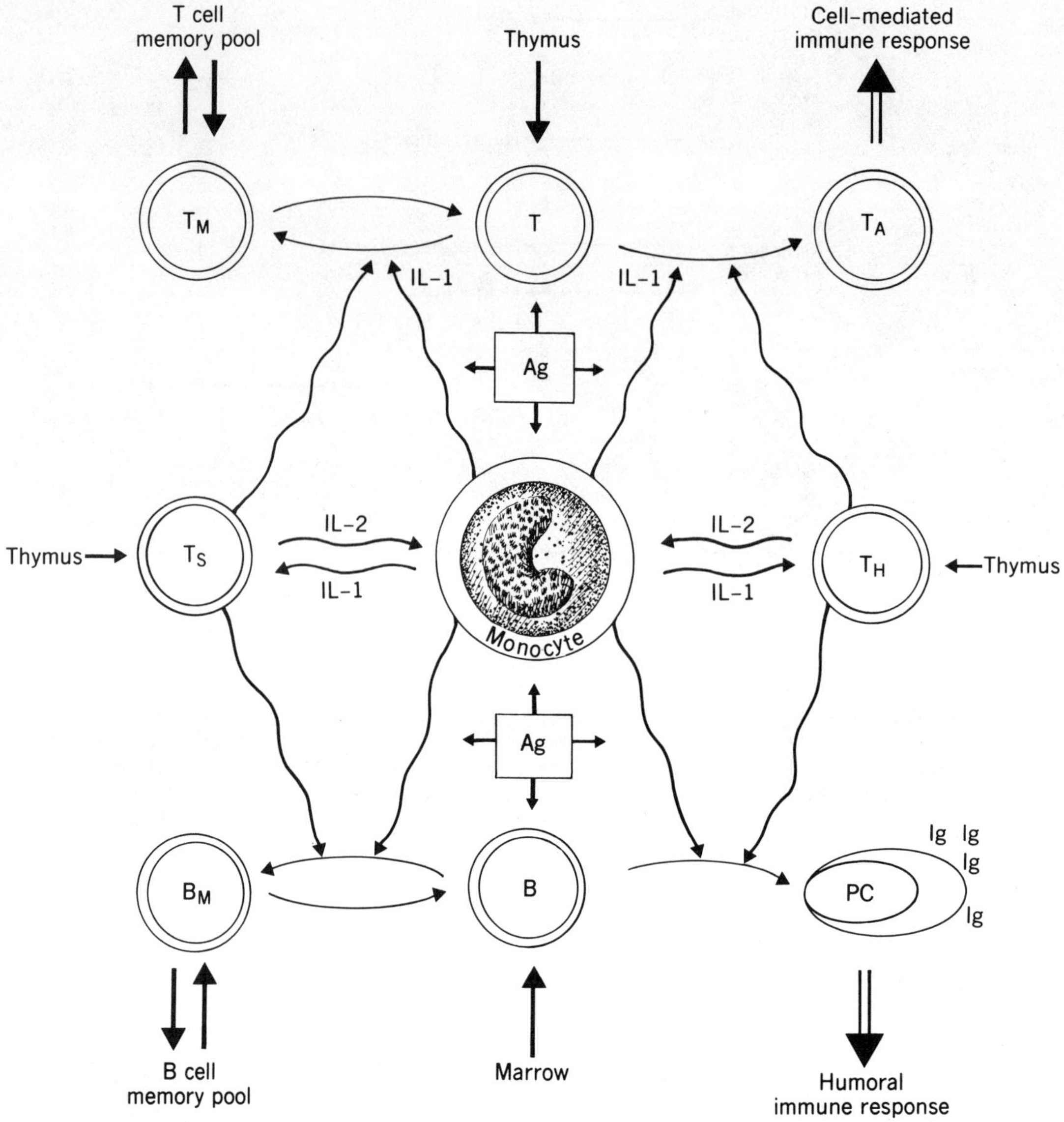

Figure 4-2. Schematic of interactions between antigen, immunocompetent mononuclear leukoycyes, and their soluble secretory products (interleukins) in regulating humoral and cell-mediated immune responses.

fetal–maternal interface. In addition, serum factors produced during pregnancy and circulating in the mother's blood are capable of down-regulating the MLR against paternal and even unrelated alloantigens.

Maternal and Fetal Immune Cells

A number of studies[71,86,89,90,99] have examined maternal blood for static and sequential changes in leukocyte populations during pregnancy. A fairly consistent pattern has emerged (Table 4-2). Absolute numbers of maternal neutrophils and monocytes increase during pregnancy, as do their numbers relative to the numbers of lymphocytes. T lymphocytes usually decrease relative to B lymphocytes and sometimes may undergo an absolute decrease. The ratio of helper:suppressor T cells usually decreases due to a consistent decrease in helper T cells, sometimes accompanied by an increase in T suppressor cells. The implication is that

TABLE 4-2. LEUKOCYTE POPULATIONS IN MATERNAL AND FETAL BLOOD DURING PREGNANCY

Leukocyte Population	Maternal Blood[71,86,89,90,99]	Fetal Blood[86]
Neutrophil	↑	NT
Monocyte	↑	↑
T lymphocytes	↓	↓
T helper	↓	→
T suppressor	↑	↓
T/B ratio	↓	↓
B lymphocytes	→	↑

NT—Not tested.
↑—Increase.
↓—Decrease.
→—No significant change.

down-regulation of lymphocyte-mediated immunologic functions occurs during pregnancy.

Less information is available on the relative numbers of leukocyte populations in fetal blood. For one thing, it is not clear what the most appropriate control population should be. Compared with normal, nonpregnant adult controls, newborn babies have significantly fewer total T cells, fewer suppressor T cells, more B lymphocytes, and more monocytes.[86]

Fetal lymphocytes can be detected circulating in maternal peripheral blood.[81] Furthermore, fetal lymphocyte clones may establish themselves and survive in the mother for extended periods of time.[6,81] At present, there is no way of knowing what long-term effects this cross-colonization of the mother's and infant's bone marrows might have. It has been suggested that graft-versus-host reaction may occur due to such cell transfer.[40]

Cell-Mediated Immune Response

Mononuclear leukocytes from pregnant women respond poorly to microbial antigens.[11] Beginning with nearly normal proliferation in response to Candida albicans or streptokinase / streptodernase in the first trimester, a progressive attenuation is noted by the third trimester. It eventually returns to normal in the postpartum period. This effect is considered intrinsic to the cells and is not dependent upon the presence of pregnancy serum. Similar results have been seen with tetanus toxoid, mumps, and tuberculin.

The effect of pregnancy on mitogen-induced blastogenesis by maternal leukocytes is more variable. Although a few investigators failed to find a pregnancy-related change in the mitogen-induced blastogenesis, the majority observed a significant decrease, as compared with nonpregnant controls or with postpartum values from the same individuals.[11,31,104] The depressive effect can be attributed to the cells themselves,[23] but autologous pregnancy serum may also be responsible.[31,105]

Lymphocytes from normal adult controls are more responsive to mitogens than are cells from neonates. Lymphocytes from premature infants exhibit greater proliferative responses than do cells from term infants. More surprising, the response of cells from infants delivered by cesarean section is greater than the mitogenic response of cells from vaginally delivered infants.[70] The physiologic reasons for these differences are not known.

Studies that have examined the MLR of pregnancy cells cultured in the absence of pregnancy serum have led to differing conclusions, probably because of methodologic differences. Two studies, using a one-way MLR, failed to detect induction of any alloantigen-specific sensitization or tolerance during pregnancy.[13,55] In contrast, another study found inhibition of the maternal-to-fetal and maternal-to-paternal MLRs.[43] The explanation may relate, in part, to different degrees of fetal cell inactivation of the maternal response.

In two-way MLR studies, where each cell population is allowed to proliferate in response to the other, the maternal–fetal MLR is consistently reduced.[30] Fetal cells proliferating in that setting produced suppressor cells which prevented maternal cell proliferation.[18,64] Fetal cells even inhibited proliferation of maternal cells when separated from them by a membrane which prevented direct cell-to-cell contact.[65] The low molecular weight factor that crossed the artificial membrane was nonspecific. Prostaglandin E_2 could be responsible for this effect, since PGE_2 is known to cause inhibition of PHA-induced leukocyte proliferation. Maternal lymphocytes are 100-fold more sensitive to PGE_2 than are fetal lymphocytes.[46]

Fairly convincing evidence indicates maternal sensitization to paternally derived antigens during pregnancy. By the 16th week of pregnancy, cytotoxic cells specific for fetal lung tissue are present in the maternal circulation.[96] The same cell preparations fail, however, to show any cytolytic effect on semiallogeneic amniotic cells or allogeneic fibroblasts. Maternal blood contains a cytotoxic cell population specific for the HLA-DR antigens of the father.[36] Maternal leukocytes also produce antigen-specific blocking factors which prevent maternal lymphocytes from recognizing or reacting against fetal HLA-DR-bearing cells. A third mechanism that may contribute to a low reactivity of maternal cells aganst fetal antigens is the production of suppressor factors by the fetal cells.[65] There is little information available regarding suppressor cells in human pregnancy, but murine studies strongly support their involvement in averting fetal allograft rejection.[16,20]

A dramatic illustration of pregnancy suppression of cellmediated immunity comes from a study of T lymphocyte colony formation during human pregnancy.[87] Peripheral blood mononuclear leukocytes stimulated with PHA were seeded on agar plates. Blood from nonpregnant individuals produced an average of 2000 colonies, but colony production from the blood of pregnant subjects was inhibited by more than 95%. The effect was apparently cell mediated because it occurred in the absence of pregnancy serum factors.

A different cellular mechanism for reduced immunologic responsiveness during pregnancy is suggested by other work.[86] Compared with normal nonpregnant women, there was a significant decrease in helper T cells in the first trimester that persisted through delivery, but normalized within 3–5 months postpartum.

Evidence for both B cell and T cell surface membrane alterations during pregnancy has been reported.[51] The changes are maximal by the l6th week of gestation and resolve completely by the second week postpartum. The importance of surface membrane alterations to tolerance of the fetal allograft is unknown, but surface membrane alterations can also be induced by alpha-fetoprotein and are seen in a limited number of non-pregnancy-related clinical disorders.

The functions of polymorphonuclear phagocytes are also altered during pregnancy. The ability of polymorphs to respond to a chemotactic stimulus (C5a) and to phagocytose bacteria is impaired when contrasted with neutrophils from nonpregnant individuals.

HUMORAL IMMUNITY

Normal Humoral Immune Mechanisms

Immunoglobulins (Ig) are produced by B lymphocytes and plasma cells in response to antigen. Structurally, Ig consists of two large (heavy) and two smaller (light) protein chain components. The heavy chains determine the Ig class (IgG, IgM, IgA, etc.), whereas both light and heavy chains contribute to the antibody specificity. The structurally variable region is abbreviated F(ab) because, when cleaved from the rest of the molecule, that fragment contains the antigen binding site. The structurally more constant region, the Fc fragment, interacts with Fc receptors on the surfaces of monocytes and with complement proteins. Ig molecules exist in families that can be classified in two ways. They can be viewed as a group of antibodies, all having the same antigen specificity (dictated by the variable region) but having different Fc structures or isotypes. Alternatively, they can be seen as members of an Ig class such as IgG, IgM, IgA, IgD, or IgE with different antigenic specificities. Each class within a family has unique properties due to structural differences in the Ig constant portion. IgG, IgM, and IgA normally circulate in peripheral blood. IgA is the primary Ig found in secretions from the nasal mucous membranes and the gut. IgE preferentially binds to tissue cells and contributes importantly to allergic responses.

A conformational change occurs in an Ig molecule following contact with specific antigen. That change opens up the site for interaction with the first complement component (C1). Activation of C1 on the surface of the Ig molecule initiates a series of enzymatic reactions that involves nine or more complement protein molecules. The end result may be damage to a target cell membrane or more effective phagocytosis of circulating immune complexes. Small molecular weight fragments cleaved from the complement proteins are responsible for anaphylaxis (C3a and C5a) and neutrophil chemotaxis (C5a).

IgG antibodies can cross the placenta and can enter the fetal circulation, but IgM and IgA antibodies cannot.[72] The transfer of IgG antibody appears to protect the neonate from subsequent infection. Alloantibodies specific for fetal antigens are prevented from crossing the fetal circulation by being bound to fetal antigens on the maternal side.

The humoral immune response is only minimally altered in pregnant women. Serum IgG and IgA levels decrease by 25–30% during normal pregnancy, whereas IgM levels show no consistent change. In contrast, IgG levels increase with parity, suggesting that greater levels of alloantibody are produced in women multiply exposed to fetal antigens.

The levels of most complement components increase during pregnancy as if they are responding in a phase-reactant manner. That is not true, however, for the first few components of the classical pathway which are known to interact with immune complexes. The lower levels of C1 may be due to complement activation because a product of C3 activation (C3d) is elevated in the serum of third trimester normal pregnant women as compared with healthy nonpregnant controls. Complement activation may be occurring at the maternal-fetal junction as alloantibodies or blocking factors react specifically with fetal antigen. The low levels of early classical complement pathway components are even more significant when compared with the elevated levels of the later components. It suggests both a substantial activation of complement during pregnancy and a limitation of activation to the early components.

Circulating immune complex levels decrease during normal pregnancy,[72,79] but not in pregnancy complicated by preeclampsia, where immune complexes are substantially increased.[72,79] One potential explanation for decreasing quantities of immune complexes in pregnancy is a factor in serum that apparently increases the rate at which normal neutrophils phagocytose immune complexes.[76]

Simple measurement of total Ig levels is not a sensitive gauge of the humoral immune response to pregnancy. Although there is limited information available regarding specific antibody production during pregnancy, rheumatoid factor decreases in pregnant rheumatoid arthritis patients[66] and anti-insulin antibody levels are lower in pregnant diabetics than in age-matched, nonpregnant diabetic controls.[24] Even in animal models, the effect of pregnancy on specific antibody production is unclear. Levels of serum antibody in pregnant animals are lower than in nonpregnant controls, especially during the second and third trimesters, but the number of antibody-forming cells is increased in pregnant animals.[26,78]

Pregnant women immunized to tetanus toxoid during the third month of pregnancy have been examined for production of IgG and IgM anti-tetanus antibodies at months 3, 5, and 9. The results of the study suggested that humoral immunity to specific antigens is not substantially impaired during pregnancy.[38]

The infants of the immunized mothers had substantial levels of anti-tetanus IgG antibody at birth, consistent with transplacental passage of specific IgG from the mother, but they also had substantial levels of specific IgM anti-tetanus antibody, implying a response of the fetal immune system to the antigen used for immunizing the mothers. Since the antigen-specific cell-mediated immune response was also elevated in the infants of the immunized mothers, it can be concluded that infants can be immunized by antigens injected into the mothers during pregnancy.

Maternal antibodies are formed with apparent specificity toward paternal histocompatibility antigens present in the fetus.[41] Unfortunately, the same blocking mechanism impairs the maternal immune responses against growth of hydatidiform moles which proliferate rapidly because of their ability to immunologically imitate a growing fetus.

Some evidence suggests that an immune response is generated by the fetus against maternal antigens. Cord serum contains antibody specific for maternal T and B lymphocytes and maternal blood contains antibodies directed against paternal cell antigens.[17] It is not clear what effect an anti-maternal immune response by the fetus would have on fetal survival.

IMMUNOREGULATION BY SERUM PROTEINS

Pregnancy Serum or Plasma

Plasma from pregnant women is capable of substantially inhibiting the MLR between mother and infant. The same plasma also inhibits the MLR between unrelated donor pairs. Plasma prepared from cord blood inhibits the MLR between mother and fetus nearly as well as does maternal serum but is ineffective at modulating the MLR of unrelated pairs. The magnitude of the inhibition increases with gestational age, reaching a maximum at the time of delivery and then decreasing to control levels within a few days postpartum (Russell, I. J., Nakamura, T., Dauphinee, M., Vipraio, G., and Talal, N.: Unpublished data). Other studies[9,62] have confirmed those observations. There is no relationship between the magnitude of MLR inhibition and the outcome of pregnancy.[9] The MLR-inhibitory activity of pregnancy serum appears to be separable into two components—one about the size of IgG and the other smaller than albumin (Russell, I. J., Nakamura, T., Dauphinee, M., Vipraio, G., and Talal, N.: Unpublished data).

It would be of great interest to identify the factor or factors responsible for the inhibitory effect of pregnancy serum on the immune response and to know whether the serum-mediated effects are physiologically important to maintenance of the fetal allograft. Seventeen serum proteins have now been specifically iden-

TABLE 4-3. IMMUNOINHIBITORY SERUM FACTORS

Protein	Molecular Weight $(\times 10^{-3})$	Carbohydrate %	Nonpregnant Blood Levels	Peak Levels in Pregnancy	Peak Week Pregnancy	Immuno inhibitory	Generation of Suppressor Cells
Chorionic gonadotropin	39	30	<10 IU/ml	100 IU/ml	8–12	Y/N	Yes
Alpha-1-acid glycoprotein (AAG)	41	45	400–1000 μg/ml	1000–2500μg/ml	—	Yes	Possible
Alpha-fetoprotein (AFP)	70	5	<40 ng/ml	500 ng/ml	28–30	Y/N	Yes
Immunoglobulin (Ig)	150	—	—	—	—	Yes	NT
Pregnancy associated globulin (PAG)	350	10	10 μg/ml	1000 μg/ml	34	Yes	NT
Alpha-2-macroglobulin (A2M)	725	—	250 mg/ml	—	—	Yes	Probable

NT = Not tested.

Y/N = Yes/No: Considerable difference of opinion exists.

tified with the pregnant state in normal women.[44] The characteristics of several of those immunoinhibitory proteins are presented in Table 4-3.

Alpha-Fetoprotein

Alpha-fetoprotein (AFP) is a small glycoprotein, synthesized by fetal liver, that crosses the placenta into the maternal circulation starting around the 12th week of gestation. Maternal levels may reach 300 ng/ml in the third trimester of pregnancy but drop sharply at parturition.[8] Murine AFP is considered to be a modulator of the immune response.[8,53,60,61] The influence of AFP on the human immune system is less clear because some investigators find inhibition like that seen in the murine system,[3,68,103] whereas others show no measurable effect that can be attributed to AFP.[3,67,85,101] One possible explanation for the discrepancy is that AFP can exist in several variant forms[85] and is sensitive to inactivation by variations in the methodology of preparation.[3]

Alpha-1-Acid Glycoprotein

The serum concentration of this glycoprotein increases as a phase reactant during conditions of inflammation, pregnancy, and cancer.[102] Alpha-1-acid glycoprotein sharply inhibits MLR, an action directed toward the responder population. It is possible that suppressor cell activity is also enhanced by alpha-1-acid glycoprotein.

Immunoglobulin

Fetal antigens derived from the father induce alloantibody production by the mother's immune system. Such antibodies from multiparous females have provided the antisera that have been very effectively used in histocompatibility typing.[14,50] Multiparous serum, containing antibodies specific for a single histocompatibility antigen, is added to one of nearly 100 wells containing the cells of an individual to be typed. Other sera with different specificities are added to the remaining wells and are incubated for a period of time to allow the antibodies to bind to the cells before a source of hemolytic complement is added. A positive match between the histocompatibility antigen on the surface of the typing cell and an antibody in the maternal serum leads to complement-mediated lysis of the cell membrane.

This observation demonstrates that maternal antibodies to paternal histocompatibility antigens are capable of activating hemolytic complement and perhaps causing fetal cell injury. Apparently, cytotoxic antibodies are produced quite early, even in primiparous pregnancies, because they have been demonstrated in maternal blood as early as 6½ weeks of gestation.[100]

It has been proposed that antibody to histocompatibility antigens of the father serves an important role in protecting the fetus from injury by blocking the immune response of the mother.[12,73,74] IgG isolated from pregnancy serum is capable of reproducing the blocking effect of whole serum and IgG eluted from the placenta has a similar activity.[74] It is proposed that the IgG blocking factor is physiologically significant because women who deliver normal term pregnancies produce the factor in their serum, whereas women who experience idiopathic spontaneous abortions fail to do so.[73] Apparently, cell-mediated immunity directed against fetal histocompatibility antigens is blocked when the antibody binds to the surface antigen and prevents its recognition by immunocompetent cells.

Although it is clear that a humoral immune response is generated by the mother against fetal alloantigens, it is not certain that those antibodies are responsible for the immunoinhibitory effect of pregnancy serum or even of its IgG fraction. Buckley and coworkers[12] carefully examined the mechanism by which four alloimmune plasmas blocked immune responses. They found that the plasmas were inhibitory of both autologous and homologous lymphocytes responding to PHA, pokeweed mitogen, candida antigen, and allogeneic cells in the one-way MLR. The blocking activity was not dependent on lymphocytotoxic injury to immunocompetent cells because it was fully effective in the absence of hemolytic complement.

Some studies have concluded that the most likely mechanism responsible for the blocking effect is a modification of the responding cells rather than an antigen-masking effect on the stimulator cells.[12] Others suggest that pregnancy serum exerts inhibitory effects on both the stimulator and responder cells.[34] Although these studies do not entirely clarify the relationship of immunoglobulins to tolerance of the fetal allograft, they do indicate a potential role of the humoral immune response in protection of the fetus.

Pregnancy-Associated Globulin

Pregnancy-associated alpha$_2$-glycoprotein (PAG) is a high molecular weight molecule. Plasma concentrations of PAG increase during pregnancy and during administration of exogenous estrogen.[94] Serum levels of this protein begin to rise gradually during the first trimester of pregnancy, peak in the third trimester, and fall precipitously after delivery. PAG is found on the surface of lymphocytes and is produced by them during in vitro stimulation with estrogen. Inhibition of the MLR by PAG has been consistently reported. Its mechanism of action is not entirely clear, but it appears to involve a cell surface complex of Fc receptors, B$_2$-microglobulin, and Ia antigen.[56] Physiologic concentrations of PAG somehow block the availability of surface Fc receptors on monocytes such that they are unavailable for reaction with the Fc portion of aggregated IgG attached to the surface of erythrocytes.[69] Similarly, PAG blocks availability of monocyte surface DR antigens to specific antibody. Antisera directed specifically against MLR determinants almost completely eliminate subsequent uptake of PAG on the cell surface.[94]

This observation suggests a possible interrelationship between PAG and the alloantibodies generated during pregnancy. The manner in which this interaction would be uniquely fetoprotective is not apparent. Low levels of maternal PAG in the first trimester may be associated with increased frequency of spontaneous abortion.[94] In contrast, pregnancy can be successful even though PAG levels are unmeasurable at term.

Human Chorionic Gonadotropin

Human chorionic gonadotropin (hCG) is a relatively small glycoprotein. The concentration of hCG in plasma begins to rise during the first week of pregnancy, peaks at 6–12 weeks, and then declines gradually thereafter. Early studies using variably purified preparations of hCG found MLR-inhibitory activity and even generation of suppressor cell activity.[32,33] More recently,[57] that activity has been attributed to a small molecular weight contaminant of crude hCG. The small molecular weight inhibitor, which remains unidentified, exhibited characteristics for an immunomodulator, including nontoxicity, inhibitory activity at low concentrations, activity in a wide range of immune systems, and reversibility when removed from the cell culture milieu.[59]

Early Pregnancy Factor

One argument against the importance of pregnancy-associated protein factors in the immunologic tolerance of pregnancy is that most are not produced in measurable amounts until long after implantation of the blastocyst has occurred. Recently, however, an activity, referred to as early pregnancy factor (EPF), has been detected within hours after fertilization and before implantation of the embryo.[58] This material, which was originally detected using the rosette-inhibition test, has since been shown to inhibit adoptive transfer of contact sensitivity in vivo after a brief incubation with early pregnancy factor in vitro.[63] EPF has been fractionated into two components, one 24,000 daltons and the other approximately 50,000 daltons. Both are immunosuppressive, but the mechanism of action is unknown.

Immunoregulation by Hormones

The concentrations of several steroidal hormones increase substantially during pregnancy. Their interactions with the immune system are still incompletely understood, but there is growing evidence that they do influence immune function. The question remains whether those effects occur at physiologic hormone concentrations. Available evidence indicates that they do not and, thus, the steroidal hormones are probably not responsible for the immunosuppressive effects of pregnancy serum.[48,80,84] It is quite likely, however, that tissue concentrations in the region of the placenta are much higher than they are in the peripheral blood, so regional effects remain a possibility.

Corticosteroids

Corticosteroid hormones given in pharmacologic doses may have profound effects on the subpopulations of mononuclear leukocytes circulating in the peripheral blood. This effect is largely due to redistribution of those cells to lymphoid organs.[82] Hydrocortisone, in supraphysiologic concentrations, is capable of dramatically inhibiting the MLR but, unlike estrogen and progesterone, appears to have some immunoinhibitory activity in the concentrations present in the serum during pregnancy.[80] The effects of corticosteroids on monocyte–macrophage function include inhibition of phagocytic activity and reduction of functional membrane receptors for the Fc portion of IgG and for the C3 molecule.[82]

To exhibit its effect on the MLR in vitro, cortisol must be present in the culture early. The effect is, thereafter, not reversible by washing the cells free of unbound hormone.[21] Corticosteroid levels increase nearly twofold during pregnancy due to increased levels of free cortisol and of cortisol binding proteins.[47] Unlike progesterone and estrogen, most of the circulating serum cortisol is produced in the maternal adrenal gland rather than in the placental–fetal complex. It is possible, however, that increased corticosteroid concentrations may exist at the placental surface, since a transcortin-like protein with immunosuppressive properties has been detected in trophoblastic extracts.[75] The most convincing evidence against cortisol being the important immunoinhibitory factor in pregnancy serum is the fact that there is no relationship between cortisol concentration and immunoinhibitory activity.[48]

Estrogens

There is less information to implicate estrogens directly in the immunoinhibitory process of pregnancy.

It is fairly clear that the immunoinhibitory effect of pregnancy serum is not due to estrogen because it has no effect at physiologic serum concentrations.[80] Despite that, it is difficult to exclude estrogen from importance in protection of the fetus. The placenta synthesizes estrogens and secretes them into both the maternal and fetal circulations,[97] therefore local tissue concentrations may be much higher than those measured in serum or even in intervillous blood.

Progesterone

The evidence for a physiologic immunoinhibitory effect of progesterone during pregnancy is more substantial. Progesterone is synthesized and secreted by trophoblastic cells so that tissue concentration in the placenta is substantially higher than its concentration in peripheral blood. Progesterone is clearly important to the maintenance of the pregnant state, since it alone will maintain pregnancy following removal of the corpus luteum early in gestation.[88] Progesterone binds to uteroglobulin which allows it to maintain high levels in the uterine fluids where, among other activities, it inhibits uterine contractions. Despite demonstrated regional immunoinhibitory changes induced by progesterone, it is still likely that the physiologic concentrations of progesterone in blood are insufficient to explain the immunoinhibitory effects of pregnancy serum.[80]

Physical Barriers in Pregnancy

The concentration of immunoinhibitory factors may be substantially higher at the placental interface, producing a chemical barrier. The placenta and the uterus also have the potential to serve as physical barriers between mother and fetus.

The Placenta Despite the acknowledged existence of humoral and cellular immunoinhibitors in pregnancy serum, it is quite possible that the major factor protecting the fetus from immunologic rejection by the mother is the placental barrier.[15] The various inhibitory activities observed in the blood of pregnant females may be merely a "downstream reflection" of a functionally important inhibitory role carried out in the region of the placenta. The placenta is a highly vascular structure of fetal origin uniquely designed for exchange of nutrients from the mother and waste products from the infant. Its ability to accomplish efficient exchange is due, in part, to its large surface area resulting from innumerable chorionic villi that invade the uterine decidua like the roots of a tree seeking water. The surface of the villus is covered by a layer of syncytiotrophoblast cells. Under them is a layer of cytotrophoblast cells surrounding the mesenchymal core which is laced with fetal capillaries. The decidual plate on the maternal side is composed of peripheral blood leukocytes, endometrial stromal cells, and decidual cells which develop from hormone-stimulated endometrial stromal cells.[52]

The placenta, rather than the fetus itself, is the graft which becomes adherent to maternal tissue and avoids immunologic rejection despite its allogeneic origin. Early attempts to explain survival of the placenta proposed that it lacked alloantigens and thus was not immunogenic. This theory has been discounted, however, because Class I histocompatibility antigens (HLA-A,B in humans) have been found on the surface of cytotrophoblastic cells in animals[15,52] and in humans.[91] These antigens are exposed to the maternal circulation and are subject to attack by specific monoclonal antibodies and by cells.[15] Careful measurements have failed to demonstrate Class II (Ia,DR) antigens on the surface of trophoblastic cells. In contrast to cytotrophoblast cells, syncytiotrophoblast cells lack definable HLA antigens. Although DR antigen-bearing cells are not found on the fetal side of the placenta, they are present on maternal decidua.[7] Despite the absence of DR antigens on trophoblast cells, multiparous females do develop anti-DR antibodies, perhaps as a result of exposure to fetal leukocytes at the time of delivery.

The Class I HLA antigens on cytotrophoblast cells are present in low numbers, which would tend to decrease their immunogenicity. In addition, their sparse distribution on the surface of cells decreases the likelihood that cross-linking by antibody will occur and trigger complement activation. The presence of fetal antigens in low numbers on the surface of placental cells does, however, provide a mechanism by which anti-fetal antibodies can be selectively removed from the IgG fraction passing into the fetal circulation.[15] There is a rapid turnover of antibodies bound to the surface of these cells, indicating that bound antibody is endocytosed, digested intracellularly, and then released back into the maternal circulation as fragments.

Although it is not uncommon for fetal cells to find their way into the maternal circulation, the reverse transfer must be an extremely rare event. The rare exception to this generalization could have dire consequences, such as the establishment of graft-versus-host disease with cells of maternal origin pitted against fetal histocompatibility antigens.[52] Therefore, the placenta seems to be a good barrier to passage of maternal lymphocytes into the fetal circulation. It was noted above that fetal cells effectively suppress the proliferation of maternal leukocytes in vitro and thus provide at least one fail-safe mechanism for inactivation of any maternal lymphocytes that find their way across the placenta.

The Uterine Cavity. Another mechanism by which an immune response against the fetal allograft may be prevented is immunologic isolation of the uterine cavity. Labeled lymphocytes placed in the endometrial cavity do not appear in the lymph nodes that drain the uterus, whereas lymphocytes placed within the myometrium do. Thus, fetal antigens within the uterine cavity are less likely to be immunogenic because of their location. Table 4-4 summarizes this and other mechanisms of immunomodulation in pregnancy compared with methods available for immunologic manipulation. The intrusion of natural killer (NK) cells and other cytotoxic lymphocytes into fetal circulation may also be blocked by specific cytotoxic NK-like fetal cells and by IgM antibody in cord blood which has specificity for killer T cells.[15]

TABLE 4-4. THE CLASSICAL MEANS OF MANIPULATING IMMUNE RESPONSES AND SIMILAR MECHANISMS OPERATING IN GESTATION THAT MAY CONTRIBUTE TO MATERNAL–FETAL IMMUNOLOGICAL COEXISTENCE

Means of Manipulating Immune Responses	Similar Mechanisms Operating in Gestation
1. Immunologically privileged sites of grafting	1. The decidualized uterus as a privileged site for grafting
2. Immunologically privileged tissues	2. Trophoblast as an immunologically privileged tissue
3. Immunologic tolerance	3. Pregnancy-induced specific hyporesponsiveness to paternal antigens
4. Immunologic enhancement	4. Production of blocking antibody during pregnancy
5. Immunosuppression	5. Nonspecific immunosuppressive properties of pregnancy proteins and placental hormones
6. Blocking T and B cell immune responses with excess antigen	6. Antigen shedding by the trophoblast
7. Blocking T and B cell immune responses with antigen–antibody complexes	7. Antigen–antibody complex production during pregnancy
8. Suppressor T lymphocytes	8. Suppressor T lymphocyte production during pregnancy

Source: Beer, A. E. and Billingham, R. E.: Maternal immunological recognition mechanisms during pregnancy. In: Maternal Recognition of Pregnancy. Excerpta Medica, Amsterdam (CIBA Found. Symp. 64), 1978, pp 293–322.

Protective Alloimmunity

A recent observation remains incompletely understood but is probably quite important. Women who have repeated spontaneous abortions can have successful pregnancies after they have been vaccinated with white blood cells from their husbands or even with cells from pooled random donors. This suggests that alloimmunization is somehow protective of the fetal–placental allograft. Indeed, an immune response by the mother against fetal antigens may be imperative to survival of the fetal allograft. Too great a similarity between maternal and paternal alloantigens may well be one cause of recurrent fetal wastage.[29]

The decidua and its constituent cells may participate actively in the immunoregulatory process at the placental interface by facilitating communication between immunocompetent cells.[52]

Resistance to Infection

As noted above, humoral immunity remains relatively intact during pregnancy, whereas cell-mediated immunity, as measured by MLR and mitogen stimulation, is consistently inhibited or suppressed during pregnancy. The same appears to be true for humoral and cell-mediated immune responses to microbial antigens in vitro. The mother and the fetus are co-sensitive to a wide variety of antigens. In most cases, when the mother is sensitized to a particular antigen, the infant is also sensitized.[37]

Bacterial Infections

Not much information exists regarding the frequency of common bacterial infections in pregnancy. Most of them are probably adequately handled by the humoral immune system and polymorphonuclear leukocyte phagocytosis. There is evidence, however, that *M. leprae* infections, which are ordinarily controlled by cell-mediated mechanisms, are adversely affected by pregnancy.[5,25]

An evaluation of the in vitro blastogenic response of lymphocytes from pregnant and nonpregnant females to a number of bacterial antigens such as *Chlamydia trachomatis*, streptococci, and tetanus demonstrated decreased lymphocyte transformation to all of these antigens during pregnancy as compared with the postpartum period and with nonpregnant controls. This observation is not trivial, because all the individuals, pregnant and nonpregnant, had active *C. trachomatis* at the time of study.[11]

Viral Infections

Cell-mediated immune response to rubella virus[95] and to cytomegalovirus[1,35] is consistently lower in pregnant than in nonpregnant females and lower during pregnancy than it is postpartum in the same individuals. Cell-mediated response against cytomegalovirus is depressed during pregnancy despite normal or even elevated antibody titers to the pertinent viral antigens. Infants can develop active cytomegalovirus infection and display reduced cell-mediated immune responses against the virus despite adequate levels of humoral antibody, some of which is passively acquired from the mother. Humoral antibody levels to herpes simplex, measles, rubella, and influenza A viruses did not change during pregnancy.[4]

Polyoma virus infections may activate during pregnancy, as evidenced by rising titers of specific antibody.[22] Pregnant patients with reactivation of virus infection exhibit higher cell-mediated immunity against viral antigens than do pregnant patients without reactivation. In fact, available data suggest that selective activation or derepression of certain latent viruses occurs during pregnancy.[93]

Fifty-three percent of pregnant women with five to nine previous pregnancies showed viral antigen-specific leukocyte activation, whereas only 15% of pregnant patients with fewer than five pregnancies and only 3% of nonpregnant multiparas exhibited such a response.[93] There was no difference in the response of these three groups to baboon C-particle virus or simian sarcoma virus.

Opportunistic Infections

Although there is evidence from animal studies that pregnant and lactating females are more susceptible to protozoan and helminthic infestations, the only available evidence in humans is an increased prevalence of infection with *Plasmodium falciparum* in areas where malaria is endemic.[10]

Preeclamptic Toxemia

Circumstantial evidence suggests that preeclampsia may represent a form of maternal rejection of the fetal allograft. One hypothesis suggests that preeclampsia results from exposure to paternal alloantigens carried by the fetus before there has been adequate presensitization to those antigens. Presensitization is proposed to occur as a result of prolonged exposure to alloantigens on the father's sperm during the weeks or months prior to conception. However, preeclampsia usually affects young primigravidas who, as a group, are less likely than are multiparas to have had prolonged exposure to paternal alloantigens before conception. Similarly, when preeclampsia occurs in multigravidas, it usually follows the introduction of new histocompatibility antigens with a change of mate.[28,39] There is an unusually high occurrence of homozygosity of HLA antigens in preeclamptic women and a higher-than-expected husband–wife HLA compatibility. What that means, in terms of an immune response against the fetus, is not clear, because the main abnormality found in MLR studies on preeclamptic females is a decreased response of paternal-against-maternal cells.[77]

Malignancy

The relationship between pregnancy and malignant tumors may not be immediately apparent, but there is some logic in considering them together. In fact, many similarities exist between the apparent mechanisms for nonrejection of the fetus and nonrejection of malignancy.[77] In both situations, blocking antibodies of the IgG class have been implicated in protecting the graft or tumor from destruction by cell-mediated immune surveillance. In addition, the dedifferentiation of malignant tumors results in production of many of the primitive protein antigens normally secreted during pregnancy.

The development of persistent trophoblastic proliferation in the form of hydatidiform mole may result from a continued presence of blocking antibody which prevents the total rejection of the conceptus at the time of an otherwise spontaneous abortion of the fetus.[92] It is also apparent that immunologic or other changes that occur during pregnancy have long-term tumor-related effects. For example, the risk of breast malignancy is modified by the parity of the affected individual.[45] Likewise, the incidence of melanoma is approximately equal in males and females, as it is in multiparas and virgin females, but the prognosis for survival is much better among women with a prior pregnancy.[42] Perhaps exposure to embryonic antigens during pregnancy enhances the anamnestic response to tumor neoantigens.

Conclusions

Despite much investigative effort, the critical factors responsible for protection of the fetal allograft are still not known with confidence. It would appear that humoral immunity is not substantially altered during pregnancy, but that cell-mediated immunity is decreased, both specifically and nonspecifically. This decrease in cell-mediated immunity may be induced by immunoinhibitory serum proteins, by steroidal hormones, or by suppressor cells. The placenta also provides a physical, though semipermeable, barrier to immunologic attack on the fetus. The immunoinhibition demonstrable in maternal peripheral blood may reflect active processes occurring at the fetal-maternal interface. There is evidence to suggest that immunologic recognition of the fetus by the mother is important to prevent allograft rejection, as may occur in preeclampsia. This down-regulation of the immune response during pregnancy carries with it a potential risk to the mother in the form of increased susceptibility to infection and to some forms of malignancy.

REFERENCES

1. Agatsuma, Y., Fitzpatrick, P., Lele, A., Kaul, A., and Ogra, P.L.: Cell-mediated immunity cytomegalovirus in pregnant women. *Am. J. Reprod. Immunol.* **1**:174–179, 1981.
2. Alpert, E., Dienstag, J. L., Sepersky, S., Littman, B., and Rocklin, R.: Immunosuppressive characteristics of human AFP:. Effect on tests of cell-mediated immunity and induction of human suppressor cells. *Immunol. Commun.* **7**:163–185, 1978.
3. Auer, I. O. and Kress, H. G.: Suppression of the primary cell-mediated immune response by human alpha-fetoprotein in vitro. *Cell. Immunol.* **30**:173–179, 1977.
4. Baboonian, C. and Griffiths, P.: Is pregnancy immunosuppressive? Humoral immunity against viruses. *Br. J. Obstet. Gynaecol.* **90**:1168–1175, 1983.
5. Barnetson, R. S., Bjune, G., and Duncan, M. E.: Evidence for a soluble lymphocyte factor in the transplacental transmission of T-lymphocyte responses to *Mycobacterium leprae*. *Nature* **260**:150–151, 1976.
6. Beer, A. E., Billingham, R. E., Head, J. R., and Parmely, M. J.:. Possible influence of maternal-to-perinatal cell transfer on the development of host defenses. In: *Development of Host Defenses*. M. D. Cooper and D. H. Dayton (Eds.). New York, Raven Press, 1977, pp. 251–271.
7. Bell, S. C. and Billington, W. D.: Anti-fetal alloantibody in the pregnant female. *Immunol. Rev.* **75**:5–30, 1983.
8. Bischof, P., Lauber, K., Girard, J. P., Herrmann, W. L., and Sizonenko, P. C.: Circulating levels of pregnancy proteins and depression of lymphoblastogenesis during pregnancy. *J. Clin. Lab. Immunol.* **12**:93–96, 1983.
9. Bissendon, J. G., Ling, N. R., and Mackintosh, P.: Suppression of mixed lymphocyte reactions by pregnancy serum. *Clin. Exp. Immunol.* **39**:195–202, 1980.
10. Bray, R. S. and Anderson, M. J.: Falciparum malaria and pregnancy. *Trans. R. Soc. Trop. Med. Hyg.* **73**:427–431, 1979.
11. Brunham, R. C., Martin, D. H., Hubbard, T. W., Kuo, C. C., Critchlow, C. W., Cles, L. D., Eschenbach, D. A., and Holmes, K. K.: Depression of the lymphocyte transformation response to microbial antigens and to phytohemagglutinin during pregnancy. *J. Clin. Invest.* **72**:1629–1638, 1983.
12. Buckley, R. H., Schoff, R. I., and Amos, D. B.: Blocking of autologous and homologous leukocyte responses by human alloimmune plasmas: A possible *in vitro* correlate of enhancement. *J. Immunol.* **108**:34–44, 1972.
13. Carr, M. C., Stites, D. P. and Fudenberg, H. H.: Cellular immune aspects of the human fetal–maternal relationship. III. Mixed lymphocyte reactivity between related maternal and cord blood lymphocytes. *Cell. Immunol.* **11**:332–341, 1974.
14. Ceppellini, R. and Van Rood, J. J.: The HLA system. I. Genetics and molecular biology. *Semin. Hematol.* **11**:233–251, 1974.
15. Chaouat, G., Kolb, J. P., and Wegmann, T. G.: The murine placenta as an immunological barrier between the mother and the fetus. *Immunol. Rev.* **75**:31--60, 1983.
16. Chaouat, G., Monnot, P., Hoffman, M., and Chaffaux, S.: Regulatory mechanisms of cell-mediated immunity in allogeneic pregnancy. *Am. J. Reprod. Immunol.* **1**:18–22, 1980.
17. Chardonnens, X. and Jeannet, M.: Immunobiology of pregnancy:. Evidence for a fetal immune response against the mother. *Tissue Antigens* **15**:401–406, 1980.
18. Chaudhuri, J.P. and Zang, K. D.: Mitosis of maternal lymphocytes in the presence of fetal cells: Possible implication in prenatal diagnosis from fetal blood samples. *Hum. Genet.* **34**:307–310, 1976.
19. Chiu, F. M., Mortensen, R. F., Osmond, A. P., and Gewur, H.: Interactions of alpha-l-acid glycoprotein with the immune system. I. Purification and effects on lymphocyte responsiveness. *Immunology* **32**:997–1005, 1977.
20. Clark, D. A., McDermott, M. R., and Szewczuk, M. R.: Impairment of host-versus-graft reaction in pregnant mice. II. Selective suppression of cytotoxic T-cell generation correlates with soluble suppressor activity and with successful allogeneic pregnancy. *Cell. Immunol.* **52**:106–118, 1952.
21. Clemens, L. E., Stites, D., and Siiteri, P. K.: In vitro suppression of human lymphocyte transformation by progesterone. *Gynecol. Invest.* **8**:20, 1977.
22. Coleman, D. V., Gardner, S. D., Mulholland, C., Fridiksdottir, V., Porter, A. A., Lilford, R., and Valdimarsson, H.: Human polyomavirus in pregnancy. A model for the study of defence mechanisms to virus reactivation. *Clin. Exp. Immunol.* **53**:289–296, 1983.
23. Daunter, B., Khoo, S. K., and Mackay, E. V.:

Lymphocyte response to plant mitogens. *Gynecol. Oncol.* **8**:198–203, 1979.

24. Dixon, P. D. and Dixon, K.: Immunological responses in pregnancy. *Br. Med. J.* **4**:361–363, 1972.
25. Duncan, M. E., Pearson, J. M., Ridley, D. S., Melsom, R., and Bjune, G.: Pregnancy and leprosy: The consequences of alterations of cell-mediated and humoral immunity during pregnancy and lactation. *Int. J. Lepr.* **50**:425–435, 1982.
26. Fabris, N.: Immunological reactivity during pregnancy in the mouse. *Experientia* **29**:610–612, 1973.
27. Fauci, A. S., Masur, H., Gelman, E. P., Markham, P. D., Hahn, B. H., and Lane, H. C.: The acquired immunodeficiency syndrome: An update. *Ann. Int. Med.* **102**:800–813, 1985.
28. Faulk, W. P. and Fox, H.: Disorders of the reproductive system. In: *Immunology in Medicine, A Comprehensive Guide to Clinical Immunology,* 2nd Edition. E. J. Holborow and W. G. Reeves (Eds.). New York, Grune & Stratton, 1983, pp. 348–352.
29. Faulk, W. P. and McIntyre, J. A.: Immunological studies of human trophoblast: Markers, subsets and functions. *Immunol. Rev.* **75**:139–175, 1983.
30. Finn, R., St. Hill, C. A., Davis, J. C., Hipkin, L. J., and Harvey, M.: Feto-maternal bidirectional mixed lymphocyte reaction and survival of fetal allograft. *Lancet* **2**:1200–1202, 1977.
31. Fujisaki, S., Mori, N., Sasaki, T., and Maeyama, M.: Cell-mediated immunity in human pregnancy: Changes in lymphocyte reactivity during pregnancy and postpartum. *Microbiol. Immunol.* **23**:899–908, 1979.
32. Fabris, N., Piantanelli, L., and Muzzioli, M.: Differential effect of pregnancy or gestagens on humoral and cell-mediated immunity. *Clin. Exp. Immunol.* **28**:306–314, 1977.
33. Fuchs, T., Hammarstrom, L., Smith, C. I. E., and Brundin, J.: *In vitro* induction of murine suppressor T cells by human chorionic gonadotrophin. *Acta Obstet. Gynecol. Scand.* **59**:355–359, 1980.
34. Gatti, R. A., Svedmyr, E. A. J., Leibold, W., and Wigzell, H.: Characterizing of a serum inhibitor of MLG reactions. III. Specificity: HLA-related antibodies. *Cell. Immunol.* **15**:432–451, 1975.
35. Gehrz, R. D.: Immunology and the host response to viral infection. *Clin. Obstet. Gynecol.* **25**:545–554, 1982.
36. Genetet, N., Genetet, B., Amice, V., and Fauchet, R.: Allogeneic responses in vitro induced by fetomaternal alloimmunization. *Am. J. Reprod. Immunol.* **2**:90–96, 1982.
37. Gill, T. J., III and Repetti, C. F.: Immunologic and genetic factors influencing reproduction. *Am. J. Pathol.* **95**:465–570, 1979.
38. Gill, T. J., III, Repetti, C. F., Metlav, L. A., Rabin, B. S., Taylor, F. H., Thompson, D. S., and Cortese, A. L.:. Transplacental immunization of the human fetus to tetanus by immunization of the mother. *J. Clin. Invest.* **72**:987–996, 1983.
39. Gleicher, N., Deppe, G., and Cohen, C. J.: Common aspects of immunologic tolerance in pregnancy and malignancy. *Obstet. Gynecol.* **54**:335–342, 1979.
40. Grogan, T. M., Broughton, D. D., and Doyle, W. F.: Graft-versus-host reaction (GVHR). A case report suggesting GVHR occurred as a result of maternofetal cell transfer. *Arch. Pathol.* **99**:330–334, 1975.
41. Hanaoka, J. and Takeuchi, S.: Individual specificity of blocking antibodies in molar and normal term placenta-bound IgG. *Am. J. Reprod. Immunol.* **3**:119–123, 1983.
42. Hersey, P., Morgan, G., Stone, D. E., McCarthy, W. H., and Milton, G. W.: Previous pregnancy as a protective factor against death from melanoma. *Lancet* **1**:451–452, 1977.
43. Herva, E. and Tiilikainen, A.: Mixed lymphocyte culture reactions at delivery and in the puerperium: Effects of parity, HLA antigens and maternal serum. *Acta Pathol. Microbiol. Scand.* **35**:333–344, 1977.
44. Horne, C. H. W. and Nisbet, A. D.: Pregnancy proteins, a review. *Invest. Cell. Pathol.* **2**:217–231, 1979.
45. Janerich, D. R.: The influence of pregnancy on breast cancer risk: Is it endocrinological or immunological? *Med. Hypotheses* **6**:1149–1155, 1980.
46. Johnsen, S. A. Olofsson, A., Green, K., and Olding, L. B.: Strong suppression by mononuclear leukocytes from cord blood of human newborns on maternal leukocytes associated with differences in sensitivity to prostaglandin E2. *Am. J. Reprod. Immunol.* **4**:45–49, 1983.
47. Kalland, T.: Alterations of antibody response in female mice after neonatal exposure to diethylstilbestrol. *J. Immunol.* **124**:194–198, 1980.
48. Kasakura, S.: Is cortisol responsible for inhibition of MLC reactions by pregnancy plasma? *Nature* **246**:496–497, 1973.
49. Kirtland, H. H., Mohler, D. N., and Horowitz, D.: A methyl dopa inhibition of suppressor-lymphocyte function: A proposed cause of hemolytic anemia. *N. Engl. J. Med.* **302**:825–832, 1980.
50. Kissmeyer-Nielsen, F. and Thorsby, E.: Human transplantation antigens. *Transplant Rev.* **4**:1–176, 1970.
51. Kosower, N. S. and Shomrat, R.: Diminished capping of lymphocytes from pregnant women. *Am. J. Reprod. Immunol.* **4**:91–94, 1983.
52. Lala, P. K., Chatterjec-Hasrouni, S., Kearns, M., Montgomery, B., and Colavincenzo, V.: Immunobiology of the feto-maternal interface. *Immunol. Rev.* **75**:87–116, 1983.
53. Lu, C. K., Changelian, P. S., and Unanue, E. R.: Alpha-fetoprotein inhibits macrophage expression of Ia antigens. *J. Immunol.* **132**:1722–1727, 1984.

54. Moller, G. (Ed.): Role of macrophages in the immune response. *Immunol. Rev.* **40**:3–255, 1978.
55. Moore, M. P., Sargent, I. L., Ting, A., and Redman, C. W.: Maternal cell-mediated immunity in pregnancy—lymphocyte responses of mothers and their non-pregnant HLA identical sisters to paternal HLA. *Clin. Exp. Immunol.* **54**:91–94, 1983.
56. Morito, T., Nakamura, T., Nakai, H., Tanimoto, K., Horiuchi, Y., and Juji, R.: Close association of human mixed lymphocyte culture antigen, Ia-like antigen and Fc receptor. *Int. Arch. Allergy Appl. Immunol.* **57**:521–528, 1978.
57. Morse, J. H.: The effect of human chorionic gonadotrophin and placental lactogen on lymphocyte transformation *in vitro. Scand. J. Immunol.* **5**:779–787, 1976.
58. Morton, H., Rolfe, B., Clunie, G. J. A., Anderson, M. J., and Morrison, J.: An early pregnancy factor detected in human serum by the rosette inhibition test. *Lancet* **1**:394–397, 1977.
59. Muchmore, A. V. and Blasese, R. M.: Immunoregulatory properties of fractions from human pregnancy urine: Evidence that human chorionic gonadotrophin is not responsible. *J. Immunol.* **118**:881–886, 1977.
60. Murgita, R. A.: The immunosuppressive role of alpha-fetoprotein during pregnancy. *Scand. J. Immunol.* **5**:1003–1014, 1976.
61. Murgita, R. A., Andersson, L. C., Sherman, M. S., Bennich, H., and Wigzell, H.: Effects of human alpha-fetoprotein on human B and T lymphocyte proliferation *in vitro. Clin. Exp. Immunol.* **33**:347–356, 1978.
62. Nakamura, T., Persellin, R. H. and Russell, I. J.: Induction of suppressor cell activity by human pregnancy serum. *Am. J. Reprod. Immunol.* **4**:133–138, 1983.
63. Noonan, F. P., Halliday, W. J., Morton, H., and Clunie, G. J.: Early pregnancy factor is immunosuppressive. *Nature* **278**:649–651, 1979.
64. Olding, L. B., Mursita, R. A., and Wigzell, H.: Mitogen-stimulated lymphoid cells from human newborns suppress the proliferation of maternal lymphocytes across a cell-impermeable membrane. *J. Immunol.* **229**:1109–1114, 1977.
65. Onander, A. M. and Olding, L. B.: Easily suppressed lymphocytes and absence of cytotoxic antibody. *Am. J. Reprod. Immunol.* **2**:254–259, 1982.
66. Ostensen, M., Lundsren, R., Husby, G., and Rekvis, O. P.: Studies on humoral immunity in pregnancy: Immunoglobulins, alloantibodies and autoantibodies in healthy pregnant women and in pregnant women with rheumatoid disease. *J. Clin. Lab. Immunol.* **11**:143–147, 1983.
67. Papiha, S. S., Wajner, M., and Wasstaff, T. I.: Inhibition of lymphocyte transformation by serum from pregnant women: Lack of correlation with levels of alpha-fetoprotein. *Biol. Neonat.* **43**:109–117, 1983.
68. Peck, A. B., Murgita, R. A., and Wigzell, H.: Cellular and genetic restrictions in the immunoregulatory activity of alpha-fetoprotein. III. Role of the MLC-stimulating cell population in alpha-fetoprotein-induced suppression of T cell-mediated cytotoxicity. *J. Immunol.* **128**:1134–1140, 1982.
69. Persellin, R. H. and Rhodes, J.: Inhibition of human monocyte Fc receptor and HLA-DR antigen expression by pregnancy alpha-2 glycoprotein. *Clin. Exp. Immunol.* **46**:350–354, 1981.
70. Pittard, W. B., III, Miller, K., and Sorensen, R. U.: Normal lymphocyte responses to mitogens in term and premature neonates following normal and abnormal intrauterine growth. *Clin. Immunol. Immunopathol.* **30**:178–187, 1984.
71. Plum, J., Thiery, M., and Sabbe, L.: Distribution of mononuclear cells during pregnancy. *Clin. Exp. Immunol.* **31**:45–49, 1978.
72. Pope, R. M., Yoshinoya, S., Rutstein, J., and Persellin, R.H.: Effects of pregnancy on immune complexes and rheumatoid factors in patients with RA, rheumatoid arthritis. *Am. J. Med.* **74**:973–979, 1983.
73. Rocklin, R. E., Kitzmiller, J. L., Carpenter, C. B., Garvoy, M. R., and David, J. R.: Maternal–fetal relation: Absence of an immunologic blocking factor from the serum of women with chronic abortions. *N. Engl. J. Med.* **295**:1209–1213, 1976.
74. Rocklin, R. E., Kitzmiller, J. L., and Garvoy, M. R.: Maternal–fetal relation. II. Further characterization of an immunologic blocking factor that develops during pregnancy. *Clin. Immunol. Immunopathol.* **22**:305–315, 1982.
75. Rocklin, H. E., Kitzmiller, J. L., and Kaye, M. D.: Immunobiology of the maternal-fetal relationship. *Ann. Rev. Med.* **30**:375–404, 1979.
76. Rosenthal, M.: Enhanced phagocytosis of immune complexes in pregnancy. *Clin. Exp. Immunol.* **28**:189–191, 1977.
77. Sargent, I. L., Redman, W. G., and Stirrat, G. M.: Maternal cell-mediated immunity in normal and pre-eclamptic pregnancy. *Clin. Exp. Immunol.* **50**:601–609, 1982.
78. Sasaki, K. and Ishida, N.: Diminished immune response in pregnant mice. *J. Exp. Med.* **116**:391–392, 1975.
79. Schena, F. P., Manno, C., Selvassi, L., Loverro, G., Bettocchi, S., and Bonomo, L.: Behaviour of immune complexes and the complement system in normal pregnancy and pre-eclampsia. *J. Clin. Lab. Immunol.* **7**:21–26, 1982.
80. Schiff, R. I., Mercier, D., and Buckley, R. H.: Inability of gestational hormones to account for the inhibitory effects of pregnancy plasmas on lymphocyte responses in vitro. *Cell. Immunol.* **20**:69–80, 1975.
81. Schindler, A. M. and Martin-du-Pan, R.: Prenatal diagnosis of fetal lymphocytes in the maternal blood. *Obstet. Gynecol.* **40**:340–346, 1972.
82. Schreiber, A. D.: Clinical immunology of the corticosteroids. *Prog. Clin. Immunol.* **3**:103–114, 1977.

83. Siesal, F. P.: Functional ontogeny of human lymphoid cells as a factor in maternal-fetal tolerance. *Am. J. Reprod. Immunol.* 1:65–68, 1981.

84. Skinnider, L. F. and Laxdal, V.: The effect of progesterone, oestrogens and hydrocortisone on the mitogenic response of lymphocytes to phytohaemagglutinin in pregnant and non-pregnant women. *Br. J. Obstet. Gynaecol.* **88**:1110–1114, 1981.

85. Soubiran, P., Mucchielli, A., Kerckaert, J. P., Bayard, B., and Masseyeff, R.: Stimulatory effect of human alpha-fetoprotein and its molecular variants on in vitro-induced lymphocyte blastogenesis. *Scand. J. Immunol.* **10**:179–186, 1979.

86. Sridama, V., Pacini, F., Yang, S-L., Moawad, A., Reilly, M., and DeGroot, L.J.: Decreased levels of helper T cells: A possible cause of immunodeficiency in pregnancy. *N. Engl. J. Med.* **307**:352–356, 1982.

87. Stahn, R., Fabricius, H., and Hartleitner, W.: Suppression of human T-cell colony formation during pregnancy. *Nature* **276**:831–832, 1978.

88. Stites, D. P. and Siiteri, P. K.: Steroids as immunosuppressants in pregnancy. *Immunol. Rev.* **75**:117–138, 1983.

89. Strelkauskas, A. J., Davies, I. J., and Dray, S.: Longitudinal studies showing alterations in the levels and functional response of T and B lymphocytes in human pregnancy. *Clin. Exp. Immunol.* **32**:531–539, 1978.

90. Sumiyoshi, Y., Gorai, I., Hirahara, F., Tanaka, K., and Minasuchi, H.: Cellular immunity in normal pregnancy and abortion: Subpopulations of T lymphocytes bearing Fc receptors for IgG and IgM. *Am. J. Reprod. Immunol.* **1**:145–149, 1981.

91. Sunderland, C. A., Redman, C. W. G., and Stirrat, G. M.: HLA A,B,C antigens are expressed on nonvillous trophoblast of the early human placenta. *J. Immunol.* **127**:2614–2615, 1981.

92. Takeuchi, S.: Immunology of spontaneous abortion and hydatidiform mole. *Am. J. Reprod. Immunol.* **1**:23–28, 1980.

93. Thiry, L., Spreher-Goldberger, S., Bossens, M., and Neuray, F.: Cell-mediated immune response to simian oncornavirus antigens in pregnant women. *J. Natl. Cancer Inst.* **60**:527–532, 1978.

94. Thomson, A. W. and Horne, C. H. W.: Biological and clinical significance of pregnancy-associated alpha-2-glycoprotein (alpha-1-pAG). A review. *Invest. Cell. Pathol.* **3**:295–301, 1980.

95. Thong, Y. H., Steele, W., Vincent, M. M., Hensen, S. A., and Bellanti, J. A.: Impaired in vitro cell-mediated immunity to rubella virus during pregnancy. *N. Engl. J. Med.* **289**:604–606, 1973.

96. Timonen, T. and Saksela, E.: Cell-mediated anti-embryo cytotoxicity in human pregnancy. *Clin. Exp. Immunol.* **23**:462–470, 1976.

97. Tulchinsky, D.: Placental secretion of unconjugated estrone, estradiol and estriol into the maternal and the fetal circulation. *J. Clin. Endocrinol. Metab.* **35**:1079–1087, 1973.

98. Unanue, E. R.: Antigen-presenting function of the macrophage. *Ann. Rev. Immunol.* **2**:395–428, 1984.

99. Valdimarsson, H., Mulholland, C., Fridriksdottir, V., and Coleman, D. V.: A longitudinal study of leukocyte blood counts and lymphocyte responses in pregnancy: A marked early increase of monocyte–lymphocyte ratio. *Clin. Exp. Immunol.* **53**:437–443, 1983.

100. Van der Werf, A. J.: Are lymphocytoxic iso-antibodies induced by the early human trophoblast? *Lancet* **1**:595, 1971.

101. Wajner, M., Papiha, S. S., and Wasstaff, T. I.: Response of human peripheral blood lymphocytes in the presence of cord sera: Relationship of lymphocyte transformation with number of pregnancies and levels of alpha-fetoprotein. *Clin. Exp. Immunol.* **52**:381–386, 1983.

102. Winzler, R.: Glycoproteins in disease. In: *Glycoproteins of Blood Cells and Plasma*, 1st Edition. G. A. Jamieson and T. J. Greenwalt (Eds.). Philadelphia, J. B. Lippincott, 1971, pp. 204–214.

103. Yachrin, S., Shani, K., and Lester, E. P.: Further studies on the mechanism of suppression of human lymphocyte transformation by human alpha-fetoprotein. *J. Allergy Clin. Immunol.* **65**:127–135, 1980.

104. Yamoto, T., Hirata, H., Tanisuchi, H., Kawai, Y., Uematsu, A., and Sugiyama, Y.: Lymphocyte transformation during pregnancy; an analysis using whole-blood culture. *Obstet. Gynecol.* **55**:215–219, 1980.

105. Yu, V. Y., Waller, C. A., Maclennan, I. C., and Baum, J. D.: Lymphocyte reactivity in pregnant women and newborn infants. *Br. Med. J.* **75**:428–432, 1975.

5

DIAGNOSIS OF PREGNANCY

The diagnosis of pregnancy is usually suspected because of the patient's symptoms. The suspicion may be reinforced or weakened by the physical findings. In many instances, especially very early in pregnancy, the diagnosis is then confirmed or excluded by using ancillary methods.

We shall first consider the clinical diagnosis of pregnancy and then the ancillary methods of diagnosis. The discussions of the clinical findings will reproduce the original descriptions of the classic physical signs of pregnancy. These descriptions demonstrate, first, that some phenomena are immutable, and second, that our forebears were very astute observers and were able to clearly describe their observations.

CLINICAL DIAGNOSIS OF PREGNANCY

Symptoms in the First Trimester

When the patient presents soon after her first missed period, the history and physical examination are useful in suggesting that she is pregnant but cannot establish that she is indeed pregnant. All the signs and symptoms of pregnancy that can be elicited during the first trimester (and some that are noted during the last two trimesters) are suggestive rather than diagnostic of the presence of pregnancy. The symptoms and signs commonly noted in early pregnancy are the following:

Amenorrhea. Amenorrhea is very suggestive of pregnancy in women who are sexually active, not using contraception, and whose menstrual pattern has previously been regular. However, many causes of amenorrhea are unrelated to pregnancy, so that the diagnosis of pregnancy cannot be established because of this symptom alone. The presence of other common symptoms of pregnancy, none in themselves diagnostic, tends to strengthen the supposition of pregnancy.

About 5% of multiparas and a much smaller percent of primigravidas note a single episode of bleeding that appears to be a menstrual period, after conception has occurred. Conversely, most women who complain of some painless vaginal bleeding in early pregnancy carry their pregnancies to term.

Nausea and Vomiting (Hyperemesis Gravidarum). These symptoms occur in the first trimester but do not usually appear until the end of the first month after the missed period. Nausea and vomiting generally last for 6–8 weeks. About half of pregnant women probably experience some degree of nausea and vomiting, but definitive data are not available. Nausea and vomiting of pregnancy usually occur early in the day and improve as the day goes on, but this pattern is not invariable. Nausea and vomiting may be due to many causes other than pregnancy, so that the presence of these symptoms is suggestive rather than diagnostic.

If the nausea and vomiting become severe enough to cause weight loss and dehydration, the symptom complex then becomes a pathologic entity, designated hyperemesis gravidarum.

The cause of nausea and vomiting of pregnancy is unknown. A psychosomatic component is suspected. In addition, because hyperemesis is frequently associated with trophoblastic tumors and multiple pregnancy, a hormonal component has been suspected. Those endocrine functions measured, which include anterior pituitary and adrenal cortical function and measurements of hCG, estrogen, and progesterone, are within normal limits; however, an element of hyperthyroidism may be present[4] (see also Chapter 36).

Fatigue and/or Lassitude. These symptoms, in some form, occur in many pregnant women. The lack of specificity weakens their diagnostic import.

Breast Symptoms. Many pregnant women become aware of tingling of their nipples and engorgement of their breasts which is painful in varying degree as one of the earliest symptoms of pregnancy. These symptoms usually disappear by the end of the third month. Breast symptoms may be due to other causes, such as hormonal changes and psychic influences.

Urinary Symptoms. Frequency and nocturia begin early in the first trimester, before the uterus has enlarged significantly and, therefore, are probably due to hormonal effects on the bladder. Frequency generally disappears or is markedly ameliorated by the end of the first trimester.

Constipation. Many pregnant women complain of constipation starting early in pregnancy and persisting to term. This symptom is nonspecific and can be elicited from many women who are not pregnant.

Signs in the First Trimester

Breast Changes. During the first two months of pregnancy the breasts become fuller and enlarged. This is due to vascular engorgement. Nipple and areolar changes may also be noted. Pigmentation of these structures may become more obvious and intra-areolar papillae may become more prominent (Fig. 5-1). The characteristic "puffy turgescence" of the nipples and areolae and hypertrophy of the intra-areolar sebaceous glands (tubercles of Montgomery) are readily recognized by the end of the second month, whereas the deepened pigmentation generally occurs later.[17] Montgomery's description emphasized the areolar structures, as the following excerpts demonstrate:[17]

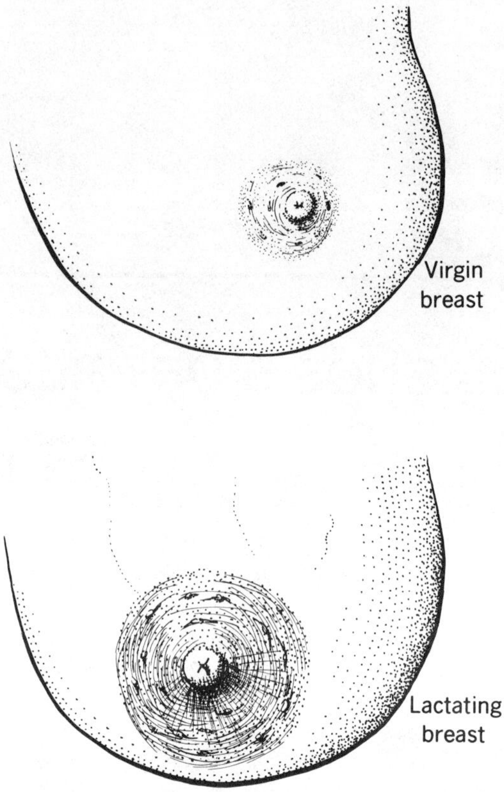

Figure 5-1. Changes in the areola and nipple, accompanied by hypertrophy of the intra-areolar sebaceous glands (tubercles of Montgomery).

> These changes do not take place immediately after conception, but occur in different persons after uncertain intervals: we must therefore consider, in the first place, the period of pregnancy at which we may expect to gain any useful information from the condition of the areola. I cannot say positively what may be the earliest period at which this change can be observed, but I have recognised it fully at the end of the second month, at which time the alteration in colour is by no means the most observable, but the puffy turgescence (though as yet slight) not alone of the nipple but of the whole of the surrounding disk, and the development of the little glandular follicles are the objects to which we should principally direct our attention, the

colour at this period being in general little more than a deeper shade of rose or flesh colour slightly tinged occasionally with a yellowish or light brownish hue.

In the centre of the coloured circle the nipple is observed partaking of the altered colour of the part and appearing turgid and prominent, while the surface of the areola, especially that part of it which lies more immediately around the base of the nipple, is studded over and rendered unequal by the prominence of the glandular follicles, which, varying in number from twelve to twenty, project from the sixteenth to the eighth of an inch. . . .

These follicles or tubercles of the areola, although by many considered merely as sebaceous glands, have really a much more important character, and more intimate connexion with the peculiar structure and function of the breasts, and hence might naturally be expected to display an active sympathy in any condition of the system which called into action the peculiar function of these organs, which is the secretion of milk for the support of the new being, for which purpose certain previous changes in the glands and ducts are necessary. Now it appears that these areolar tubercles are intimately connected with the lactiferous tubes, some of which can be traced into them and opening on their summit, so that in pregnant women a sero-lactescent fluid may be often distinctly perceived issuing from them, and in nurses they have been observed to pour forth drops of perfect milk.

It appears that . . . each of these follicles is, in common with the nipple and surrounding areola, furnished with very small sebaceous glands which lie around its base, the ducts of which, from one to four in number, are found opening on the surface of the tubercle.

Uterine Changes. One of the earliest changes detectable in the pregnant uterus is a soft localized enlargement of the fundus over the implantation site. Implantation is usually eccentric. The implantation site is generally located high on the posterior or anterior wall, near to one or the other sidewalls of the uterus. Occasionally, implantation is more centrally spaced. If implantation is eccentric, the soft prominence is near the cornua on the side of the implantation, so that the uterus is asymmetrically enlarged. These facts, which have been amply demonstrated by modern ultrasonography, again confirm the clinical astuteness of our predecessors. Witness the following descriptions. First, by Piskacek[18] (Fig. 5-2), who wrote:

Through my studies I could determine the following: One can in the beginning of pregnancy, often already in the fifth week after the beginning of the last period, sometimes earlier, make the observation that the uterus has become asymmetric. This asymmetry consists of the fact that one side-half appears larger to the bimanual feeling fingers than the corresponding other half. The enlargement of the one side can exceed the other by a great deal. If one looks closer at the larger half it becomes clear, that in most cases the cornua is also enlarged. One can determine a rounding on this point of the uterus. I will call it projection which spreads out upwards and to the side and besides either to a larger degree forward or backwards or to a lesser degree towards the front and backwards.

If one tests the level difference between the projected and not projected cornual region then one can determine, that the upper border of the projected part depending on the pregnancy length stands considerably higher than the part of the fundus uteri, which belongs to the unprojected cornua.

At the same time with the projection one can in most cases feel a furrow which towards the middle and upwards borders the projection. One can trace the furrow as a shallow, in many cases, as a deep furrow . . . .

One feels the furrow on the fundus on the border between the projected cornua and the not projected part of the other side . . . the furrow which is located on the front or backward wall of the uterus is always a continuation of the one located in the fundus if such is present . . . .

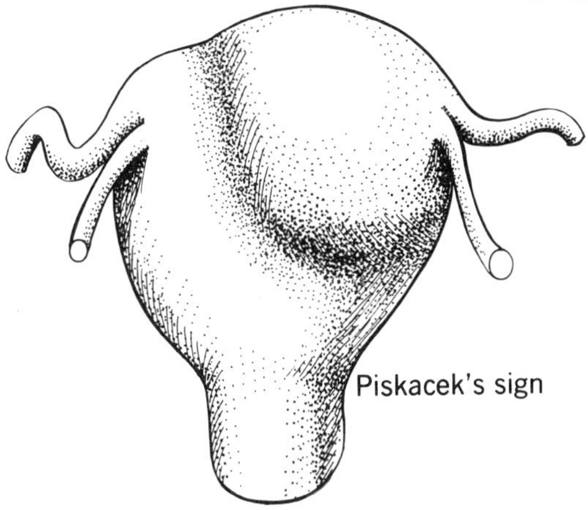

Figure 5-2. Piskacek's sign consists of asymmetric enlargement of the pregnant uterus, due to enlargement of the cornual region over the implantation site.

A slightly different description of the changes in uterine contour (Fig. 5-3) was provided by von Braun,[23] who wrote:

The most important symptom of early detection of pregnancy is the change in consistency of the uterus which is emphasized by many authors, and according to the author's experiences, especially the unusual shape of the uterus which will be seen with careful examination.

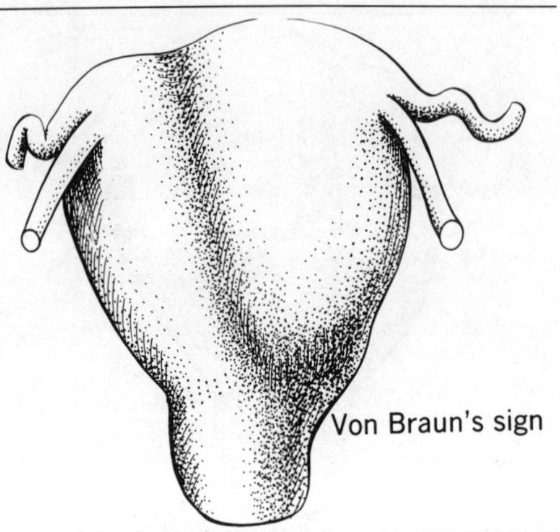

Figure 5-3. Von Braun's sign is slightly different from Piskacek's sign. Von Braun emphasized a clear longitudinal groove, dividing the corpus uteri into two parts of different size and consistency.

The special shape of the uterus is that it seems to be thicker on one side than on the other, at the end of the first and the beginning of the second month. One side sometimes is twice as thick as the other one. If one can call the two unlike parts horns, which does not correspond to the original meaning of this word, we find that the thicker horn shows a different consistency. It appears to be softer while the other one is almost like a normal uterus. The softer area of the uterus extends to the other half across the midline of the uterus. On the border of both dissimilar horns, the difference in consistency can be felt particularly at the front, as a clear longitudinal sulcus, which is pushed to one side so that it divides the corpus uteri into two parts of different size. At the same time the fundus seems to be irregular, slightly pulled in to form a saddle shape, in this way the saddle lies against the thinner horn.

Von Braun's sign can be detected at about 5 weeks. Later in pregnancy uterine symmetry is restored. The corpus becomes more spherical and softens. Uterine enlargement is obvious to the experienced examiner by 8–10 weeks.

In addition to the changes in the corpus, the lower uterine segment and the cervix also change during the first trimester. The earliest change in the lower segment consists of a circumscribed softening in the midline, just below the corporocervical junction (Ladin's sign) (Fig. 5-4). Ladin's description of the finding[13] follows:

This sign consists of a circular elastic area situated in the median line of the anterior surface of the body of the uterus, just above the junction of body and cervix, that is to say, at the isthmus of the uterus; this area varies in size according to the duration of pregnancy, and offers to the palpating finger the distinct sensation of fluctuation. It can frequently be made out as early as the fifth week, when the area is the size of a fingertip; but it can always be felt in the sixth week, when it is somewhat larger. As pregnancy advances, this area increases in size in a crescentic manner, and extends upward toward the fundus until the third month of pregnancy, when nearly the entire anterior body of the uterus presents a fluctuating, cystic feel to the examining finger.

The change in the consistency is observed in the anterior wall when the pregnant uterus is in the normal position or slightly retroverted; in extremely retroverted or retroflexed uteri the elastic area is found in the posterior wall, but the sign is usually felt a week or so later than in uteri in the normal position.

The sign is obtained by bimanual palpation, which is a requisite in eliciting it; while the uterus is fixed by counter-pressure with the external hand, the anterior wall of the uterus, from the tip of the cervix to the fundus, is palpated with the internal finger or fingers, and if early pregnancy exists, the elastic, fluctuating area will be felt in the spot indicated above.

Ladin's sign is detectable at about the sixth week but is not invariably present and can be missed even when present. Slightly later in pregnancy, one can detect a more generalized softening of the lower uterine segment (Fig. 5-5). This sign was first described by Reinl in 1884[19] as follows:

Last winter, in Professor Hegar's gynecology clinic, I had the opportunity of acquainting myself with a new and excellent sign of the early months of pregnancy.

This consists in the demonstration of an unusual softness, flexibility, and thinning of the lower uterine segment, that is, of the part directly above the insertion of the uterosacral ligaments.

This finding is not only demonstrable when the rest of the uterus feels firm, as is often the case, but also very definitely when it is soft and elastic.

Also, in the latter case it is always possible to compress the lower uterine segment, to actually thin it out with the finger, and so to differentiate it from the upper part of the uterus, while it still clearly differs in consistency from the cervix below. The pliability and laxness of these parts can be so extensive that one may be in doubt as to whether any connection exists between the cervix and the larger abdominal or pelvic mass.

We know of no condition which can produce findings similar to pregnancy; solid tumors certainly do not, and hemato- and hydro-metra present no diagnostic difficulties. Our sign can therefore be used with confidence for the differential diagnosis of pregnancy.

This remarkable development results from the fact that the lower uterine segment becomes the most attenuated and elastic part of the entire uterus during pregnancy; therefore, as one can easily demonstrate,

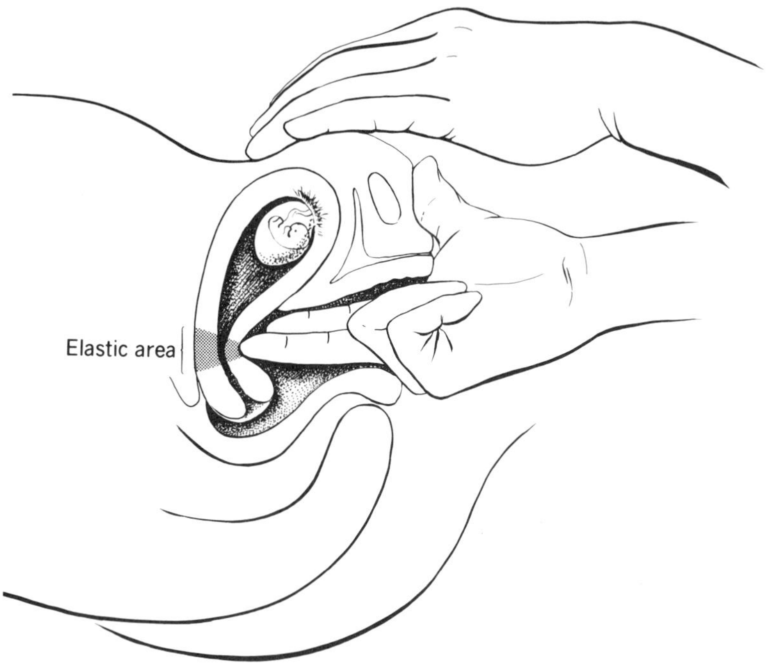

Figure 5-4. Ladin described an elastic area offering decreased resistance to palpation located just above the corporocervical junction.

it is possible, after displacing the uterus upward, to grasp the lower segment between the fingers of the vaginal and abdominal hands, compress it, and completely thin it out.

Absence of this sign does not, however, exclude pregnancy by any means, for one can easily imagine that with chronic infarction of the lower uterine segment pregnancy could occur without this change being demonstrable.

Now known as Hegar's sign, this physical finding has stood the test of time and, in the hands of an experienced examiner, is highly indicative of pregnancy because few other conditions can cause it to appear.

The prominent changes in the cervix are alterations of consistency and color. From about the fourth week, a progressive softening which changes the consistency of the cervix from one that approximates that of the tip of the nose to one reminiscent of the consistency of the lip is noted. The cyanosis begins at about the fourth week and deepens as pregnancy progresses.

Vaginal Changes. The most prominent early change noted in the vagina and at the introitus is cyanosis. Although others noted and described this sign before Chadwick, his report popularized the finding, which is now designated as Chadwick's sign.[6] The following excerpts from Chadwick's article convey the essence of his findings:

> The color begins as a pale violet in the early months, becomes more bluish as pregnancy advances, until it often assumes finally a dusky, almost black, tint; this last is familiar to every obstetrician. It is not due to pigmentation, but to an hypertrophy of the venous plexuses in the mucous membrane of the vagina (or a dilatation of the minute veins), induced by the afflux of blood to the uterus under the stimulus of pregnancy. The predominance of the veins in this location could alone account for the bluish color; moreover, when, toward the end of pregnancy, the color is most intense, varicose veins are plainly visible in the labia and in the legs.
>
> Almost all speak of the violet color as seen on the collum uteri, on the whole extent of the vagina, and consequently requiring the use of a speculum; now, while I do not claim that the change is not perceptible throughout the whole extent of the vagina and collum uteri, I do maintain that it is equally manifest at the introitus vaginae when the labia are simply separated by the fingers. After satisfying myself on this point by numerous investigations with the speculum, I was consequently able to dispense with that instrument, and thus render the sign more generally and easily applicable.

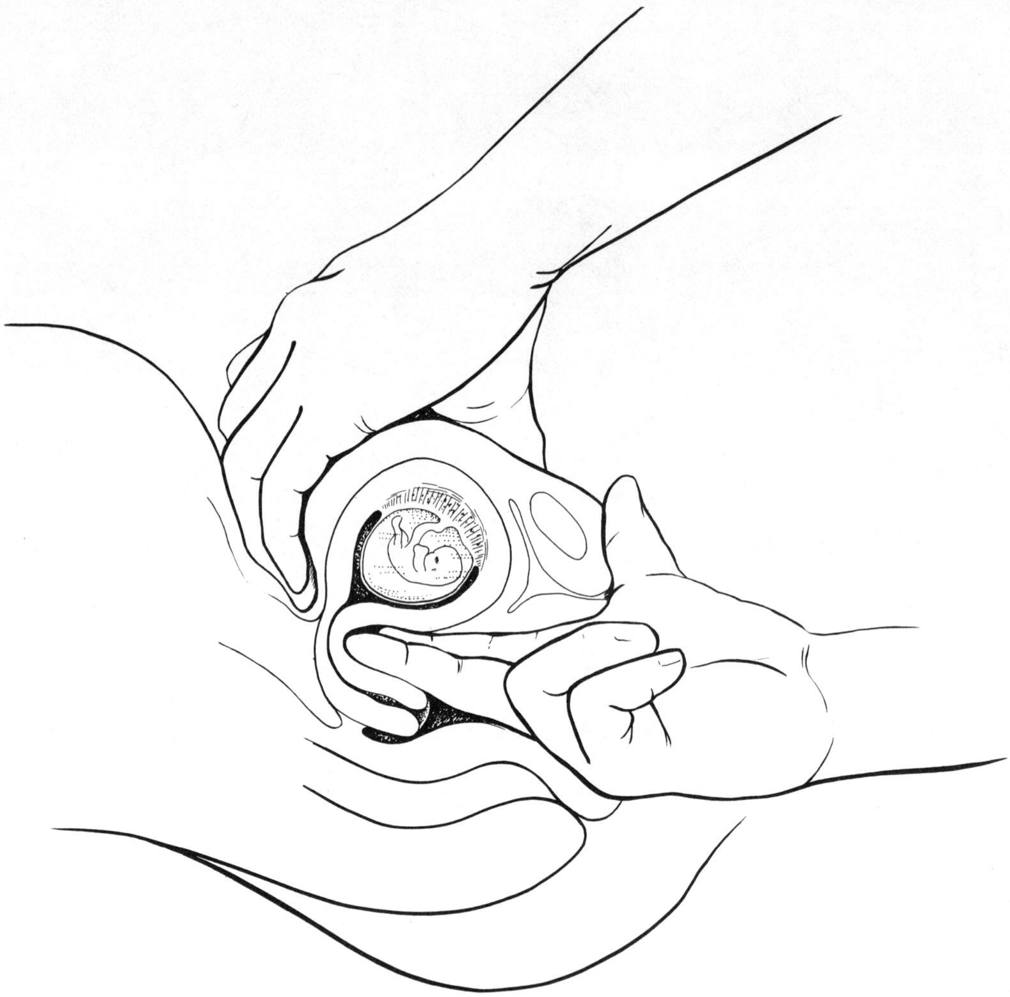

Figure 5-5. Hegar's sign, described by Reinl, occurs later in pregnancy than does Ladin's sign and consists of a generalized softening of the lower uterine segment.

Symptoms in the Last Two Trimesters

The most significant new symptom that occurs in the latter two-thirds of pregnancy is quickening. This perception of fetal movements is usually noted during the 17th week after the last menstrual period. The popular idea that multiparas generally appreciate quickening somewhat earlier, due to their previous experience of the sensation of fetal movement, or due to earlier contact of the uterus with the abdominal wall in multiparas, has recently been challenged by a study that demonstrated no significant difference in the time at which quickening was perceived in multiparas or primigravidas.[11] Although the perception of quickening is only suggestive of pregnancy, palpation of fetal movements by the examiner is diagnostic (see below).

Dermatologic Changes. Cutaneous manifestations are also prominent in later pregnancy (see Chapters 3 and 28). The pigmentation of the linea alba which often begins late in the first trimester intensifies, especially in patients with dark complexions. Chloasma gravidarum, which begins about the 16th week, is noted by 50%–70% of pregnant women, especially in brown-eyed brunettes. Striae gravidarum, seen on the abdomen, breasts, and thighs, appear in about 90% of pregnant women during the second trimester. In some patients, vascular telangiectases develop. These vascular "spiders" are caused by the high estrogen levels of pregnancy.

Backache. As discussed in Chapter 3, many pregnant women complain of backache, due primarily to the increased lordosis of pregnancy.

Signs in the Last Two Trimesters

Enlargement of the Abdomen. After the 16th week of pregnancy, abdominal enlargement becomes apparent in many pregnant women, as the uterus rises out of the pelvis and into the abdomen. Abdominal enlargement is generally more pronounced in multiparas than in primigravidas. The difference is due to diastasis recti and less muscle tone in the multiparous women. Enlargement of the abdomen, even when progressive, is not proof positive of pregnancy, because other intra-abdominal masses can cause abdominal enlargement, as can pseudocyesis.

Progressive uterine enlargement, especially when accompanied by progressive changes in uterine shape from asymmetrical to globular to elongation is highly suggestive, if not truly diagnostic, of pregnancy.

Uterine Contractions. Uterine contractions can be detected as early as the third month of pregnancy but are more frequent, and thus more likely to be appreciated by the examiner, in the last two trimesters. These contractions were described by John Braxton Hicks in 1871.[9] His original description has not been improved upon, as the folowing excerpts demonstrate:

> But after many years' constant observation, I have ascertained it to be a fact that the uterus possesses the power and habit of spontaneously contracting and relaxing from a very early period of pregnancy, as early, indeed, as it is possible to recognize the difference of consistence—that is, from about the third month.
>
> If, then, the uterus be examined without friction or any pressure beyond that necessary for full contact of the hand continuously over a period of from five to twenty minutes, it will be noticed to become firm if relaxed at first, and more or less flaccid if it be firm at first. It is seldom that so long an interval occurs as that of twenty minutes; most frequently it occurs every five or ten minutes, sometimes even twice in five minutes. However, in some cases I have found only one contraction in thirty minutes. The duration of each contraction is generally not long, ordinarily it lasts from two to five minutes. When the uterus is irritable or has been irritated it lasts longer than this; under particular circumstances . . . it may assume an almost continuous action analogous to that which is noticed after long obstructed labour.
>
> In a general way the pregnant woman is not conscious of these contractions of the uterus, but sometimes she will remark that she has a tumour in her lower abdomen, thinking it a constant thing; but another will observe that she has a swelling sometimes, but which vanishes at other times. But occasionally it happens that the uterus is more than usually sensitive, and that the contractions are accompanied by pain; and then on examination it is found that each pain she complains of is co-incident with a contraction.
>
> For the last six years and upwards I have made use of the intermittent action of the uterus as the principal symptom upon which I have depended in the diagnosis of pregnancy. I am not aware that I have been less successful than the others in determining the existence of pregnancy; on the contrary, I have felt myself at an advantage in the possession of an additional sign to make up the deficiency or temporary inapplicability of the others; as, for instance, when external noise prevents the heart sounds from being heard.

Although the detection of these contractions enhances the probability that an intrauterine pregnancy is present, an absolute diagnosis cannot be made on this basis, because the uterus may contract in the absence of pregnancy, for example, due to foreign bodies or myomas.

Ballottement. Ballottement may be performed through either the abdominal wall or the vaginal wall. The sign is elicited by placing two fingers upon the abdomen, or into the anterior vaginal fornix. A sharp push is given against the uterus, after which the fingers remain in their original position. Shortly after the sharp pressure has been applied, a fetal part floats against the examiner's fingers (Fig. 5-6). Ballottement of fetal parts can be detected in the fourth month of pregnancy. This sign is useful, but not infallible, because such things as pedunculated myomas, ovarian tumors, and ascites can mislead the examiner.

Uterine Souffle. The uterine souffle is not diagnostic of pregnancy, because it may be heard in association with any entity that causes an increased supply of blood to the uterus. The souffle is a blowing murmur, which is synchronous with the woman's pulse, and is heard best

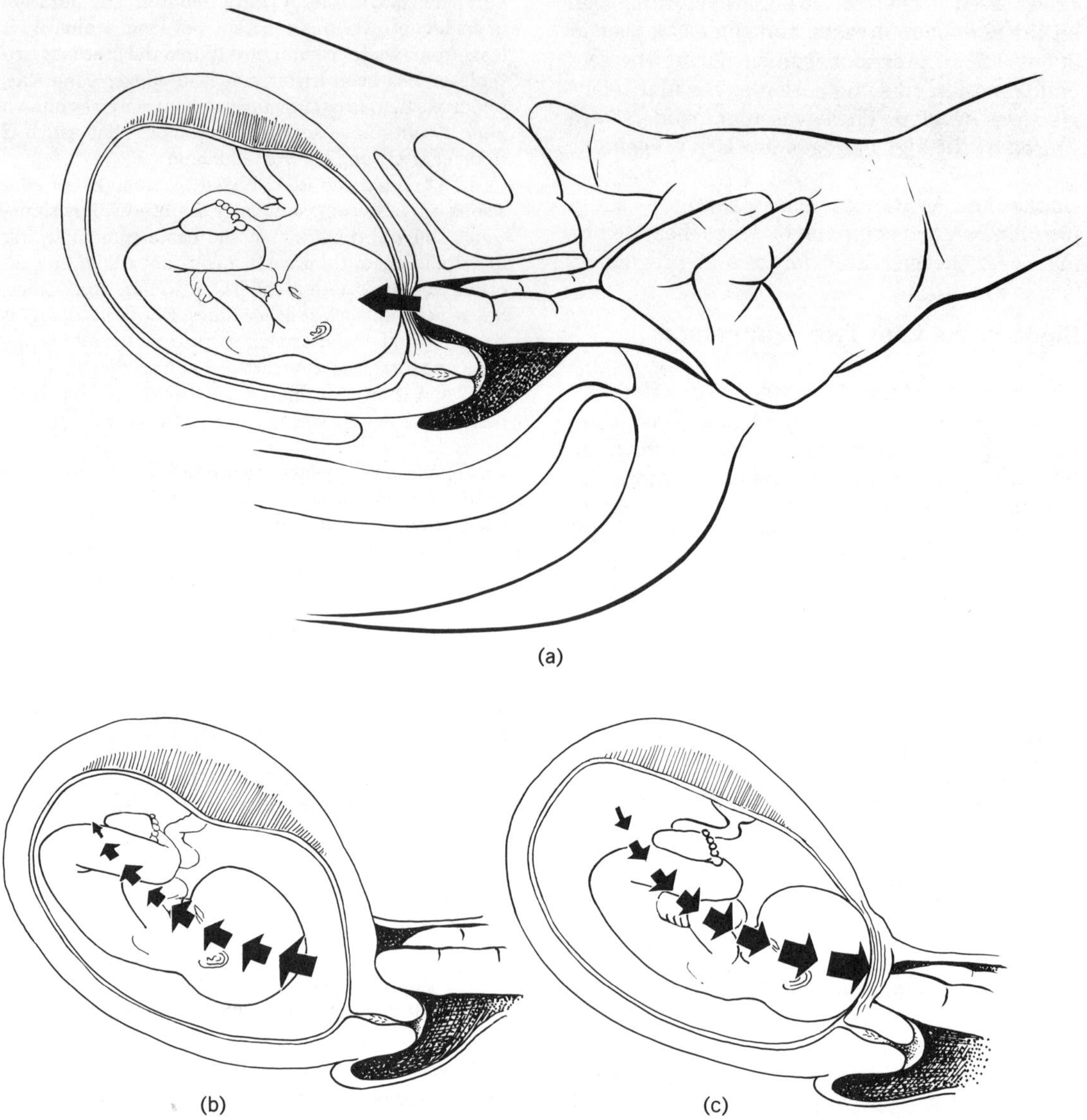

(a)

(b)

(c)

Figure 5-6. Ballottement is elicited by pushing sharply against the uterus. The fingers remain in place. Shortly after the impelling push, the fetal part floats against the examiner's fingers.

just above the symphysis pubis. The souffle is usually detectable after the start of the fifth month of pregnancy and is caused by maternal blood flow through the uterine vessels.

Palpation of Fetal Parts and Fetal Movements. At the end of the fourth month it becomes possible to feel fetal parts through the abdominal wall, especially in slender women. Myomas can mimic fetal parts, so to establish a positive diagnosis of pregnancy, it is necessary to palpate distinct fetal parts, such as the head, the breech or the extremities. If, at the same time, the examiner notes active fetal movements, the diagnosis is clear. Fetal movements become obvious in many women by the sixth month, and in virtually all women by the seventh month.

Hearing the Fetal Heart. The fetal heart rate can be heard, with the aid of a fetoscope, during the 18th–19th weeks of pregnancy.[11] At the 18th week, the fetal heart is best heard just above the pubic symphysis. As pregnancy progresses the location at which the fetal heart is most audible varies with the presentation and position of the fetus. Classic descriptions state that the fetal heart rate is usually 120–140 beats per minute and is a double sound, reminiscent of a ticking watch heard through a pillow. The rate in any individual normal pregnancy may vary from the range of 120–140 beats per minute.

DIFFERENTIAL DIAGNOSIS OF PREGNANCY

The differential diagnosis of presumed pregnancy includes all entities that cause the symptoms and signs detailed above as presumptive evidences of pregnancy.

Differential Diagnosis in the First Trimester

Symptoms. The differential diagnosis of amenorrhea includes all causes of secondary amenorrhea such as hypothalamic amenorrhea, amenorrhea secondary to nutritional disorders, exercise, Asherman's syndrome, or systemic diseases. If a positive β-hCG pregnancy test is obtained, these causes can be eliminated. Hematometra, another cause of amenorrhea, may be associated with an enlarging abdominal tumor. Nausea and vomiting are nonspecific symptoms which can be due to anything from emotional upsets to infections and gastrointestinal disorders. Fatigue is also a nonspecific symptom that can be due to a variety of causes. Pain and tingling in the breasts may be due to several conditions such as fibroadenosis, mastitis, hormonal imbalance, and premenstrual tension syndrome. Frequency of urination may be due to cystitis, cystocele, external pressure on the bladder, or emotional problems. Constipation is also a nonspecific symptom which is not useful in the differential diagnosis of pregnancy.

Signs. Among the first trimester signs of pregnancy are breast, uterine, and vaginal changes. Lactation can be associated with a variety of causes ranging from exogenous medications through pituitary adenomas and to idiopathic galactorrhea. Changes in the size and shape of the uterus can be due to benign uterine tumors such as leiomyomas or adenomyosis and to hematometra or pyometra secondary to cervical stenosis. Leiomyomas are the commonest cause of growth of the nonpregnant uterus. Generally the irregular contours and firm consistency of the myomatous uterus help to distinguish it from the pregnant uterus. Various adnexal masses, particularly when in close proximity or adherent to the uterus, can also give the impression of a pregnant uterus. Changes in the coloration of the vagina and cervix can occur in the late luteal phase, or under the influence of exogenous hormones, or in association with any intra-abdominal condition that interferes with drainage from the pelvic veins.

Differential Diagnosis in the Second Trimester

Symptoms. The major new symptom in the second trimester is quickening. A sensation of quickening may be volunteered by patients with pseudocyesis. Pseudocyesis usually develops in women who have an intense desire for pregnancy. These patients present many of the signs and symptoms of pregnancy, including amenorrhea, nausea and vomiting, urinary frequency, breast pain, and quickening. The false impression of quickening is usually due either to increased peristalsis or to voluntary contracting of the abdominal musculature.

Signs. Signs of pregnancy in the second trimester include enlargement of the abdomen, changes in uterine size and contour, uterine contractions, the placental souffle, ballottement and palpation of fetal parts, and auscultation of the fetal heart.

The appearance of an enlarged abdomen can be due to pseudocyesis, excessive weight gain, various pelvic and abdominal tumors, ascites, ventral hernias, or relaxation of the abdominal wall. Palpation of uterine contractions is extremely useful in differential diagnosis because no other entity gives the same sensation as does a clearly palpable contraction. Ballottement of fetal parts and palpation of fetal parts can be deceptive, since other conditions, such as a freely mobile ovarian or other adnexal mass, or a pedunculated myoma, may give the impression of being ballotteable. Irregularity of a myomatous uterus could give the examiner the illusion of palpating fetal small parts. However, if both these observations can be made at the same time, the diagnosis of pregnancy is strengthened. The placental souffle can be due to any entity that increases blood flow to the uterus. However, detection of the fetal heartbeat, at a rate distinctly different from the maternal heart rate, is a positive sign of pregnancy.

DETERMINATION OF PARITY

Under some circumstances, the obstetrician may find it necessary to determine whether the pregnant patient is in her first pregnancy or has had previous advanced pregnancies and/or deliveries.

A group of physical findings suggest that the patient has had a previous pregnancy: The breasts in multiparous women are more pendulous than they are in primigravidas and the nipples may be more prominent. In brunettes, pigmentation of the nipple and areola may persist from a previous pregnancy. The abdominal wall is more relaxed in a multipara. The skin of the abdomen may be loose and pendulous. In addition to the pink striae gravidarum which are associated with the present pregnancy, old striae gravidarum which are silvery white in appearance are usually present.

The cervix of a primigravida may be softened, but generally remains closed until the last few weeks of pregnancy. The external cervical os in a primigravida is circular or slightly oval. In multiparas, it is generally a transverse slit. In our experience, this has been the most reliable sign of a previous delivery. The vagina of the primigravida is narrower and the rugae are well developed. In a multipara, the vagina is roomier and the rugae, especially on the posterior wall, are less prominent. The labial opening of primigravidas is generally narrow, with the labia opposed to each other. The hymenal ring is usually present in primigravidas. In multiparas, the vulvar opening is larger, the frenulum is absent, and the hymenal remnants are replaced by the carunculae myrtiformes.

ANCILLARY AIDS TO DIAGNOSIS OF PREGNANCY

Doppler Effect Instrumentation

One of the most widespread applications of ultrasonics in pregnancy diagnosis is the utilization of instruments which are based upon the Doppler phenomenon. When an ultrasonic wave is reflected from a stationary object, the frequency of the reflected wave is equal to the frequency of the incident wave. In contrast, if the wave is reflected from an object that is moving along the axis of the incident wave, the frequency of the reflected wave is altered. Movements of the object away from the wave lengthen the wavelength of the reflected wave, thus decreasing frequency. Movement of the object toward the source shortens the wavelength of the reflected wave, thereby increasing frequency. This principle has been used in the design of fetal heart detectors, which are, in a sense, highly sensitive fetoscopes. They are designed to cancel out all frequencies except the Doppler-shift differences between the frequencies of the incident and reflected wave. Thus the frequency of the tones heard varies with the fetal heartbeat. These detectors can identify the fetal heartbeat consistently at 12 weeks of pregnancy and thus provide early direct evidence of pregnancy.

Gray Scale Ultrasound

Gray scale ultrasonography can detect the presence of a gestation sac in early pregnancy by demonstrating an echogenic circular or ovoid rim surrounding a transonic area. In pregnancies destined to be successful, real-time ultrasonic evaluation may reveal a gestational sac as early as 21 days after ovulation. A well defined sac can be measured by 28 days after ovulation in all successful pregnancies. At 28 days, the mean diameter of the gestational sac ranges from about 8 to 18 mm. By 45 days' gestation, fetal heart motion can be detected in 100% of pregnancies that are to be successful. At that time, the diameter of the gestational sac ranges from about 20 to 35 mm. Fetal heart movements are detectable in 100% of normal pregnancies when the mean diameter of the gestational sac is 30 mm or more.[2]

Pregnancy Tests

Although a variety of pregnancy tests have been developed since the initial bioassay reported by Ascheim and Zondek,[1] all pregnancy tests currently in routine use are based upon the detection of the effects or presence of hCG. The hCG molecule shares a common alpha subunit with several other hormones, but the beta subunit is relatively specific for each hormone. Antibodies have been raised which selectively recognize the beta subunit.[22] hCG is detectable in the sera of all pregnant women by 4 weeks after the last menstrual period (2 weeks after ovulation). During the first 8 weeks of pregnancy, serum concentrations of hCG increase exponentially. During the first 3–4 weeks of pregnancy, the urinary excretion curve for hCG parallels the serum concentration curve.[7] Three classes of hCG-based pregnancy tests are available. They are immunoassays (IA), radioimmunoassays (RIA), and radioreceptor assays (RRA) (Table 5-1).

Immunoassays. The immunoassays are performed on urine. They are either slide tests or tube tests. In either form, these tests rely on an antigen–antibody reaction (Fig. 5-7). Several drops of the patient's urine are mixed with serum containing antibodies to hCG derived from animals immunized against hCG. In the second step of the test, either erythrocytes coated with hCG or latex particles coated with hCG are added to the urine–serum mixture. If hCG is present in the patient's urine, it binds all the anti-hCG antibodies added in Step 1. The added hCG-coated particles (latex or erythrocytes) therefore see no free anti-hCG antibodies and remain in suspension. If the patient's urine contains no hCG or too little hCG to bind the available antibodies added in Step 1, the free antibodies bind to the erythrocytes or latex particles, thus causing them to clump and agglutinate. The presence of clumping or agglutination thus signifies that the patient's urine did not contain hCG, and the pregnancy test is read as negative.

Because anti-hCG antibodies cross-react with LH, most of the immunologic tests have been adjusted to lower the sensitivity enough to avoid obtaining a false positive reaction caused by the high LH concentrations found in perimenopausal women and at midcycle in cycling women.

The slide tests employ latex particles and are rapid and easy to perform. These tests can detect hCG in the urine in concentrations as low as 500–4000 mIU/ml depending upon the brand of pregnancy test kit used. They are not very reliable until at least 2 weeks after the missed period. The tube tests employ either latex particles or erythrocytes (hemagglutination inhibition). They are more sensitive than slide tests and take 1–2 hours to perform. The tube tests can detect hCG in urine at concentrations which range from 150 to 1000 mIU/ml.[3] The most sensitive tube tests are capable of detecting pregnancy with high accuracy 15 days after ovulation.

In summary, slide tests are rapid and simple to perform, but those that generate fine particles may be difficult to interpret. The presence of blood or protein interferes with the accuracy of most of the urine tests which may yield false positive results in a significant percentage of patients with proteinuria, especially if the protein concentration is more than 50 mg/100 ml of urine. Therefore, it is prudent to test the urine for protein and to check with the manufacturer concerning the amount of interference from protein expected with the test system being used. The tube tests take longer to perform but are easier to read. For office use in routine pregnancy diagnosis, a rapid slide test is adequate. This can be backed up with one of the sensitive macroflocculative tube tests for situations where the result of the slide test does not fit with the clinical impression.

Radioimmunoassay. In the RIA, a specified quantity of radioiodinated hCG is added to an aliquot of the patient's serum. Then anti-βhCG antibodies are added. The hCG in the patient's serum competes with the radiolabeled

TABLE 5-1. AVAILABLE PREGNANCY TESTS

	Immunoassays				
	Slide Tests	Tube Tests	New Tube Tests	RIA	RRA
Specimen	Urine	Urine	Urine	Serum	Serum
Indicator	Latex	Latex or erythrocytes	Latex or erythrocytes	Labeled hCG	Membrane receptors
Time to perform	2 min	1.5–2 h	1.5–2 h	1–3h	1h
Sensitivity	1000–4000 mIU/ml	500–1000 mIU/ml	200–250 mIU/ml	3–30 mIU/ml	200 mIU/ml
Time accuracy	6 weeks after LNMP	6 weeks after LNMP	4 weeks LNMP	First week of pregnancy	4 weeks after LNMP

How hCG-detecting pregnancy tests work.

Urine containing hCG

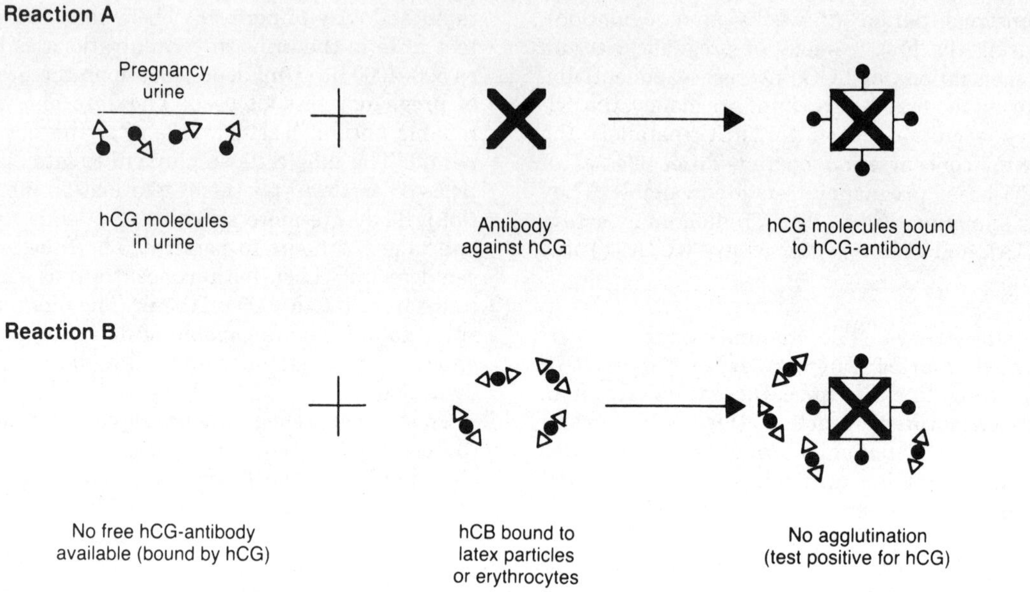

Urine suspected of containing hCG is mixed with a solution having antibody against hCG. If the urine does contain hCG, the hCG molecules are bound to the antibody (reaction A); when hCG attached to latex particles or erythrocytes is added (reaction B), because all the antibody against hCG was consumed in reaction A, *no* agglutination takes place.

Urine containing no hCG

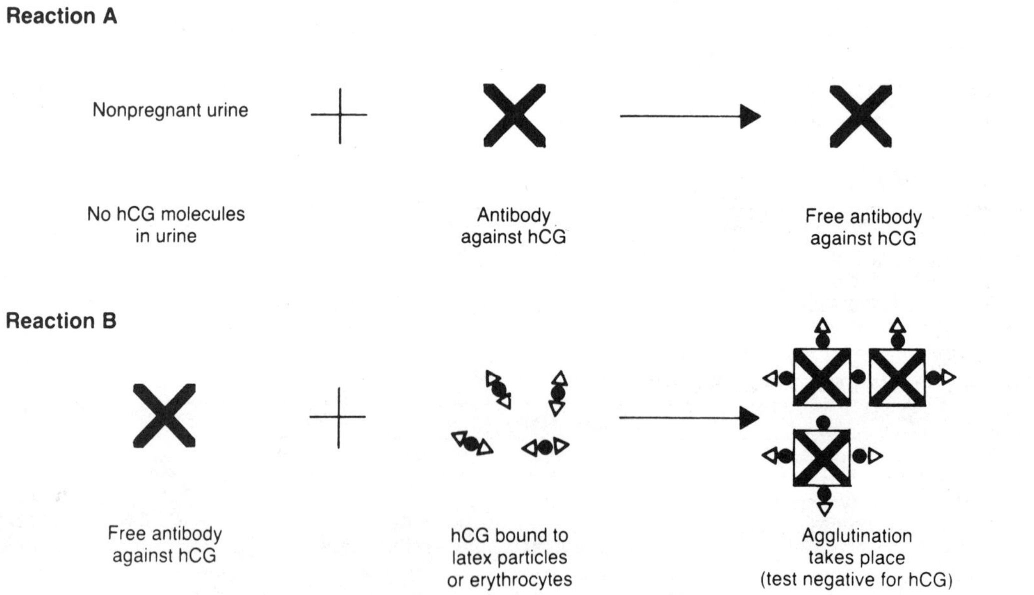

If the urine contains no hCG, binding of the antibody against hCG cannot occur (reaction A): the antibody is thus available (reaction B) to bind to the hCG attached to the latex particles or erythrocytes, and agglutination takes place.

hCG for the antibodies. Thus, the quantity of bound labeled hCG decreases in direct proportion to the amount of unlabeled hCG present in the patient's serum. RIA kits commercially available for the detection of hCG in serum or plasma can detect hCG at levels of 15–30 mIU/ml and detect pregnancy during the second week of gestation with high accuracy. RIA techniques require equipment and technical expertise. They are more expensive and take longer to perform. However, the sensitivity, specificity, and quantitation offered by the RIA overcome the disadvantages in certain clinical situations.

Radioreceptor Assays. Radioreceptor assays are, in a sense, bioassays. These tests employ radiolabeled hCG along with membrane receptors usually prepared from corpora lutea of cows. The test is based on the binding of intact hCG to the membrane receptor.[16] Cross-reaction with LH, which binds to the same receptors, limits the specificity of this assay. To avoid this, assay kits are set to a sensitivity of 200 mIU/ml serum and can diagnose pregnancies before the first missed menses. The RRA commercial kit now available allows measurement of hCG in 1 hour and is comparable to the newer tube tests in accuracy.

A variant of the immunoassay is the enzyme-linked immunoabsorbent assay (ELISA). This technique can be used in either immunoassays or receptor assays for hCG. In these assays, the antigen is labeled with an enzyme, instead of with radioactivity. When incubated with the appropriate substrate, the enzyme yields a quantifiable color change. These assays are sensitive and specific and avoid some of the drawbacks inherent in the use of radioisotopes.[3]

Other proteins that appear to be specific to pregnancy have also been utilized in the diagnosis of pregnancy. These include human placental lactogen (hPL), pregnancy-specific β_1-glycoprotein (PSBG), also designated swangerschafts-spezifische β_1-glykoprotein (SP_1), trophoblast-specific betaglobulin (TBG), and pregnancy associated plasma protein (PAPP-C). Like hCG, hPL and PSBG are synthesized by the syncytiotrophoblast. During the first trimester of pregnancy, serum concentrations of all three proteins correlate with each other.[5] At this moment, neither hPL nor PSBG is likely to replace hCG in routine pregnancy testing.

Others[20] have utilized the presence of an early pregnancy factor (EPF) which appears in the maternal circulation within hours of fertilization. This immunosuppressive factor is thus detectable prior to implantation. The Rosette Inhibition Test is utilized to detect the modified maternal lymphocytic activity induced by EPF. The clinical utility of the Rosette Inhibition Test is still unresolved.

Turbid sera and the presence of high lipid concentrations or hemolysis may interfere with the accuracy of the serum assays.

Pregnancy tests do not reveal the source of any detected hCG, although *quantitative* RIA for β-hCG can help in establishing the likelihood of ectopic versus intrauterine gestation, when used in conjunction with diagnostic sonography. Throughout the first trimester of pregnancy, the increase in serum concentrations of hCG is closely correlated with the rate of increase in trophoblastic mass.[5] During the first 60 days of normal pregnancy, hCG levels double every 1.2–2.2 days. The rise in hCG levels is quite consistent from patient to patient and can be utilized to determine gestational age. After 60 days' gestation, hCG values vary widely and cannot be utilized to estimate gestational age.[14,15]

Ultrasonography and quantitative hCG measurements can be used together to identify approximate gestational age of normal pregnancies and to identify abnormal pregnancies. In successful pregnancies, a well defined gestational sac can be identified when the β-hCG is greater than 1000 ng/ml (5700 mIU/ml).[2] A clear intrauterine gestational sac, characterized by an echogenic rim surrounding a transonic area, should be present in all normal pregnancies when the serum hCG level is above

Figure 5-7. Urine suspected of containing hCG is mixed with a solution having antibody hCG. If the urine does contain hCG, the hCG molecules are bound to the antibody (reaction A); when hCG attached to latex particles or erythrocytes is added (reaction B), because all the antibody against hCG was consumed in reaction A, no agglutination takes place. If the urine contains no hCG, binding of the antibody against hCG cannot occur (reaction A); the antibody is thus available (reaction B) to bind the hCG attached to the latex particles or erythrocytes, and agglutination takes place. (From Duenhoelter, J. H.: Pregnancy tests—evaluating and using them. *Contemp. OB/GYN* **19**:239–248, 1982, by permission of Medical Economics Company.)

6500 mIU/ml. Absence of an intrauterine gestational sac at this level of hCG is highly suggestive of an ectopic pregnancy, and the presence of the gestational sac with hCG levels below 6000 mIU/ml suggests an abnormal pregnancy.[8,12] If repeat hCG titers fail to demonstrate appropriate doubling times, the suspicion of an abnormal pregnancy is strengthened.

DIAGNOSIS OF FETAL DEATH

In early pregnancy, the most frequent indication that fetal death has occurred is that the uterus fails to grow. When cessation of uterine growth is noted, a pregnancy test should be done. If one obtains two negative pregnancy tests, utilizing the sensitive tests discussed

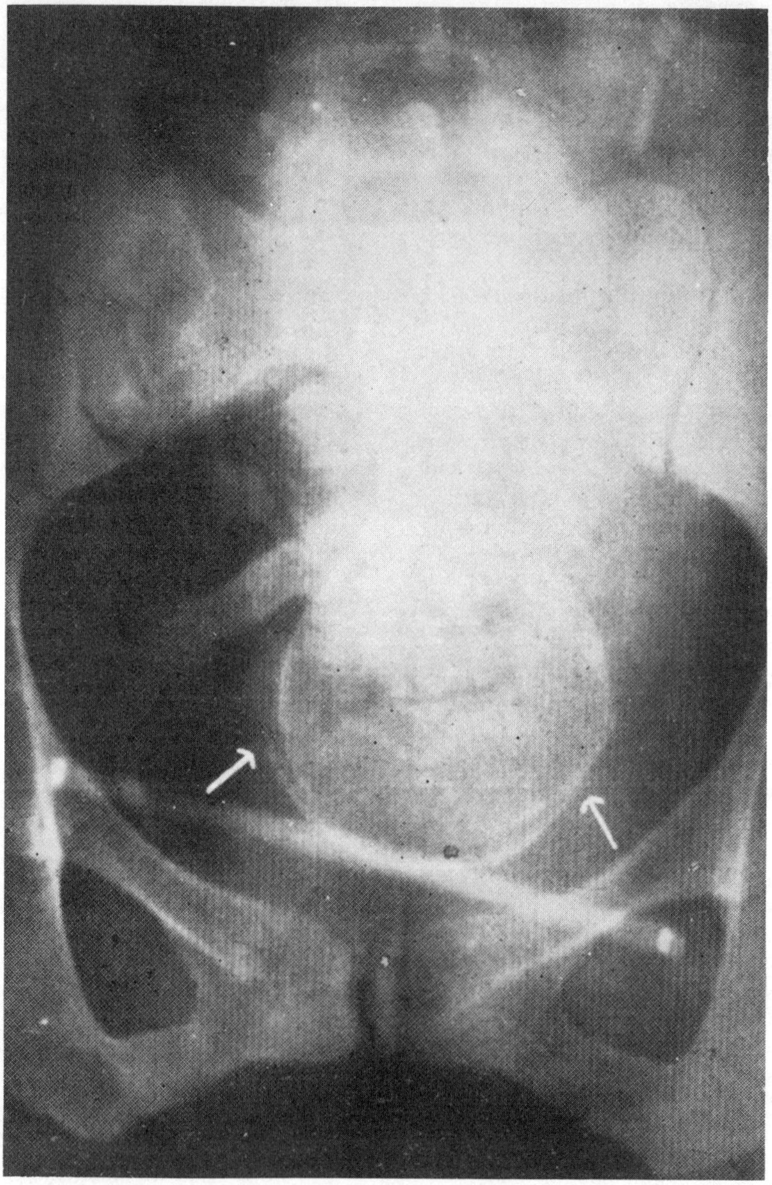

Figure 5-8. Spalding's sign consists of an overlapping of the bones of the fetal skull. However, this sign may be seen in a living fetus, during labor, or associated with scant amniotic fluid. (Reprinted from Spalding, A. B.: A pathognomonic sign of intra-uterine death. *Surg. Gynecol. Obstet.* **34:**754–757, 1922,[21] by permission of *Surgery, Gynecology and Obstetrics.*)

above, the diagnosis of fetal death is strongly supported. In the latter half of pregnancy, the most frequent occurrence leading to the suspicion of fetal demise is that the mother notices that the fetal movement has stopped. The fetal heart tones cannot be identified, even using a Doppler-effect instrument. The absence of a fetal heartbeat and fetal movements can be confirmed with real-time ultrasonography.

Finally, the aspiration of brownish, turbid amniotic fluid, when amniocentesis is done in a clinical setting suggestive of fetal death in utero, is supportive of that diagnosis. Some of the clinical signs and symptoms of pregnancy discussed earlier may begin to wane.

If real-time ultrasonography, which is the method of choice to detect fetal heartbeats and fetal movements, is not available, one may utilize roentgenography. Roentgenograms may show evidence of fetal death, but they are dependent upon postmortem changes in the fetus. Roentgenographic signs of fetal death include the classic Spalding's sign (overlapping of the skull bones), gas in the fetal circulation, exaggeration of the curvature of the fetal spine, or extreme angulation of the fetal spine. Spalding described his finding in 1922[21] as follows:

In the Women's Clinic of Stanford University we have, during the past few months, made positive diagnoses of intra-uterine death by the aid of X-ray pictures of the foetal skull, and from a review of the literature this seems to be an original observation.

It seems that very shortly after intra-uterine death, the brain tissue shrinks, which produces a typical overlapping of the foetal skull bones. This overlapping of the foetal skull bones seems to be pathognomonic of the condition of the intra-uterine death and gives a picture quite different from the overlapping produced by molding.

With the X-ray, the decreased size of the foetal head from the postmortem shrinking can be determined because the cranial bones remain nearly the same size and shape. As the head shrinks, the bones overlap at times to an astonishing distance. The radius of curvature of the shrunken head becomes obviously smaller than that of the unchanged cranial bones. When both the above changes are noted in the X-ray picture it seems justifiable to conclude that the child is dead and such has been our experience in the X-ray study of 21 babies *in utero.* In this series, 3 babies were dead and presented the typical finding; 18 were alive, of which 17 showed no changes in the X-ray picture of the foetal head and the suture lines. One baby showed marked overlapping of the skull bones due to molding caused by a long first stage of labor, but in spite of this overlapping, the skull bones showed no disproportion in relation to the bulk of the contents of the skull. (Fig. 5-8)

Spalding's sign is not seen until the fetus has been dead for at least several days, and often for two to three weeks. On occasion, the skull of a live fetus may give a false appearance similar to Spalding's sign.

Gas in the fetal vascular system is a more specific sign of fetal death. The gas is usually located in the heart and larger arteries, but is also seen in smaller vessels, especially in the liver and the spleen. The gas is largely composed of nitrogen. Gas in the fetal circulation is the most common roentgenographic sign of fetal death.[10]

Increased curvature and angulation of the fetal spine occur after maceration of the viscera and spinous ligaments. When severe, these signs indicate fetal demise, but lesser curvatures of the spine can be seen in the living fetus.

REFERENCES

1. Ascheim, S. and Zondek, B.: Eid und hormon *Klin. Wochenschr.* **6**:1321–1322, 1927.
2. Batzer, F. R., Weiner, S., Corson, S. L., Schlaff, S., and Otis, C.: Landmarks during the first forty-two days of gestation demonstrated by the beta-subunit of human chorionic gonadotropin and ultrasound. *Am. J. Obstet. Gynecol.* **146**:973–979, 1983.
3. Batzer F. R.: Early pregnancy detection: Past, present, future. In: *Fertility Control.* S. L. Corson, R. J. Derman, and L. B. Tyrer (Eds.). Boston/Toronto, Little, Brown and Co., 1985, pp. 41–60.
4. Bouillon, R., Naesens, M., Van Assche, F. A., De Keyser, L., De Moor, P., Renaer, M., De Vos, P., and De Roo, M.: Thyroid function in patients with hyperemesis gravidarum. *Am. J. Obstet. Gynecol.* **143**:922–926, 1982.
5. Braunstein, G. D., Rasor, J. L., Engvall, E., and Wade, M. E.: Interrelationships of human chorionic gonadotropin, human placental lactogen, and pregnancy-specific β_1-glycoprotein throughout normal human gestation. *Am. J. Obstet. Gynecol.* **138**:1205–1213, 1980.
6. Chadwick, J. R.: The value of the bluish coloration of the vaginal entrance as a sign of pregnancy. *Trans. Am. Gynecol. Soc.* **2**:399–418, 1886.
7. Corson, S. L., Batzer, F. R., and Schlaff, S.: A comparison of serial quantitative serum and urine tests in early pregnancy. *J. Reprod. Med.* **26**:611–614, 1981.
8. Ghorashi, B. and Gottesfeld, K. R.: The Gray Scale appearance of the normal pregnancy from 4 to 16 weeks of gestation. *J. Clin. Ultrasound* **5**:195–201, 1977.
9. Hicks, J. B.: On the contractions of the uterus throughout pregnancy: Their physiological effects and their value in the diagnosis of pregnancy. *Trans. Obst. Soc. Lond.* **13**:216–231, 1871.

10. Holm, O. F.: The roentgenological signs of intrauterine foetal death. *Acta Obstet. Gynecol. Scand.* **36**:58–74, 1957.
11. Jimenez, J. M., Tyson, J. E., and Reisch, J. S.: Clinical measures of gestational age in normal pregnancies. *Obstet. Gynecol.* **61**:438–443, 1983.
12. Kadar, N., DeVore, G., and Romero, R.: Discriminatory hCG zone: Its use in the sonographic evaluation for ectopic pregnancy. *Obstet. Gynecol.* **58**:156–161, 1981.
13. Ladin, L. J.: Signs of early pregnancy. *Med. Crec.* **143**:294–296, 1936.
14. Lagrew, D. C., Wilson, E. A., and Fried, A. M.: Accuracy of serum human chorionic gonadotropin concentrations and ultrasonic fetal measurements in determining gestational age. *Am. J. Obstet. Gynecol.* **149**:165–168, 1984.
15. Lagrew, D. C., Wilson, E. A., and Jawad, M. J.: Determination of gestational age by serum concentrations of human chorionic gonadotropin. *Obstet. Gynecol.* **62**:37–40, 1983.
16. Landesman, R. and Saxena, B. B.: Results of the first 1000 radioreceptor assays for the determination of human chorionic gonadotropin. *Fertil. Steril.* **27**:357–368, 1976.
17. Montgomery, W. F.: *An Exposition of the Signs and Symptoms of Pregnancy, the Period of Human Gestation, and the Signs of Delivery.* London, Sherwood, Gilbert and Piper, 1837.
18. Piskacek, L.: Über die Frühdiagnose der Gravidität. *Wien. Med. Wochenschr.* **54**:877, 942–948, 1904.
19. Reinl, C.: Ein neues scheres diagnostischen Zeichen der Schwangerschaft in der ersten Monaten. *Prag. Med. Wochenschr.* **9**:253–254, 1844.
20. Smart, Y. C., Fraser, I. S., Roberts, T. K., Clancy, R. L., and Cripps, A. W.: Fertilization and early pregnancy loss in healthy women attempting conception. *Clin. Reprod. Fertil.* **1**:177–184, 1982.
21. Spalding, A. B.: A pathognomonic sign of intrauterine death. *Surg. Gynecol. Obstet.* **34**:754–757, 1922.
22. Vaitukaitis, J. L., Braunstein, G. D., and Ross, G. T.: A radioimmunoassay which specifically measures human chorionic gonadotropin in the presence of human luteinizing hormone. *Am. J. Obstet. Gynecol.* **113**:751–758, 1972.
23. von Braun, R.: Über Frühdiagnose der Gravidität. *Centralbl. Gynäk.* **13**:488–495, 1899.

6

ANTEPARTUM CARE

Antepartum (prenatal) care comprises those medical, educational, and psychological efforts made during the entire gestation to the end that the pregnant woman and her fetus arrive at term in good health, well prepared for parturition. Three specific tasks are clearly identified:

- Prevention, early detection, and treatment of obstetrical complications
- Diagnosis and treatment of medical and surgical disorders
- Preparation of the patient and her family for the birth experience and parenthood

Fetal and neonatal morbidity and mortality, intrauterine growth retardation, premature birth, and maternal mortality are significantly altered by the quality of prenatal care. Antepartum care also has great utility in aiding the mother to develop self-confidence and to trust the people caring for her. Amounting to but 10–20% of the financial cost of obstetrical services, high-quality antepartum care provides a rich return on the investment.

This chapter describes the initial clinical evaluation, using a problem list and risk assessment format which is followed by an outline of subsequent observations and procedures. Sections then follow on emotions and attitudes, nutrition, employment and work, and common complaints and questions. A discussion of learning objectives and curricula of courses of antepartum education precede a section on the special problem of adolescent pregnancy which concludes the chapter.

The large amount of information collected from a patient during the antepartum course is best recorded in a specially prepared and consistent format. Computerization has been useful as a method of keeping data current, avoiding omissions, consolidating information, and making data available in different locations. Such a record-keeping system is seen in Fig. 6-1a–c.

GLOSSARY

Several commonly used terms, phrases, and numerical codes are defined below. Most of the definitions are taken from *Obstetric–Gynecologic Terminology*, edited for The American College of Obstetricians and Gynecologists by Dr. Edward C. Hughes, and published by F. A. Davis in 1972.

Reproductive History

Gravida (gravid, gravidity). A woman who is pregnant.

Nulligravida—Never pregnant.

Primigravida (*gravida 1*)—Pregnant once.

Multigravida—Pregnant two or more times.

Parity. The state of having given birth to one or more live or dead infants weighing 500 grams or more, or from a pregnancy of 20 weeks' duration or more. The term excludes current pregnancies. Multiple births, that is, a set of twins, should be considered one parity.

ANTEPARTUM DATA BASE HISTORY PART I

NAME ______________________ PHONE ____________

ADDRESS ______________________ ZIP CD ____________

CLINIC (1) ______________ DATE RECORD INITIATED (2) ____________

BEXAR COUNTY HOSPITAL DISTRICT

NAME | ADDRESS | ZIP CD | PHONE

AGE (3)	(4)	MENSES	LMP (5)	EDD (6)	RELIGION
	P TERM PRE AB L	ONSET CYCLE FLOW	MO DAY YEAR	MO DAY YEAR	

INTAKE NOTES

PREGNANCY CONFIRMED TEST		BP	WT	DIET SUPPLEMENT GIVEN	APPT FOR PHYSICAL EXAM DATE	PLACE	TIME	WILL BREAST FEED	PVT MED RECORDS
DATE	DATE								

EDUCAT./INST./DRUGS GIVEN

HEALTH SINCE CONCEPTION — "CHECK ONLY IF POSITIVE AND EXPLAIN ON THE LINES BELOW"

WNL (7)	N/V (8)	VAG. BLD. (9)	FEBRILE ILL (10)	X-RAYS (11)	PREGNANCY PLANNED	URINARY COMPLAINTS

DRUGS (PRESCRIP & NON PRESCRIP INCLUDING OC'S ______________________

PAST OBSTERICAL HISTORY — "CHECK AND EXPLAIN ALL POSITIVES"

	METHOD OF DELIVERY	COMPLICATIONS OF PREVIOUS PREGNANCY		MEDICAL SURG. HIST.	FAMILY HISTORY
NO PREVIOUS PREGNANCIES (12)	PREV DEL NONE (22)	NONE (33)	# FET DEATHS (47)	WNL (50)	WNL (65)
# PREVIOUS PREGNANCIES (13)	#VAG DELIVERY (23)	ANEMIA (34)	# NEON DEATH (48)	ABN PAP (51)	ALLERGIES (66)
DATE LAST PREG ENDED MO YR (14)	#SPON DEL (24)	DIABETES (35)	CONG ANOM (49)	ALLERGIES (52)	BLEEDING (67)
B W LARGEST CHILD g(15)	#FORCEPS (25)	HYPERTENS (36)	LIST CAUSES OF DEATH AND ANOMALIES	ANEMIA (53)	BREAST CANCER (68)
B W SMALLEST CHILD g(16)	#BREECH (26)	INCOMP CX (37)		BLEEDING DISORDER (54)	CONG HEARING LOSS (69)
ABORTIONS	#VAC EXTR (27)	MULT GEST (38)		BLOOD TRANS (55)	DIABETES (70)
#SPONT (17)	#C SECTION (28)	PL ABRUPTIO (39)		DIABETES (56)	MENTAL RETARD (71)
# INDUCED (18)	#LC TRANS (29)	PL PREVIA (40)		EPILEPSY (57)	MULT GEST (72)
# SUCTION (19)	#LC VERT (30)	PP HEM (41)		PHLEBITIS (58)	NEURO DIS (73)
# IV INJ (20)	#CLASSICAL (31)	PREM LABOR (42)		HT DIS (59)	SICKLE CELL DIST (74)
#OTHER (21)	RHO GAM GIVEN (32)	TROPH DIS (43)		Hi BP (60)	OTHER (75)
		UTI (44)		STD (61)	
		ECTOPIC (45)		SURGERY (62)	
		OTHER (46)		UTI (63)	
				OTHER (64)	

FAMILY PLANNING	NUTRITIONAL HISTORY	SOCIAL HISTORY
PREV EXP / WANTS: OC S ☐ ☐, IUD ☐ ☐, BARRIER ☐ ☐, STERILIZ ☐ ☐, NATURAL ☐ ☐	WT CHANGE THIS PREGNANCY — (+ OR -) ______ LBS ______ WKS GESTATION; NO NUTRITIONAL DEFICIENCY ☐; DEFICIENCIES IN: CALORIES ☐ VITAMIN A ☐; CALCIUM ☐ VITAMIN C ☐; PROTEIN ☐ FOOD FADS ☐	S M W D S; DESCRIBE USE OF ALCOHOL, TOBACCO, MARIJUANA AND OTHER SUBSTANCES; YRS. EDUC. COMPLETED; FOOD STAMPS; OCCUPATION; OTHER SOCIAL PROBLEMS
PREV DIFFICULTIES		

EXPLAIN POSITIVES AND LIST HOSPITALIZATION AND OPERATIONS ______________________

LAB ORDERED CHECK IF ORDERED: CBC ☐ UA ☐ UC ☐ STS ☐ BLD GRP ☐ RUEBELLA ☐ SONAR ☐ OTHER ☐ IRREG ANTIBODY ☐

SIGNATURES MED STUDENT ____________ NURSE ____________ PHYSICIAN ____________

MEDICAL RECORDS FORM
BCHD 276-1 REV 3/84 [ ] INPATIENT [ ] OUTPATIENT IP 318 OP 050

Figure 6-1. (a) Demographic and historical data. The numbers in parentheses are for computer input.

CLINIC ____________

DATE EXAM PERFORMED (76) ______ MO. ______ DAY ______ YR

PRES. WT (77) ____________ HEIGHT (78) ____________

NON PREG. WT. (79) ________ B.P. (80) ________

PULSE ________ TEMP. ________

ANTEPARTUM DATA BASE PHYSICAL EXAM PART II

	NORMAL	ABNORMAL	DESCRIBE ABNORMALITIES
HAIR & SKIN	☐	☐	
ORAL CAVITY	☐	☐	
EYES & EARS	☐	☐	
NECK	☐	☐	
BREASTS	☐	☐	
AXILLAE	☐	☐	
LUNGS	☐	☐	
HEART	☐	☐	
BACK	☐	☐	
EXTREM.	☐	☐	

ABDOMEN DESCRIBE SCARS AND MASSES ____________

UTERUS (CM ABOVE PUBIS) (81)								CONSISTENCY:		TENDERNESS:	
FETUS: PRESENTATION (>28 Wks.)	CEPH		BR		TRANS		FETAL HEART:	RATE		LOCATION	

PELVIC EXAMINATION

VUL/VAG. WNL		CERVIX - WNL		CORPUS	RECTO VAGINAL	
VULVOVAGINITIS		DES ABN		COMP. WITH (82) ______ WKS	WNL	☐
TRICH		POLYP		GESTATION	HEMORRHOIDS	☐
YEAST		CERVICITIS		OTHER	MASSES	☐
HERPES		CONDYLOMA		ADNEXA: WNL ☐	BLOOD	☐
OTHER		LACERATION		ABNORMAL ☐	OTHER	☐
CONDYLOMA		OTHER				
OTHER ABN						

PROCEDURES: PAP		G.C. CULTURE		OTHER CULTURE		WET PREP	

EXTREMITIES

DESCRIBE ABNORMALITIES ____________

CONSULT/REFERRALS ____________

SIGNATURE

STUDENT ____________ NURSE ____________ PHYSICIAN ____________

Figure 6-1. (b) Data from the physical examination—also computer compatible.

ANTEPARTUM DATA BASE SUMMARY AND FLOW SHEET PART III

AGE	P				DATE OF EXAM			INITIAL EDD		
		TERM	PRE	AB	LC	MO	DAY	YR.	MO	DAY	YR

(83) REVISED EDD			INITIAL RISK EVALUATION — CIRCLE ONE	
MO	DAY	YR	(84) **MAT** LO MED HI	(85) **FETAL** LO MED HI

INITIAL LAB RESULTS

HGB+(86) ______ HCT (87) ______ UA (88) ______ UC (89) ______ STS (90) ______

BG/RH (91) ______ IRG/AB (92) ______ RUB (93) ______ GC (94) ______ PAP (95) ______

INITIAL PROBLEM LIST	INITIAL PLANS/ORDERS	NURSES NOTES
(96) IUP ______ weeks by dates		
(97)		
(98)		
(99)		
(100)		
(101)		
(102)		
(103)	Ret. to ______ Clínic in ______ wks.	

COURSE OF PREGNANCY

VISIT DATE (YR)												
WEEKS GEST.												
BLOOD PRESSURE												
WEIGHT												
PRESENTATION (AFTER 28 WKS.)												
FHT (AFTER 20 WKS.)												
EDEMA												
URINE A/S												

SONAR RESULTS / DATES

OTHER

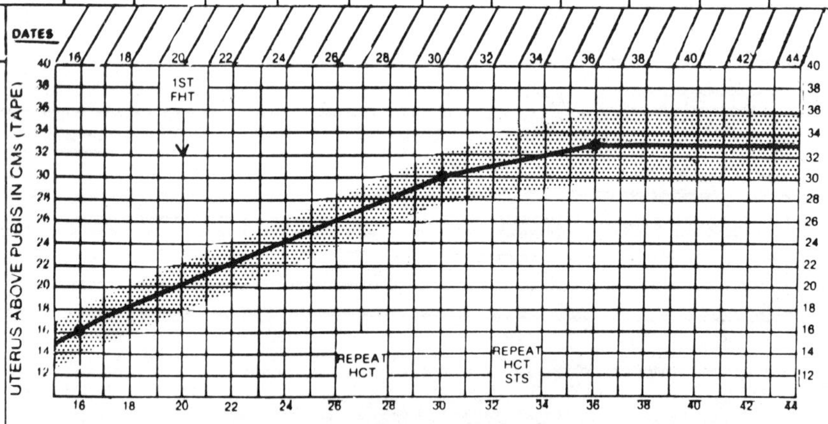

SIGNATURES
STUDENT ______ NURSE ______ PHYSICIAN ______

MEDICAL RECORDS FORM
BCHD 276-3 3/84 [ ] INPATIENT [ ] OUTPATIENT IP 318 OP 050

Figure 6-1. (c) Summary and flowsheet. The shaded graph represents the usual pattern of uterine growth. Other data from subsequent visits are recorded on progress notes and entered into the computer data base.

Nullipara—A woman who had never had a pregnancy extending past 20 weeks. Nulliparas may have previously had one or more pregnancies terminated prior to 20 weeks.

Primipara—A woman who has completed and delivered only one pregnancy extending past 20 weeks' gestation.

Multipara—A woman who has delivered two or more pregnancies extending past 20 weeks.

Parturition. The process of giving birth—labor and delivery.

Parturient. A woman in the process of giving birth.

Terms Describing the Pregnancy Length

Period of gestation. The number of completed weeks of pregnancy between the first day of the last normal menstrual period and the date in question.

Trimester. A pregnancy may be divided into three trimesters:

First trimester—LMP through 14 weeks.

Second trimester—15 through 28 weeks.

Third trimester—29 through 42 weeks.

Term pregnancy. A pregnancy which has continued through 37 weeks' duration.

Preterm pregnancy—A pregnancy which has progressed past 20 weeks but has not completed 37 weeks.

Post-term pregnancy—A pregnancy which has continued past 42 completed weeks. The terms "prolonged pregnancy" and "postdate pregnancy" are often used as synonyms.

Puerperium. The period of 42 days following birth.

Puerpera. A woman who has given birth during the previous 42 days.

Terms Applied to the Fetus

Gestational age. The estimated age of the fetus calculated from the first day of the last normal menstrual period.

Intrauterine growth retardation (IUGR). A phrase indicating that intrauterine growth is believed to be less than "normal." *Small for gestational age (SGA)* is applied to the delivered child and indicates that the newborn is in the lowest tenth percentile or less for birth weight for any given gestational age.

Lightening. The sensation by the pregnant woman that the fetus has descended or "dropped" into the pelvis. It may occur at any time in the last 4–8 weeks and is usually associated with less upper abdominal pressure—hence "lightening" or "less heavy." The process usually occurs slowly, therefore the interpretation of the word as "struck by lightning" is incorrect.

Quickening. The perception by the pregnant woman of fetal movement. It may be noted first between the 16th and 20th week.

Multiple pregnancy. The state of being pregnant with two or more fetuses.

Premature newborn (preterm newborn, "premie"). An infant born between the 20th and 37th completed weeks of pregnancy. The unreliability of the history of pregnancy duration has resulted in the common acceptance of prematurity or a premature newborn as a newborn with a birth weight less than 2500 grams. Many infants with such birth weights, however, are not premature, and many newborns delivered at 35 weeks weigh more than 2500 grams. A better term for the newborn under 2500 grams is "low-birth-weight infant" (LBWI).

Post-term newborn. An infant born after the completion of 41 (some say 42) weeks of pregnancy.

Postmature newborn (postmaturity). A term describing the syndrome of a newborn having certain placental, nutritional, and cutaneous changes thought to be due to dysfunction or insufficiency of the placenta. The newborn may or may not be post-term.

Viability. Used to describe the status of fetal development believed to be sufficient for extrauterine existence.

Numerical Codes

It is common to codify the number of past pregnancies into various sequences.

The four-digit code. For example, "P (pregnancy) 4-2-1-5." The four digits stand for (1) term pregnancy, (2) preterm pregnancy, (3) abortion, and (4) living children (T.P.A.L.). Multiple pregnancies count as one; living children means children currently living and has no particular obstetrical significance.

The five-digit code. For example, "P (pregnancy) 7-4-2-1-5." The additional digit is the first in the sequence and is merely the total number of pregnancies, that is, the sum of the second, third, and fourth items. In both the four- and five-digit codes, current pregnancies are not considered. In the examples above, the woman has been pregnant seven times, four of which were term, two of which were preterm, and one of which ended in abortion. Of the seven pregnancies, she has five living children.

Two- or three-digit code. The two- or three-digit code uses the abbreviations for gravidity and parity and includes a current pregnancy, for example, Gr4,P2,A1. This would indicate the patient is currently pregnant, has had two pregnancies progress to at least 20 weeks and one terminate prior to 20 weeks. At times the code is written with only two digits, for example, Gr4,P2.

In all these systems, no distinction is made between induced abortion and spontaneous abortion or between liveborn or stillborn fetuses. Ectopic pregnancies are included according to their duration—almost always with the abortions.

INITIAL EVALUATION

The first interview and examination of the pregnant woman and the interpretation of the data obtained are extremely important for successful medical supervision of pregnancy. The impact of gestation on the health of the patient, as well as the effect of any general health problems on the course and outcome of the pregnancy, is assessed from the initial data. The relationships between the patient and her husband and those who will care for her through the stressful and emotional exeriences begin and take a major direction at the first encounter. It is necessary that a sufficient amount of time be allotted to assure that good information is obtained and that the patient's physical and mental needs are recognized and recorded.

The initial evaluation has three main elements:

- Collection of a data base from the medical history, the physical examination, and certain laboratory tests
- Interpretation and assessment of the data specifically determining duration of the pregnancy, nutritional status, all current potential problems, and the outcome risk for mother and baby
- The making of a plan to initiate indicated diagnostic and therapeutic measures and arranging for the next visit

Collection of a Data Base

The initial evaluation involves the collection and recording of considerable information, the interpretation of these data by the formulation of a problem list and a risk assessment, and putting into motion selective screening procedures to augment the original data base. A tentative plan for continued observations is also made. It is useful to highlight abnormal findings as they are recorded, for they will form the basis of the problem list.

The Medical History. An effort is made to identify past and current events which might influence the course and outcome of the pregnancy. Special attention is directed toward health status since conception (febrile illnesses, vaginal bleeding, medications, weight changes, nausea and vomiting, emotional distress, and exposure to toxic agents). A 24-hour dietary recall is obtained for nutrition assessment. All previous pregnancy experiences are recorded in detail and clinical records are obtained if the data are not clear. Of particular prognostic significance are repeated spontaneous abortions, previous fetal deaths (stillbirths), low-birth-weight infants, birth injuries, congenital anomalies, medical illness (anemia, diabetes, UTIs, hypertension), multiple gestation, postpartum hemorrhage, malpresentation, and cesarean section.

Health status and events prior to conception are recorded as they may bear on the pregnancy (drug allergies and reactions, hospitalizations, bleeding tendencies, and communicable and chronic diseases). The family history notes especially breast cancer, fraternal twinning, diabetes, bleeding tendencies, and congenital illnesses. Evidence of financial, marital, and occupational difficulties should be sought. The use of drugs, including alcohol and tobacco, is recorded quantitatively. Single patients should have an opportunity to discuss adoption and all may need information regarding child care, food stamps, and the use of community agencies for assistance. In early pregnancy, an opportunity to discuss abortion should be available to all patients.

The Physical Examination. Blood pressure, pulse, height, and weight are recorded for every patient. Temperature and respiratory rates may be obtained, when indicated. Observation of the skin and scalp and an examination of the organs of special sense should be performed. Breasts and axillae should be examined for masses and tenderness. Areolar glands are quite prominent in pregnancy and a white, watery secretion from the nipple is normal. Inverted nipples should be brought out by palpation and the patient encouraged to practice this in preparation for breast feeding. The heart rate, rhythm, and sounds should be noted. A faint systolic murmur at the base is normal in pregnancy, but other murmurs may be abnormal and may require further evaluation. Patients with asthma or other pulmonary diseases should be given a careful lung examination. Surgical scars on the abdomen should be noted and the operation recorded. If the uterus is palpated in the abdomen (normally this is possible after 10–12 weeks gestation), it should be measured with a tape measure from the symphysis pubis to the highest point (Fig. 6-2). Fetal heart tones may be detected at 10–12 weeks gestation with ultrasound equipment and after 20 weeks with a head stethoscope. Fetal parts usually can be identified after 28 weeks. Palpable masses other than the uterus should be described as to location, consistency, tenderness, size, and mobility. The extremities should be evaluated for edema, varicosities, and deep tendon reflexes.

The pelvic examination should look particularly for changes associated with pregnancy. Vulvar varicosities, previous episiotomy scars, edema, inflammatory lesions, ulcers, and masses are noted. Congenital cysts in the upper vagina and the presence of vaginal septa may be noted in patients with no previous pregnancies. Inclusion cysts from previous episiotomies and lacerations may be seen in the outer one third of the vagina, posteriorly. Signs of inflammation and a symptomatic discharge call for a wet smear of the vaginal secretions to identify the specific type (see Chapter 27). The cervix should be observed for epithelial lesions, lacerations, and dilatation and effacement. A small circumoral ectropion is normal in pregnancy. Large cervical lacerations, usually at three and nine o'clock, should be described if these extend to the vaginal vault. A gonorrhea culture may be ob-

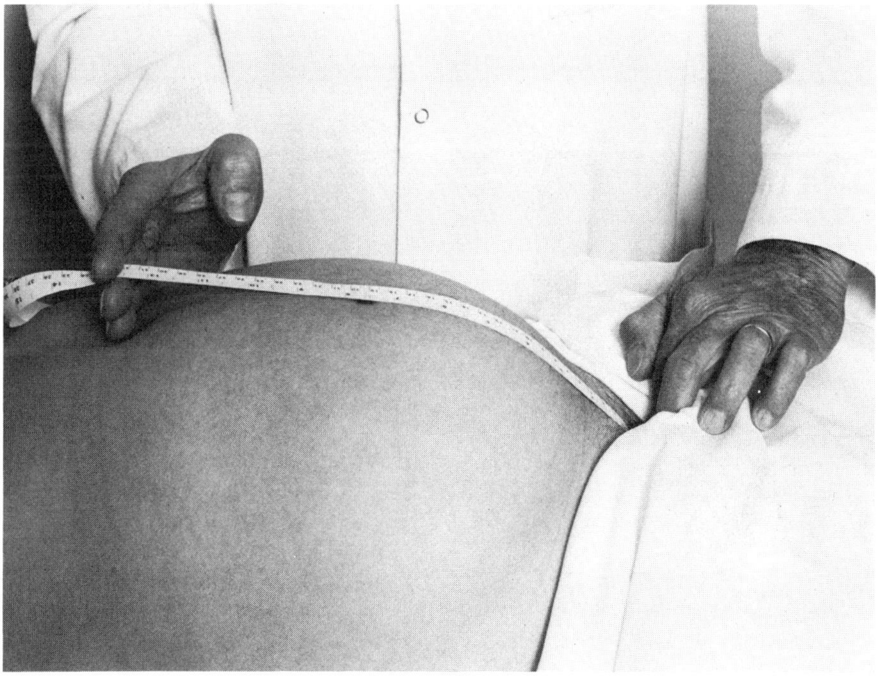

Figure 6-2. The uterus is measured from the top of the pelvic symphysis (L hand) to the top of the fundus. The tape does not follow the convexity downward, but rather is extended craniad to a point directly over the highest part of the uterus (R hand).

tained from the endocervix in high-risk patients and a cervical Papanicolaou (pap) smear should be taken. The size, shape, position, and consistency of the uterus should be described. Some asymmetry of the corpus is normal in the first 12–14 weeks, but marked asymmetry may indicate a myoma, an interstitial pregnancy, or a bicornis unicollis uterus. A uterus that fills the pelvis is characteristic of a 12–13 week gestation. Early in pregnancy, the ovaries and fallopian tubes retain their usual positions, but, by 16 weeks, may be felt in the lower abdomen or flank. Enlargements may be best recognized at the time of the abdominal examination. Adnexal masses greater than 3 x 3 cm are abnormal. A rectovaginal examination is used to evaluate the rectum and the posterior pelvis. Manual pelvimetry is uncomfortable and imprecise, and pelvic capacity has no decision-making significance until the onset of labor or when termination of pregnancy is necessary. For these reasons, manual pelvimetry is best deferred until the results are relevant and prompt feedback is possible (see Chapter 7).

Laboratory Tests. All patients require a CBC, serological test for syphilis (STS), blood group, Rh factor and irregular antibody screen, urinalysis, gonorrhea culture, and pap smear. The rubella immune status may be available from previous examination, but, if not, is necessary. Many clinics do a urine culture or use a reagent strip for leukocytes and nitrites. Other tests may be performed for screening purposes. Clinics that screen for tuberculosis usually use skin testing prior to a chest x-ray.

Interpreting the Data Base

Duration of Pregnancy and Establishing an Estimated Date of Delivery (EDD). At the initial evaluation, the presence of pregnancy is confirmed (see Chapter 5) and the duration of gestation and EDD are calculated. When menses have not occurred following a previous pregnancy, when a long period of amenorrhea preceded the conception, or when discrepancies appear very early in pregnancy (before 12 weeks), uterine size on three consecutive examinations—each 2–3 to three weeks apart—may be used to establish the EDD. Sonography is most helpful when two examinations are performed 2–3 weeks apart between the 18th and 30th week or when the procedure is done by a skilled sonographer prior to the 12th week. It is difficult to fix an accurate EDD from physical examination alone when first attempted after 14 weeks. Once an EDD has been established, abnormalities of uterine size can be noted by comparison to the normal for the period of gestation. A discrepancy may lead to the diagnosis of growth retardation, multiple gestation, or polyhydramnios. The EDD should be changed only in the last 12 weeks and only after all evidence indicates that the problem is an error in dates and not a disturbance inside the uterus. Reasons for a change in the EDD should be clearly documented.

A Nutrition Assessment. An evaluation of nutritional status should be made. Items to be considered include nutritional history (24-hour dietary recall, level of information, attitudes), findings in the physical examination, prepregnancy weight compared with present weight, and hemoglobin (Hb) and hematocrit (Hct). Risk factors which may be overlooked include food fads, therapeutic diets, substance abuse, repeated pregnancies, poverty, and adolescence.[22] Based on these data, any nutritional problem can be defined and a plan prepared.

Formulation of a Problem List. After the data base is completed, relevant problems should be recorded. A problem may be a diagnosis (pregnancy, diabetes), a physical finding (heart murmur), a historical item (previous stillbirth), a laboratory value (positive STS), or a condition (uterus large for dates). Items in the problem list should have an implication for the health of the mother and baby and should be such as to modify the course of pregnancy, labor, delivery, and postpartum period, or to require diagnostic or therapeutic measures. Problems should be recorded in a prominent location where they will be seen at each subsequent visit. The space available for problems should be sufficient to permit later additions. As a rule, each problem should be listed separately; however, it may be useful at times to combine certain items to avoid unnecessary duplication, for example, dysuria, frequency, and hematuria may be readily combined as one problem, because the assessment and evaluation will call for the same measures. In combining problems, care must be taken that important issues are not obscured. A diagnosis should not be recorded until confirmed. The diagnosis and duration of pregnancy should be the first item listed with others following in order of significance.

Risk Estimation. Using the problem list, an estimation of the risk of the pregnancy can be made. This is a prognosis statement but helps to assure that the patient's needs are met. Risk assessment should be undertaken at each visit to appreciate the impact of new problems promptly. It must be recognized that many complications of late pregnancy, labor, delivery, and the puerperium will not be foreseen or predicted. An assessment of "low risk" must not lead to complacency. It is wise to make separate risk assessments for the fetus–neonate and the mother. For example, there is little maternal risk in an incompetent cervix or Rh isoimmunization, whereas the risk to the fetus may be great. On the other hand, both mother and fetus are at increased risk in chronic hypertension or when the mother is over 35 years of age. It is also possible to estimate the severity of risk. For example, a class III cardiac patient is at much greater maternal risk than a patient with a previous cesarean section. Several systems have been developed which award points for intensity of risk. The score then may be compared to a table of relative risks.[10,17] We do not believe it necessary to take this quasiquantitative approach, but it is imperative to recognize the additive effect of multiple problems, such as diabetes complicated by urinary tract infection or chronic hypertension. Most patients are readily classified into low-, medium- or high-risk groups. The estimate of risk must be clearly recorded, readily available, and easily changed. Coding with colored tape has proved useful in some clinics.

Making the Plan

Each problem requires a diagnostic/therapeutic plan, the sum of which gives the direction for the supervision and monitoring of the pregnancy. Selective screening for various genetic, metabolic, and infectious diseases is initiated, clinical records from other institutions and physicians are ordered for later review, and therapy of intercurrent problems is begun. The plan also includes the appointment date for the next visit. A typical problem list and plan might be:

Problem 1:	Intrauterine pregnancy, 14 weeks by dates and size
Plan:	Nutritional supplement and advice. Registered for Prenatal Classes beginning September 5
Problem 2:	Previous cesarean section
Plan:	Obtain clinical records from Dr. _______ and _______ Hospital, Chicago, Illinois
Problem 3:	Asymptomatic bacteruria
Plan:	Ampicillin, 500 mg b.i.d. for 10 days. Repeat urine culture in 3 weeks
Problem 4:	Positive family history of diabetes
Plan:	Do GTT 28–30 weeks of pregnancy
Return visit:	August 24, 1984

SUBSEQUENT CARE

Clinical Observations

Following initial evaluation, the patient is seen at intervals, depending on the problem list and the plans. For low-risk patients, the typical schedule is every 4 weeks during the first 28 weeks, every 2–3 weeks from 28 to 36 weeks, and weekly thereafter. Most patients who begin their prenatal care in the first trimester have 12–15 office visits.

At each visit, the problem list, risk assessment, and plans are reviewed, an interval history is obtained, and results of diagnostic and therapeutic efforts previously ordered are recorded. Physical examination and laboratory work are performed.

The Physical Examination

- Blood pressure
- Weight
- Abdominal exam
  - Fetal outline by abdominal palpation after 28 weeks
  - Measurement of the uterine fundus above the symphysis, using a tape measure
  - Presence and location of the fetal heart tones, identifying the method used
- Extremities
  - Presence of edema and the quality of the deep tendon reflexes
  - Description of varicose veins or other skin lesions
- Other observations are made at the patient's request or as indicated on the basis of the original problem list. A pelvic examination is not routinely done but should be performed for symptoms and at 40 weeks.

The Routine Laboratory Work

- Urinalysis, using a reagent strip, for albumin, sugar, leukocytes, and nitrites
- Hb and Hct determinations at 24 and 36 weeks
- Repeat STS at 34 weeks
- Other laboratory work as indicated by the problem list

Anticipated Landmarks

- Systolic and diastolic blood pressures often fall slightly at 14–16 weeks, returning to prepregnancy or early-pregnancy level at 30–34 weeks.
- An increase in weight at a rate of approximately 2 pounds per month.
- The uterine fundus will grow regularly, achieving 20 cm (± 2 cm) at 20 weeks and 30 cm (± 2 cm) at 30 weeks, not to exceed 36 cm. The fundal height usually is equal to the weeks of gestation from 18 to 30 weeks. This rule is not valid in patients weighing more than 200 pounds.
- The fetal heart may be heard very early by Doppler, but rarely prior to 20 weeks by stethoscope.
- The fetal head and breech usually can be outlined by 30 weeks.
- Some edema of the ankles and feet is common.
- The Hct may decrease 1–3 points between 20 and 34 weeks and then return to higher levels as the effect of hemodilution disappears.

Using the added data base, the problem list is modified by deleting those no longer relevant and adding new ones. Risk assessment also may require modification. The progress note should be completed with explicit plans concerning orders and a date for return.

Preterm Evaluation

At the 33rd or 34th week visit, the prenatal course to date should be reviewed to answer the following questions:

- Is this patient in optimum condition to experience labor and delivery or cesarean section?
- If not, what remains to be done to achieve that goal?
- Are final plans for hospitalization and admission clear?
- Is the type of pain relief program planned for labor and delivery agreed upon and recorded in the antepartum record?
- Have copies of the antepartum record been sent to the hospital to be available when needed?

Some physicians provide their patients with a data card to carry with them which contains blood group and Rh factor, last Hct, EDD, and any other information which might be required in an emergency.

EMOTIONS AND ATTITUDES

It is not surprising that pregnancy may induce many manifestations of psychological lability. The first pregnancy, especially, is a stressful event, often reawakening old problems. Pregnant women need emotional support and turn to those whom they have found helpful in the past, including physicians and other health care personnel. Pregnancy may have the effect of enhancing healthy relationships with attendants who are sympathetic and understanding. The pregnant state often stimulates learning with good retention.

Several emotional changes occur normally and may be anticipated. Exploration of these feelings can be therapeutic to patients and can often provide useful information to physicians and nurses during the prenatal period.

Ambivalence

Most women have feelings of both wanting and not wanting a pregnancy, whether it is planned or unplanned. Even when the pregnancy is planned, motivation for becoming pregnant may be variable, inconstant, or neurotic. Personal, medical, and economic circumstances at the time of diagnosis of pregnancy and at delivery affect this ambivalence. It is important for the patient to understand that feelings of ambivalence are normal.

Anxiety

Fears of a malformed infant, death or damage to herself, doubts about her ability to handle the pain of labor and delivery, and other less well defined concerns are common. These anxieties may be manifested in sleeping and eating disturbances, irritability, and frequent crying. Opportunity should be allowed for discussion of these fears and the mother should be told that these fears are common to almost all pregnant women.

Introspection

Early in pregnancy, the patient views the pregnancy as a part of herself, that is, a growing organ. She is concerned about the derangement of her bodily appearance and function. Physical symptoms of pregnancy tend to heighten this concern, and conflict between the patient and her environment is often apparent at this time. After 18–20 weeks, when perceived fetal movements define the pregnancy in more separate and "baby" terms, patients usually will feel much better physically and psychologically. At this time, they may develop concerns about the normality of the baby and about their own health. Interest in events surrounding the end of pregnancy, such as labor, delivery, and care of the newborn, increases. Near term, most women are impatient to have the pregnancy over, for they feel awkward and uncomfortable. They are anxious to hold and examine their babies, wear other clothes, and return to their nonpregnant state. Many women pregnant for the first time express concerns about their ability to care for the newborn, whereas multiparas may be concerned about the effect of the new baby on older children.

Marital Tensions

Increased concern about herself and her physical symptoms, as well as fatigue, may cause the woman to become less interested in the concerns of her husband. This especially may be true in love-making and coitus, where misinformation and fear may inhibit intimacy. As a result, husbands experience jealousy, anger, and hostility, mingled with pride, anticipation, and happiness, thus becoming confused and frustrated. Patients need insight into these phenomena. Acting out of this tension by unusual or even destructive behavior may be prevented by education and discussion.

Resources for Coping

Loved ones who share both the problems and the excitement of the pregnancy are a significant resource. Family and friends can bring helpful external support. Increased contact with health care personnel should result in growing confidence in the skills and compassion of the care-givers. A conscious effort should be made to identify environmental strengths and weaknesses and to react appropriately to them. Explanation, reassurance, and education are essential to the development of self-confidence. Gentle candor and support by the care team are useful in building good patient-provider relationships. Physicians must avoid developing dependence in the patient, but rather should encourage the patient's self-confidence.

NUTRITION

Information about maternal nutrition and maternal/fetal health is derived from observations from "normal" pregnancy,[15] newborn growth and development,[12] data from periods of marked caloric deprivation of populations,[12] clinical and experimental observations in various disorders,[19] histologic examination of human placentas,[19] birth and organ weights of newborns,[14] and bench research utilizing animal species.[15,24] Ethical considerations preclude some human investigations and many gaps in our knowledge remain. However, enough is known to permit individuals and society to follow nutritional practices likely to result in favorable outcome of pregnancy.

Growth and development of the fetus and placenta plus anatomic and physiologic maternal changes demand about 28–30,000 kcal during a 40-week gestation.[12] When provided by appropriate dietary intake, this is manifested by an 11–12 kg weight gain, 45% of which is conceptus. When caloric intake is reduced, maternal tissues supply fetal needs as long as possible. Fetal growth is inhibited under conditions of marked deprivation and consumption of all available maternal resources. A gain of about 4 kg should occur during the first 20 weeks of a normal pregnancy, with the remaining 7–8 kg occurring in the second half. Reckoned by trimester, weight gain should be 2 kg, 4 kg, and 5 kg in the first, second, and third, respectively.

The food sources of these calories vary considerably throughout the world. The increased protein mass at term may be as much as 1 kg,[9] so that some additional usable protein appears to be needed. For most pregnant women in the United States, a modest increase (300 calories/day) in the usual diet is sufficient to assure adequate caloric and protein intake.[15]

Minerals

Fetal and placental needs for iron total 300 mg at term and the expanded maternal red cell mass requires another 500 mg. Scott and Pritchard[20] estimate that this necessitates about 7.3 mg iron/day, mostly from exogenous sources. Fetal bone development at term will have utilized about 30 g of calcium.[18] Although calcium absorption may be increased in pregnancy, the National Research Council advises an increase in dietary intake of this mineral throughout pregnancy.[16] This may be provided in natural foods or by supplementation. The trace elements magnesium, phosphorus, potassium, sodium, and zinc are necessary for health and are present in the normal diet of most North Americans. Insufficient or excessive amounts of iodine may produce thyroid disorders. The efficacy and safety in pregnancy of fluoride administration for dental reasons has not been proved.

Supplementation

The normal diet of North Americans provides sufficient amounts of all vitamins, with the possible exception of folic acid. A small supplement of additional vitamins probably is neither harmful nor useful. If dietary folic acid is to be augmented, 0.4 mg/day should be sufficient. For most individuals, supplementation with 30–60 mg of elemental iron and 0.4 mg of folic acid is adequate. In unusual circumstances, a gram of calcium and additional vitamins may be needed.

Table 6-1 gives the National Research Council's recommended daily allowances for good nutrition in pregnancy.

Clinical Problems

A nutritional assessment should be made at each visit. The Hb and Hct may be repeated at 28 and 34 weeks.

Variations of Maternal Weight. A considerable range in weight gain appears to be compatible with a nutritionally sound mother and newborn. Presuming adequate caloric intake, maternal weight gain occurs in response to the growing conceptus. Weight loss or persistent failure to gain weight may be due to an inadequate diet, an abnormal conceptus, increased maternal metabolic demands from infection or thyroid dysfunction, severe nausea, vomiting, or any combination of these.

Failure to gain in a patient who is signifi-

TABLE 6-1. RECOMMENDED DAILY ALLOWANCES FOR YOUNG ADULT NONPREGNANT, PREGNANT, AND LACTATING WOMEN

Nutrient and Unit	Nonpregnant	Pregnant	Lactating
Energy (kcal)	2000	+300	+500
Protein (g)	44	+30	+20
Vitamin A (mg RE)	800	+200	+400
Vitamin D (μg)	5	+5	+5
Vitamin E (mg and TE)	8	+2	+3
Vitamin C (mg)	60	+20	+40
Thiamine (mg)	1.0	+0.4	+0.5
Riboflavin (mg)	1.2	+0.3	+0.5
Niacin (mg)	13	+2	+5
Vitamin B_6 (mg)	2	+0.6	+0.5
Folacin (mg)	400	+400	+100
Vitamin B_{12} (μg)	3.0	+1.0	+10
Calcium (mg)	800	+400	+400
Phosphorus (mg)	800	+400	+400
Magnesium (mg)	300	+150	+150
Iron (mg)	18	+30–60*	+30–60*
Zinc (mg)	15	+5	+10
Iodine (μg)	150	+25	+50

* This intake cannot be met by the iron content of habitual American diets; the use of a supplement is recommended.

Source: Nutrition Services in Perinatal Care. Report of Committee on Nutrition of the Mother and Preschool Child, Food and Nutrition Board, Assembly of Life Sciences, National Research Council. Washington, DC, National Academy Press, 1981, p. 5. Reprinted from "Nutrition Services in Perinatal Care," 1981, with permission of the National Academy Press.

cantly underweight at the onset of pregnancy is ominous.[5] When uncorrected, reduced fetal weight can be anticipated. The impact is lessened if the problem can be corrected in the third trimester.[14] Failure to gain weight by women who are overweight at the onset of pregnancy has little effect on fetal organ weight. This suggests that the diets contain sufficient essential nutrients to assure normal fetal growth and that excess caloric demands are satisfied by maternal stores. Intentional weight loss during pregnancy and lactation is probably unwise, even for the obese. An intake of high-quality nutrients may permit stabilization of weight at its initial level, producing what is, in effect, a loss of 5–6 kg.

Weight gain in excess of 10–12 kg is common. When distributed throughout the pregnancy and not associated with symptoms, little difficulty is expected, other than perhaps a large infant. It is unlikely that more than 1 kg gain in a week can be due to caloric intake, so rapid weight gain often indicates fluid retention in maternal tissues or within the uterus.

Adolescence The recommended daily allowance for pregnancy is increased by 300 calories in adolescents.[16] This may be useful if conception occurs soon after the menarche, but otherwise probably is not necessary. Microcytic hypochronic anemia is encountered commonly from dietary or menstrual causes. Rarely an anemia in adolescence may herald a more serious underlying disorder, such as leukemia or chronic renal disease.

Effort. The energy cost of working in pregnancy is related to the patient's weight and not to the pregnancy itself.[21] Patients whose work does not include weight bearing probably require a normal intake. Excessive weight bearing may need to be supported by additional calories.

Pica. Obsessive craving of certain foods is experienced by many women. Ingestion of starch and clay is not infrequent, nor is the use of shaved or chipped ice. Most of these cravings are compatible with good nutritional status. When extreme, gastrointestinal disorders may result and evidence of insufficient intake of calories and iron may become apparent.

Drug Abuse. The fetal effects of certain drugs are considered in Chapter 14. Heroin, in particular, often results in marked reduction of caloric intake, which would be first noted as absolute or relative weight loss. Alcohol abuse may also be associated with nutritional deficiencies.

EMPLOYMENT AND WORK

The increase in the number of women employed outside their home and the rapidly expanding varieties of jobs filled by women have resulted in great interest in the interrelationship between pregnancy and employment.[7,8,11] It is projected that, in 1985, about 38 million women, aged 16–44, are in the U.S. labor force.[23] This large involvement has produced many issues:

- The impact of work and the workplace on the status of the reproductive health of women (the ability to conceive, the demands of the employment on the pregnancy)
- The effect of work and the workplace on fetal growth and development
- The impact of pregnancy and the postpartum period on ability to perform the job
- The impact on individual rights regarding employment and advancement by limitations and restrictions imposed in an effort to reduce hazards to the pregnant woman and her fetus
- Support for the pregnant employee and her spouse in terms of maternity leave, return to work, and provisions for breast-feeding
- Employee insurance coverage for obstetrical and neonatal services

Few published materials offer hard data on many of these questions. Much common wisdom is based on intuitive, cultural, and anecdotal impressions which may or may not be valid. Until careful studies provide firm data, statements must be tentative and inclined toward safety for the patient and her fetus/newborn.[3,6] Physicians, however, should avoid slanting their recommendations to gain nonmedical benefits for the patient.

Clearly, most recommendations concerning health problems in pregnancy must be made on a case-by-case basis. "Normal" pregnancy and "usual" work should be compatible until the onset of labor. Some conditions may require a temporary respite and others may demand a prolonged period away from the job. The indications for absence from work may be maternal (cardiopulmonary vascular illnesses, infection, painful disorders, and severe anemia) or fetal (previous late abortion and premature labor,

TABLE 6-2. GUIDELINES FOR CONTINUATION OF VARIOUS LEVELS OF WORK DURING PREGNANCY

Job Function		Week of Gestation
Secretarial and light clerical		40
Professional and managerial		40
Sitting with light tasks		
Prolonged	(>4 h)	40
Intermittent		40
Standing		
Prolonged	(>4h)	24
Intermittent	(>30 min/h)	32
	(<30 min/h)	40
Stooping and bending below knee level		
Repetitive	(>10 times/h)	20
Intermittent	(<10, >2 times/h)	28
	(<2 times/h)	40
Climbing		
Vertical ladders and poles		
Repetitive	(≧4 times/8 h shift)	20
Intermittent	(<4 times/8 h shift	28
Stairs		
Repetitive	(≧4 times/8 h shift)	28
Intermittent	(<4 times/8 h shift)	40
Lifting		
Repetitive	>23 kg	20
	<23, >11 kg	24
	<11kg	40
Intermittent	>23 kg	30
	<23, >11kg	40
	<11 kg	40

certain abnormalities of the uterus, intrauterine growth retardation, and concern about teratogenic substances). The AMA's council on scientific affairs recently published guidelines for continuation of various levels of work during pregnancy (Table 6-2, Ref. 19).

Industrial substances known to produce fetal and maternal effects include lead, mercury, certain organic compounds (dioxin, PCDs, etc.), and halogenated hydrocarbons. Environmental hazards of note are ionizing radiation, microorganisms, and waste anesthetic gases. Radiant energy from microwaves, lasers, and television does not appear to have unique risks apart from its ability to burn. (Chapter 14 discusses teratogenic agents in greater detail.)

Return to work after delivery depends on the job and the mother. In most circumstances, return to work four weeks after delivery is satisfactory. When maternity leave is not reimbursable and when fiscal concerns are uppermost, parturients may return to work earlier. Cesarean section and other complications may delay resumption of employment for longer than four weeks. Many businesses provide opportunity for breast-feeding mothers to return to work and still nurse.

COMMON COMPLAINTS/QUESTIONS*

Gastrointestinal

Constipation. Dietary changes, insufficient fluid intake to meet the greatly increased demands of pregnancy, and decreased intestinal motility may all contribute to constipation in pregnancy. Patients need to understand that constipation means hard, inspissated stools, not less frequent bowel movements of normal consistency. Education and retraining are the foundations of treatment of constipation. Patients should be reminded to respond to the urge for

*By permission of John Wiley & Sons, Inc. This section is reproduced with minor changes from Gibbs, R. S. and Gibbs, C. E., Ambulatory obstetrics, a clinical guide. In: *Clinical Obstetrics,* New York, John Wiley & Sons, 1979.

bowel movement promptly and to increase daily intake of fluid (other than milk), pulpy fruit, and a bran cereal. Low-pressure tap-water enemas may be administered during the first 28 weeks but should be reserved for impaction. Bowel lubricants, laxatives, and stool softeners are usually not necessary.

Indigestion. Upper abdominal distress described as "heartburn" or indigestion is probably due to a mild lower esophagitis related to a small hiatal hernia or to reflux of gastric secretions. Typically, the distress is worse late at night or after lying down. Treatment of indigestion should be with a mild antacid. Persistent distress, pain, or bleeding demands evaluation for gallbladder disease, peptic ulcer, and other serious disorders.

Nausea and Vomiting. Nausea and vomiting are common problems characteristically seen in the first trimester and are usually noted when the stomach is empty. Occasionally, symptoms are severe enough to result in dehydration and weakness. Objective evidence of severity includes weight loss, urinary concentration, and ketonuria. Poor skin turgor, tachycardia, and dry tongue also may be noted on physical examination. When abdominal pain occurs with vomiting, or when symptoms are noted after 16 weeks, other conditions should be suspected (see Chapter 5).

Management depends on the degree of dehydration. When no dehydration is present, frequent small meals, avoidance of citrus and dairy products, and eating crackers with water prior to getting out of bed in the morning may be helpful. No drug is specifically approved by the FDA as an anti-emetic in pregnancy. The phenothiazines and trimethobenzamide are used in severe forms of the disorder associated with dehydration and ketonuria. Rehydration by intravenous fluids may be necessary several times during the course of a pregnancy.

Vascular

Hemorrhoids. Dilatation of the external hemorrhoidal veins occurs during pregnancy because of vascular engorgement in the pelvis. Dilatation may produce itching, pain, or bleeding and the patient may notice a lump at the anus. Often edematous skin is stretched over the dilated hemorrhoidal vein, but occasionally a clot can be palpated or visualized in the vein. Treatment is directed toward reducing constipation, avoiding straining at bowel movement, and relieving acute complaints. Itching is best relieved by a 10–15-minute sitz bath daily followed by local application of zinc oxide ointment which also may be used after each bowel movement. Topical anesthetics are usually unnecessary. Acute pain is best treated by more frequent sitz baths. Over-the-counter preparations of compresses and ointments may be useful. A clot in the external hemorrhoidal vein may be removed under local anesthetic through a small incision over the convexity of the clot. Bleeding is very slight and relief is prompt and dramatic. Sitz baths for 15 minutes three times a day should follow thrombectomy for three or four days.

Varicose Veins. Varicose veins of the extremities are to be distinguished from the small purplish skin veins noted in both pregnant and nonpregnant patients. Varicose veins are subcutaneous, often 1 cm or more in diameter, and may run a tortuous course for several inches. Below the knee, they are posterior and medial. In the thigh, they follow the course of the saphenous vein anteriormedially to join the femoral. They also may be seen posteriorly in the upper thigh and buttocks. Although the varicose veins often preexist the pregnancy, the increased venous pressure and circulating blood volume of pregnancy result in considerable enlargement as early as 12 or 14 weeks. Varicose veins of the vulva are rarely apparent prior to pregnancy but may become visible and palpable in one or both vulva. The veins themselves do not transluminate, but they may be apparent when a light is placed behind the vulva.

Varicose veins may produce discomfort in the legs and vulva, but ulceration is uncommon. Inflammation in one or more segments of the vein occurs and is manifested by redness, tenderness, swelling, and increased temperature. Vulvar varicosities may result in considerable blood loss and in hematoma formation at delivery. It probably is best to cut an episiotomy through a part of the varicosity rather than to risk rupture and hematoma formation.

Treatment of varicose veins is directed toward relieving discomfort and preventing thrombophlebitis. This may be done by compressing the veins when they are empty by elastic stockings or elastic bandages extending from the foot to about mid-thigh. For varicosities higher in the leg, in the buttocks, or in the vulva, special leotard-like garments are available. Application of heat, anti-inflammatory analgesics, and perhaps heparin are successful in treatment of phlebitis in a varicosity.

Neuromuscular

Backache. Low backache is frequent in late pregnancy and usually is due to increased lumbar lordosis (the so-called "pride of pregnancy") as the abdomen enlarges. Occasionally, radiation of pain to the posterior leg in the sciatic distribution occurs, but neurologic abnormalities are rare. Treatment is rest on the side on a firm mattress plus appropriate exercises to reduce lordosis by tilting the pelvis anteriorly (tucking the buttocks in; forward thrust of the pelvis). Proper shoes with good support and low heels are useful, as is a lifting maternity girdle (may be purchased at a maternity lingerie shop or a surgical supply house). Backache that does not respond or that is associated with fever or urinary tract symptoms requires further evaluation. X-rays of the spine should not be taken during pregnancy unless absolutely necessary.

Headaches. Headaches arise from many causes during pregnancy. Those associated with any of the following need careful evaluation: visual disturbances, vomiting, blood pressure more than 140/90 or other signs of toxemia, vertigo and falling, loss of consciousness and fainting, involuntary muscle movements, and persistence of headache despite use of mild analgesics. Mild generalized and topical headaches with no other symptoms can be treated symptomatically. Drugs that contain no aspirin are preferable. Prostaglandin inhibitors are not approved for use in pregnancy.

Leg Cramps. Strong and painful contractions of the calf muscles may occur late in pregnancy. They often appear at night and result in loss of sleep and an aching, tender leg for two or three days. The cause is uncertain. Some authorities believe that the cramps are due to a disturbance in the serum calcium:phosphorus ratio. They suggest restoration of the balance by decreasing phosphorus absorption with the use of antacid gels after meals. Other management includes wearing proper shoes, elevating the legs when sitting, and taking mild sedatives at bedtime. Pregnant women also may experience diffuse aching in the thighs not associated with cramps. Although this usually is due to postural changes, it is necessary to consider thrombophlebitis of the femoral system.

Hygiene

Bathing and Skin Care. Daily baths are important in preventing skin infections. Both tubs and shower stalls are hazardous sites and care must be taken to prevent falls. Water does not enter the vagina during bathing unless the introitus is anatomically abnormal. Following bathing, nonscented oils may be applied to the skin of the abdomen, breasts, and thighs in an effort to reduce striae formation.

Coitus. Vaginal bleeding, threatened abortion, labor, and ruptured membranes are unequivocal contraindications to coitus. The effect of orgasm on uterine contractility possibly leading to premature labor is uncertain. Coitus may be uncomfortable in the latter three months of pregnancy. Couples may be advised of alternative coital positions and noncoital sexual practices. Maternal deaths have been reported from air embolism during cunnilingus.

Douches. Douches are not useful except when prescribed by a physician for a specific time and purpose. They should almost always be avoided in pregnancy by utilizing other treatment methods and agents.

Physical Activity and Exercises. A daily exercise program is useful for neuromuscular preparation for childbirth as well as to maintain good psychological feelings. Normal pregnant women are able to maintain activities to which they are accustomed, including swimming and dancing. Disagreeable signs or symptoms following usual exercise should prompt consultation with a physician. Women who previously have not exercised regularly may be encouraged to walk daily but should not initiate new activities which could create difficulties.

Travel. Advice about travel should be based on the state of health of the patient at the time of the proposed travel. The greatest hazard to normal patients is being in an unfamiliar place when medical care is needed. Commercial air travel produces no problems. Long periods of sitting, as in an auto or a bus, may result in considerable edema of the lower extremities and some pelvic discomfort, so that it is wise to walk about for 10–15 minutes every 2 hours. Travel into countries with endemic diseases should be avoided if possible and, if not, precautionary measures must be taken. Immunization with dead virus vaccines is safe[4] and prophylactic antibiotics against enteritis may be helpful. Restriction of travel is appropriate for patients with recurrent spontaneous abortion and premature labor, and for patients with serious medical disorders.

PATIENT EDUCATION PROGRAMS

The purpose of prenatal education programs is to develop the patient's self-confidence for coping with the stresses of pregnancy and parenthood. Special programs, such as psychoprophylaxis (Lamaze), although essentially training efforts, also increase self-confidence. Other benefits of prenatal classes include improved health awareness in the community, a more satisfactory use by the patient of health care personnel and facilities, perhaps a shorter and less uncomfortable labor, and, for some, a rewarding psychological and emotional experience. Inclusion of the father of the child is beneficial, for it usually enhances relationships and helps to resolve his feelings of being peripheral to the pregnancy. Sources of curriculum materials for prenatal classes include the American College of Obstetricians and Gynecologists, the American Academy of Pediatrics, the Bureau of Maternal and Child Health of state health departments, and the U.S. Department of Health and Human Services. Several companies that manufacture pharmaceuticals and baby foods also provide curriculum materials. Information unique to the particular institution where labor and delivery will be conducted should be prepared for the patients. Sensitivity to cultural values and customs is required in selection, use and development of teaching materials.

Basic Curriculum Content

Physiology of Menstruation and Conception

- Effects of ovarian hormones on endometrium
- Timing of ovulation in relationship to ovarian hormone production and menstruation
  Site and timing of fertilization
  Site of production of sperm and the relationship among sperm, semen, and ejaculation

Physiology of Pregnancy, Labor, and Delivery

- Major events in fetal growth and development
- Functions of the placenta, membranes, and fluid
- Significant events in labor, delivery, and the puerperium
- Important danger signs and what should be done for each

Family Planning

- Methods of family planning
- Reasons for pregnancy spacing and the risk of pregnancy after age 35

Health Maintenance in Pregnancy

- Recommended exercise programs during pregnancy and the puerperium
- Variations in bowel function during pregnancy
- Recommended sexual activity
- Recommended work activity
- Preparation for breast-feeding and bottle-feeding

Nutrition

- Categories of nutrients, giving three foods for each
- Recommended daily caloric intake and normal weight gain pattern of pregnancy
- Usual food sources and servings of protein, vitamin A, vitamin C, and iron

The Hospital Experience

- Location of the admission area and the procedures for admission to the hospital for delivery
- Appearance and general activities of the labor and delivery rooms and the nursery
- Planned program of pain relief
- Postpartum and nursery procedures regarding maternal and infant bonding and baby feeding

Baby Care

- Principles of breast- and bottle-feeding
- Discussion of the advantages and disadvantages of breast-feeding
- Relaxation while breast-feeding

- Nutrition during lactation
- Position of mother and baby for breast-feeding
- Care of the nipples
- Preparation of the breasts for breast-feeding and manual expression
- Recognition of complications that warrant medical treatment

Bathing the Baby

- Why and where
- Equipment and material
- Techniques

Newborn Health Care

- Immediate postnatal care
- Cord care
- First check-up
- Immunizations
- Signs and symptoms of illness; when and where to take the baby for care
- Giving medicines

Normal Patterns of Development

- Normal body, hand, language, and social development from birth to 24 months
- Recognition of slow development
- Demonstration of techniques of developing motor skills

Special Programs (Hypnosis, "Natural Childbirth," Lamaze)

These programs are designed to assist women in labor and delivery by reducing the need for narcotics and by increasing active participation. The programs are similar in structure and content. Training is given during the latter part of pregnancy and usually consists of five to nine sessions, offered subsequent to the basic material described above. Emphasis is on developing pain-reducing techniques, including muscle relaxation, breathing exercises, abdominal and back massage, and various postures and positions. For hypnosis, trance induction and release are practiced; in psychoprophylaxis, particular attention is paid to the relationship among the patient, her husband (or other coach), and the birth attendant.

Early in the development of these techniques, it was hoped that pain could be eliminated and that analgesics could be avoided. This has not been achieved with most patients, but the benefits of these training programs are so great that patients should be encouraged to participate. Concurrently, patients should be assured that whatever they require for pain relief will be administered. The presence of a trained and informed partner in the labor and delivery rooms can be very helpful to the patient and to those who care for her. Success or failure, therefore, should not be measured by anyone by the degree of analgesia obtained and drugs avoided, but, rather, by the satisfaction the patient and her coach have with the effort she made.

ADOLESCENT PREGNANCY

Adolescent pregnancy is defined as a gestation terminating prior to maternal age 18. This is a major social problem in the United States. The health care professions should be eager to assist in dealing with it wherever possible.[1] A great deal has been written in the past 15 years reviewing the issue from every aspect. The purpose of this section is to emphasize the opportunities presented by the antepartum period to prevent complications, sequelae, and recurrence.[2]

Pathology of Adolescent Pregnancy

Obstetrical problems such as pregnancy-induced hypertension, premature labor, low-weight births, stillbirths, and dystocia are increased in adolescent pregnancy. This increase is directly related to the care received by these individuals, rather than being inherent in adolescence itself. When delay, neglect, and noncompliance are the rule, complications can be anticipated. When care begins early and is complied with, results in terms of maternal and perinatal morbidity and mortality can be expected to be as good as those of a similar, but slightly older population.

Coexistent social pathology may be much more serious and much more difficult to deal with satisfactorily. Social and psychological factors may have led to the pregnancy or may result in some secondary gain to the adolescent. Even more consequential, however, may be the loss of self-esteem, isolation from peers, academic dropout, and vocational limitations.

Management

Antepartum care offers time, place, and opportunity to confront the issues and problems positively. Prenatal care should be easily accessible with a minimum of red tape and should be given in a professional, kind, but nonpatronizing fashion. The young woman (and the father of the child, when possible) should be encouraged to participate in the care as much as they are willing to. The medical care itself differs very little from that given to other nulliparas, with perhaps a bit more emphasis on nutrition and hygiene, and ample opportunity for questions and discussion of anxieties and fears. In some populations, substance abuse and venereal disease may occur with increased frequency. The physician should be alert for evidence of these problems.

Mobilization of community resources often falls to the doctor's office or clinic. Psychological, academic, and vocational concerns must be dealt with. Mental health centers are useful in bringing insight into the factors that may have prompted conception and in helping the young woman to reestablish self-confidence and self-esteem. Most school systems now have programs which allow adolescents to stay in school throughout pregnancy and afterward. If a continued academic program is rejected by the patient, vocational training is often available through public schools or other agencies. As pregnancy continues, most of these young women become quite concerned about their responsibilities as mothers. Teenage parent support groups often are useful in helping them to prepare themselves for parenthood.[13]

During this process, the importance of assuming responsibility for their sexual practices and the means of avoiding unwanted pregnancies must be clearly conveyed. The antepartum and immediate postpartum periods offer excellent opportunities to lay the foundation for the prevention of recidivism.

REFERENCES

1. Alan Guttmacher Institute: The Teenage Pregnancy: The Problem That Hasn't Gone Away. New York, 1981.
2. American College of Obstetricians and Gynecologists: Adolescent Perinatal Health. A Guidebook for Services. Chicago, IL, American College of Obstetricians and Gynecologists Task Force on Adolescent Pregnancy, 1979.
3. American College of Obstetricians and Gynecologists: Guidelines on pregnancy and work. Rockville, MD, U.S. Department of Health, Education and Welfare, Public Health Service, Centers for Disease Control, National Institute for Occupational Safety and Health. 1977.
4. American College of Obstetricians and Gynecologists: Immunization during pregnancy. Chicago, IL, American College of Obstetricians and Gynecologists Technical Bulletin No. 64, May 1982.
5. Brown, J. E., Jacobson, H. N., Askue, L. H., and Peick, M. G.: Influence of pregnancy weight gain on the size of infants born to underweight women. Obstet. Gynecol. **57**:13–17, 1981.
6. Council on Scientific Affairs: Effects of pregnancy on work performance. JAMA **251**:1995–1997, 1984.
7. Edelin, R., Feldberg, R., Glenn, E. N., Kahne, H., Mitchell, D., Mittenthal, P., Murphy, I., O'Farrell, B., Parrish, D., Ryser, C., Seidman, A., and Wofford, J.: Working women: A study of women in paid jobs. Boulder, CO, Westview Press, 1978.
8. Feinstein K. W. (Ed.): Working Women and Families. Beverly Hills, CA, Sage Publications, 1979.
9. Gibbs, C. E. and Seitchik, J.: Nutrition in pregnancy. In: Modern Nutrition in Health and Disease, 6th Edition. R. S. Goodhart and M. E. Shils (Eds.). Philadelphia, Lea & Febiger, 1980, pp. 743–751.
10. Hobel, C. J., Hyvarinen, M. A., Okada, D. M., and Oh, W.: Prenatal and intrapartum high-risk screening. I. Prediction of the high-risk neonate. Am. J. Obstet. Gynecol. **117**:1–9, 1973.
11. Hunt, V. R., Lucas-Wallace, K., and Manson, J. M.: Work and the Health of Women. Boca Raton, FL, CRC Press, 1979.
12. Hytten, F. E. and Leitch, I.: The Physiology of Human Pregnancy, 2nd Edition, Chap. 15. Boston, Blackwell Scientific Publications, 1971, pp. 440–460.
13. McGee, E. A.: Too Little, Too Late: Services for Teenage Parents. A working paper. New York, The Ford Foundation, October 1982.
14. Naeye, R. L., Blanc, W., and Paul, C.: Effects of maternal nutrition on the human fetus. Pediatrics **52**:494–503, 1973.
15. National Research Council: Maternal Nutrition and the Course of Pregnancy. Committee on Maternal Nutrition, Food and Nutrition Board, National Academy of Sciences, 1970.
16. National Research Council: Recommended Dietary Allowances, 9th Edition, 1980, p. 130.
17. Nesbitt, R. E. L. and Aubry, R. H.: High-risk obstetrics. II. Value of semiobjective grading system in identifying the vulnerable group. Am. J. Obstet. Gynecol. **103**:972–985, 1969.
18. Pitkin, R. M.: Calcium metabolism in pregnancy: A review. Am. J. Obstet. Gynecol. **121**:724–737, 1975.
19. Resnik, R.: Maternal diseases associated with abnormal fetal growth. J. Reprod. Med. **21**:315-318, 1978.
20. Scott, D. E. and Pritchard, J. A.: Anemia in pregnancy. Clin. Perinatol. **1**:491–506, 1974.

21. Seitchik, J.: Unpublished data.
22. Task Force on Nutrition: Assessment of maternal nutrition. A.C.O.G., The American Dietetic Association, 1978.
23. United States Bureau of Labor Statistics: Handbook of Labor Statistics. Washington, DC, U.S. Government Printing Office, 1980.
24. Winick, M.: Nutrition and Fetal Development. New York, John Wiley & Sons, 1974.

7

NORMAL LABOR

Normal labor (eutocia) is defined by timely progress in cervical dilatation and descent and expulsion of the fetus after clinically apparent regular uterine contractions have begun. The definition of timely progress varies with circumstances. In general terms, however, normal labor should last not less than three hours nor more than 18 hours. Labors less than three hours long are termed *precipitate* and are said to be associated with increased perinatal morbidity and mortality. A labor that lasts more than 18 hours is considered *prolonged.* The definition of the duration of normal labor also varies with the parity of the *parturient* (woman in labor). Labor is shorter in the multipara than in the primigravida.

Identification of the time of onset of clinically significant regular uterine contractions is often very difficult. Thus, as discussed later, a combination of the state of cervical dilatation and uterine contractions is used to identify, sometimes in retrospect, the time of onset of labor.

UTERINE CONTRACTILITY

Uterine contractions are the primary determinants of the progress of labor. Other factors considered in this chapter and in Chapters 22 through 26 influence progress and sometimes are dominant. However, in most labors, the most important factor is uterine activity.[17]

Uterine contractions are clinically detectable as early as the third month of gestation. For most of pregnancy, these contractions are weak and are localized to small regions of the uterus, rather than generalized over the entire corpus. During the last trimester, strong contractions, similar to those observed in labor, are detectable by the examiner. However, they are usually painless and frequently are not perceived by the woman. The localized, although strong, contractions help to prepare the cervix for labor but do not cause progressive rapid dilatation because they are uncoordinated and lack fundal dominance.[2] Multiparous women perceive Braxton Hicks contractions (see Chapter 5 for original description) earlier in gestation than do primigravidas, who usually do not perceive painful contractions until several hours before labor actually begins.

The transition from Braxton Hicks contractions to the contractions of true labor is gradual, rather than abrupt. The mechanism by which the contraction pattern changes to a labor pattern is unknown. Historically, it was believed that uterine contractility in labor was organized geometrically. The contractile impulse was said to originate in a pacemaker site in the region of the fundus or cornua. The stimulus then speads in a descending direction from the fundus down. However, we now know that "pacemaker" function can wander from cell to cell and is not restricted to any specific group of cells. Uterine muscle is "syncytial," that is, the contractile wave is myogenic, and spreads directly from cell to cell without the benefit of an intrinsic neural mechanism. For reasons which are incompletely understood, when labor begins the contractions become coordinated and spread over the entire myometrium. As labor progresses, a gradient of contractile force is established from the fundus downward to the lower uterine segment, due largely to the greater concentration of contractile elements in the fundus as compared to the lower segment. The intensity of the contractile force of the fundus increases as normal labor progresses. The differential in force between the fundus and the midportion of the uterus (fundal dominance) increases, because the increase in contractile force of the midportion is proportionately less than the increase in contractile force of the fundus. Contractile activity in the lower uterine segment, weak at the onset of labor, becomes even weaker as labor progresses. These phenomena lead to a division of the uterus into two segments—an actively contractile upper uterine segment and a relatively passive lower uterine segment.

As labor continues, the fundal and mid-uterine regions thicken and the lower uterine segment thins and dilates. These phenomena are secondary to the ability of uterine smooth muscle to adjust its length-tension relationships. In the active upper segment of the uterus, after each contraction the myofibrils do not return to their precontraction resting length, but rather assume a shorter postcontraction resting length. At the new resting length, the myofibrils are able to maintain the same tension and to relax and contract with the same efficiency as they did at the previous longer resting length. Thus, the myofibrils of the active segment become progressively shorter and thicker with each contraction.

In contrast, the lower uterine segment is progressively pulled upward around the presenting part. To effect this, the muscle fibers of the lower uterine segment lengthen after each contraction, and maintain tension and the ability to contract and to relax at progressively longer resting lengths. As the lower uterine segment progressively lengthens and dilates, the myometrium thins markedly. The junction of the thickened active segment and the thinned passive segment is marked by a ridge of muscle that can be palpated around the internal circumference of the uterus. This ridge is designated the *physiologic retraction ring.*

The lower uterine segment which is formed from the lower half of the corpus (also termed the isthmus) is bounded inferiorly by the cervix. The normal cervix prevents expulsion of the fetus until labor occurs. As discussed below, the cervix remains functionally closed until late in pregnancy.

THE PELVIC FLOOR

The pelvic floor or pelvic diaphragm is formed by the levator ani and coccygeus muscles that meet in the midline. It is covered by the parietal layer of endopelvic fascia. Viewed from above, it appears as a hammock of muscle sweeping down from the pelvic brim, investing urethra, vagina, and rectum. There are two gaps in the muscular diaphragm. The anterior gap is bridged by the *urogenital diaphragm* and transmits the urethra and vagina. The posterior gap transmits the rectum and the anal canal.

The levator ani muscles are divided into three segments, which form the major part of the pelvic diaphragm. The coccygeus muscle completes the pelvic diaphragm posteriorly. The pubococcygeus muscle can be further divided into three parts: the pubourethralis, which skirts the urethra and blends with its intrinsic muscular coat; the pubovaginalis, which inserts into the lateral and posterior walls of the vagina; and the puborectalis, which forms a loop around the anorectal junction and is inserted into the lateral and posterior walls of the anal canal. The iliococcygeus and ischiococcygeus muscles complete the lateral parts of the pelvic floor (Fig. 7-1).

The pelvic floor has inherent tone and reflexly responds to changes in intra-abdominal pressure. The pubococcygeus is traversed by the urethra, vagina, and rectum and functions to support the vagina, the uterus (indirectly), and the bladder, urethra, and rectum. The pubovaginalis (bulbocavernosus) muscles also act as a sphincter for the vagina. The puborectalis muscle controls descent of fecal material and acts as an auxiliary sphincter for the anal canal.

The endopelvic fascia is reflected off the pelvic viscera. It is a continuation of the transversalis fascia of the anterior abdominal wall. Where these organs pierce the pelvic floor, tubular fibrous investments are carried upward from the endopelvic fascia to form tightly fitting collars that blend with the outer muscular coats of the organs. A blend of endopelvic fascia, connective tissue, and the outer muscular coats of the various organs gives rise to the ligaments of support. The fascia between pubis and urethra is known as the pubourethral fascia; between pubis and cervix, the pubocervical fascia; be-

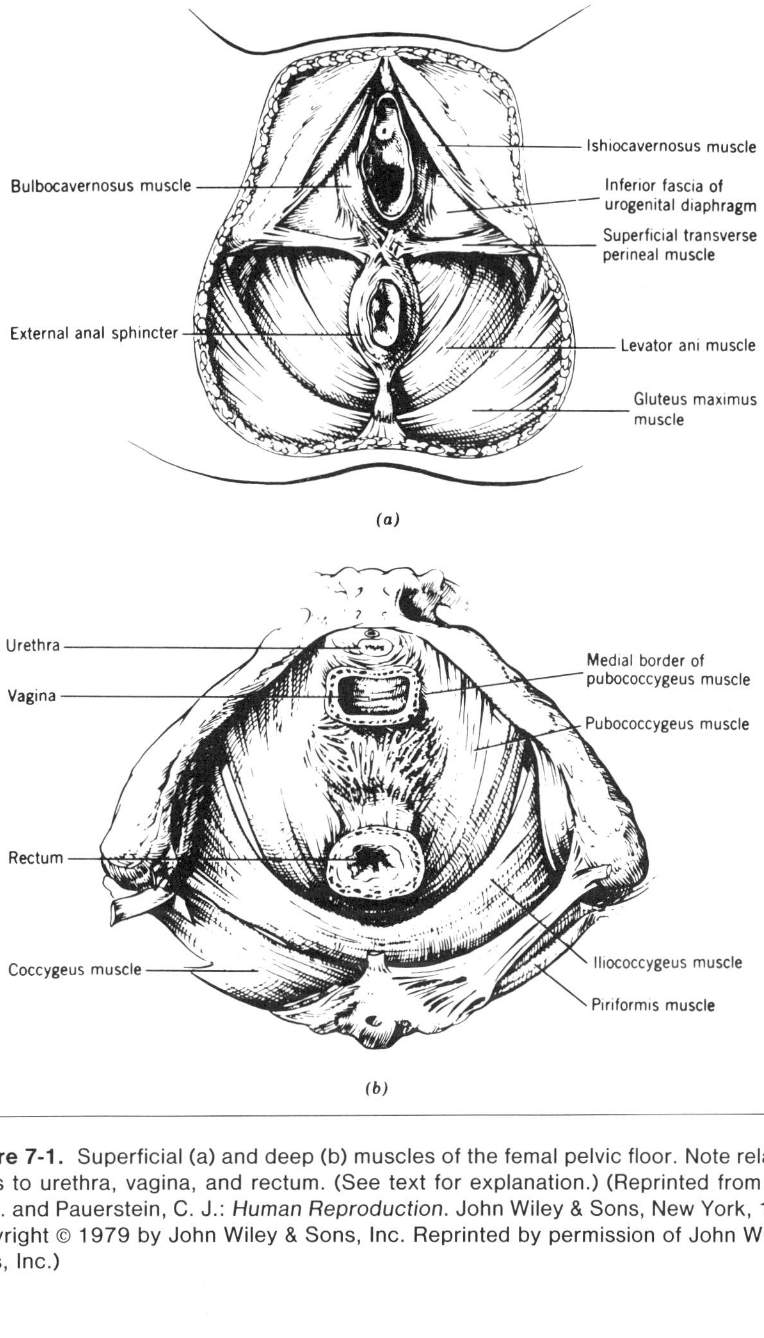

Figure 7-1. Superficial (a) and deep (b) muscles of the femal pelvic floor. Note relationships to urethra, vagina, and rectum. (See text for explanation.) (Reprinted from Huff, R. W. and Pauerstein, C. J.: *Human Reproduction.* John Wiley & Sons, New York, 1979. Copyright © 1979 by John Wiley & Sons, Inc. Reprinted by permission of John Wiley & Sons, Inc.)

tween bladder and vagina, the vesicovaginal fascia; between rectum and vagina, the rectovaginal fascia. The condensations of tissue on the lateral aspects of the isthmus of the uterus extending to the lasteral pelvic wall are called the *cardinal ligaments.* The condensations extending from the posterior aspect of the uterine isthmus to the sacrum are the uterosacral ligaments. The vesical, uterine, and rectal layers of endopelvic fascia are continuous with the fascia of the pelvic diaphragm, the obturator fascia, the iliac fascia, and the transversalis fascia.

The resistance and shape of the pelvic floor play an important role in facilitating rotation and flexion of the presenting part during labor. As the presenting part descends, the anterior portion of the pelvic floor is pressed outward against the pubic symphysis. The posterior portion is stretched into a thin-walled tube. The perineal body, normally about 5 cm thick, becomes thinned to about 0.05 cm, as it is displaced downward by the presenting part's pressure on the vulva, which stretches and thins the contiguous levator ani fibers.

THE BONY PELVIS

General

The bony pelvis is made up of four bones, which meet at four articulations (Fig. 7-2). The two innominate bones are joined to each other in front at the symphysis pubis, and to each side of the sacrum at the sacroiliac joints. The sacrum and coccyx are joined at the sacrococcygeal joint. The obstetrician is concerned only with that portion of the pelvis which lies below the linea terminalis. This portion has been designated the *true* pelvis, because it is the bone-defined tunnel that the infant must traverse at birth. However, the journey is not similar to a train passing through a straight tunnel of uniform bore, but instead involves descending and rotating through a canal which first describes a fairly straight line and then a curvilinear path. This pathway is dictated by the pelvic architecture which is the consequence of walking upright.

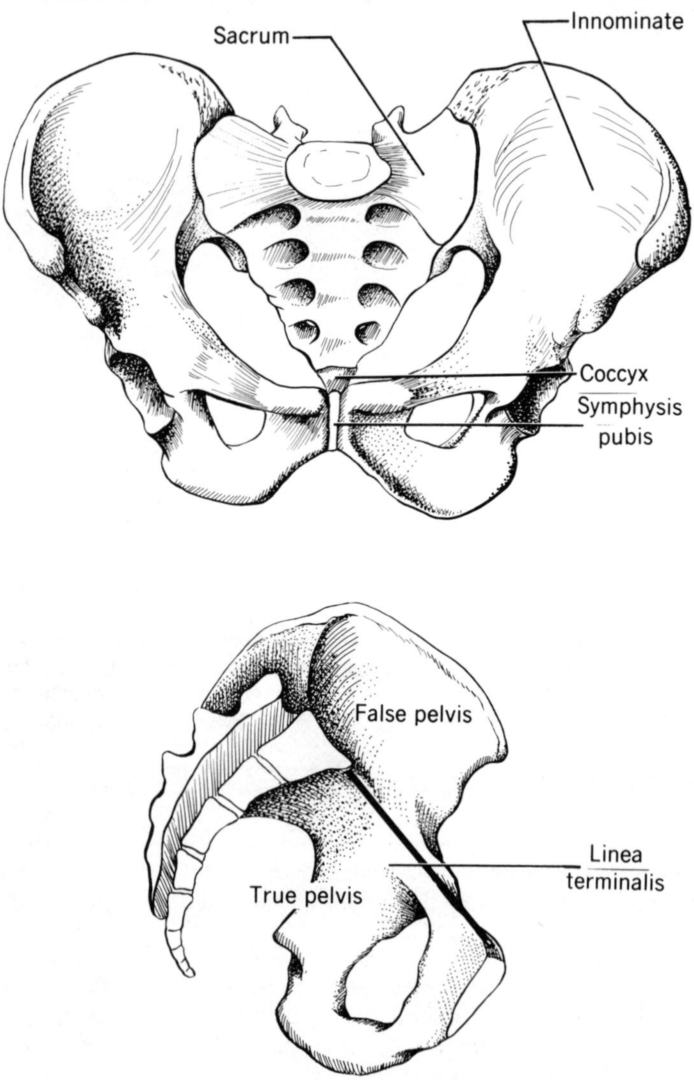

Figure 7-2. The bony pelvis. (See text for description.)

Both the size and the configuration of the pelvis influence the difficulty or ease with which the pelvis can be negotiated by the presenting part. The pelvic configurations encountered in practice are variants of four basic pelvic configurations described by Caldwell and Moloy[3] (Fig. 7-3) (Table 7-1). This classification is of great value in guiding the clinician to the features to look for on pelvic examination. However, the real utility of the Caldwell–Moloy classification is in the interpretation of x-ray pelvimetry. Most modern obstetricians do not utilize x-ray pelvimetry, except for the evaluation of the pelvis in breech presentation (see Chapter 24).

To understand the journey through the birth canal, we will follow the baby's head through an obstetrically ideally shaped *(gynecoid)* pelvis of adequate dimensions. The course that the pre-

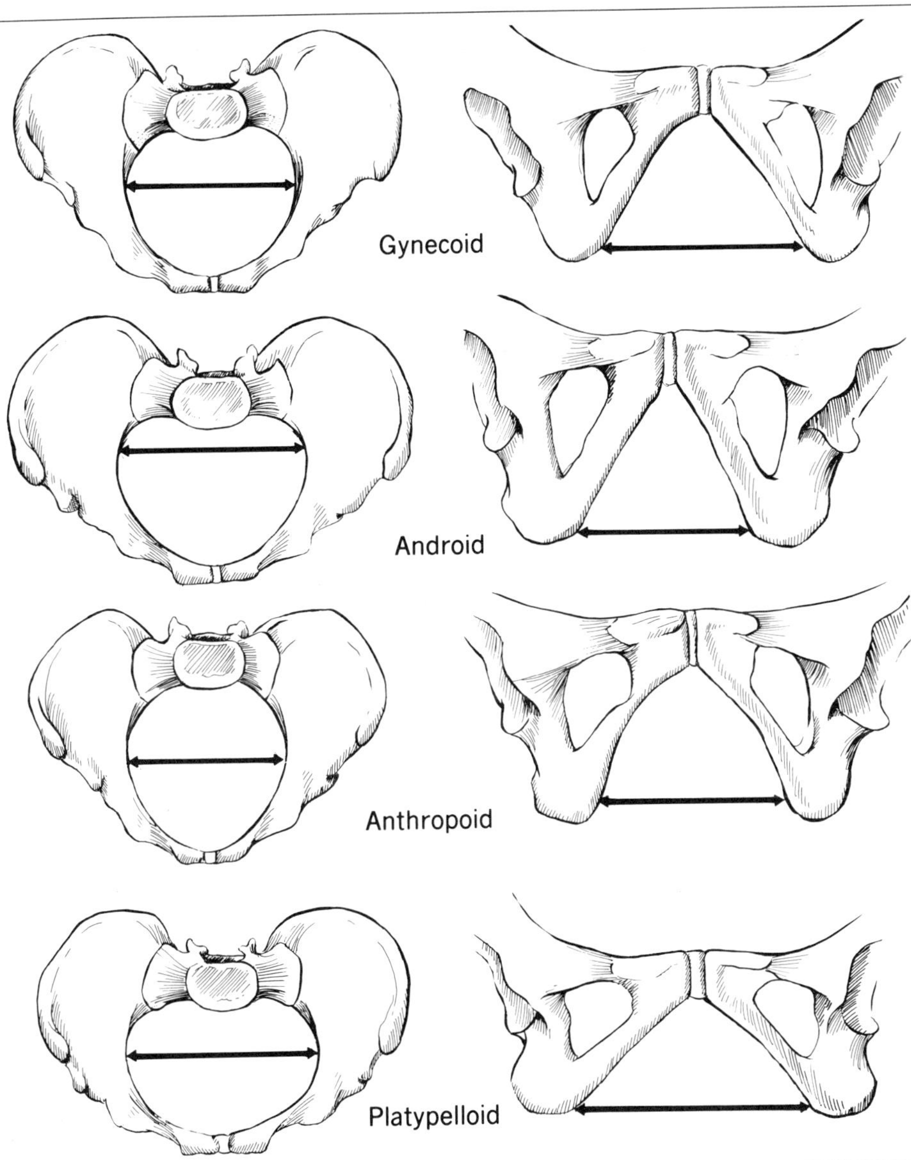

Figure 7-3. The four basic pelvic configurations described by Caldwell and Moloy. The major factors in classifying a pelvis are shape of the pelvic inlet, slope of the side walls, and character of the subpubic arch.

TABLE 7-1. CHARACTERISTICS OF THE FOUR BASIC PELVIC TYPES DESCRIBED BY CALDWELL AND MOLOY[3]

	Gynecoid	Android	Anthropoid	Platypelloid
Forepelvis	Wide	Narrow	Narrow	Wide
Side walls	Straight	Convergent	Divergent	Straight
Inclination of sacrum	Medium	Forward (lower third)	Backward	Forward
Sacrosciatic notch	Medium	Narrow	Wide	Narrow
Ischial spines	Not prominent	Prominent	Not prominent	Not prominent
Subpubic arch	Wide	Narrow	Medium	Wide
Bone structure	Medium	Heavy	Medium	Medium

senting part must follow is called the *pelvic axis* (Fig. 7-4). The upper portion moves downward in an approximately straight line until the level of the ischial spines is reached. At that point, the trajectory changes to a curvilinear path, forward and downward.

In its descent, the presenting part successively encounters the pelvic inlet, the midplane, and the pelvic outlet.

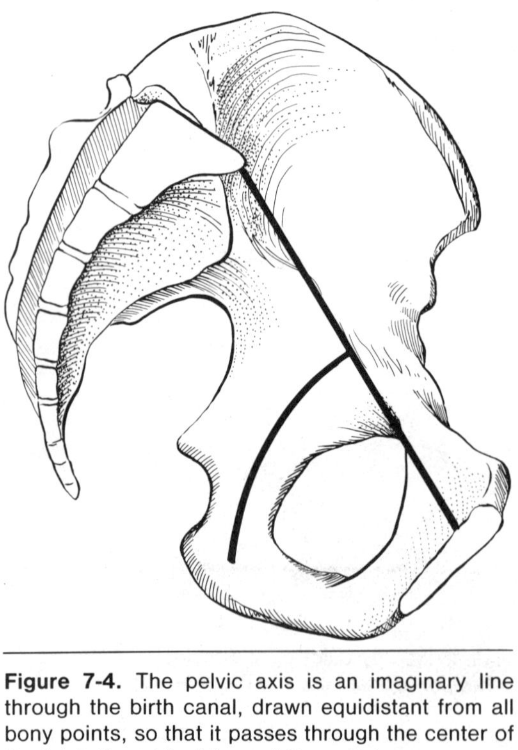

Figure 7-4. The pelvic axis is an imaginary line through the birth canal, drawn equidistant from all bony points, so that it passes through the center of the inlet, the midpelvis, and the outlet.

The Inlet. The inlet is bounded anteriorly by the upper portion of the symphysis pubis, posteriorly by the upper sacrum, and laterally by the iliopectineal lines (Fig. 7-5). The plane of the inlet of the gynecoid pelvis may be visualized as a horizontal ovoid in that the average longest transverse diameter (13.5 cm) is greater than the average longest anteroposterior diameter (11.0 cm). This latter diameter, called the *obstetric conjugate,* is measured from the middle portion of the sacral promontory to that point on the posterior superior aspect of the symphysis pubis which is closest to the sacrum. The obstetric conjugate is the narrowest anteroposterior diameter that the presenting part must negotiate to enter the inlet. The obstetric conjugate may be measured directly by roentgenography or estimated clinically, as detailed below.

The Midpelvis. The midpelvic plane is bounded anteriorly by the lower edge of the symphysis pubis, laterally by the ischial spines, and posteriorly by the sacrum, at the interface of the fourth and fifth sacral vertebrae (Fig. 7-6). The anteroposterior diameter, measured from the lower border of the symphysis pubis, through the level of the ischial spines to the junction of the fourth and fifth sacral vertebrae, measures 12.0 cm. The transverse diameter, which is the distance between the ischial spines (interspinous diameter) measures about 10 cm.

The Outlet. The outlet is described, not as a single plane, but rather as two planes (Fig. 7-7). The base of each plane is a line drawn between the ischial tuberosities. This transverse or intertuberous diameter is about 11.0 cm long. The apex of the anterior triangle is the subpubic

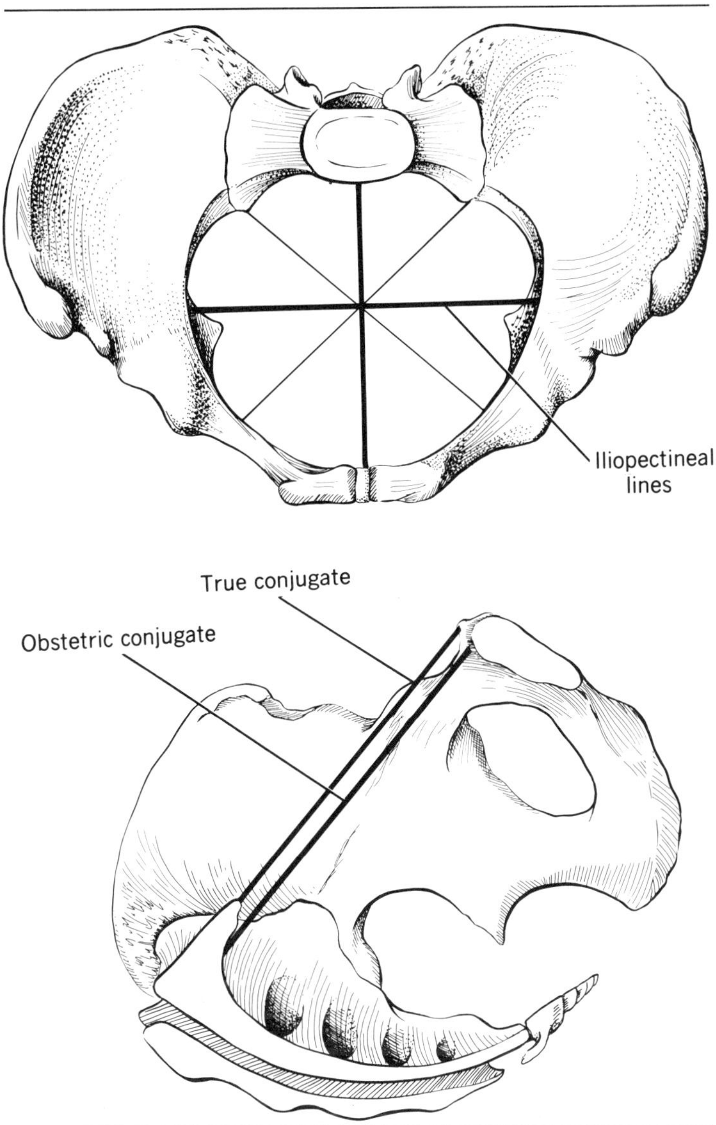

Figure 7-5. The plane of the inlet. (See text for description.)

angle, and its sides are bounded by the ischial tuberosities. The anterior saggital diameter, which is the distance from the subpubic angle to the midpoint of the intertuberous diameter, measures 6.0 cm.

The apex of the posterior triangle is at the sacrococcygeal joint, and its sides are bounded by the sacrotuberous ligaments. The posterior sagittal diameter, which is measured from the midpoint of the intertuberous diameter to the sacrococcygeal junction, averages about 7.5 cm in length.

The anteroposterior diameter of the outlet is about 11.5 cm long and is the distance from the inferior margin of the symphysis pubis to the sacrococcygeal joint.

In the *gynecoid* pelvis, the pelvic side walls are fairly parallel to each other, the sacrum is well curved, the ischial spines are not prominent, and the subpubic arch is wide, as evidenced by a subpubic angle of at least 90°.

Clinical Evaluation

Clinical examination reveals the width of the subpubic angle and the shape of the subpubic

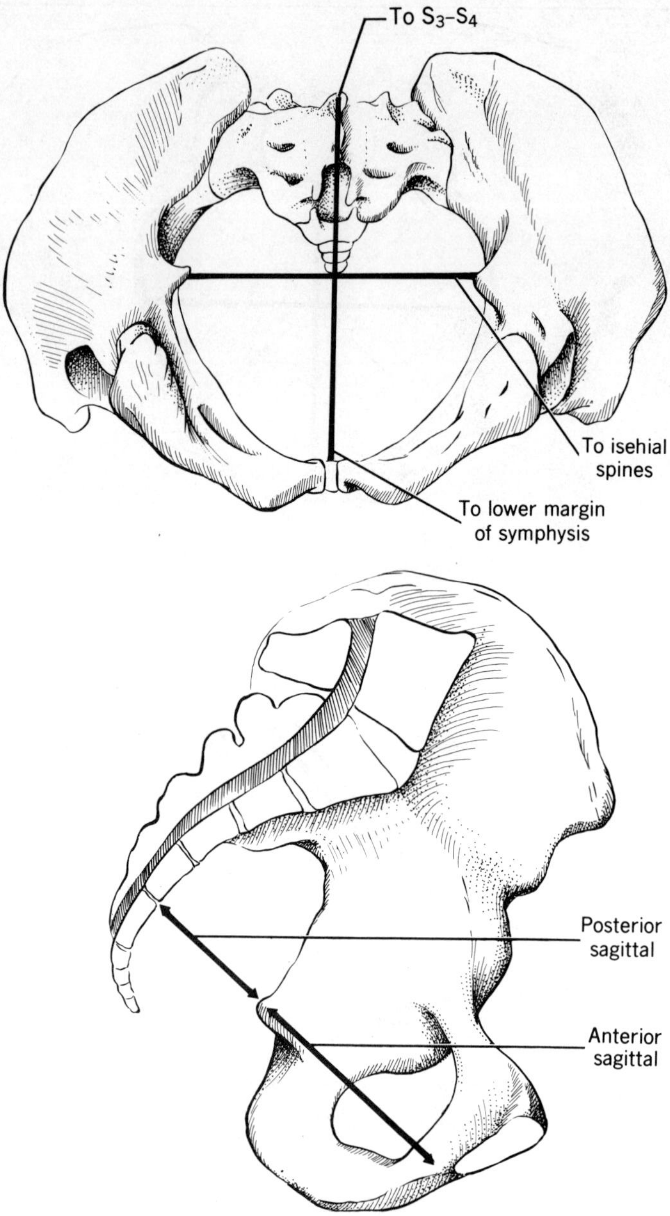

Figure 7-6. The plane of the midpelvis. (See text for description.)

arch. The width and shape of the sacrosciatic notch can be estimated, and the prominence of the ischial spines can be determined by following the sacrospinous ligaments to their ischial attachments. Only two of the pelvic diameters can be ascertained by clinical examination. The first of these, the anteroposterior diameter of the inlet, called the obstetric conjugate, is determined indirectly.

The Inlet. Estimation of the obstetric conjugate: The obstetric conjugate is measured by first estimating the diagonal conjugate (Fig. 7-8). To do so, the index and second fingers are held together and brought upward on the sacrum until the promontory is reached by the second finger. At this point, the examining hand is elevated until the index finger contacts the pubic arch. This point is marked with the other hand. The examining hand is removed from the vagina, and the distance between the tip of the second finger and the point marked on the index finger is measured. The obstetric conjugate is then estimated by subtracting either 1.5 or 2.0

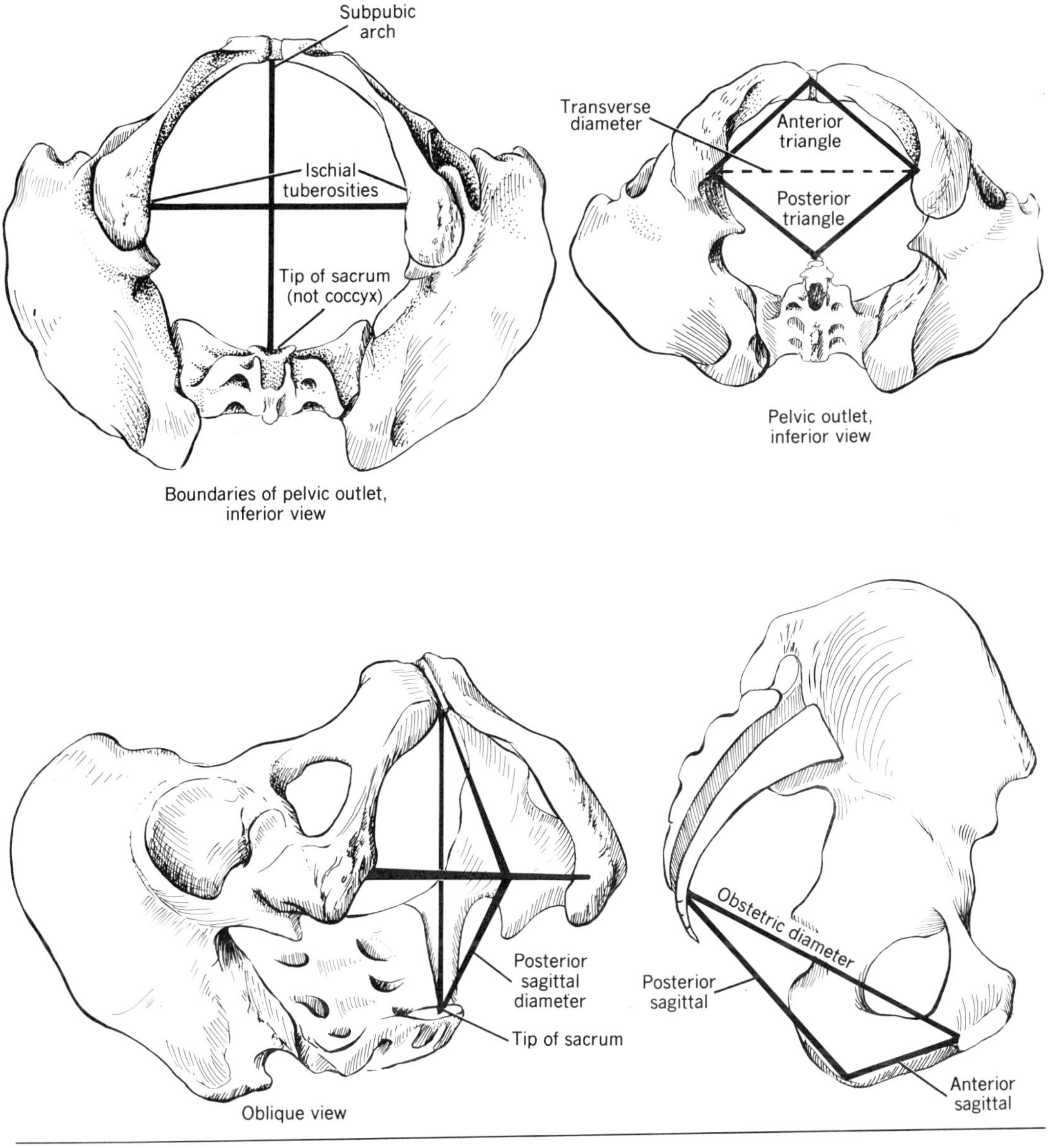

Figure 7-7. The plane of the outlet. (See text for description.)

cm from the diagonal conjugate, depending upon the angle of inclination of the symphysis pubis. A diagonal conjugate of 11.5 cm or greater thus implies that the obstetric conjugate is 10.0 cm or more, and therefore normal.

The measurement of the diagonal conjugate and of the derived obstetric conjugate is not nearly as precise as the above statements imply. Radiographic comparison of the diagonal and obstetric conjugates reveals a mean difference of 1.2 cm, but the differences range from 0.2 to 2.5 cm. The obstetric conjugate is greater than 10.0 cm in 75% of patients in whom the clinical diagonal conjugate is measured as less than 11.5 cm. Conversely, in 5% of patients in whom the diagonal conjugate is measured as 11.5 cm or more, the obstetric conjugate is actually 10.0 or less. Most important, 90% of patients whose diagonal conjugates are less than 11.5 deliver vaginally with no difficulty.[12]

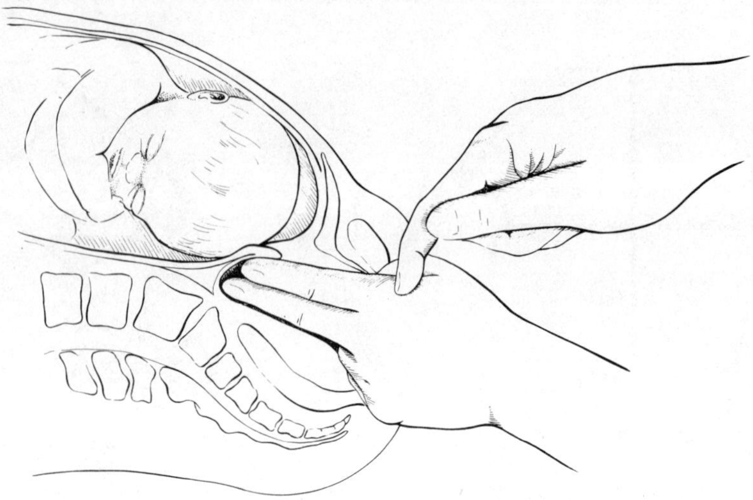

Figure 7-8. Measuring the diagonal conjugate of the inlet. (See text for description.)

The practical implication of these data and other supporting reports is that measurement of the diagonal conjugate is useful only to detect the extremely contracted inlet. Clinical evaluation of pelvic configuration is useful in understanding the mechanism of normal labor and the causes of prolonged or arrested labor. In practice, when dealing with cephalic presentations, the best test of the adequacy of the pelvis is a trial of labor. Exceptions to this statement will be noted in subsequent chapters.

The Midpelvis. Pelvic shape greatly influences the ease or difficulty with which the midpelvis is negotiated by the presenting part. If the basic pelvic configuration is gynecoid or platypelloid and the midplane measurements are adequate, the midpelvis will nearly always be readily negotiated. Even in larger pelves, android and anthropoid configurations increase the difficulty significantly.[13] The adequacy of the midpelvis cannot be ascertained by clinical examination.

In the past, formulas dependent upon measurements of midpelvic diameters obtained by x-ray pelvimetry were utilized in attempts to predict the ease with which the presenting part would traverse the midpelvis. However, none of these formulas offer absolutely reliable predictions. For practical purposes, if the interspinous diameter is more than 9.0 cm and the posterior sagittal diameter of the midplane is above 4.6 cm, the midpelvis usually is readily traversed by the presenting part. This dictum is modified by pelvic configuration, as noted above.[11] In cephalic presentations, trial of labor is still the best test of midpelvic adequacy.

The Outlet. The adequacy of the outlet can be readily measured by physical examination. The key diameters are the intertuberous and the posterior sagittal. Unfortunately, the accuracy of clinical estimations, when compared with actual measurements made by x-ray pelvimetry, is poor.[10] However, an anteroposterior diameter of the outlet which is more than 10.5 cm is seldom associated with difficult deliveries.[14]

Clinical evaluation of pelvic measurements offers only a tentative prognosis for the success or failure of labor. Clinical evaluation of pelvic architecture helps the physician to understand the mechanisms of labor and to predict some of the problems encountered in labor. In cephalic presentations, the best indicator of the relative adequacy of the pelvis is a trial of labor. In breech presentation, where the decision to allow labor mst be made early, x-ray pelvimetry offers valuable guidance. However, in evaluating the films, as much attention should be paid to the morphology of the pelvis as to the measurements.

THE FETUS

The fetal head is the most important part of the fetus during the journey through the birth canal, because it is the largest and most rigid portion of the fetus. The skull is composed of the cranium, the face, and the base. The bones of the face and the base are well fused and well ossified. Thus they are not malleable or moldable. In contrast, the bones of the cranium (or vault) are not well ossified; they are thin and are joined only by membrane at the sutures (Fig. 7-9). The vault is made up of five bones: two frontal bones, two parietal bones, and the occipital bone. The parietal bones meet in the midline at the sagittal suture and meet the occipital bones at the lambdoidal suture. A triangular space is left open at the juncture of the sagittal and lambdoidal suture. This triangular space is designated the posterior fontanelle or lambda and is a landmark used to determine fetal presentation and position. The frontal bones are joined anteriorly at the frontal suture and meet the parietal bones at the coronal suture. The juncture of the frontal and parietal bones is not completed at birth, leaving a 2 x 3 cm diamond-shaped space called the anterior fontanelle or bregma. The presence of the anterior fontanelle facilitates molding of the head during descent through the pelvis and also provides a useful landmark.

Important landmarks on the skull are:

- The *vertex*, which is the region on the top of the cranium bordered in front and back by the anterior and posterior fontanelles and by the parietal bosses laterally. The vertex, by definition, is that portion of the fetal head that is encountered by the examiner's fingers when the head is fully flexed.

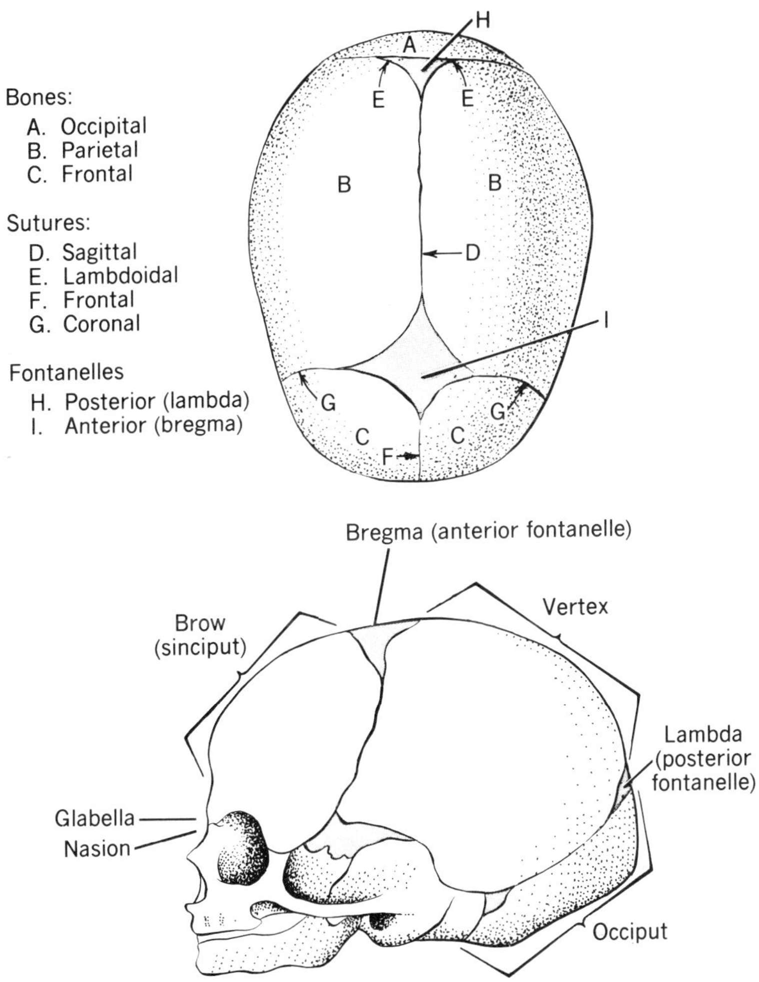

Figure 7-9. Bones and landmarks of the fetal head. (See text for description.)

- The *occiput*, which is the region below the lambdoidal sutures and is composed entirely of the occipital bone.
- The *bregma*, which is the anterior fontanelle. Partial deflexion of the fetal head causes the bregma, instead of the vertex, to present itself to the examining fingers.
- The *glabella*, which is the elevated area between the orbital ridges.
- The *brow* or sinciput, which lies between the coronal sutures above and the glabella and orbital ridges below.
- The *nasion*, or root of the nose, which is just inferior to the glabella.

The important diameters of the fetal head are demonstrated in Fig. 7-10. The biparietal diameter, which is 9.5 cm, is the largest transverse diameter. The bitemporal diameter is the distance between the temporal bones. Measuring about 8.0 cm, this is the smallest transverse diameter. The suboccipitobregmatic diameter, which averages 9.5 cm, measured from the junction of the neck and the occipital bone to the center of the anterior fontanelle, is the presenting anteroposterior diameter of the head in true vertex presentation, when the head is fully flexed.

Progressive extension of the head presents increasingly large diameters, until a brow presentation is reached. A military position, or bregmatic presentation, brings the occipitofrontal diameter of 11.5 cm into play. This diameter is measured from the occipital prominence to the glabella. Further extension to a brow presentation causes the occipitomental diameter of 13.5 cm to present. This diameter is measured from the vertex to the chin. The pelvis cannot accommodate such a large diameter, unless the pelvis is huge or the head is very small, as in prematurity or microcephaly. Thus, there is no normal mechanism for delivery of a brow presentation. When the head is fully extended, so that the chin (mentum) presents, the effective diameter is the submentobregmatic diameter, which is measured from the junction of the mandible and the neck to the bregma and averages 9.5 cm. As will be discussed in Chapter 25, mentum (also called *face*) presentations can deliver vaginally.

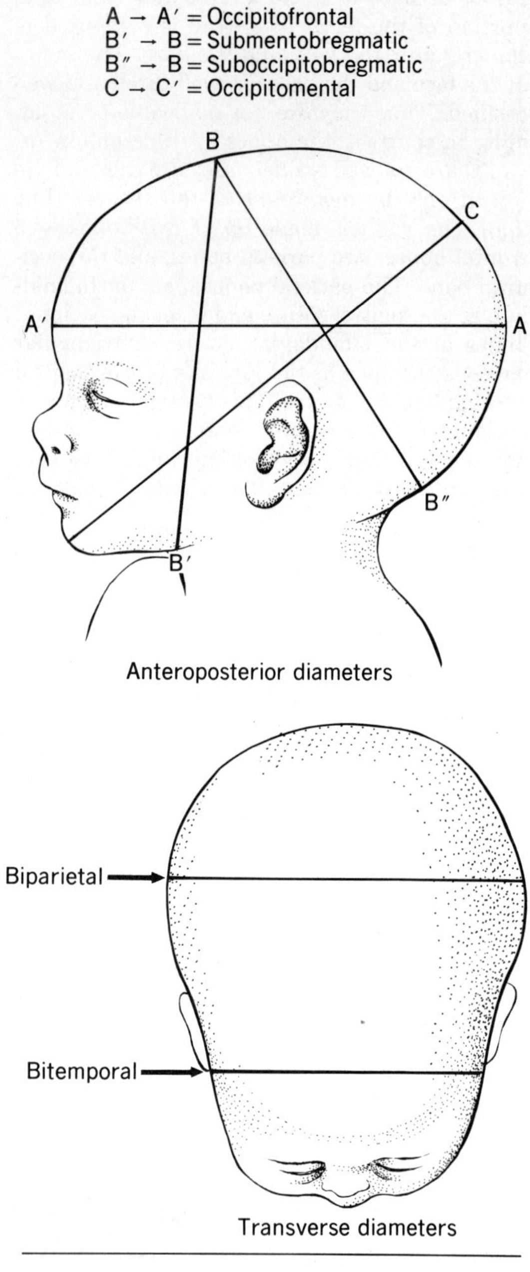

Figure 7-10. Important diameters of the fetal head. (See text for description.)

FETOPELVIC RELATIONSHIPS

The fetal head must descend along the pelvic axis and, at the same time, must rotate to accommodate the appropriate diameters of the head to the pelvic diameters. Progress in descent is ascertained by clinical examination, using the ischial spines as the pelvic reference point and the presenting part as the fetal reference point. To this end, the following conventions are utilized.

Presentation

This refers to the fetal pole that presents at the pelvic inlet. There are three presentations: cephalic, or head first; breech, which denotes that the feet or buttocks present at the inlet; and shoulder, which means that the back or abdomen is presenting.

Lie

The first two presentations, cephalic and breech, are associated with *longitudinal lie*, in which the maternal and fetal long axes are parallel to each other. Shoulder presentations are associated with *transverse* or *oblique* lie, in which the long axis of the fetus is perpendicular or oblique to that of the mother.

Position

The position of the fetus is the relationship of a designated point on the presenting part to the walls of the maternal pelvis. For this purpose, the pelvis, looked at from below, is divided into quadrants, based on maternal anatomic relations. Those on the right side of the mother are called right, those toward her back are called posterior, and so forth (Fig. 7-11). The designated reference point is then located, and the position noted as on the coordinates of a map. For example, if the reference point is the chin or mentum, and it is located in the right anterior maternal quadrant, the position is right mentum anterior or RMA. Should the reference point be located directly in line with the transverse diameter, it is designated as either right or left mentum transverse (RMT or LMT). Should it be aligned directly in the anteroposterior diameter, the position is then mentum anterior (MA) or mentum posterior (MP). Thus, each designated reference point can be placed in one of eight locations: anterior, posterior, right transverse, left transverse, right anterior, left anterior, right posterior, or left posterior. Other reference points in cephalic presentations are: occiput (OA, OP, ROT, LOT, ROA, LOA, ROP, LOP), bregma, and brow. Occiput is designated when the head is fully flexed. As noted above, the bregma and the brow present as the head becomes more deflexed, and the chin or mentum presents when the head is completely deflexed.

The reference point in breech presentation is the sacrum (SA, SP, RST, LST, RSA, LSA, RSP, LSP). The fetal reference point for a transverse or oblique lie is the acromion or scapula, but the maternal reference points employ a somewhat different convention (see Chapter 25).

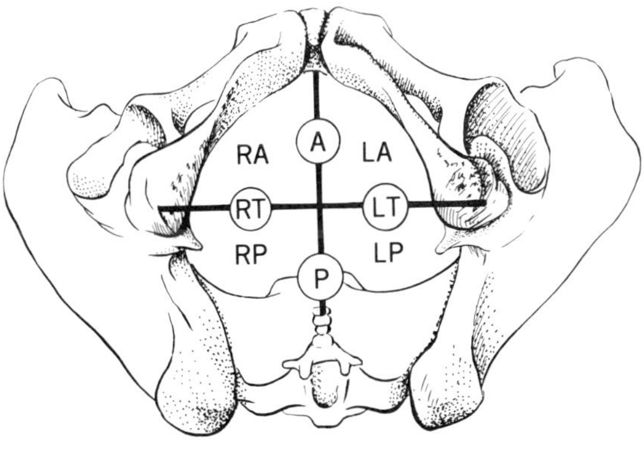

A = Anterior
P = Posterior
RT = Right transverse
LT = Left transverse
RA = Right anterior
RP = Right posterior
LA = Left anterior
LP = Left posterior

Figure 7-11. Relationships of presenting part to maternal pelvis. (See text for description.)

Presenting Part

The presenting part is the part of the fetus first touched by the examining fingers during pelvic examination

Attitude

This term refers to the relationship of the fetal parts to each other. For example, as described above, the attitude of the fetal head may vary from full flexion to extreme extension.

To illustrate the use of the above terms, refer to the situation depicted in Figure 7-12. The *lie* is longitudinal, the *presentation* is cephalic, and, because the *attitude* is full-flexion, the *presenting part* is the vertex. The designated reference point is the occiput. Because the occiput is located on the mother's right side in the anterior quadrant, the *position* is designated right occiput anterior (ROA).

When labor begins, or in some instances prior to labor, the presenting part enters the pelvis. In cephalic presentations the anteroposterior diameter, the longest diameter of the head, is generally directed into the longest diameter of the inlet. Thus, in most instances, the

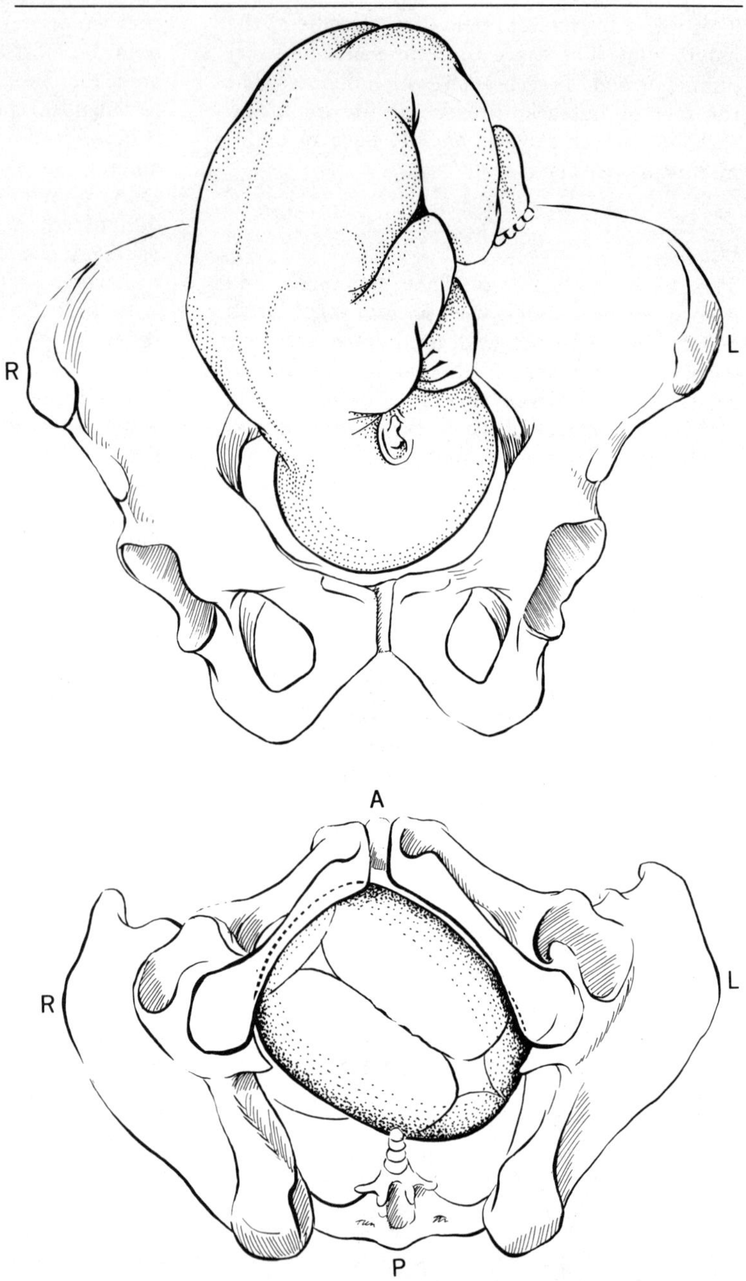

Figure 7-12. Diagram showing presentation and position. The lie is longitudinal, the presentation is cephalic, the presenting part is the vertex, the position is ROA.

head enters the inlet in a transverse position. The head then continues descent in this position at least until *engagement* occurs.

The definition of engagement in cephalic presentation is that the biparietal diameter has successfully negotiated the plane of the inlet. Because of the shape of the fetal head, the examiner can infer that the biparietal diameter has passed the inlet when the vertex has reached the level of the ischial spines. This inference is based upon the generalization that the distance from the spines to the plane of the inlet is about 5 cm, whereas the distance from the vertex to the biparietal diameter is 4.5 cm or less. The location of the presenting part with reference to the ischial spines is designated the *station* of the presenting part. By convention, the level of the ischial spines is called station 0 (Fig. 7-13). The level of the inlet, 5 cm above the spines, is designated station minus 5. The station 1 cm below the inlet is station minus 4, and so forth. The stations below the spines are also 1 cm apart and are numbered from plus 1 to plus 5, which is the perineum. These relationships vary with the depth of the individual pelvis, but the convention is useful in the clinical analysis of labor.

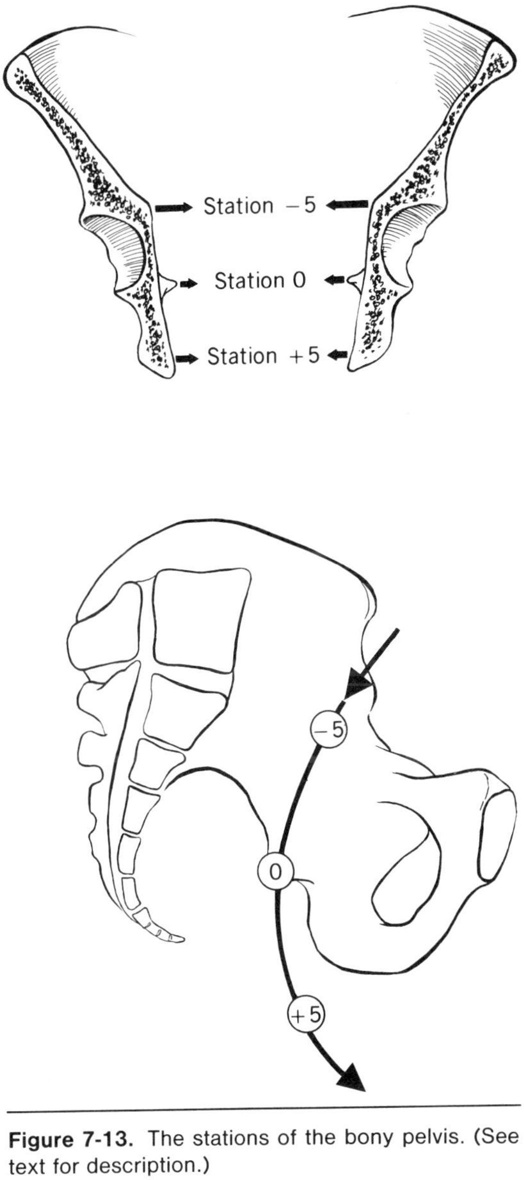

Figure 7-13. The stations of the bony pelvis. (See text for description.)

In practice, two major problems are encountered. First, the examiner must judge the station of the bony skull and not the soft tissue, which may be quite thick if a large *caput succedaneum* has formed. The examiner must gain experience in judging the thickness of edematous scalp that intervenes between the examining finger and the bony skull.

The second problem is that the inference of engagement in cephalic presentations by locating the presenting part (the vertex) at or below the level of the spines only holds when the head is well flexed. We noted earlier that progressive extension from vertex to brow presentation brings progressively larger fetal diameters into play. An additional consequence of deflexion is that the presenting part is farther away from the biparietal diameter. Thus, in mentum presentation, the biparietal diameter is above the inlet when the chin is at station 0, because the distance from the face to the biparietal plane (7 cm) exceeds the distance from the spines to the plane of the inlet (5 cm) (Fig. 7-14). The likelihood that engagement has occurred can be estimated on examination. In addition to touch diagnosis of the presenting part, engagement is likely if the sacral hollow is well filled and the sacrum is two-thirds covered by the head, and if three-fourths of the width of the symphysis is covered by the head. This clinical observation is the consequence of the normal mechanisms involved in engagement and descent. Engagement in primigravidas usually occurs during the last few weeks of pregnancy, prior to the onset of labor. In multiparas, engagement often occurs after the onset of labor.

The head usually enters the pelvis with the posterior parietal bone presenting. The posterior parietal prominence descends past the sacral promontory while the anterior parietal bone is still above the plane of the inlet. This presentation is termed *posterior asynclitism* and is diagnosed by feeling the sagittal suture in an eccentric position, closer to the symphysis pubis than it is to the sacrum. Thus, the biparietal plane is obliquely related to the plane of the inlet. With labor, the head descends, with the posterior parietal bone in contact with the sacrum. Lateral flexion then moves the sagittal suture toward the sacrum, and the anterior parietal prominence slips past the pubis to enter the pelvis. The obliquity is thus corrected and synclitism is restored, with the sagittal suture now equidistant from the sacrum and the symphysis (Fig. 7-15).

Sometimes the anterior parietal bone is most

dependent, with the sagittal suture located closer to the sacrum than to the symphysis. In this event, termed *anterior asynclitism*, the anterior parietal prominence descends past the symphysis to enter the pelvis. Lateral flexion occurs in the direction of the symphysis, allowing the posterior parietal bone to rotate over the sacral promontory to enter the pelvis. Asynclitism, of either variety, allows a diameter of less than 9 cm to enter the pelvis, rather than the biparietal diameter of 9.5 cm. This mechanism can be very important, particularly if the head is larger than average or the inlet borderline.

As the head is entering the pelvis, pelvic resistance normally causes increased *flexion* of the head, so that the chin is tucked in closer to the chest and the occiput is lower than the bregma, which is lower than the sinciput. Thus, the smaller occipitobregmatic diameter is substituted for the occipitofrontal diameter.

As the flexed head descends, it also rotates. The inlet may be visualized as a horizontal oval, in which the transverse diameter exceeds the anteroposterior diameter. Therefore, the head enters the pelvis with the occiput transverse. As the head descends into the midpelvis, it encounters not the transverse oval of the inlet, but rather a vertical oval in which the anteroposterior diameter is longer than the transverse diameter. Therefore, the head rotates to bring its anteroposterior diameter into congruence with the anteroposterior diameter of the midplane. During this process, called *internal rotation*, the occiput usually rotates anteriorly, toward the symphysis pubis. Although rotation begins, and is often complete, by the time the head contacts the pelvic floor, it is likely that the configuration of the muscles of the pelvic floor influences anterior rotation of the occiput. In some instances the occiput rotates toward the sacrum rather than the pubis (occiput posterior position). Internal rotation generally occurs after full dilatation of the cervix, during the second stage of labor.

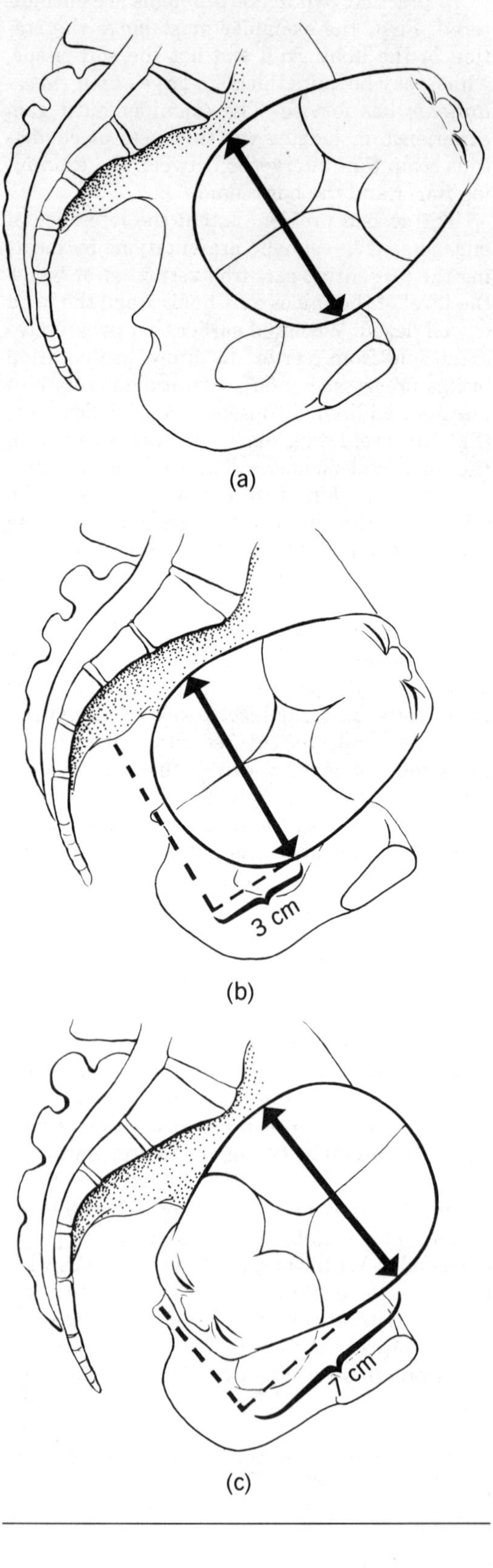

Figure 7-14. Effect of deflexion attitudes on the influence of engagement. (a) When the lowermost level of the head is several centimeters above the ischial spines, it is not engaged. (b) In the absence of excessive caput formation when the lowermost portion of the flexed head is at the level of the spines, engagement has occurred. (c) In contrast, when a face presentation has reached the level of the spines, the biparietal diameter has not negotiated the inlet.

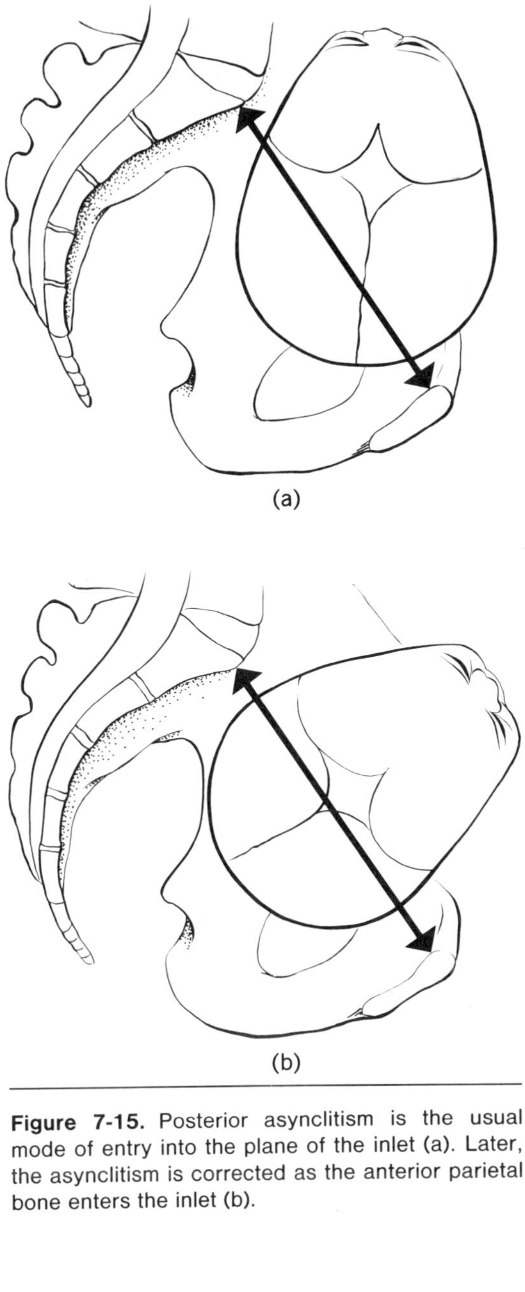

Figure 7-15. Posterior asynclitism is the usual mode of entry into the plane of the inlet (a). Later, the asynclitism is corrected as the anterior parietal bone enters the inlet (b).

Delivery occurs by *extension* of the head, which is the resultant of the pelvic floor offering resistance to the head, which is being forced downward by uterine contractions and voluntary pushing. The occiput descends to contact the bottom of the pubic symphysis. After this occurs, the occiput acts as a fulcrum, and the resultant forces cause extension of the head. More and more of the head becomes visible between the labia, as detailed below.

CLINICAL COURSE OF LABOR

Clinical convention, but not biologic reality, divides labor into three stages. During the *first stage* of labor, the cervix dilates and effaces. The first stage begins with the first true labor pain and ends when the cervix is fully (10 cm) dilated. The end of the first stage of labor is much easier to define than is the onset.

The *second stage* of labor is the stage during which the presenting part descends through the birth canal. It begins when the cervix is fully dilated and ends when the baby is delivered.

The *third stage* of labor begins after the delivery of the baby and ends with the delivery of the placenta.

The hour immediately after delivery of the placenta is sometimes called the *fourth stage* of labor.

The pregnant patient should be advised to report to the hospital if any of the following occur:

Bleeding. Any active bleeding, whether slight or heavy, is an indication for the patient to report to the hospital for evaluation. (See Chapter 15.) However, the blood-tinged mucus discharge ("bloody show"), while a harbinger of labor, is not in itself an indication for the patient to report to, or to remain in, the hospital.

Ruptured Membranes. The patient should also be advised that rupture of the membranes, an event which might manifest itself as slow leakage of fluid from the vagina or as a gush of fluid from the vagina, mandates her going to the hospital for evaluation. Should the presence of ruptured membranes be confirmed (see Chapter 17), the patient should be admitted to the hospital for further evaluation.

Uterine Contractions. Patients should be informed that uterine contractions occurring 10 minutes apart or less for one hour are an indication for reporting to the hospital.

When the patient presents to the hospital, her prenatal records should be available on the labor and delivery suite. If she has not been seen previously, a complete obstetrical history should be taken.

With the prenatal records in hand, or the history completed, three key questions must be addressed: (1) Is the patient in labor? (2) Are any abnormalities present? (3) How imminent is delivery? To this end, an obstetrical examination is performed. In the absence of bleeding or ruptured membranes, it is useful to begin with a sterile transvaginal digital examination. The introitus is sprayed or cleansed with an antiseptic, the labia majora are separated widely with the index and middle fingers of the one hand, and the index and second fingers of the other hand, clad in a sterile glove, are introduced into the vagina. The examination should initially determine the effacement and dilatation of the cervix. Next, the position of the cervix relative to the axis of the birth canal should be noted. If the cervix is at the midline or anterior and within easy reach, labor has either already begun or will begin from a "ripe" cervix. Should the cervix be far posterior, either labor has not yet begun or the patient is in very early labor. The next things to be decided are the fetopelvic relationships. Presentation, position, presenting part, attitude, and station should be determined.

After completing the pelvic examination, the remainder of the physical examination should be performed if delivery is not near. (See Chapter 6.)

Next, abdominal examination is undertaken to estimate the size of the baby and to determine the baby's position by utilizing Leopold's maneuvers, which are designed to answer four questions in turn (Fig. 7-16): (1) Which fetal pole is in the uterine fundus? (2) To which maternal side is the fetal back? (3) Where is the cephalic prominence with relationship to the fetal small parts? (4) Which fetal part is presenting at the pelvic inlet? The maneuvers were originally described by Leopold and Pantzer[15] as follows:

> First Manipulation—The hands approach each other at the finger tips, then the palms of the hands are laid across the abdomen of the woman. After that the palms slide gently and uniformly upward over the entire pregnant uterus as far as the fundus, thus defining its position in relation to the navel and ensiform cartilage. This manipulation determines at the same time whether the child lies vertical or transverse, whether the head or breech lies in the fundus, the size of the child, and how far pregnancy has advanced.
>
> Second Manipulation—Both extended hands move from the ensiform cartilage to the sides of the abdomen and are laid flat one on each side of the uterus. One hand will feel the small parts, the other the long, large cylinder which corresponds to the child's back. In this manipulation the finding of the child's back is facilitated by placing one hand flat on the median line of the abdomen and pressing the uterus gently backward. Thereby the liquor amnii is pressed toward one side, and the child's back toward the other, nearer to the abdominal walls, (where it) can thus be felt very easily with the other hand.
>
> Third Manipulation—The right or left hand spreads its fingers as wide apart as possible, and with the thumb and tip of the middle finger, seizes the presenting part of the child just above the pelvic inlet. In order to be able to properly seize the head already engaged in the pelvic inlet in primiparae, it should be sought in the direction of the pelvic cavity with the tips of the thumb and middle finger. In multiparae the hand and finger tips are held more horizontally in order to seize the head which now stands higher in the uterus. For facilitating this manipulation in multiparae especially, the other hand, lying upon the fundus of the uterus, presses against the presenting part of the child. If the presenting part is hard and round, it can only be the head which feels like a hard ball and may be moved hither and thither. The breech appears much softer and more uneven.
>
> If the presenting head or breech is felt uncommonly covered, indistinct, and somewhat softer than usual, the suspicion is justified that the placenta lies in the lower uterine segment. If no presenting part can be detected, the head should be sought in the side of the uterus. This effort will usually succeed if the uterus is gently palpated with short strokes of the fingers of one hand. The head will then make short jerking movements.
>
> The third manipulation is of great value in all cases where the presenting part, head or breech, remains either in or above the pelvic inlet. If however–as often occurs in primiparae during the last few weeks of pregnancy or in the course of labor—the presenting part is found already in the cavity or outlet of the pelvis, then the
>
> Fourth Manipulation is of importance. In this it is best for the examiner to stand at the side of the bed, his back turned toward the face of the parturient. The finger tips of both hands now enter slowly and gently from above along the sides of the pelvis into its cavity. Should the tension of the abdominal walls render this manipulation difficult, it may be greatly facilitated by causing the parturient to draw her thighs somewhat upward, to place her heels together, and to separate her knees. When the head is low, one feels distinctly that a hard, round part of the child fully occupies the pelvis, and the more prominent forehead on one side can be readily distinguished from the less prominent nape of the neck on the opposite side. . . .

The fourth maneuver is of no value when the presenting part is floating. However, when the presenting part is in the pelvis, identification of the cephalic prominence (described above as "the more prominent forehead") indicates whether the head is flexed or deflexed. If the head is flexed, the cephalic prominence is felt on the same side as the small parts. If the head is deflexed, the cephalic prominence is felt on the same side as the back.

After completing the physical examination, one next determines whether or not the patient is in active labor. This determination is made by

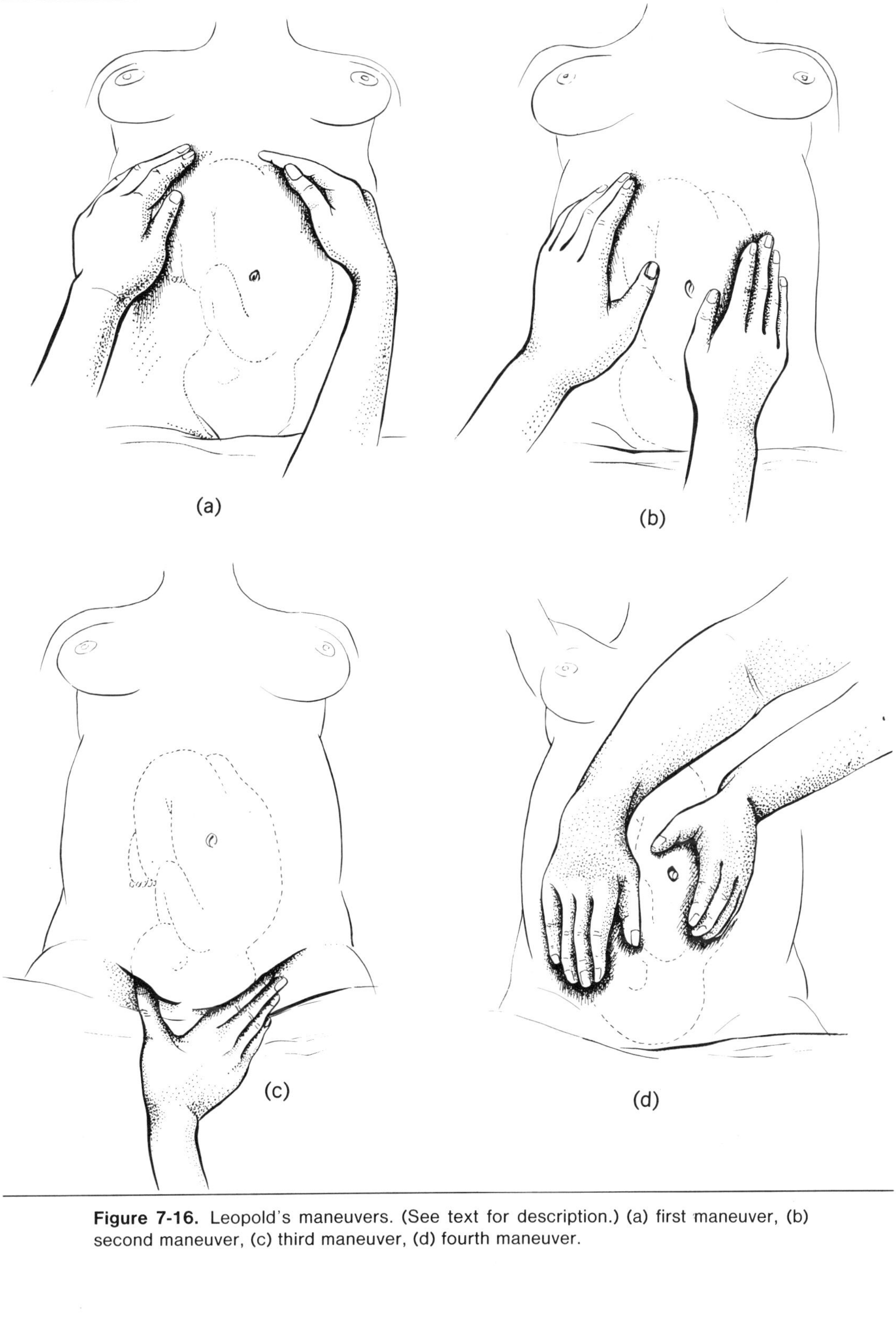

Figure 7-16. Leopold's maneuvers. (See text for description.) (a) first maneuver, (b) second maneuver, (c) third maneuver, (d) fourth maneuver.

observation of frequency and intensity of contractions and changes in effacement and dilatation.

In many hospitals, it is customary to shave the pudenda of the patient admitted in labor and to administer an enema. Review of the literature, as well as clinical experience, reveals no rational basis for these maneuvers. Although it may be necessary at delivery to shorten the pubic hair with a scissor in order to expose the perineum for episiotomy and repair, neither a perineal shave nor an enema are necessary to the conduct of normal labor and delivery.

Progress during labor is best followed by plotting cervical dilatation against time, on semilogarithmic paper (Fig. 7-17). It is often difficult to distinguish between true and false labor, and it is often impossible to identify prospectively the moment that true labor actually begins. In general, the contractions of true labor may be distinguished from those of false labor by the following criteria: The contractions of true labor occur at regular intervals. The intervals between contractions gradually become shorter. As time passes, the intensity of each contraction increases and the perceived pains radiate throughout the lower abdomen and into the back. The contractions of true labor cause progressive cervical dilatation and cannot be stopped by sedating the patient. In contrast, the irregular contractions of false labor or prelabor do not lead to significant cervical dilatation. They occur at irregular intervals. The interval between contractions remains approximately the same as does the intensity of contractions. The pain is perceived chiefly in the abdominal region. The contractions can be stopped or diminished in frequency by sedation.

Because it can be difficult to pick the moment when the contractions of false labor or prelabor transition to those of true labor, various devices are used to designate the time that labor begins. One method dates the onset of labor by asking the patient to identify the time when either contractions began to occur at regular intervals or the time when they changed to the character she is experiencing in labor. Friedman devised a method for following labor by plotting, on square-ruled graph paper, cervical dilatation (on the ordinate) against time in hours (on the abscissa). The onset of labor is dated from the onset of "regular" uterine contractions, as defined above. When one uses these definitions, a sigmoid curve is characteristically obtained. This curve shows a *latent phase* followed by an *acceleration phase* followed by a *deceleration phase*.[7] The latent phase begins with the onset of labor contractions and ends with the beginning of the active phase. The active phase begins when the rate of cervical dilatation begins to accelerate. The active phase ends at full dilatation with the onset of the second stage of labor. The slope of the line plotted during the latent phase is nearly flat, reflecting changes in the cervix and lower uterine segment preparatory to the onset of rapid cervical dilatation. The active phase is further divided into the *acceleration phase* (the onset of the active phase), the nearly linear *phase of maximal slope*, and the *deceleration phase* which ends the active phase (Fig. 7-18).

As might be imagined, the latent phase shows wide variations in length, because its time of onset depends upon the patient's estimate of when regular contractions began.

Other clinicians and uterine physiologists have attempted to avoid this problem by not considering the latent phase at all in their graphic analysis. Rather than attempting to tell from the contraction pattern when the latent phase began and ended, these observers define all contractions prior to cervical dilatation of 3 cm as "prelabor." When this definition is used, a plot of cervical diltation in active labor against time on a semilogarithmic scale results in a straight line. If the labor plot is begun at 3 cm of cervical dilatation, no deceleration phase is noted.[8]

The first stage of labor is completed within 8 hours in primigravidas, and within 6 hours in multiparas. A useful rule of thumb is that at least 1 cm of cervical dilatation should be accomplished per hour. A first stage of labor that lasts 12 or more hours is abnormal. The second stage of labor is completed in less than 1 hour in most instances. More than 2 hours in the second stage, in the presence of active contractions, is considered to be an abnormally prolonged second stage.

Although the progress of labor is largely determined by uterine activity, cervical compliance is also very important. The contractions of active labor arise at some location in the fundus and spread downward over the corpus and lower uterine segment. As labor progresses, the frequency of contractions increases. At the very onset of labor, contractions may occur at 20-minute intervals. In active labor, three to five contractions occur in a 10-minute interval. Contractions occurring 2 minutes apart are frequently observed in advanced labor. The resting pressure between contractions (tonus) is 5–10

BEXAR COUNTY HOSPITAL DISTRICT

COURSE OF LABOR

ADMISSION TIME:____:____

INPATIENT CHART

DATE

Begin plot on admission at "0" hours.

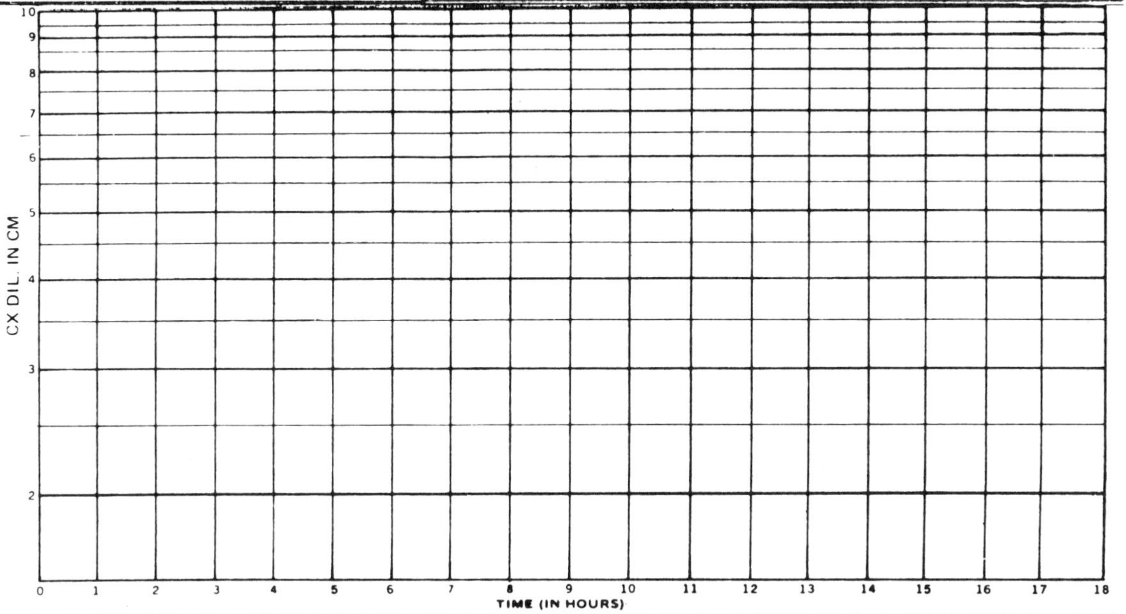

DATE	HOUR	MEMB	CONTRACTION			FH	CERVIX		FETUS		RECORD ALL EXAMS, MED., OBS.	INITIALS
			Freq.	Durat.	Int.		Eff.	Dil.	Pos	Sta.		

ONSET OF LABOR: Date:__/__/__time:___ ONSET OF SECOND STAGE: Date:__/__/__time:___

OXYTOCIN STARTED
Date:__/__/__time:_____
OXYTOCIN DISC.
Date:__/__/__time:_____

CHART ORDER #
IP OP
N OB
321 361

MEDICAL RECORDS FORM
BC# 162 3/79

INPATIENT CHART

Figure 7-17. Form used to chart progress in labor.

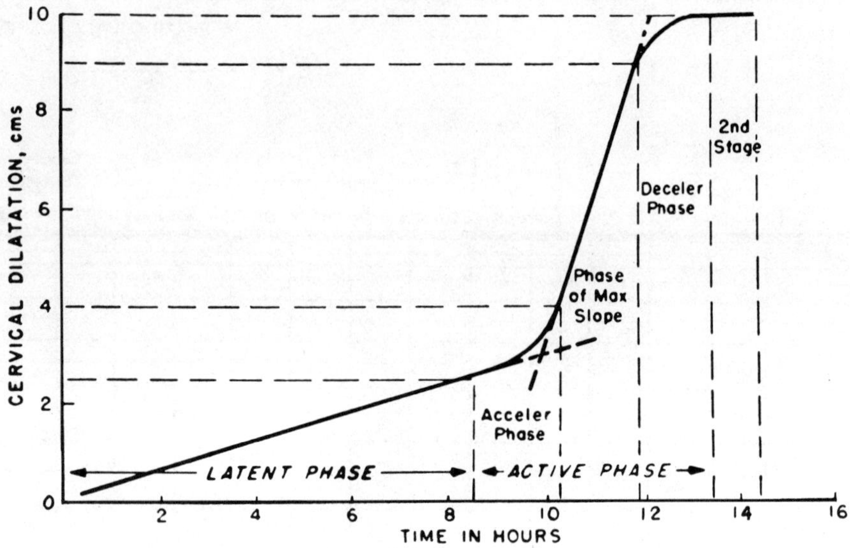

Figure 7-18. Labor curves constructed from 500 nulliparous labors by Friedman.[7] (See text for explanation.) (Reprinted with permission of the American College of Obstetricians and Gynecologists from Friedman, E. A.: Primigravid labor. A graphicostatistical analysis. *Obstet. Gynecol.* **6**:567–589, 1955.)

mmHg, and the amplitude of contractions (maximum increase above resting pressure) is usually 30–50 mmHg. Contractions with intensity below 24 mmHg are associated with slow progress, and those below 15 mmHg with no progress.[2] As labor advances, the average amplitude of contractions also increases.

The examiner can readily evaluate the frequency of contractions and can estimate the amplitude. The hand straddles the fundus with the palm flat against the uterus. As the contraction reaches a peak, the examiner attempts to indent the uterus by compressing an area of its surface between the thumb and opposing fingers. With experience, especially if one has had the opportunity to feel contractions that are also being monitored via an intra-amniotic catheter connected to a pressure transducer, an examiner can learn to judge the approximate amplitude of contractions. By noting the time from the onset of the contraction to its disappearance, the duration of the contraction is recorded. Clinical evaluation of onset and disappearance of a contraction correlates quite well with direct measurements of changes in intrauterine pressure.

The fetal heart rate should be counted, either by auscultation with a stethoscope designed for that purpose (fetoscope) or with an ultrasound transducer that utilizes the Doppler effect to detect the fetal heart. The best time to monitor the fetal heart rate is just after a contraction. The normal fetal heart rate is 120–160 beats per minute. The fetal heart rate should be recorded every 15 minutes during the first stage of labor and every 5 minutes during the second stage of labor.

The effectiveness, or efficacy, of labor is determined by the rate at which the cervix effaces and dilates. This, in turn, depends upon the state of the cervix at the onset of labor. During pregnancy, the cervix must change from a closed tube, which prevents the uterine contents from being extruded, to a very soft and compliant ring that is sufficiently distensible to allow the infant to pass through it. Moreover, these changes must occur at the appropriate time in gestation. If they occur too soon, pregnancy wastage is noted—the "incompetent os" syndrome. If, on the other extreme, the uterus contracts powerfully against an "unripe" cervix, uterine rupture or cervical detachment can occur. "Ripening" of the cervix describes changes which include softening, increased effacement, increased distensibility (compliance), and partial dilatation. Ripening is the final step in a sequence of cervical changes in pregnancy that begin with increased vascularization and hypertrophy in early pregnancy. Hypertrophy is followed by softening of the cervix in the second half of pregnancy. However, this softening is not accompanied by increased compliance.[16]

Ripening results from biochemical changes in the cervix. The cervix is composed of fibroblasts, which secrete collagen and a ground substance composed of glycosaminoglycans and glycoproteins. The collagen fibers are imbedded in the ground substance. The nonpregnant cervix is about 80% collagen, in contrast to the cervix at full dilatation, which is about 50% collagen. It appears that collagen is destroyed and replaced by increased mucopolysaccharides of the ground substance.[5] It is likely that prostaglandins $F_{2\alpha}$ and E_2 are involved in the ripening process.

During the last trimester, the cervix becomes partially *effaced* and partially dilated. These changes are continuations of the changes that occur throughout pregnancy. The cervical canal is 2–3 cm long at the start of the third trimester. *Effacement* refers to the progressive shortening of the cervical canal until it is obliterated. Although the fully effaced cervix, especially in a primigravida, may be only a few millimeters thick, thinning of the cervix is neither necessary to, nor synonymous with, effacement (Fig. 7-19). Judgment of the degree of effacement is based upon estimating what percent of the original length of the cervix has been incorporated into the lower uterine segment. Thus, when the cervix is 4/5 of its original length, it is 20% effaced. Full or complete effacement means that the lower segment is of uniform thickness, from the lateral aspects to the external os. The fully effaced cervix of a multipara is usually much thicker than the fully effaced cervix of a primipara. During the last four weeks of pregnancy, the cervix progressively effaces. Nulliparas are more effaced than multiparas at any given time prior to labor. The average nullipara enters labor 70% effaced, and the average multipara is about 60% effaced. Cervical dilatation also begins prior to the onset of labor. Cervical dilatation of 1–3 cm is seen in a majority of multiparous patients at 6 months of gestation, and in 15% of primigravidas.[6] The mean cervical dilatation increases from about 1 cm 4 weeks prior to delivery to more than 2 cm during the 3 days immediately prior to labor. Upon admission in early labor, the average nullipara's cervix is dilated 2.5 cm and the average multipara's cervix is dilated 3.5 cm.[8]

Most of the work performed by the contracting uterus in the first stage of labor is directed

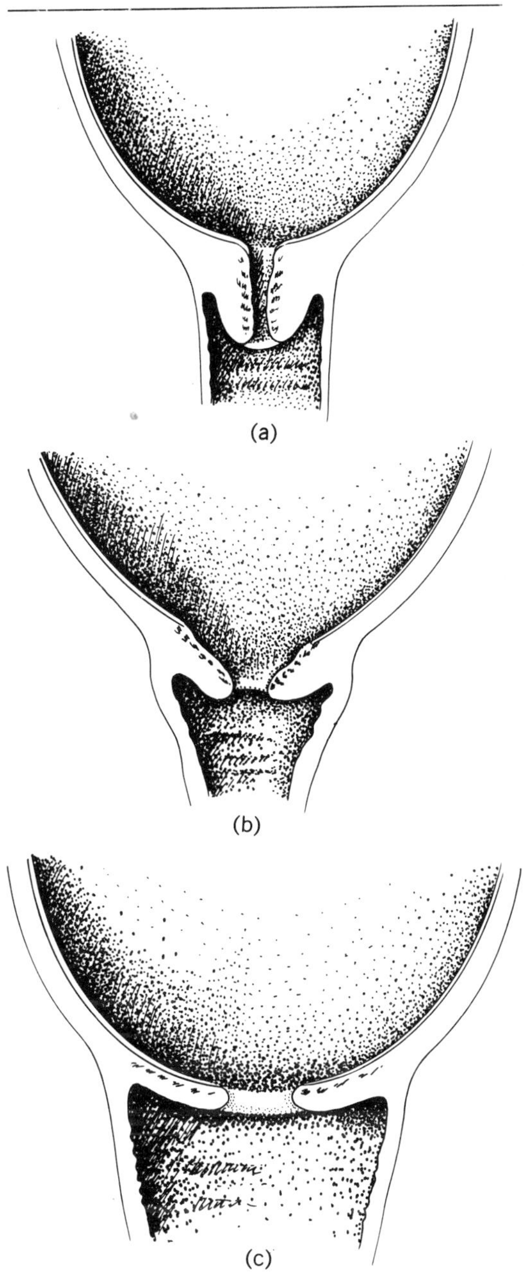

Figure 7-19. At the end of pregnancy, the cervical canal is 2–3 cm long (a). During prelabor and labor, the cervical canal progressively effaces (b). Finally, the cervical canal is obliterated and the lower segment is of uniform thickness (c).

toward progressive effacement and dilatation of the cervix. Thus, it follows that the more effacement and dilatation accomplished prior to the onset of active labor, the less work the uterus must do to accomplish complete effacement and full dilatation. The state of the patient's cervix at the onset of labor thus correlates with the duration of the labor, whether spontaneous or induced. Therefore, various methods of "scoring" the state of the cervix have been presented in the literature.[1]

During the first stage of labor, the lower uterine segment is pulled upward and outward over the presenting part, as the upper segment progressively shortens. The presenting part does not descend significantly until the cervix is fully dilated. After full dilatation, the uterine supporting structures anchor the cervix anteriorly (pubocervical fascia), laterally (cardinal ligaments), and posteriorly (uterosacral ligaments). These structures prevent the cervix from rising higher than the plane of the inlet. Thereafter, uterine contractions cannot pull the cervix any further up, and, instead, the fetus is forced downward into the birth canal.

Other factors that influence the duration of labor include parity, the "fit" of the presenting part against the cervix, and, in cephalic presentations, the position of the head. If one records intrauterine pressure, measures the maximum pressure attained by each contraction from the onset of labor to full dilatation (variously referred to as maximum amplitude or intensity in the literature), and sums these maximum pressures, "uterine work" in labor can be calculated.[4] Less uterine work is required to attain full dilatation in multiparas than in primigravidas; less uterine work is necessary to achieve full dilatation when the head is anterior than when it is in the transverse or posterior position. Good mechanical apposition of the head to the birth canal increases the rate of cervical dilatation in response to a given amount of uterine work. Some instances of failure of progressive cervical dilatation are due to a contracted pelvic inlet preventing the head from coming into close apposition with the lower segment. In breech or transverse positions, the intact membranes serve as a hydrostatic stimulus to the lower uterine segment. When the membranes rupture, dilatation slows or stops, unless the presenting part comes into close and even contact with the lower segment.

Progress in descent and dilatation is ascertained by performing sterile vaginal examinations at regular intervals. If labor is progressing normally, an hourly examination is sufficient. The position and station of the presenting part, the status of the membranes, and the effacement and dilatation of the cervix should be recorded immediately after the examination is completed. It is very important that notes of the examination, as well as notes of other events, include the date and time and are signed. The first stage ends at full dilatation.

After full dilatation, a reflex occurs, probably mediated by the pressure of the presenting part against the birth canal. With the onset of each contraction, the patient grunts and "bears down," tensing all her muscles and utilizing her abdominal musculature to exert pressure on the uterus. The contractions of the second stage are stronger than those of the first stage. They occur every 1.5–2 minutes and last 60–100 seconds. The membranes usually rupture during the second stage but may rupture during the first stage (see also Chapter 22).

During the second stage the presenting part descends to reach the vulva. In cephalic presentations, the head distends the perineum, and the fetal scalp can be seen at the vulva with a contraction. The perineum becomes progressively distended with successive contractions, and the ovoid of fetal scalp visible between the labia becomes larger and more circular (Fig. 7-20).

After each contraction, the head rides upward slightly, so that the visible ovoid of fetal scalp is smaller. Successive contractions enlarge the opening until *crowning*, the stretching of the vulvar opening to encircle the largest diameter of the fetal head, occurs.

Primigravidas should be moved from the labor room to the delivery room when the presenting part is distending the perineum with each contraction. Multiparous patients should be moved to the delivery room when they are 6–8 cm dilated. Meticulous aseptic technique is essential in the delivery suite. Personnel should wear, in addition to clean scrub suits or scrub gowns, shoe covers, masks, and caps.

The position for delivery varies among cultures. In many cultures, the parturient assumes some varient of the upright position, such as kneeling, squatting, sitting or standing. These positions allow more effective use of the muscles of the abdomen to increase intraabdominal pressure. These positions make asepsis and controlled delivery more difficult, however.

In England, the lateral recumbent position is popular. This position avoids compression of the vena cava, and thus avoids the *supine hypotensive syndrome*, and allows controlled delivery of the head and avoidance of lacerations.

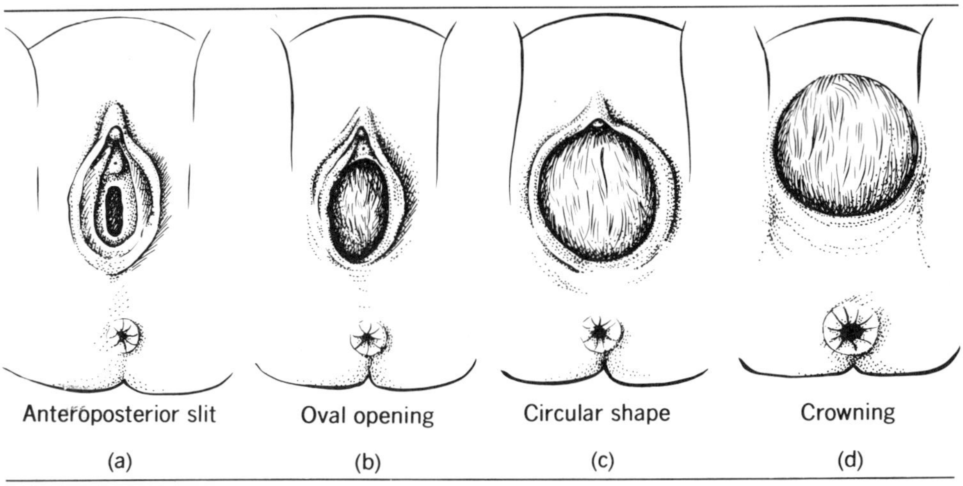

Figure 7-20. Progressive changes in the vulvar opening. The slit-like opening becomes first ovoid, then circular. (See text for details.)

The drawback is that this is a difficult position for management of lacerations and complications of the third stage of labor.

In our delivery rooms, we utilize a semisitting position. The patient is placed on her back, with her legs in stirrups and her buttocks at the lower edge of the delivery table. Our delivery tables have adjustable backs, which we raise to an angle of 30°–45°, adjusted to the patient's comfort (Fig. 7-21). This position increases the efficiency of the expulsive forces over those in the classic dorsal lithotomy position and main-

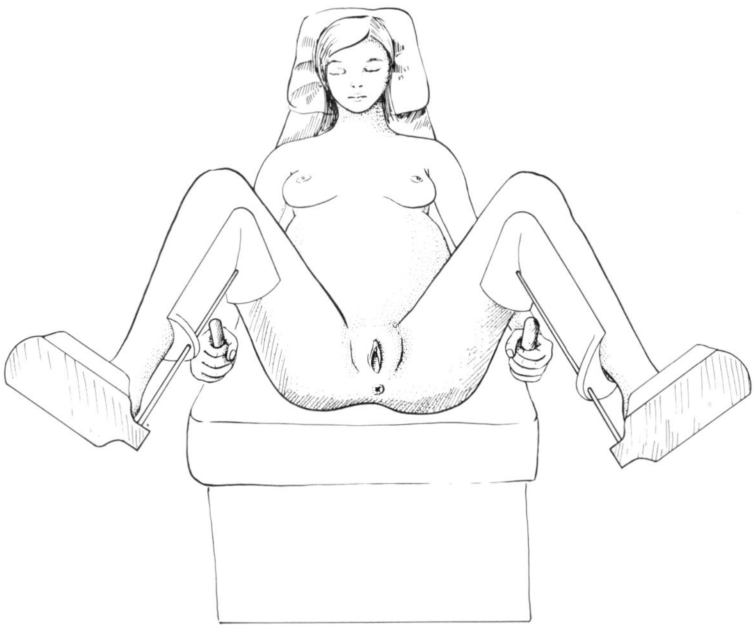

Figure 7-21. Semisitting position used for most deliveries in Medical Center Hospital of The University of Texas Health Science Center at San Antonio.

tains all the advantages of the latter position, allowing asepsis, ready auscultation of the fetal heart, ease of providing anesthesia, and permitting controlled delivery, the use of forceps, episiotomy and repair, and efficient management of the third stage.

After the patient assumes this position, the vulva, inner thighs, and lower abdomen are thoroughly washed with an antiseptic solution, which is then blotted. Sterile drapes are then utilized under the patient's buttocks and to cover the legs and abdomen to the midchest.

After the patient is prepared for delivery, a vaginal examination is performed to evaluate presentation, position, station, cervical dilatation, and state of the membranes.

In multiparous patients, one may elect to deliver the patient without doing an episiotomy. If so, when the head distends the vulva so much that crowning is imminent, it is useful to use the thumb and fingers of one hand to press downward on the occiput to increase flexion. At the same time, the opposite hand, protected by a towel that covers the rectum, lifts the chin upward and forward (Fig. 7-22). The technique was described by its originator, Ferdinand von Ritgen,[18] in 1855 as follows:

> With the three fingers of one hand against the occiput, holding the head back, the four fingers of the other hand are placed with their tips against the posterior perineum, behind the anal orifice, near the tip of the coccyx, and on either side of the medial raphe. During the interval between contractions, preferably right after the cessation of a contraction, inward and upward pressure usually encounters the infant's chin, gliding it forward, while the three fingers on the occiput result in anterior extension of the head, which occurs slowly about the fulcrum of the neck, at the lower border of the pubic symphysis. Both hands are held motionless as soon as a contraction begins and until it is over. Immediately afterward, the pressure is resumed against the chin. As the latter gradually advances, the external pressure on it must also advance, from the posterior perineum to the anal orifice and finally to the anterior perineum, until the chin is delivered across the transverse ligament. The external pressure should be applied somewhat laterally to the median raphe, so that one parietal boss can be delivered through the introitus before the other, this more effectively ensuring against a tear than when both bosses protrude through the introitus simultaneously.

Ritgen's maneuver allows a controlled delivery of the head; the slow extension of the head protects the perineum from laceration. Modern obstetrical practice favors protection of the perineum (and probably the head) in delivery of primigravidas and many multiparas, by performing prophylactic episiotomy. Episiotomy should be performed before the muscles of the pelvic floor have been stretched excessively, and yet close enough to delivery to avoid excessive

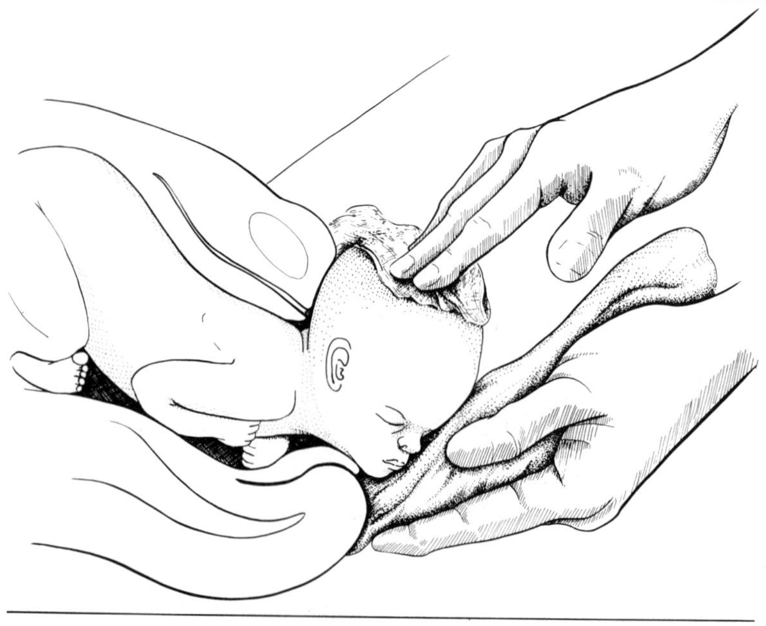

Figure 7-22. Ritgen's maneuver. (See text for description.)

blood loss from the episiotomy. Most clinicians perform the episiotomy when 2–3 cm of fetal scalp is visible at the introitus between contractions. Although either median or mediolateral episiotomy may be done, most obstetricians favor median episiotomy except in specific circumstances (see Chapter 43).

The sinciput descends along the sacral curve, and the bregma, forehead, nose, mouth, and chin are sequentially delivered over the perineum. Soon after the head is delivered, it rotates 45° toward the transverse diameter (OA to LOA or to ROA). This *restitution* restores the normal relationship between the head and the shoulders because the shoulders had remained in the oblique diameter, while the neck had twisted to allow the head to rotate directly anterior.

The shoulders descend through the pelvis in the oblique diameter. Upon contact with the pelvic floor, the anterior shoulder rotates from the anterior oblique to the direct anteroposterior diameter. The head accompanies this rotation and rotates from the right or left oblique to the right or left transverse.

The anterior shoulder comes into close contact with the inferior margin of the symphysis, and becomes a fulcrum, just as the occiput did earlier. The posterior shoulder is then delivered over the perineum by lateral flexion. The remainder of the body follows without difficulty.

The physician controls the delivery of the infant's body. A useful way is to use the hand that is on the side corresponding to the infant's back to hold the infant's shoulder. The infant's head rests on this hand. As delivery of the body proceeds, the opposite hand is substituted, and the hand originally placed on the shoulder now slides down the infant's back to the junction of legs and torso. The middle finger is placed between the thighs, while the palm and remaining digits support and control the legs and buttocks. The baby is held against the examiner's lap while the cord is clamped.

The third stage of labor, which begins after delivery of the baby and ends with delivery of the placenta, usually begins with escape of the remaining amniotic fluid. The uterine fundus is palpable just below the umbilicus. The third stage of labor requires two separate, but related, processes—separation of the placenta and expulsion of the placenta. The shearing of the placenta from its uterine attachments usually occurs 2–3 minutes after delivery. Placental separation is signaled by the uterine fundus rising above the umbilicus, and a greater length of umbilical cord protruding from the vulva, usually accompanied by an increase in vaginal bleeding. At this point the uterus should be palpated. If it is firm, the examiner may push downward on the fundus and, at the same time, exert steady gentle traction on the umbilical cord with the other hand. Although some authorities have stated that traction on the cord might cause uterine inversion (see Chapter 47), this has not been documented. Indeed, the only problem associated with cord traction is that, if one pulls too hard, the cord breaks, and there is nothing to pull on thereafter.

If the placenta has not separated by the time that the physician has finished with the infant, several options are available. In the absence of active bleeding, one may simply wait for placental separation to occur. The amount of time that one is willing to wait varies greatly from place to place. In our own clinic, we wait about 20 minutes. In the presence of active bleeding, or after an appropriate interval of waiting, manual removal of the placenta may be performed (Fig. 7-23). One hand is placed upon the abdomen to steady the uterus. The other hand is held with the fingers extended and overlapped to be as narrow as possible and is inserted into the vagina and then carefully and slowly through the cervix into the corpus of the uterus. The cord is palpated, and followed to its origin at the placenta. Next, the placental edge is located, and the cleavage plane between placenta and uterus is entered. The ulnar margin of the hand is inserted into this plane, with the palmar surface of the fingers in contact with the maternal side of the placenta. The placenta is then separated from the uterus with a side-to-side shearing motion. After the entire placenta has been separated from the uterus, it is grasped in the hand and withdrawn.

If no cleavage plane can be located, or if an area of tenacious adherence of the placenta to the uterine wall is encountered, attempts at manual removal should be stopped at once, because no attempt should be made to remove a *placenta accreta* manually (see also Chapter 47).

Most obstetricians routinely administer ecbolic agents in the immediate puerperium. The agents used are oxytocin, or ergonovine maleate, or some combination of oxytocin and an ergot derivative. The timing and route of administration also vary. There is little rationale for routine use of ecbolic agents. The average blood loss associated with normal delivery is about 500 ml, most of which is lost during the first hour. Clinicians have come to believe that

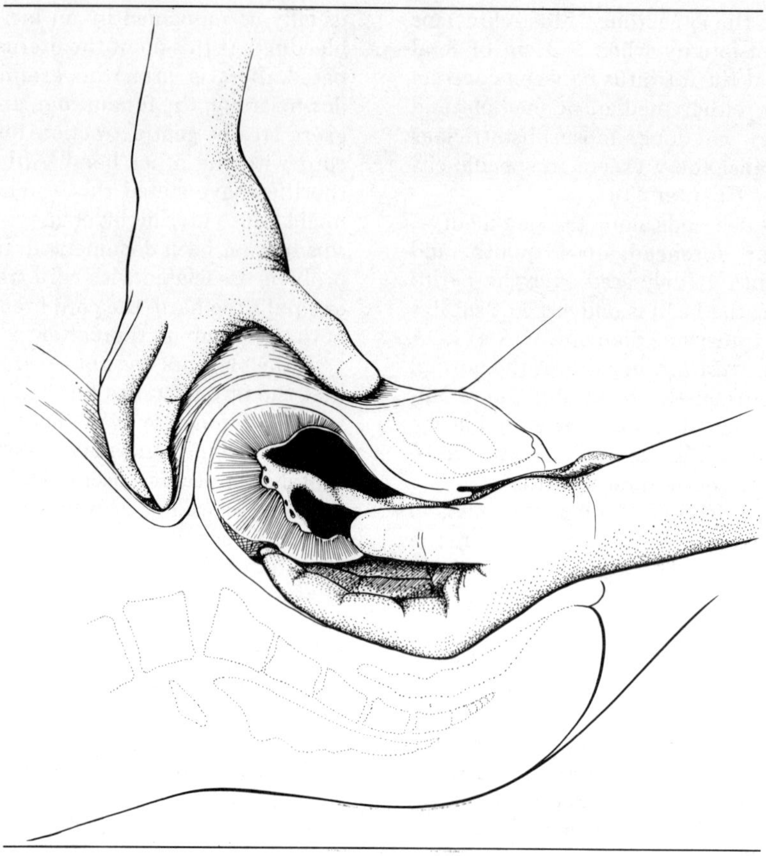

Figure 7-23. Manual removal of the placenta. The placenta edge is located, and the cleavage plane between the placenta and the uterus is entered. (See text for description.)

the amount of blood lost is related to the rapidity of placental separation. Many obstetricians also believe that puerperal hemostasis is obtained by the uterus maintaining a state of tonic contracture for several hours postpartum. Because of these beliefs, various drugs and manipulations have been utilized to accelerate placental detachment and expulsion and to maintain the puerperal uterus in a contracted state.

In reality, neither of these assumptions is justified. Several studies have shown that shearing of the placenta from its uterine attachment occurs within 2–3 minutes after delivery. Furthermore, the normal puerperal uterus does not remain tonically contracted. The uterus continues to contract intermittently immediately postpartum, with two major changes from the pattern seen late in the first stage of labor. The frequency of contractions decreases, so that 1 hour after delivery, they occur about half as often as they did in the late first stage. The intensity of contractions increases progressively during the first 20–30 minutes after delivery, to reach values above those seen in the first stage of labor. Both intensity and frequency gradually diminish during the early puerperium. Contractions may occur as infrequently as 4/hour with resting pressures (tonus) as low as 5 mmHg, yet no increased blood loss occurs in such patients, whether or not they have received an oxytocic agent. Thus, postpartum uterine hemostasis is independent of sustained uterine contracture.[9] Such studies suggest that routine postpartum use of ecbolic agents may be quite unnecessary, a conclusion that many experienced obstetricians have reached on purely clinical grounds. (See also Chapter 47.)

REFERENCES

1. Bishop, E. H.: Pelvic scoring for elective induction. *Obstet. Gynecol.* **24**:266–268, 1964.

2. Caldeyro Barcia, R. and Alvarez, H.: Abnormal uterine action in labour. *J. Obstet. Gynaecol. Br. Emp.* **59**:646–656, 1952.
3. Caldwell, W. E. and Moloy, H. C.: Anatomical variations in the female pelves and their effect in labor with a suggested classification. *Am. J. Obstet. Gynecol.* **26**:479–504, 1933.
4. Cibils, L. A. and Hendricks, C. H.: Normal labor in vertex presentation. *Am. J. Obstet. Gynecol.* **91**:385–395, 1965.
5. Danforth, D. N.: Early studies of the anatomy and physiology of the human cervix and implications for the future. In: *Dilatation of the Uterine Cervix: Connective Tissue Biology and Clinical Management*, F. Naftolin and P. G. Stubblefield (Eds.). New York, Raven Press, 1980, pp. 3–15.
6. Floyd, W. S.: Cervical dilatation in the mid-trimester of pregnancy. *Obstet. Gynecol.* **18**:380–381, 1961.
7. Friedman, E. A.: *Labor, Clinical Evaluation and Management.* New York, Appleton-Century-Crofts, 1967, pp. 27–41.
8. Hendricks, C., Brenner, W. E., and Kraus, G.: Normal cervical dilatation pattern in late pregnancy and labor. *Am. J. Obstet. Gynecol.* **106**:1065–1082, 1970.
9. Hendricks, C. H.: Uterine contractility changes in the early puerperium. *Clin. Obstet. Gynecol.* **1**:125–144, 1968.
10. Kaltreider D. F.: The contracted outlet. *JAMA* **154**:824–827, 1954.
11. Kaltreider, D. F.: Criteria of midplane contraction. What is their value? *Am. J. Obstet. Gynecol.* **63**:392–399, 1952.
12. Kaltreider, D. F.: The diagonal conjugate. *Am. J. Obstet. Gynecol.* **61**:1075–1086, 1951.
13. Kaltreider, D. F.: Pelvic shape and its relation to midplane prognosis. *Am. J. Obstet. Gynecol.* **63**:116–121, 1952.
14. Kaltreider, D. F.: The prediction and management of outlet dystocia. *Am. J. Obstet. Gynecol.* **67**:1049–1066, 1954.
15. Leopold, G. and Pantzer, M. E. C.: Die Beschränkung der inneren und die groösstmoögliche Verwerthung der aüsseren Untersuchung in der Geburtshülfe. Vierter Beitrag zur Verhütung des Kindbettfiebers mit einem Rückblicke auf das Jahr 1889. *Arch. Gnäek. (Berl.)* **38**:330–366, 1890.
16. Liggins, G. C.: Ripening of the cervix. *Semin. Perinatol.* **2**:261–271, 1978.
17. O'Driscoll, K., Foley, M., and MacDonald, D.: Active management of labor as an alternative to cesarean section for dystocia. *Obstet. Gynecol.* **63**:485–490, 1984.
18. Ritgen, F. von: Ueber sein Dammschutz verfahren. *Monatsschr. Geburtsk. Frauenkrankh.* **6**:321–347, 1855.

8

ANALGESIA AND ANESTHESIA FOR NORMAL LABOR AND DELIVERY

This chapter presents recent developments in obstetrical analgesia and describes innovations in the field. The subject matter is divided into sections dealing with systemic analgesia for labor, regional analgesia, general anesthesia for labor and cesarean section, and effects of anesthesia on neonatal neurobehavior.

Substances administered to women in labor have access to both maternal and fetal tissues and are distributed widely among maternal and fetal fluids and tissues according to their individual characteristics. Transfer of drugs across the placenta is largely by simple diffusion. Passage is flow dependent and affected significantly by protein binding,[25] drug molecular weight, degree of ionization, fat solubility, and acid–base balance.

Reduction in maternal blood levels of drug occurs through metabolism and elimination via the kidney and/or the liver. Fetal drug elimination occurs by rediffusion into the maternal circulation and through direct fetal metabolism. In general, fetal metabolic pathways are poorly developed. For this reason, drugs trapped in the fetal circulation at delivery may exert prolonged effects on the newborn.[20]

SYSTEMIC ANALGESIA FOR LABOR

During the past three decades, meperidine has achieved preeminence as a systemic analgesic during labor. It is generally preferred over morphine because it produces less nausea and vomiting and appears to accumulate less readily in the fetal brain. Intravenous administration has largely superseded intramuscular administration because smaller doses may be given i.v., and systemic effects may be titrated more precisely.

Meperidine crosses the placenta rapidly. It has been recovered from the fetus within 2 minutes of maternal administration. Equilibrium may be achieved within 6 minutes,[51] reaching typical umbilical cord to maternal vein concentration ratios of 0.75:0.90.[52] Plasma protein binding is approximately 64%.[34] The elimination half-life of meperidine in the infant is 18.1 hours, seven times longer than the maternal elimination half-life of 2.42 hours.[8] This appears to be due to physiologically impaired neonatal hepatic metabolism.

Meperidine is metabolized in the liver through *N*-demethylation to produce normeperidine. Meperidinic acid is also produced as the product of hydrolysis. Normeperidine has significant analgesic properties and toxicity greater than or equal to that of the parent compound, meperidine.[5,35,36] Following exposure of the mother to multiple doses of meperidine during labor, both meperidine and normeperidine accumulate continuously in fetal tissues. Normeperidine levels of 60% or more of the total active drug can be present in fetal blood at the time of delivery.[37] The greatest neonatal excretion of meperidine occurs when the maternal drug administration to delivery interval is 2–3 hours. Maximum normeperidine excretion occurs when drug administration to delivery intervals exceed 4 hours.[35,36]

Meperidine produces maternal hypoventilation and hypoxia when administered. In labor, maternal PO_2 increases with uterine contractions and falls 20–50% when measured between contractions. After administration of as little as 50 mg of meperidine, maternal PO_2 falls by an additional 10% or more.[30] In the presence of borderline fetal asphyxia, this drop in PO_2 could significantly increase fetal acidosis.

Butorphanol, a synthetic parenteral analgesic with mixed agonist-antagonist properties, offers potential advantages as an analgesic for the laboring woman. It is five times as potent as morphine, 20 times as potent as pentazocine, and 40 times as potent as meperidine.[15] It crosses the placenta rapidly and is promptly distributed to fetal and maternal tissues. Protein binding is 80%. Metabolism is by dealkylation, hydroxylation, and conjugation in the liver. The metabolites of butorphanol are inactive. Excretion is primarily renal, with a small contribution from the biliary system. Two milligrams of butorphanol produce a degree of respiratory depression similar to that caused by 10 mg of morphine. Doubling the butorphanol dosage augments respiratory depression only slightly, whereas a substantial increase is produced by 20 mg of morphine. Butorphanol may thus offer a significant advantage over meperidine and morphine.[33,45]

Placental transmission of butorphanol occurs readily with a mean umbilical venous to maternal ratio of 0.84 being achieved within 1.5–3.5 hours after intramuscular administration.[39] Cervical dilation and Apgar scores are equivalent with meperidine and butorphanol, but the latter provides superior maternal analgesia.[49] In summary, butorphanol provides good pain relief, produces inactive metabolites, and appears to cause minimal maternal and neonatal respiratory depression when utilized for labor analgesia.

The following principles for the use of systemic analgesia during labor are recommended: (1) Since the total dosage of administered narcotic and the time from administration to delivery are critical factors governing transfer of drug to the fetus, use the smallest dosage possible, administered as near to the time of delivery as practical. (2) Repetition of dosage should be kept to a minimum to avoid accumulation of drug and drug metabolites in the fetus. (3) Intramuscular administration should be avoided because of uncertainty of absorption and because relatively large doses are needed to produce satisfactory maternal analgesia. (4) Recommended drugs and i.v. dosages include meperidine, 25 mg, or butorphanol, 1 mg, administered, when possible, within 2 hours of delivery. (5) Administration should be timed so that the maximum infusion of the drug occurs during a uterine contraction when placental perfusion is minimal. Although a drug administered to the mother may be eliminated promptly and completely from her system, it may be trapped for a considerable period in her fetus and newborn.

REGIONAL ANALGESIA FOR LABOR

Pharmacology

The local anesthetic molecule consists of three parts: (1) a lipophilic aromatic group, (2) a tertiary or secondary amino group, and (3) an ester or amide intermediate chain. Of the four drugs used commonly in obstetric anesthesia, 2-chloroprocaine and tetracaine are ester-linked drugs, and lidocaine and bupivacaine are amide-linked drugs. Metabolism of the ester drugs is accomplished through rapid hydrolysis by plasma cholinesterases. 2-Chloroprocaine is the most rapidly metabolized and has a maternal serum half-life of 21 seconds and a fetal serum half-life of 43 seconds.[19] Tetracaine is a long-acting ester drug of considerable potency and toxicity. It is used primarily for spinal anesthesia. Of the amide drugs, lidocaine is the shortest acting and least toxic. Bupivacaine has a slower onset of action, but the duration of action is considerably longer than that of the other drugs. Onset and duration of action for all drugs are related to the concentration.

The availability of a local anesthetic drug for distribution to the fetoplacental unit depends upon several factors, including maternal protein binding, uterine blood flow, total blood concentration, peak concentration, maternal tissue uptake, maternal and fetal metabolism and excretion, and concomitant administration of epinephrine to reduce drug absorption.[50]

Bupivacaine has considerable cardiotoxicity.[18] Cardiac arrests have been reported in women being prepared for cesarean section under epidural analgesia with bupivacaine. These have been associated chiefly with the use of the 0.75% concentration of this drug. The FDA has withdrawn approval for this concentration of bupivacaine. Following bupivacaine-induced cardiac arrest, immediate delivery by cesarean section may enhance maternal cardiac venous return by reducing aorta–caval compression by the pregnant uterus, thus facilitating resuscitation.[41]

Bupivacaine cardiotoxicity is related to its binding to cardiac muscle tissue in high concentration.[24] Acidosis exacerbates the cardiotoxic effects of bupivacaine.

The healthy fetus is able to tolerate significant amounts of local anesthetic drug in its bloodstream and tissues. However, in the presence of fetal acidosis, the tolerance to these compounds and their metabolites is reduced.

Pudendal and Paracervical Block (PCB)

In performing pudendal block, relatively large quantities of local anesthetics are used. The drugs of choice are 1% lidocaine, 0.5% bupivacaine, and 1% or 2% 2-chloroprocaine. The technique of pudendal block is straightforward[6] (Fig. 8-1). After the patient has been prepped and draped and is in the lithotomy position, the Iowa trumpet is placed into the vagina so that the ring of the trumpet is over the thumb of the left hand and the bead at the tip is at the tip of the second finger. The left maternal ischial spine is palpated. The end of the trumpet is placed at the spine over the insertion of the left sacrospinous ligament. A long pudendal needle which has been previously marked such that no more than 1 cm may project beyond the tip of the trumpet, is inserted into the trumpet. The tip of the needle is passed into the vaginal mucosa overlying the sacrospinous ligament just posterior and medial to the tip of the ischial spine. A submucosal wheal is made by injecting a small amount of local anesthetic solution. The needle is then advanced through the sacrospinous ligament near its attachment to the ischial spine. Constant pressure is applied to the plunger while the needle is advanced through the ligament. A sudden loss of resistance occurs when the tip of the needle penetrates the ligament and enters the space posterior to it where

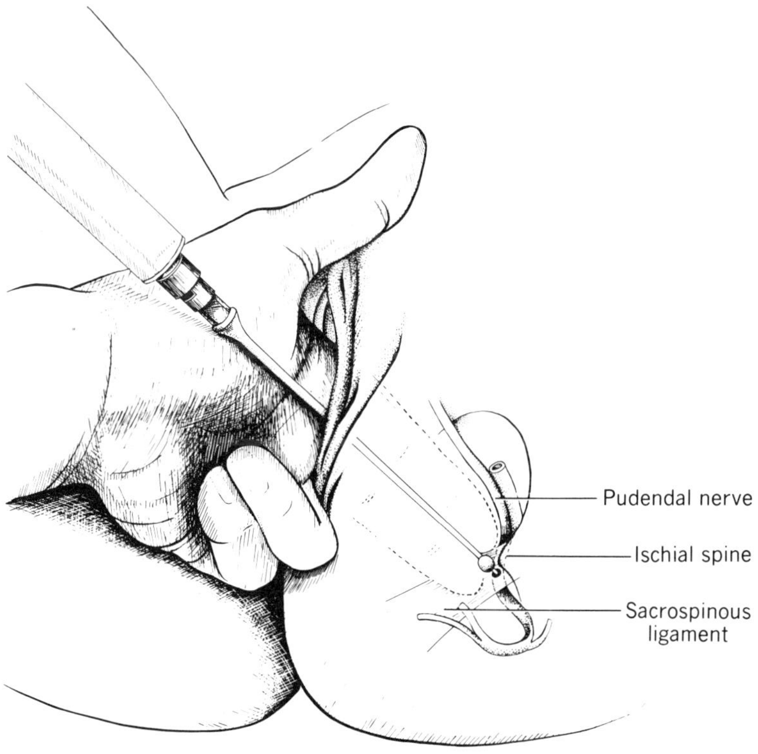

Figure 8-1. Technique of pudendal block. The ischial spine is located by palpation, and the trumpet is placed over the insertion of the sacrospinous ligament. See text for detailed description.

the pudendal nerve and its accompanying vessels are located. Aspiration is then carried out. If aspiration yields arterial or venous blood, the needle should be withdrawn slightly and aspiration repeated. If no blood is obtained, 3–5 ml of local anesthetic solution is injected. The needle is then withdrawn to the vaginal mucosa and reinserted. Another 3 ml of local anesthetic solution is injected. The needle is then withdrawn. To block the right pudendal nerve, the operator's right hand is inserted into the vagina as the left manipulates the syringe. No more than 20 ml of local anesthetic solution should be used to block both pudendal nerves.

A significant advantage of pudendal block is that the administration-to-delivery interval is short, thus minimizing fetal drug accumulation. Only in the event of a direct intravascular injection will the fetus acquire significant quantities of local anesthetic drug. Retropsoas and subgluteal abscesses can follow pudendal block and PCB analgesia. This diagnosis should be suspected in any parturient in whom hip pain and fever subsequently develop.

PCB remains a highly controversial technique. Obstetricians without access to epidural analgesia often rely heavily on this technique for pain relief during the first stage of labor. The chief complication is post-PCB bradycardia. This occurs from 3 to 10 minutes following injection. Incidence appears to be related to type of drug, its concentration, and volume of injection. Although the cause of bradycardia has not been definitively ascertained, evidence is accumulating that fetal hypoxia is responsible. In vitro studies using isolated uterine artery segments demonstrated that arterial segments constrict when exposed to local anesthetic drugs.[9] This response of the uterine vasculature should result in reduced uterine blood flow upon exposure to circulating blood levels of local anesthetic drugs. In vivo studies in gravid ewes[21] demonstrate significant reductions in uterine blood flow when this vascular bed is exposed to local anesthetics. Human fetal scalp PO_2 declines 5 minutes after injection of 200 mg of 1% lidocaine.[4] This supports a hypoxic etiology for post-PCB bradycardia.

The principal drugs employed for PCB are lidocaine, 1%; bupivacaine, 0.25%; and 2-chloroprocaine, 1%. There are disadvantages to all three. Bupivacaine produces the longest duration of analgesia but is not approved for this indication by the FDA. 2-Chloroprocaine produces adequate, though brief, analgesia with a mean duration of only 39 minutes.[60] Lidocaine is intermediate and in the author's view remains the preferred agent.

Paracervical block utilizes the same Iowa trumpet guide employed in pudendal block.[6] (Fig. 8-2). The patient should be in the lithotomy position, preferably in the delivery room. The injection can also be done in the labor room, though with more difficulty. The Iowa trumpet is grasped in the same manner as for pudendal block and is inserted into the left or right lateral vaginal fornix. The cervix should be between 4 and 8 cm dilated. Prior to 4 cm of dilatation, the block is apt to inhibit labor, whereas after 8 cm of dilatation, the block is technically difficult and carries an increased risk of accidental injection into the fetal scalp. The injection is made at three to four o'clock in the left vaginal fornix. The long needle, prepared so that no more than 3 mm can extend beyond the tip of the trumpet, is then inserted into the trumpet. With this system, only mucosal penetration is achieved. Once the mucosa is penetrated, aspiration is accomplished. If no blood is returned, approximately 6 ml of local anesthetic solution is injected. The trumpet and needle are now directed to the right vaginal fornix, at the eight to nine o'clock position. Mucosal penetration is accomplished with the needle and 6 ml of local anesthetic solution is injected.

The following guidelines are offered for prophylaxis of post-PCB bradycardia[10]: (1) The drug must be used in low concentration, in low volume, and without added epinephrine (1% lidocaine, 6–8 ml each side, is preferred). (2) Superficial injection should be utilized. Needle penetration to a depth of greater than 5 mm should be avoided. (3) Bupivacaine should probably be avoided because its effects on uterine blood flow and myometrial contractility appear to be more significant and prolonged than those of the other agents.

Subarachnoid Block Analgesia

The chief advantage of this regional block is that only small doses of local anesthetic drug need be administered. For example, 30 mg of lidocaine produces excellent analgesia for vaginal delivery. The disadvantages include hypotension, respiratory arrest, and postspinal headache. Lidocaine and tetracaine are the time-honored drugs for spinal analgesia. Recently, bupivacaine has been evaluated as an alternative. Bupivacaine, 0.5% in 8% glucose

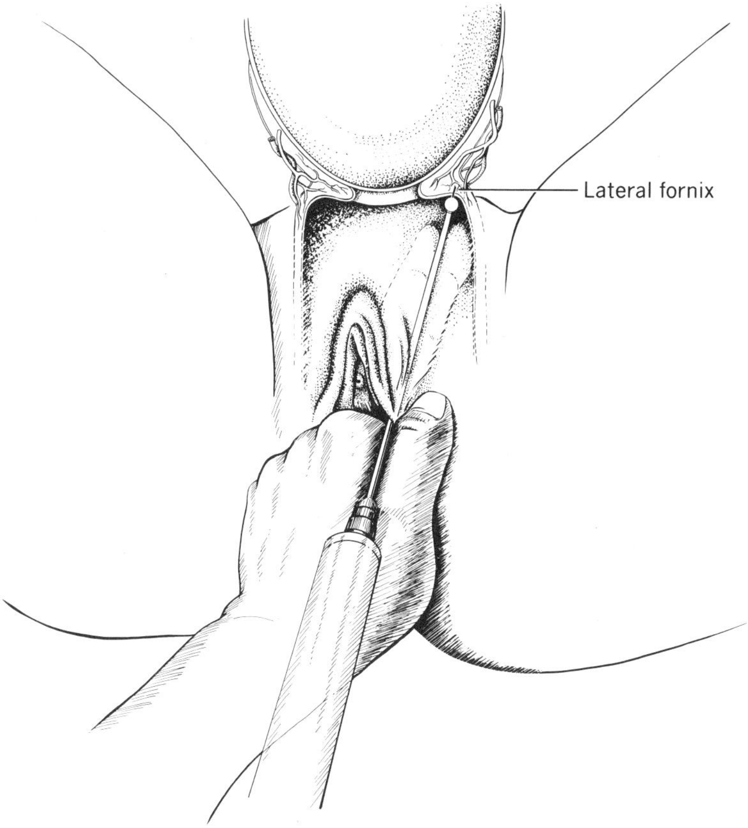

Figure 8-2. Technique for paracervical block. The drawing shows the proper placement of the needle guide.

solution, has been utilized at a dose varying from 7.5 mg to 10 mg, depending upon the height of the patient. With this concentration of bupivacaine there is a less profound motor block than with tetracaine. Hyperbaric bupivacaine is apparently a safe and efficacious drug for establishing spinal anesthesia for cesarean section.[53]

Recently, efforts have been made to achieve analgesia for labor utilizing intrathecal opiates. Injection of 1 or 2 mg of morphine intrathecally after cervical dilation of at least 3 cm is achieved completely relieves the pain of labor within 15–60 minutes. Analgesia persists for 8–11 hours. Arterial blood pressure, heart rate, pin prick sensation, and motor power are unchanged during the period of analgesia. Side effects are somnolence, pruritus, nausea, and vomiting. These can be effectively reversed with naloxone.[2] Similar results are obtained with the administration of 1 mg of synthetic beta-endorphin intrathecally.[48] This approach holds promise for the future.

Lumbar Epidural Analgesia (LEA)

LEA is not a single technique. Its effects differ depending upon the drug, method of administration, and volume and concentration of anesthetic agent employed. One often hears that "epidural analgesia" produces hypotension, or prolongs labor, or mandates the use of forceps. In some cases these are valid criticisms. However, selection of the optimal drug dosage and technique of administration nearly eliminates these problems. LEA is rapidly becoming the most widely used form of regional block analgesia for relief of pain during labor and delivery. The most popular drugs for LEA are bupivacaine, 0.125–0.5%; lidocaine, 1–2%; and 2-chloroprocaine, 1–2%. Mepivacaine, formerly the drug of choice for LEA, accumulates in fetal tissues and in the amniotic fluid, resulting in increased toxicity for the newborn.[7] Its use has been largely abandoned. Most anesthesiologists prefer 0.25% bupivacaine (5–7 ml) for LEA during the first stage of labor. Although occasional "spotty" sensory blockade occurs with this low concentration, this disadvantage is offset by the relative lack of motor impairment. 2-Chloroprocaine is generally preferred for delivery analgesia, although 1% or 2% lidocaine is also popular. 2-Chloroprocaine has a rapid onset of action, producing a profound motor blockade which increases pelvic relaxation, thus facilitating delivery. Mean maternal blood levels 30 minutes after administration of 20 mg of bupivacaine for segmental LEA were less than 0.2 ηg/ml and fetal scalp blood levels were less than 0.05 ηg/ml. The fetal–maternal ratio for bupivacaine was approximately 1:5 during labor. Maternal hypotension correlates with fetal bradycardia, but fetal blood level of bupivacaine does not.[32]

To eliminate the postinjection peaks of local anesthetic drug and to reduce maternal and fetal concentrations, many anesthesiologists now employ continuous administration of local anesthetic solutions for LEA. The technique involves the initial epidural administration of a 2–10 ml loading dose of bupivacaine, 0.25–0.5%, followed by continuous infusion at a rate of 5–10 ml per hour. The lowest effective concentration of bupivacaine should be infused for the shortest possible time.

Continuous infusions of bupivacaine, 2-chloroprocaine, and lidocaine have no significant effect on baseline fetal heart rate (FHR) or uterine activity. Although late and variable FHR decelerations are noted more frequently in the bupivacaine group, neurologic and adaptive capacity scores do not differ among the three groups of neonates. No neonates in the experimental group score lower than a control group of neonates whose mothers do not receive analgesia for labor and delivery.[1]

Since narcotics administered epidurally do not produce sympathetic blockade and its associated hypotension, several recent studies have been carried out to evaluate this form of analgesia for labor. In general, it appears that morphine administered in the epidural space produces poor labor analgesia[29,52] and gains rapid access to the maternal circulation, and thus is available for transfer to the fetus. Maternal and fetal respiratory depression have been reported[57] and postpartum emesis is common.[12] Because of these unfavorable experiences with morphine, other narcotics have been investigated.

Many obstetricians believe that LEA slows labor. The literature both supports and refutes this view. Because of the presence of many confounding variables, and due to the difficulty in securing satisfactory controls, few adequate studies exist. In general, LEA does not appear to significantly prolong the first stage of labor. However, the second stage is prolonged, largely because of decreased voluntary expulsive forces. Thus, the rate of forceps delivery is increased. The forceps rate can be reduced by allowing adequate duration of the second stage of labor, during which the parturient employs voluntary bearing down efforts in conjunction with uterine contractions. Full perineal analgesia should be avoided until crowning of the presenting part occurs.

LEA increases the incidence of abnormal FHR patterns such as late decelerations.[38,55] However, many of the changes are transient. FHR changes may be associated with transient uterine hypertonus during the second stage of labor arising in association with oxytocin administration. Oxytocin should be used judiciously and in conjunction with careful monitoring when employed with LEA.

LEA exerts a beneficial effect on oxygen consumption ($\dot{V}O_2$) and minute ventilation ($\dot{V}E$) between and during uterine contractions in the first stage of labor.[23] During contractions before LEA, $\dot{V}O_2$ and $\dot{V}E$ increased by 43% and 75%, respectively, whereas following LEA there was no significant increase in either parameter during contractions. During contractions with pushing, $\dot{V}O_2$ and $\dot{V}E$ were 25% and 31% lower, respectively, in patients having LEA, compared with those having no analgesia or sedation. The increase in $\dot{V}O_2$ and $\dot{V}E$ in labor is apparently primarily due to pain associated with uterine contractions.

GENERAL ANALGESIA FOR LABOR

General analgesia is infrequently used during labor. The popularity of the methoxyflurane inhaler has diminished since discovery that overdosage with this agent could cause high output renal failure. Entonox, a 50%:50% mixture of N_20 and 0_2, is still popular in Great Britain but has not found acceptance in the United States.

GENERAL ANESTHESIA FOR LABOR AND CESAREAN SECTION

General anesthesia is rarely indicated for vaginal delivery. It is largely restricted to difficult breech or twin delivery. The mask techniques of the past, utilizing ether or cyclopropane, have given way to endotracheal anesthesia. In an effort to reduce the degree of newborn depression, light anesthesia techniques utilizing systemic analgesics and muscle relaxants have evolved. In the United States, the most popular general anesthesia technique utilizes sodium thiopental, 3–5 mg/kg, as the induction agent, followed by succinylcholine, 40–100 mg, to facilitate tracheal intubation. N_20 in 0_2 is used to maintain analgesia until delivery of the fetus has been accomplished. Preoxygenation with 100% oxygen is utilized to increase oxygen stores in the lungs. In the presence of fetal distress, utilization of 100% oxygen until delivery of the infant is encouraged. Under general anesthesia, when the maternal $Pa0_2$ is raised from 100 to 300 torr, umbilical vein PO_2 is raised from approximately 30 torr to approximately 50 torr.[52] Until recently, the improvement in fetal oxygenation with increasing maternal $Pa0_2$ was thought not to continue with increases of $Pa0_2$ above 300 torr. However, women breathing 100% oxygen during cesarean section under LEA demonstrate an increase of umbilical venous PO_2 to 57 torr when a maternal $Pa0_2$ of 523 torr is achieved. This decreases the average time to sustained respirations of the newborn from approximately 40 seconds, with mothers breathing room air, to 12 seconds when breathing 100% O_2.[51]

To reduce the likelihood of aspiration of gastric contents, cricoid pressure is utilized to compress the esophagus just as the patient loses consciousness following induction of anesthesia. Pressure is maintained until the endotracheal tube has been inserted and its cuff inflated.

After delivery of the infant, additional analgesia may be provided in the form of intravenous narcotics such as morphine, meperidine, and fentanyl, or via inhalational agents such as halothane, enflurane, and isoflurane.

Effects of enflurane and ketamine on fetal acid–base balance have been studied by Downing et al.[17] Enflurane, by causing vasodilatation and uterine relaxation, enhances maternal to fetal transplacental exchange. This beneficial effect is not observed with ketamine anesthesia. When used for cesarean section, enflurane decreases maternal blood pressure by 10–15% after anesthetic induction. Apgar scores, blood gases, and acid–base balance followed normal patterns. Enflurane is rapidly transferred from mother to fetus but is quickly eliminated by the newborn once respiratory function is established.[14]

The principal complications of general anesthesia are hypertension, associated with endotracheal intubation, and aspiration of vomitus. Hypertension related to endotracheal intubation is exaggerated in the presence of preeclampsia or underlying hypertensive disease. Systolic blood pressure may increase as much as 100 torr immediately following tracheal intubation. The hypertension is transient, usually lasting less than 10 minutes. When hypertensive patients receive general anesthesia with endotracheal intubation, blood pressure must be monitored closely, preferably by direct intraarterial measurement. Intravenous trimethaphan, sodium nitroprusside, hydralazine, and nitroglycerin have been used in an effort to ablate the hypertensive response. Because of its rapid action and arteriolar vasodilating properties, sodium nitroprusside seems preferable. Although some authors report no fetal or newborn toxicity with its use,[58] placental transfer and fetal toxicity due to cyanide accumulation have been documented.[39]

Aspiration symptoms in association with general anesthesia for delivery have received much attention in recent years. The pH of gastric contents is less than 2.5 in more than 50% of obstetrical patients, rendering them susceptible to extensive pulmonary damage with aspiration.[59] Since virtually all laboring gravidas have gastric fluid volumes greater than 25 ml, all must be considered at risk for aspiration. Antacids have been advocated for routine administration during labor in an effort to elevate the gastric fluid pH. This should reduce the incidence of Mendelsohn's syndrome, but particulate antacid solutions themselves have severe toxicity when administered directly into the lungs of dogs.[22] In an effort to avoid administration of particulate antacids, use of 0.3 molar sodium citrate has been proposed. Glycopyrrolate, 0.4–0.6 mg, administered intramuscularly 40–120 minutes before induction of anesthesia significantly increases gastric fluid pH.[3] Two new drugs, cimetidine and ranitidine, histamine H2 receptor antagonists, may also prove to be of value. These drugs inhibit gastric acid secretion. Metoclopramide, which increases gastric emptying by promoting peristalsis and relaxation of the pyloric sphincter, may prove useful. It appears that routine prophylactic administration of cimetidine or ranitidine, supplemented with sodium citrate prior to induction of anesthesia, is appropriate management.

REGIONAL ANALGESIA FOR CESAREAN SECTION

Because of the complications related to the use of general anesthesia for cesarean section, regional block analgesia is becoming more commonplace. It has been estimated that 13–15% of true maternal deaths are attributable to anesthesia.[55] The majority of these have been associated with general anesthesia. The chief reasons for the advantage of regional analgesia over general anesthesia are avoidance of aspiration of gastric contents, because the patient remains awake, and the reduced risk of hypoxia because oxygen in high concentration may be administered.

Spinal Analgesia for Cesarean Section

Spinal analgesia for cesarean section is still in general use. If hypotension can be avoided through the adminstration of a vascular preload, neonatal acid–base derangements are rare. Prehydration should consist of 1000–1500 ml of Ringer's lactate solution, and uterine displacement should be utilized to prevent the supine hypotensive syndrome. Dextrose-containing solutions should not be used for vascular preload, because neonatal hypoglycema may occur when more than 20 g of intravenous glucose is administered immediately prior to delivery.

Contraindications to spinal anesthesia for cesarean section include patient refusal, maternal fever and/or local lumbar infection, coagulation disorders, hypovolemia, congenital heart disease with intracardiac shunts, and some forms of neurologic disease.

Epidural Analgesia for Cesarean Section

Epidural analgesia for cesarean section has been gaining in popularity. The most commonly used technique employs bupivacaine, 0.5%, administered by an epidural catheter with a two-stage injection to obtain a complete sensory block from S5 to T4. Transient hypotension is not uncommon with analgesia to this level, even when preoperative fluid loading with 1000–1500 cc of balanced electrolyte solution is employed. The patient should be tilted to the left after administration of the local anesthetic and should remain in this position until after delivery of the placenta.

Obesity may influence the cephalad spread of analgesia.[24] The level of analgesia is positively correlated with the body mass index and with body weight. Reduced dosage should be utilized in obese obstetrical patients.

A comparison of bupivacaine, 2-chloroprocaine, and etidocaine for epidural analgesia for cesarean section has demonstrated excellent results with both bupivacaine and 2-chloroprocaine.[15] Etidocaine was proved unsatisfactory, because the sensory block was inadequate in most patients.

Studies comparing epidural analgesia with general anesthesia for cesarean section show no significant advantage of either technique in terms of fetal heart rate patterns, newborn acid–base balance, 1 and 5-minute Apgar scores, and time to sustained respiration.

Maternal hemodynamics, including cardiac output, are altered relatively little during epidural analgesia as compared to changes demonstrable with general anesthesia and spinal analgesia. For this reason, patients with cardiac disease who do not have intracardiac shunting are generally anesthetized for cesarean section with lumbar epidural block. However, if uncorrected maternal hypotension occurs, Apgar scores may be lowered and fetal acidosis appears.

Placental blood flow does not decrease significantly during cesarean section under lumbar epidural analgesia. Maternal blood pressure decreases significantly if an intravenous preload &100 ml/kg body weight) is not administered. In contrast, maternal blood pressure remains stable if a preloading infusion is utilized. Intervillous blood flow increases temporarily in patients receiving vascular preload. This does not differ significantly from intervillous blood flow in patients who are not given an epidural block.

In summary, there is little difference in neonatal outcome depending upon whether general anesthesia or epidural anesthesia is utilized for cesarean section. Although some studies suggest that maternal morbidity is less following LEA for cesarean section, neonatal acid–base values and Apgar scores are not influenced. The author's preference is for LEA, which, when used with suitable vascular preload and lateral displacement of the uterus, offers safe analgesia for cesarean section. The risks of aspiration and hypoxia, which account for the principal mortality associated with general anesthesia, are thus avoided.

EFFECTS OF ANALGESIA/ANESTHESIA ON NEONATAL NEUROBEHAVIOR

Although the Apgar scoring system provides information concerning the biochemical and respiratory status of the newborn infant, subtle changes which might be produced by obstetrical anesthesia cannot be appreciated with this test. To evaluate more subtle changes, a battery of "neurobehavioral" tests have appeared. These include the Bayley Scales, the Brazelton Neonatal Behavioral Assessment Scale (NBAS), the Scanlon Early Neonatal Behavioral Scale (ENNS), and various others which evaluate the infant's motor behavior, ability to alter state of arousal, ability to respond to a variety of external events, and ability to suppress meaningless or obtrusive stimuli.[13] Of these tests, the Brazelton NBAS is the most comprehensive but has largely been supplanted by the Scanlon ENNS, which is shorter and less complex. The latter test utilizes 15 individual observations of primary reflexes, muscle tone, and decremental response to stimulation. The test takes 4–10 minutes to administer and does not require that the infant be awakened for the purpose of the examination.

Systemic Analgesia

The effects on the newborn of narcotics administered during labor have been studied extensively but remain controversial. Although not all studies are in accord, in general, meperidine adversely affects neurobehavioral performance in the early neonatal period. The deleterious effect is related to the cumulative dose of meperidine administered and to the cord blood levels of meperidine. It appears that all narcotics are capable of producing neonatal depression and also subtle changes in neurobehavior. These changes appear to be dose related.

Regional Analgesia

Pudendal block is an effective means of producing perineal analgesia for delivery. Most physicians think that pudendal block is an innocuous procedure, without neonatal side effects. Neurobehavioral evaluations were obtained 5 and 25 hours following delivery in 55 infants whose mothers were given either bupivacaine, mepivacaine, or 2-chloroprocaine for pudendal block analgesia. No significant effects of these agents on infant neurobehavior were noted except for a significant difference in response to pin prick, the infants whose mothers had received mepivacaine having the best decrement to pin prick scores. Relatively high newborn capillary blood levels of bupivacaine (0.15 μg/ml) were noted in this study, but no detectable neurobehavioral changes could be attributed to this drug.[53]

Paracervical block analgesia does not produce neonatal neurobehavioral changes but decreases muscle tone immediately after birth. However, improvement occurs with age.

Because, with epidural analgesia for labor and delivery, significant quantities of local anesthetic drug may be transferred to the fetus, efforts have been made to evaluate the neurobehavioral status of infants born to mothers receiving epidural analgesia. Relatively few neonatal neurobehavioral effects can be ascribed to epidural analgesia for labor and delivery. However, effort should be made to achieve segmental blocks with low concentrations of local anesthetic agents to minimize any possible effects of large doses.

General Anesthesia

When general anesthesia is employed for delivery, the neonatal neurobehavioral status is influenced by the drugs utilized, their dosage, the duration of their administration, and the interval from induction of anesthesia to delivery. Neonatal neurobehavioral tests following vaginal delivery under ketamine, sodium thiopental, and epidural analgesia were evaluated by Hodgkinson et al.,[29] who first used the Scanlon neurobehavioral test administered on the first and second days of life to evaluate 275 neonates divided among these three groups. The greatest percentage of high scores for overall assessment, tone, rooting, sucking, Moro response, placing, alertness, and decrement to pin prick were obtained in infants born to mothers receiving lumbar epidural analgesia with 2-chloroprocaine. The lowest scores were obtained after thiopental usage for general anesthesia. Those following the use of ketamine were intermediate. In a follow-up study,[27] the work was extended to include infants born by cesarean section. Spinal analgesia with tetracaine was compared to general anesthesia with sodium thiopental or ketamine. Similar results were obtained, the infants born to mothers receiving spinal anesthesia receiving higher scores. Others[28] found no significant differences in neonatal acid-base values and Apgar scores in infants of mothers who received epidural lidocaine analgesia, compared to those whose mothers received general anesthesia with sodium thiopental, nitrous oxide, and oxygen. No significant differences were noted in neurobehavioral scores, although, if maternal hypotension occurred due to epidural analgesia, weak rooting and sucking reflexes were noted in the newborns during the first two days of life. All babies born of high-risk obstetrical patients exhibited abnormal neurologic activity, as evidenced by either depression of muscle tone and reflexes or abnormalities of all the tested variables.

The addition of low doses of halogenated anesthetic agents to general anesthesia for cesarean section does not adversely affect the neonatal acid-base status, Apgar score, and neurobehavioral status of infants at 2 and 25 hours of age.[55] Also, inhalational agents used to provide analgesia for vaginal delivery do not cause significant changes in neonatal neurobehavior.[57]

The significance of neurobehavioral derangements measured in the early neonatal stage and later remains uncertain. Although there have been some suggestions of subsequent retarded development of cognitive or motor skills, other studies reveal only minor neurobehavioral changes and no adverse long-term effects of obstetric anesthesia or analgesia.

Until this situation is clarified, it is wise to follow the recommendation of the American Academy of Pediatrics Committee on Drugs.[11] Until further studies become available, "it would be advisable to avoid the use of drugs or drug dosages that are known to produce significant changes in neurobehavior of the infant. This statement does not mean that the patient in labor should be denied reasonable relief of pain by analgesic or anesthetic agents, but rather that the minimum effective dose of these agents should be administered when indicated."

REFERENCES

1. Abboud, T. K., Afrasiabi, A., Sarkis, F., Daftarian, F., Nagappala, S. Noueihed, R., Kuhnert, B. R., and Miller, F.: Continuous infusion epidural analgesia in parturients receiving bupivacaine, chloroprocaine, or lidocaine—Maternal, fetal, and neonatal effects. *Anesth. Analg.* **63**:421–428, 1984.
2. Baraka, A., Noueihid, R., and Hajj, S.: Intrathecal injection of morphine for obstetric analgesia. *Anesthesiology* **54**:136–140, 1981.
3. Baraka, A., Saab, M., Salem, M. R., and Winnie, A. P.: Control of gastric acidity by glycopyrrolate premedication in the parturient. *Anesth. Analg.* **56**:642–645, 1977.
4. Baxi, L. V., Petrie, R. H., and James, L. S.: Human fetal oxygenation following paracervical block. *Am. J. Obstet. Gynecol.* **135**:1109–1112, 1979.
5. Belfrage, P., Boreus, L. O., Hartvig, P., Irestedt, L., and Raabe, N.: Neonatal depression after obstetrical analgesia with pethidine: The role of the injection–delivery time interval and of the plasma concentrations of pethidine and norpethidine. *Acta Obstet. Gynecol. Scand.* **60**:43–49, 1981.
6. Bonica, J. J.: Pudendal block and local anesthesia of the perineum. In: *Principles and Practice of Obstetric Analgesia and Anesthesia*, Vol. 1. Philadelphia, F. A. Davis, 1967, pp. 487–506.
7. Brown, W. U. Jr., Bell, G. C., Weiss, J. B., and Alper, M. H.: Mepivacaine in amniotic fluid following maternal epidural anesthesia. *Anesthesiology* **47**:384–386, 1977.
8. Caldwell, J. and Noatrianni, L. J.: Disposition of pethidine in childbirth (letter). *Br. J. Anaesth.* **50**:307–308, 1978.
9. Cibils, L. A.: Response of human uterine arteries to local anesthetics. *Am. J. Obstet. Gynecol.* **126**:202–210, 1976.
10. Cibils, L. A. and Santonja-Lucas, J. J.: Clinical significance of fetal heart rate patterns during labor. III. Effect of paracervical block anesthesia. *Am. J. Obstet. Gynecol.* **130**:73–100, 1978.
11. Committee on Drugs, American Academy of Pediatrics: Effect of medication during labor and delivery on infant outcome. *Pediatrics* **62**:402–403, 1978.
12. Crawford, J. S.: Forum: Experiences with epidural morphine in obstetrics. *Anaesthesia* **36**:207–209, 1981.
13. Dailey, P. A., Baysinger, C. L., Levinson, G., and Shnider, S.M.: Neurobehavioral testing of the newborn infant. In: *Clinics in Perinatology Symposium on Obstetric Anesthesia and Analgesia*, Vol. 9, No. 1. T. H. Joyce (Ed.). Philadelphia, W. B. Saunders Co., 1982, pp. 191–214.
14. Datta, S., Corke, B. C., Alper, M. H., Brown, W. U., Jr., Ostheimer, G. W., and Weiss, J. B.: Epidural anesthesia for cesarean section: A comparison of bupivacaine, chloroprocaine, and etidocaine. *Anesthesiology* **52**:48–51, 1980.
15. Del Pizzo, A.: A double-blind study of the effects of butorphanol compared with morphine in balanced anaesthesia. *Can. Anaesth. Soc. J.* **25**:392–397, 1978.
16. Dick, W., Knoche, E., and Traub, E.: Clinical investigations concerning the use of Ethrane for cesarean section. *J. Perinat. Med.* **7**:125–133, 1979.
17. Downing, J. W., Houlton, P. J. C., Brock-Utne, J. G., and Buley, R. J. R.: The contrasting effects of enflurane on transplacental exchange after methodhexitone and ketamine induction of anaesthe-

sia for caesarean section. *Anaesth. Intensive Care* **6**:239–242, 1978.

18. Eisler, E. A., Thigpen, J. W., Shnider, S. M., Halpern, S. H., Brookshire, G. L., and Levinson, G.: Bupivacaine cardiotoxicity in normal and acidotic rabbits. Presented at the SOAP Fifth Scientific Session, April 14, 1984, San Diego, CA, p. 41.
19. Finster, M., Perel, J. M., Hinsvark, O. N., and O'Brien, J. E.: Pharmacodynamics of 2-chloroprocaine (Nesacaine), an ester-type local anesthetic. The Fourth European Congress of Anesthesiology, Madrid, Spain. New York, American Elsevier, 1974, p. 189 (Abstract 456).
20. Fishburne, J. I., Jr.: Systemic analgesia during labor. In: *Clinics in Perinatology Symposium on Obstetric Anesthesia and Analgesia*, Vol. 9. T. H. Joyce (Ed.). Philadelphia, W. B. Saunders Co., 1982, pp. 29–53.
21. Fishburne, J. I., Jr., Greiss, F. C., Jr., Hopkinson, R., and Rhyne, A. L.: Responses of the gravid uterine vasculature to arterial levels of local anesthetic agents. *Am. J. Obstet. Gynecol.* **133**:753–761, 1979.
22. Gibbs, C. P., Schwartz, D. J., and Wynne, J. W.: Antacid pulmonary aspiration in the dog. *Anesthesiology* **51**380–385, 1979.
23. Hagerdal, M., Morgan, C. W., Sumner, A. E., and Gutsche, B. B.: Minute ventilation and oxygen consumption during labor with epidural analgesia. *Anesthesiology* **59**425–427, 1983.
24. Halpern, S. H., Eisler, E. A., Shnider, S. M., Shapiro, D. A., Levinson, G., and Rosen, M. A.: Myocardial tissue uptake of bupivacaine and lidocaine after intravenous administration in normal and acidotic rabbits. Presented at the SOAP First Scientific Session, April 13, 1984, San Diego, CA, p. 22.
25. Hamshaw-Thomas, A. and Reynolds, F.: Materno-fetal drug exchange across the rabbit placenta. Presented at the SOAP First Scientific Session, April 13, 1984, San Diego, CA, p. 19.
26. Hodgkinson, R. and Husian, F. J.: Obesity and the cephalad spread of analgesia following epidural administration of bupivacaine for cesarean section. *Anesth. Analg.* **59**:89–92, 1980.
27. Hodgkinson, R., Bhatt, M., Kim, S. S., Grewal, G., and Marx, G. F.: Neonatal neurobehavioral tests following cesarean section under general and spinal anesthesia. *Am. J. Obstet.* Gynecol. **132**:670–674, 1978.
28. Hollmen, A.I., Jouppila, R., Koivisto, M., Maatta, L., Pihlajaniemi, R., Puukka, M., and Rantakyla, P.: Neurologic activity of infants following anesthesia for cesarean section. *Anesthesiology* **48**:350–356, 1978.
29. Hodgkinson, R., Marx, G. F., Kim, S. S., and Miclat, N. M.: Neonatal neurobehavioral tests following vaginal delivery under ketamine, thiopental, and extradural anesthesia. *Anesth. Analg.* **56**:548–553, 1977.
30. Huch, A.: Maternal hypoxaemia after pethidine. *J. Obstet. Gynaecol. Br. Commonw.* **81**:608–614, 1974.
31. Hughes, S. C., Rosen, M. A., Shnider, S. M., Abboud, T. K., Stefani, S. J., and Norton, M.: Maternal and neonatal effects of epidural morphine for labor and delivery. *Anesth. Analg.* **63**:319–324, 1984.
32. Jouppila, R., Jouppila, P., Kotiniemi, L., Puolakka, J., Puukka, M., and Puukka, R.: Maternal and foetal plasma bupivacaine concentrations in labour with segmental epidural analgesia. *Ann. Chir. Gynaecol.* **67**:190–194, 1978.
33. Kallos, T. and Caruso, F. S.: Respiratory effects of butorphanol and pethidine. *Anaesthesia* **34**:633–637,1979.
34. Klotz U., McHorse, T. W., and Wilkinson, G. R.: The effect of cirrhosis on the disposition and elimination of meperidine in man. *Clin. Pharmacol. Ther.* **16**:667–675,1974.
35. Kuhnert, B. R., Kuhnert, P. M., and Tu, A. L.: Meperidine and normeperidine levels following meperidine administration during labor. I. Mother. *Am. J. Obstet. Gynecol.* **133**:904–908, 1979.
36. Kuhnert, B. R., Kuhnert, P. M., and Tu, A. L.: Meperidine and normeperidine levels following meperidine administration during labor. II. Fetus and neonate. *Am. J. Obstet. Gynecol.* **133**:909–914, 1979.
37. Kuhnert, B. R., Philipson, E. H., Kuhnert, P. M., and Syracuse, C. D.: Exposure of mother, fetus and neonate to meperidine and normeperidine following multiple doses during labor. Presented at the SOAP First Scientific Session, April 13, 1984, San Diego, CA, p. 17.
38. Lavin, J., Samuels, S., and Miodovnik, M.: The effect of chloroprocaine hydrochloride and bupivacaine as epidural anesthetics on the fetal heart rate. Abstracts of the 28th Annual Meeting of the Society for Gynecologic Investigation, St. Louis, MO, 1981, p. 79 (Abstract 132).
39. Lewis, P. E.: Placental transfer and fetal toxicity of sodium nitroprusside. *Gynecol. Invest.* **8**:46, 1977.
40. Maduska, A. L. and Hajghassemali, M.: A double-blind comparison of butorphanol and meperidine in labour: Maternal pain relief and effect on the newborn. *Can. Anaesth. Soc. J.* **25**:398–404, 1978.
41. Marx, G. F.: Cardiopulmonary resuscitation of late-pregnant women. *Anesthesiology* **56**:156, 1982.
42. Marx, G. F. and Mateo, C. V.: Effects of different oxygen concentrations during general anaesthesia for elective caesarean sections. *Can. Anaesth. Soc. J.* **18**:587–593, 1971.
43. Merkow, A. J., McGuinness, G. A., Erenberg, A., and Kennedy, R. L.: The neonatal neurobehavioral effects of bupivacaine, mepivacaine, and 2-chloroprocaine used for pudendal block. *Anesthesiology* **52**:309–312, 1980.

44. Moir, D. D.: Editorial—Maternal mortality and anaesthesia. *Br. J. Anaesth.* **52**:1–3, 1980.
45. Nagashima, H., Karamanian, A., and Malovany, R.: Respiratory and circulatory effects of intravenous butorphanol and morphine. *Clin. Pharmacol. Ther.* **19**:738–745, 1976.
46. Niv, D., Rudick, V., Chayen, M. S., and David, M. P.: Variations in the effect of epidural morphine in gynecological and obstetric patients. *Acta Obstet. Gynecol. Scand.* **62**:455–459, 1983.
47. Nybell-Lindahl, G., Carlsson, C., Ingemarsson, I., Westgren, M., and Paalzow, L.: Maternal and fetal concentrations of morphine after epidural admnistration during labor. *Am. J. Obstet. Gynecol.* **139**:20–21, 1981.
48. Oyama, T., Matsuki, A., Taneichi, T., Ling, N., and Guillemin, R.: β-Endorphin in obstetric analgesia. *Am. J. Obstet. Gynecol.* **137**:613–616, 1980.
49. Quilligan, E. J., Keegan, K. A., and Donahue, M. J.: Double-blind comparison of intravenously injected butorphanol and meperidine in parturients. *Int. J. Gynaecol. Obstet.* **18**:363–367, 1980.
50. Ralston, D. H. and Shnider, S. M.: The fetal and neonatal effects of regional anesthesia in obstetrics. *Anesthesiology* **48**:34–64, 1978.
51. Ramanathan, S., Gandhi, S., Arismendy, J., Chalon, J., and Turndorf, H.: Oxygen transfer from mother to fetus during cesarean section under epidural anesthesia. *Anesth. Analg.* **61**:576–581, 1982.
52. Rothberg, R. M., Rieger, C. H. L., and Hill, J. H.: Cord and maternal serum meperidine concentrations and clinical status of the infant. *Biol. Neonate* **33**:80–89, 1978.
53. Santos, A., Pedersen, H., and Finster, M.: Spinal anesthesia with bupivacaine for cesarean section. Presented at the SOAP Seventh Scientific Session, April 15, 1984, San Diego, CA, p. 51.
54. Schifrin, B.: Fetal heart rate pattern following epidural anesthesia and oxytocin infusion during labor. *J. Obstet.* Gynaecol. Br. Commonw. **79**:332–339, 1972.
55. Shnider, S. M., Abboud, T., Levinson, G., Wright, R. G., Kim, S., Henriksen, E., Hughes, S. C., Roizen, M. F., and Johnson, J.: General anesthesia for cesarean section: Maternal and fetal norepinephrine levels and neonatal neurobehavioral status. *Anesthesiology* **53**:S302, 1979.
56. Shnider S. M., Way, E. L., and Lord, M. J.: Rate of appearance and disappearance of meperidine in fetal blood after administration of narcotic to the mother. *Anesthesiology* **27**:227–228, 1966.
57. Stefani, S. F., Hughes, S. C., Shnider, S. M., Abbaud, T., Henriksen, E., Williams, V., and Johnson, J.: Neonatal neurobehavioral effects of inhalational analgesia for delivery. *Anesthesiology* **53**:S314, 1979.
58. Strauss, R. G., Keefer, J. R., Burke, T., and Civetta, J. M.: Hemodynamic monitoring of cardiogenic pulmonary edema complicating toxemia of pregnancy. *Obstet. Gynecol.* **55**:170–174, 1980.
59. Taylor, G. and Pryse-Davies, J.: The prophylactic use of antacids in the prevention of the acid-pulmonary-aspiration syndrome (Mendelsohn's Syndrome). *Lancet* **1**:288–291, 1966.
60. Weiss, R. R., Nathanson, H. G., and Tehrani, M. R.: Paracervical block with 2-chloroprocaine. *Anesth. Analg.* **56:709**–716, 1977.

9

THE PUERPERIUM

The puerperium traditionally is defined as the interval from delivery until the anatomic and physiologic changes of pregnancy have resolved. Because of the manner in which most institutions schedule postpartum appointments, it has been customary to state that the puerperium extends six weeks from the day of delivery. This is arbitrary, however, because some physiologic changes of pregnancy resolve before six weeks, whereas others persist beyond that time.

The puerperium is a period of momentous physical, social, and emotional change for the patient and her family. The woman is intensely concerned about her own health and that of her newborn infant. Therefore, it is a period in which obstetricians have a unique opportunity to positively influence patients' attitudes toward medical care.

This chapter discusses the clinical management of patients in the immediate postpartum period and the anatomic and endocrinologic changes that occur in the female reproductive system in preparation for resumption of normal cyclic menses, and contraception and sterilization.

CLINICAL CARE OF THE PUERPERAL PATIENT

Following delivery, the patient should remain under intensive surveillance for several hours until her vital signs are stable, uterine bleeding has stabilized, and the effects of any anesthetic have resolved. During this period, a dilute solution of oxytocin (10–20 units in 1000 cc of carrier solution) may be infused to prevent uterine atony. Mechanical massage of the uterine fundus may accomplish this same effect and obviates the need for intravenous infusion.

Once the patient's condition is stable, she may be transferred to the postpartum ward. She is then allowed to gradually resume full activity. During the time that the patient remains in the hospital, she should be evaluated for evidence of infection and excessive vaginal bleeding. She should be examined to be certain that her episiotomy is well approximated and that a paravaginal hematoma has not formed and should be questioned to be certain that she is voiding normally.

The length of time that the patient remains in the hospital depends upon several factors, including type of delivery, support systems at home, occurrence of postpartum complications, clinical course of the neonate, and institutional practices. At present, there is a strong trend toward decreasing the length of postpartum hospitalization. Many institutions discharge patients within 48 hours of delivery. Routine early discharge, however, is suitable only for the reliable, well-motivated patient who has had an uncomplicated hospital course and who has an excellent support structure at home.

Prior to leaving the hospital, the parturient should receive detailed counseling concerning infant care and contraception. The effects of lactation upon menstrual and endocrine function should be reviewed. Certain forms of contraception, such as barrier methods, may be instituted immediately upon discharge from the hospital. The use of oral contraceptives or the intrauterine contraceptive device should be delayed until later in the puerperium.

The best guideline to resumption of activity for an uncomplicated patient is her own sense of well-being. She should be encouraged to resume usual activities when she believes that her strength permits. Many of the restrictions imposed upon patients are arbitrary and have no basis in scientific fact. The patient should be cautioned specifically, however, to report immediately any episode of heavy vaginal bleeding or sustained fever and any difficulties related to the care and feeding of the infant.

The timing of the postpartum appointment varies among different institutions. Most problems related to breast-feeding, infant care, maternal infection, and maternal hemmorrhage are apparent within the first two weeks of the puerperium. Therefore, some medical centers schedule follow-up appointments at this time. When insertion of an intrauterine contraceptive device is anticipated or interval sterilization is planned, an appointment at six or eight weeks postpartum may be more appropriate.[40]

ANATOMIC AND PHYSIOLOGIC ALTERATIONS

Cardiovascular System

During pregnancy, dramatic changes occur in the maternal cardiovascular system.[16] (See Chapters 3 and 31.) Cardiac output during labor and delivery increases over and above the increases due to pregnancy itself. Early in the first stage of labor, cardiac output increases by approximately 15% above prelabor baseline. Late in the first stage, cardiac output rises to 30% above baseline. In the second stage of labor, cardiac output may be as much as 45% above baseline levels. During each of these time periods, cardiac output increases by an additional 15% in association with contractions.

In the first hour after delivery, cardiac output ranges from 30% to 65% above prelabor baseline. Thereafter, it declines progressively. Approximately 50% of the return to nonpregnancy levels of cardiac output occurs by the end of the second postpartum week. By six weeks after delivery, cardiac output has returned to normal nonpregnant levels.

Blood volume also decreases progressively after delivery. The average blood loss associated with vaginal delivery is 500–600 cc. Cesarean delivery usually results in blood loss of 1000–1100 cc. Preeclampsia, chorioamnionitis, multiple gestation, placenta previa, and abruptio placentae are the principal conditions associated with excessive blood loss at either vaginal or abdominal delivery. By the third postpartum day, approximately 16% of the blood volume increase associated with pregnancy has resolved. Heart rate, blood pressure, and total body water usually return to nonpregnant levels by the end of the first week.

Urinary Tract

Renal blood flow, glomerular filtration rate, filtration fraction, and creatinine clearance increase during pregnancy. By six weeks postpartum, these physiologic increases in renal function have resolved. In contrast, certain anatomic alterations in the urinary tract take longer to return to normal. Dilation of the renal calyces and ureters may persist for up to three months after delivery. Approximately 20% of women experience incomplete emptying of the bladder immediately after delivery, and some require catheterization.[16] Instrumentation of the bladder in association with stasis in the upper tracts predisposes to urinary tract infection. Puerperal patients should be questioned carefully about symptoms suggestive of cystitis or pyelonephritis.

Uterine Involution

At term, the uterus weighs approximately 1000 grams and receives almost 20% of maternal cardiac output. Immediately after delivery, the uterus is approximately 20–24 weeks size. By the end of the third postpartum day, the uterus has decreased to 12–14 weeks size, and by the completion of the second postpartum week, to 10 weeks size. Six weeks postpartum, the uterus has returned to its nonpregnant size and configuration. At this point, it weighs 70–100 grams and receives less than 1% of cardiac output.

Uterine involution begins immediately following delivery of the fetus and placenta. The initial process of involution is enhanced by administration of oxytocin and by mechanical massage of the uterine fundus. Lactation may hasten subsequent involutional changes. Abnormalities in uterine involution may be responsible for delayed postpartum hemorrhage. Infection, retained placental tissue, uterine anomalies, and trophoblastic disease are the principal entities that should be considered in the differential diagnosis of uterine subinvolution.

Within the uterus, changes occur in the endometrium.[5,53] The placental site is initially covered by a fresh blood clot. Beneath the clot is a layer of tissue composed of decidual cells and primitive endometrial glands. Polymorphonuclear leukocytes and monocytes are present in both the clot and the underlying endomyometrium. Prominent vascular changes occur in the area beneath the placental attachment site. Arterial and venous channels become occluded by fibrin deposition and assume a hyalinized appearance. As a result of these vascular alterations, extensive necrosis develops, resulting in sloughing of the superficial layer. This effluent is recognized clinically as lochia.

Some decidual cells and primitive glandular cells remain, however. By the seventh postpartum day, mitotic figures are recognized in the glandular epithelium. Ultimate regeneration of the placental site depends upon proliferation of reserve cells in the decidua basalis and ingrowth of new glandular and stromal cells from the adjacent endometrium. By six to eight weeks postpartum, the previous placental site cannot be identified by gross or microscopic examination.

In the endometrium distant from the placental site, regenerative activity increases progressively during the first week postpartum. Initially, there is extensive infiltration of the endometrium by polymorphonuclear leukocytes. The leukocytic infiltration usually resolves within the first 10 days of the puerperium and is replaced by an infiltrate composed of lymphocytes and plasma cells. The infiltrates may persist as long as three to four months postpartum. These infiltrates do not represent infection, but rather the normal reparative process.

By the fourth day after delivery, mitosis is evident within the glandular epithelium. By the seventh postpartum day, a new surface epithelium has formed. By the 15th day, early proliferative changes are apparent. At the end of the second month after delivery, the endometrium should be completely restored. The earliest time that secretory endometrium has been documented is the 44th day after delivery.

RESUMPTION OF OVULATION AND MENSTRUATION

Immediately following delivery, serum hCG concentrations begin to decrease. By the end of the second week postpartum, hCG has been cleared from the circulation.

FSH and LH concentrations are low during the first 14 days of the puerperium.[6,37,46,50] By 15 days after delivery, serum concentrations of both gonadotropins increase to normal follicular phase levels. The low levels of gonadotropins in the immediate postpartum period appear to be due to decreased GnRH secretion by the hypothalamus. Although administration of a GnRH agonist at this time will restore gonadotropin secretion, the pattern of gonadotropin secretion may not be normal.[10,54] The response of FSH to GnRH normalizes before that of LH.[28,31]

Ovarian refractoriness to relatively low circulating gonadotropin levels also may be responsible for the delay in return of normal ovulatory and menstrual function. This refractoriness can be overcome by administration of gonadotropins.[65]

The exact mechanism of hypothalamic and ovarian suppression in the puerperium is not understood. High serum levels of prolactin may be at least partially responsible. In lactating and nonlactating women, the gradual rise in gonadotropin levels coincides with the decline in prolactin concentration. Baseline prolactin levels remain elevated, and menses and ovulation are delayed for a longer period of time in lactating as compared to nonlactating women. Finally, administration of bromocriptine to nonlactating postpartum women results in a prompt significant decrease in prolactin concentration and increase in FSH levels.[52]

In nonlactating women, the mean interval to resumption of menses is 59 days. The mean time until first ovulation is 73.5 days. Approximately 40% of women ovulate prior to their first menses (Fig. 9-1).

In lactating women, the time until first menses and ovulation is delayed beyond that observed for nonlactating patients (Fig. 9-2). The duration of hypothalamic–pituitary–ovarian suppression varies directly with the duration of lactation. Individuals who breast-feed for less than one month usually resume menses and ovulation within 75 days. In women who lactate beyond one month, the average interval to first ovulation is 112 days. Ovulation before the end of the ninth postpartum week is unusual. Beyond that time, however, ovulation occurs with increasing regularity even though the woman is lactating. Approximately 60% of first menses in lactating women are preceded by ovulation. Therefore, after the first nine weeks of the puerperium, breast-feed-

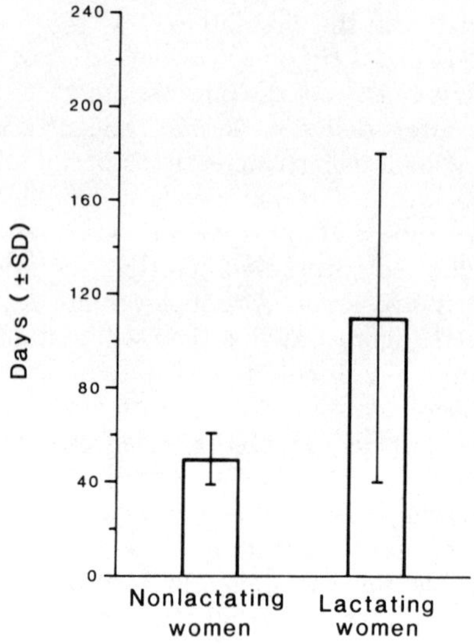

Figure 9-1. Mean length of time until ovulation in puerperal patients.

ing does not offer secure protection against pregnancy.[17,46]

LACTATION

Physiology of Lactation

A variety of changes occur in the maternal breast during pregnancy in preparation for lactation.[60,61] Mammary glandular tissue increases as a result of formation of new lobuli and hypertrophy of preexisting lobular–alveolar structures. Epithelial cells proliferate most actively in areas adjacent to fat lobules. As pregnancy advances, fat is progressively replaced by glandular tissue. Ductule and alveolar proliferation are accompanied by a concurrent increase in the blood supply to the breast. New capillaries form around the developing lobuli, and preexisting vessels increase in diameter. Ductule proliferation is mediated primarily by the effects of estradiol. Progesterone, in turn, promotes alveolar proliferation and development. The final differentiation of mammary epithelial cells into mature milk cells is controlled by prolactin. Relatively normal concentrations of cortisol, insulin, thyroid hormone, and growth hormone also must be present for normal milk synthesis and secretion to occur (Fig. 9-3).

Serum prolactin concentrations increase steadily throughout pregnancy, reaching a maximum of 200–400 ng/ml near term. Despite high prolactin levels, lactation does not occur because high concentrations of estradiol and progesterone inhibit the interaction between prolactin and its receptors on the alveolar cell membranes.

The critical stimulus for synthesis and secretion of milk is the sharp decrease in serum progesterone and estradiol concentrations immediately following delivery. Breast engorgement usually occurs on the third or fourth postpartum day when sex steroid levels have declined sufficiently that the action of prolactin on the mammary epithelial cell is no longer inhibited. Until that time, only colostrum is produced. Colostrum is a thin watery secretion containing minerals, proteins, fat droplets, lymphocytes and monocytes, and desquamated epithelial cells.

While serum estradiol and progesterone concentrations are decreasing, prolactin levels are also diminishing. By the end of the first postpartum week, the basal serum prolactin level in a nursing mother is approximately 100 ng/ml, although suckling causes large transient in-

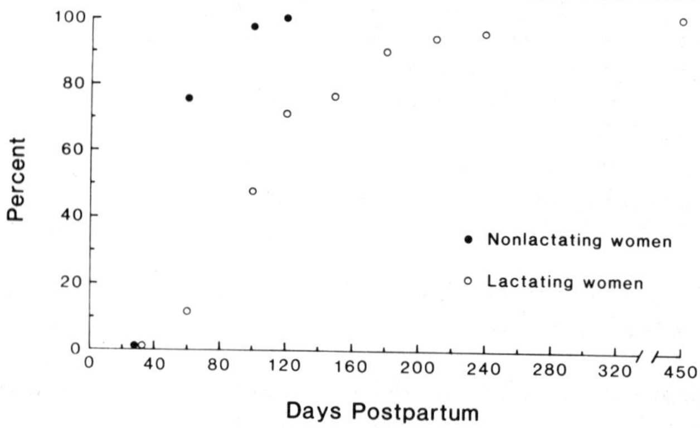

Figure 9-2. Cumulative percentage of women ovulating at selected intervals postpartum.

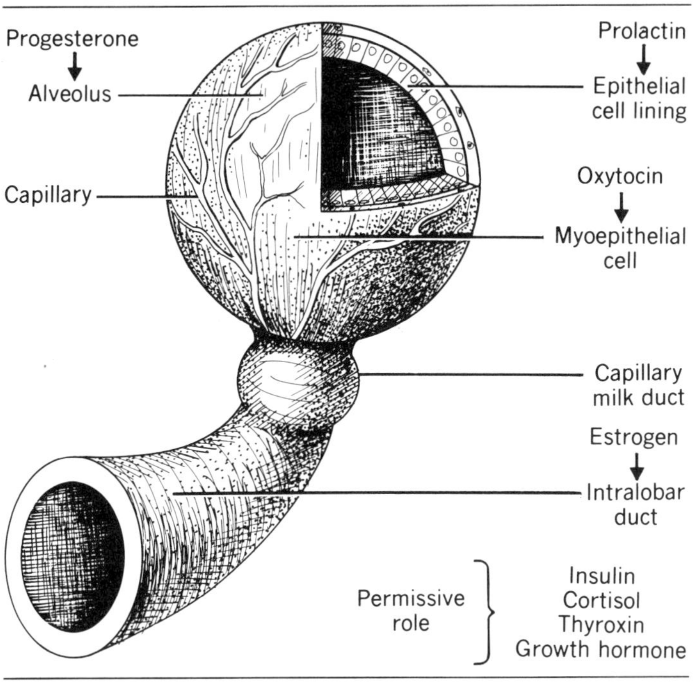

Figure 9-3. Physiology of lactation. Schematic diagram illustrates the effects of specific hormones in preparing the breast for lactation.

creases in prolactin secretion. By 8–12 weeks postpartum, basal prolactin levels decline further to 40–50 ng/ml. Ten to 20-fold increases in prolactin concentration still occur in association with suckling. After 12–16 weeks, basal prolactin levels have returned to normal, but transient increases still occur coincident with nursing.

Actual ejection of milk from the breast results from an intricate physiological process that depends upon chemical and neuronal stimuli (Fig. 9-4).[55] When the suckling infant grasps the maternal nipple, tactile neurons in the areola are stimulated. Stimulatory input is transmitted through the sensory nerve roots of T4, 5, and 6 to the paraventricular and supraoptic nuclei of the hypothalamus. In turn, these centers synthesize oxytocin, which is transported to the posterior pituitary and released into the systemic circulation. Oxytocin stimulates the myoepithelial cells of the breast to contract, which promotes emptying of milk from the alveoli into the ductules and ejection of milk from the major ducts. This neural–hormonal pathway also can be activated by the presence of the child or by the sound of its cry.

Advantages of Breast-Feeding

Milk is composed primarily of water, lactose, fat, protein, and minerals.[2] Human and cow's milk differ in many respects, most notably in protein composition (Tables 9-1 and 9-2).[30] The principal protein components of human milk are the whey proteins, substances that do not precipitate in the stomach. The predominant proteins of cow's milk are caseins, which give milk its characteristic color and which precipitate as curds under the acid conditions of the stomach.

There are several sound reasons to encourage mothers to breast-feed.[6,29,62] Although nursing is not absolutely necessary for effective bonding, breast-feeding can facilitate mother–infant interaction. Breast milk is an inexpensive, readily available source of nutrition. With the possible exception of iron and vitamins C and D, human milk provides all the essential nutrients that the infant needs for almost the entire first year of life. This economic consideration is especially compelling in indigent patients, both in the United States and in developing countries.

In addition to the social, emotional, and economic advantages of breast-feeding, medical benefits are associated with lactation. During the first three months postpartum, lactation offers reasonably secure protection against pregnancy. Breast-feeding also offers protection for the infant against food allergy because cow's milk protein is one of the principal causes of allergic reaction in infants. Approximately 1% of bottle-fed infants develop such an allergy.

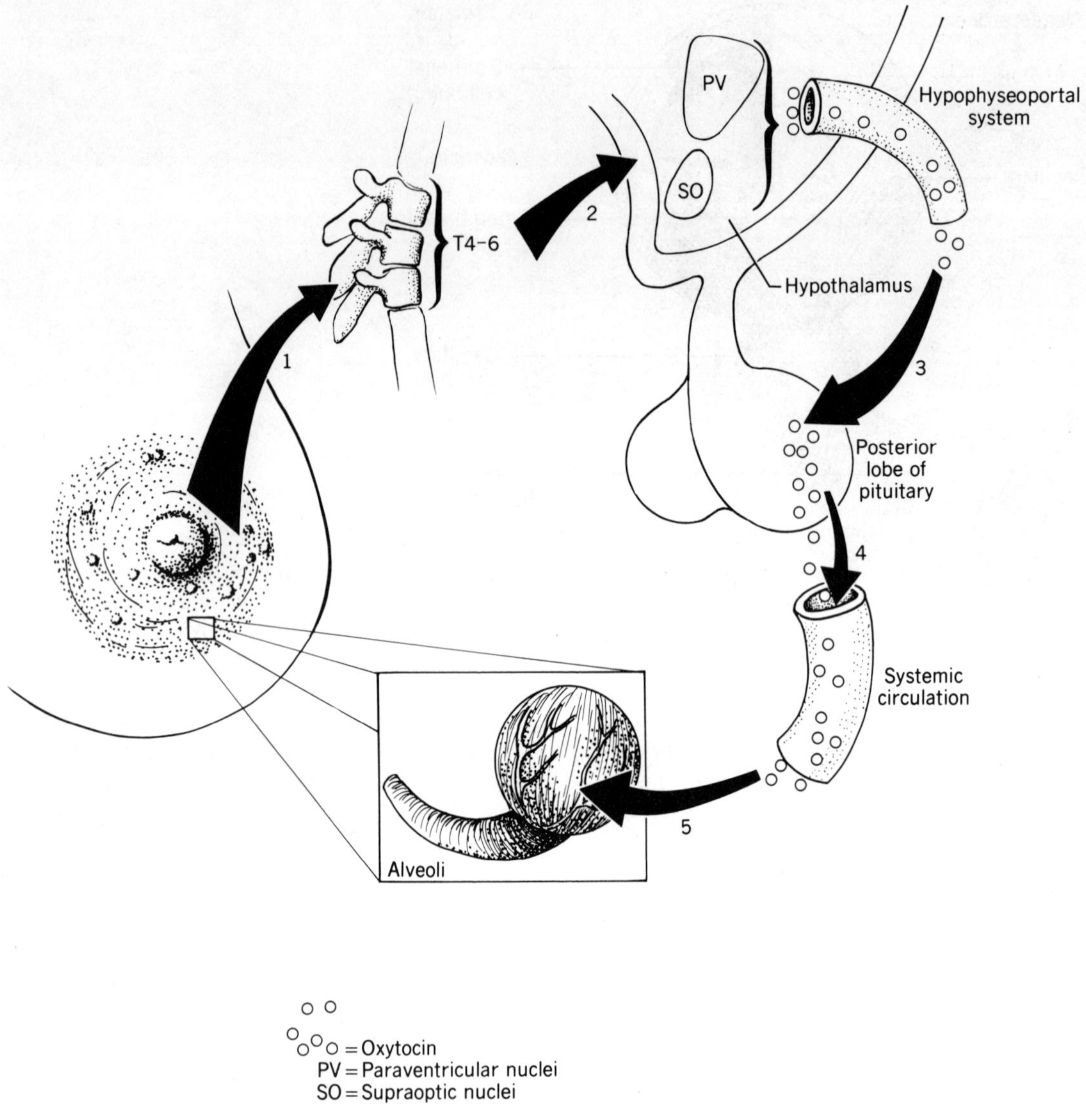

Figure 9-4. Physiology of milk ejection. (1) Sensory input from stimulation of tactile receptors in nipple and areola is transmitted by sensory components of T4–6 to the spinal cord and then upward to the hypothalamus. (2) Supraoptic (SO) and paraventricular nuclei (PV) synthesize oxytocin which is transmitted via hypophyseoportal system to the posterior lobe of the pituitary (3). Posterior pituitary then releases oxytocin into the systemic circulation (4). Oxytocin acts upon myoepithelial cells in the alveoli and small ductules of the breast to cause milk ejection (5).

Most importantly, breast-feeding enhances the infant's immunity against infection. Unlike cow's milk, human milk contains appreciable quantities of lysozyme, lactoferrin, and secretory IgA. These proteins are important in protecting the young infant against microorganisms that enter the host via the gastrointestinal tract. A statistically significant decrease in respiratory illnesses, otitis media, necrotizing enterocolitis, and diarrheal illnesses is seen in breast-fed infants as compared to bottle-fed infants.[18]

Successful breast-feeding requires a commitment of time and physical energy on the part of the mother. The most serious obstacles to successful lactation are maternal fatigue and emotional stress. During the early puerperium,

TABLE 9-1. COMPOSITION OF HUMAN COLOSTRUM, MATURE HUMAN MILK, AND COW'S MILK*

Component	Human Colostrum	Mature Human Milk	Cow's Milk
Water (g)	87	87	87
Total solids (g)	13	13	13
Protein (g)	7.9	1.1	3.5
Fat (g)	1.3	4.5	3.7
Lactose (g)	3.2	6.8	4.9
Mineral content (g)	0.6	0.2	0.7
Sodium (mg)	92	15	58
Potassium (mg)	55	55	138
Chloride (mg)	117	43	103
Calcium (mg)	31	33	125
Magnesium (mg)	4	4	12
Phosphorus (mg)	14	15	100
Iron (mg)	0.09†	0.15†	0.10†
Vitamins (μg)			
A	89	53	34
C	4400	4300	1600
D	—	0.03†	0.06†
Riboflavin	30	43	157
Nicotinic acid	75	172	85
Thiamine	15	16	42

* Concentration per 100 ml.
† Poor source of nutrient.
Source: Adapted from Jenness, R.: The composition of human milk. *Semin. Perinatol.* **3**:225, 1979.

when breast-feeding is being established, the new mother should be relieved of responsibilities other than care of the newborn. She should be encouraged to rest as much as possible between infant feedings. When nursing the baby, she should retire to a quiet area of the home so that she is not distracted from her interaction with the neonate. It is particularly important for the lactating woman to adhere to the principles of good nutrition. Tables 9-3 and 9-4 summarize the increased nutrient requirements of lactating women.[30]

TABLE 9-2. PROTEIN CONTENT OF HUMAN COLOSTRUM, MATURE HUMAN MILK, AND COW'S MILK*

Component	Human Colostrum	Mature Human Milk	Cow's Milk
Proteins (% of total protein)			
Casein	—	40	82
Whey	—	60	18
Major whey protein (mg)			
Alpha-lactalbumin	333	263	40
Lactoferrin	384	168	—
Lysozyme	34	42	—
Albumin	36	52	23
IgA	364	142	40

* Concentration per 100 ml.
Source: Adapted from Jenness, R.: The composition of human milk. *Semin. Perinatol.* **3**:225, 1979.

TABLE 9-3. ESTIMATED INCREASED NUTRIENT REQUIREMENTS OF LACTATING WOMEN*

Nutrient	Net Increase (per day)
Calories	+ 500 kcal
Protein	+ 20 g
Calcium	+ 400 mg
Phosphorus	+ 400 mg
Magnesium	+ 150 mg
Iron	+ 30–60 mg
Zinc	+ 10 mg
Iodine	+ 50μg

* Increased requirements relative to recommended daily allowances (RDA) for nonlactating women.
Source: Adapted from The Committee on Nutrition of the American Academy of Pediatrics: Nutrition and lactation. *Pediatrics* **68:**435–441, 1981. Reproduced by permission of *Pediatrics.*

Approximately 60% of women in the United States initially breast-feed their infants. The percentage of nursing mothers has increased by almost 100% since the late 1970s. Counseling by health care personnel, particularly obstetricians, is influential in shaping women's attitudes about breast-feeding.[64] Similarly, hospital practices such as rooming-in that promote early mother–infant contact are important in fostering interest in breast-feeding. In view of the many benefits to mother and infant that result from breast-feeding, such efforts on the part of health care personnel should continue.

Mastitis

Mastitis, the most frequent complication associated with nursing, occurs in up to 10% of lactating women. Mastitis usually is caused by *Staphylococcus aureus*, an organism of normal skin flora in many women. Its entry into the ductule system of the breast is facilitated when the nipples become dry and fissured.

Symptoms of mastitis include high fever, chills, malaise, and pain in the affected breast. Physical examination usually demonstrates an erythematous, tender, indurated area in one breast in association with tender axillary lymphadenopathy. Drainage from the affected breast may be frankly purulent. In some instances the infection progresses to abscess formation.

Diagnostic evaluation begins with a thorough physical examination to exclude other causes of puerperal fever such as acute pyelonephritis, endometritis, pneumonia, and viral syndrome. A sample of milk from the affected breast should be collected for Gram stain and culture. In patients who appear seriously ill, blood cultures should be obtained to rule out the presence of staphylococcal bacteremia. (See Chapter 38.)

Over 90% of strains of *Staphylococcus aureus* are resistant to penicillin G. Therefore, the antibiotic of choice is one of the anti-staphylococcal penicillins. Most women with puerperal mastitis can be managed as outpatients. Inpatient management is indicated in women who appear seriously ill, in individuals who do not respond promptly to oral antibiotic therapy, and in patients who have a breast abscess. Women with the latter complication require antibiotic therapy and surgical drainage. It is not necessary to discontinue nursing during treatment for mastitis. Failure to empty the engorged

TABLE 9-4. ESTIMATED INCREASED VITAMIN REQUIREMENTS OF LACTATING WOMEN*

Vitamin	Net Increase (per day)
A	+ 400.0 μg retinol equivalents
D	+ 5.0 μg
E	+ 3.0 mg tocopherol equivalents
C	+ 40.0 mg
Thiamine	+ 0.5 mg
Riboflavin	+ 0.5 mg
Niacin	+ 5.0 mg niacin equivalents
B_6	+ 0.5 mg
Folacin	+ 100.0 μg
B_{12}	+ 1.0 μg

* Increased requirements relative to recommended daily allowances (RDA) for nonlactating women.
Source: Adapted from The Committee on Nutrition of the American Academy of Pediatrics: Nutrition and lactation. *Pediatrics* **68:**435–441, 1981. Reproduced by permission of *Pediatrics.*

breast regularly may, in fact, interfere with effective treatment of the underlying infection.

Suppression of Lactation

It is not absolutely necessary to suppress lactation in patients who do not desire to breast-feed. These women should be advised that breast engorgement and discomfort resolve spontaneously within several days even though no medication is administered. During the period of time that their breasts are distended, patients should be advised to wear a comfortable brassiere for support and to avoid nipple stimulation. They should use small doses of analgesics such as acetaminophen or aspirin to control pain.

The drug of choice to suppress lactation is bromocriptine mesylate. This dopamine agonist produces a rapid decrease in serum prolactin concentration. The recommended dose is 2.5 mg orally, twice daily, for 14 days. The principal side effects of bromocriptine mesylate are headache, vertigo, nausea, and postural hypotension. One or more of these symptoms occur in up to 28% of patients. Untoward reactions are most likely during the first three days of therapy.

Prior to the introduction of bromocriptine mesylate, steroid hormones, usually combinations of an estrogen and testosterone, were used to suppress lactation. Such agents no longer should be employed for this indication. They have not been consistently effective in suppressing lactation and there is an increased incidence of thromboembolism in women who receive these agents in the immediate puerperium.[19] Although the absolute incidence of this disorder is low, the relative risk of thromboembolism may be increased up to 10-fold in women treated with estrogen/testosterone combinations.

Administration of Drugs to the Nursing Mother

Virtually any medication administered to the mother may pass from maternal plasma into breast milk. Factors that favor transfer of a drug into breast milk include low molecular weight, low degree of protein binding, and high lipid solubility. As a general rule, less than 2% of the total dose of a drug administered to the mother is excreted into breast milk. In order to minimize the neonate's exposure to medication, the mother should attempt to arrange her schedule so that she takes her medication after feeding her infant. This helps to ensure low maternal drug concentrations at the time of the next feeding.

Although the amount of drug secreted into breast milk is very low, there are certain situations where even these low concentrations may be harmful to the neonate. The drugs of most concern are anti-neoplastic agents, iodide, radionuclides, and lithium. Use of any of these agents absolutely contraindicates breast-feeding.[4]

EMOTIONAL CHANGES DURING THE PUERPERIUM (See Chapter 42)

The postpartum period is distinguished by marked fluctuations in mood. In the immediate puerperium, the new mother typically feels elated that the long-awaited baby has arrived and that it is healthy. However, upon returning home, she frequently experiences a sharp emotional let-down. She may feel overwhelmed and exhausted by the expenditure of emotional and physical energy necessary to care for the newborn. Such feelings may be particularly prominent in the woman who has other small children requiring supervision and attention. The woman also may feel physically unattractive to her partner and isolated from friends whose careers are oriented outside the home. Increasing irritability, tearfulness, loss of libido, and sleep and appetite disturbances are the usual symptoms displayed by women with the "postpartum blues." Disturbances in cognitive function also may occur.

Forty to 60% of otherwise normal, healthy women experience brief episodes of postpartum depression.[23] In the vast majority, depression is mild and shortlived. Most women can be effectively treated by the obstetrician and concerned family members. The former should offer reassurance that the symptoms experienced by the patient are common to many new mothers. The latter should help with household tasks so that the new mother has time to rest and relax. Once the infant has established a regular sleeping and eating schedule, the patient and her partner should be encouraged to enjoy an occasional evening away from the demands of childcare.

Three to 4% of parturients experience a severe postpartum depression that warrants intensive therapy.[23] Such a disorder is particularly likely to occur when the pregnancy was unplanned and unwanted and when the marital union is unstable. Single mothers are at greatest risk for severe postpartum depression. Women who have a history of depressive illness unrelated to pregnancy have a 20–30% incidence of postpartum depression. Patients with a prior history of postpartum depression have a recurrence risk of 30–50% with subsequent pregnancies.

Patients with severe postpartum depression typically experience an overwhelming sense of sadness. Decreases in appetite and libido are prominent. Sleep disturbances may take the form of either insomnia, characterized by early-morning wakefulness, or hypersomnia. Fatigue, loss of energy, loss of memory, and inability to concentrate may occur. The patient may lose interest in her physical appearance and may cease to participate in activities that she previously enjoyed. Patients may become preoccupied with feelings of worthlessness and may begin to experience suicidal ideation. Some may contemplate harming their newborn infant.

The etiology of severe postpartum depression is not completely understood. In some instances, environmental factors clearly are responsible for the depressive symptoms. In other instances, the depression may be related to biochemical changes in the central nervous system. One theory currently under investigation is that fluctuating estrogen levels postpartum alter the concentration of serotonin receptors in the brain. The changes in serotonin concentration, in turn, may be responsible for the alterations in mood.[22] Another theory is that transient thyroid dysfunction may result in a depressive reaction.

Patients with severe depression symptoms should be referred for complete psychiatric evaluation. In most instances, the disorder can be treated with antidepressant medication and supportive counseling. Family members must be enlisted in the effort to provide nonjudgmental emotional support to the woman. In rare instances, electroconvulsive therapy may be indicated.

Many women at risk for severe postpartum depression can be identified antepartum if the obstetrician elicits a detailed social and medical history.[9] Patients are at increased risk for puerperal depression when one of the following conditions is present.

- Patient and spouse are experiencing marital difficulty.
- Patient is single or separated.
- Patient has previous history of postpartum depression.
- Pregnancy is unplanned and unwanted.

Patients judged to be at high risk should be offered supportive counseling by the obstetrician early in pregnancy. Appropriate referrals to social service agencies, adoption agencies, and marriage counseling centers should be made promptly so that the patient may attempt to resolve her personal and social problems prior to delivery.

FAMILY PLANNING

Reversible Contraception

In 1980, there were more than six million pregnancies in the United States. Over 50% of these pregnancies were unplanned. In some instances, the women did not desire pregnancy at all. In other situations, the pregnancy was poorly timed. One-half of the unintended pregnancies were terminated by legal abortion. In some cities in the United States, there is one legal abortion for every liveborn infant.[32]

The economic, social, and medical expense associated with inconsistent family planning is immense. Therefore, it is incumbent upon the obstetrician to provide the patient with complete counseling concerning contraception before she is released from the hospital.

Selection of a method of contraception should be based upon several considerations. First, and most important, should be the expressed desires of the patient. If the patient does not feel comfortable with a particular method of contraception, she will not use it consistently and thus will be exposed to risk of unwanted pregnancy. The patient's opinions will depend upon her prior contraceptive experience, previous counseling from health-care providers, and her moral and religious convictions. The second consideration is the physician's assessment of the patient's level of education, medical sophistication, and motivation. Barrier methods or the rhythm method are not optimal choices in young, poorly educated, and poorly motivated patients. On the other hand, such methods may be eminently satisfactory for intelligent, well-motivated women with regular menstrual cycles and stable sexual relationships.

Another important consideration is the projected frequency of the patient's sexual contact. Barrier methods may be quite acceptable to the woman who has infrequent sexual exposure. Oral contraceptives or the IUCD may be better alternatives for the patient who has frequent sexual contact and who desires secure protection from pregnancy. The final consideration in selection of contraceptive technique is the patient's medical and surgical history. There are several definite contraindications to use of oral contraceptives and the IUCD. There are few, if any, medical contraindications to use of barrier methods or natural planning methods.

Oral Contraceptives

Combination Pills

Formulation. Combination oral contraceptives contain an estrogen and a progestin. The estrogen component is either mestranol or ethinyl estradiol. Mestranol differs from ethinyl estradiol only in that it is methylated at the third carbon position (Fig. 9-5). Mestranol is converted to ethinyl estradiol through demethylation in the liver. Considerations of relative potency of these two estrogens are not usually of clinical importance.

Combination pills may be divided into three main groups in accordance with their estrogen content.

- High-dose estrogen (80–100 μg)
- Intermediate-dose estrogen (50 μg)
- Low-dose estrogen (30–35 μg)

The incidence of many of the major and minor side effects of oral contraceptives varies directly with the total estrogen content of the pill.

Several different synthetic progestins are found in combination oral contraceptives (Fig. 9-6). The most commonly used progestins, in order of decreasing potency, are norgestrel, norethindrone acetate, and norethindrone. These substances are derivatives of the C-19 compound, nortestosterone, not the C-21 compound progesterone. Certain of the major side effects of oral contraceptives, particularly the metabolic derangements, are directly related to the total progestin concentration in the pill.

Mechanism of Action. The contraceptive effect of the combination pill depends upon suppression of gonadotropin secretion and, hence, ovulation. The progestin component primarily suppresses LH secretion, whereas the estrogen component suppresses FSH. The estrogen component also stabilizes the endometrium to prevent breakthrough bleeding and potentiates the action of the progestational agent.

Efficacy. The combination pill is the most secure of the reversible methods of contraception. The theoretical incidence of failure is 0.1%. The actual observed incidence of failure is 1– 2%. Failures occur primarily because patients fail to restart their next cycle of pills on schedule. Ovarian suppression is therefore not complete and ovulation occurs.

Common Side Effects. The most common side effects associated with use of combination oral contraceptives are listed in Table 9-5. Whereas each of these effects is important to the individual patient, they are unlikely to pose a serious threat to the woman's health. The first four complications are most likely to occur during the initial two to three months of therapy and usually resolve by the end of that time.

Breakthrough bleeding also is particularly likely to occur in the first three months of use. The incidence is increased in women using low-dose estrogen pills due to inadequate estrogen stimulation of the endometrium. Breakthrough bleeding usually resolves by the end of the third cycle. If the bleeding does not resolve spontaneously, it can be managed by supplementing the pill with low doses of estrogen (ethinyl estradiol, 20 μg). Administration of supplemental estrogen should be continued until bleeding resolves.

Chloasma may occur during oral contracep-

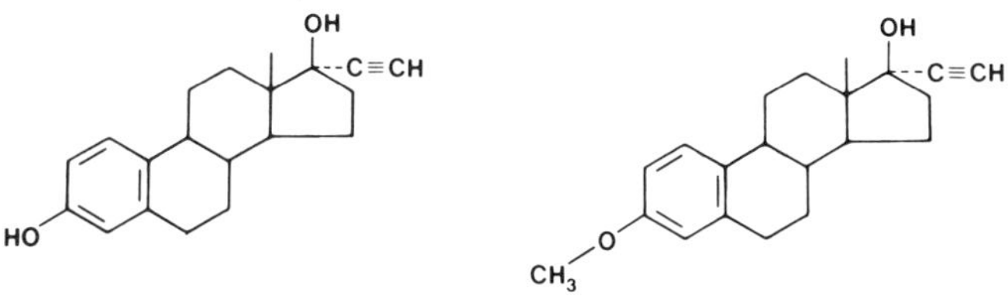

Ethinyl estradiol

Mestranol

Figure 9-5. Estrogen components of combination oral contraceptives.

PROGESTIN COMPONENT OF COMBINATION ORAL CONTRACEPTIVES

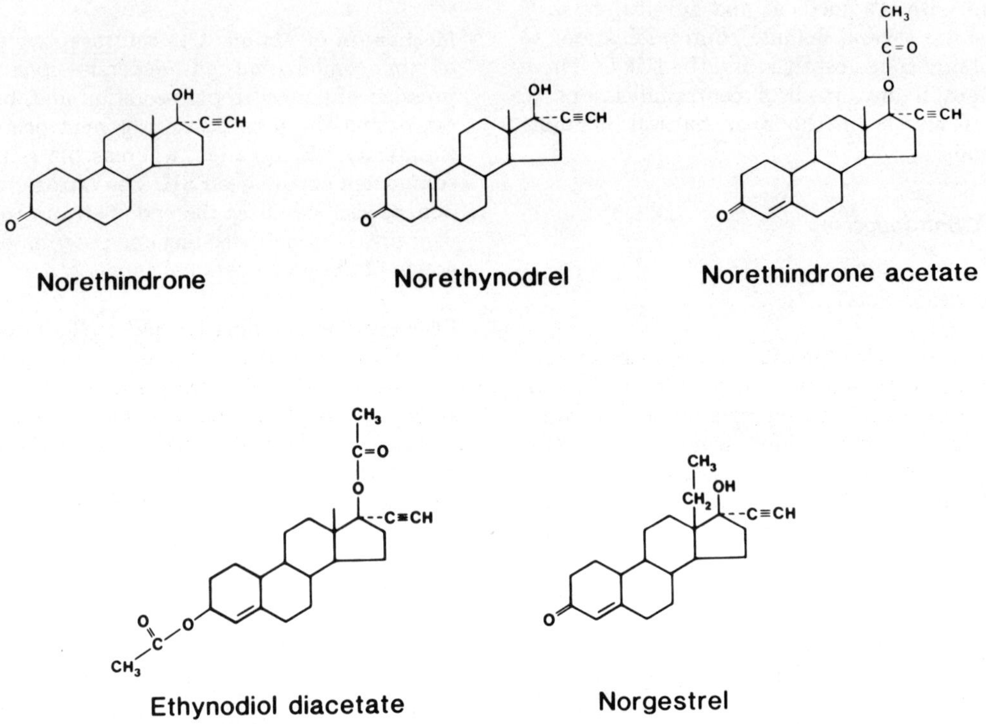

Figure 9-6. Progestin components of combination oral contraceptives.

tive therapy. Upon discontinuation of the pill, the pigmentation may decrease but may not resolve completely. This problem is not a serious medical complication, but it can be quite distressing to the individual patient.

Major Side Effects

THROMBOEMBOLISM. The incidence of deep venous thrombosis in the leg is increased fourfold in women who use oral contraceptives as compared to age-matched controls who do not use the pill. The incidence of superficial thrombophlebitis of the leg is increased twofold. The presence of varicose veins does not increase the risk of deep or superficial thrombophlebitis. The incidence of thromboembolism varies directly in proportion to the total estrogen concentration of the pill.

Although the relative risk of venous thrombosis is increased in oral contraceptive users, the absolute incidence of this complication is quite low. For users of the 50 μg pill, the incidence of venous thrombosis is approximately 1:1200 users per year. The incidence of thromboembolism appears to be even lower in patients who use the lower-dose estrogen preparations.[49,55]

TABLE 9-5. COMMON SIDE EFFECTS ASSOCIATED WITH USE OF ORAL CONTRACEPTIVES

Nausea and vomiting
Fluid retention
Weight gain
Breast tenderness
Breakthrough bleeding
Chloasma

CEREBROVASCULAR ACCIDENT. Women with a history of vascular headaches may experience an exacerbation upon use of the pill. Vascular headaches also may appear for the first time in pill users. More importantly, in women using oral contraceptives, the incidence of thrombotic and hemorrhagic stroke is increased threefold and twofold, respectively, compared to age-matched controls. The absolute incidence of cerebrovascular accident, however, is very low: less than 1:10,000 users per year.[15]

MYOCARDIAL INFARCTION. The risk of myocardial infarction is increased in pill users. The relative risk varies with age and smoking history. Most of the excess risk of myocardial infarction is concentrated in women above age 35 who smoke and who have other risk factors for coronary artery disease such as hypertension, obesity, hyperlipidemia, and diabetes. Nonsmoking women under the age of 35, who are in good general health and who take the low-dose pills, are extremely unlikely to have any serious cardiovascular complication.[27,38,39,56,57]

METABOLIC DERANGEMENTS. Both the estrogen and progestin components of the pill alter carbohydrate metabolism.[55] The sex steroids lower concentrations of insulin receptors, thus increasing peripheral resistance to the action of insulin. Approximately 15–40% of women taking the pill develop an abnormal glucose tolerance test. These alterations in carbohydrate metabolism are readily reversible upon discontinuation of the medication.

Oral contraceptives containing 50 μg of estrogen cause increases in serum LDL, VLDL, cholesterol, and triglyceride concentrations. Such changes in lipid metabolism tend to increase the risk for coronary artery disease. The low-dose pills cause lesser increases in LDL and VLDL and simultaneously increase HDL-cholesterol concentrations. The latter alteration appears to offer a protective effect against coronary atherosclerosis. This beneficial alteration in lipid concentration is due to a lowering of both the estrogen and progestin concentration in the newer pills.

The estrogen component of oral contraceptives increases hepatic synthesis of transcortin. Although the concentration of total and free cortisol is increased in women using the pill, the pituitary–adrenal axis functions normally in response to stress. Similarly, the estrogen in the pill increases hepatic synthesis of thyroid binding globulin. Accordingly, the serum concentration of total T4 increases and the T3-resin uptake decreases. Free T4 concentrations remain normal.

BILIARY TRACT FUNCTION. Cholestatic jaundice is one of the major gastrointestinal complications of oral contraceptive therapy.[15] Although the incidence of this side effect is very low, it is particularly likely to occur in women with a history of cholestatic jaundice of pregnancy. Therefore, such women should not receive oral contraceptives.

Hepatocellular adenoma, another serious hepatic complication, occurs in approximately 1 in 250,000 pill users. Although histologically benign, the tumor can enlarge to the point of rupture and can cause exsanguinating hemorrhage.[3,21,40,43]

The annual incidence of cholelithiasis in women of all ages is approximately 158 per 100,000. The relative risk of gallbladder disease is increased twofold by oral contraceptives. The increase in cholelithiasis occurs primarily because estrogen induces alterations in cholesterol and bile salt solubility that favor precipitation of cholesterol crystals. In addition, the progestin component of the pill may cause some degree of biliary stasis, which also predisposes to stone formation.[8]

The incidence of acute pancreatitis is increased in women who use oral contraceptives. In some women, pancreatic inflammation results from biliary tract obstruction due to cholelithiasis. In some, pancreatitis is the direct result of hyperlipidemia. In others, pancreatitis appears to result from the inhibitory effect of progesterone on the secretory ducts of the pancreas.

HYPERTENSION. Hypertension develops in approximately 5% of women who have used oral contraceptives containing 50 μg or more of estrogen for 5 years. The incidence of hypertension in patients using the low-dose pill appears to be significantly lower. When hypertension does occur, it is associated with alterations in the renin–angiotensin system. The characteristic abnormalities are increased plasma renin substrate, plasma renin activity, and aldosterone concentrations. Although pill-related hypertension usually is reversible, the elevated blood pressure may not resolve for 3–6 months after discontinuation of oral contraceptives.[34]

Women who develop hypertension while on the pill are not at greater risk of experiencing preeclampsia during a subsequent pregnancy and individuals who have had preeclampsia are not at increased risk for developing hypertension while on the pill.

POSTPILL AMENORRHEA. This complication occurs in less than 1% of patients. It is most likely to develop in women who have a prior history of oligomenorrhea or amenorrhea. Most individuals resume normal ovulatory cycles within 3 months after discontinuing oral contraceptives.

DEVELOPMENT OF MALIGNANCY. There is no consistent evidence that use of oral contraceptives increases the subsequent risk of breast or cervical cancer.[12,55] Preexisting benign fibrocystic disease of the breast, in fact, usually improves in women using oral contraceptives.[43,50] The risk of ovarian cancer and endometrial cancer actually is reduced in women who have used the pill. In a recent multicenter study, investigators from the Centers for Disease Control observed a relative risk of ovarian cancer of 0.6 in pill users as compared to nonusers. The relative risk of endometrial cancer was 0.5.[13,14]

PRESCRIBING THE COMBINATION PILL. One of the sub-50 μg pills is the most appropriate choice for the majority of women. These agents combine a high degree of efficacy with a remarkably low incidence of serious side effects. Of the sub-50 μg pills, the optimal formulation would appear to be the one with the lowest concentration of both estrogen and progestin. Prior to prescribing the pill, the physician should make certain that there are no absolute or relative contraindications to its use (Tables 9-6 and 9-7). The physician should document in the medical record that the patient has been counseled about the principal complications associated with use of oral contraceptives. A complete physical examination should be performed and cervical cytology obtained. Specific laboratory studies such as hematocrit, lipid profile, glucose, or liver function tests should be ordered if indicated by the patient's medcial history.

As a general rule, administration of oral contraceptives should be delayed until approximately two weeks postpartum. The primary reason to delay is that use of estrogen-containing compounds in the immediate puerperium may be associated with an increased incidence of thromboembolism. Once contraceptive therapy is begun, the patient should return for reevaluation within three months. At this time, she should be questioned about any side effects related to the pill and about her routine for administering the medication. Any errors in timing of administration should be corrected. Use of 28-pill packets, which contain 21 active pills and 7 inert pills, may be helpful in insuring that patients use their medication properly.

TABLE 9-6. ABSOLUTE CONTRAINDICATIONS TO USE OF ORAL CONTRACEPTIVES

Estrogen-dependent tumor (breast cancer, endometrial cancer)
Pregnancy
History of thromboembolism
Undiagnosed uterine bleeding
Ischemic heart disease
Severe liver disease
History of obstructive jaundice in pregnancy
Congenital hyperlipidemia

TABLE 9-7. RELATIVE CONTRAINDICATIONS TO USE OF ORAL CONTRACEPTIVES

Vascular headaches
Hypertension
Insulin-dependent and non-insulin-dependent diabetes mellitus
Uterine leiomyoma
Severe depression
Seizure disorder
Sickle cell disease or sickle cell C disease
Cigarette smoking and age >35 years

Triphasic Oral Contraceptives. At the present time, three triphasic preparations are available in the United States. Two of these formulations provide for varying amounts of norethindrone (0.5–1.0 mg) at different phases of the cycle in combination with a fixed amount of ethinyl estradiol (35 μg). The third preparation contains varying amounts of levonorgestrel (0.05–0.125 mg) in combination with varying concentrations of ethinyl estradiol (30–40 μg).

The primary objective in developing these new agents was to reduce the total steroid content of the pill, particularly the progestin component. A secondary objective was to reduce the incidence of midcycle breakthrough bleeding and amenorrhea. Multicenter investigators have confirmed that the triphasic preparations are comparable in efficacy to the fixed-dose low-estrogen pills. There is no definitive evidence at present, however, that there are fewer side effects associated with use of the triphasic agents.

Progestin-Only Pills (Minidose Pills). The progestin-only pills currently available in United States contain either norethindrone or norgestrel. These agents do not consistently suppress ovulation. Rather, their contraceptive action depends upon two effects. They cause changes in cervical mucus that interfere with sperm transport. They also cause histologic changes in the endometrium that render it unreceptive to ovum implantation.

The progestin-only pills are indicated primarily for the woman who has a medical contraindication to use of combination oral contraceptives or the intrauterine contraceptive device and who does not wish to use barrier methods. The minidose pills have two serious disadvantages that limit their usefulness even in these situations. They have a relatively high incidence of failure compared to combination oral contraceptives (2–8% versus 1%) and approximately 30–40% of women using these agents experience troublesome breakthrough bleeding. Unexpected heavy bleeding is, in fact, the most common reason cited for discontinuation of the minidose pills.

Intrauterine Contraceptive Device. Intrauterine contraceptive devices (IUCD) are classified into two types: nonmedicated and medicated. The two most commonly used nonmedicated IUCDs are the Saf-T-Coil^{R} and the Lippes Loop^{R}. The latter device is produced in four different sizes, from smallest (size A) to largest (size D). The most frequently used medicated IUCDs contain either copper (copper T and copper 7) or progesterone (Progestasert^{R}) (Fig. 9-7). A recent review article provides an excellent description of the specific design features of these devices.[59]

All IUCDs share a common principal mechanism of action. Their contraceptive effect is considered to be due primarily to induction of an inflammatory reaction in the endometrium that interferes with implantation of the fertilized ovum. The progesterone-containing IUCD exerts both a mechanical and a hormonal effect that renders the endometrium unfavorable for ovum implantation. The copper in the copper T or copper 7 enhances the inflammatory reaction in the endometrium and also may be directly cytolytic to the blastocyst and endometrial cells.[45] The fact that the IUCD inhibits implantation, but not necessarily conception, may be an important consideration for some individuals, and this fact must be explained to the patient.

The IUCD provides an excellent method of contraception for the multiparous patient who has a stable sexual relationship and no history

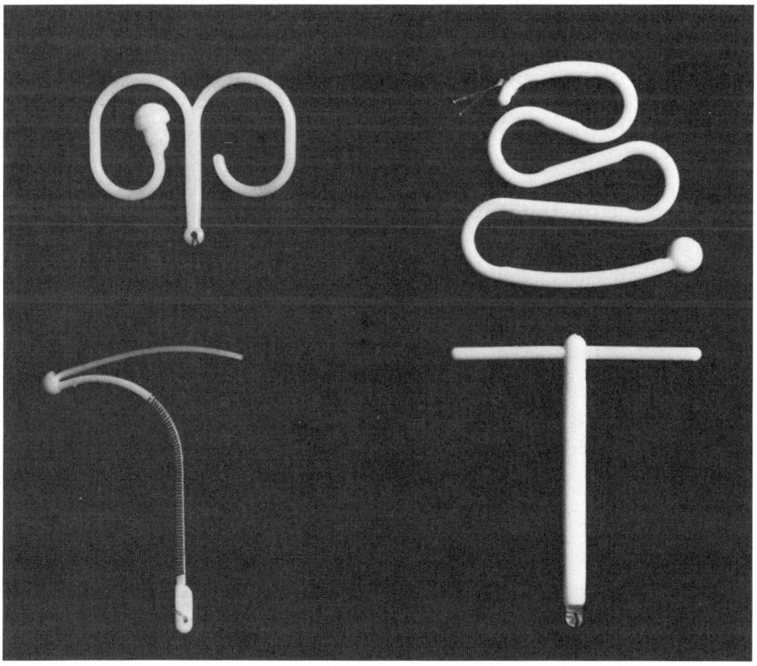

Figure 9-7. Photographs of four of the most commonly used IUCDs. From left to right: Saf-T-Coil®, Lippes Loop®, Copper-7®, Progestaset®.

TABLE 9-8. RELATIVE CONTRAINDICATIONS TO USE OF AN INTRAUTERINE CONTRACEPTIVE DEVICE

Suspected intrauterine pregnancy
History of pelvic inflammatory disease
History of severe dysmenorrhea
History of menorrhagia
History of ectopic pregnancy
Unexplained genital tract bleeding
Suspicion of gynecologic malignancy
Stenosis of the endocervical canal
History of septic abortion or puerperal endometritis within the past three months
Abnormality of the endometrial cavity that is incompatible with structure of the IUCD

of menstrual dysfunction. In such individuals it can be expected to have a high retention rate. There are limitations and contraindications to its use, however (Table 9-8).

There are few differences among IUCDs with respect to either efficacy or complications. The one significant difference is the length of time that the device may remain in place. The nonmedicated devices, in theory, can be used indefinitely. The medicated devices need to be removed at periodic intervals: one year for the Progestasert^R and three years for the copper-containing devices.

Complications associated with use of the IUCD are listed in Table 9-9. The most frequent untoward effects are increased menstrual bleeding and dysmenorrhea, which occur in approximately 5–15% of IUCD users. Excessive bleeding and dysmenorrhea can be minimized by administering prostaglandin synthetase inhibitors at the time of menses. In approximately 5–10% of cases the IUCD is either spontaneously expelled or causes sufficient bleeding and pain that the patient requests removal.

TABLE 9-9. COMPLICATIONS ASSOCIATED WITH USE OF AN INTRAUTERINE CONTRACEPTIVE DEVICE

Increased menstrual bleeding
Intermenstrual bleeding
Dysmenorrhea
Expulsion
Pelvic inflammatory disease
Embedding
Perforation of fundus or cervix
Accidental pregnancy

Perforation of the uterine fundus is a rare, but potentially serious, complication of the IUCD. Fundal perforation usually occurs coincident with insertion of the device. It is more common with devices that are inserted by the "push-out" as opposed to the "pull-back" technique. Perforation of the cervix may occur at the time of insertion of the IUCD or after the device has been in place for some time. In the latter instance, perforation typically occurs because the device becomes displaced from its fundal position, resulting in pressure of the stem of the device against the endocervical canal.

Perforation of either the fundus or cervical canal usually is asymptomatic. The diagnosis is considered because the string of the IUCD no longer is accessible to the patient or the examiner. When symptoms are present, the two most common are pelvic pain and irregular bleeding. Ultrasonography is the most reliable way to determine whether an IUCD is intra- or extrauterine. Hysteroscopy is also of value in confirming intrauterine location of a displaced IUCD and in removing the device. Medicated IUCDs that become dislodged into extrauterine locations should be removed by laparoscopy or laparotomy. From a purely medical point of view, there does not appear to be any harm in allowing nonmedicated IUCDs to remain intraperitoneal. Medical-legal considerations may dictate their removal, however.

The two most serious complications associated with the IUCD are infection and accidental pregnancy. Several investigations have confirmed a strong relationship between the IUCD and increased risk of acute salpingitis.[22] The relative risk of salpingitis associated with use of the IUCD is four to nine times that experienced by age-matched controls who do not use the IUCD. Independent of other risk factors for infection, the annual incidence of acute salpingitis among IUCD users is 1–2%.

The failure rate associated with the IUCD is 1–3% per year. In women who experience method failure, there is an increased incidence of ectopic pregnancy. There also is increased risk of spontaneous abortion. In some series, the incidence of spontaneous abortion in IUCD-related pregnancies has been as high as 40–50%.[59] Moreover, a high percentage of the abortions occur because of infection, some of which result in maternal mortality.[11] For these reasons, the IUCD should be removed as soon as pregnancy is diagnosed. If this is not possible, the patient should be counseled about the increased risk of spontaneous abortion and infection and should be offered the option of pregnancy termination.

Diaphragm. The diaphragm is a rubber device composed of a dome and a rim. The rim encases a metal spring, which may have one of three configurations. The selection of a specific type of spring is based upon the contour of the patient's vagina and the position of the uterus. When pelvic anatomy is normal, either the coiled or flat spring is acceptable. The arcing-spring diaphragm should be considered when the uterus is markedly ante- or retroverted or when mild degrees of cystocele or uterine prolapse are present.

To be most effective, the diaphragm should be used in conjunction with a spermicidal cream or jelly. The spermicide should be applied along the rim and inside the dome prior to insertion of the diaphragm. The patient may insert the device with her fingers or with a plastic applicator. Figure 9-8 illustrates the correct position of the diaphragm within the vagina. When the diaphragm is in place, the patient should be able to void freely, and she should not be consistently aware of its presence. The proper method for insertion of the device should be demonstrated in the physician's office and the obstetrician should insure that the patient can insert and remove the device easily.

The patient should leave the diaphragm in place for a minimum of six hours after intercourse. Removal of the device too soon may decrease the amount of spermicide to such a point that sperm can survive in the vagina. Douching within six hours of intercourse may also have this effect.

If more than six hours have elapsed since insertion of the diaphragm, a second application of the spermicide is necessary before intercourse. The diaphragm need not be removed; additional spermicide may be applied intravaginally with an applicator. Another application of spermicide is indicated each time intercourse is repeated. This is necessary regardless of the length of time the diaphragm has been in place.

When used correctly, the diaphragm provides an excellent combination of safety and efficacy. The incidence of accidental pregnancy associated with the diaphragm is 5–12%.[19] The only serious complication resulting from use of the diaphragm is the rare occurrence of toxic shock syndrome. Pressure ulcers in the upper vaginal vault and/or cervical erosion also may

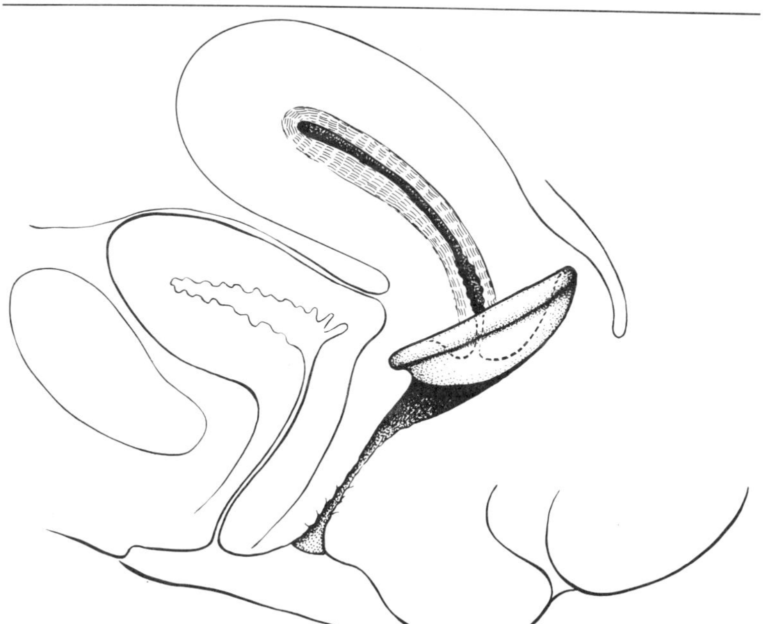

Figure 9-8. Illustration demonstrates the correct position of diaphragm within the vagina. The rim is held in place against the muscular vaginal wall, and the dome completely covers the cervical os.

develop in some patients. The principal disadvantage of the diaphragm is that it may be inconvenient and aesthetically displeasing for the patient to use and it may detract from the spontaneity of the sexual experience. The latter difficulty may be lessened by encouraging the patient to insert the device at a time remote from the act of intercourse. Alternatively, the sexual partner can be instructed to insert the diaphragm during foreplay.

Contraceptive Sponge. Development of the contraceptive sponge began in 1976. In 1983, the Food and Drug Administration granted final approval of the device as a nonprescription contraceptive. The sponge is made of polyurethane and is 5.5 cm in diameter and 2.5 cm thick. It is impregnated with 1 g of the spermicide nonoxynol 9. It also contains small amounts of preservatives such as citric, sorbic, and benzoic acids. Its pH is in the range of 4–5. The contraceptive effect of the sponge is due primarily to sustained release of spermicide. Approximately 125 mg of nonoxynol 9 is liberated into the upper vaginal vault during 24 hours.[20]

The sponge should be inserted in the same manner as the diaphragm. A small indentation on one side of the sponge is intended to assure correct placement against the cervix. A polyester retrieval loop is attached to the other side of the device to facilitate removal.

The sponge should be left in place for a minimum of six hours after intercourse. It provides continuous protection against pregnancy for 24 hours. After removal, it should be discarded. The sponge may be used while the woman is menstruating but should not be utilized simply as a tampon.

There are few serious complications associated with use of the contraceptive sponge. As with the diaphragm, isolated patients have developed toxic shock syndrome while the sponge was in place. More common problems encountered by users of the sponge include breakage of the retrieval loop, fragmentation of the sponge, and vaginal itching.

A recent multicenter study compared the contraceptive sponge to the diaphragm for efficacy and convenience. Cumulative one-year pregnancy rate was higher in sponge users (17%) than in diaphragm users (12.5%). Sponge users were more likely to discontinue use of the device because of vaginal irritation. Despite the slightly higher failure rate, however, certain features of the sponge were attractive to patients. It was easy to use and was not inordinately messy. It did not require fitting in a physician's office, and it could be purchased without a prescription. In addition, it provided continuous protection against pregnancy for 24 hours regardless of the number of episodes of intercourse.[20]

Contraceptive Foams, Creams, and Jellies. The contraceptive effect of foams, creams, and jellies is mediated by the spermicide nonoxynol 9. These preparations should be inserted into the upper vaginal vault against the cervix shortly before intercourse. Insertion is facilitated by use of a plastic applicator.

No serious side effects are associated with use of these agents. They may, however, cause localized burning and irritation in the vagina and penile irritation in the sex partner. The suppository preparations also may not disperse evenly. In addition, they are messy and may detract from the spontaneity of sex. Failure rates associated with use of spermicidal peparations alone are in the range of 5–15%. The incidence of failure is decreased if the male concurrently uses a condom.

"Natural" Family Planning Techniques. The natural family planning methods estimate the time of ovulation by observation of the calendar, the basal body temperature, or the physical properties of cervical mucus. These methods are particularly appealing to individuals whose religious convictions prevent them from utilizing one of the contraceptive methods described above. They are most effective in well-motivated women who have regular menstrual cycles. In such patients, failure rates range from 5% to 15%. In women who do not have regular monthly cycles, failure rates may be higher.

When using the calendar method of rhythm, the woman estimates the time of ovulation by subtracting 14–16 days from the length of her usual cycle. She then abstains from intercourse for approximately four days before and four days after the estimated day of ovulation. The range of six to eight days is selected to account for monthly variations in the time of ovulation. For example, in a patient who has a regular monthly cycle of 28 days, the expected day of ovulation is day 12–14. Therefore, this individual would abstain from sexual intercourse from day 10 to day 18 in order to be as secure in her contraception as possible.

Measurement of basal body temperature may provide a more precise estimate of the time of ovulation. When utilizing this method of contraception, the woman should record her oral temperature each morning before arising from bed. Ovulation typically occurs when the basal temperature curve decreases slightly and then rises to a higher plateau.

The patient also may estimate the time of ovulation by noting when the mucus begins to increase in amount and viscosity. These changes in the physiochemical properties of cervical mucus are mediated by the estradiol surge associated with ovulation and are precisely the changes that physicians attempt to observe when performing postcoital tests or artificial insemination.

Sterilization

Some women may request sterilization at cesarean section or immediately following vaginal delivery. Tubal ligation does not increase the incidence of complications associated with cesarean childbirth, nor does it prolong the operative time significantly. Sterilization can also be accomplished safely during the two or three days that the patient remains hospitalized after vaginal delivery. The operation may be performed under general, regional, or local anesthesia.[42]

Prior to performing sterilization, the obstetrician must insure that the neonate has been evaluated by the attending pediatrician and that no obvious anomalies are present. In addition, the obstetrician should be certain that the patient has been counseled concerning alternative methods of reversible contraception, likelihood of surgical failure, and prospects for reversal of the procedure. The physician should identify patients at high risk for subsequently requesting reversal and consider delaying sterilization in these women until a later time. The risk factors are young age, low parity, and unstable marital situation.

Pomeroy and Modified Pomeroy Technique. The Pomeroy procedure is the most frequently performed tubal ligation in the United States. This operation was first described by Bishop and Nelms[7] who credited Ralph Pomeroy with origination of the technique. They urged widespread adoption of the procedure because of its simplicity, safety, and security.

The operation is simple to complete and is associated with very few serious complications. It can be easily performed at cesarean delivery and in the immediate puerperium. Reported failure rates range from 1/200 to 1/400 for procedures performed either at the time of cesarean delivery or immediately postpartum.[24,25] The one exception to these statistics is the report by Prystowsky and Eastman of one failure in 57 Pomeroy procedures (1.7%) performed at the time of cesarean section. Their observed incidence of failure for puerperal procedures was 1/340, a figure in keeping with other reports.[46]

A commonly used modification of the Pomeroy procedure is illustrated in Fig. 9-9.[24] It differs from the original description of the operation in that a single, rather than double, ligature is employed. The initial step of the procedure is to elevate the midportion of the tube with an atraumatic clamp. A single suture of 0-chromic or 0-plain catgut is tied securely around the tube, and a portion of the knuckle is excised. Over a period of 10–14 days, the suture resorbs, and the ends of the tubes separate. The larger the original knuckle of tube, the greater will be the ultimate separation between the severed ends of the tubes.

A second modification of the Pomeroy procedure is illustrated in Fig. 9-10.[23] In this operation, the tube is ligated in two separate locations, and the intervening portion of tube is excised. The rationale for this modification is that it insures prompt, wide separation of the two ends of the tube and, in theory at least, reduces the risk of fistula formation. At the present time no prospective, randomized investigation has demonstrated this modification to be superior to either the original Pomeroy technique or other modified procedures.

Uchida Procedure. The Uchida procedure was developed by Hajime Uchida of Ishikawa, Japan.[60] A modification of Uchida's original operative technique is illustrated in Fig. 9-11. The tube is grasped in its midportion and a dilute solution of epinephrine (1:100,000) in saline is injected beneath the serosa. The serosa then is excised, exposing the muscularis of the tube. The tube is doubly ligated with 0-chromic and a 5 cm segment is excised. Thereafter, the proximal end of the tube is inverted between the leaves of the broad ligament and the distal end is left exteriorized. The defect in the visceral peritoneum then is oversewn.

The principal advantage of the Uchida procedure is the very low failure rate. Over a 28-year period, Uchida[60] personally performed more than 20,000 operations and reported no apparent failures. Unfortunately, he did not provide detailed follow-up of his patients, and

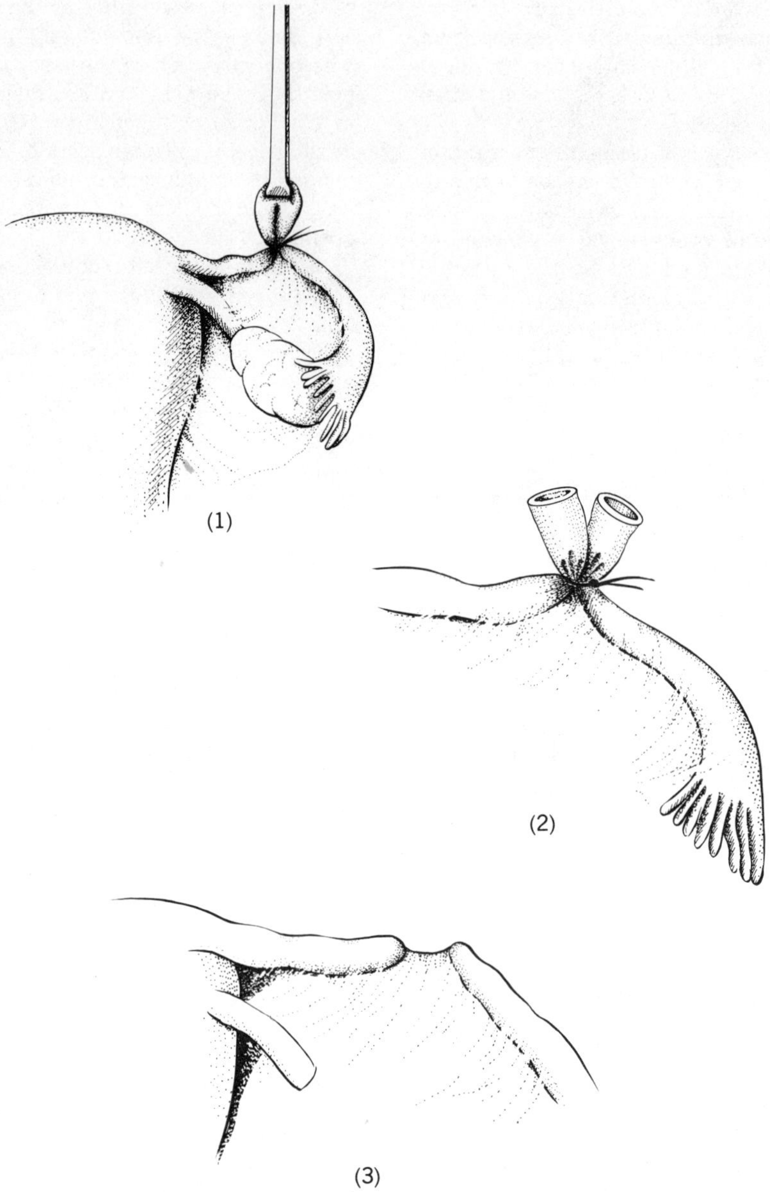

Figure 9-9. Pomeroy technique. (1) Formation and ligation of knuckle of tube with 0-plain or 0-chromic suture. (2) Excision of portion of tube. (3) After resorption of suture, ends of tube are separated.

there are no other large series to compare with his.

There are two major disadvantages to the Uchida procedure. First, because such a long segment of tube is removed, the potential for reversal may not be as good as with other methods of tubal occlusion. Second, the operation is more difficult to perform than the Pomeroy technique. Therefore, the procedure may be associated with increased blood loss and increased operating time.

Oxford Procedure. The Oxford technique has been popularized by Stallworthy and Williams.[24] The basic principle of the technique is to remove a small segment of the tubal isthmus

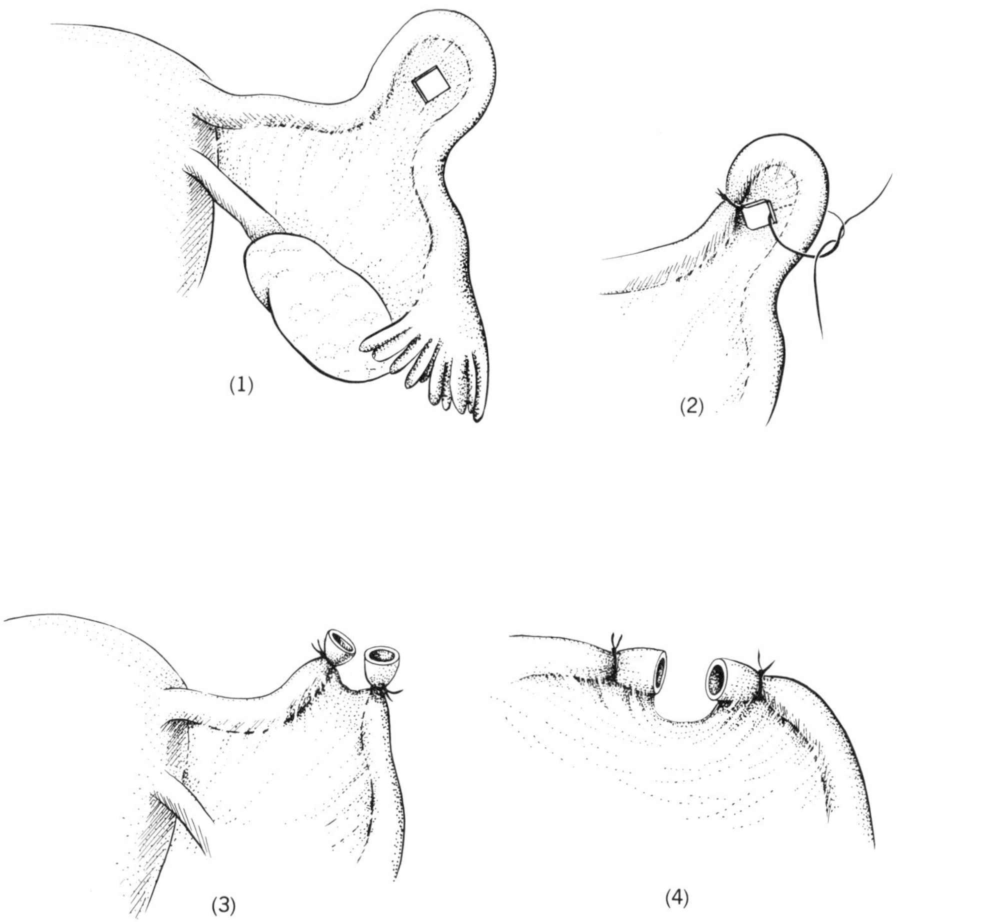

Figure 9-10. Modified Pomeroy technique. (1) Avascular window is created in mesosalpinx. (2) Two separate sutures of 0-plain or 0-chromic are passed through the window in mesosalpinx. Each end of tube is ligated. (3) Portion of tube is excised. (4) Ends of tube are separated from one another immediately rather than at the time the suture resorbs.

and then separate the severed ends of the tube by interposing the round ligament. The procedure illustrated in Fig. 9-12 incorporates modifications proposed by Green and Laros.[24] At a point approximately 1.5 cm from the cornua, the tube is doubly ligated with 0-chromic suture. A 5 mm segment of the isthmic portion of tube is then excised. The distal ligature on the proximal end of the tube is left long and is threaded beneath the round ligament. The two ends of the suture then are tied together, thus anchoring the proximal tube behind the round ligament. The distal segment of tube is brought in front of the round ligament and secured in this position by incorporation into the previous ligature.

The failure rate of the Oxford technique is comparable to that of the Pomeroy procedure. The principal advantage of this technique is its potential for reversal because such a small segment of the tube is destroyed. More than 70% of patients have successful term pregnancies after reversal of the Oxford procedure.[24] The major disadvantage is its technical complexity and the requirement for more extended operative exposure. These considerations make the technique less suitable for an operation performed through a small infraumbilical incision.

Irving Procedure. This procedure first was described by Frederick Irving[26] in 1924. It is illustrated, with slight modification, in Fig. 9-13. The initial step of the operation is to doubly ligate and divide the tube approximately 4 cm

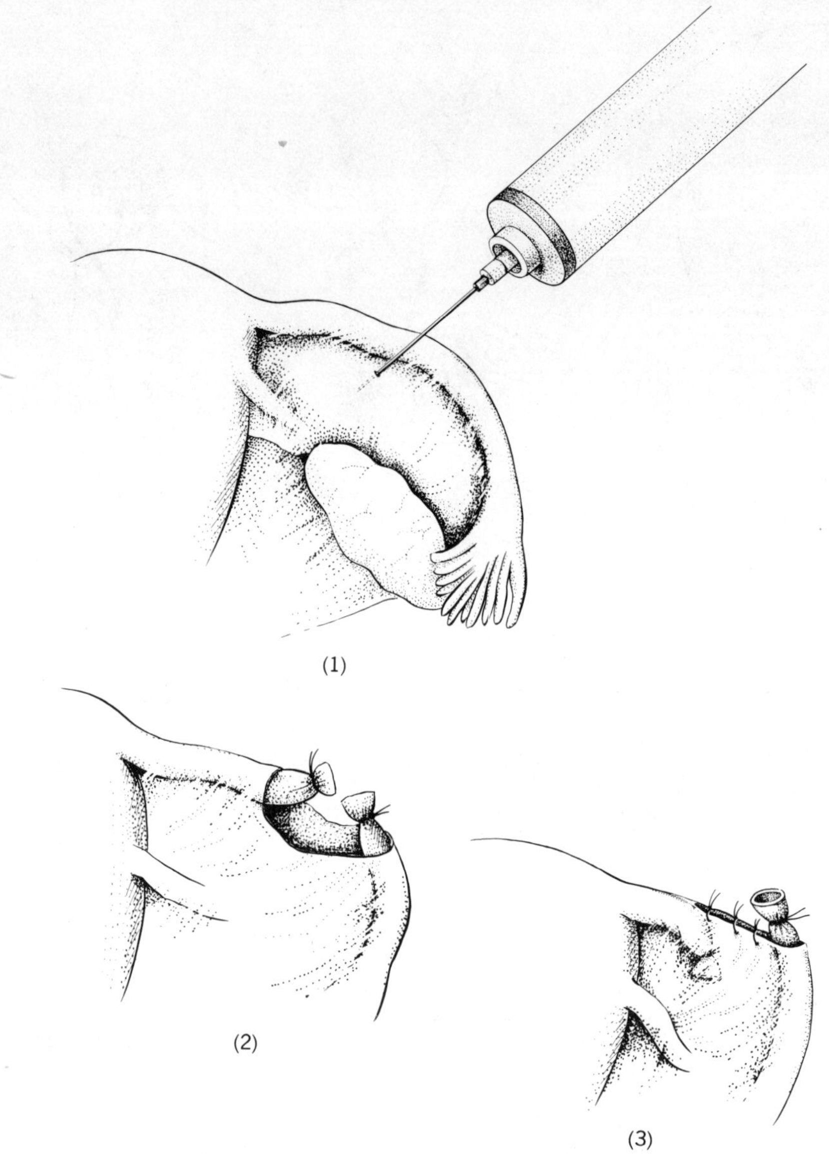

Figure 9-11. Uchida technique. (1) Dilute solution of epinephrine is injected into serosa of tube. (2) Muscularis of tube is exposed. Tube is doubly ligated with 0-chromic. It then is divided approximately 5 cm from cornua and segment is removed. (3) Proximal end of tube is buried within broad ligament. Distal end is exteriorized and peritoneum is oversewn.

from the cornua. The distal ligature on the proximal tube should be left long and threaded onto a curved needle. Sharp dissection then is used to free the tube from the underlying mesosalpinx. At this point, a small tunnel, 2 cm in length, is created in the myometrium just above the insertion of the round ligament. The long suture attached to the proximal tube is threaded through the tunnel and the tube is guided into the myometrium. When the suture is tied, the tube becomes anchored within the myometrial tunnel. The myometrial defect is then closed with a figure-of-8 suture.

The major advantage of the Irving procedure

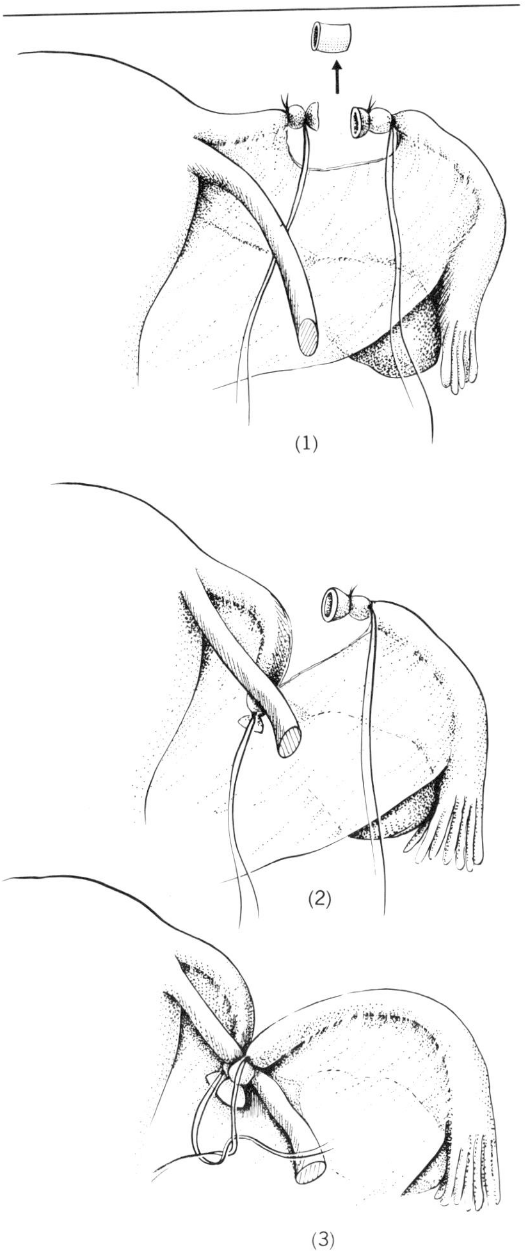

Figure 9-12. Oxford technique. (1) A 5 mm segment is removed from isthmus of tube. Each end of tube is doubly ligated with 0-chromic suture. (2) Distal ligature on proximal end of tube is passed beneath the round ligament. The two ends of the suture are tied to one another, anchoring the tube behind the round ligament. (3) Distal end of tube is brought anterior to round ligament. Distal suture on this portion of tube is tied.

is its high degree of efficacy. To date, there have been only two isolated reports of pregnancy after sterilization by the Irving technique.[24] The disadvantages of the operation are its technical difficulty, poor potential for reversal, increased blood loss, and increased operative time. In addition, because greater operative exposure is required, the procedure is not well suited to the postpartum period.

Kroener Procedure. This procedure was developed by William F. Kroener and was described by his son in 1969.[33] The essential principle of the operation is to resect the fimbriated end of the fallopian tube (Fig. 9-14). The first step of the procedure is to isolate the fimbria. A suture of 0-silk then is placed around the tube, proximal to the fimbria. The ligature is tied, taking care to include the fimbria ovarica in the tie. A second ligature then is placed around the tube, proximal to the first, and tied. Once both ligatures are secure, the fimbria is excised.

The advantage of the Kroener procedure is its simplicity. It is suitable for cesarean delivery and for the immediate postpartum period. Its principal disadvantages are a high incidence of failure and poor potential for reversal. In his original series, Kroener[33] reported no failures in 140 patients. However, other investigators have reported failure rates ranging from 0.9% to 3%, which is higher than those associated with the Pomeroy, Uchida, or Irving procedures.[35,57]

Tubal Occlusion by Clip or Ring. Some investigators have performed tubal occlusions in the immediate postpartum period under laparoscopic visualization. In such procedures, a spring-loaded plastic clip or ring is applied to the isthmic portion of the tube. Although laparoscopy is an excellent technique for interval sterilization, it has at least two disadvantages when employed in the immediate puerperium. First, proper placement of the laparoscope can be extremely difficult because of the enlarged uterus. The incidence of uterine perforation during postpartum laparoscopic procedures may be as high as 2%.[24] Second, there appears to be a high incidence of failure when these devices are used immediately postpartum. A 10% incidence of failure occurred when the Bleier clip was applied under direct vision at the time of cesarean delivery. The incidence of failure was 8.2% when the clip was applied through the laparoscope in postpartum patients.[1] A 13.6% incidence of failure has been noted in a similar group of pa-

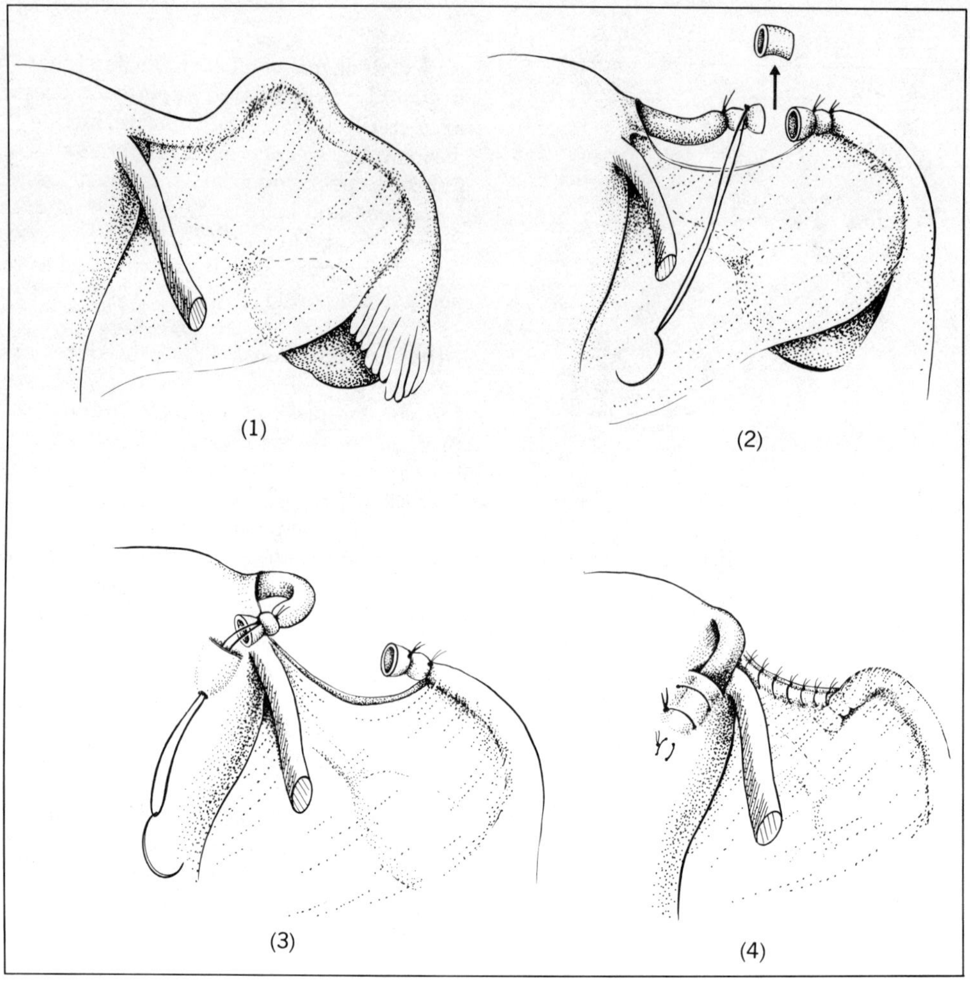

Figure 9-13. Irving technique. (1) Midportion of tube is elevated. (2) A 5 mm segment is removed from isthmus. Both ends of tube are doubly ligated with 0-chromic. (3) Myometrial tunnel is created on anterior uterine wall medial to insertion of round ligament. Distal suture on proximal end of tube is threaded into a needle and passed through the tunnel. (4) Suture is exteriorized and tied. Proximal end of tube is fixed securely within tunnel by additional sutures.

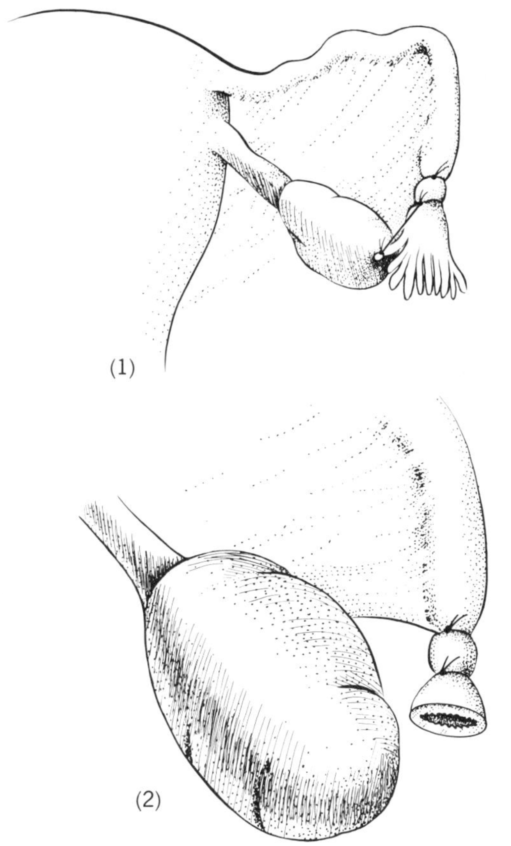

Figure 9-14. Kroener technique. (1) Two sutures of 0-silk are placed proximal to fimbria, incorporating the fimbria ovarica. (2) Fimbria is excised.

tients.[35] One of the major factors responsible for the high failure rate may be that, immediately after delivery, the tubes are enlarged and edematous and thus may not be effectively occluded by the plastic devices. Laparoscopic tubal occlusion should not be employed in the postpartum period because of the technical difficulties associated with this procedure and the high incidence of failure.

REFERENCES

1. Adelman R.: High failure rate of a plastic tubal (Bleier) clip. *Obstet. Gynecol.* **64**:721–724, 1984.
2. American Academy of Pediatrics—Committee on Nutrition. Nutrition and lactation. *Pediatrics* **68**:435–441, 1981.
3. Antoniades, K., Campbell, W. N., Hecksher, R. H., Kessler, W. B., and McCarthy, G. E.: Liver cell adenoma and oral contraceptives. *JAMA* **234**:628–629, 1975.
4. Anderson, P. O.: Drugs and breast feeding. *Semin. Perinatol.* **3**:271–278, 1979.
5. Anderson, W. R. and Davis, J.: Placental site involution. *Am. J. Obstet. Gynecol.* **102**:23–33, 1968.
6. Andreassen, B. and Tyson, J. E.: Role of the hypothalamic-pituitary-ovarian axis in puerperal infertility. *J. Clin. Endocrinol. Metab.* **42**:1114–1122, 1976.
7. Bishop, E. and Nelms, W. F.: A simple method of tubal sterilization. *N.Y. State J. Med.* **30**:214–216, 1930.
8. Bennion, L. J., Ginberg, R. L., Garrick, M. B., and Bennett, P. H.: Effects of oral contraceptives on the gallbladder bile of normal women. *N. Engl. J. Med.* **294**:189–192, 1976.
9. Braverman, J. and Roux, J. F.: Screening for the patient at risk of postpartum depression. *Obstet. Gynecol.* **52**:731–736, 1978.
10. Canales, E. S., Zarate, A., Garrido, J., Leon, C., Soria, J., and Schally, A. V.: Study on the recovery of pituitary FSH function during puerperium using synthetic LRH. *J. Clin. Endocrinol. Metab.* **38**:1140–1142, 1974.
11. Cates, W., Ory, H. W., Rochat, R. W., and Tyler, C. W.: The intrauterine device and deaths from spontaneous abortion. *N. Engl. J. Med.* **245**:1155–1159, 1976.
12. Centers for Disease Control: Long-term oral contraceptive use and the risk of breast cancer. *JAMA* **249**:1591–1595, 1983.
13. Centers for Disease Control: Oral contraceptive use and the risk of ovarian cancer. *JAMA* **249**:1591–1595, 1983.
14. Centers for Disease Control: Oral contraceptive use and the risk of endometrial cancer. *JAMA* **249**:1600–1604, 1983.
15. Collaborative Group for the Study of Stroke in Young Women: Oral contraception and increased risk of cerebral ischemia or thrombosis. *N. Engl. J. Med.* **288**:871–877, 1973.
16. Creasy, R. K. and Resnick, R. (Eds.): *Maternal-Fetal Medicine. Principles and Practice.* Philadelphia, W. B. Saunders Co., 1984.
17. Cronin, T. J.: Influence of lactation upon ovulation. *Lancet* **2**:422–424, 1968.
18. Cunningham, A. S.: Morbidity in breast-fed and artificially fed infants. *J. Pediatr.* **90**:726–729, 1977.
19. Daniel, D. G., Campbell, H., and Turnbull, A. C.: Puerperal thromboembolism and suppression of lactation. *Lancet* **2**:287–289, 1967.
20. Edelman, D. A., McIntyre, S. L., and Harper, J.: A comparative trial of the Today contraceptive sponge and diaphragm. *Am. J. Obstet. Gynecol.* **159**:864–876, 1984.
21. Edmondson, H. A., Henderson, B., and Benton, B.: Liver-cell adenomas associated with use

of oral contraceptives. *N. Engl. J. Med.* **294**:470–472, 1976.

22. Flesh, G., Weiner, J. M., Corlett, R. C., Boice, E., Mishell, D. R., and Wolf, R. M.: The intrauterine contraceptive device and acute salpingitis. *Am. J. Obstet. Gynecol.* **135**:402–408, 1979.
23. Garvey, M. J. and Tollefson, G. D.: Postpartum depression. *J. Reprod. Med.* **29**:113–115, 1984.
24. Green, L. R. and Laros, R. K.: Postpartum sterilization. *Clin. Obstet. Gynecol.* **23**:647–659, 1980.
25. Husbands, M. E., Pritchard, J. A., and Pritchard, S. A.: Failure of tubal sterilization accompanying cesarean section. *Am. J. Obstet. Gynecol.* **107**:966–967, 1974.
26. Irving, F. C.: A new method of insuring sterility following cesarean section. *Am. J. Obstet. Gynecol.* **8**:335–337, 1924.
27. Jain, A. K.: Cigarette smoking, use of oral contraceptives, and myocardial infarction. *Am. J. Obstet. Gynecol.* **126**:301–307, 1976.
28. Jeppsson, S., Rannevik, G., and Kullander, S.: Studies on the decreased gonadotropin response after administration of LH/FSH-releasing hormone during pregnancy and the puerperium. *Am. J. Obstet. Gynecol.* **120**:1029–1034, 1974.
29. Jelliffe, D. B. and Jelliffe, E. F. P.: "Breast is best:" Modern meaning. *N. Engl. J. Med.* **297**:912–915, 1977.
30. Jenness, R.: The composition of human milk. *Semin. Perinatol.* **3**:225–240, 1979.
31. Keye, W. R. and Jaffe, R. B.: Changing patterns of FSH and LH response to gonadotropin-releasing hormone in the puerperium. *J. Clin. Endocrinol. Metab.* **42**:1133–1138, 1976.
32. Klein, L.: To have or not to have a pregnancy. *Obstet. Gynecol.* **65**:1–4, 1985.
33. Kroener, W. F.: Surgical sterilization by fimbriectomy. *Am. J. Obstet. Gynecol.* **104**:247–251, 1969.
34. Laragh, J. H.: Oral contraceptive-induced hypertension—nine years later. *Am. J. Obstet. Gynecol.* **126**:141–147, 1976.
35. Lean, T. H., Vengadasalam, D., and Cole, L. P.: A comparison of the clip and ring techniques for laparoscopic sterilization of post-abortion and postpartum patients. *Int. J. Gynaecol. Obstet.* **16**:150–156, 1978.
36. Mabray, C. R., Malinak, L. R., and Flowers, C. E.: Tubal sterilization. *Obstet. Gynecol.* **36**:204–207, 1970.
37. Madden, J. D., Boyar, R. M., MacDonald P. C., and Porter, J. C.: Analysis of secretory patterns of prolactin and gonadotropins during twenty-four hours in a lactating woman before and after resumption of menses. *Am. J. Obstet. Gynecol.* **132**:436–441, 1978.
38. Mann, J. I., Vessey, M. P., Thorogood, M., and Doll, R.: Myocardial infarction in young women with special reference to oral contraceptive practice. *Br. Med. J.* **2**:241–244, 1975.
39. Mann, J. I. and Inman, W. H. W.: Oral contraceptives and death from myocardial infraction. *Br. Med. J.* **2**:245–248, 1975.
40. May, E. T., Christopherson, W. M., Mahr, M. M., and Williams, H. C.: Hepatic changes in young women ingesting contraceptive steroids. *JAMA* **235**:730–732, 1976.
41. Mishell, D. R. and Roy, S.: Copper intrauterine contraceptive device event rates following insertion 4 to 8 weeks postpartum. *Am. J. Obstet. Gynecol.* **143**:29–33, 1982.
42. Munson, A. K. and Scott, J. R.: Postpartum tubal ligation under local anesthesia. *Obstet. Gynecol.* **39**:756–758, 1972.
43. Nissen, E. D., Kent, D. R., Missen, S. E., and McRae, D. M.: Association of liver tumors with oral contraceptives. *Obstet. Gynecol.* **48**:49–55, 1976.
44. Ory, H., Cole, P., MacMahon, B., and Hoover, R.: Oral contraceptives and reduced risk of benign breast diseases. *N. Engl. J. Med.* **294**:419–422, 1976.
45. Oster, G. and Salgo, M. P.: The copper intrauterine device and its mode of action. *N. Engl. J. Med.* **293**:432–438, 1975.
46. Perez, A., Vela, P., Masnick, G. S., and Potter, R. G.: First ovulation after childbirth: The effect of breastfeeding. *Am. J. Obstet. Gynecol.* **114**:1041–1047, 1972.
47. Prystowsky, H. and Eastman, N. J.: Puerperal tubal sterilization. *JAMA* **158**:463–467, 1955.
48. Reyes, F. I., Winter, J. S. D., and Faiman, C.: Pituitary–ovarian interrelationships during the puerperium. *Am. J. Obstet. Gynecol.* **114**:589–594, 1972.
49. Royal College of General Practicioners: Mortality among oral-contraceptive users. *Lancet* **2**:727–733, 1977.
50. Said, S. A. H. and Wide, L.: Serum levels of FSH and LH following normal parturition. *Acta Obstet. Gynecol. Scand.* **52**:361–365, 1973.
51. Sartwell, P. E., Arthes, F. G., and Tonascia, J. A.: Epidemiology of benign breast lesions: Lack of association with oral contraceptive use. *N. Engl. J. Med.* **288**:551–554, 1973.
52. Seki, K., Seki, M., and Okumura, T.: Serum FSH rise induced by CB-154 in postpartum women. *J. Clin. Endocrinol. Metab.* **39**:206–208, 1974.
53. Sharman, A.: Postpartum regeneration of the human endometrium. *J. Anat.* **87**:1–14, 1953.
54. Sheehan, K. L. and Yen, S. S. C.: Activation of pituitary gonadotropic function by an agonist of luteinizing hormone-releasing factor in the puerperium. *Am. J. Obstet. Gynecol.* **135**:755–758, 1979.
55. Speroff L., Glass, R. H., and Kase N. G.: *Clinical Gynecologic Endocrinology and Infertility,* 3rd Edition. Baltimore, Williams & Wilkins, 1983.
56. Stadel, B. V.: Oral contraceptives and cardiovascular disease. I. *N. Engl. J. Med.* **305**:612–618, 1981.

57. Stadel, B. V.: Oral contraceptives and cardiovascular disease. II. *N. Engl. J. Med.* **305**:672–677, 1981.
58. Tappan, J. G.: Kroener tubal ligation in perspective. *Am. J. Obstet. Gynecol.* **115**:1053–1057, 1973.
59. Tatum, H. J.: Clinical aspects of intrauterine contraception. *Fertil. Steril.* **28**:325, 1977.
60. Uchida, H.: Uchida tubal sterilization. *Am. J. Obstet. Gynecol.* **121**:153–158, 1975.
61. Vorherr, H.: Hormonal and biochemical changes of pituitary and breast during pregnancy. *Semin. Perinatol.* **3**:193–198, 1979.
62. Whitehead, R. G.: Nutritional aspects of human lactation. *Lancet* **1**:167–169, 1983.
63. Weinstein, L.: Breast milk—a natural resource. *Am. J. Obstet. Gynecol.* **136**:973–975, 1980.
64. Winikoff, B. and Baer, E. C.: The obstetrician's opportunity: Translating "breast is best" from theory to practice. *Am. J. Obstet. Gynecol.* **138**:105–117, 1980.
65. Zarate, A., Canales, E. S., Sonia, J., Ruiz, F., and MacGregor, C.: Ovarian refractoriness during lactation in women: Effect of gonadotropin stimulation. *Am. J. Obstet. Gynecol.* **112**:1130–1132, 1972.

10

THE NEWBORN INFANT

This chapter provides basic information about the neonate, particularly those neonatal events that are influenced by the obstetrician.

THE HEALTHY NEONATE

Growth and Development of the Fetus

From conception to adulthood, growth and development are a continuum. Specific events take place at specific times along this continuum. The rate of growth or type of development (chemical growth, embryogenesis, organogenesis) varies. (See Chapter 2.) From conception to birth, the weight of the human conceptus increases 6 billion times. Cell number multiplies to 2000 billion. Water, protein, fat, and mineral content of the fetal body increases 1–2 billion-fold each. The chemical development of the fetus is best categorized as an expansion of body water compartments and a deposition of proteins, minerals, and fats. The relative proportions of these constituents in relation to body weight change as the fetus matures. Actively acquired components (proteins, fats, extracellular minerals, and water) progressively replace extracellular water and minerals (Fig. 10-1).[10] This rapid rate of growth requires a continuous supply of energy and of essential "building blocks" which the fetus is unable to synthesize. The essential elements for growth are some amino acids, fatty acids, and minerals, most of which are provided by the mother to the fetus through the placenta, which also removes metabolic wastes from the fetus. It is possible that amniotic fluid also contributes to fetal nutrition. Cell and organ development parallels the chemical growth of the fetus. Cells increase in number and size and differentiate to fulfill specific functions. New tissues are formed and organs develop into systems that will ultimately allow the organism to lead an independent life. Most organ formation occurs in the first trimester of the pregnancy, but additional maturation is required for some organs (lung, brain). The brain continues to grow and mature for about two years after birth.

Normal intrauterine growth patterns during the second half of pregnancy can be estimated from measurements obtained at birth on infants of known gestational ages. Curves for weight, length, and head circumference during fetal life have been constructed and variations related to different environmental, ethnic, and socioeconomic back grounds have been recognized (Fig. 10-2)[21,27,38] Although the Denver grid is the commonly used reference, it is not appropriate for all areas or all ethnic populations in the United States. A major drawback of these graphs is that they assume that the prematurely delivered neonate is "normal" if he has no congenital malformation and that the birth weight is representative of the weight of other fetuses who remain in utero at that stage of gestation. All weight curves approach linearity between 28 and 38 weeks of gestation, at which time the fetus gains an average of 26 g daily. Birth weight–gestational age curves allow classification of neonates into various groups of clinical importance (Fig. 10-3). A neonate whose gestational age, calculated from the first day of the

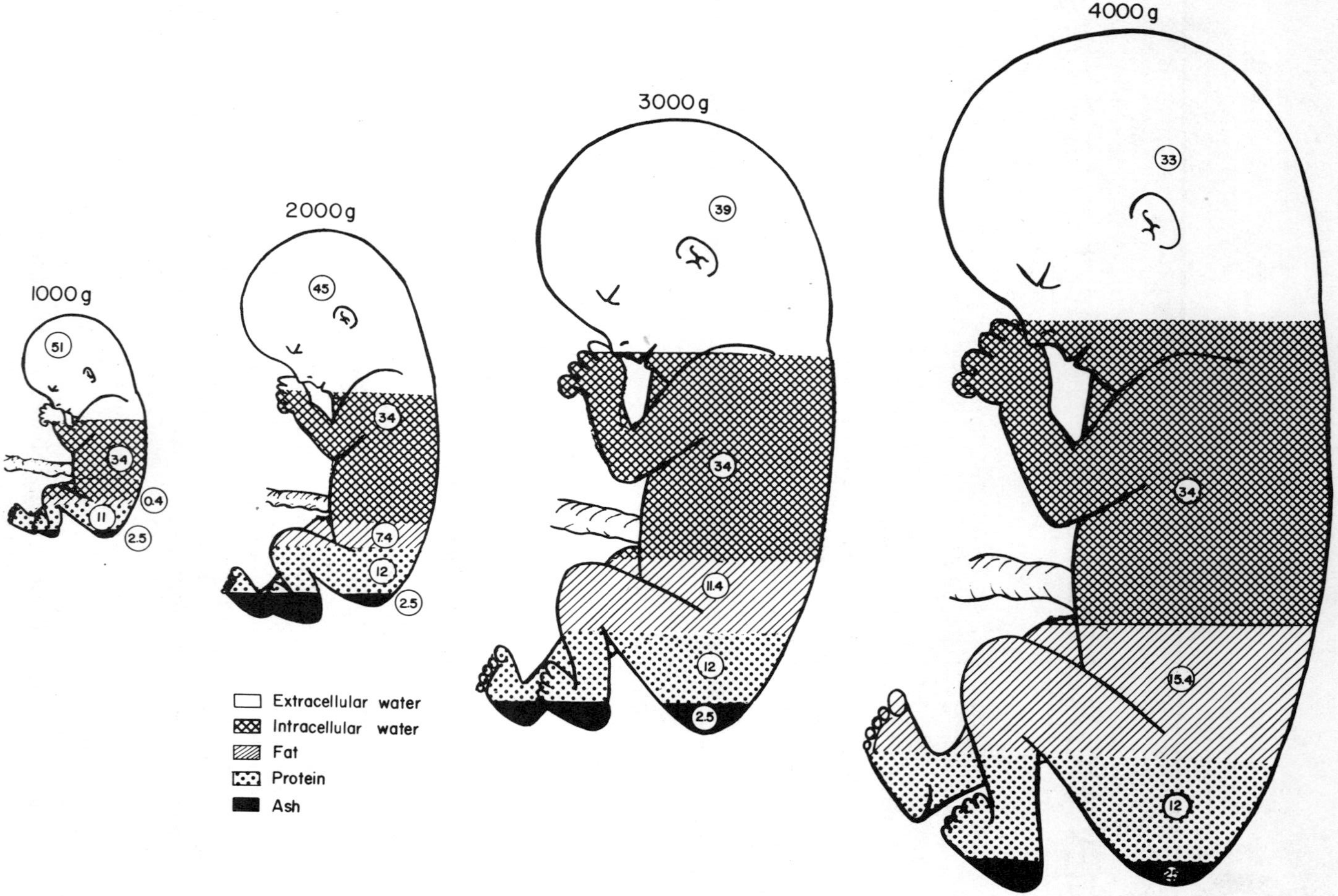

Figure 10-1. Body composition of average fetuses of various weights. Figures in each area show the proportion (%) of body weight occupied by each constituent. (Reprinted from Brans, Y. W. and Cassady, G. Fetal nutrition and body composition. In: Total parenteral nutrition: premises and promises. H. Ghadimi (ed.) Philadelphia, John Wiley and Sons, 1975, pp. 301–333, by permission of John Wiley & Sons, Inc.)

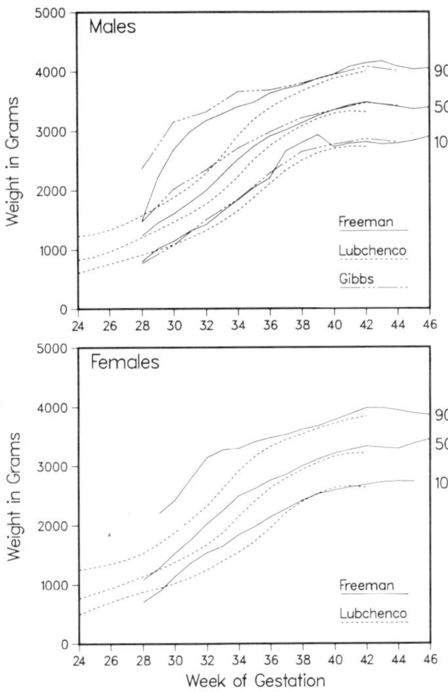

Figure 10-2. Birth weight vs. gestational age in male (top) and female (bottom) neonates delivered at high altitude (Denver, CO, ———), delivered at sea level of low socioeconomic status (Atlanta, GA; whites, ------; and delivered at sea level of low socioeconomic status in Hispanic population (San Antonio, TX, — ---).

last menstrual period, is equal to or greater than 37 completed weeks but less than 42 completed weeks is a *term neonate.* A neonate whose gestational age is less than 37 completed weeks is a *preterm* neonate, and one whose gestational age is 42 completed weeks or greater is *post-term.* Likewise, neonates whose birth weights are between the 10th and 90th percentiles (inclusive) for a given gestational age and population characteristics are called *appropriate for gestational age* or normally grown. Neonates whose birth weight exceeds the 90th percentile are termed *large for gestational age* or macrosomic. Neonates whose birth weights are below the 10th percentile are termed *small for gestational age* or intrauterine growth retarded.

Organ Function in Utero

Most fetal organs function much the same as they function in newborn babies. Major exceptions are the liver, the lungs, and the heart.

The Gastrointestinal Tract. Although most nutrients required for fetal growth are acquired through the placenta, the gastrointestinal tract of the fetus is functional very early in gestation. Fetal swallowing of amniotic fluid can be demonstrated as early as 12 weeks' gestation. That the fetus not only swallows amniotic fluid but also contributes to the removal of proteins from the amniotic fluid is suggested by the higher protein concentrations found in the amniotic fluid of fetuses whose swallowing mechanism is impaired (anencephaly, hydrops) or whose gastrointestinal tract is interrupted (esophageal atresia, duodenal atresia).[52] Swallowing of proteins along with amniotic fluid has been demonstrated in both humans and animals by infusion of foreign or labeled proteins or amino acids into the amniotic cavity. Not only do the labeled substances disappear from the amniotic fluid, but the label appears within hours in the gastrointestinal tract of the living fetus.[24] The rate of disappearance of each amino acid from amniotic fluid is characteristic of that amino acid.[53] Studies of intra-amniotic injection of radioactively labeled serum proteins in Rhesus monkeys suggest that proteins are absorbed intact by the fetal intestine.[8] The exact route of absorption of individual amino acids is still contested. They could be swallowed and absorbed

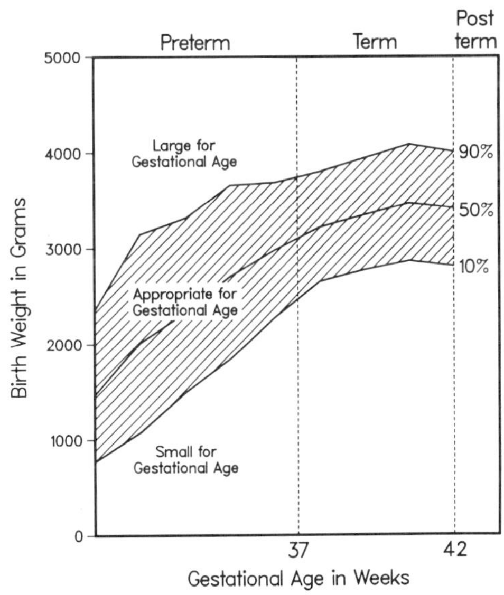

Figure 10-3. Definitions based on birth weight and gestational age superimposed on unpublished data from Gibbs.

by the gut, but they could also be absorbed through permeable fetal membranes, the placenta, or the umbilical cord. The permeability of the fetal membranes to amino acids is very low and could not account for the rapid clearance of amino acids from amniotic fluid.[29] Transfer of amino acids and proteins from amniotic fluid to maternal blood and then to the fetus could conceivably take place via the placenta, but the bulk of evidence suggests that this route is not significant. Transfer of amino acids to the fetus may also take place via the umbilical cord. Human experiments suggest that the disappearance of amino acids from amniotic fluid is too rapid to be explained solely by fetal swallowing.[29] The half-life of methionine in Rhesus monkey amniotic fluid is 1.1 days, which is consistent with fetal swallowing being the principal clearance mechanism, but not the only one. The absorbed amino acids are utilized for protein synthesis. Amniotic fluid proteins may provide as much as 17% of a human fetus' daily protein intake.[50]

Unabsorbed nutrients and digestive secretions accumulate in the intestine until birth.

The Brain. In humans, most cerebral development takes place before birth. Two-thirds of all brain cells are formed prior to the 40th gestational week. Most neuronal multiplication occurs prior to the fifth gestational month. Thereafter most activity consists of glial cell multiplication and synaptic organization. Glial cell multiplication is most active from 35 to 40 weeks of gestation.

The Kidneys. Although the placenta is the major organ for removal of fetal metabolic wastes and for regulation of water and electrolyte homeostasis during fetal life, renal function begins during the 9th week of gestation. As the fetus matures, renal function per unit of body mass increases as does the efficiency of tubular reabsorption of electrolytes.[39] The urine thus formed makes an increasingly larger contribution to amniotic fluid volume as gestation progresses. At term, all nephron units are in place. No new nephrons are formed in postnatal life. However, the kidney does not fully mature until about a year after birth. In the meantime, tubular and glomerular functions are limited, impairing the infant's ability to tolerate loading stresses, and limiting the capacity to conserve substances such as amino acids, phosphate, and bicarbonate.[18] Renal maturation is more a function of postnatal age than of gestational age.

The Liver. There are two major functional differences between the fetal and neonatal liver. Until close to term, the liver is the major producer of fetal red blood cells. Under normal circumstances, this function decreases sharply in the last month of intrauterine life. Secondly, the fetal liver lacks glucuronyltransferase and is thus unable to conjugate bilirubin. This is a protective mechanism in utero because conjugated bilirubin would be unable to leave the fetus through the placenta as effectively as unconjugated bilirubin does.

The Lungs and Fetal Breathing Movements. Although the basic architecture of the lungs is visible by the 15th postmenstrual week, four major developments are needed before the lungs can become fully operational. First, the bronchial tree must continue to subdivide into even smaller bronchioles and finally into an alveolar system. Second, the alveolar system must develop a close anatomic and functional interrelation with the capillary bed. Both of these developments occur around 26–28 weeks of gestation.[55] Third, some of the cells lining the alveolar wall must differentiate into type II pneumocytes. These cells, which are large and contain lamellar osmiophilic cytoplasmic inclusions, are responsible for surfactant synthesis. They too first appear at 27–28 weeks of gestation. Finally, sufficient surfactant must be synthesized by and released from the type II pneumocytes to maintain alveolar stability when air breathing begins. Under normal conditions, this final step in lung maturation occurs between 34 and 37 weeks of gestation. Surfactant or dipalmitoyllecithin is a tensioactive phospholipid that counteracts the physical forces that would otherwise compel the alveoli to collapse completely at the end of expiration, thus greatly increasing the work of breathing. The major component of surfactant is lecithin or phosphatidylcholine (Fig. 10-4), although some minor components play a major role in stabilizing the alveoli, especially phosphatidylglycerol.[54] Thanks to surfactant, once air breathing begins, a functional residual capacity progressively develops. The alveoli expand and contract, but never empty completely.

Breathing movements, once thought to determine the beginning of postnatal life, occur as early as 11 weeks of gestation. The human fetus spends at least 30% and possibly as much as 60–80% of his time "breathing" at a rate of 40–70 per minute. Although these respiratory movements are shallow, some exchange of

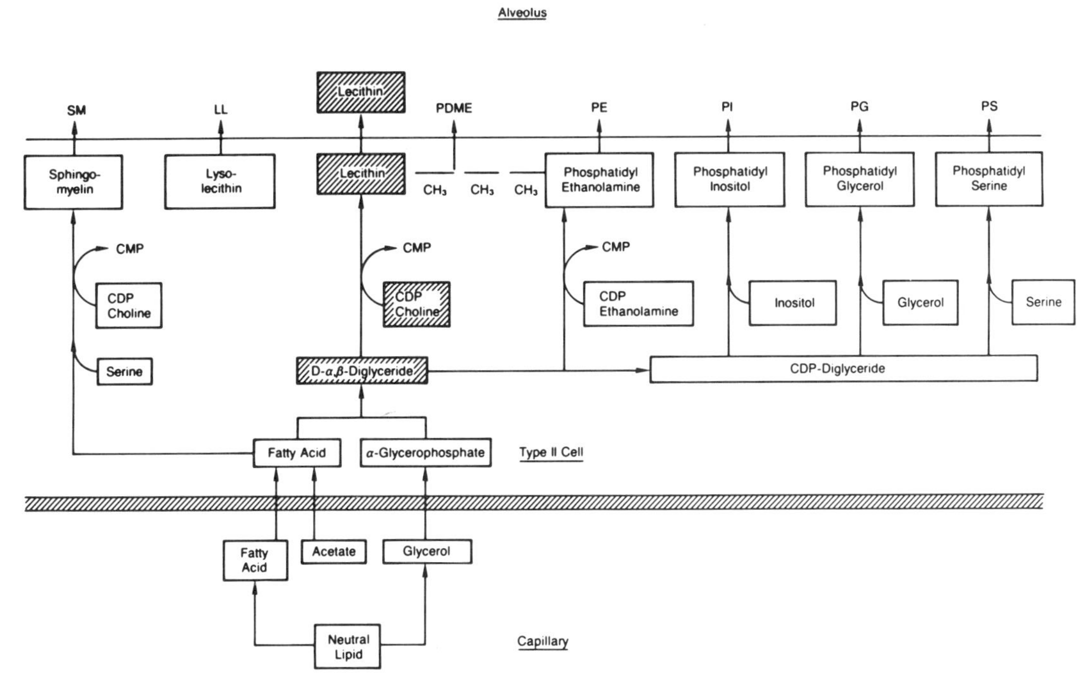

Figure 10-4. Biosynthesis of pulmonary surfactant. The main pathway is shaded.

fluid takes place between alveolar and amniotic fluid.

The Heart and Circulation. In the fetus, the gas exchange function of the lungs is fulfilled entirely by the placenta (Fig. 10-5). Arterialized blood (oxygen tension or $PO_2 \sim 30$ torr) flows from the placenta through the umbilical vein and the ductus venosus into the inferior vena cava, where it admixes with venous blood returning from the lower part of the body (resulting $PO_2 \sim 26$ torr). As it enters the right atrium, blood from the inferior vena cava is directed preferentially through the foramen ovale into the left atrium. From there it passes into the left ventricle, the aortic arch, and into all organs except the lungs. The pulmonary circulation is a low-flow, high-pressure system that receives only about 10% of total blood volume. As venous blood returning from the upper portion of the body enters the right atrium through the superior vena cava, it is directed preferentially toward the right ventricle. Blood leaves the right ventricle through the main pulmonary artery and rejoins the aorta via the ductus arteriosus. Thus, the fetal ventricles work in parallel and not in series as they do postnatally. Venous blood returns to the placenta through the aorta, internal iliac arteries, and umbilical arteries ($PO_2 \sim 20$ torr).

Transition to Extrauterine Life

At term birth, the gastrointestinal tract, the brain, the kidneys and, to a degree, the liver are ready to function. The transition from intrauterine to extrauterine life involves mostly cardiopulmonary adaptation and thermoregulation.

For many weeks before birth, the chest has "practiced" breathing movements and the pulmonary alveoli have filled with fluid. As the baby is delivered, two series of phenomena take place. Clamping of the cord produces a drop in arterial PO_2 and a rise in arterial carbon dioxide tension (PCO_2). The combination of PaO_2s below 15–20 torr and $PaCO_2$s above 65 torr triggers gasping which, in concert with neurosensory (touch, light, noise, cold) and proprioceptive (gravity) stimuli causes breathing to begin and air to enter the alveoli. Because of the properties of surfactant, each successive breath requires less alveolar opening pressure and leaves an increasing functional residual capacity at the completion of expiration. The recoil of the chest as it exits the genital canal facilitates

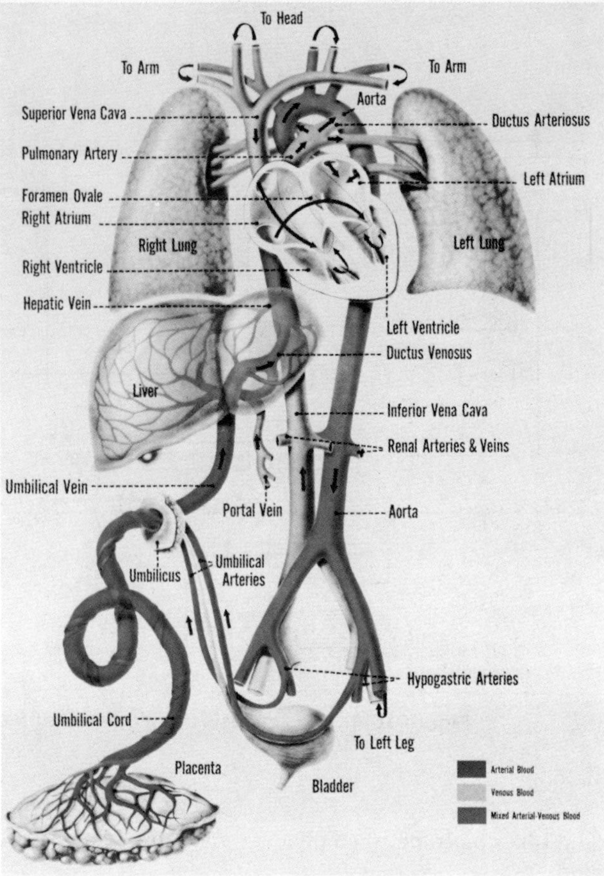

Figure 10-5. Fetal circulation. (Reprinted with permission of Ross Laboratories, Columbus, OH 43216, from Clinical Education Aid #1, G157, © 1978, Ross Laboratories.)

air entry into the lungs and expansion of the alveoli against the forces of surface tension at the air–liquid interface in the alveoli.[46] As air enters the lungs, the lungs expand and for the first time large amounts of blood enter the pulmonary circulation. Residual alveolar fluid is reabsorbed into the capillaries and lymphatic ducts. Pulmonary vascular resistance drops, increasing venous return to the left atrium. The resulting increase in left atrial pressure causes the foramen ovale to close within minutes. The absence of placental blood return functionally closes the ductus venosus, although it may remain anatomically patent for several days. Finally, decreases in pulmonary vascular resistance concurrent with increases in systemic vascular resistance transiently reverse the flow of blood through the ductus arteriosus, which now shunts from left to right. Within 12–24 hours, the ductus arteriosus closes. Postnatal circulation, with the ventricles functioning in series rather than in parallel, is established.

Thermal regulation, which for 40 weeks was ensured by the maternal organism, is now taken over by the neonate. In response to catecholamine stimulation, the neonate burns brown adipose tissues, located mostly subcutaneously around the shoulder girdle and upper spinal cord, and heat is generated. Because of the neonate's inability to generate heat by increasing muscle activity (shivering) and to lose much heat by sweating, thermal stresses are not uncommon and must be watched for in the first few days.

Within the first few days after birth, the kidneys improve their ability to retain water and to concentrate urine. This is at least partially due to an increase in urea concentration in the glomerular filtrate as the neonate reaches an anabolic state. Finally, substrate-induced enzymes

TABLE 10-1. APGAR SCORE

Sign	0	1	2
Heart rate	Absent	Slow	>100/min
Respirations	Absent	Weak cry; hypo ventilation	Good, strong cry
Muscle tone	Limp	Some flexion	Active motion
Reflex irritability (response to suctioning)	No response	Grimace	Cough or sneeze
Color	Blue or pale	Body pink; extremities blue	Completely pink

such as glucuronyltransferase and intestinal disaccharidases (lactase, sucrase, maltase) become active.

Evaluation of the Neonate

Careful evaluation of the neonate at birth and shortly after birth is the key to identifying problems that may affect the baby's postnatal course. This evaluation includes three major areas: Apgar scoring, physical examination, and assessment of gestational maturity.

Apgar Score. This method was devised to describe the condition of the neonate at birth. The indices are the heart rate, respiratory rate, muscle tone, reflex irritability, and color. Each of these signs is graded 0 (worst), 1, or 2 (best) (Table 10-1).[7] A total score of 10 is optimum, although seldom attained at 1 minute; a total score of 3 or less is usually indicative of infants in poor condition. Although the score was designed to be obtained exactly 1 minute after birth, it has become customary to score at both 1 and 5 minutes after birth. There are a number of pitfalls: (1) The timing of the scoring is critical; in order to be useful, the score must be determined *exactly* 1 and 5 minutes after birth. An automatic timing device is particularly valuable. (2) Personnel biases influence the score: midwives tend to give higher scores than obstetricians, whereas obstetricians tend to give higher scores than anesthesiologists, nurse anesthetists, pediatricians, or delivery room nurses. (3) The 1 minute Apgar score gives the best impression of the neonate's condition at birth and correlates with acid-base status of the neonate, and the 5 minute score generally correlates best with neonatal mortality and morbidity. The most important use of the Apgar score is to allow someone who was not present at delivery to reconstruct a picture of what the baby was like. The change in score from 1 to 5 minutes provides an index of the success of resuscitative measures. (4) Resuscitative measures, if indicated, should under no circumstances be delayed until the 1 minute Apgar score has been determined.

Physical Examination. A physical examination should be performed as soon as possible after birth and a complete prenatal history obtained from the baby's mother. Special emphasis should be put on findings that may place the baby at risk of complications. Systematic inspection of the neonate is usually more informative than palpation, percussion, and auscultation.

Assessment of Gestational Maturity. Gestational age is usually expressed as time elapsed since the first day of the mother's last normal menstrual period. This estimate, although weakened in accuracy by the variability of the preovulatory phase, is *the best single* clinical estimate of fetal maturity available. Menstrual age is generally accepted as *the standard of reference* for other methods.

A variety of parameters correlate with gestational age. The medical world is divided historically and geographically concerning the value of these parameters. The French rely heavily on neurological parameters, whereas the Anglo-Saxon school prefers observation of external body characteristics. The former is best exemplified by the scheme of Amiel-Tison which selects such variables as passive and active tone and reflex activity to predict gestational age.[6] Electroencephalograms, often employing evoked responses to sensorial stimuli and measurements of nerve conduction velocity, have been used in attempts to quantify neurological maturity. Electroencephalographic patterns of intrauterine growth retarded neonates by any of these methods are comparable, with some minor discrepancies, to those of their normally grown gestational peers. These sophisticated laboratory techniques require expertise in interpretation and are of limited clinical utility.

Physical observations are easily available, but have definite limitations. Anthropometric measurements, taken singly or in combinations, are of limited value as all are affected in varying degrees by the quality of intrauterine growth. Head circumference is least affected and is therefore the best predictor of fetal maturity. The biparietal diameter as determined ultrasonically, although little used by pediatricians, is extensively employed by obstetricians to determine maturity. (See Chapter 12.)

A number of external somatic characteristics have been carefully studied. These include skin texture, color, opacity, and edema; texture of hair; hardness of skull; number of plantar skin creases; formation and firmness of external cartilage of the ear; breast size and nipple formation; and character and pigmentation of external genitalia. Taken separately, these characteristics correlate only moderately with gestational age, but, except for breast size, are little affected by quality of intrauterine growth. Combinations of several characteristics taken together allow estimation of gestational age with an accuracy of about ± 3 weeks. The studies of Dubowitz and associates provided a widely used and valuable clinical scheme that uses both neurological and external characteristics.[17] When carefully performed, the resulting score correlates highly with gestational age (±2 weeks: Gestational age $= \frac{\text{Score}}{4} + 25$, $r = 0.93$.)

Roentgenological evidence of epiphyseal maturity is a poor predictor of gestational age. Though presence of the distal femoral epiphysis indicates maturity, its absence has no meaning. Moreover, bone maturity is retarded in intrauterine growth retardation. A number of laboratory chemical parameters correlate with gestational age, but none, taken separately, can better the prediction obtained from an accurate clinical examination using the Dubowitz scheme. Alpha-1-fetoprotein levels and reticulocyte counts are potentially interesting, since they seem to be independent of the quality of intrauterine growth.

In summary, the scheme developed by Dubowitz and associates is useful in clinically estimating gestational age. The degree of precision increases with the clinician's proficiency. Gestational age, estimated from an accurate menstrual history, remains the single most valuable clinical tool in estimating fetal maturity and is the standard of reference for all other techniques. For the most part, these studies have involved white babies. Extension of the results to black infants must be made tenuously. The number of skin creases on the sole of the foot has been shown to be different at similar gestational ages in white and black babies.[12] The black fetus may mature faster, both neurologically and physically.[58]

Care of the Neonate in the Delivery Room

Even when no resuscitation is required, the most crucial steps in the care of all newly born babies is to maintain body temperature and to clear the airway of foreign matter. This should take, at most, one or two minutes. When the baby is dry, warm, and breathing comfortably, the parents can become acquainted with their new child. Prophylactic care of the eyes and umbilical cord, administration of vitamin K, and proper identification of the neonate are usually done in the delivery room, but they may await transfer to the recovery room or "transitional" nursery.

Thermoregulation. The temperature of most delivery rooms is regulated for the benefit of the physicians and nurses rather than in the interest of the parturient, let alone the baby. Unless active steps are taken to prevent it, the neonate's body temperature falls rapidly. Coming out of the warm amniotic fluid into the cold delivery room may be equated to stepping from a hot shower into an air-conditioned bathroom, except that the neonate is unable to generate heat by shivering and has a disproportionate surface area in relation to body weight. A mild degree of asphyxia also tends to delay the chemical thermogenetic response. The neonate left in cold room air loses 4.5 °C within one minute; whether the baby is wet or dry makes little difference. Recovery takes more than 30 minutes.[16] If the neonate is dried immediately and wrapped in a blanket, the temperature still falls to about 34 °C but increases to 36 °C within 10 minutes. Placement under a source of radiant heat does not prevent a drop of 1.5 °C in body temperature, but the recovery within 10 minutes is more effective. The best way to handle the neonate is to dry him off immediately under

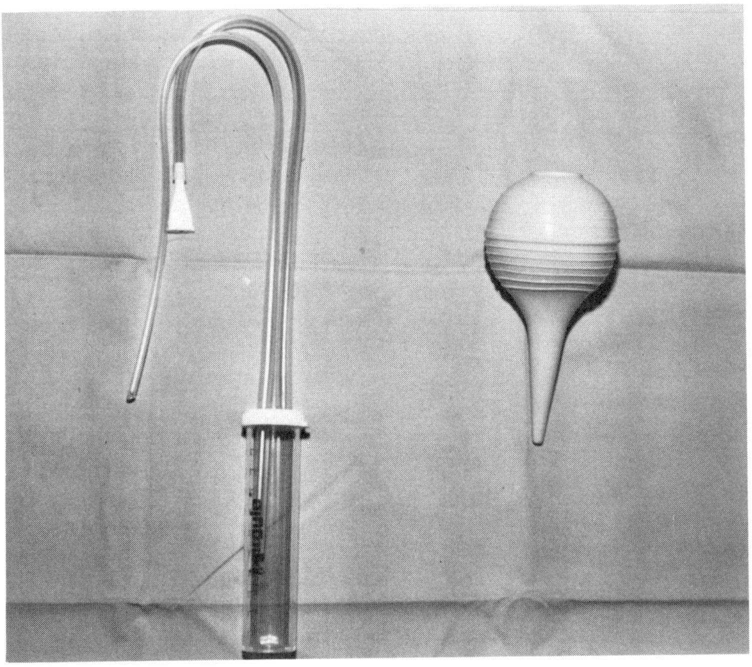

Figure 10-6. Airway suction apparatus: bulb syringe (right) and DeLee trap (left).

a radiant warmer; in that case the temperature remains around 37°C. Although old-fashioned heat lamps ae better than nothing, a modern radiant warmer should be part of the furnishings of all delivery rooms.

Clearing of Airway. At birth, the neonate's mouth, nose, and pharynx are usually obstructed by secretions, mucus, and maternal blood. Gentle suctioning with a bulb syringe (Fig. 10-6, right) is usually sufficient to clear the mouth and nose. Sometimes a DeLee trap (Fig. 10-6, left) is needed to clear the hypopharynx. Vigorous suctioning or use of a suction catheter should be avoided as they might produce severe vagal reflexes with apnea and bradycardia. The mouth should always be suctioned first. Suctioning the nose is irritating and may induce reflex aspiration; aspiration of foreign material into the lungs will result if the mouth has not been cleared first.

Eye Care. Gonococcal ophthalmia neonatorum remains a threat to the eyesight of neonates. Acceptable prophylactic agents include 1% silver nitrate solution, 0.5% erythromycin ophthalmic ointment or drops, and 1% tetracycline ophthalmic ointment or drops. Erythromycin and tetracycline have the additional advantage of offering prophylaxis against chlamydia ophthalmia neonatorum. All these drugs are available in single-dose ampules or tubes. One of them should be given shortly after birth (within one hour) to all neonates. The eyelids and surrounding skin are cleaned carefully with sterile cotton which may be moistened with sterile water. Two drops of the prophylactic agent are instilled into each conjunctival sac, different ampules being used for each eye. If antibiotic ointment is used, a thin line of ointment, at least half an inch long, is spread along the junction of the bulbar and palpebral conjunctivae of the lower lid. The eyelids are manipulated to ensure the spread of drops or ointment. After one minute, excess solution or ointment is gently wiped from the eyelids and the surrounding skin. The eyes need not be irrigated with either water or normal saline, as this procedure does not reduce the incidence of chemical conjunctivitis. Infants born to mothers known to be infected with agents that cause ophthalmia neonatorum should receive systemic as well as prophylactic therapy.

Cord Care. Since the umbilicus frequently becomes the first area of the body to become colonized with staphylococci, it has become popular to apply an antimicrobial agent to the umbilicus and cord stump. No single method of cord care has proved superior in preventing colonization and disease. Triple dye (brilliant green, proflavine hemisulfate, and crystal violet) is most effective in inhibiting staphylococcal colonization if applied shortly after birth to the cord stump and one inch of skin around the umbilicus. Single-use applicators are available. Data suggest that triple dye may actually increase colonization rates with group B β-hemolytic streptococci, so caution is indicated in areas of the country where group B β-hemolytic streptococcus is prevalent. Silver sulfadiazine is less effective than triple dye against staphylococci but may be more effective against group B β-hemolytic streptococci. A single application of either antimicrobial is sufficient and does not hamper later attempts at catheterizing umbilical vessels. However, if the umbilicus needs to be disinfected for umbilical vessel catheterization, the antimicrobial agent should be reapplied after the procedure. The practice of keeping the umbilicus moist "to facilitate catheterization" should be discouraged. It is unnecessary and may actually promote microbial colonization.

Tetanus Prophylaxis. In rare instances where the umbilical cord has not been severed with a sterile instrument or when there is doubt how the cord was cut, prophylaxis against neonatal tetanus with 250 units of human tetanus immune globulin, injected intramuscularly, is advisable.[2]

Vitamin K. For the prevention of vitamin K-dependent hemorrhagic disease, every neonate should receive a single intramuscular dose of 0.5–1.0 mg of vitamin K_1 (phytonadione) within one hour of birth.[3]

Skin Care. Cleansing of the skin should be delayed until the neonate's temperature has been stabilized. Fresh water or a mild, nonmedicated soap (preferably in single-use containers) can be used to remove blood and meconium. Antiseptic soaps, especially those containing hexachlorophene, are contraindicated except during certain epidemics, as they may be reabsorbed through the skin and cause cerebral damage.

Identification of the Neonate. Two identical bands indicating the mother's name, hospital admission number, the neonate's sex, and the date and time of birth should be placed on the wrist or ankle of the baby while still in the delivery room. These identification bands should be checked by both the nurses and the physician before the neonate leaves the delivery room and when he is admitted to the nursery. When the neonate is shown to the mother, she should be asked to verify the information on the identification bands and the sex of the neonate. Footprinting and fingerprinting are not recommended. They are neither cost-effective nor usually of sufficient quality to be acceptable as proof of identification in a court of law.

Parent–Infant Bonding: An Environmental View of Childbirth. Great strides have been made during the past 20 years toward improving the psychological and physical environment for childbirth.[34] The decreased use of general anesthesia and opiate analgesia and their replacement by regional or local anesthesia, even for elective cesarean sections, allow the mother to relate to her newborn baby from the moment of birth. There is a trend toward keeping the neonate with his mother as much as possible, in contrast to the total separation of 6–12 hours followed by only short encounters at feeding for 3 or 4 days that were in vogue 15 years ago. Rooming-in of the baby with the mother or at least unrestricted access of the mother to her baby is encouraged. Fathers are allowed to participate during labor and delivery, and they, too, may experience the thrill of seeing their baby delivered. Indeed, the pendulum has probably swung too far. "Consumer activism" has led to a recrudescence of home deliveries in the unproven belief that delivery in the home environment, with the participation of the entire family, is even more likely to strengthen parent–infant bonds. The American health care delivery system is not geared toward safe handling of home deliveries and such practice should be discouraged. In an attempt to provide an acceptable alternative, an increasing number of hospitals are offering "birthing rooms" for deliveries where no complications are anticipated. Birthing rooms are usually combined labor and delivery rooms with comfortable and pleasant furniture and subdued noise and lighting levels replacing the sterile, cold environment of the usual labor and delivery rooms. The equipment necessary for mother and baby (gas outlets, vacuum, resuscitation equipment) is present, but hidden from view. From a neonatologist's point of view, this is an excellent alternative, provided that the baby is never endangered by the environment.

Klaus and Kennell[34] compared the effect of extended early contact between mother and baby to what, in the early 1970s, was traditional care. Traditional contact involved giving the mother a glimpse of her baby in the delivery room, brief contact and identification 6–12 hours after birth, and visits of 20–30 minutes every 4 hours for bottle feeding. Extended contact included all these steps plus nude body contact between mother and baby under an overhead heating panel for one hour within the first three hours after birth and five hours of contact every afternoon for three days after delivery. A month later, mothers who had had extended contact with their babies were more reluctant to leave their babies with someone else, they stood and watched more carefully while the physician examined their babies, they showed greater soothing behavior, and they had more eye-to-eye contact with their babies. Other studies have supported these observations. However, some authors have criticized these studies for not differentiating between bonding and attachment.[25] According to them, bonding is a unidirectional (from parent to infant) and rapid process (within the first hours or days after birth) facilitated by physical contact. Attachment, on the other hand, is a bidirectional, reciprocal process between mother and infant that develops gradually during the first year of extrauterine life and is influenced by psychological variables. It may be that stronger bonding facilitates the attachment process, but this is unsupported by objective data.

Care of the Neonate in the Nursery

Nutrition. Four major questions come to mind when discussing feeding of neonates: When? How? What? What indicates optimal nutrition? The answer to the last question is generally an appropriate rate of weight gain, that is, a rate that allows the baby's weight to remain at least on the growth curve achieved in utero and preferably on the 50th percentile line. A neonate born at term loses about 5% of birth weight over the first three or four days before starting to gain weight. The nature of this weight loss is not completely defined, but partly represents a loss of body water and partly a loss of brown fat used for thermoregulation. The *quality* of weight gain must also be considered. The infant of a diabetic mother or a hydropic neonate may be larger and heavier than average, but the excess is due to fat in the former case and to water in the latter. Quantitatively, these babies may appear "better" than average. Qualitatively, they reveal marked metabolic imbalance. No good studies of body composition have been performed on these babies, but anecdotal data suggest that they may actually be deficient in body proteins. Neonates whose intrauterine growth was retarded are smaller and lighter at term than their normal gestational peers and have an excess of water and a lack of proteins.

Finally, some feeding techniques or formulas produce water retention instead of (or in addition to) tissue accretion and may appear "better" to the casual observer because they yield faster rates of weight gain. A more appropriate end point would be the rate of tissue accretion, but this cannot be easily measured.

Normal mature babies learn to regulate their own nutritional intake soon after birth, voicing hunger loudly and sucking to satiety if left to their own devices. These babies thus illustrate some of the basic principles of feeding.

When to Feed. In our society, we allow babies a resting or fasting period of a few hours, during which they presumably recover from the shock of birth. In developing countries, neonates commonly suckle within half an hour after delivery without suffering any harm such as aspiration of milk into the lungs. Neonates who tend to become hypoglycemic, such as infants of diabetic mothers, are often fed within the first four hours without problems. In our experience, normal newborn babies may be fed safely within 2–3 hours after birth.

The practice of waiting eight hours before initiating feedings should be reevaluated. Early feedings reduce wastage of fat and glycogen reserves and limit the rise of serum bilirubin, presumably by reducing the enterohepatic reabsorption of bilirubin. Intestinal motility is decreased in the fasting neonate, and conjugated bilirubin excreted with biliary fluids stagnates in the intestinal lumen. This gives bacterial flora and enzymes greater opportunity to unconjugate bilirubin. Unconjugated bilirubin is thus reabsorbed into the blood stream and contributes to overloading an immature liver.

What and How to Feed. The main concern at the time of the first feeding is to avoid regurgitation and aspiration pneumonitis. The first feeding should always be to test the neonate's pharyngeal coordination and patency of the upper gastrointestinal tract. The use of 5% or

10% dextrose in water for this purpose should be discouraged. Dextrose and milk have similar irritating effects on the bronchoalveolar epithelium, whereas sterile water is less damaging. The first feeding should always be with sterile water. Isotonic saline would probably be preferable physiologically, as the bronchial tree has been exposed to amniotic fluid throughout fetal life, but it is not palatable.

Beginning with the second feeding, breast milk or artificial formulas may be used. There is no need to start with dilute formula. Standard dilutions of 67 k cal/dl (20 kcal/oz) are well tolerated from the beginning. The value of higher concentrations for normal mature babies is doubtful when they are fed ad libitum. Infants usually compensate for higher concentration by reducing volume intake.

The relative advantages of breast milk versus formulas based on cow's milk have been debated for many years. The possible benefits of human milk fall into four categories: nutritional, immunologic, psychological, and economic. There are few differences in quantitative composition between human milk and formulas, but there are qualitative differences that may be important. In human milk, whey proteins predominate (60%) whereas casein (82%) predominates in two of the three most commonly used formulas. The importance of the whey/casein ratio for digestibility of milks is not clear. More important, probably, is the larger concentration of cysteine and lesser content of methionine in human milk. Because neonates have little cystathionase at birth (the enzyme that converts methionine to cystine), methionine may accumulate and is neurotoxic. Human milk also contains taurine, a neurotransmitter that is important for brain growth, whereas formulas contain little or none. Human milk contains unsaturated fatty acids that are more readily absorbed than the saturated fatty acids of cow's milk and it contains lipase to boost fat digestibility. Whether these differences in composition really affect the nutritive value of formulas remains debatable.

Immunologic properties of human milk, though undeniably present, are even more theoretical. Human milk contains various cells and substances that may protect the recipient against infections: macrophages, immunocompetent lymphocytes, opsonins, lactoferrin, and immunoglobulins, especially IgAs.[20] Whether breast-feeding actually protects neonates against infections is questionable. Studies showing this to be true were either performed in the United States in the first decades of the 20th century when home refrigeration was not generally available, or performed in underdeveloped countries where lack of hygiene and refrigeration may have contributed to the results. The question of whether human milk protects against infections or formulas contain infectious organisms has not been answered. There is no doubt that, in underdeveloped countries, formula increases morbidity and mortality from infections. Whether it does so in Europe and North America is questionable.

It is possible that breast-feeding enhances maternal–infant bonding and attachment, but this remains to be demonstrated. Certainly, no woman should be made to feel guilty if she cannot or does not wish to breast-feed.

Economic reasons are probably the best argument for breast-feeding in certain sectors of society. Breast milk is free, whereas formula can strain the family budget. Even a working mother can continue to feed her own milk to her baby if she empties her breasts regularly and refrigerates the milk in clean containers. Employers are becoming increasingly aware of the need to provide the opportunity for doing so. Unfortunately, formula feeding has become somewhat of a status symbol in the very strata of society where breast-feeding would be most helpful financially. This idea should be discredited.

In summary, the current resurgence of interest in breast-feeding should be encouraged.[1] The major advantage may be economic, although there may also be nutritive, psychological, and immunological advantages. There are very few absolute contraindications to breast-feeding. The American Academy of Pediatrics has published an extensive review of drugs and chemicals that are excreted into human milk and their possible effects on the baby.[4]

Stools and Urine. Ninety percent of newborn babies pass meconium within the first 24 hours; most do so within 36 hours. If by that time no meconium has appeared, it is imperative to investigate the reason, which could be functional or anatomical. Meconium, the dark stools that have accumulated during fetal life, contains desquamated epithelial cells from the intestinal tract, mucus, epidermal cells, lanugo, digestive enzymes, and bile pigments. After three to four days, the stools assume the light yellow appearance and characteristic odor of neonate's stools.

Ninety-three percent of neonates pass urine within 24 hours of birth, and over 99% do so within 48 hours. Failure to do so requires investigation.

Circumcision. Circumcision is common in the United States. Arguments about its usefulness are often emotional rather than scientific. There is no medical indication for routine circumcision of neonates, nor is there any need to attempt to retract the foreskin daily. Many foreskins do not retract completely until the child is two years of age: 25% of foreskins are retractable by six months, 50% by one year, 80% by two years, and 90% by four years.[23] If circumcision is performed, it should be done after the first 12–24 hours of the neonatal period and not during the postnatal stabilization period. Although the time-honored custom is to circumcise babies without the benefit of anesthesia based on the mistaken belief that "neonates do not feel pain" this practice is barbaric. Regional anesthesia of the penile dorsal nerve is easy to achieve and should be encouraged.

Screening for Inborn Errors of Metabolism. All neonates should be screened for hyperphenylalaninemia (which includes phenylketonuria) and congenital hypothyroidism. In some states, screening has been extended to galactosemia, histidinemia, and homocystinuria. Blood samples should be obtained after at least 24 hours of milk feedings.

Length of Stay in the Nursery. Most mothers remain in the hospital for 48–72 hours after an uncomplicated delivery, although in selected populations with well-structured programs for home visits, discharge from the hospital as early as 12–24 hours is safe. Every effort should be made to discharge the baby at the same time as the mother, although third-party payers frown on the practice of keeping a neonate in the hospital in excess of 3 days if the only reason is the mother's need to remain longer in the hospital. In general, it is preferable for healthy neonates to spend at least 24 hours in the hospital.

Admission of Outborn Neonates to a Nursery. There is no need to handle outborn neonates differently from their inborn peers. The days when outborn neonates were automatically treated with antibiotics and placed in isolation are past. It is important to find out where the baby was born, who cut the umbilical cord and how. If the cord was not severed with a sterile instrument, tetanus prophylaxis is indicated, as it is when there is uncertainty on how the cord was cut. Antibiotics may be indicated if a baby was delivered in a dirty environment, such as the floor of a public place.

Team Approach to Perinatal Care

One of the most important developments in recent years has been increasing collaboration and communication between perinatologists (obstetricians), neonatologists, and obstetrical anesthesiologists before and after a baby's birth. Precise information about the mother's health and the course of pregnancy is important to the care of the baby. Follow-up about the neonate's health is important to the obstetrician and the obstetrical anesthesiologist to gauge efficacy of their handling of the mother during pregnancy, labor, and delivery. Important decisions involving the mother–fetus pair are often best taken collegially, to the benefit of all concerned.

THE NEONATE WITH PROBLEMS

Perinatal Asphyxia and Resuscitation in the Delivery Room

Perinatal asphyxia is the result of some problem during fetal life, labor, and/or delivery which delays the onset of respiration. Postmaturity, pregnancy-induced hypertension in the mother, maternal hypotension, placental abruption, bleeding from placenta previa or vasa previa, cord compression, and maternal sedation in the four hours prior to delivery are common causes of perinatal asphyxia. Monitoring of uterine contractions, fetal heart rate, and fetal scalp pH often provide warning signs of asphyxia and its severity as well as the probable cause for it. The asphyxiated baby is easy to recognize: he is limp, pale or cyanotic, and apneic. The pathophysiology of asphyxia is schematized in Fig. 10-7. Once this situation is observed, time is of the essence. For each minute that the baby is not breathing, arterial pH drops by 0.1 unit and arterial $PaCO_2$ increases by 10 torr; within one minute, PaO_2 is zero, leading to a state of mixed respiratory and metabolic acidosis. Although asphyxia is commonly classified as moderate or severe on the basis of the one-minute Apgar score (moderate: score 4–7; severe: score 0–3), such classification is only useful for retrospective analysis. There is no time to wait for the one-minute Apgar score in order to decide what to do. Resuscitation schemes based on Apgar scores are dangerous and useless.

There are five steps to successful resuscitation:

1. Evaluate the baby.
2. Ensure thermoregulation.

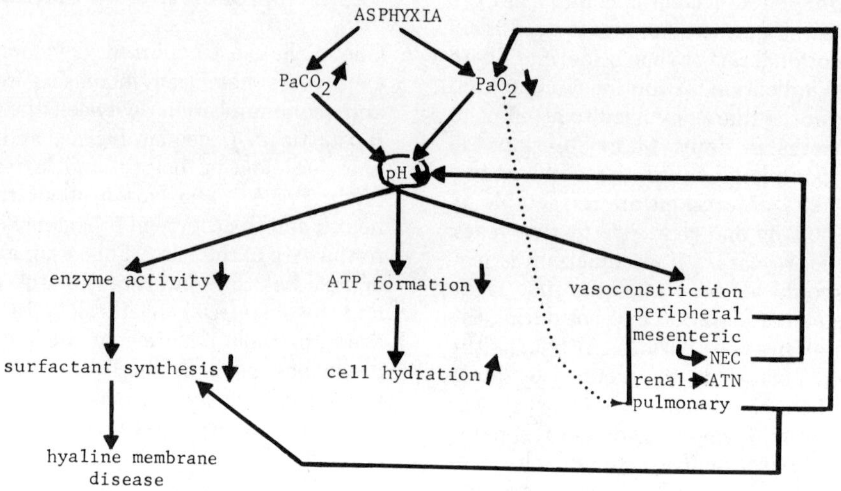

Figure 10-7. Pathophysiology of perinatal asphyxia.

3. Clear the airway.
4. Establish breathing.
5. Maintain circulatory support.

The first three steps are followed in all deliveries, even when the baby is not asphyxiated. They can and should be performed simultaneously and should usually take no more than 30 seconds. Evaluation is particularly important to estimate gestational maturity and to identify major congenital malformations (in some cases resuscitation is not indicated), to judge whether anemia is present, and to recognize the presence of meconium.

Clearing the airway (mouth first, then nose) often triggers reflex respiratory movements. If it does not, the baby must be ventilated with a bag and mask. The baby's head should be positioned in the midline and in a neutral position (Fig. 10-8). Either flexion or hyperextension of the neck may produce compression of the trachea. A mask of proper size and shape that fits

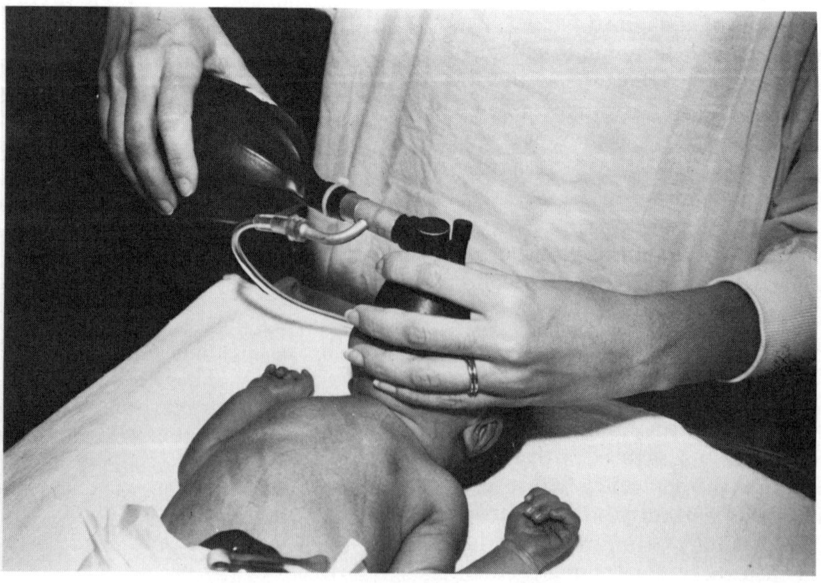

Figure 10-8. Proper positioning of bag and mask for neonatal ventilation.

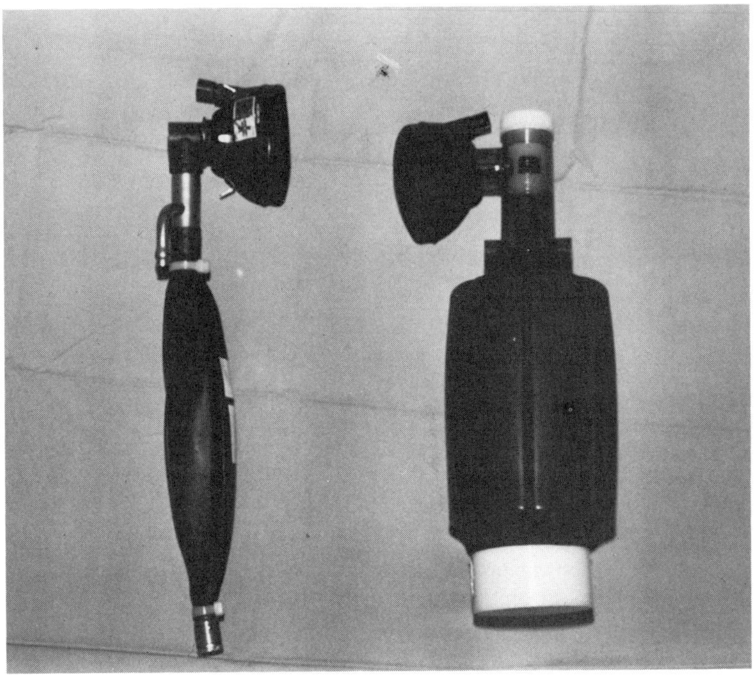

Figure 10-9. Types of ventilation bags: self-inflating (right) and anesthesia-type bag (left).

snugly over the mouth and nose of the baby is essential. The jaw should be supported with two or three fingers to prevent the tongue from slipping back and obstructing the airway. Two types of bags are used. Self-inflating bags (Fig. 10-9, right) are easier to use, but they do not deliver 100% oxygen and they often have a built-in valve that limits inflation pressures. Since the bag re-inflates automatically, leaks are difficult to detect and a close watch must be maintained on the baby's chest to make sure that it is inflating. "Anesthesia" bags (Fig. 10-9, left) require more experience to use but are more effective. They provide 100% oxygen. Inflation and deflation pressures may be adjusted by the squeezing pressure and by the tightening of the exhaust tube. If the mask does not fit tightly over the baby's face or there is a leak elsewhere in the system (e.g., the bag is not connected to a source of gas), the bag does not inflate. Enough pressure should be applied on the bag to produce a visible, but not excessive rise of the chest wall. The rate should be 40–60 per minute. It is advisable to place an orogastric tube to prevent distension of the stomach. If the baby's heart rate does not rise above 120 per minute within 60 seconds of ventilation with bag and mask, endotracheal intubation should be performed. Successful intubation requires that the head be kept in a neutral position and that a proper laryngoscope blade (0 or 1; straight, not curved) and endotracheal tube of correct size and shape (2.5, 3.0, 3.5, or 4.0) be used (Fig. 10-10). Use the largest tube that will fit the trachea without forcing so that no leaks develop around the tube. Straight endotracheal tubes are less traumatic than the Cole tubes that have a narrowed tip. Use of stylets or obturators to "stiffen" the tube is unnecessary and potentially dangerous. One must not push the tube too far into the trachea, thereby selectively intubating one of the main stem bronchi and inflating only one lung. Detection of equal breath sounds on both sides of the chest usually suffices to position the tube until radiological verification can be obtained.

Ventilating through a correctly placed endotracheal tube usually results in an immediate increase in heart rate. If bradycardia persists despite adequate ventilation, cardiac massage is necessary. Unless the baby is very big, or the operator has small hands, this is best accomplished by compressing the heart at a rate of 100–120 per minute between both thumbs placed on the middle third of the sternum and the other fingers placed on the spine (Fig. 10-11). Another method is to depress the middle third of the sternum with the second and third fingers (Fig. 10-12). Either technique minimizes

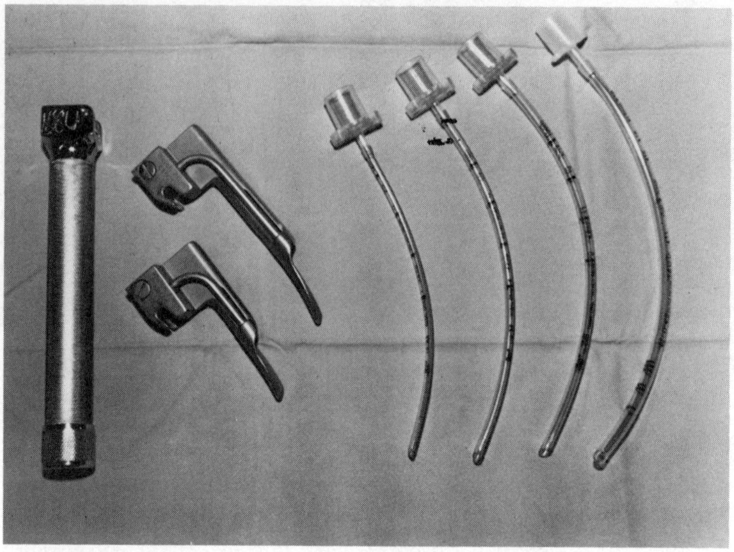

Figure 10-10. Intubation equipment: laryngoscope with 0 and 1 straight blades and 2.5, 3.0, 3.5, and 4.0 mm straight endotracheal tubes.

the risk of organ trauma (liver, spleen) or rib fractures.

Medications are seldom required during resuscitation in the delivery room. When needed, they should be injected intravenously directly into the umbilical vein or through a catheter placed in an umbilical vessel.

Naloxone. Naloxone, at a dosage of 0.005–0.01 mg/kg, is useful to reverse respiratory depression secondary to maternal sedation with narcotics. The duration of action may be shorter than that of the narcotic. The neonate should be observed closely for the possibility of recurring respiratory depression. If this should occur, a second dose of Naloxone may be given.

Epinephrine. Epinephrine, although often used in asystolic or bradycardic neonates (1 ml of 1/10,000 dilution) in an attempt to increase

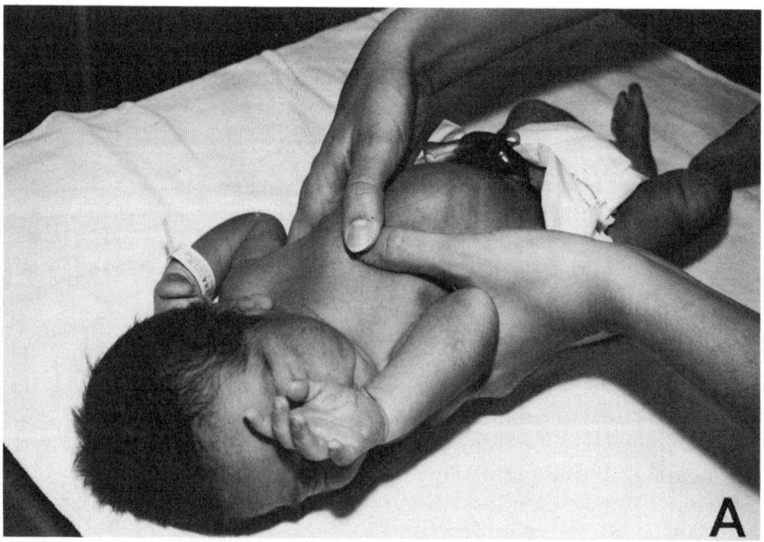

Figure 10-11. Demonstration of cardiac massage: two-hand technique.

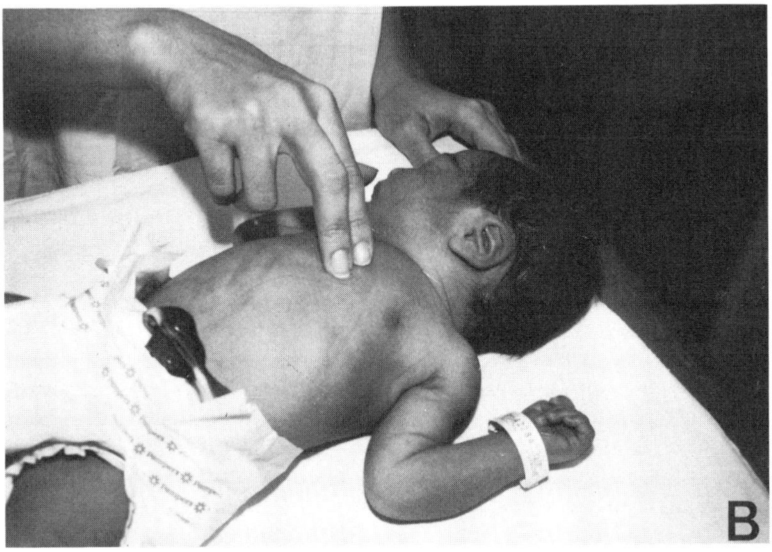

Figure 10-12. Demonstration of cardiac massage: one-hand technique.

myocardial contractility and heart rate, is not recommended. Most neonates who are bradycardic at birth are so because of hypoxia and acidosis which interfere with cellular production of ATP and impair the Na^+/K^+ pump which keeps Na^+ and water outside the cells and K^+ inside. The result is myocardial cells bloated with water. Treatment consists of correcting hypoxia and acidosis to reestablish myocardial function. Epinephrine and other cardiac stimulants are unlikely to improve the function of a waterlogged myocardium. Moreover, an asphyxiated neonate is already in a state of intense vasoconstriction. Blood flow is reflexly shunted away from "less vital" organs such as the lungs, kidneys, gastrointestinal tract, muscles, and skin to benefit the brain and heart. By increasing vasoconstriction, epinephrine may favor the development of acute tubular necrosis and necrotizing enterocolitis. If cardiac stimulation is needed, isoproterenol is a better drug to use since it also has vasodilatory properties (0.5 μg/kg/min). In this case, fluids usually should be given to prevent hypotension.

Sodium Bicarbonate. If the baby responds promptly to resuscitative measures, there is no urgency to administer bicarbonate. It is best to check acid-base status once the baby is stable in the nursery and to correct metabolic acidosis as needed. If prolonged resuscitation is needed and the heart rate delays its return to normal, bicarbonate (2–5 mEq/kg diluted 1:2 with sterile water and injected at a rate of 1 mEq per minute) may partially correct pH and improve myocardial function as well as decrease pulmonary vascular resistance. Bicarbonate should *never* be administered unless ventilation is well established. Bicarbonate given to a baby whose $PaCO_2$ is elevated would be transformed to CO_2, which would further elevate $PaCO_2$, and paradoxically lower pH.

Dextrose. An asphyxiated baby consumes calories and tends to become hypoglycemic. In prolonged resuscitative efforts, dextrose (0.5 g/kg as a 25% solution over 5 minutes) will provide calories and prevent depletion of glycogen reserves. Rapid infusion of either bicarbonate or dextrose must be avoided as they produce a sharp rise in serum osmolality which may contribute to intracranial hemorrhage, especially in small preterm neonates.

Albumin. Hypovolemia is a frequent complication of severe asphyxia. Blood transfusion (uncrossmatched 0 negative blood from the blood bank or maternal blood) is the treatment of choice. Albumin is not recommended because its intravascular life is short and it has only minimal effect on blood pressure and blood volume. In preterm babies with hyaline membrane disease, albumin accumulates in pulmonary macrophages and may impair oxygen diffusion in the lung.

Anemia and meconium aspiration offer special problems in neonatal resuscitation. Anemia may result from hemolysis during fetal life (erythroblastosis fetalis) or bleeding from the fetus into his mother, into a twin, or into his environment. Since blood volume and hematocrit are linearly related in the neonate, anemia is compounded by hypovolemia. Such babies often do not breathe at birth and will not breathe spontaneously until the anemia is corrected. It is imperative to provide blood as rapidly as possible. The most readily available source is usually the baby's mother: 10–20 ml/kg of the baby's estimated body weight is drawn from a mother's vein into a heparinized syringe and infused into the baby over five to ten minutes. Usually the baby will start breathing spontaneously as blood is pushed in and may be extubated by the time the transfusion is completed.

In meconium aspiration, the neonate should, if possible, be prevented from breathing until the meconium has been cleared from the airway. To be effective, meconium removal must take place before meconium particles have been aspirated into small bronchi and alveoli. This can best be accomplished in two steps. First and most important, the obstetrician must suction the baby's mouth and nose clear of meconium with a bulb syringe or a DeLee trap as soon as the head is delivered, while the chest is still compressed in the birth canal. Then, after delivery of the baby, the umbilical cord should be severed immediately. The baby should be intubated with as large an endotracheal tube as possible. The resuscitator sucks on the tube through a face mask while withdrawing the tube. Intubation and suction are repeated until no more meconium can be removed. The absence of meconium on the vocal cords at direct laryngoscopy does not preclude the presence of meconium in the trachea. Intubation should be performed whenever thick meconium is present in amniotic fluid. Washing the lungs with saline is not recommended: it recovers no more meconium than dry suctioning and, if meconium produces a ball-valve effect, it may be difficult to recover the fluid. This double-suction technique has drastically reduced morbidity and mortality from meconium aspiration syndromes.

After resuscitation, the neonate should be observed closely in the neonatal intensive care unit. A chest radiograph should be obtained to rule out the presence of air leaks, meconium, and rib or clavicle fractures. Arterial blood gases, plasma glucose and calcium, and hematocrit should be checked. The baby should be observed for signs of cerebral, renal, and gastrointestinal dysfunction. Feedings should be initiated with caution as asphyxia may have compromised the intestine and may predispose to necrotizing enterocolitis.

Abnormal Duration or Quality of Intrauterine Life

Prematurity. Because of its many complications, prematurity remains the major cause of neonatal morbidity and mortality. The frequency and severity of the complications of prematurity increase as gestational maturity decreases (Table 10-2). Each of these will be discussed in greater detail later in this chapter.

Postmaturity. Along with the greater risk of dying in utero before or during labor (of uteroplacental insufficiency?), the main complication of postmaturity is related to the meconium aspiration syndrome.

Small for Gestational Age. Small for gestational age neonates account for 10% of the total neonatal population. Possible causes for delayed intrauterine growth are many. (See Chapter 20.) Small for gestational age neonates do not tolerate the birth process as well as their normal size peers. In the delivery room, special attention to thermoregulation is in order, since these babies lack substrates for thermogenesis. Perinatal asphyxia, polycythemia, hypoglycemia and hypocalcemia, and necrotizing enterocolitis are well known complications. Adverse long-term sequelae are more common than in appropriate for gestational age neonates, but the cause of delayed fetal growth is an important determinant for this.

Large for Gestational Age. Large for gestational age neonates also comprise one-tenth of the neonatal population. (See Chapter 20.) Complications of this condition include polycythemia with the risk of multi-organ hypoxia from decreased oxygen delivery (seizures, respiratory distress, renal vein thrombosis, necrotizing enterocolitis), hyperbilirubinemia, and metabolic problems (hypoglycemia, hypocalcemia, hypomagnesemia). Hypoglycemia is particularly frequent. All large for gestational age neonates must be assumed to be infants of diabetic mothers until proved otherwise. Since hypoglycemia is usually asymptomatic, yet may be harmful to the brain, it is wise to follow a care-

TABLE 10-2. COMPLICATIONS OF PREMATURITY

CEREBRAL IMMATURITY
Intracranial Hemorrhages
Bilirubin Encephalopathy
RETINAL IMMATURITY
Retrolental Fibroplasia
PULMONARY IMMATURITY
Hyaline Membrane Disease
Oxygen therapy → bronchopulmonary dysplasia
Respiratory therapy → air leaks
Patent Ductus Arteriosus
Cardiovascular Instability (diving reflex)
INTESTINAL IMMATURITY
Necrotizing Enterocolitis
METABOLIC IMMATURITY
Hyperglycemia
Hypoglycemia
Hypocalcemia ⟩ → Osteopenia/rickets → fractures
Hypovitaminosis D ⟩
Hyponatremia
LIVER IMMATURITY
Cholestasis
RENAL IMMATURITY
Acute Tubular Necrosis

ful schedule for monitoring plasma glucose and treating even asymptomatic hypoglycemia (Fig. 10-13). It has become customary to treat plasma glucose levels less than 40 mg/dl. If, however, plasma glucose levels have not fallen below 40 mg/dl by the fourth hour after birth, they are unlikely to do so later and monitoring may be discontinued. Because of the large size of the baby, there is an increased risk of birth trauma. Infants of diabetic mothers, whatever their size, also have a somewhat greater incidence of congenital malformations, but no specific pattern emerges.

Respiratory Problems

Hyaline Membrane Disease (Respiratory Distress Syndrome—Type I). Hyaline membrane disease results from birth before the mechanisms for synthesis of surfactant are fully developed. In the absence of surfactant or in the presence of insufficient amounts of surfactant, pulmonary alveoli are unstable and progressively become atelectatic (Fig. (10-14). Arterial oxygenation decreases, carbon dioxide is retained, and pH declines. These events not only further impair the production of surfactant but produce pulmonary vasoconstriction, damage to the alveolar lining, and exudation of a fibrinous material into the alveoli. A vicious circle is thereby established. The best prevention is bringing a premature neonate into extrauterine life without cold, hypoxic, and acidotic stresses.

Three major advances have occurred in the past 15 years to help deal effectively with this syndrome and diminish its morbidity and mortality: the application of continuous airway pressure or, for a neonate who requires mechanical ventilation, the maintenance of a positive end expiratory pressure; the use of steroids antenatally in attempts to induce the development of the surfactant synthesis system; and replacement therapy with natural, artificial, or synthetic surfactants. This latter technique is experimental but promising.

Application of continuous positive airway pressure to the premature neonate with hyaline membrane disease[26] is largely responsible for the dramatic decrease in mortality from this syndrome. Its function is depicted in Fig. 10-15, as are its complications. With careful monitoring of the infant, complications are rare in the present state of experience with the technique. The key is to avoid the transmission of excessive positive pressure to the mediastinum when lung compliance begins to improve (two to five days after birth).

Equally exciting has been the discovery that certain drugs administered to the mother prior to delivery of a premature baby can induce early maturation of the surfactant system.

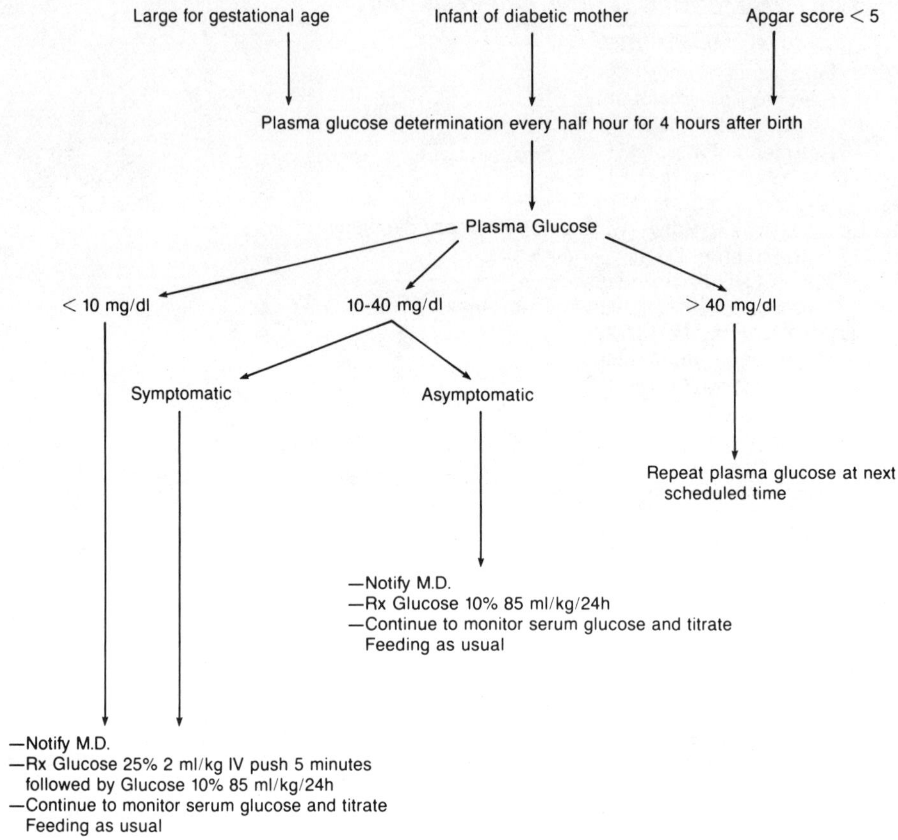

Figure 10-13. Monitoring and treatment of hypoglycemia.

Steroids (betamethasone) have been studied most extensively in humans, but heroin, thyroid hormone, and various β-sympathomimetic agents (hexoprenaline, isoxsuprine, and ritodrine) have also been found to be effective in human or animal models. Betamethasone is effective if the fetus can be exposed to it for at least 24 hours and preferably for 48 hours prior to delivery. Fetuses less than 34 weeks appear to be more responsive than those 34 weeks or older, but the latter less commonly develop hyaline membrane disease. Side effects appear minimal. The major question is the duration of effectiveness: once turned on, do the surfactant-synthesizing systems remain turned on, or, assuming that premature labor can be stopped, is it necessary to re-expose the fetus to the drug periodically to maintain effective surfactant synthesis? Further studies are needed to answer this question.

The possibility of replacing deficient surfactant by instillation of a natural surfactant or of a substitute into the trachea of a premature neonate has intrigued scientists for years. They have used "natural" surfactants (substances purified from the product of lung lavage of an animal of the same species as the recipient), "synthetic" surfactants (products manufactured from commercially available chemicals), and "artificial" surfactants (products purified from the product of lung lavage of an animal of a species other than the recipient to which have been added a variety of pure chemicals). Various replacement substances and modes of administration of those surfactants have been tried, including aerosolisation, ultrasonic nebulization, intratracheal instillation, pharyngeal deposition, or by blowing powder into the lungs.

At present, the weight of experimental evidence suggests that the administration of approximately 1.1 mg of phosphatidylglycerol per gram of lung or of 53 mg of surfactant per kg of

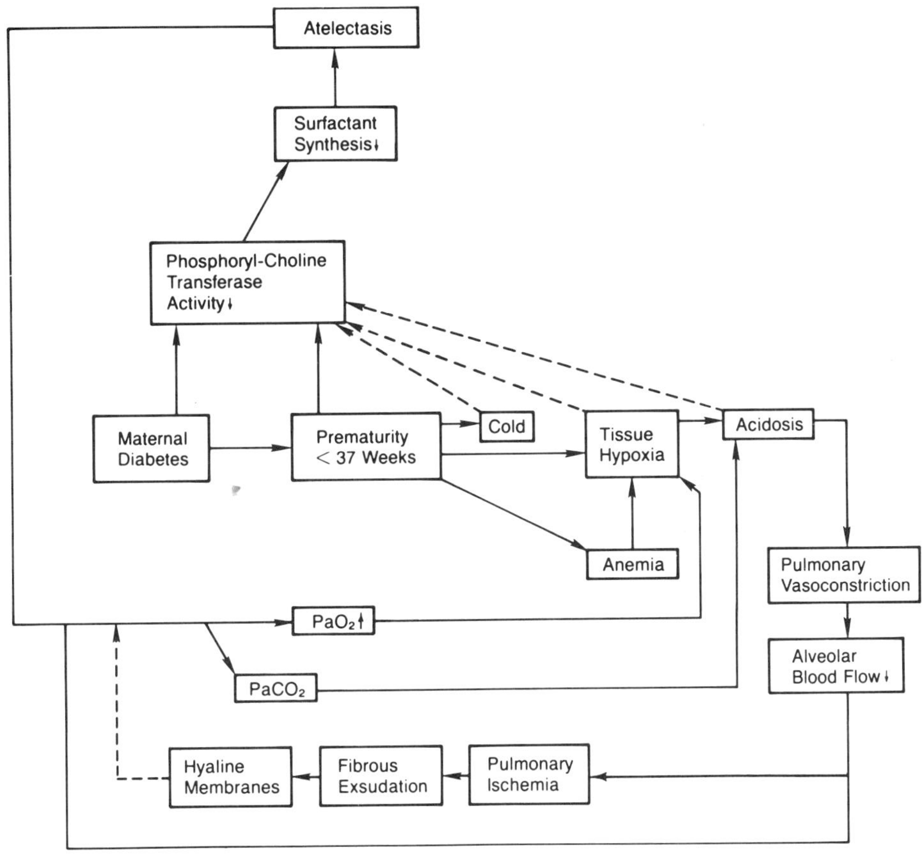

Figure 10-14. Pathophysiology of hyaline membrane disease.

body weight may have beneficial effects in the treatment of hyaline membrane disease. The preferred route of administration seems to be by tracheal instillation. Natural surfactants seem to have a slight edge over synthetics. The future will have to tell us whether species specificity is important. Attention will be given to substances free of proteins capable of inducing immunological reactions. It appears likely that surfactant replacement therapy will be available shortly.

Transient Tachypnea (Respiratory Distress Syndrome—Type II, Wet Lung Syndrome). This syndrome occurs most often in term or large premature neonates who have been heavily sedated during labor or who were born by cesarean section. Maternal diabetes also predisposes to this problem. It results from a delay in clearing lung alveolar fluid after delivery. Although the symptoms may mimic those of hyaline membrane disease, they are usually far milder. Most neonates recover completely within the first 24 hours.

Aspiration Syndromes. Neonates who aspirate meconium or, more rarely, amniotic fluid free of meconium may have severe disease (Fig. 10-16). A few still die from it. These are mostly fetuses who suffered severe enough asphyxia to start gasping in utero and who aspirate large amounts of meconium into their alveoli before delivery. Not much can be done in this situation except to support the neonate until he can expel the meconium. The most dire complication is the so-called "persistent fetal circulation" syndrome in which severe acidosis and hypoxia produce intense vasoconstriction of pulmonary arterioles. The lung reverts to its fetal state with poor perfusion. Most of the blood shunts right to left through the ductus arteriosus or the

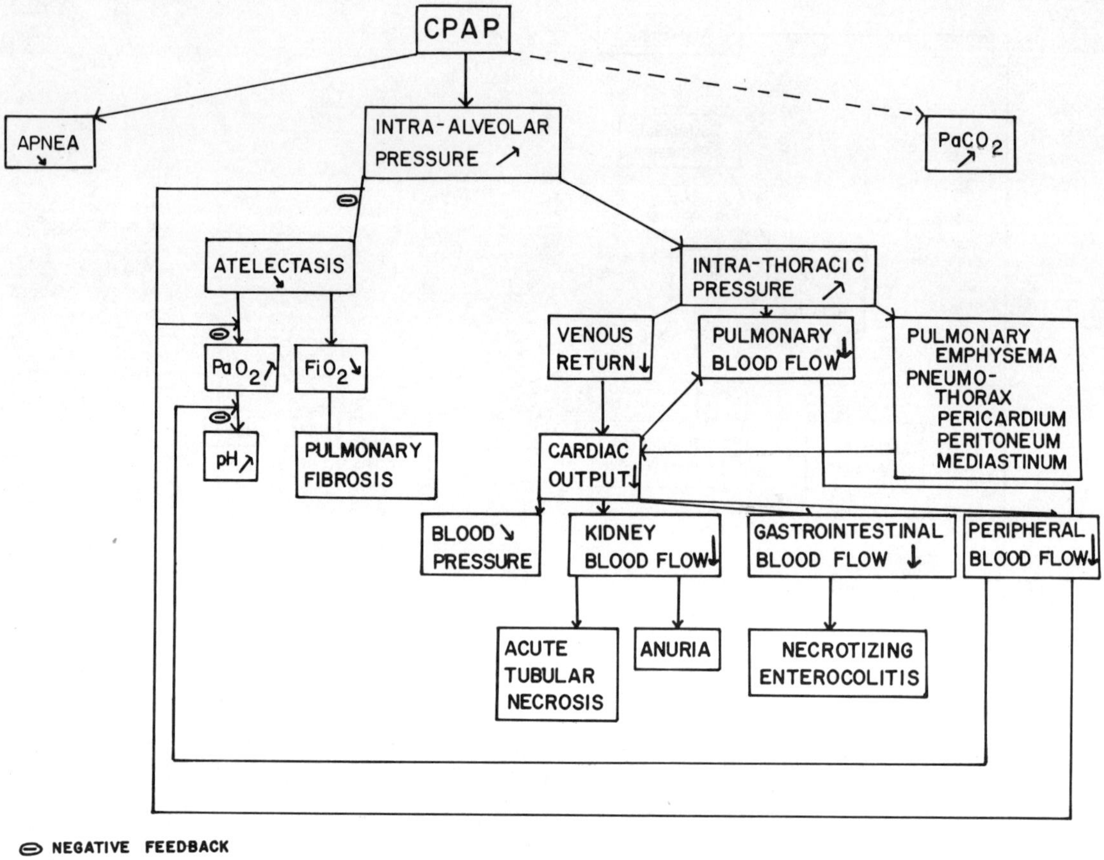

Figure 10-15. Mechanism of action and complications of continuous positive airway pressure.

foramen ovale. The kidneys and brain have usually suffered asphyxia too. Persistent fetal circulation, acute tubular necrosis, and seizures offer a grim prognosis.

Hyperbilirubinemia

Most neonates develop some hyperbilirubinemia ("physiologic jaundice"). In term babies, total serum bilirubin seldom exceeds 6–7 mg/dl, whereas in preterm neonates the rise of bilirubin is exacerbated and prolonged. Among the many circumstances in which hyperbilirubinemia exceeds the limits of a physiologic occurrence, two most pertinent to obstetricians are fetal isoimmunization (see Chapter 21) and breast milk jaundice. The etiology of breast milk jaundice is not clear. Its occurrence should not preclude continuation of breast milk feedings because the hyperbilirubinemia is self-limited. Postnatal management of the isoimmunized fetus is outlined in Fig. 10-17. No strictly objective criteria indicate when and how to treat hyperbilirubinemia to avoid bilirubin-induced encephalopathy (kernicterus).

Necrotizing Enterocolitis

Necrotizing enterocolitis is one of the most common, and most deadly, complications of prematurity, especially of the premature neonate weighing 1500 g or less. Unfortunately, it is not confined to the tiny baby and occasionally strikes apparently healthy term neonates as well. The pathogenesis is poorly understood. Figure 10-18 schematizes our present understanding of this disease.[13] Of the three main pathophysiologies involved—nutrition, infections, and intestinal ischemia—the latter appears to play the leading role. Any factor that diminishes oxygen delivery to the intestine may initiate necrotizing enterocolitis. These factors

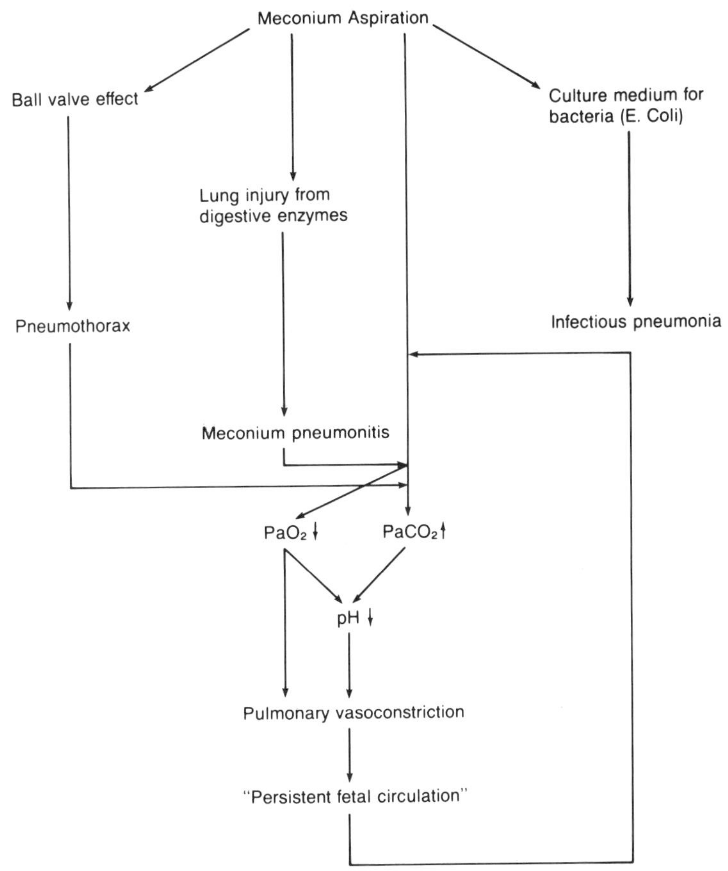

Figure 10-16. Pathophysiology of meconium aspiration.

include restriction of mesenteric blood flow (cardiac malformation, double volume exchange transfusions through a catheter lodged in the portal system, patent ductus arteriosus, polycythemia, diving reflex secondary to perinatal asphyxia), mesenteric flow of anemic blood, or interference with mesenteric capillary blood flow by hypertonic feedings. Since formulas of whatever tonicity are diluted to isoosmolality in the stomach, feeding of hypertonic formula draws fluid from the mesenteric capillary bed in order to dilute it. The resulting fluid shifts can cause repeated episodes of hypoxemia in intestinal cells. The role of infections has been mostly inferred from animal experiments which probably have little bearing on the human situation. The role of nutrition seems to be more important. Although it was once thought that breast milk protected against necrotizing enterocolitis, this has not been confirmed. The use of hypertonic formulas is on the decline and more progressive and careful feedings of small premature neonates, backing off at the slightest suspicion, seems to have reduced the incidence of necrotizing enterocolitis. The order of the day for small premature neonates appears to be parenteral nutrition until respiratory stabilization, followed by enteral feedings in increasing small increments with reversion to parenteral nutrition at the first sign of intolerance.

Retrolental Fibroplasia

Retrolental fibroplasia is thought to be the result of exposing the retina of premature babies to excessive arterial oxygen tension (PaO_2). "High" PaO_2 may produce vasoconstriction of retinal vessels, followed by neovascularization of the retina, retinal hemorrhage, proliferation of vessels in the vitreous, and, finally, retinal detachment and blindness.[22] Unfortunately, in immature neonates, even careful monitoring of

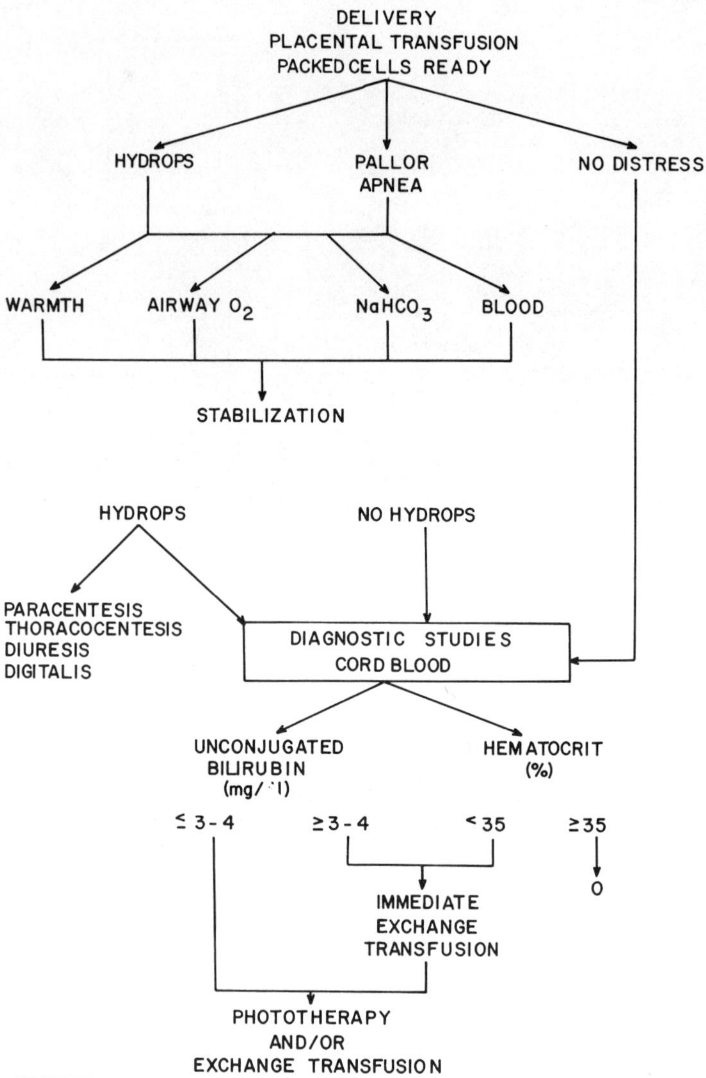

Figure 10-17. Schematic postnatal management of the isoimmunized fetus.

PaO_2, maintaining it between 60 and 100 torr, does not preclude the development of retrolental fibroplasia. As larger numbers of very small premature babies survive, the incidence of retrolental fibroplasia rises also. Attempted prophylaxis of this condition with vitamin E remains controversial.[49] Treatments, including cryotherapy, scleral buckling, and laser surgery, have had unimpressive results.

Intracranial Hemorrhage

Intracranial hemorrhages are a major source of morbidity and mortality in premature neonates, especially those weighing less than 1500 grams. Roughly half of neonates with birth weights of 500–1500 grams bleed intracranially. Most of them do so within the first three postnatal days, even though they may have had no prior requirement for ventilatory assistance and sometimes even no need for supplemental oxygen. The causes of this hemorrhaging are uncertain. Theories have implicated disseminated intravascular coagulation, birth trauma, capillary fragility, increase in intracranial pressure from pneumothoraces and shunts through the ductus arteriosus, sudden increases in serum osmolality following injection of hypertonic bicarbonate or dextrose, and others. Diagnosis has been enhanced by the availability of sector ultrasono-

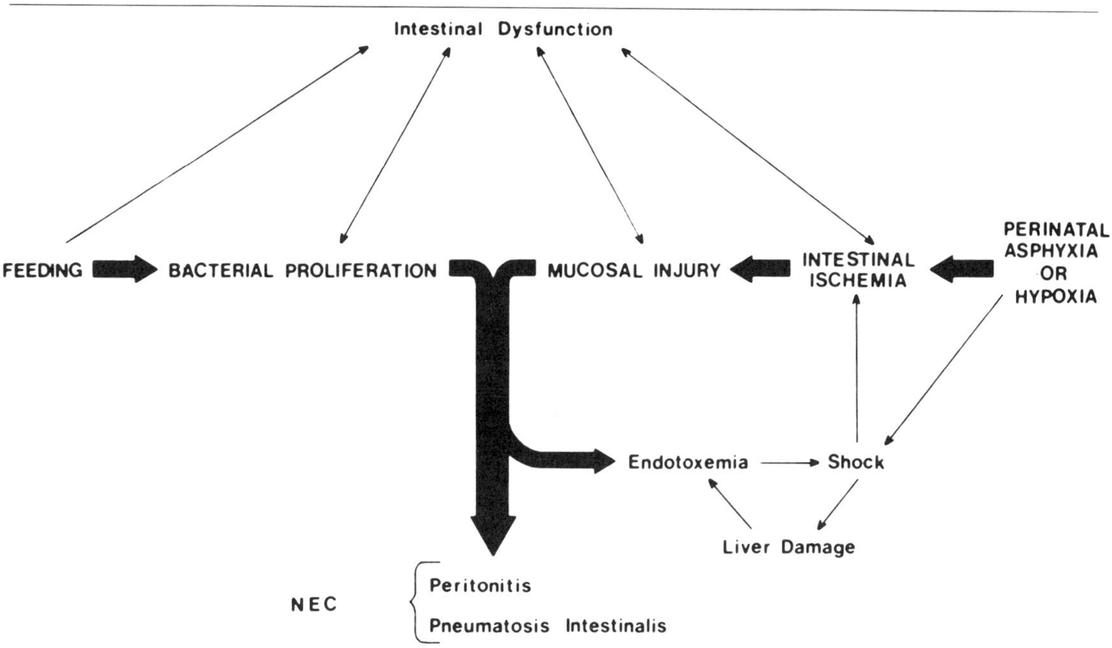

Figure 10-18. Pathophysiology of necrotizing enterocolitis. Bold type indicates factors of primary importance. (Reprinted from Brown, E. G. and Sweet, A. Y.: Neonatal Necrotizing Enterocolitis. New York, Grune & Stratton, 1980, by permission of authors and Grune & Stratton, Inc., publishers.)

grams. The sequelae of this problem are as varied as its possible causes (Fig. 10-19). The long-term impact remains to be determined. Small premature babies (less than 1500 grams) should be handled gingerly. Rapid administration of hypertonic substances should be prohibited. Minimal handling helps to prevent sporadic increases in blood pressure that may affect cerebral circulation. Pneumothoraces should be avoided. Patent ductus arteriosus should be treated promptly or even preventively by surgery or prostaglandin antagonists. Parents should not be told that their tiny baby who is doing very well is out of danger until several days have passed and the presence of an intracranial hemorrhage has been ruled out by ultrasonography.

Anemia and Polycythemia

Abnormalities of the red cell and blood volume are so common, so easy to treat, and so potentially devastating if therapy is withheld, that a hematocrit should be performed in every newborn infant. Anemia at birth has already been discussed. Its opposite, polycythemia, can also produce serious, sometimes life-threatening, insults to the brain, heart, lungs, kidneys, and intestines. Whenever the volume of red cells exceeds a certain proportion of the circulating blood volume, sludging of red cells may occur and may impair circulation to various organs. In vitro measurement of blood viscosity offers the most convenient estimate of sludging and of the risk of oxygen ischemia. In most nurseries, viscosity determinations are not routinely available; therefore, hematocrit levels are relied upon for diagnosis of this syndrome. The difficulty has been to define a hematocrit value that identifies neonates with hyperviscosity and minimizes the number of either false negative or false positive results. Other areas of contention include the site of blood sampling for hematocrit determination (whether from a small peripheral vein or from a large central vein), whether all neonates at risk or only symptomatic ones need to be treated, and whether preventive treatment of neonates at risk affects the incidence of short- and long-term complications. Based on our own work, the scheme depicted in Fig. 10-20 has evolved for monitoring and treatment of polycythemia. It is currently in use in our nurseries. Infants of diabetic mothers, small for dates neonates, and babies with trisomy 21

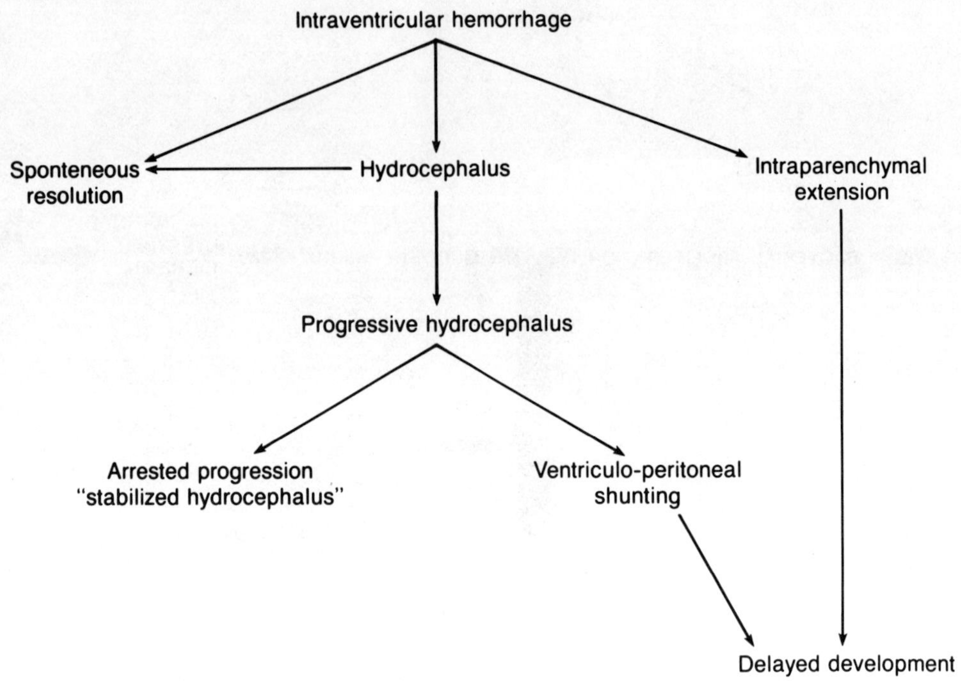

Figure 10-19. Progression of intraventricular hemorrhage.

are particularly at risk for polycythemia. Treatment is by partial exchange transfusion, that is, exchanging whole blood for plasma or a plasma equivalent in order to bring the hematocrit down to a desired level according to the formula:

$$\text{Exchange volume (in ml)} = \frac{\text{Observed hematocrit-desired hematocrit}}{\text{observed hematocrit}} \times \text{birth weight} \times \text{blood volume}$$

where the observed hematocrit is that measured in the umbilical vein, the desired hematocrit is usually 55%, and the blood volume is assumed to be 85–90 ml/kg.

Substance Abuse in Pregnancy

Abuses that have received attention in the press include maternal drug addiction, smoking, caffeine, and alcohol ingestion.

Narcotic Addiction. Although many drugs given to or taken by mothers, including pentazocine, phenobarbital, diazepam and related substances, amphetamines, gluthetimide, propoxyphene, and ethchlorvynol, have been shown to produce withdrawal symptoms in the neonate, maternal narcotic addiction is by far the most common cause of neonatal withdrawal symptoms. In general, the severity of withdrawal symptoms in the newborn correlates directly with the dosage of narcotics taken by the mother.[28] The onset of symptoms occurs most frequently in the first 24 hours but may be delayed up to four days. In case of methadone withdrawal, however, symptoms have occasionally been delayed by as long as two to four weeks[31] and their severity is related to the total dose of methadone ingested by the mother during the last 12 weeks of pregnancy, the maternal dose of methadone at delivery, and the intrapartum serum methadone levels.[28] Central nervous system irritability heralds the withdrawal symptoms: tremors, hyperactivity, constant and shrill crying, incessant activity, and sometimes seizures. Gastrointestinal symptoms include vomiting and diarrhea, yet apparent hunger. Respiratory symptoms may include apneic spells, sneezing, and cyanosis. Skin lesions over points of contact with bedding are not uncommon.[56] There has been a great deal of controversy over the relative effects of heroin and me-

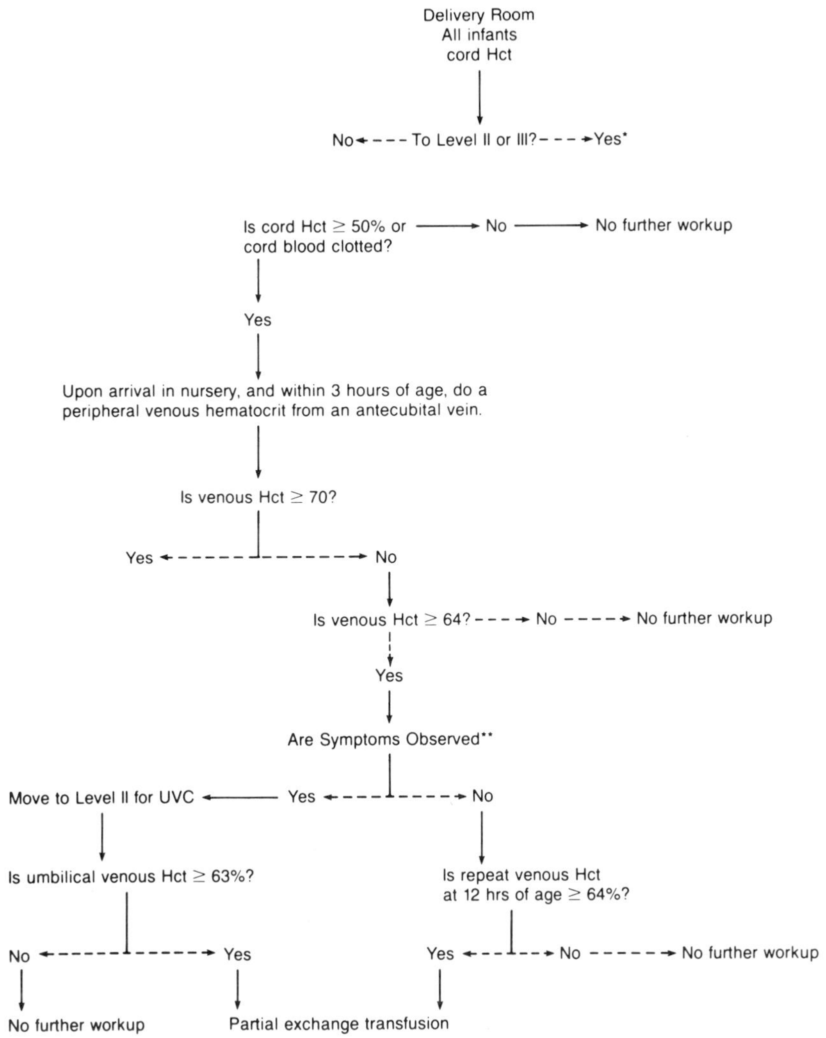

Figure 10-20. Monitoring and management of polycythemia. Infants of diabetic mothers, growth-retarded infants, and Trisomy 21 who are admitted directly to LII who have cord hct ≧50% or when cord blood is clotted, should have venous hct soon after admission. If venous hct is ≧70%, UVC should be done immediately. If venous hct is between 64 and 70%, infant is observed for symptoms or laboratory findings such as hypoglycemia or hyperbilirubinemia. If symptomatic (symptoms are lethargy, tachypnea, tachycardia, abdominal distention, tremors, or convulsions), immediate UVC and blood sampling is done. If asymptomatic, venous hct is repeated at 12 hours. Venous hct at 12 hours ≧64% should receive a UVC. Management following UVC is as shown in the algorithm.

thadone. At low to high dosages (10–160 mg/day), methadone produces more severe withdrawal symptoms, more frequent seizures, more hyperbilirubinemia, and more hyaline membrane disease than does heroin.[62] Methadone also increases fetal stress response.[63] At low dose, methadone appears to delay physical growth of the neonate during the first three to four months, with an acceleration of growth pattern in the following months.[15] In this country, however, there is as yet no legal alternative to attempting detoxification of the pregnant woman, even if it harms her fetus. Empirically, however, it appears that the low methadone maintenance dosages used at the present time have few ill effects on the fetus and neonate compared to the rather high dosages that were in vogue 10 years ago. Treatment of withdrawal symptoms in the neonate is best achieved by the use of paregoric or tincture of opium (6 drops every 4 hours orally to begin with) or chlorpromazine (0.5–1.0 mg/kg every 6 hours i.m. or orally).[47,56] Paregoric offers the most flexibility and is the drug of choice. Phenobarbital takes too long to reach a steady state and diazepam has the disadvantage of being dissolved in propylene glycol, a substance that interferes with albumin binding of bilirubin.

Maternal Smoking. There is no question that maternal cigarette smoking is associated with a reduction in birth weight.[41,42,56] The reduction in birth weight correlates directly with the number of cigarettes smoked.[56] It appears that the mechanism for the decreased fetal weight is a direct effect of cigarette smoke on decreasing intervillous blood flow in the placenta.[36,45] Stunting of intrauterine growth appears to be reversible if smoking is stopped early in pregnancy. Other fetal effects have been less well established, such as decreased Apgar scores[30] and increased incidence of polycythemia,[40] of cleft lip and palate,[19] and of abortions.[35] The precise mechanism of the noxious effects of cigarette smoking has not been established beyond doubt. In the present state of knowledge, however, it would be wise to recommend that pregnant women refrain from smoking.

Caffeine. Though much publicized in the lay press and media, the effects of caffeine on the fetus are yet to be determined. Caffeine is present in coffee, tea, colas and other carbonated beverages, cocoa, chocolate, and over-the-counter medications for cold, allergy, headaches, diuretics, and stimulants.[44] It is estimated that the average pregnant woman consumes 144 mg of caffeine per day.[44] Two cups of coffee (or 200 mg of caffeine) are sufficient to increase catecholamine production to the point of causing vasoconstriction of blood flow in uterine and intervillous placental vessels.[32,37] This could theoretically produce intrauterine growth retardation if the insult is repeated often enough. In animals, various mutagenic and teratogenic effects have been described, but never in humans.[44] On the other hand, in a large study of over 12,000 women, no effects have been found after controlling for smoking, other habits, demographic data and, medical history.[37] The safest recommendation at this time appears to be to limit caffeine consumption during pregnancy, but there seems to be no need to prohibit its use altogether on the basis of available information.

Alcohol. Exposure to alcohol during fetal life may have deleterious effects for the fetus and neonate, although detectable effects are rare. They may range from withdrawal symptoms shortly after birth to a fetal alcohol syndrome which is estimated to affect approximately 2% of neonates born to mothers who take alcohol during the pregnancy.[56] (See Chapter 20.)

Birth Injuries* (in Collaboration with Rajam S. Ramamurthy, M.D.†)

The incidence of birth trauma has declined in recent years owing to advances in obstetrics and to increased use of cesarean section. Trauma occurs in 2–7 per 1000 live births and is seen more frequently in infants weighing more than 2500 grams than in those below that weight. Early reports attributed a high percentage of neonatal mortality to birth injury; trauma still accounts for 2% of all neonatal deaths.

Soft Tissue Injuries

Bruising and Ecchymoses. These may be seen over the presenting part and are often severe in prolonged, difficult labor and in abnormal fetal presentations. Bruising and ecchymoses are due to suffusion of blood secondary to venous congestion. Common examples are swelling and discoloration of the legs in footling breech, of the gluteal region and external genitalia in frank breech, and of the face in face presentation. Actual bleeding may be present in the soft tissue and petechiae are often seen. The swelling generally disappears in 24–48 hours. Absorption of bilirubin from breakdown of red blood cells may

* Parts of this section are reprinted verbatim with the permission of the authors and publishers of Ramamurthy, R. S. and Pyati, S. P.: Birth injuries and acquired injuries in neonatal intensive care. In: *Atlas in Perinatology.* S. Aladjem and D. Vidyasagar (Eds.). Philadelphia, W. B. Saunders Co., 1982, pp. 239–253.

† Associate Professor, Department of Pediatrics, The University of Texas Health Science Center at San Antonio, San Antonio, Texas.

result in delayed and prolonged hyperbilirubinemia, depending on the amount of extravasated blood. Early phototherapy may be of some benefit.

Petechiae. The occurrence of petechiae over the forehead and face may be evidence of a tight cord around the fetal neck. When the lesions progress or are seen in many parts of the body, other causes of thrombocytopenia and petechiae must be considered.

Subconjunctival Hemorrhages. These are seen in 20% of infants, may occur after normal delivery, and require no treatment. However, when the conjunctivae appear swollen, possible injury to other structures in the eye should be ruled out by thorough examination.

Lacerations. Lacerations may be caused by a scalpel blade during cesarean section, by scissors during an episiotomy, by sampling of blood from the fetal scalp for pH monitoring, or rarely by forceps. Laceration and edema of the neonatal vulva may occur in frank breech presentations. Unless there is free bleeding, no attempt should be made to suture a laceration in the delivery room. The suturing should be done as early as possible under sterile conditions using fine (7-0) nylon suture. Small lacerations may require merely an adhesive bandage. Lacerations of areas likely to be soiled with feces and urine should be well protected. It is preferable for lacerations of the face to be treated by a plastic surgeon to obtain better cosmetic results.

Necrosis of Subcutaneous Fat. Areas of circumscribed induration due to subcutaneous fat necrosis may be seen in infants more than three to four days old. Locations are commonly the back and buttock, occasionally the thigh, the cheek, and other parts. The overlying skin is of normal color or red.

When large areas are involved, there are local tenderness and warmth. The margin is well defined and feels firm on palpation. Biopsy of these areas shows endothelial swelling and perivascular inflammation in the subcutaneous fat. At a later stage, necrosis of the fat occurs. Occasionally calcification may be seen. The most common etiology is trauma during delivery; others are hypoxemia, excessive chilling, and ischemia. This condition must be differentiated from scleredema, which is seen in very sick infants and has a grave prognosis. Other differential diagnoses are cellulitis, lipogranulomatosis, and panniculitis.

No treatment is required for subcutaneous fat necrosis. Even extensive lesions gradually soften and disappear in 6–8 weeks. Atrophy is sometimes seen at the site of injury, as is secondary infection.

Injury to the Sternocleidomastoid. A 1–2 cm mass near the middle of the sternocleidomastoid muscle may be noticed a few days to two weeks after birth. When torticollis is seen on the same side, the condition is called congenital torticollis, muscular torticollis, or sternomastoid fibroma. The injury is thought to be either intrauterine or acquired at delivery. A hematoma forms in the belly of the muscle and later becomes fibrosed. The infant holds the head to one side. Differential diagnosis includes true deformities of the spine, such as Klippel–Feil syndrome and Sprengel's deformity.

In the past, steroids and sclerosing solutions were injected into the mass. The best approach, however, is not to manipulate the mass in any manner and to keep the head turned to the opposite side as much as possible. Complete recovery is usually seen in two to three months. If it does not heal spontaneously, surgical correction may be necessary.

Scalp Abscesses. Scalp abscesses have been reported as an occasional complication of fetal monitoring, especially in cases where amniotic infections coexisted. The incidence has been estimated at 0–0.4%.[48] Symptoms may be observed as early as the first postnatal day and as late as 3 weeks after birth, but most lesions are apparent by the third or fourth day. The best prevention is not to reuse scalp electrodes, even after adequate sterilization, and to shave routinely the area of the scalp surrounding the site of electrode implantation and to disinfect the area with an iodophor.

Head Injuries. The head, being the most common presenting part, is subjected to more trauma during birth than any other part of the body.

Caput Succedaneum. The presenting part of the fetus' head, which in most cases is the vertex, is usually edematous and elongated owing to the pressure exerted on it during descent through the pelvis. Under normal circumstances the caput should disappear in 24 hours. Following prolonged and difficult labor, there is excessive molding of the skull bones, severe edema, and discoloration of the scalp. If this is seen in a pale, shocky infant, even in the presence of a normal hematocrit, subaponeurotic bleeding should be suspected. As much as 50–150 ml of blood may be lost beneath the aponeurosis of the scalp. Attention should be given to immediate correction of volume loss and then to correction of hematocrit. Radiography may reveal fractures. Prolonged severe hyperbilirubinemia is a late manifestation of this lesion and may require several exchange transfusions. The blood should not be aspirated for fear of introducing infection. Even the severe forms of caput succedaneum resolve without sequelae unless there is associated intracranial hemorrhage.

Cephalhematomata. Actual hemorrhages under the periosteum of skull bones, cephalhematomata occur in 0.4–2.5% of all newborns and are more frequent over the parietal bones. Primiparous delivery and application of forceps are predisposing factors. The incidence is about 33% in mid-forceps delivery, 4% in low-forceps delivery, and 1.7% in delivery without forceps.

Swelling is limited to the margins of skull bones and does not cross suture lines because the periosteum is attached to the edges of the bones. Cephalhematomata become more prominent a day after birth when edema of the rest of the scalp subsides. They are nontransilluminant, nonpulsatile, and noncompressible; these features differentiate them from other swellings on the head such as hemangiomas and meningoencephaloceles.

Significant blood loss with shock occurs rarely as a complication of a cephalhematoma. Skull fractures are seen in approximately 10% of cases. Routine skull radiographs for all infants with cephalhematomata are not practiced in our unit. Radiographs are obtained only if there is evidence of excessive blood loss, altered activity, or suspicion of a depressed fracture of the skull. Delayed hyperbilirubinemia due to absorption of bilirubin from enclosed hemorrhage is perhaps the most common complication.

No therapy is necessary. The mother should be informed about the lesion and advised not to massage it or to apply anything over it. The majority of cephalhematomata disappear in 2–8 weeks. Occasionally a permanent calcified nodule persists for several years.

Fractures of the Skull. Early reports quote an incidence of 30% for fractures of the skull in association with cephalhematomata. The current incidence is only 10%, which probably reflects improved obstetric techniques and a decrease in high-forceps and mid-forceps deliveries. Most fractures are linear and occur radially from the margin of the bone, following the planes of cleavage. Occasionally a portion of the bone becomes depressed with no actual break in the bone. Linear fractures of the parietals are the most common form of skull fracture seen. Very rarely in breech deliveries, when the squamous portion of the occipital bone hooks under the symphysis pubis, the basal portion breaks away from it as traction is applied to deliver the head. This injury is invariably fatal owing to tearing of the venous sinuses that run along the bone.

Diagnosis of skull fracture is made radiographically. Depressed fractures may be seen on contour views only. Very commonly, the inexperienced eye mistakes suture lines, vascular grooves, and "ripple lines" representing soft tissue folds for fracture, and vice versa. Most linear fractures heal without complication. Radiographs taken 8–10 days later show a shell of bone over the hematoma, which may persist for several months.

Rarely, permanent cyst-like spaces are left between the inner and outer tables of the bone. Leptomeningeal cysts may occur secondary to protrusion of a portion of meninges into the fracture site. Such cysts grow larger, so this condition may be recognized by rapid head growth.

Depressed fractures are treated by manual elevation of the bone or by vacuum suction. Otherwise, the depressed portion of the bone may exert pressure on the underlying brain and lead to atrophy.

Intracranial Hemorrhage. Two factors are operative in the etiology of intracranial hemorrhage: trauma and hypoxia. On the basis of the location of the hemorrhage, either or both causes may be considered. In the full-term baby, subdural hemorrhage in the neonatal period is almost exclusively due to trauma. Primary subarachnoid hemorrhages are due to trauma in term infants and to trauma or hypoxia in preterm infants. Periventricular, intraventricular, and intracerebral hemorrhages are predominantly caused by hypoxia. Only the traumatic types of intracranial hemorrhage are discussed here.

Subdural hemorrhage is directly related to cephalopelvic disproportion. The use of vacuum extraction is a factor in the increased incidence of intracranial hemorrhage, and in cephalhematoma, retinal hemorrhage, electroencephalographic abnormalities, permanent brain damage, and death. (See Chapter 44.)

There are three locations at which tearing of the dura leads to hemorrhage. The clinical manifestations, management, and outcome vary depending on the location of the hematoma.

Tentorial tears occur when there is excessive molding of the head and fronto-occipital elongation. The hemorrhage is infratentorial. When it is massive, symptoms are present at birth. Early signs are coma, unequal pupil size, skew deviation of the eyes, absence of doll's eye response, nuchal rigidity, and opisthotonus. As the brain stem is compressed, the pupils become dilated and fixed, and, finally, respiratory arrest occurs. The rapid progression of symptoms in tentorial tears makes surgical evacuation impossible, and death is the rule. The occasional survivors develop hydrocephalus.

Laceration of the falx cerebri occurs when there is extreme fronto-occipital elongation, as in face and brow presentations. Blood accumulates in the longitudinal cerebral fissure. Bilateral cerebral signs may be present. However, most of the findings are related to the infratentorial extension of the clot. As with tentorial tears, the rapid progression of symptoms precludes surgical evacuation of the clot.

Hemorrhage over the convexity of the brain occurs secondary to rupture of the bridging veins entering the superior saggital sinus. This may be due to extreme vertical molding of the skull or to fracture of the skull. Rupture of the bridging veins is often seen at autopsy as an incidental finding. If significant bleeding compresses the cerebral cortex or if there is contusion of the cortex, seizures may occur on the second day of life. Focal signs such as hemiparesis and lateral deviation of the eyes are present. The classic sign is unilateral paralysis of the third cranial nerve due to herniation of the temporal lobe through the tentorial opening. In symptomatic infants, hemorrhage over the convexities should be removed by subdural tap. Minimal asymptomatic hemorrhage occasionally progresses to chronic subdural effusion. Bulging fontanel, rapidly growing head, and failure to thrive should prompt suspicion of this problem. Repeated subdural taps and, occasionally, surgical removal of the pseudomembrane that forms around the hematoma may be required to evacuate a chronic subdural effusion. Hemorrhage over the convexity has a good prognosis. Nearly 80% of affected infants are normal at follow-up. Very rarely, seizures and hydrocephalus may be seen.

Full-term infants may occasionally develop a primary subarachnoid hemorrhage following trauma. Seizures occurring on the second day of life in infants appearing normal in the interictal period should make one suspect subarachnoid bleeding. Infants with minimal symptoms have a 90% chance of being normal.

Computerized tomography is the most valuable diagnostic procedure for all forms of intracranial hemorrhage. X-rays of the skull are useful only in the presence of fractures. Subdural tap may be useful. Although a negative tap does not rule out intracranial hemorrhage, the presence of increased numbers of red cells, a protein level in excess of 120 mg/dl, and hypoglycorrhachia in the context of historical and clinical evidence are highly suggestive of hemorrhage.

Leak of Cerebrospinal Fluid. This is a very rare complication reported after fetal monitoring via a scalp electrode. Cerebrospinal fluid drainage usually ceases spontaneously within 3 days, but application of collodion may hasten resolution of the problem. One of three neonates reported with this complication developed meningitis, but the relationship between the leak and the infection was uncertain.[57]

Injuries to Peripheral Nerves

Facial Palsy. Infranuclear facial palsy is usually seen after prolonged labor in which the head rests on the sacrum for a long time or after difficult forceps deliveries. It may also be due to contralateral injury to the brain following fracture of a temporal bone. Rarely, bilateral facial paralysis is due to absence of the nucleus (Möbius syndrome); this is associated with abducens paralysis. In central facial paralysis only the lower portion of the face is involved, the eye and forehead being spared.

The weakness is noticed at the time of birth and is more apparent when the patient is made to cry. Absence of the nasolabial fold, wrinkling of the forehead, slight prominence of the cheek, impaired closure of the eye on the affected side, and drawing of the mouth to the opposite side when stimulated constitute the spectrum of signs in this paralysis. As an isolated finding in some infants, one corner of the mouth fails to move downward and outward during crying. This is due to congenital absence of the depressor angulus oris muscle.

No specific therapy is indicated for the majority of cases. Sucking should be observed to ensure that there is no excessive dribbling from the corner of the mouth. The eye should be protected with methylcellulose drops, and an eye patch should be applied if necessary. The majority of cases show improvement in three to four days. Patients should be examined at around 10 days of age, when a nerve excitability test may differentiate true nerve degeneration from neurapraxia (edema of the nerve), which resolves in four to six weeks. Other electrodiagnostic tests may be done depending on the progress. Most infants with traumatic facial paralysis recover. Even when there is evidence of nerve degeneration in the initial stages, regeneration occurs at the rate of about 2.5 cm a month.

Brachial Plexus Palsy. This condition, as most other trauma, is often seen in large infants following difficult delivery of the shoulders. It has also been reported in association with uneventful spontaneous deliveries. It may be due to avulsion of the roots of the brachial plexus during traction on the head to deliver the shoulders in normal presentation or to stretching of the brachial plexus in breech presentation. Three types of palsies are seen. The first is *Erb's palsy*, in which muscles supplied by nerve roots C5 and C6 are involved. The Moro reflex is asymmetrical. The arm hangs limp at the side of the body, is adducted and internally rotated at the shoulder, and is pronated at the elbow with the wrist flexed ("waiter's tip" posture). The second is *Klumpke's paralysis*, in which the C8 to T1 roots are involved. It is rarely seen as an isolated injury and is thought to occur from stretching of the lower plexus nerve against the coracoid process of the scapula during attempts to deliver the shoulder. The flexor and extensor muscles of the wrist and the intrinsic muscles of the hand are weak. The grasp reflex is impaired. The third type, *combined paralysis*, is more common than Klumpke's paralysis. The entire arm is involved. Absence of sweating, atrophy of the hand muscles, sensory impairment on the ulnar side of the hand, and Horner's syndrome on the affected side due to involvement of sympathetic fibers from T1 may be present. Fracture of the clavicle, fracture and dislocation of upper humeral epiphyses, fracture of the shaft of the humerus, and injury to the cervical spine should all be considered in the differential diagnosis of any paralysis of the arm.

During the first few days after birth, the arm should be held in a position of rest. Most infants show recovery within two to three weeks. When gradual improvement is seen, passive exercises to abduct and extend the shoulder, supinate the arm, and extend the wrists must be taught to the parents. The patient should be seen regularly until full recovery is accomplished. Electromyography is useful to evaluate the extent of damage and to estimate prognosis; starting at two to three weeks, it should be done periodically. Infants should be encouraged to use their affected arms, because they can become unaware of their hands otherwise. Even in the mildest forms of paralysis, winging of the scapula, abduction of the shoulder, or lack of supination may persist.

Paralysis of the Phrenic Nerve. Paralysis of the phrenic nerve may be associated with brachial plexus palsy and may appear following breech deliveries. The cervical roots of C3, C4, and C5 are involved, resulting in paralysis of the diaphragm on the affected side. Presenting signs include tachypnea, cyanosis, and apnea. The diaphragm does not move down on inspiration, so the abdomen does not become prominent during inspiration. Bilateral diaphragmatic paralyses are rare. Breath sounds may be absent and atelectasis may be present on the affected side. Diagnosis is established by fluoroscopy, which shows abnormal elevation of the affected side and seesaw movement of the two sides during respiration. Radiography may reveal elevation of the diaphragm. Differential diagnosis includes all other types of neonatal respiratory distress.

In the majority of cases, recovery is complete in four to six weeks. The infant should be positioned on the affected side to allow the normal side to move freely. If recovery is slow and complications such as recurrent pneumonia in the atelectatic lung occur, surgical plication or excision of a portion of the diaphragm is performed to tighten the diaphragm to allow the lung to expand. Prognosis after such surgery is good.

Injuries of the Spinal Cord. More than 100 cases of spinal cord injuries during the birth process have been reported in the world literature. The lesion varies from localized hemorrhage in the anterior cornua to complete destruction of the spinal cord at one or more vertebral levels. Spinal cord lesions are seldom associated with dislocation or fracture of vertebral bodies. One-third of spinal lesions occurring after breech deliveries are secondary to spontaneous delivery and two-thirds are associated with extraction. After cephalic presentation, more than half the cases occur in the absence of unusual traction. Two-thirds of infants with spinal lesions die; 50% of them have anatomically proven transection of the spinal cord at one or more levels. Whatever the fetal presentation, lesions most often affect the cervical and upper two thoracic levels. The most common site of lesions is from the level of the fifth cervical vertebra to the first thoracic vertebra after breech presentation and from the level of the first to the sixth cervical vertebra after cephalic presentation.

Hyperextension of the head in footling breech presentation (see Chapter 24) appears to be a particularly dangerous position. Vaginal delivery resulted in spinal or vertebral lesions in about 25% of such infants, whereas only 4% of those delivered by cesarean section had dislocation of the first to third cervical vertebrae without spinal lesion. Cesarean section appears to be the method of choice for delivering the fetus with a hyperextended head, although transection of the cord can occur in utero.[14]

Fractures

Fracture of the Clavicle. The most common fracture encountered in the newborn period, fracture of the clavicle is usually detected during the initial examination when palpation of the clavicle is routinely done. Rarely, snapping of the bone may be heard or felt by the obstetrician while delivering the shoulder. If the fracture is complete, the two fragments grate against each other and a crepitus is felt under the fingers. This may be painful and the infant may not move the arm on that side. Associated brachial palsy may be present. Routine radiographs are not necessary. The situation must be explained to the mother with particular emphasis on formation of callus, which appears as a knot over the clavicle in about seven to ten days. No therapy is necessary if the fragments of bone are not dislocated. If the fragments are dislocated, bracing of the shoulder with a figure-of-eight bandage may be helpful.

Fracture of Long Bones. The humerus and femur are the most commonly fractured long bones. Lack of movement of the extremity may be the earliest sign. Not much soft tissue reaction occurs, and local redness, tenderness, and swelling, if present, are minimal. Fractures through epiphyseal lines are difficult to diagnose, and dislocations should be considered in differential diagnosis. Management is usually immobilization by splints and elastic bandage for two to three weeks until substantial callus has formed. Healing occurs rapidly, in three to eight weeks.

Injuries to Abdominal Organs. Injuries to abdominal organs sometimes follow breech deliveries. The most commonly damaged internal organ is the liver. The adrenal glands, kidneys, gastrointestinal tract, and spleen are occasionally involved. Hemorrhage, the most immediate complication of abdominal organ rupture, may not be recognized early enough and may result in shock and death. Mortality ranges from 0.9% to 9.6%.

Rupture of the liver and rupture of the spleen tend to occur in large infants who have hepatosplenomegaly from various causes. Liver rupture is usually subcapsular. Tachycardia and pallor may be early signs when the hemorrhage is beneath the capsule. Over the next few hours, the hepatic capsule becomes tense and ruptures. This leads to further hemorrhage, hypovolemia, and shock. Free bleeding into the peritoneal cavity may gravitate to the inguinal region, producing bluish discoloration. If there is severe bleeding, discoloration of the abdominal wall may be seen. Radiographs may show free fluid. In the case of splenic rupture, exaggeration of mucosal folds of the greater curvature of the stomach may be seen in about half the cases.

The large size of the fetal adrenals predisposes them to birth injury. Neonatal adrenal hemorrhage may not produce any symptoms. Autopsies reveal that adrenal rupture occurs much more frequently than is clinically recognized. Prolonged jaundice is perhaps the most common sign. Other signs such as abdominal mass, pallor, shock, vomiting and diarrhea, hypoglycemia, and findings suggestive of adrenal insufficiency may be present. Diagnosis is established radiologically. Differential diagnosis includes kidney masses, Wilms' tumor, and neuroblastoma.

Correcting hypovolemia and shock is most urgent in managing severe intra-abdominal hemorrhage. Blood transfusion may be needed even if the hematocrit is normal. With acute blood loss there is a time lag before the hematocrit drops. After the infant is stabilized, diagnostic procedures such as radiographs and aspiration of the peritoneal cavity may be done. Early surgical intervention may be life-saving for many of these neonates.

Fetal Infections

With the exception of syphilis, bacterial infections of the fetus are most commonly associated with prolonged rupture of the membranes or chorioamnionitis. (See Chapters 17 and 38.) This discussion will be limited to the TORCH infections—toxoplasmosis, syphilis, rubella, cytomegalovirus, herpes, and hepatitis—with emphasis on prevention. Infections with these organisms are difficult to differentiate on the basis of symptomatology—hence reference to a TORCH syndrome. Most often, there are no symptoms at birth. Occasionally, the sole symptom that draws attention is intrauterine growth retardation. Rarely, a full-blown syndrome may be present, which may include microcephaly or hydrocephalus, intrauterine growth retardation with proportionate decreases in weight, length, and head circumference or hydrops fetalis, pancytopenia, hepatosplenomegaly, pneumonia, petechiae, jaundice, bony abnormalities, and congenital malformations. It was once hoped that elevated levels of IgM in cord blood might allow screening of neonates at risk for TORCH infections, but the incidence of false positive results is too high. However, in small for gestational age babies, neonates with congenital malformations, and neonates with suspicious symptoms, IgM levels may be useful to determine whether or not to pursue a diagnosis of fetal infection.

Toxoplasmosis. Toxoplasma gondii is acquired either by consuming undercooked meat or by contact with feces of cats. (See Chapter 38.) Neonates with symptoms of congenital toxoplasmosis should be treated to prevent further tissue invasion and destruction, but damage done prenatally is irreversible. There is no need to isolate a neonate with congenital Toxoplasma infection.

Rubella. (See Chapter 38.) There is no treatment for the neonate with congenital rubella syndrome. The neonate should be isolated from his peers.

Cytomegalovirus (CMV). (See Chapter 38.) Most babies born with congenital CMV infections are asymptomatic at birth, but long-term sequelae may be devastating. Hearing losses (13–65%), language (82%) and learning disabilities, and mental retardation leading to school failures are not uncommon. Contrary to most other viral infections, permanent immunity is not always conferred by the primary infection. Reinfection of previously infected women has been known to lead to sequential cases of congenital CMV infection in two consecutive siblings infected in utero. There is no effective treatment for congenital CMV infection, but the neonate should be isolated from his peers.

Herpes Simplex. (See Chapter 38.) Neonates delivered of women with genital herpes simplex infection are at risk of developing herpes infection themselves, with death or severe neurologic sequelae being the rule. Herpes does not cross the placenta and infection occurs only during delivery or after rupture of the membranes. Neonates at risk should be isolated from their peers, but not from their mothers, provided the mothers have been instructed in hand washing and gown wearing. Breast-feeding is permissible if the mother has no herpetic lesions in the area of the breasts. Mothers with herpes labialis or stomatitis should be instructed to wear a mask and not to kiss or nuzzle their babies until the sores have cleared.

Hepatitis B. As is the case for herpes, hepatitis B virus (HBV) probably does not cross the placenta, but infection of the neonate occurs at the time of birth. About 90% of infants whose mothers are positive for both hepatitis B surface antigen (HBsAg) and hepatitis B e antigen (HBEAg) will become infected and most will become permanent carriers. (See Chapter 34.) If the mother is HBsAg positive, the neonate should receive hepatitis B immune globulin (HBIG 0.5 ml, intramuscularly) as soon as possible after birth and a first dose of HBV vaccine (10 μg or 0.5 ml) prior to discharge from the hospital. Second and third doses of HBV vaccine (10 μg or 0.5 ml each) should be given one and six months after the first dose. Neonates born to mothers who are HBsAg-positive should be handled by a gloved attendant, but there is no need to isolate the baby. Their blood should be handled with proper precautions. Breast-feeding should be allowed. Susceptible personnel who are likely to be exposed to blood from HBV-infected infants or mothers should receive 20 μg (1 ml) of HBV vaccine. Household members and sexual contacts of those who are HBsAg-positive should receive HB vaccine if, after testing, they are negative for antigen and antibody.[5]

Hepatitis A. Neonates of mothers who have hepatitis A infection during pregnancy should not receive immune globulins. If the maternal infection occurs at delivery or during the postpartum period, the neonate should receive 0.02 ml/kg of immune globulin intramuscularly as soon as the diagnosis is made. The neonate does not need to be isolated.[3]

Syphilis. Pregnant women should be screened for syphilis at the first prenatal visit, at delivery, and at any time exposure to an infected partner occurs or suspicious lesions develop. Serologic tests for syphilis should be performed on cord blood of neonates for whom the results of maternal tests are unavailable or questionable. A reactive VDRL or fluorescent treponemal antibody absorption (FTA-ABS) test on cord or neonatal blood does not necessarily indicate that the neonate is infected, since passive transfer of antibodies occurs through the placenta. An IgM FTA-ABS test is more specific. Although a positive test is diagnostic for congenital syphilis, a negative test does not rule it out. In follow-up of an asymptomatic baby, VDRL tests may be repeated periodically. If the reaction is caused by passive immunization, the titers should decline and become negative by three to four months, postnatally. If the baby is infected, titers will not decrease or will rise. If adequate follow-up is in doubt, it is safer to treat the baby on suspicion alone. A neonate with congenital syphilis does not need to be isolated unless he is symptomatic.

Tuberculosis. Transplacental tuberculosis is rare, but, when it occurs, is very severe and often fatal. More often neonatal tuberculosis is acquired after birth from a mother or other family member with active but undiagnosed and untreated tuberculosis. If the mother with tuberculosis is undergoing chemotherapy, the neonate should receive prophylactic isoniazid therapy. If the mother is not receiving adequate therapy at the time of delivery, the neonate should be separated from his mother until therapy is initiated. BCG vaccine should be reserved for the rare situations where the baby will be exposed to uncontrollable tuberculosis in the environment. After BCG injection, the baby should be separated from his environment until skin tests for tuberculosis turn positive (3-4 weeks).

Perinatal Mortality and Quality of Survival

In the last 10-15 years, "adjusted" fetal and neonatal mortality rates (i.e., rates obtained after exclusion of babies weighing less than 500 grams) have declined by more than half in the United States.[11] This lowering of mortality rates has been accompanied by a change in emphasis toward improvements in birth-weight-specific perinatal mortality rates and has shifted the focus of attention toward babies of increasingly low birth weights.

A recent survey of rates and causes of perinatal mortality over a 6-year period in Medical Center Hospital in San Antonio, encompassing over 38,000 births, demonstrated that the trends observed in our hospital are representative of those reported from similar institutions. Adjusted perinatal and fetal mortality rates were 16.1 and 7.8 per 1000 births, respectively. Adjusted neonatal mortality rate was 8.5 per 1000 live births. Perinatal mortality struck babies weighing 500-1499 grams particularly heavily. Within this group, infants weighing 1000 grams or more had a much lower mortality rate.

With the advent of neonatal intensive care, the ability to maintain very low-birth-weight neonates alive for 28 days has improved dramatically. However, these babies often do not survive very long beyond the neonatal period. About 15% of liveborn neonates in this weight range suffer postneonatal deaths. Statistics for survival of liveborn babies 500-999 grams appear to be a great deal better than they really are if postneonatal deaths are not included.

One-third of all stillbirths cannot be explained by either maternal or fetal pathologic conditions. Chronic or acute fetal anoxia and maternal pathologic conditions each account for about one-fifth of stillbirths. Fetal anoxia is most commonly due to placental abruption, followed by cord accidents. The most common maternal pathologic conditions are diabetes and preeclampsia/eclampsia, followed by chorioamnionitis and incompetent cervix. Inappropriate fetal growth is commonly reflected as intrauterine growth retardation and postmaturity. Seven percent of stillbirths are due to congenital malformations, with anencephaly in the lead.

Immaturity without specific pathologic conditions is blamed for 30% of neonatal deaths. Congenital malformation incompatible with life is the second leading cause of death, followed closely by hemorrhages, mostly intracranial. Systemic infection and hyaline membrane disease account for, respectively, 10% and 8% of neonatal deaths. Hyaline membrane disease, once the leading cause of death, is now fifth.

Close scrutiny of the causes of perinatal deaths sheds little hope of further improvements in perinatal survival within the immediate future. More than half of perinatal deaths (40% of fetal deaths and 63% of neonatal deaths) are due to causes for which no effective therapy exists. One-third of fetal losses occur in the absence of any detectable maternal or fetal pathologic condition. One of every five perinatal deaths is associated with congenital malformations incompatible with life or idiopathic hydrops fetalis. Almost one-third of neonatal deaths are due to extreme immaturity, especially pulmonary immaturity. Although progress has been made in devising pharmacologic means of stopping premature labor, overall impact on the number of deliveries at less than 28 weeks of gestation has been disappointing. Intracranial hemorrhages, the etiology of which remains elusive, claim one of six lives during the neonatal period and more later from complications of posthemorrhagic hydrocephalus. If a serious impact is to be made on perinatal mortality in the 1980s and 1990s, priority should be given to four areas. (1) Prenatal care must be improved in order to decrease the impact of maternal diseases, such as preeclampsia and diabetes, on the fetus; to decrease problems such as abruptio placentae and cord accidents; and possibly to decrease the number of unexpected fetal deaths. More effective systems for the delivery of prenatal care might allow the obstetrician to detect signs of impending premature labor and to delay birth until maturation has further progressed. (See Chapter 18.) (2) More effective means must be devised to stop or delay premature labor, especially prior to 30 weeks' gestation. (3) The riddle of intracranial hemorrhages must be solved. (4) Diagnosis and treatment of perinatal infections must be improved.

It is not sufficient for a baby to survive; the goal should be intact survival. The prognosis for high-risk neonates has improved in recent years. The data must be considered cautiously because follow-up studies have not been of sufficient duration (mostly two to five years) to allow solid conclusions. Neonates severely asphyxiated at birth (Apgar score below 3) have about an 80% chance of being normal, provided that adequate resuscitative measures are promptly undertaken. The one serious exception is the small for gestational age baby. In one preliminary study, three of three term small for gestational age neonates with severe asphyxia had very low developmental quotients later in childhood. Neonates requiring mechanical ventilation have an 85% chance of being normal at two to nine years. One third of those with some neurological sequelae are only mildly affected. Very low birth weight, small for gestational age neonates (less than 1500 grams) are similar to appropriate for gestational age neonates of similar birth weight in physical, neurological, and mental development up to two years of age.[59] Finally, very low-birth-weight neonates, in general, tend to develop physically as well as full-term neonates, provided correction is made for their prematurity. They have an 80% chance of being normal neurologically and their intelligence–developmental quotients are usually comparable to those of their term peers. Neurosensory losses have been reported with varying degrees of frequency: 25% for vision, 3–29% for hearing, 65% for speech. More troublesome is a recent preliminary report suggesting that 68% of very low birth-weight neonates who had been identified as normal on the basis of standard testing showed evidence of significant learning deficits by age six to eight.[61] These deficits are in perception of and ability to copy various shapes (including letters and numbers). More information is needed before the neuro-intellectual future of very small premature neonates can be judged unequivocally. With rising survival rates come increasing incidences of retrolental fibroplasia and intraventricular hemorrhages, problems that affect long-term development.

Cost Effectiveness of Intensive Perinatal Care

In an era of increasing concern about the cost of medical care to society, it is fitting to end this chapter with a discussion of the cost and benefits of perinatal intensive care. A recent analysis based on the probability of death or damage indicated that fetuses of 25 weeks' gestation and above have a greater than 50% probability of intact survival. Perinatal intensive care and intervention for fetal reasons appear justified at or after 25 weeks, but perhaps not for younger fetuses.[43] Cost effectiveness studies of neonatal intensive care have been limited to neonates weighing 500–1500 grams at birth. In 1978, hospital costs for a neonate weighing less than 1000 g at birth averaged $14,236 (range: $72 to $124,-627) for nonsurvivors and $40,287 (range: $10,-

744 to $106,050) for survivors.[51] Society has to carry the financial burden and must be the final judge of the justification for neonatal intensive care. More complex financial analyses based on total medical costs over expected lifetime as well as potential earnings have disagreed with each other. One study concluded that any neonate weighing less than 1500 grams at birth will be a net economic burden on society,[9] whereas another estimated that neonates weighing 900 grams or more are "net earners," whereas those below 900 grams are "net losers" and are a burden on society.[60] Thus, on strictly financial grounds, intensive care of neonates weighing less than 900 grams may not be justified. Other factors must be considered, including the feelings of parents and relatives of a surviving baby and future advancements in medical knowledge that may reduce both mortality and morbidity. Society has chosen to support many other programs such as chronic renal dialysis, transplantation and geriatric programs. They too are a drain on financial resources. Decisions concerning priorities will have to be reappraised periodically as knowledge advances.

REFERENCES

1. American Academy of Pediatrics: Policy statement based on task force report: The promotion of breast feeding. *Pediatrics* **69**:654-661, 1983.
2. American Academy of Pediatrics: *Report of the Committee on Infectious Diseases*, 1982.
3. American Academy of Pediatrics and American College of Obstetricians and Gynecologists: *Guidelines for Perinatal Care*, 1983.
4. American Academy of Pediatrics Committee on Drugs: The transfer of drugs and other chemicals into human breast milk. *Pediatrics* **72**:375-384, 1983.
5. American Academy of Pediatrics Committee on Infectious Diseases: Prevention of hepatitis B virus infection. *Pediatrics* **75**:362-364, 1985.
6. Amiel-Tison, C.: Neurological evaluation of the maturity of newborn infants. In: *Status of the Fetus. Report of the 2nd Ross Conference on Obstetric Research.* Columbus, OH, Ross Laboatories, 1971, pp. 274-281.
7. Apgar, V.: A proposal for a new method of evaluation of the newborn infant. *Curr. Res. Anesth. Analg.* **32**:260-267, 1953.
8. Bangham, D. R., Hobbs, K. R. and Tee, D. E. H.: Transmission of serum proteins from fetus to mother in the Rhesus monkey. *Lancet* **2**:1173-1174, 1960.
9. Boyle, M. H., Torrance, G. W., Sinclair, J. C., and Horwood, S. P.: Economic evaluation of neonatal intensive care of very-low-birthweight infants. *N. Engl. J. Med.* **308**:1330-1337, 1983.
10. Brans, Y. W. and Cassady, G.: Fetal nutrition and body composition. In: *Total Parenteral Nutrition: Premises and Promises.* H. Ghadimi (Ed.). New York, John Wiley & Sons, 1975, pp. 301-333.
11. Brans, Y. W., Escobedo, M. B., Hayashi, R. H., Huff, R. W., Kagan-Hallet, K. S., and Ramamurthy, R. S.: Perinatal mortality in a large perinatal center: Five-year review of 31,000 births. *Am. J. Obstet. Gynecol.* **148**:284-289, 1984.
12. Brett, E. M.: The estimation of foetal maturity by the neurological examination of the neonate. In: *Clinics in Developmental Medicine*, Vol. 19. Lavenham, Lavenham Press, 1965, pp. 105-115.
13. Brown, E. G. and Sweet, A. Y.: *Neonatal Necrotizing Enterocolitis.* New York, Grune & Stratton, 1980.
14. Chapman, G. P., Weller, R. 0., Normand, J. C. S., and Gibbens, D.: Spinal cord transection in utero. *Br. Med. J.* **2**:398, 1978.
15. Chasnoff, I. J., Hatcher, R., and Burns, W. J.: Early growth patterns of methadone addicted infants. *Am. J. Dis. Child.* **134**:1049-1051, 1980.
16. Dahm, L. S. and James, L. S.: Newborn temperature and calculated heat loss in the delivery room. *Pediatrics* **49**:504-513, 1972.
17. Dubowitz, L. M. S., Dubowitz, V., and Goldberg, C.: Clinical assessment of gestational age in the newborn infant. *J. Pediatr.* **77**:1-10, 1970.
18. Edelmann, C. M. and Spitzer, A.: The kidney. In: *The Physiology of the Newborn Infant.* C. A. Smith and N. M. Nelson (Eds.). Springfield, IL, Charles C. Thomas, 1976, pp. 416-458.
19. Ericson, A., Källén, B., and Wersterholm, P.: Cigarette smoking as an etiologic factor in cleft lip and palate. *Am. J. Obstet. Gynecol.* **135**:348-351, 1979.
20. Fleischman, A. R. and Finberg, L.: Breast milk for term and premature infants—optimal nutrition? *Semin. Perinatol.* **3**:397-405, 1979.
21. Freeman, M. G., Graves, W. L., and Thompson, R. L.: Indigent Negro and Caucasian birth-weight gestational age tables. *Pediatrics* **46**:9-15, 1970.
22. Friendly, D. S.: Eye disorders in neonates. In: *Neonatology.* G. B. Avery (Ed.). Philadelphia, J. B. Lippincott, 1981, pp. 1128-1143.
23. Gairdner, D.: The fate of the foreskin: A study of circumcision. *Br. Med. J.* **2**:1433-1437, 1949.
24. Gitlin, D., Kumate, J., Morales, C., Noriega, L., and Arevalo, N.: The turnover of amniotic fluid protein in the human conceptus. *Am. J. Obstet. Gynecol.* **113**:632-645, 1972.
25. Goodman Campbell B. B. and Taylor P. M.: Bonding and attachment: Theoretical issues. *Semin. Perinatol.* **3**:3-13, 1979.
26. Gregory, G. A., Kitterman, J. A., Phibbs, R. N., Tooley, W. H., and Hamilton, W.K.: Treatment of

the idiopathic respiratory distress syndrome with continuous positive airway pressures. *N. Engl. J. Med.* **284**:1333–1340, 1971.
27. Gruenwald, P.: Growth of the human fetus. I. Normal growth and its variations. *Am. J. Obstet. Gynecol.* **94**:1112–1132, 1966.
28. Harper, R. G., Solish, G., Feingold, E., Gersten-Woolf, N. B., and Sokal, M. M.: Maternal ingested methadone, body fluid methadone, and the neonatal withdrawal syndrome. *Am. J. Obstet. Gynecol.* **129**:417–424, 1977.
29. Heller, L.: Intrauterine amino acid feeding of the fetus. In: *Parenteral Nutrition in Infancy and Childhood.* New York, Plenum Press, 1974, pp. 206–213.
30. Hingson, R., Gould, J. B., Morelock, S., Kayne, H., Heeren, T., Alpert, J. J., Zuckerman, B., and Day, N.: Maternal cigarette smoking, psychoactive substance use, and infant Apgar score. *Am. J. Obstet. Gynecol.* **144**:960–966, 1982.
31. Kandall, S. R. and Gartner, L. M.: Late presentation of drug withdrawal symptoms in newborns. *Am. J. Dis. Child.* **127**:58–61, 1974.
32. Kirkinen, P., Jouppila, P., Koivula, A., Vuori, J., and Puuka, M.: The effect of caffeine on placental and fetal blood flow in human pregnancy. *Am. J. Obstet. Gynecol.* **147**:939–942, 1983.
33. Klaus, M. H., Jerauld, R., Kreger, N. C., McAlpine, W., Steffan, M., and Kennel, J. H.: Maternal attachment: Importance of the first postpartum days. *N. Engl. J. Med.* **286**:460–464, 1972.
34. Klaus, M. H. and Kennell, J. H.: *Maternal-Infant Bonding.* St. Louis, C. V. Mosby, 1976.
35. Kline, J., Steinz, A., Susser, M., and Warburton, D.: Smoking: A risk factor for spontaneous abortion. *N. Engl. J. Med.* **297**:793–796, 1977.
36. Lehtovirta, P. and Forss, M.: The acute effect of smoking on intervillous blood flow of the placenta. *Br. J. Obstet. Gynaecol.* **85**:729–731, 1978.
37. Linn, S., Schoenbaum, S. C., Monson, R. R., Rosner, B., Stubblefield, P. G., and Ryan, K. J.: No association between coffee consumption and adverse outcomes of pregnancy. *N. Engl. J. Med.* **306**:141–145, 1982.
38. Lubchenco, L. O., Hansman, C., Dressler, M., and Boyd, E.: Intrauterine growth as estimated from liveborn birth-weight data at 24–42 weeks of gestation. *Pediatrics* **32**:793–800, 1963.
39. McCrory, W. W.: *Developmental Nephrology.* Cambridge, MA, Harvard University Press, 1972.
40. Meberg, A., Hägas, P., Sardes, H., and Foss, O. P.: Smoking during pregnancy—hematological observations in the newborn. *Acta Paediatr. Scand.* **68**:731–734, 1972.
41. Meberg, A., Sarde H., Foss 0. P., and Stenwig J. T.: Smoking during pregnancy—effects on the fetus and on thiocyanate levels in mother and baby. Acta Paediatr. Scand. **68**:547–552, 1979.
42. Meyer, M. B.: How does maternal smoking affect birth weight and maternal weight gain? *Am. J. Obstet. Gynecol.* **131**:888–893, 1978.
43. Milligan, J. E. and Shennan, A. T.: Perinatal intensive care: Where and how to draw the line. *Am. J. Obstet. Gynecol.* **148**:499–503, 1984.
44. Morris, M. B. and Weinstein, L.: Caffeine and the fetus: Is trouble brewing? *Am. J. Obstet. Gynecol.* **140**:607–610, 1981.
45. Naeye, R. L.: Effects of maternal cigarette smoking on the fetus and placenta. *Br. J. Obstet. Gynaecol.* **85**:732–737, 1978.
46. Nelson, N. M.: Respiration and circulation after birth. In: *The Physiology of the Newborn Infant.* C. A. Smith and N. M. Nelson (Eds.). Springfield, IL, Charles C. Thomas, 1976, pp. 117–262.
47. Neumann, L. L. and Cohen, S. N.: The neonatal narcotic withdrawal syndrome: A therapeutic challenge. *Clin. Perinatol.* **2**:99–109, 1975.
48. Okada, D. M. and Chow, A. W.: Neonatal scalp abscess following intrapartum fetal monitoring: Prospective comparison of two spiral electrodes. *Am. J. Obstet. Gynecol.* **127**:875–878, 1977.
49. Phelps, D. C.: Vitamin E and retrolental fibroplasia in 1982. *Pediatrics* **70**:420–425, 1982.
50. Pitkin, R. M. and Reynolds, W. A.: Fetal ingestion and metabolism of amniotic fluid protein. *Am. J. Obstet. Gynecol.* **123**:356–363, 1975.
51. Pomerance, J. J., Ukrainski, C. T., Ukra, T., Henderson, D. H., Nash, A. H., and Meredith, J. L.: Cost of living for infants weighing 1,000 grams or less at birth. *Pediatrics* **61**:908–910, 1978.
52. Queenan, J. T., Gadow, E. B., Bachner, P., and Kubarych, S. F.: Amniotic fluid proteins in normal and kRh-sensitized pregnancies. *Am. J. Obstet. Gynecol.* **108**:406–414, 1970.
53. Renaud, R., Kirschtetter, L., Koehl, C., Boog, G., Brettes, J. P., Schumacher, J. C., Vincendon, G., Willard, D., and Gandar, R.: Amino-acid intra-amniotic injections. In: *Recent Progress in Obstetrics and Gynaecology, Proc. VII World Cong. Obstet. Gynecol. (Moscow 1973).* Amsterdam, Excerpta Medica, 1974, pp. 234–256.
54. Scarpelli, E.: *The Surfactant System of the Lung.* Philadelphia, Lea & Febiger, 1968.
55. Stahlman, M. T. and Gray, M. E.: Anatomical development and maturation of the lungs. *Clin. Perinatol.* **5**:181–196, 1978.
56. Stevenson, R. E.: *The Fetus and Newly Born Infant: Influence of the Prenatal Environment.* St. Louis, C. V. Mosby, 1977.
57. Turbeville, D. F. and McCaffree, M. A.: Fetal scalp electrode complications: Cerebrospinal fluid leak. *Obstet. Gynecol.* **54**:469–470, 1979.
58. Vincent, M. and Hugon, J.: Relationships between various criteria of maturity at birth. *Biol. Neonate* **4**:223–279, 1962.
59. Vohr, B. R., Oh, W., Rosenfield, A. G., and Cowett, R. M.: The preterm small-for-gestational age infant: A two year follow-up study. *Am. J. Obstet. Gynecol.* **133**:425–431, 1979.
60. Walker, D. J. B., Feldman, A., Vohr, B. R., and Oh, W.: Cost-benefit analysis of neonatal inten-

sive care for infants weighing less than 1000 grams at birth. *Pediatrics* **74**:20–25, 1984.

61. Widmayer, S. M., Bauer, C. R., Figueredo, M., and Milham, J.: Developmental sequelae of premature birth in school age children. *Clin. Res.* **30**:909A, 1982.
62. Zelson, C., Lee, S. J., and Cassalino, M.: Neonatal narcotic addiction: Comparative effects of maternal intake of heroin and methadone. *N. Engl. J. Med.* **289**:1216–1220, 1973.
63. Zuspan, F. P., Gumpel, J. A., Mejia-Zelaya, A., Madden, J., and Davis, R.: Fetal stress from methadone withdrawal. *Am. J. Obstet. Gynecol.* **122**:43–46, 1975.

PART II

ABNORMAL OBSTETRICS

SECTION A
ANTEPARTUM AND INTRAPARTUM EVALUATION OF THE FETUS

11

FETAL MONITORING

The stillbirth rate has gradually declined during the past 20 years. In 1960 the rate was 16.1/1000 births, and in 1980, 9.2/1000 births.[34] This decline can be attributed to a number of factors, one of which is more accurate surveillance of the fetus during the antenatal period and labor. Prior to 1960, the fetus could be said to be alive or dead on the basis of perceived fetal activity by the mother and the presence or absence of a fetal heart beat heard when listening over the mother's abdomen with a fetoscope. Fetal distress in labor was diagnosed when the fetal heart rate decreased at the end of a uterine contraction. The development of continuous fetal heart rate monitoring allowed the health care team to assess fetal health more accurately. The cause of a given heart rate change could be ascribed much more definitively, thus allowing the physician or nurse to prescribe more rational therapy. Because no test is perfect and continuous fetal heart rate monitoring is no exception, other biophysical and biochemical tests of fetal well-being have been developed. Some, but not all, of the other methods of monitoring the fetus will be discussed in this chapter.

HISTORY OF FETAL MONITORING

Fetal movement has been utilized since antiquity to signal the presence or absence of fetal life. It was not until 1650 that Le Goust stated in an ode that his friend Marsac had noted that the fetus jumps, turns, twirls, and moves about freely and is able to change its position frequently and that its heart beats "comm'un traquet" (like a mill clapper).[32] Nothing more was heard about fetal heart sounds until Mayor of Geneva mentioned in a talk that he had heard the fetal heart while trying to listen for fetal movement. The first published report of fetal heart sounds was written by Jacques Kergaradec, a French physician, who, being a close friend of Laennec, was interested in using Laennec's new instrument, the stethoscope. While listening for fetal movement, he heard the fetal heart. This work was first presented to the Academy of Medicine in Paris in 1822, when he stated, "From the variations that have arisen in the beats of the fetal heart, will it not be possible to judge the state of the health or disease of the fetus?" This prophetic work was published as an appendix to Laennec's second edition of his *Treatise on Mediate Auscultation*.

An Irish physician, John Ferguson, had visited Laennec and saw him confirm pregnancy using the stethoscope. He introduced the technique to Dublin in 1827. In 1826, Robert Collin became the Master of the Rotunda. One of his assistants was Evory Kennedy, who became an expert in the use of the stethoscope in pregnancy. He wrote a monograph entitled *Observations on Obstetric Auscultation*, published in 1833. This monograph delineated the definition of fetal distress, a fetal heart rate less than 100 or greater than 160 beats per minute, criteria which were used for many years.

Phonocardiography was invented in 1880. The first tracing of fetal heart sounds was made by Pestalozza in 1881. Though many investigators in the period from 1920 to 1950 recorded the fetal heart using electronic techniques, it remained for Edward Hon[11] to develop methods for continuous recording of the fetal heart rate. The continuous tracing of the heart rate enabled Hon to describe a series of patterns of heart rate changes that could be attributed to specific causes, permitting the physician to use specific therapies to ameliorate fetal distress.

INSTRUMENTATION

The patterns of fetal heart rate change are related to uterine contractions. Thus, any instrumentation utilized must be able to monitor and record continuously both the fetal heart rate and the uterine activity. The essential components required to accomplish the objective include a transducer to sense fetal cardiac activity, a transducer to pick up uterine activity, a signal processor that will convert the fetal signal to heart rate, and a strip-chart recorder and/or oscilloscope to record uterine pressure and heart rate. For convenience, each of these components will be discussed separately, although they must perform together when used clinically.

Several types of transducer have been, or are being, used to pick up the fetal heart. The oldest, as mentioned above, is the stethoscope which has been modified into a fetoscope by placing the bell at the end of a rod which is either hand-held or placed on the head. The purpose of the rod is to remove fingers, which tend to dampen the fetal heart sound, from the bell. The disadvantage of the fetoscope is that the signal received cannot be fed to any form of counting mechanism other than the human mind. Thus, obtaining a continuous heart rate is impossible. This is not meant to imply that the fetoscope is totally obsolete. It still is used effectively in certain situations such as routine antepartum visits and in labor in the low-risk patient who does not wish to be connected to the continuous fetal heart rate monitoring unit.

The transducer usually used for continuous fetal heart rate monitoring is ultrasonic. An electric current applied to a piezoelectric crystal of quartz causes a high frequency sound to be generated. The sound is directed toward the beating fetal heart, which causes a shift in the frequency of the reflected sound (the Doppler shift). This shift is picked up by a receiving crystal and returned to the central processor as a series of electrical signals. One disadvantage of ultrasonic signals is that they are electrically "dirty" and thus until recently were difficult to convert to an exact fetal heart rate. In addition, the signal is lost whenever the fetus moves, and to restore it requires moving the transducer.

The next most frequently used transducer is a spiral electrode. It is attached directly to the fetal scalp and records an electrocardiogram from the fetus. The electrical signal obtained is very "clean" and thus easy to count. However, the membranes must be ruptured to apply the electrode, and the spiral wire does penetrate the fetal scalp. This penetration is followed by a local abscess in about 4–7 cases of every 1000 scalp electrodes applied.[15] The abscess is usually easily treated by local incision and drainage, plus parenteral antibiotics. Another problem with the penetrating aspect of the scalp electrode is that improper placement may injure the fetus. The electrode has been reported to have been applied to the eye, nose, and other areas in which scarring from the application may prove injurious.[15] It is vital that the person applying the electrode make certain that either the fetal scalp or buttock is presenting.

Two infrequently used methods of obtaining the fetal heart beat are phonocardiogram and abdominal electrodes. The former uses a sensitive microphone to pick up the fetal heart sound. However, there are many other sounds in the pregnant abdomen, such as bowel sounds and fetal movements. These extraneous sounds will also be counted, giving an incorrect fetal heart rate. Maternal abdominal electrodes may be used to obtain fetal electrocardio graphic signals. A fetal electrocardiograph will be obtained in 60–90% of the patients, with the higher percentage obtained in patients close to term. The difficulty with this technique is that maternal electrocardiographic signals are received by the same electrodes. They are of much larger amplitude than is the fetal ECG and occasionally are coincidental with it. These factors make it very difficult to count the fetal heart rate from this transducer.

The electrical signals received from one of the above transducers are amplified and then fed to a counting unit, a cardiotachometer. The cardiotachometer divides the time between any two succeeding beats by 60 to obtain the instantaneous rate. In some instances the electrical signals are preconditioned to remove electrical noise, or computer logic is used in an effort to achieve an accurate representation of the instantaneous heart rate. The rate may be electrically averaged over a few seconds in order to obtain a smooth written record. It is necessary to understand exactly how a given monitor processes signals if the records are to be interpreted accurately.

The output of the cardiotachometer is then fed to an oscillograph where the heart rate is recorded, usually on heat-sensitive paper. The paper is divided into two major units (channels). The bottom channel is used to record the output from the uterine pressure transducer, and the top channel records the output of the cardiotachometer. The lower channel has a vertical height of 40 mm with 20 equally spaced divisions electronically calibrated to measure a pressure between 0 and 100 mmHg. The upper channel usually has a vertical height of 70 mm with 21 equally spaced divisions calibrated to a heart rate between 30 and 240 beats per minute. The standard paper speed of most recorders is 3 cm per minute; however, some units have a toggle switch that permits a paper speed of 1 cm per minute. The recorder is housed in a cabinet which usually has a small oscilloscope that displays the fetal heart signal being received by the cardiotachometer. There is also a small speaker in the cabinet that emits an audible beep with each beat of the heart. The speaker can be turned off. The persistent beeping is frequently annoying to both patient and medical personnel. Some of the newer units have added a printed time on the oscillograph paper, and some have the ability to print other messages such as medication given.

Recording of uterine activity is important for two reasons. First, the periodic changes in fetal heart rate are related to uterine contractions, as discussed below. Second, it is important to assess uterine activity when evaluating failure to progress in labor. The most common method used to evaluate uterine activity is with an external transducer (tocodynamometer) placed over the uterine fundus and held in place with a belt. This transducer measures a uterine contraction. However, the recorded pressure correlates poorly with the pressure developed by the uterus. The same is true of the resting pressure (tonus). This type of transduction really indicates only the frequency and duration of the uterine contractions. The only accurate way to measure resting tonus and maximal intrauterine pressure is to utilize an indwelling catheter connected to a strain gauge. The catheter and strain gauge are filled with saline, to form a closed pressure system.

The combined output of the heart rate monitor and the pressure transducer are recorded (Fig. 11-1). This permits the medical personnel monitoring the labor to view the fetal heart rate, the heart rate variability, the resting uterine pressure, and the maximum pressure

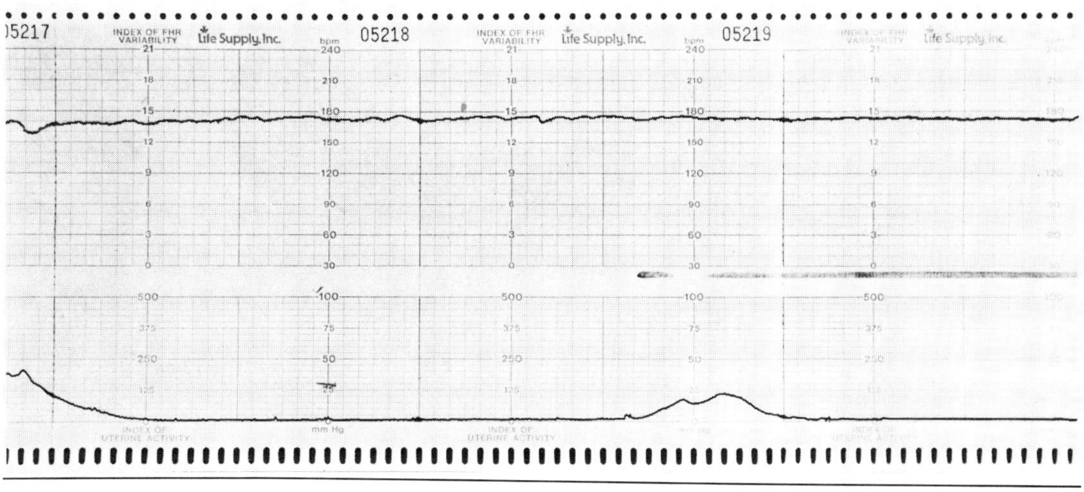

Figure 11-1. Fetal tachycardia, decreased short-term variability with some but decreased long-term heart rate variability.

achieved with each uterine contraction on a continuous basis.

INTERPRETATION OF FETAL HEART RATE

The heart rate can arbitrarily be divided into three areas: baseline rate, variability, and periodic changes.

Baseline

Baseline heart rate is defined as that rate which is present when the fetus is not being subjected to an acute stress. The baseline rate is the result of the intrinsic rate of the heart plus modifications imposed by the sympathetic and parasympathetic nervous systems. A change in baseline heart rate occurs when a new baseline has been established for 1, 10, or 15 minutes.[5,12,30] This wide variation in definition of the time necessary for a change in baseline rate is probably due to which factor or factors were considered in making the definition. For example, if the observers were looking at a change in baseline rate in response to a maternal stimulus, such as having the mother breathe a 15% oxygen mixture and looking for tachycardia, the response time is about 7–10 minutes.[10] However, this response time includes maternal circulation, placental transfer, and fetal response. If one looks at the response time of the fetal heart rate to a change in fetal state, the elapsed time is only 2–3 minutes.[29] However, most fetal state changes last at least 5–10 minutes. Because this is probably the most frequent reason for a change in baseline, the original definition of 10 minutes to define a new baseline is reasonable.[12]

The baseline rate tends to change with fetal state, in general being slightly faster during state 2F (like REM sleep) (Table 11-1).[29] However, these changes may be inconsistent, and do not usually take the heart rate outside of its normal baseline rate of 120–160 beats per minute. Prior to the time that states of the fetus become well defined (36–38 weeks in the human),[29] fetal heart rate may accelerate for prolonged periods with fetal breathing or fetal movement. These activity patterns usually last less than 10 minutes, however. Thus, by strict definition, the accompanying heart rate increase would be periodic and designated an acceleration rather than a baseline change. The major changes in baseline are bradycardia, defined as a baseline rate of less than 120 beats per minute, and tachycardia, defined as a baseline rate of greater than 160 beats per minute.

Bradycardia

Spontaneous bradycardia occurs when there is no known etiology for it and the fetus is well. The heart rate in these instances is seldom below 100 beats per minute, as though this fetus had a lower set point. In contrast, the baseline heart rate is usually less than 100 beats per minute when hypoxic bradycardia occurs. Beat-to-beat variability is also absent with hypoxic bradycardia. This type of bradycardia frequently precedes imminent fetal death and is an indication for immediate delivery.

Fetal bradycardia can also be the result of a fetal heart block. This is a third-degree block (complete disassociation between the auricles and ventricles) in almost every instance.[40] The frequency of congenital heart disease is high (30%),[40] thus a very thorough ultrasound evaluation using M-mode should be performed in these cases. Maternal collagen disease is another frequent cause of congenital heart block. Sixty-three percent of 22 children with congeni-

TABLE 11-1. FETAL ACTIVITY STATES

Fetal State	1F*	2F†	3F	4F
Eye movements	Absent	Present	Present	Present
Body and extremity movement	Incidental	Periodic	Absent	Continuous
Heart rate accelerations	Isolated	Frequent	Absent	Large, long
Heart rate variability	Low	Increased	Increased	—

* State 1F is like quiet sleep.
† State 2F is like REM sleep.
Source: Nijhuis, J. G., Martin, C. B. and Prechtl, H. F. R.: Behavioral states of the human fetus. In *Continuity of Neural Functions from Prenatal to Postnatal Life.* H. F. R. Prechtl (ed.). London: S. I. M. P. with Blackwell Scientific; Philadelphia: Lippincott, 1984, pp. 65–77.[29]

tal heart block were delivered from mothers who had clinical evidence of collagen disease.[23] Maternal antinuclear antibody Ro (SS-A) in the serum plus immunoglobulin and complement deposition in the atrial appendage were demonstrated in an infant with congenital heart block.[17] These findings have been confirmed in two other infants with positive immunoglobulin and complement staining in all cardiac tissues.[42] Whenever fetal heart block is documented, a complete maternal study for the presence of collagen disease is necessary. The fetal heart rate is generally quite low, 20–80 per minute, when complete heart block is present. The diagnosis can be made definitively if disassociation between the fetal P and QRS complexes is seen on an abdominal electrocardiogram. Another method of diagnosis is use of real-time ultrasound to demonstrate atrioventricular disassociation. Therapy in this situation is conservative since the fetuses do well in the absence of congenital heart disease.

Drugs may also induce fetal bradycardia. Any compound that can cause maternal bradycardia and that crosses the placenta will cause fetal bradycardia. A beta blocker given to control maternal essential hypertension is the drug most frequently responsible for maternal and fetal bradycardia. To date, no untoward fetal side effects have been observed when the mother was taking a beta blocker. Maternal hypothermia is a rare cause of fetal bradycardia.

There are groups of heart rate changes that some would call bradycardias but others would term decelerations. In some instances they fit the definition of bradycardia in that the cardiac slowing lasts longer than 10 minutes, but usually the heart rate has returned to normal in less than 10 minutes. There are two groups in this category—one spontaneous and one iatrogenic. Spontaneous prolonged decelerations most frequently occur during labor but may also occur during the antepartum period. There is usually a sudden decrease in the heart rate, frequently to less than 100 beats per minute. The heart rate stays reduced for 1–10 or more minutes and suddenly returns to normal. The etiology of the decrease is uncertain, but it is presumed that fetal hypoxia is associated. Some fetuses delivered following prolonged decelerations in labor are depressed. However, the majority are not. Prudence requires that one either prove that the fetus is alright with scalp sampling, or that one assume the worst, hypoxia, and deliver the fetus after two to three prolonged decelerations. Although prolonged decelerations are infrequently noted antepartum, as many as 50% of fetuses who demonstrate this pattern during antepartum testing have fetal distress during labor.[4] These patients should therefore be delivered or should be tested on a daily basis, if delivery is not opted for. The second type of prolonged deceleration is iatrogenic and is associated with paracervical block. The incidence was 26% in one study.[6] The heart rate was less than 110 but not below 60 beats per minute. The onset of bradycardia was 1.2–12.2 minutes following paracervical block, and the duration of bradycardia was 2.0–32.3 minutes. In general, fetuses are not depressed if they are delivered after the paracervical block bradycardia has abated. Fetuses delivered during the bradycardia have a tendency to be depressed. Thus, if bradycardia occurs, the mother should be given supplemental oxygen and the fetus allowed to recover in utero before delivery.

Tachycardia

Fetal tachycardia (Fig. 11-1) can be caused by a variety of things, including fetal hypoxia, maternal fever, amnionitis, maternal hyperthyroidism, fetal anemia, and drugs given to the fetus, such as beta sympathomimetic agents and parasympathetic-blocking drugs. Fetal hypoxia is the most serious cause of fetal tachycardia. The degree of hypoxia is usually mild. The heart rate is seldom above 180 beats per minute. Even though the hypoxia is usually minimal, tachycardia, particularly if ominous periodic changes are associated with it, should alert the physician that the fetus is being stressed. If fetal scalp blood sampling is not available, pregnancy interruption is indicated when fetal tachycardia is accompanied by late decelerations, even in the presence of some heart rate variability.

Maternal infection is perhaps the most frequent cause of fetal tachycardia. When the infection is in a site other than the uterus, the tachycardia is due to maternal fever. The mother is the heat sink for the fetus, which is usually about 0.5 °C hotter than the mother. As the mother's temperature goes up, so does that of the fetus, and fetal tachycardia develops. In some instances, particularly in the presence of amnionitis, fetal tachycardia develops before maternal fever.

Two classes of drugs, the parasympatholytics characterized by atropine and the beta sympathomimetic drugs used to inhibit labor, result in fetal tachycardia.

A supraventricular tachycardia can develop.

Heart rate usually exceeds 180 beats per minute, which may be continuous or intermittent. The major problem with a continuing tachycardia is the possibility of congestive heart failure. However, the fetus seems more resistant to heart failure than does the newborn with the same heart rate. Attempts to treat the fetus by digitalizing the mother, and thus the fetus, have met with varying degrees of success. In one instance, fetal cardioversion was reported using fetal umbilical cord compression under ultrasound guidance.[22] When the tachycardia persists, the fetus should be delivered if at term or carefully observed for signs of cardiac failure using real-time ultrasound when premature.

An unusual baseline variant is the sinusoidal pattern, which may be observed during either the antepartum period or labor. It is one of the most frequently misdiagnosed patterns, because strict definitions are not followed. This is an extremely ominous pattern in the absence of alphaprodine given to the mother. It is very important that it be properly diagnosed. Sinusoidal pattern displays an undulating baseline with a frequency of 2–5 cycles per minute. The cycles have an amplitude of at least 5 beats per minute, there is no short-term variability, and the pattern is continuous (Fig. 11-2).[24] The two most common errors are making the diagnosis in the presence of short-term variability or in the presence of a pattern that is intermittent. The pseudosinusoidal patterns are usually benign, whereas true sinusoidal patterns usually are associated with severe fetal anemia or hypoxia.

HEART RATE VARIABILITY

The time between any two succeeding beats of the heart in a well-oxygenated fetus is seldom the same, thus if one plots the instantaneous heart rate, the baseline appears to be irregular. This is called beat-to-beat variability of the heart rate or short-term heart rate variability. There is also a longer-term heart rate variability which occurs with a frequency of 3–6 cycles per minute. This type of variability also occurs in the well-oxygenated fetus. Normal heart rate variability is a difference of from 6 to 25 beats per minute; a change of 2–6 beats per minute is reduced variability; and, if beat-to-beat varia-

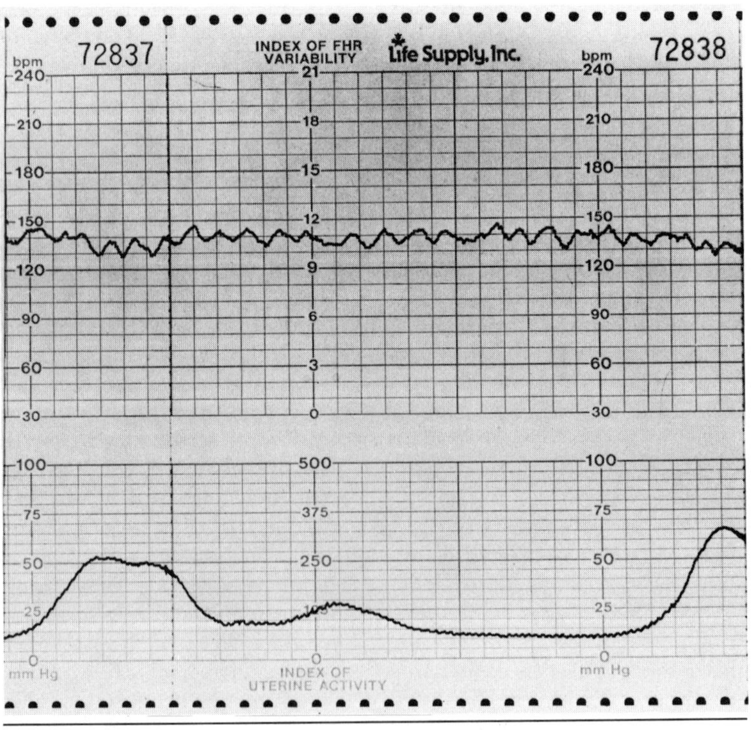

Figure 11-2. Sinusoid heart rate.

tion is less than 2 beats per minute, variability is considered to be absent.

The variability of the heart rate involves the interaction of several components: the central nervous system, the sympathetic and parasympathetic nervous systems, and the heart itself. Alteration of variability can be caused by a change in one or several of these components.

An intact central nervous system is required for normal fetal heart rate variability. Both short- and long-term variability seem to be reduced in the anencephalic fetus who has a medulla, a midbrain, and a reduced cerebral cortex.[43] Loss of cortex and midbrain reduces long- and short-term variability even further. The most complete loss is seen in the absence of cortex, midbrain, and medulla. Loss of the cervical spinal cord does not seem to further decrease variability. Additional evidence that the cerebral cortex plays a role in variability is provided by the change in variability associated with a change in fetal state. There is a significant association between fetal somatic and eye movements and fetal heart rate variability.[29]

The effect of the nervous system on variability is predominantly mediated via the parasympathetic system, although there is some evidence of a minor role for the sympathetic system. The contributions of these two branches of the nervous system have been studied using pharmacologic blockers or stimulators in animal models. Parasympathetic blockade with atropine significantly reduces short-term variability. Blocking the beta sympathetic system with propranolol reduces long-term variability, and stimulation of the alpha sympathetic system with phentolamine reduces the R-R interval. Combined blockade with all three agents reduces short- and long-term variability.[21]

Assuming that a fetus is neurologically intact, a variety of factors may influence fetal heart rate variability. These include fetal state, movement, temperature, oxygenation, and drugs.

Fetal state is the factor which most frequently changes heart rate variability. State 1F (like quiet sleep) in the fetus is accompanied by a significant reduction in heart rate variability, and state 2F (like REM sleep) is accompanied by a significant increase (Table 11-1).[29] Sleep cycles are established in the human fetus after 36 weeks of gestation. They occur with a periodicity of 30–70 minutes. The fetus spends roughly 50% of its time in each state.

Changes in respiratory rate, blood pressure, and temperature affect the variability of the heart rate in the adult. There is reason to believe that similar modifications of the variability in the fetus accompany alterations in fetal breathing, blood pressure, and temperature.

Drugs given the mother that traverse the placenta can significantly alter fetal heart rate variability. The most frequently used drugs that seem to have an impact are narcotics, sedatives, tranquilizers, and beta blockers. All these drugs decrease variability in varying degrees, depending primarily on the dosage of the drug given.

Perhaps the most important factor affecting variability is oxygenation of the fetus. Acute and moderate fetal hypoxia increases fetal heart rate variability. In experimental animals, variability does not decrease markedly until the hypoxia is prolonged or extremely profound (preterminal). This is probably also true in the human fetus. The difficulty in a clinical situation is to distinguish (in the absence of pharmacologic agents) between the hypoxic fetus and one which is simply in quiet sleep. Two points may be helpful. First, the sleeping fetus changes state within a maximum of 80 minutes.[2] Second, the sleeping fetus usually has some variability, whereas the chronically hypoxic fetus may have none.

PERIODIC HEART RATE CHANGES

The periodic changes in the fetal heart rate usually are related to uterine contractions. Periodic changes in heart rate include three types of deceleration (early, late, and variable) and acceleration of the heart rate.[12]

Early Decelerations

Early decelerations begin within the first half of the uterine contraction as uterine pressure is increasing (Fig. 11-3). The decline in the heart rate is gradual. The lowest rate is seldom less than 100 beats per minute. The etiology of this heart rate change is compression of the fetal head. The mechanism by which compression of the fetal head causes a decrease in heart rate is a reduction in cerebral circulation which reduces oxygen supply to the brain. This reduction in oxygen supply activates the cardiodeceleratory center in the brain, which acts through the vagus nerve to slow the heart. Because the oxygen supply interruption is mild, intermittent, and temporary, there is no damage to the

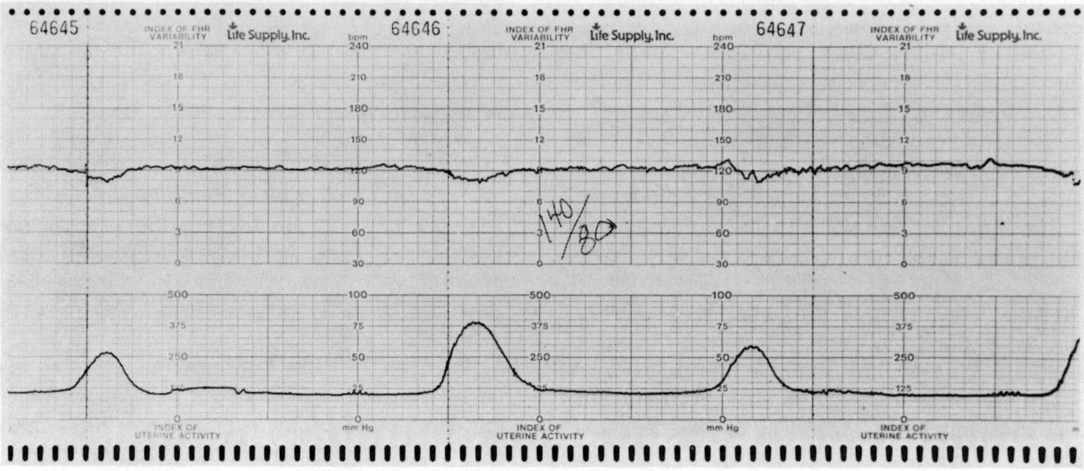

Figure 11-3. Early decelerations.

fetal central nervous system. Early decelerations are not ominous.

Late Decelerations

Late decelerations usually begin at or after the peak of the uterine contraction. They, like early decelerations, have a slow onset and gradual recovery, thus appearing like inverse uterine contractions (Fig. 11-4). Late decelerations are divided into mild, moderate, and severe, according to their depth of deceleration. Mild late decelerations do not go below 100 beats per minute, moderate late decelerations display a minimum heart rate between 60 and 99 beats per minute, and severe late decelerations have a minimum heart rate that is less than 60 beats per minute. Late decelerations are the result of an interruption of the fetal oxygen supply at the uteroplacental interface.

Because the amount of oxygen available in the umbilical venous blood is the resultant of the oxygen content of the maternal arterial blood, the maternal blood flow through the intervillous space, and the amount of trophoblastic surface available for transfer, a problem in any of these areas may cause late decelerations. A significant decrease in maternal arterial blood oxygen saturation rarely occurs; however, if the mother has cyanotic congenital heart disease or

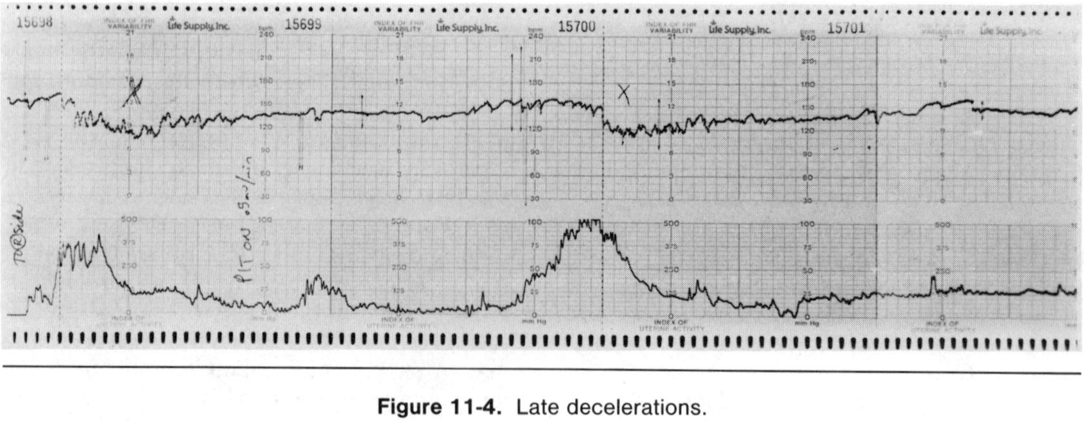

Figure 11-4. Late decelerations.

severe pulmonary disease, maternal oxygen saturation may be low enough to have a fetal effect. The incidence of fetal growth retardation and fetal wastage is significantly increased in the presence of maternal cyanotic heart disease. Occasionally the mother may have acute[1] episodes of hypoxia that cause fetal decelerations, for example, an eclamptic seizure.

Reduction of fetal oxygenation due to an interruption in maternal blood supply to the intervillous space may be acute or chronic or a combination of the two. A temporary reduction or cessation of blood flow through the intervillous space occurs with each uterine contraction. When the fetus is normally oxygenated, and contractions last no longer than 90 seconds and occur with a frequency of no greater than one every 2 minutes, the fetal arterial oxygen tension seldom goes below 18–20 torr, the threshold for the development of late decelerations.[26] When uterine activity is so frequent or prolonged that fetal oxygen tension decreases to a value less than 18 torr, late decelerations occur. The therapy is straightforward: decrease uterine activity. This can frequently be easily accomplished by turning off exogenously given oxytocin. When uterine polysystole or hypertonia is spontaneous and not the result of premature separation of the placenta, intravenous administration of a betamimetic such as ritodrine at a dose of 100 μg per minute may be beneficial. Anytime that the fetus is living in a reduced oxygen environment, it is important to have the mother breathe 100% oxygen, which elevates maternal arterial PO_2 and may result in an increase in fetal oxygenation.

Maternal hypotension is another cause of maternal intervillous blood flow reduction. This is most likely to occur in the inadequately hydrated laboring patient who receives conduction anesthesia. It can usually be prevented by giving the patient 1000 cc of crystaloid before conduction anesthesia is administered. If the patient still develops hypotension following anesthesia, additional fluid (500 cc) may be given. The patient's legs should be elevated to induce an autotransfusion. Ephedrine, 10–20 mg i.v., may be administered. (See Chapter 8.)

Intrinsic maternal uterine vascular disease, such as maternal hypertension, may result in reduction in intervillous space blood flow. When this baseline reduction is compounded by the further decrease associated with each uterine contraction in labor, late decelerations occur. It would seen reasonable in this situation to use vasodilators to improve uterine blood flow, but the uterine vascular bed in late pregnancy does not respond to vasodilators. Giving the hypertensive mother a vasodilator dilates other vascular beds and further diverts blood flow from the uterus, compounding the problem.

Reduction of placental surface area available for oxygen transfer occurs as a result of placental infarctions, a frequent accompaniment of chronically reduced uterine blood flow. However, it can occur with apparently normal uterine blood flow.

The mechanisms of late decelerations are: The reduction in oxygen supply to the fetus activates chemoreceptors located in the fetal aortic arch and the central nervous system. The peripheral chemoreceptors' message of decreased oxygen tension is relayed to the central nervous system where activation of the cardiodeceleratory center in the brain stem occurs. Activation of the cardiodeceleratory center results in a decrease in heart rate through afferent impulses conducted down the vagus nerve, which shifts the signal generation of the sinoatrial node to a more peripheral part of the node where the electrical impulse is generated more slowly. When hypoxia becomes more intense and prolonged, the myocardium itself becomes depressed and heart rate decreases further. During the early phase of fetal hypoxia, the peripheral and visceral vessels constrict and the cardiac and cerebral vessels dilate, causing a redistribution of cardiac output favoring intact fetal survival. It is not known how long the human fetus can tolerate any specific level of hypoxia before irreversible brain damage occurs; however, studies in the monkey fetus may offer guidelines. Complete asphyxia of the monkey fetus for a period exceeding 14 minutes results in irreversible damage to the fetal brain stem. This damage is in most instances incompatible with continuing life. Moderate hypoxia (oxygen tension of less than 15 torr) for more than 3 hours is associated with damage to the cerebral cortex compatible with long-term neurologic sequelae.[25]

VARIABLE DECELERATION

The onset of variable decelerations occurs at any time during the uterine contraction (Fig. 11-5). Variable decelerations are characterized by a rapid slowing of the heart rate and a rapid recovery. These decelerations, like late deceler-

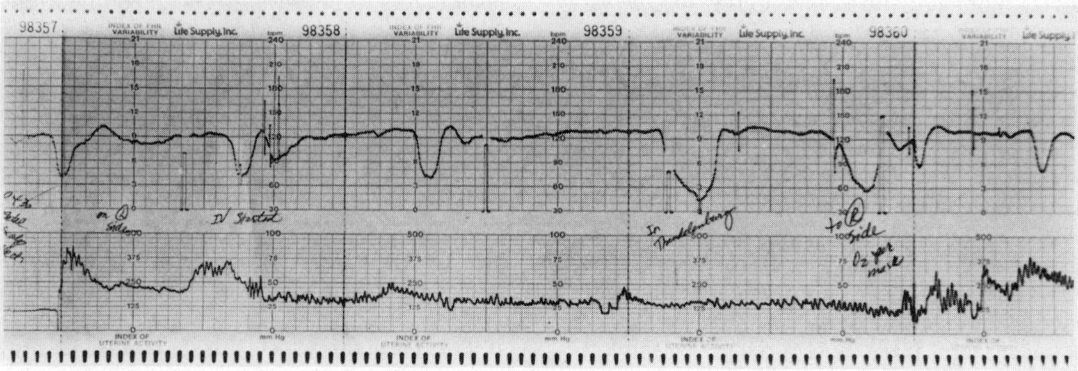

Figure 11-5. Variable decelerations.

ations, are classified as mild, moderate, and severe on the basis of the depth and duration of the decelerations (Table 11-2).

Variable decelerations are thought to be due to compression of the umbilical cord. When the membranes are intact, compression may happen when oligohydramnios is present (i.e., in growth-retarded or postdate fetuses). The majority of significant cord compression patterns occur during labor after the membranes have been ruptured. In this situation, the cord may be compressed between the fetus and the uterus or may become entangled with fetal parts —arms, legs, or neck. When the cord is compressed, the fetal oxygen supply is interrupted. The ensuing fetal bradycardia may be on the same basis as explained above for late decelerations or may have a slightly different mechanism. When the umbilical arteries are compressed, fetal hypertension results. Fetal hypertension can activate fetal baroreceptors to cause bradycardia in the same manner as does activation of chemoreceptors.

Therapy is to attempt to disentangle fetus, cord, and mother by first making certain that the cord has not prolapsed, and then by changing the mother's position. The first step is to turn the mother from back to side, or if she is on her side, to her opposite side. If these maneuvers do not help, placing the mother in the knee-chest position occasionally will.

ACCELERATIONS

Accelerations, or increases in fetal heart rate, may also occur, generally in association with fetal movement. Occasionally fetal movement may be instigated by uterine contractions, resulting in a pattern of periodic accelerations.[38] The presence of such a pattern is generally reassuring.

FETAL SCALP BLOOD SAMPLING

An important technique for evaluation of the fetus during labor was developed by Saling.[39] It consists of obtaining microquantities of blood from the fetal scalp during labor. The acid–base

TABLE 11-2. VARIABLE DECELERATIONS

Type	Minimum Heart Range	Duration
Mild	Any depth not <80/minute	<30 seconds any duration
Moderate	<80/minute	Any duration
Severe	<70/minute	>60 seconds

In some instances there may be an acceleration immediately preceding or following the abrupt slowing or recovery of the heart rate. This overshoot phenomenon is felt by some authors to indicate a more significant hypoxia in the fetus, as is a gradual rather than abrupt recovery of the heart.

status of the fetal blood is then measured. Since an oxygen-deprived fetus rapidly develops metabolic acidosis, scalp blood sampling would seem to be an excellent way to determine which fetus is truly distressed.

The test can only be performed when the cervix is dilated 3 cm or more and the membranes can be safely ruptured. An endoscope is first placed in the vagina and through the dilated cervix. The observer should be able to view the fetal presenting part, which must be either the fetal scalp or buttock if blood sampling is to be done. When the presenting part has been adequately visualized, it should be cleansed of amniotic fluid with a dry cotton swab. A small incision is then made, using the depth-calibrated razor blade furnished with the scalp sampling kit. This incision is best made at the beginning of a contraction unless the fetus is experiencing variable decelerations, in which case the puncture should be made when the heart rate has been normal for 30–45 seconds. The droplet(s) of blood which forms at the incision site is collected in a preheparinized glass capillary. The capillary is sealed with putty and, using a magnet, a preintroduced iron filing is run back and forth in the capillary to mix the blood with the heparin. The capillary tube is placed in an ice bath until pH or buffer base can be determined. This should be accomplished promptly. The values from scalp blood correlate well with those of fetal carotid artery blood in the absence of severe edema of the fetal scalp. Factors that can significantly interfere with an accurate evaluation using this method are air bubbles in the collected specimen, clotting of the blood, amniotic fluid in the specimen, and alkalosis or acidosis of the mother. Air has a much lower PCO_2 and higher PO_2 than does fetal blood. When the sample of fetal blood has more than 25% bubbles, it may significantly affect the pH determination. Amniotic fluid has a low pH (about 7.00) compared to fetal blood, thus, if there is much amniotic fluid contamination of the sample, it may be falsely acidotic. Maternal acidosis and alkalosis can be reflected in the fetus, so it is important to obtain a specimen of maternal venous blood collected without stasis for determination of maternal blood pH if there is any suspicion of maternal acidosis or alkalosis (i.e., a hyperventilating mother or one who has had a long, active labor).

A fetal scalp sample should be taken whenever the physician is uncertain whether or not fetal distress exists. The technique is useful in the following circumstances: mixed heart rate patterns; late decelerations with moderate beat-to-beat variability; mild late decelarations with absent variability; severe late decelerations with good variability; moderate and severe variable declerations with variability and meconium staining of the amniotic fluid, or oligohydramnios; and as soon as possible in labor when the patient's pregnancy has gone beyond 42 weeks and she has either meconium staining of the amniotic fluid or oligohydramnios. The scalp stimulation test mentioned below should be used first in the above circumstances. If this results in an acceleration of the fetal heart, scalp sampling is not necessary.

The fetal scalp pH is normally about 7.30 during the first stage of labor, decreasing somewhat during the second stage of labor to 7.25 at delivery. This value is usually slightly higher than the umbilical arterial blood pH. (Incidentally, it is always wise to obtain a sample of umbilical artery and vein blood following delivery when fetal distress is suspected or when the newborn is depressed at birth.) Fetal scalp blood pH values greater than 7.25 are considered normal. When a normal value is obtained, a repeat scalp pH should be obtained only if the distress pattern persists or becomes more marked. When the same pattern persists, repeat the procedure in 30–60 minutes. If the pattern becomes worse, repeat it immediately. A pH value between 7.20 and 7.24 is moderate acidosis, which requires repeat sampling in 15–30 minutes. When there is a downward trend in pH, delivery is indicated. A pH less than 7.20 is definite acidosis and delivery is indicated unless the sample is significantly contaminated with amniotic fluid or the mother is markedly acidotic. In the former case, a repeat sample should be taken immediately, and in the latter, the maternal sample should answer the question.

Not all hospitals are equipped to do scalp pH. However, kits are available, as are pH meters designed expressly for this technique, so it could be available on any delivery service. Its principal value is in reducing the frequency of cesarean section for fetal distress by demonstrating a normal pH in the presence of a worrisome fetal heart rate tracing.

CLINICAL USE OF FETAL INTRAPARTUM MONITORING

Since continuous fetal heart rate monitoring has become readily available, a vigorous discussion has been conducted as to the efficiency of fetal monitoring and about who should be monitored. Several uncontrolled, and therefore potentially biased, studies have demonstrated reduced perinatal mortality in infants monitored intrapartum.[7,16,31] Some of these studies have distinguished between high- and low-risk infants. In at least one of the studies[28] there appeared to be a reduction in perinatal mortality when the high-risk infant was continuously monitored and an increase in mortality when the low-risk infant received the same management. Several studies[8,9,13] utilizing a prospective randomized choice of patients for either continuous or intermittent fetal monitoring failed to show a difference in either perinatal mortality or morbidity. The number of patients was too small to demonstrate a difference even if one existed. A recent study,[18] which was prospective, randomized, and included both low- and high-risk patients, showed increased perinatal morbidity (higher seizure rate) in a group of infants managed throughout labor using intermittent auscultation compared to those continuously monitored electronically. There was no difference in perinatal mortality in the two groups of infants. Since there were over 6000 babies in each group, the likelihood that one will lower perinatal mortality by using continuous monitoring is low. However, it must be noted that the management by intermittent auscultation in this study was optimal (i.e., listening to the fetal heart rate every 15 minutes during the first stage of labor and after every contraction during the second stage of labor). None of the studies to date enlighten us as to which patients must be continuously monitored during their labor. They point somewhat strongly toward monitoring the high-risk patient and less strongly toward monitoring the low-risk patient. Many patients have a strong preference to be or not to be monitored continuously. The patient should be told the risks and benefits of the two types of monitoring, keeping in mind the importance of the nursing personnel if one is to use intermittent monitoring.

There are two potential risks of continuous fetal monitoring. The first and most important is an increase in cesarean section rate when continuous monitoring is used.[8,28] This is due to increases in the rates of both fetal distress and of failure to progress in labor. The increase due to the latter indication is difficult to explain and is not found in all studies. That of the former can be significantly reduced by using fetal scalp sampling to assist in establishing the diagnosis of true fetal distress.[8]

The majority of patients can be continuously monitored using external techniques—ultrasound for fetal heart rate and tocodynamometer for uterine contractions. It must be remembered that certain inaccuracies are inherent in these techniques. One cannot rely upon the measurement of fetal heart rate variability unless it is absent, and uterine contractions cannot be quantitated either in terms of tonus or the maximum amplitude. One also must make certain that the ultrasound transducer is directed toward the fetal heart and must recognize that each time the fetus moves, the heart rate may be lost. Recently, attempts have been made to overcome one of the flaws in external monitoring, inaccurate recording of variability by using autocorrelation techniques. In many instances, this seems to produce records similar to internally recorded tracings, particularly in the antepartum period, although it must be realized that some data are rejected.

When there is a need for more accurate representation of fetal heart rate variability, a scalp electrode should be used provided that the cervix is 2–3 cm dilated and that the membranes can be ruptured safely. An intrauterine catheter should be used whenever there is a need to accurately assess uterine activity (e.g., failure to progress in labor and/or the use of oxytocin to induce or stimulate labor).

Pregnancy should be terminated when further habitation in the intrauterine environment may damage the fetus. The challenge is to know when damage is about to occur and to attempt to prevent it. The principal damage that may occur is due to lack of oxygen. When the fetus becomes hypoxic, increases in brain and heart blood flow occur as a result of cerebral and cardiac arterial vasodilation. This tends to sustain oxygen delivery to these two vital organs until the hypoxia is sufficient to substantially reduce cardiac contractility. At this point, adequate perfusion of the heart and brain can no longer be maintained. We know from animal[25] and human[14] studies that late, prolonged, and severe variable decelerations are associated with significant hypoxia. The degree and duration of hypoxia cannot be inferred from the type of decelerations. Heart rate variability may assist the clinician in making the diagnosis. Significant reduction in variability may indicate profound and/or prolonged hypoxia as described previously. Another method of assessing the severity of hypoxia is to examine fetal acid–base balance using fetal scalp sampling, as described above.

Therapy of fetal hypoxia depends on understanding the mechanisms involved in its production. When the maneuvers previously described fail to correct an ominous fetal heart rate pattern, the physician must decide whether emergency delivery of the fetus is necessary. This decision should be based on the actual or suspected degree of fetal hypoxia, the fetal age, and the time required to do a cesarean section.

The degree of fetal hypoxia can be estimated from fetal scalp blood pH, because hypoxic fetuses resort to anaerobic metabolism and thus develop acidosis. If the fetal scalp blood has a pH of less than 7.20, one can assume fetal hypoxia. Since not everyone has the capability to do fetal scalp sampling, other criteria may be used to judge fetal hypoxia. It has recently been shown that when the fetus responds with acceleration of the heart rate to scalp pressure or pinching, its pH is not less than 7.20.[3] Unfortunately, the reverse is not true. Not all fetuses who do not accelerate their heart rate are acidotic. Thus it is sometimes necessary to rely on the heart rate alone to determine acidosis. A general guideline is that the term infant should be delivered within 60 minutes of recognition of an ominous pattern. For example, a fetus with baseline tachycardia, absent variability, and severe late decelerations requires immediate delivery. Any pattern of late decelerations with absent variability requires immediate delivery. The guideline should also be modified by fetal age. The premature fetus, particularly one estimated to weigh less than 1500 grams, should be delivered at the first sign of fetal distress. The above philosophy increases the section rate for fetal distress, perhaps unnecessarily, since at least 50% of fetuses delivered emergently using these guidelines will have normal Apgar scores. However, until more accurate methods of fetal diagnosis are available, it seems better to subject the mother to the risk associated with cesarean section rather than to continue labor in the presence of hypoxia.

ANTEPARTUM TESTING

Evaluation of the fetus during the antepartum period was minimal until the advent of continuous fetal heart rate monitoring. Intermittent auscultation allowed only knowledge of whether the fetus was alive or dead. Pose et al.[33] and Ray et al.[35] developed a significant test for antepartum evaluation of the fetus when they stimulated uterine contractions and looked for late decelerations of the fetal heart rate as an indicator of fetal hypoxia. Later, the development of the nonstress test, the kick count, and the biophysical profile added new methods of evaluating the fetus during the prenatal period.

Testing should be started whenever one becomes concerned about fetal well-being and treatment of the fetus is feasible. The primary indications for testing and the usual age at which to commence testing are listed in Table 11-3.

The contraction stress test is performed by having the patient sit in a reclining chair or lie comfortably in bed. It is important to assure that the patient has no supine hypotension. A Doppler ultrasound transducer and tocodynamometer are connected to the patient's abdomen and fetal heart rate, uterine contractions, and fetal activity are recorded for about 30 minutes. If spontaneous uterine contractions are

TABLE 11-3. INDICATION FOR ANTEPARTUM TESTING

Indication X/wk	Type Test*	Date to Start	Frequency
Post dates	Stress test	41½–42 weeks	1
	Ultrasound		1
IUGR	NST	When diagnosed	1
	Ultrasound		1/Q 2–3
Diabetes	NST/CST	32	1
Preeclampsia	NST	When diagnosed	2
Decreased fetal movement	NST	When diagnosed	1
Previous stillbirth	NST	30–32 weeks	1
Rh	CST	28–32 weeks	1

* All these may be modified if using the kick count, which should be done once weekly to 32 weeks, then 3x a week until delivery.

not present with a frequency of 3 per 10 minutes, or if the spontaneous contractions which are present are not associated with late decelerations of the heart rate, the uterus can be stimulated. The most common way of stimulating the uterus is by giving a constant infusion of intravenous oxytocin, starting at a dose of 0.5 mU per minute and doubling the dose every 15–30 minutes until either 3 contractions per 10 minutes are achieved or all contractions present are associated with late decelerations. Recently, some units have induced uterine activity by stimulating the nipples of the breasts using a warm wash cloth. If no late decelerations are seen in the entire strip and the uterine contraction frequency is 3 per 10 minutes the test is negative and the fetus should be able to safely tolerate another week in utero. If there are any late decelerations on the tracing, even the most subtle (Fig. 11-6), the test is called suspicious and should be repeated the following day. When the contractions have persisted for 30 minutes and late decelerations follow 50% or more of the contractions, regardless of contraction frequency, or when late decelerations follow all contractions and the contraction frequency is 3 per 10 minutes, the test is positive (Fig. 11-7). When the uterine contraction frequency exceeds 3 per 10 minutes, or a contraction lasts longer than 90 seconds with an associated late deceleration of fetal heart rate, hyperstimulation has occurred and the test should be repeated the following day. Infrequently, a sinusoidal pattern is seen. A true sinusoidal pattern, in the absence of alphaprodine administration is indicative of severe fetal anemia or hypoxia. Prolonged decelerations of the heart rate occasionally occur either spontaneously or in response to a uterine contraction. This is an ominous sign and mandates continuous monitoring of the patient for the next few hours and a repeat test the following day.

The nonstress test is the most widely used antepartum fetal assessment test. A normal fetus has frequent heart rate accelerations associated with fetal movement.[37] During REM sleep the normal fetus accelerates its heart rate by 20 beats per minute for at least 20 seconds twice during a 20 minute period (Fig. 11-8). A fetus who meets these criteria is called reactive and one who does not, nonreactive. Since the fetus spends up to one-half of its time in quiet sleep, the majority of nonreactive fetuses are simply asleep. Drugs, prematurity, and hypoxia are also associated with fetal nonreactivity.

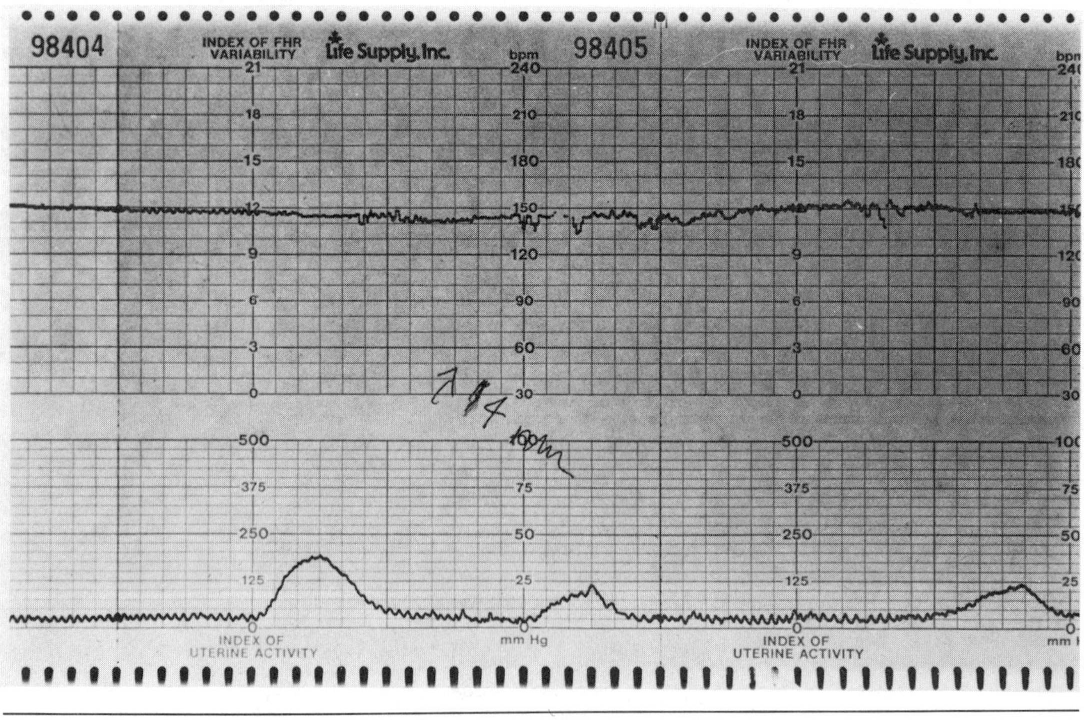

Figure 11-6. Suspicious CST.

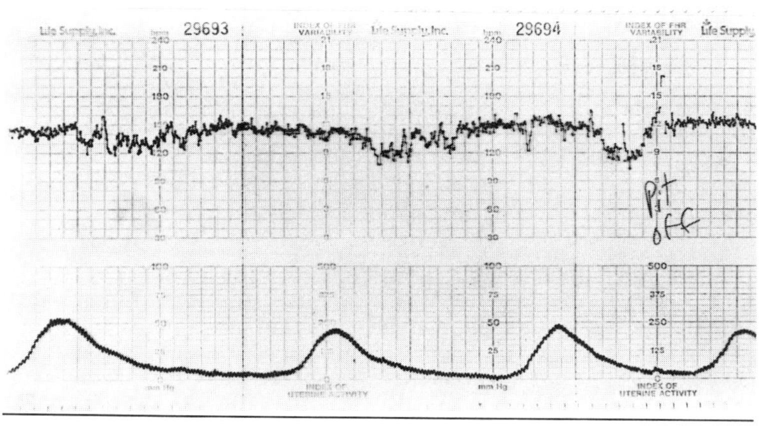

Figure 11-7. Positive CST.

The test is performed by placing an ultrasonic transducer to record fetal heart rate and a tocodynamometer on the maternal abdomen to record fetal activity. Usually reactivity is seen in the first 30 minutes of recording. If this does not occur, some advocate either shaking the fetus through the mother's abdominal wall or feeding the mother in the belief that an increase in fetal glucose will change fetal state. Neither increased fetal glucose[36] nor shaking[44] changes fetal state. Recent attempts to shorten the testing time using acoustic stimulation seem encouraging.[41] In this instance, an artificial larynx is placed on the maternal abdomen, a mixed sound emitted, and fetal reactivity determined.

Interpreting both the stress and nonstress test can be enhanced by knowing the variability of the heart rate. In the past, one could not rely on the presence of variability obtained from an external Doppler-derived tracing. As noted earlier, the ultrasound signal is such that artificial variability may be introduced. The new autocorrelation techniques offer promise that variability may be correctly interpreted from these tracings.

Stress and nonstress tests are frequently used in tandem when testing high-risk fetuses. The nonstress test is used as the primary surveillance, performed once or twice a week. If the nonstress test is nonreactive, a stress test is done. When either test alone indicates a hypoxic fetus, the incidence of false positive results is as high as 50%. However, when both tests indicate fetal distress, the false positive rate is low.

When the fetus shows any signs of hypoxia

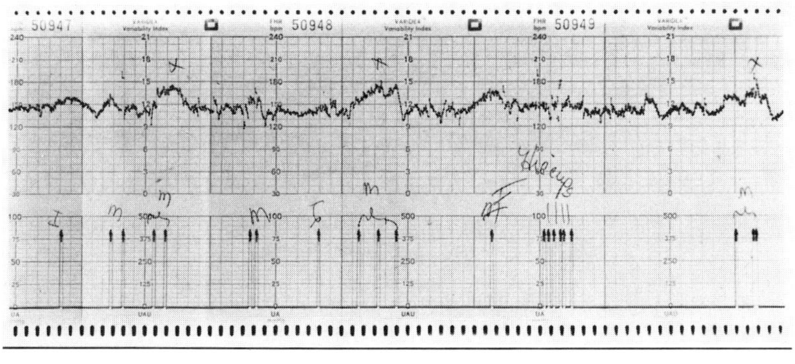

Figure 11-8. Reactive NST.

TABLE 11-4. BIOPHYSICAL PROFILE

Nonstress Test	Reactive (Score 2)	Nonreactive (Score 0)
Fetal breathing	One episode of 60 sec during a 30 min recording	< episode every 30 min
Fetal movement	3 gross movements in 30 min	<3/30 min
Fetal tone	Full flexion of body, head, and extremities	Extension
Amniotic fluid volume	>1 cm pocket in vertical diameter	1 cm or less

and is at 36 weeks or more in gestation, accompanied by pulmonary maturity, delivery is indicated. One should attempt vaginal delivery if the membranes can be ruptured and a scalp electrode attached. If the fetus is less than 36 weeks and fetal pulmonary maturity is present, delivery should be accomplished only if the fetus is nonreactive and has a positive contraction stress test. If pregnancy is continued, fetal testing should be done daily or every other day. When the fetus is less than 36 weeks, has evidence of pulmonary immaturity, and is nonreactive with a positive stress test, delivery is frequently based on the results of the biophysical profile (to be described) or delivery is postponed for 48 hours while corticosteroids are given to the continuously monitored fetus.

A fetal test rapidly growing in popularity is the daily fetal movement count. This may be done in a variety of ways. All have the patient keep a daily record of the number of fetal kicks perceived. Some have the mother count only the first 10 kicks, with anything less than 10 during the day being abnormal. Others have the mother rest for 2 hours in the afternoon or evening and count the number of episodes of fetal activity during those 2 hours; there should be at least six episodes. We favor the latter technique as it accomplishes two goals—maternal rest for 2 hours during the day and observation of fetal activity. A significantly lower fetal mortality occurs in pregnancies managed with kick counts as compared to controls not managed in this manner.[27] When an abnormal kick count is reported, a stress and/or nonstress test should be done the same day.

BIOPHYSICAL PROFILE

The biophysical profile is a method of assessing fetal health using fetal breathing, heart rate reactivity, movement, tone, and amniotic fluid volume.[20] The normal values for these parameters are given in Table 11-4. Each normal value is given a score of 2 and an abnormal value, a score of 0. When all the scores are summed, a biophysical profile score is determined. A score of 8–10 indicates a fetus in no distress; 4–5, moderate potential of distress; and 0–2, fetal distress. Manning et al.[19] feel that primary use of the test gives results which are better than using the stress and nonstress tests. However, most investigators utilize the biophysical profile as a secondary test. When the stress and nonstress tests indicate fetal distress in an immature fetus, daily biophysical profiles occasionally allow continuation of the pregnancy.

REFERENCES

1. Batson, G. A.: Cyanotic congenital heart disease and pregnancy. *J. Obstet. Gynaecol. Br. Commonw.* **81**:549–553, 1974.
2. Brown, R. and Patrick, J.: The nonstress test: How long is enough? *Am. J. Obstet. Gynecol.* **141**:646–651, 1981.
3. Clark, S. L., Gimovsky, M. L., and Miller, F. C.: The scalp stimulation test: A clinical alternative to fetal scalp blood sampling. *Am. J. Obstet. Gynecol.* **148**:274–277, 1984.
4. Druzin, M. L., Gratacos, J., Keegan, K. a., and Paul, R. H.: Antepartum fetal heart rate testing. VII. The significance of fetal bradycardia. *Am. J. Obstet. Gynecol.* **139**:194–198, 1981.
5. Freeman, R. K. and Garite, T. J.: *Fetal Heart Rate Monitoring.* Baltimore, Williams & Wilkins, 1981, p. 63.
6. Freeman, R. K., Gutierrez, N. A., Ray, M. L., Stovall, D., Paul, R. H., and Hon, E. H.: Fetal cardiac response to paracervical block anesthesia, Part 1. *Am. J. Obstet. Gynecol.* **113**:583–591, 1972.
7. Gabert, H. A. and Stenchever, M. A.: Continuous electronic monitoring of the fetal heart rate during labor. *Am. J. Obstet. Gynecol.* **115**:919–923, 1973.
8. Haverkamp, A. D., Orleans, M., Langendoerfer, S., McFee, J., Murphy, J., and Thompson, H. E.:

A controlled trial of the differential effects of intrapartum fetal monitoring. *Am. J. Obstet. Gynecol.* **134**:399–412, 1979.

9. Haverkamp, A. D., Thompson, H. E., McFee, J. G., and Cetrulo, C.: The evaluation of continuous fetal heart rate monitoring in high risk pregnancy. *Am. J. Obstet. Gynecol.* **125**:310–317, 1976.
10. Hon, E. H.: Personal communication.
11. Hon, E. H. and Hess, O. W.: Instrumentation of fetal electrocardiography. *Science* **125**:553–554, 1957.
12. Hon, E. H. and Quilligan, E. J.: The classification of fetal heart rate. *Conn. Med.* **31**:779–784, 1967.
13. Kelso, I. M., Parsons, R. J., Lawrence, G. F., Arora, S. S., Edmonds, D. K., and Cooke, I. D.: An assessment of continuous fetal heart rate monitoring in labor. *Am. J. Obstet. Gynecol.* **131**:526–532, 1978.
14. Kubli, F. H., Hon, E. H., Kazin, A. F., and Takemura, H.: Observations on fetal heart rate and pH in the human fetus during labor. *Am. J. Obstet. Gynecol.* **104**:1190–1206, 1969.
15. Ledger, W. J.: Complications associated with invasive fetal monitoring. *Semin. Perinatol.* **2**:187–194, 1978.
16. Lee, W. K. and Baggish, M. S.: The effect of unselected intrapartum fetal monitoring. *Obstet. Gynecol.* **47**:516–520, 1972.
17. Litsey, S. E., Noonan, J. A., O'Connor, W. N., Cottrill, C. M., and Mitchel, B.: Maternal connective tissue disease and congenital heart block: Demonstration of immunoglobulin in cardiac tissue. *N. Engl. J. Med.* **312**:98–100, 1985.
18. MacDonald, D., Grant A., Pereira S. M., Boylan P., and Chalmers, I.: The Dublin randomized controlled trial of intrapartum fetal heart rate monitoring. *Am. J. Obstet. Gynecol.* **152**:524–539, 1985.
19. Manning, F. A., Baskett, T. F., Morrison, I., and Lange, I.: Fetal biophysical profile scoring: A prospective study in 1,184 high-risk pregnancies. *Am. J. Obstet. Gynecol.* **140**:289–294, 1981.
20. Manning, F. A., Platt, L. D., and Sepos, L.: Antepartum fetal evaluation: Development of a fetal biophysical profile. *Am. J. Obstet. Gynecol.* **136**:787–795, 1980.
21. Martin, C. B.: Fetal heart rate variability—regulatory mechanisms. In: *Research in Perinatal Medicine*. P. W. Nathanielz and J. T. Parer (Eds.). Ithaca, NY, Perinatology Press, 1984, pp. 179–203.
22. Martin, C. B., Nijhuis, J. G., and Weijer, A. A.: Correction of supraventricular tachycardia by compression of the umbilical cord: Report of a case. *Am. J. Obstet. Gynecol.* **150**:324–326, 1984.
23. McCue, C. M., Mantakas, M. E., Tingelstad, J. B., and Ruddy, S.: Congenital heart block in newborns of mothers with connective tissue disease. *Circulation* **56**:82–90, 1977.
24. Modanlou, H., Freeman, R. K., Oritz, 0., Hinkes, P., and Pillsbury, G.: Sinusoidal fetal heart rate patterns and severe fetal anemia. *Obstet. Gynecol.* **49**:537–541, 1977.
25. Myers, R. E: Two patterns of perinatal brain damage and their conditions of occurrence. *Am. J. Obstet. Gynecol.* **112**:246–276, 1972.
26. Myers, R. E., Mueller-Heubach, E., and Adamsons, K.: Predictability of the state of fetal oxygenation from a quantitative analysis of the components of late deceleration. *Am. J. Obstet. Gynecol.* **115**:1083–1094, 1973.
27. Neldam, S.: Fetal movement as an indicator of fetal wellbeing. *Lancet* **1**(8180):1222–1224, 1980.
28. Neutra, R. R., Feinberg, S. E., Greenland, S., and Friedman, E. A.: The effect of fetal monitoring on neonatal death rates. *N. Engl. J. Med.* **299**:324–326, 1978.
29. Nijhuis, J. G., Martin, C. B., and Prechtl, H. F. R.: Behavior states of the human fetus. In: *Continuity of Neural Functions from Prenatal to Postnatal Life*. H. F. R. Prechtl (Ed.). Philadelphia, Spastics International Publications, 1984, pp. 65–77.
30. Parer, J. T.: Evaluation of the fetus during labor. *Curr. Probl. Pediatr.* **12**(6):1–58, 1982.
31. Paul, R. H., Huey, C. F., and Yeager, C. F.: Clinical fetal monitoring: Its effect on cesarean section rates and perinatal mortality. *Postgrad. Med.* **61**:160–166, 1977.
32. Pinkerton, J. H. M.: Fetal auscultation—some aspects of its history and evolution. *Irish Med. J.* **69**:363–368, 1976.
33. Pose, S. V., Escarcena, L., Althabe, 0., Schwarcz, R. L., Ibarra-Polo, A. A., Quintanilla, R., and Caldeyro-Barcia, R.: Effects of normal and abnormal uterine contractions on fetal oxygen and heart rate. In: *Effects of Labour on the Fetus and Newborn*. R. Caldeyro-Barcia, C. Mendez-Bauer, and G. S. Dawes (Eds.). Oxford, Pergamon Press, 1967.
34. Pritchard, J. A., MacDonald, P. C., and Gant, N. F. (Eds.): *Williams Obstetrics*, 17th Edition. Norwalk, CT, Appleton-Century-Crofts, 1985, pp. 1–6.
35. Ray, M., Freeman, R. K., Pine, S., and Hesselgesser, R.: Clinical experience with the oxytocin challenge test. *Am. J. Obstet. Gynecol.* **114**:1–9, 1972.
36. Richardson, B., Briggs, M. L., Toomey, C., Barry, K. J., and O'Grady, J. P.: The effect of maternal glucose administration on the specificity of the nonstress test. *Am. J. Obstet. Gynecol.* **145**:141–146, 1983.
37. Rochard, F., Schifrin, B. S., Goupil, F., Legrand, H., Blottiere, J., and Sureau, C.: Nonstressed fetal heart rate monitoring in the antepartum period. *Am. J. Obstet. Gynecol.* **126**:699–706, 1976.
38. Sadovsky, E., Rabinowitz, R., Freeman, A., and Yarkoni, S.: The relationship between fetal heart rate accelerations, fetal movements and uterine contractions. *Am. J. Obstet. Gynecol.* **149**:187–189, 1984.

39. Saling, E. and Schneider, D.: Biochemical supervision of the fetus during labor. *J. Obstet. Gynaecol. Br. Commonw.* **74**:799–811, 1967.
40. Shenker, L.: Fetal cardiac arrhythmias. *Obstet. Gynecol. Surv.* **38**:561–572, 1979.
41. Smith, D. V., Phelan, J. P., Paul, R. H., and Broussard, P.: Fetal acoustic stimulation testing: A retrospective experience with fetal acoustic stimulation test (FAS-TEST). *Am. J. Obstet. Gynecol.*, **153**:567–569, 1985.
42. Taylor, P. V., Scott, J. S., and Gerlis, L. M.: Maternal connective tissue disease and congenital heart block. N. Engl. J. Med. **312**:1328–1329, 1985.
43. Terao, T., Kawashima, Y., Noto, H., Inamoto, Y., Lin, T. Y., Sumitome, K., and Meada, M.: Neurologic control of fetal heart rate in 20 cases of anencephalic fetuses. *Am. J. Obstet. Gynecol.* **140**:201–208, 1984.
44. Visser, G. H. A., Zuckenberg, U. J., deVries, J. I., and Dawes, G. S.: External physical stimulation of the human fetus during episodes of low heart rate variation. *Am. J. Obstet. Gynecol.* **145**:579–584, 1983.

12

THE USE OF ULTRASOUND IN OBSTETRICS

Ultrasound is a universally used diagnostic modality in obstetrics and gynecology. However, at present, no data unequivocally suggest benefit from its routine use in antenatal and intrapartum care. Recently, a panel of experts under the auspices of the National Institutes of Child Health and Development published 28 indications for the use of ultrasound in obstetrics (Table 12-1).[14]

THE ULTRASOUND EXAMINATION

The data base that can be recovered from an obstetrical ultrasound examination has increased exponentially. This increase is attributed to technological advances related to dynamic (real-time) equipment which simplifies the examination and to improvement in the resolution of echograms.

However, the necessity for the sonographer to perform detailed studies on all pregnancies and to rule out all possible anomalies on every fetus is being questioned. There is concern about:

1. false negative and positive diagnoses of congenital anomalies made by nonphysician professionals or by physicians accustomed to scanning mainly normal pregnancies;
2. the increase in examination time and, by inference, ultrasonic intensity necessary for the detection of anomalies in low-risk pregnancies;
3. lack of manifestation of a number of anomalies (Table 12-2) at 16–18 weeks' gestation, a time commonly used for initial scans;
4. cost-effectiveness of testing all pregnancies for anomalies when the overall yield is small; and
5. remuneration of all these tests by third-party payers.

Because of these concerns, the ultrasound examination is presently limited to a basic or "standard study" applicable to pregnant women at low risk for anomalies; such examinations are designed to answer specific questions about the pregnancy (see below). If, during the course of a standard study, an abnormality is suspected, "second opinion" scans are recommended. By contrast, in women at high risk for birth defects, targeted imaging for fetal anomaly (TIFFA) examinations are performed initially, usually in tertiary centers, by physicians with expertise in this area.

In the standard study, data are collected regarding:

1. gestational age;
2. fetal growth and weight;
3. qualitative estimate of amniotic fluid volume;
4. placental position and grade;
5. number of fetuses;
6. presence of fetal heart motion;
7. gross fetal abnormalities, if any; and
8. presence of pelvic mass.

This chapter addresses some of the components of the standard study, the use of ultra-

TABLE 12-1. INDICATIONS OF USE OF DIAGNOSTIC ULTRASOUND SUGGESTED BY NATIONAL INSTITUTES OF HEALTH CONSENSUS CONFERENCE

Estimation of gestational age for patients with uncertain clinical dates	Suspected abruptio placentae	Suspected ectopic pregnancy
	Adjunct to external version from breech to vertex presentation	Adjunct to special procedures
Evaluation of fetal growth		Suspected fetal death
Vaginal bleeding of undetermined etiology in pregnancy	Estimation of fetal weight and/or presentation in premature rupture of membranes and/or premature labor	Suspected uterine abnormality
Determination of fetal presentation	Abnormal serum alpha-fetoprotein value	Intrauterine contraceptive device location
Suspected multiple gestation	Follow-up observation of identified fetal anomaly	Ovarian follicle development surveillance
Adjunct to amniocentesis	Follow-up evaluation of placental location for identified placenta previa	Biophysical evaluation for fetal well-being after 28 weeks of gestation
Significant uterine size/clinical dates discrepancy	History of previous congenital anomaly	Observation of intrapartum events
Pelvic mass	Serial evaluation of fetal growth in multiple gestation	
Suspected hydatidiform mole		Evaluation of fetal condition in late registrants for prenatal care
Suspected polyhydramnios or oligohydramnios	Adjunct to cervical cerclage placement	

Source: Reference 14.

sound as an adjunct to certain diagnostic and therapeutic procedures, and TIFFA examinations.

STANDARD STUDY

Gestational Age

Clinical assessment of pregnancy dates can be unreliable because in 20–40% of gravidas, the onset of the last menstrual period (LMP) is uncertain.[13] Even when the LMP is stated by the pregnant woman, the information is inaccurate, falling within a margin of 3 weeks in 90% of cases.[1]

Accurate and objective assessment of dates is essential to the management of pregnancy. First, fetal age forms the x coordinate of a variety of graphs pertaining to pregnancy (Table 12-3). Second, the degree of maturity attained is pivotal in making the decision to abbreviate a particular pregnancy for the benefit of mother or fetus. Third, reliance on only clinical methods to schedule repeat cesarean section has been associated with a high incidence of respiratory distress in the neonate.[3,21,22]

Pregnancy dates can be predicted from a number of fetal parameters including: fetal crown–rump length (CRL), biparietal diameter (BPD), femur length (FL), head circumference (HC), abdominal circumference (AC), other fetal bones, and the binocular distance. The rela-

TABLE 12-2. LIST OF ANOMALIES THAT ARE NOT APPARENT BY 16–18 WEEKS OF GESTATION, AN INTERVAL COMMONLY USED FOR INITIAL SCANS

Early hydrocephalus
Microcephalus
Some cardiac defects
Obstruction of gastrointestinal tract
Polycystic renal dysplasia, recessive form
Heterozygous achondroplasia

TABLE 12-3. LIST OF SOME GRAPHS PERTAINING TO PREGNANCY BASED ON GESTATIONAL AGE AS *X* COORDINATE

Cephalic growth, biparietal diameter, and head circumference
Growth of the abdominal circumference
Length of fetal skeletal bones
Alpha-fetoprotein

tionship of these fetal measurements to pregnancy dates from (1) 7 to 26 weeks and (2) 26 weeks to term is shown in Tables 12-4 and 12-5, respectively. A discussion of some of these parameters follows.

BPD. The BPD should be measured from the outer to the inner aspects of the parietal echoes in a plane that shows the thalamic bodies (Fig. 12-1). The variation in gestational age relative to specific BPD values increases with advancing gestation. This variation is small (7–10 days) from 14 to 26 weeks and large (±21 days) in the third trimester of pregnancy (Tables 12-4 and 12-5). Thus, for reliable estimation of dates, it is necessary to obtain the BPD by midpregnancy.

Growth Adjusted Sonar Age (GASA). In some pregnancies at risk for growth retardation or macrosomia, it may be beneficial to obtain two BPDs for evaluating dates more precisely. The rationale is based upon the fact that 90% of normal fetuses maintain the same BPD percentile rank in the interval between 20 and 33 weeks of gestation.[52,54]

The first BPD should be obtained between 20 and 26 weeks. It is used to estimate mean gestational dates (Table 12-4). The second BPD is then used to place the BPD size in a specific growth percentile bracket (Table 12-6). A large BPD, greater than the 75th percentile (>75p), translates into a less mature fetus relative to the mean estimate of dates. On the other hand, a small BPD, smaller than the 25th percentile (<25p), translates into a more mature fetus relative to mean dates (Fig. 12-2).

The method of GASA decreases or advances dates only in fetuses with large (≥75p) or small (≤25p) BPD size, respectively. Furthermore, its use theoretically reduces the 90% confidence interval governing assessment of mean dates from ±10–11 days to ±3–5 days.[52,54] The method is not intended to diagnose macrosomic or small-for-gestational-age fetuses, because such diagnoses should be based on a number of parameters including AC and HC.[51]

Smazal et al.[61] recently found that dates predicted by a single BPD are similar to those estimated by GASA. However, their study lumped all fetuses together and did not compare estimates of dates by single and paired BPD methods only in the subset of fetuses where GASA changed the fetal age assigned by the first BPD. Their accuracy of GASA was close to ±5 days. However, the accuracy of a single BPD was also approximately ±5 days, a finding not consistent with any other report.[39]

Femur Length (FL). The accuracy of the prediction of mean dates by the FL is controversial. Initial studies indicated that the variation in dates relative to specific FLs is small: ±7–10 days (2 S.D.) in the first 26 weeks of pregnancy.[25,43] However, the variance in dates predicted by FL may be as large as ±2.8 weeks (2 S.D.) throughout pregnancy.[32]

TABLE 12-4. MEAN GESTATIONAL AGE (MENSTRUAL DATES) IN WEEKS (WK) RELATIVE TO FETAL CROWN RUMP LENGTH (CRL), BIPARIETAL DIAMETER (BPD), FEMUR LENGTH (FL), HEAD CIRCUMFERENCE (HC), AND ABDOMINAL CIRCUMFERENCE (AC) IN THE FIRST TWO TRIMESTERS OF PREGNANCY

CRL		BPD and FL		HC		AC
Wk/CRL	Length/cm	Wk/BPD	Wk/FL	Wk/HC	Perimeter/cm	Wk/AC
7+	1.0–1.2			14–	8.5	
8–	1.3		14–	14	9.0	
8	1.4–1.5		14	14+	9.5	
8+	1.6–1.7		15–	15–	10.0	16–
9–	1.8		15	15	10.5	16
9–	1.9		15+	15+	11.0	16+
9–	2.0		16–	16–	11.5	17
9–	2.1		16	16	12.0	17+

TABLE 12-4. *Continued*

CRL		BPD and FL		HC		AC
Wk/CRL	Length/cm	Wk/BPD	Wk/FL	Wk/HC	Perimeter/cm	Wk/AC
9	2.2		16+	16+	12.5	18−
9+	2.3–2.4		17−	17−	13.0	18
9+	2.5		17	17	13.5	19−
9+	2.6	13+	18−	17+	14.0	19
10−	2.7	14−	18−	18−	14.5	20−
10−	2.8	14	18	18	15.0	20
10−	2.9	14+	19−	18+	15.5	20+
10	3.0	14+	19−	19−	16.0	21−
10+	3.1	15−	19	19	16.5	21
10+	3.2	15	20−	20−	17.0	22−
10+	3.3	15+	20−	20	17.5	22
10+	3.4	16−	20	20+	18.0	23−
11−	3.5	16	21−	21−	18.5	23
11−	3.6	16+	21	21	19.0	24−
11−	3.7	17−	21+	22−	19.5	24
11−	3.8	17	22−	22	20.0	25−
11−	3.9	17+	22	22+	20.5	25
11	4.0	18−	22+	23	21.0	25+
11+	4.1	18	23−	23+	21.5	26−
11+	4.2	18+	23	24−	22.0	26
11+	4.3	19−	24−	24+	22.5	27−
11+	4.4	19	24	25	23.0	
11+	4.5	19+	24+	25+	23.5	
12−	4.6	20−	25−	26	24.0	
12−	4.7	20	25	26+	24.5	
12−	4.8	20+	26−			
12−	4.9	21−	26			
12−	5.0	21	26+			
12	5.1	21+				
12	5.2	22−				
12+	5.3	22−				
12+	5.4	22				
12+	5.5	22+				
12+	5.6	23−				
12+	5.7	23				
13−	5.8	23+				
13−	5.9	24−				
13−	6.0	24				
13−	6.1	24+				
13−	6.2	25−				
13−	6.3	25				
13	6.4	25				
13+	6.5	26−				
13+	6.6	26				
13+	6.7	26+				

Note: BPD values represent composite means: Plus sign = +1 to +3 days; minus sign = −1 to −3 days: Range for CRL = ± 5 days (2 S.D), for BPD = ± 10 days (2 S.D.), and for FL = ±10 days (2 S.D.).

Source: Adapted from the following references:

Robinson, H. P. and Fleming, J. E. E.: A critical evaluation of sonar "crown-rump length" measurements. *Br. J. Obstet. Gynaecol.* **82:**702–710, 1975.

Sabbagha, R. E. and Hughey, M.: Standardization of sonar cephalometry and gestational age. *Obstet. Gynecol.* **52:**402–406, 1978.

Hadlock, F. P., Harrist, R. B., and Deter, R. L. Fetal femur length as a predictor of menstrual age: Sonographically measured. *Am. J. Roentgenol.* **138:**875–878, 1982.

Hadlock, F. P., Deter, R. L., Harrist, R. B., and Park, S. K.: Fetal head circumference: Relation to menstrual age. *Am. J. Roentgenol.* **138:**649–653, 1982.

Hadlock, F. P., Deter, R. L., Harrist, R. B., and Park, S. K.: Fetal abdominal circumference as a predictor of menstrual age. *Am. J. Roentgenol.* **139:**367–370, 1982.

TABLE 12-5. MEAN (M) AND RANGE* (R) OF GESTATIONAL AGE (MENSTRUAL DATES) IN WEEKS (WK) RELATIVE TO FETAL BIPARIETAL DIAMETER† (BPD), FEMUR LENGTH (FL), HEAD CIRCUMFERENCE (HC), AND ABDOMINAL CIRCUMFERENCE (AC) IN THE THIRD TRIMESTER OF PREGNANCY

BPD Week R	BPD Week M	Length (cm)	FL Week M	FL Week R	HC Week R	HC Week M	Perimeter(cm)	AC Week M	AC Week R
		5.1	27	±3			22.5	27−	±2
		5.2	27+	±3			23.0	27	±2
		5.3	28−	±3			23.5	28−	±2
		5.4	28	±3			24.0	28	±2
		5.5	29−	±3			24.5	29−	±2
		5.6	29	±3	±2.1	27−	25.0	29	±2
		5.7	30−	±3	±2.1	27	25.5	30−	±2
		5.8	30	±3	±2.1	28	26.0	30	±3
		5.9	30+	±3	±3.0	28+	26.5	31−	±3
		6.0	31	±3	±3.0	29	27.0	31	±3
		6.1	31+	±3	±3.0	30−	27.5	32−	±3
		6.2	32	±3	±3.0	30	28.0	32	±3
		6.3	32+	±3	±3.0	31	28.5	33−	±3
		6.4	33−	±3	±3.0	32−	29.0	33	±3
		6.5	33	±3	±3.0	32	29.5	34−	±3
		6.6	34−	±3	33−	±3.0	30.0	34	±3
		6.7	34	±3	±3.0	33	30.5	35−	±3
±2	27−	6.8	35−	±3	±3.0	34	31.0	35	±3
±2	27	6.9	35	±3	±3.0	35	31.5	36−	±3
±2	27	7.0	36−	±3	±3.0	36−	32.0	36	2.5
±2	27+	7.1	36	±3	±3.0	36	32.5	37−	2.5
±2	28	7.2	37−	±3	±2.5	37	33.0	37	2.5
±2	28+	7.3	37	±3	±2.5	38−	33.5	38−	2.5
±3	29−	7.4	38−	±3	±2.5	38	34.0	38	2.5
±3	29	7.5	38	±3	±2.5	39	34.5	39−	2.5
±3	29+	7.6	39−	±3	±2.5	40	35.0	39	2.5
±3	30−	7.7	39	±3	±2.5	41−	35.5	40−	2.5
±3	30	7.8	40−	±3	±2.5	42−	36.0	40	2.5
±3	30+	7.9	40	±3	±2.5		36.5	41−	2.5
±3	31	8.0							
±3	31+	8.1							
±3	32	8.2							
±3	32+	8.3							
±3	33−	8.4							
±3	33	8.5							
±3	33+	8.6							
±3	34	8.7							
±3	35−	8.8							
±3	35+	8.9							
±3	36	9.0							
±3	36+	9.1							
±3	37−	9.2							
±3	38−	9.3							
±3	39	9.4							
±3	40	9.5							

* Range: confidence interval for BPD is 90% and for femur, HC, and AC is 95%.

† BPD value represents menstrual dates relative to *composite* mean BPD values.

Note: Plus sign = +1 to +3 days; minus sign = −1 to −3 days.

Source: Adapted from the following references:

Sabbagha, R. E. and Hughey, M.: Standardization of sonar cephalometry and gestational age. *Obstet. Gynecol.* **52:**402–406, 1978.

Hadlock, F. P., Harrist, R. B., Deter, R. L., and Park, S. K. : Fetal femur length as a predictor of menstrual age: Sonographically measured. *Am. J. Roentgenol.* **138:**875–878, 1982.

Hadlock, F. P., Deter, R. L., Harrist, R. B., and Park, S. K.: Fetal head circumference: Relation to menstrual age. *Am. J. Roentgenol.* **138:**649–653, 1982.

Hadlock, F. P., Deter, R. L., Harrist, R. B., and Park, S. K.: Fetal abdominal circumference as a predictor of menstrual age. *Am. J. Roentgenol.* **139:**367–370, 982.

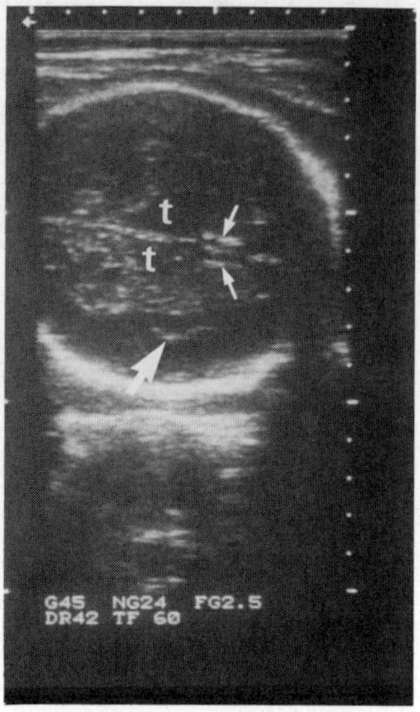

Figure 12-1. Transverse echogram of fetal head defining the anatomic plane for the biparietal diameter. The two thalamic bodies (t) on opposite sides of the midline are shown to the left of the septi pellucidi (small arrows). The latter forms the medial wall of the frontal horns of the lateral ventricles. The large arrow points to the insula (formerly thought to be the Sylvian fissure). The middle cerebral artery can be seen pulsating adjacent to the insula. The area between the insula and the distal parietal complex represents the basal ganglia which normally reflect a translucent echo pattern.

Dating by Other Parameters

Although the predictive accuracy of the HC is similar to that of the BPD, its measurement by a digitizer is more complex. The AC and the binocular distance (Fig. 12-3) are less accurate than other fetal measurements in prediction of dates.[24,31]

Choice of Parameters for Dating

Single BPD. In the second trimester of pregnancy, dates are best estimated by single BPD measurements.[8,10,62] Prior to 26 weeks' gestation, dolichocephaly or side-to-side flattening of the fetal head, which may artificially make the fetus appear to be less mature, occurs infrequently.[23] Furthermore, any change in dates resulting from some narrowing of the BPD is already built into the normal variation expected from cephalometry. Thus, routinely obtaining a cephalic index (BPD/occipitofrontal diameter) on all fetuses regardless of gestational age or the clinical condition cannot be justified. In preterm neonates, antenatal measurement of the cephalic index is inaccurate in predicting which fetus is dolichocephalic or brachycephalic.[44]

When and What to Select. In fetuses at high risk for hydrocephalus, microcephalus, and alteration in the shape of the head (likely to occur in the presence of premature rupture of the membranes or in multiple pregnancy during the third trimester), it is best to use a dimension other than BPD to estimate dates. Similarly, in fetuses at high risk for short limb dysplasia, the femur should not be considered useful for dating.

If dates estimated from menstrual history fall outside the confidence intervals predicted ultrasonically, the latter should be used for assigning the length of pregnancy. By contrast, if menstrual and ultrasonic dates are similar, either method or the average of the two estimates can be used. When the two estimates are similar, the probability of the accuracy of the end point, that is, the expected date of delivery, is enhanced (Bayes' theorem).

Averaging estimates of dates from data derived from different fetal dimensions is not scientifically sound. First, the biologic variation and measurement error for the various fetal parameters is not the same. Thus, by "averaging," equal weight is erroneously given to different fetal dimensions, compounding the error of each method and diluting the contribution of the best predictor.[5,42] Second, in the presence of asymmetric intrauterine growth retardation (IUGR), single fetal measurements such as the HC or the FL should be used, because the AC is more likely to be small. In the presence of symmetric lUGR, all dimensions are small and averaging will not improve the accuracy of dating.

Charts for Dating. A number of BPD, femur, HC, and AC charts are available. Appropriate charts are listed in Tables 12-4 and 12-5. Note that the fetal BPD chart used in Tables 12-4 and 12-5 is not significantly different from the composite mean chart. The latter is derived from a number of studies employing uniform ultrasonic methodology and combining BPD data derived from gravidas of different racial origins, but all residing in locations at or near sea level.[53] Variation in the FL, HC, and AC among different racial groups has not been extensively studied.

TABLE 12-6. BIPARIETAL DIAMETER (BPD) PERCENTILE RANKS FROM 2 TO 40 WEEKS OF GESTATION USED FOR EVALUATING CEPHALIC GROWTH AND SECOND SONAR COMPONENT OF THE GROWTH ADJUSTED SONOGRAPHIC AGE

Fetal Age (wk)	Average Fetus (>25 to <75)	Large Fetus (75 to 95)	Small Fetus (5 to 25)
29	7.4–7.7	7.8–8.3	6.8–7.3
29+	7.5–7.8	7.9–8.4	6.9–7.4
30−	7.6–7.8	7.9–8.5	7.0–7.5
30	7.7–7.9	8.0–8.6	7.1–7.6
30+	7.8–8.0	8.1–8.7	7.2–7.7
31−	7.8–8.0	8.1–8.7	7.2–7.7
31	7.9–8.1	8.2–8.8	7.3–7.8
31+	8.0–8.2	8.3–8.9	7.4–7.9
32−	8.0–8.2	8.3–8.9	7.4–7.9
32	8.1–8.3	8.4–9.0	7.5–8.0
32+	8.2–8.4	8.5–9.0	7.6–8.1
33−	8.3–8.4	8.5–9.1	7.6–8.2
33	8.4–8.5	8.6–9.1	7.7–8.3
33+	8.5–8.6	8.7–9.2	7.8–8.4
34−	8.5–8.7	8.8–9.2	7.8–8.4
34	8.6–8.8	8.9–9.3	7.9–8.5
34+	8.7–8.9	9.0–9.4	8.0–8.6
35−	8.7–8.9	9.0–9.5	8.1–8.6
35	8.8–9.0	9.1–9.6	8.2–8.7
35+	8.9–9.0	9.2–9.6	8.2–8.8
36−	8.9–9.1	9.3–9.6	8.2–8.8
36	9.0–9.2	9.3–9.7	8.3–8.9
37	9.1–9.3	9.4–9.8	8.4–9.0
38	9.2–9.4	9.5–9.9	8.5–9.1
39	9.3–9.5	9.6–10.0	8.7–9.2
40	9.5–9.6	9.7–10.1	8.9–9.4

Second sonar (a) must be done between 30 and 33 weeks because of maximal variation in fetal BPD size in this interval and prior to onset of IUGR in most cases; (b) must be done at least 6 weeks after first BPD.
Source: Modified from Sabbagha, R. E., Hughey, M., and Depp, R.: Growth adjusted sonographic age (GASA): A simplified method. *Obstet. Gynecol.* **51**:383–386, 1978. Reprinted with permission from the American College of Obstetricians and Gynecologists.

Assessment of Growth

Antenatal detection of altered fetal growth (IUGR or macrosomia) by clinical means is possible in less than 50% of growth-altered pregnancies. The reason is partly related to erroneous dates in a large number of cases. By comparison, the diagnosis of abnormal growth can be ruled out in approximately 95% and established, when present, in about 85% of pregnancies examined ultrasonically.

The ultrasonic criteria used in the evaluation of growth include:

1. biometry,
2. estimation of fetal weight,
3. dynamic assessment of fetal activity, and
4. blood velocity studies.

Biometry. The fetal dimensions frequently used to evaluate altered growth include the BPD, HC, AC, and FL. Separate charts detailing growth percentiles relative to each week of pregnancy are available. In Tables 12-6 and 12-7, the normal growth of the BPD and the femur are shown. The utilization of ratios such as HC/AC or FL/AC are generally poor in sensitivity and do not enhance the accuracy of the diagnosis of altered growth achieved by relating the size of single dimensions to normal growth curves.

Fetal Perimeters. The HC and AC can be measured in one of two ways. The first involves derivation of the circumference from two diameters obtained from the outer aspects of either the head or the trunk, as shown in Fig. 12-4. The second is by means of a digitizer that directly measures the actual perimeters. It is important to realize that HCs and ACs derived from these two methods are statistically significantly dif-

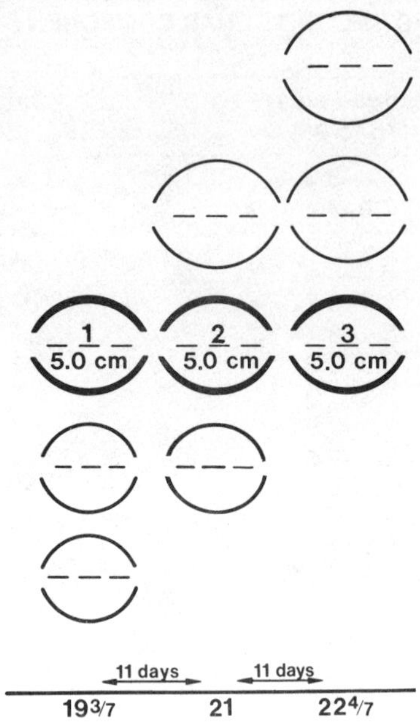

Figure 12-2. An illustration of the variability in the biparietal diameter (BPD) at a mean gestational age of 21 weeks. The three fetuses with a BPD of 5.0 cm differ in gestational age from 19 3/7 weeks to 22 4/7 weeks. However, fetus number 1 with rapid head growth and large BPD is less mature than fetus number 2 or 3. Similarly, fetus number 3 with slow cephalic growth is more mature than the other two fetuses.

ferent from each other. Therefore, separate tables should be used for each method.

When the BPD continues to fall into a normal percentile bracket, IUGR can be ruled out in more than 90% of cases.[50] On the other hand, when the BPD falls below the 25th percentile, the predictive value for IUGR is only 50%.[50] Thus, in the latter situation, the HC and the AC should be obtained in order to place the fetus in one of nine growth brackets (Fig. 12-5). Note that growth patterns 3 or 6 and 9 are at high risk for asymmetric and symmetric IUGR, respectively. By comparison, growth pattern number 1 is at high risk for macrosomia.[63] The predictive value of these patterns in identifying altered growth is about 85%.

Birth Weight. A number of formulas incorporating fetal dimensions are used for the prediction of BW. The error in BW prediction is directly proportional to the actual fetal size and varies from 14% to 20% (2 S. D.).[26]

Weiner et al.[66] published a BW formula designed for use in small fetuses:

$$BW = 94.593\,(HC) + 34.227\,(AC) - 2134.616$$

This formula, when targeted to low-birth-weight fetuses is more accurate than other formulas used for all fetuses. These authors also showed that FL improved the accuracy of BW prediction when specifically used only in fetuses with long or short femur bones.

Utilization of any of the BW formulas is useful in selected clinical situations such as pregnancies at high risk for (1) preterm labor, (2) IUGR, and (3) macrosomia. For example, in gravidas at risk for macrosomia, the accuracy of predicting a large-for-gestational-age fetus by formula is approximately 78%, whereas in low-risk pregnancies, the predictive value of the same formula drops to 57%. Nonetheless, macrosomia can be predicted with an accuracy of 89% if both the AC growth percentile and the estimate of BW (by formula) exceed the 90th percentile.[64]

Dynamic Assessment of Fetal Activity. Fetal functions that can be evaluated ultrasonically include fetal breathing movements (FBM), fetal body motion (FM), hiccups, swallowing, micturition, and eye movements. Routine observation of all of these functions can be time consuming. Additional investigations are necessary to define their sensitivity in the prediction of fetal hypoxia.

Biophysical Profile

Manning et al.[36] suggest that assessment of dynamic functions such as FBM, FM, and fetal tone (FT), as well as amniotic fluid volume (AFV), is accurately predictive of the normal and hypoxic fetus. They examine the fetus for a period of 30 minutes and assign a score of 0 if the dynamic function is absent and 2 if it is present. The biophysical scores were normal in 97.5% of fetuses studied. In the remaining fetuses the scores were either equivocal (6 or less) or abnormal (4 or less). There were only 8 intrauterine fetal deaths in structurally normal fetuses within one week of a normal biophysical score, yielding a false normal rate of 0.63/1000. They compared these data to other studies concerning the false normal rates of the contraction stress test (ST) and the nonstress test (NST), namely, 0.4/1000 and 3.2/1000, respectively.

In the interpretation of the biophysical profile, it is important to appreciate that the differ-

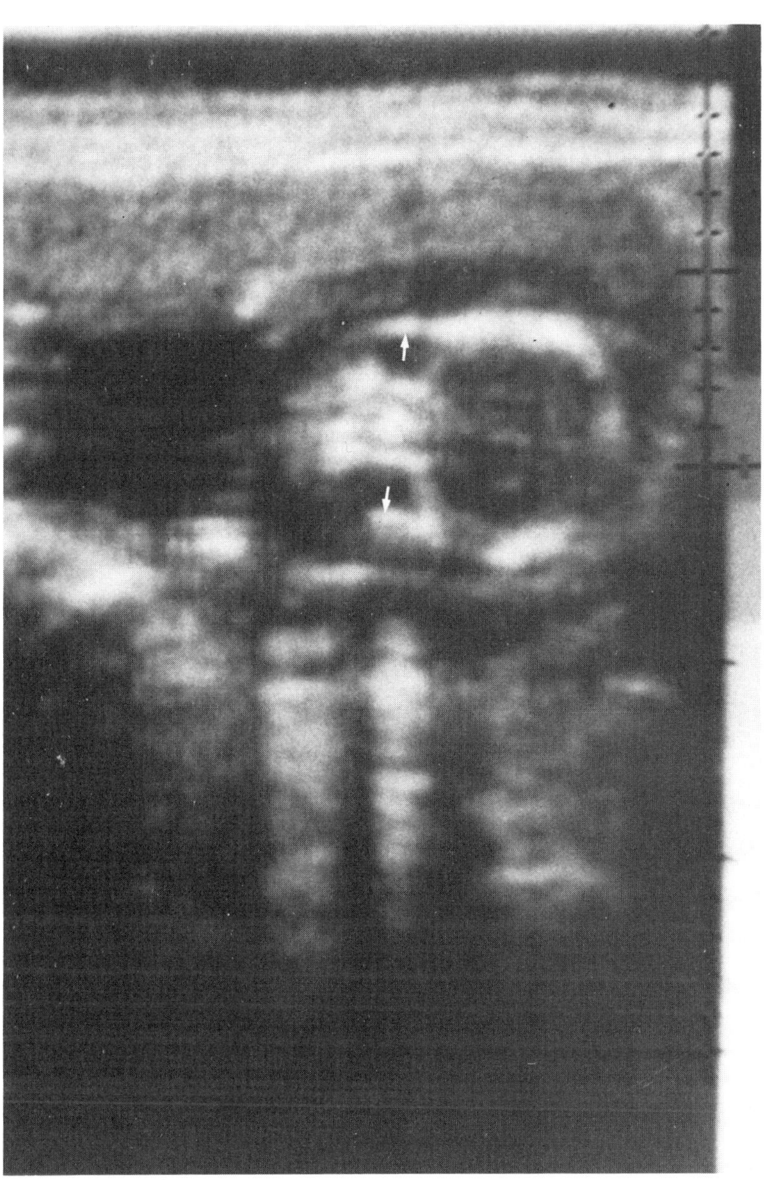

Figure 12-3. Coronal view of fetal orbits. Arrows point to the outer boundaries of the orbits used to measure the binocular distance; the measurement is used as a guideline for determining gestational age and for detection of hypertelorism or hypotelorism.

ent components are not controlled or elicited by the same mechanism.

Specifically, FBMs follow a circadian rhythm, whereas body movements do not.[45] Only FBMs are increased approximately 1.5–2 hours after maternal feeding.[37,40] Furthermore, the effects of a variety of drugs on FM may also be quite different from the effects on FBMs.[34]

Amniotic Fluid Volume (AFV)

The significance of oligohydramnios (single pockets of amniotic fluid with a diameter of 1–3 cm measured in a vertical plane) is controversial. The results of one study involving near-term pregnancies identified as high risk by previous ultrasonic biometry studies or by clinical

TABLE 12-7. THE NUMBER OF MEASUREMENTS TAKEN AND THE MEAN LENGTH ±2 S.D. OF THE ULTRASOUND FEMUR LENGTH FROM 14 WEEKS OF GESTATION TO TERM

Weeks of Gestation	Number of Measurements	Arithmetic Mean (mm)	±2 S.D. (mm)
14	31	16.6	2.5
15	28	19.9	2.3
16	28	22.0	3.0
17	35	25.2	2.9
18	30	29.6	3.1
19	32	32.4	3.1
20	27	34.8	2.5
21	29	37.5	4.1
22	23	40.9	3.9
23	33	43.5	3.6
24	38	46.4	3.5
25	33	48.0	4.6
26	39	51.1	5.0
27	37	53.0	3.2
28	39	54.4	4.1
29	28	57.3	4.3
30	48	58.7	3.8
31	50	61.5	4.5
32	52	62.8	4.2
33	41	64.9	4.6
34	41	65.7	4.4
35	59	67.7	4.8
36	56	69.5	4.6
37	51	70.8	4.3
38	46	71.8	5.6
39	34	74.2	5.1
40	28	75.4	5.6

observation indicate that oligohydramnios (amniotic fluid pocket ≤1 cm) was predictive of IUGR in approximately 89% of cases.[35]

In another study, however, oligohydramnios (amniotic fluid pocket less than 1 cm diameter) accurately predicted only 8% (8/52) of undergrown infants.[29] Other investigators found a 3.9% incidence of oligohydramnios in a large unselected population and showed that the value of the finding in predicting IUGR was 40%. However, the sensitivity of the test was only 16%.[47] These data suggest that oligohydramnios is more significant when associated with high-risk pregnancies diagnosed by clinical and/or other ultrasonic criteria.

Postdate Pregnancies. After 42 weeks' gestation, the presence of oligohydramnios increases the risk for late decelerations requiring cesarean section.[46] A retrospective study of postdate pregnancies showed that when the AFV was marginal (1–2 cm) or decreased (less than 1 cm), fetal heart rate tracings showed decelerations and bradycardia in approximately 44% and 71% of such pregnancies, respectively. The incidence of late decelerations requiring cesarean section was approximately 5% and 17% respectively, an increase over the 1% level found in postdate pregnancies with normal AFV.[46]

Blood Velocity

Doppler Shift. When an ultrasonic beam is directed at an acute angle to a moving target (e.g., blood flowing through an artery), the frequency of the echoes produced is changed. The change in frequency is known as the Doppler shift and is expressed in kilohertz (kHz), a range audible to the human ear. Blood velocity continually changes in response to the systolic and diastolic components of the cardiac cycle. As a result, an ultrasonic beam directed at an artery generates a series of Doppler shifts. These can be continually recorded by means of a Fast Fourier system, producing velocity waveforms

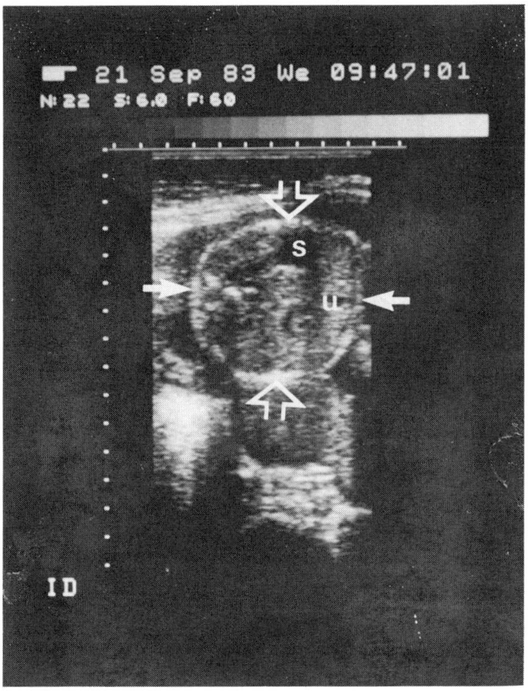

Figure 12-4. Transverse echogram of fetal abdomen showing stomach (s) and small portion of umbilical vein (u). The diameters used are perpendicular to each other and extend from the outer aspects of (a) the spine, left arrow, and anterior abdominal wall, right arrow; and (b) the widest portion of the lateral abdominal walls, open arrows.

(Fig. 12-6). In normal pregnancy, Fourier waveforms display a wide diastolic component, reflecting the low vascular resistance characteristic of the uncompromised intervillous circulation.[15,38,57] When the systolic peak of the velocity waveform (S) is divided by the end diastolic component (D), an S/D ratio is generated. Use of an S/D ratio eliminates the necessity to measure the angle between the incident beam and the blood vessel, because it remains unchanged in the cardiac cycle. In uncomplicated pregnancies, end diastolic velocity continues to increase until term, indicating progressively decreasing resistance in the placental bed. As a result, the S/D ratio declines from 2.8 to 2.2 between midpregnancy and term.[57] In pregnancies complicated by IUGR and/or hypertension with proteinuria, the end diastolic component is increased and S/D ratios as high as 3.8 at 29 weeks' gestation and 3.0 at term are observed [6,57,58]

Recently, Fleischer et al.[19] divided the weight of neonates into four percentile groups: less than 25p, 35–50p, 51–75p, and more than 75p. In the lowest weight group, the S/D ratio was significantly greater than in the other three groups. The predictive value of a positive test (S/D ratio over 3.0) was only 49%, but the sensitivity and specificity were 78% and 83%, respectively. The low predictive value of the test in complicated pregnancies may be related to

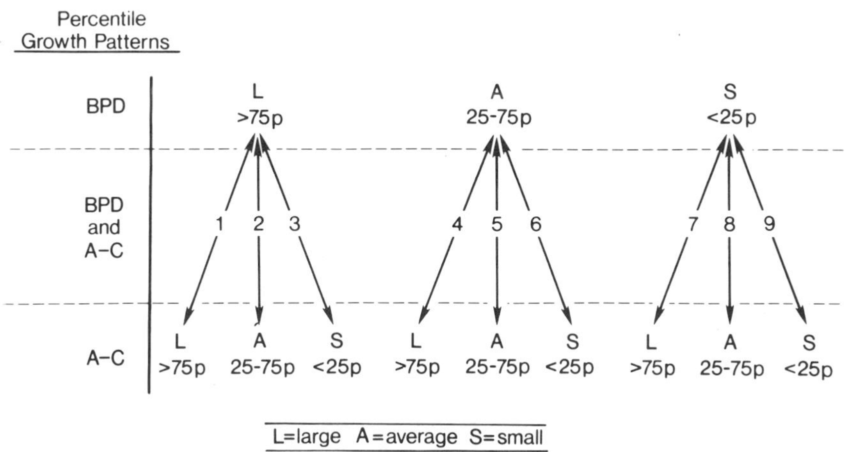

Figure 12-5. Nine fetal growth patterns noted by using both biparietal diameter (BPD) and abdominal circumference (AC) percentiles (p).

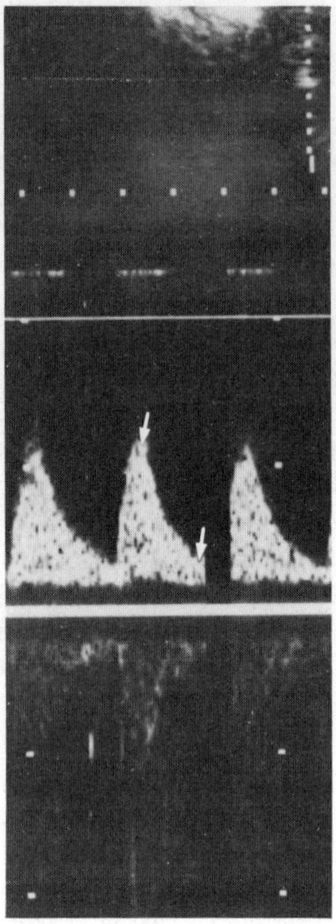

Figure 12-6. Doppler velocity waveforms produced from the umbilical artery. Arrows point to peak systole and end diastole.

compensatory mechanisms that come into play when the fetus is in jeopardy. These mechanisms are related to increases in fetal blood pressure and in extraction of oxygen and substrate.

In complicated pregnancies, elevated S/D ratios are also noted by Doppler studies of the uterine arteries. The increased vascular resistance in such pregnancies is attributed to impaired trophoblastic erosion of the spiral arteries,[6] an event which may precede (1) abnormalities in the velocity waves obtained from any of the umbilical arteries and (2) reduction in fetal head and body size.

Use of Ultrasound as a Secondary Test

Ultrasound is an invaluable adjunct in a variety of diagnostic and therapeutic procedures, including the following:

1. Amniocentesis. Ultrasound is used to define dates, assess the number of fetuses, localize the placenta, and define the most appropriate spot on the maternal abdomen for amniocentesis.
2. Chorionic Villus Sampling (CVS). In the interval of 8–12 weeks' gestation, ultrasound is used to guide the insertion of a catheter to the placenta for sampling villi. The latter are used for DNA analysis, chromosome mapping, and enzymology.[16,59]
3. Rh Disease. Ultrasound is used to (a) define dates for proper interpretation of the OD at 450 um, (b) monitor the development of fetal ascites, and (c) orient percutaneous intraperitoneal or intraumbilical needle insertion into the fetus in pregnancies requiring intrauterine transfusion. Ultrasound is useful in monitoring the degree of sensitization to the Kell antigen. In this condition, the hemolytic process may be very rapid and may result in fetal deterioration prior to any significant change in the concentration of bilirubin in the amniotic fluid.[4]
4. Fetal Pulmonary Maturity. Sonograms allow the placenta to be graded from 0 to III according to homogeneity in texture, internal densities, and undulations that start at the chorionic plate and sometimes extend to the basal plate. In grade III placentas, the undulations reach the basal plate and separate the placenta into distinct cotyledons. A grade III placenta is predictive of fetal pulmonary maturity 91–100% of the time. However, only 15% of term pregnancies show a grade III placenta, despite attainment of fetal pulmonary maturity. Thus, the clinical utility of the test is poor. In the presence of IUGR, a grade III placenta may be seen in the early part of the third trimester of pregnancy.
5. Other areas. See Table 12-1.

Targeted Imaging for Fetal Anomalies (TIFFA)

The indications for TIFFA studies include elevated amniotic fluid alpha-fetoprotein (AF/AFP), history of a previous congenital defect, suspicion of an anomaly on a standard ultrasound examination, and conditions that increase the risk for anomalies, such as IUGR, oligohydramnios, polyhydramnios, breech presentation at term, maternal diabetes mellitus, exposure to teratogens, balanced translocations, and adoption.

The Examination. The ultrasonographer performing TIFFA examinations should obtain a detailed history and should exercise patience in finding the anatomic planes that are more likely to reveal specific defects, if present. The ultrasonographer should be knowledgeable about the following:

1. The differential diagnosis of a variety of abnormal findings such as hypertelorism and hypotelorism (increase or decrease, respectively, in the normal distance between two orbits); cleft lip/palate; nonimmune hydrops; hydrocephalus; microcephalus; macrocephalus; shortlimb dysplasia; soft tissue, thoracic, or abdominal mass.
2. The association of some defects with other anomalies, for example, atrial septal defects with thanatophoric dwarfism, or macrocephaly with achondroplasia, or spina bifida with hydrocephalus.
3. Risk of recurrence of the anomaly in question.

Accuracy of TIFFA Examinations. The accuracy of TIFFA is related to the skill and experience of the ultrasonographer. However, other factors enter into the formula, the most important of which are prevalence of the anomaly in the specific geographic location, screening mandated by information in the history, a pregnancy complication necessitating additional studies, biochemical tests, and/or a standard ultrasound examination.

The predictive value of TIFFA examinations in a variety of anomalies is listed in Table 12-8.[55]

Importance of TIFFA Examinations. TIFFA examinations are essential in management of pregnancies at high risk for birth defects because when the anomaly is known, the couple can be advised about the severity of the lesion, the role of surgical correction in utero or in the neonatal period, and the option of pregnancy termination in selected cases, especially when the defect is not compatible with extrauterine life.

TABLE 12-8. ACCURACY OF TARGETED DYNAMIC IMAGING FOR FETAL ANOMALIES[55]

TIFFA	Congenital Anomaly +	Congenital Anomaly −	Total
Abnormal*	78	4	82
Normal†	3	509	512
Total	81	513	594

* Predictive value of abnormal = 78/82 or 95%.
† Predictive value of normal = 509/512 or 99%.

The information obtained by the sonographer is communicated to the referring physician so that he/she can seek appropriate consultation for in utero or neonatal therapy and can reach a decision regarding the time, place, and mode of delivery.

Specific Anomalies

Craniospinal Defects

Anencephalus. The diagnosis can be suspected by 10–12 weeks of pregnancy by careful examination of the contour of the crown–rump image. The diagnosis should be verified in the early part of the second trimester.

Hydrocephalus. Differentiation between a posterior cyst noted in Dandy-Walker syndrome and aqueductal stenosis is possible if the ventricular system is not completely dilated.[11]

Holoprosencephaly. This condition results from incomplete cleavage of the primitive forebrain. The cerebral hemispheres are separated to variable degrees. In the most severe form or the alobar variety, the falx cerebri and interhemispheric fissure are absent and there is a single ventricle (Fig. 12-7). Facial abnormalities such

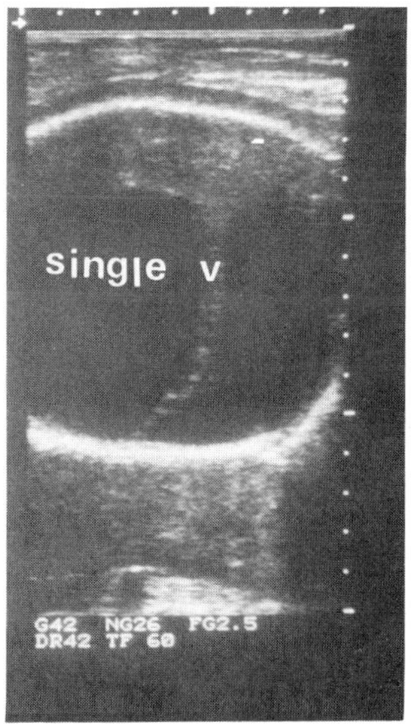

Figure 12-7. Transverse scan of fetus with holoprosencephaly. Note single ventricle with an ill-defined membrane extending across the ventricle. the proximal echoes represent reverberations.

as hypotelorism, cleft lip/palate, and cyclopia (absence of median bones of the face and single orbital cavity) are present. It is possible to differentiate this defect from both hydranencephaly and porencephalic cysts. Hydranencephaly or congenital absence of both cerebral hemispheres is secondary to bilateral internal artery occlusion early in development. Ultrasonically, the cerebrospinal fluid in the brain is seen surrounding the basal ganglia, midbrain, and cerebellum. Isolated porencephalic cysts result from in utero vascular occlusions and infarction of the brain.

Cephaloceles. The term denotes protrusion of meninges through some defect in the skull. However, the bony defect may be quite small and not visualized sonographically. A protrusion of meninges with no neurologic tissue is termed meningocele. By contrast, an encephalocele represents protrusion of meninges and brain tissue.

The abnormality can be differentiated from cystic hygroma and fetal edema by the very thin walls representing meninges, by changes in shape observed with fetal movement and attributed to flow of cerebrospinal fluid to the dependent portion of the sac, and by lack of thick multiple septa characteristic of hygromas.[56]

Microcephalus. The diagnosis is made by careful measurement of the head circumference. In this abnormality, the occipitofrontal diameter is reduced disproportionate to the reduction in the BPD. When microcephalus is suspected, the BPD is not used for dating the pregnancy. Presence of microcephalus will lead to the incorrect assumption that the fetus is less mature than it is. It is doubtful that the diagnosis of microcephalus can be made prior to 20 weeks of pregnancy.

Spina Bifida. The defect is better visualized if associated with a skin-covered meningocele (Fig. 12-8). Lesions located in the sacral area, even when less than 2 cm in diameter, may still be apparent sonographically.[55] The accuracy of a positive ultrasonic finding in diagnosing spina bifida ranges from 79% to 93%.[7,48,55] The predictive value of ultrasonographic absence of spina bifida is 98%.[55] The latter statistic is significant because a normal TIFFA study in the face of abnormal AFP and acetylcholinesterase tests strongly implies that the biochemical markers are falsely positive.[28,65]

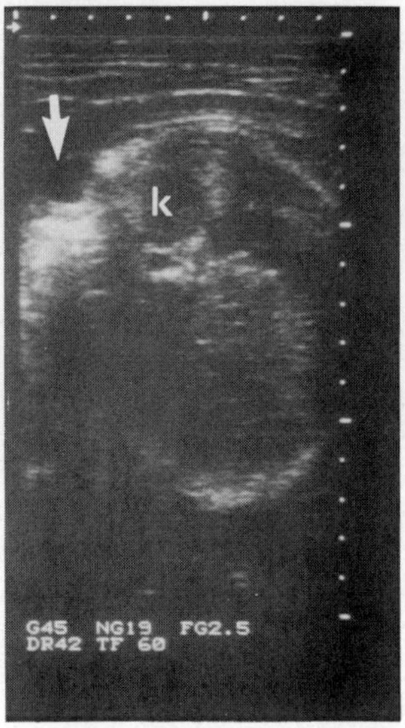

Figure 12-8. Transverse scan of fetal lumbar area showing the left kidney, arrows. The right kidney is shadowed by the spine. Single arrow points to a thin meningocele sac wall covering a V-shaped spina bifida.

Fetal Chest. Ultrasonic imaging of the fetal heart is being rapidly developed. Recognition of fetal arrhythmia and definition of the size of cardiac chambers is possible using M-mode echo-cardiography. The four chamber view can be dynamically examined and diagnoses such as atrial and ventricular septal defects as well as hypoplastic ventricles have been correctly made (Fig.12-9).[12] In some fetuses, the pulmonary and aortic outflow tracts can also be examined. However, the accuracy of ultrasound in the diagnosis of cardiac defects is not yet defined.

Fetal Abdomen. This category includes gastrointestinal (GI), renal, and pelvic abnormalities. Obstruction of the GI tract can manifest in the form of (1) esophageal atresia with absence of the stomach "bubble" normally noted in the upper abdomen; (2) duodenal atresia showing two cystic masses, the stomach and the proximal aspect of the duodenum; and (3) lower GI obstruction, showing multiple large dilated loops of bowel with very thin walls.[30]

Omphalocele can be differentiated from gastroschisis by noting one or more of the following: (1) absence of free-floating bowel in the amniotic cavity, (2) a thin sac surrounding the

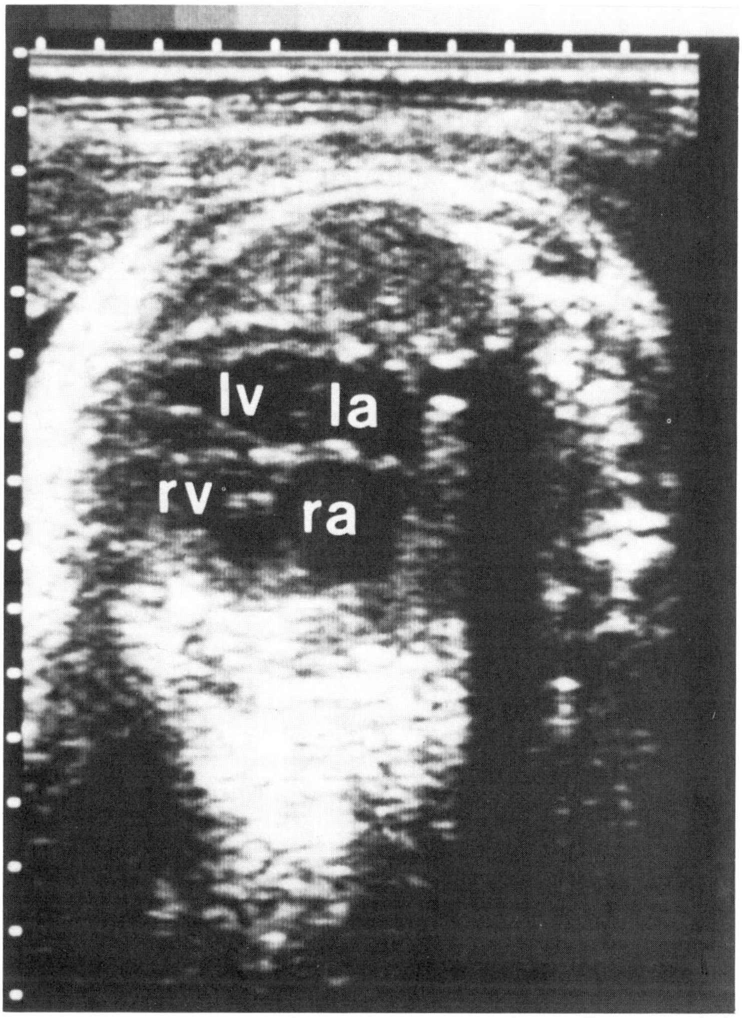

Figure 12-9. Transverse scan of fetal chest showing four-chamber view of the heart. The interventricular septum is clearly seen between the right ventricle (rv) and left ventricle (lv). The foramen ovale is closed. Note the left atrium (la) and right atrium (ra).

herniated portion of bowel, and (3) insertion of the umbilical cord in the apex of the mass (Fig. 12-10).

"GI obstruction" may not become ultrasonically apparent until the third trimester of pregnancy.[41] Approximately 30% of fetuses with duodenal atresia have abnormal karyotypes (usually trisomy 21) and 50% of those with omphalocele have other anomalies mainly involving the fetal heart and karyotype.

Renal dysplasia in the form of polycystic and multicystic disease can be differentiated from hydronephrosis. In the latter condition, obstruction to the ureteropelvic junction or dilation of the ureters is usually apparent. Polycystic renal disease (recessive form) may not become apparent until the third trimester of pregnancy.[60]

Renal agenesis remains difficult to diagnose because:

1. Imaging of the fetus is obscured by oligohydramnios.
2. Hypertrophied adrenal glands can simulate the echoes produced by the kidneys (Fig. 12-11).
3. Fat deposits in the renal bed can simulate renal echoes (fig. 12-11).

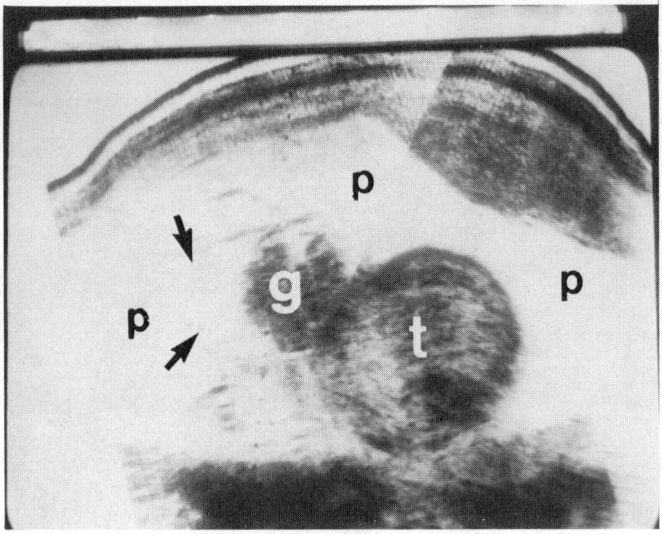

Figure 12-10. Transverse scan of fetal trunk (t) showing omphalocele (g) and thin membrane covering the gut (arrows). Polyhydramnios (p) is also noted.

4. The "furosemide challenge" has not been uniformly successful in outlining the fetal bladder, particularly in IUGR fetuses with intact kidneys.[49]

Other Anomalies

1. Short limb dysplasia can be diagnosed by comparison of fetal limb length to established standards. The diagnosis of some forms of skeletal dysplasia, such as heterozygous achondroplasia, cannot be made prior to 20 weeks' gestation.[18]
2. Abnormalities of the integument such as chronic granulomatous skin disease, harlequin ichthyosis, and epidermolysis bullosa can be diagnosed by ultrasonically directed fetoscopy.[17]
3. Facial abnormalities such as cleft lip/palate are discernible. The binocular distance is used to diagnose hypertelorism and hypotelorism (Fig. 12-3).
4. Polyhydramnios is diagnosed when a pocket of amniotic fluid, ultrasonically visualized in a vertical plane, exceeds 7–8 cm (see Fig. 12-10.).[18] Approximately 20–25% of such pregnancies are associated with

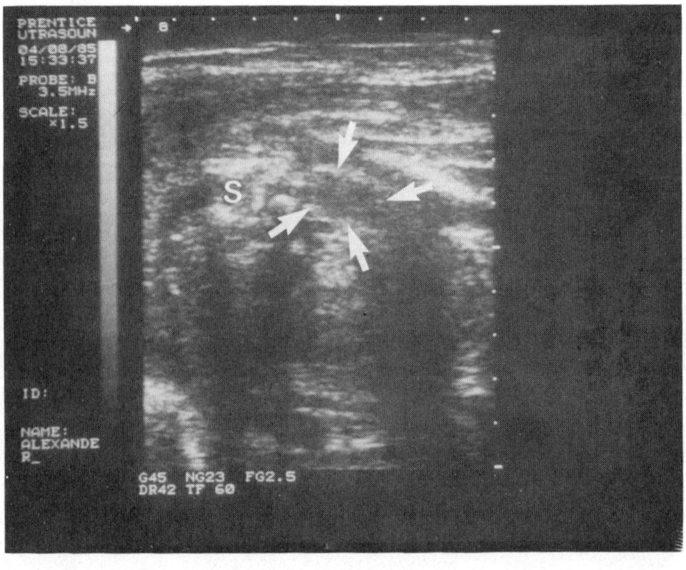

Figure 12-11. Cross section of fetal lumbar area. Note spine (s) and kidney-like echoes in a fetus with renal agenesis.

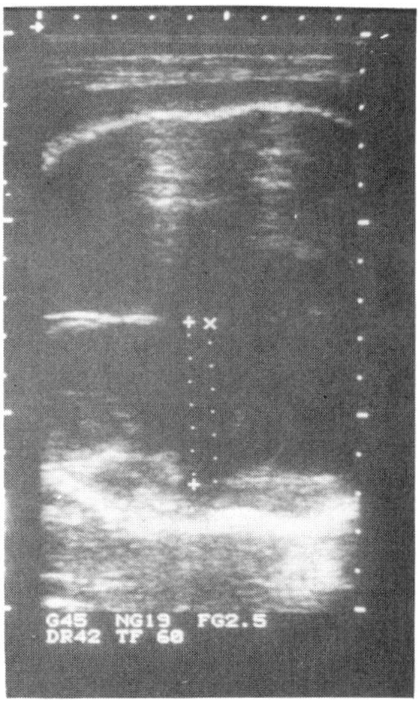

Figure 12-12. Transverse scan of fetal head in hydrocephalic fetus showing enlarged ventricle (+ signs) and hemispheric distance (x letters). The ventricular/hemispheric (V/H) ratio is abnormal: 86%.

fetal anomalies, some of which (e.g., endocardial fibroelastosis) may be difficult to diagnose by ultrasound.[55]

In Utero Surgery

Presently, a number of centers in the United States are examining, on an experimental basis, the possible benefit to the placement of in utero diversion shunts, under ultrasonic guidance. Three abnormalities lend themselves to in utero surgery: hydrocephalus, urethral obstruction, and diaphragmatic hernia.

Hydrocephalus. The diagnosis of hydrocephalus is made when the width of the lateral ventricles relative to that of the cerebral hemispheres or V/H ratio exceeds 30–35% (Fig. 12-12).[33] However, between 14 and 16 weeks' gestation, the V/H ratio normally exceeds this ratio. The diagnosis may be difficult to establish at this time in pregnancy, unless ventricular dilatation is extensive.

The selection criteria used for in utero surgery include progressive hydrocephalus, differentiation from other cystic lesions in the brain, absence of other anomalies, normal karyotype, and discovery of the condition, prior to 32 weeks' gestation. In utero surgery for hydrocephalus is not utilized at present.

Urethral Obstruction. This condition results in dilatation of the bladder, ureters, and renal pelvis. In male fetuses, the obstruction is usually secondary to a posterior urethral valve, in which case, the proximal portion of the urethra may appear dilated (Fig. 12-13).[27] In female fetuses, the condition is secondary to urethral atresia and is uncommon.

On a theoretical basis, shunting of urine from the fetal bladder to the amniotic cavity relieves the backpressure on the renal pelvis, preventing

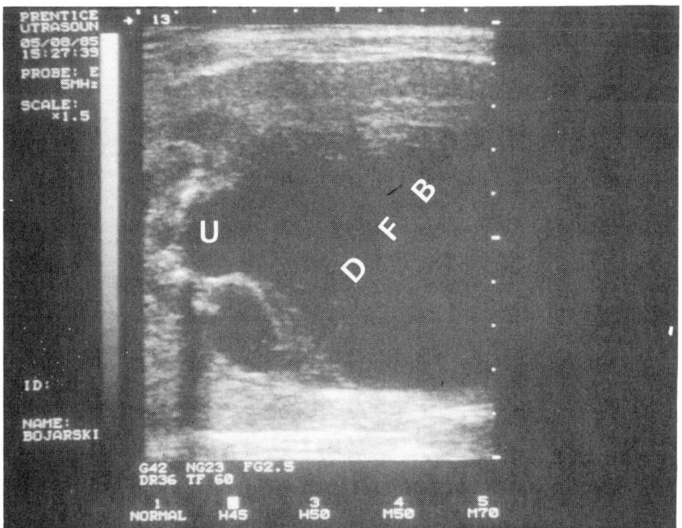

Figure 12-13. Transverse scan of lower abdomen in a fetus with posterior urethral valve obstruction. Note dilated fetal bladder (DFB) and proximal end of urerthra (u).

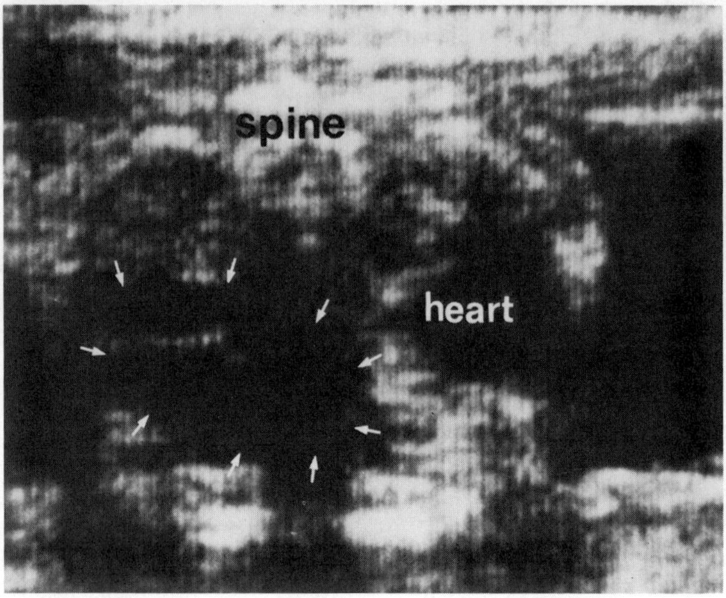

Figure 12-14. Transverse scan of fetal chest showing large cystadenomatoid malformation of the lung (arrows) and displacement of the heart (large arrow) to the right side.

destruction of renal parenchyma. The prognosis depends on a number of factors including (1) severity of oligohydramnios, (2) presence of other anomalies, and (3) whether or not shunting is instituted early enough in pregnancy to allow expansion of the chest and prevention of secondary pulmonary hypoplasia, a common cause of fetal demise.

The differential diagnosis of urethral obstruction includes a mesodermal defect of the urinary system and abdominal wall[20,55] and ureterovesical obstruction, the latter resulting in massive dilation of the ureters and hydronephrosis.[55] The benefit of shunting in either of these anomalies is not known.

Diaphragmatic Hernia. At present, in utero treatment of this abnormality is being carried out only in experimental animals. The abnormality should be differentiated from other masses in the chest such as cystic adenomatoid malformation (Fig. 12-14). In the latter condition, the "stomach bubble" is usually visualized in the upper abdomen.[2]

REFERENCES

1. Anderson, H. F., Johnson T. R., Barclay, L. M., and Flora, J..: Gestational age assessment. I. Analysis of individual clinical observations. *Am. J. Obstet. Gynecol.* **139**:173–177, 1981.
2. Asher, J. B., Sabbagha, R. E., Tamura, R. K., Luck, S., and Gerbie, A. B.: Fetal pulmonary cyst: Intrauterine diagnosis and management. *Am. J. Obstet. Gynecol.* **151**:97–98, 1985.
3. Benson, R. C., Berendes, H., and Weiss, W.: Fetal compromise during elective cesarean section. *Am. J. Obstet. Gynecol.* **105**:579–588, 1969.
4. Berkowitz, R. L., Beyth, Y., and Sadovsky, E.: Death in utero due to Kell sensitization without excessive elevation of the OD 450 value in amniotic fluid. *Obstet. Gynecol.* **60**:746–748, 1982.
5. Bowie, J. and Andreotti, R.: Estimating gestational age in utero. In: *Ultrasonography in Obstetrics and Gynecology.* P. Callen (Ed.). Philadelphia, W. B. Saunders Company, 1983, pp. 21–39.
6. Brosens, I., Dixon, H. J., and Robertson, W. B.: Fetal growth retardation and arteries of the placental bed. *Br. J. Obstet. Gynaecol.* **64**:656–664, 1979.
7. Campbell, S.: Ultrasound in obstetrics and gynaecology: Recent advances. *Clin. Obstet. Gynaecol.* **10**:475–506, 1983.
8. Campbell, S., Warsof, S. L., Little, D., and Cooper, D. J.: Routine ultrasound screening for the prediction of gestational age. *Obstet. Gynecol.* **65**:613–620, 1985.
9. Chamberlain, P. F., Manning, F. A., Morrison, I., Harman, C. R., and Lange, I. R.: Ultrasound evaluation of amniotic fluid volume. II. The relationship of increased amniotic fluid volume to

perinatal outcome. *Am. J. Obstet. Gynecol.* **150**:250–254, 1984.

10. Crane, J. P., Martin, C., Kopta, M. M., and Knight, A. B.: Accuracy of single versus multiple ultrasonic parameters in determining fetal age in timed pregnancies. Scientific Program and Abstracts of the 32nd Annual Meeting of the Society for Gynecologic Investigation, Phoenix, AZ, 1985, p. 246 (Abstract 65P).
11. Depp, R., Sabbagha, R. E., Brown, T. J., Tamura, R. K., and Reedy, N. J.: Fetal surgery for hydrocephalus: Successful in utero ventriculo-amniotic shunt for Dandy–Walker syndrome. *Obstet. Gynecol.* **61**:710–714, 1983.
12. De Vore, G. R.: Fetal echocardiography—A new frontier. *Clin. Obstet. Gynecol.* **27**:359–377, 1984.
13. Dewhurst, C. J., Beazley, J. M., and Campbell, S.: Assessment of fetal maturity and dysmaturity. *Am. J. Obstet. Gynecol.* **113**:141–149, 1972.
14. Diagnostic ultrasound imaging in pregnancy. U.S. Department of Health and Human Service. Public Health services, National Institutes of Health publication no. 84–667, 1984.
15. Eik-Nes, S. H., Brubakk, A. O., and Ulstein, M. K.: Measurement of human fetal blood flow. *Lancet* **1**:283–284, 1980.
16. Elias, S., Martin, A. O., Simpson, J. L., Sabbagha, R. E., and Gerbie, A. B.: Chorionic villus sampling for first trimester prenatal diagnosis. *Am. J. Obstet. Gynecol.* **152**:204–213, 1985.
17. Elias, S., Mazur, M., Sabbagha, R. E., Esterly, N. B., and Simpson, J. L.: The prenatal diagnosis of harlequin ichthyosis. *J. Clin. Genet.* **17**:275–280, 1980.
18. Filly, R. A., Golbus, M. S., Carey, J. C., and Hall, J. G.: Short-limbed dwarfism: Ultrasonographic diagnosis by mensuration of fetal femoral length. *Radiology* **138**:653–656, 1981.
19. Fleischer, A., Schulman, H., Farmakides, G., Bracero, L., Blattner, P., and Randolph, G.: Umbilical artery velocity waveforms and intrauterine growth retardation. *Am. J. Obstet. Gynecol.* **151**:502–505, 1985.
20. Garris, J., Kangarloo, H., Sarti, D., Sample, W. F., and Smith, L. E.: The ultrasound spectrum of prune-belly syndrome. *J. Clin. Ultrasound* **8**:117–120, 1980.
21. Goldenberg, R. L. and Nelson, K.: Iatrogenic respiratory distress syndrome. *Am. J. Obstet. Gynecol.* **123**:617–620, 1975.
22. Hack, M., Fanaroff, A. A., Klaus, M. H., Mendelawitz, B. D., and Merkatz, I. R.: Neonatal respiratory distress following elective delivery. A preventable disease? *Am. J. Obstet. Gynecol.* **126**:43–47, 1976.
23. Hadlock, F.P., Deter, R. L., Harrist, R. B., and Park, S. K.: Neonatal respiratory distress following elective delivery. A preventable disease? *Am. J. Obstet. Gynecol.* **126**:43–47, 1976.
24. Hadlock, F. P., Deter, R. L., Harrist, R. B., and Park, S. K.: Fetal abdominal crcumference as a predictor of menstrual age. *Am. J. Roentgenol.* **139**:367–370, 1982.
25. Hadlock, F. P., Deter, R. L., Harrist, R. B., and Park, S. K.: Ultrasonically measured fetal femur length as a predictor of menstrual age. *Am. J. Roentgenol.* **138**:875–878, 1982.
26. Hadlock, F. P., Harrist, R. B., Sharman, R. S., Deter, R. L., and Park, S. K.: Estimation of fetal weight with the use of head, body, and femur measurements—A prospective study. *Am. J. Obstet. Gynecol.* **151**:333–337, 1985.
27. Hobbins, J. C., Romero, R., Grannum, P., Berkowitz, R. L., Cullen, M., and Mahoney, M. Antenatal diagnosis of renal anomalies with ultrasound. *Am. J. Obstet. Gynecol.* **148**:868–877, 1984.
28. Hobbins, J. C., Venus, I., Tortora, M., Mayden, K., and Mahoney, M. J.: Stage II ultrasound examination for the diagnosis of fetal abnormalities with an elevated amniotic fluid alpha-fetoprotein concentration. *Am. J. Obstet. Gynecol.* **142**:1026–1029, 1982.
29. Hoddick, W. H., Callen, P. W., Filly, R. A., and Creasy, R. K.: Ultrasonographic determination of qualitative fluid volume in intrauterine growth retardation: Reassessment of the 1 cm rule. *Am. J. Obstet. Gynecol.* **149**:758–762, 1984.
30. Jassani, M. N., Gauerer, M. W. L., Fanaroff, A., Fletcher, B., and Merkatz, I. R.: A perinatal approach to the diagnosis and management of gastrointestinal malformations. *Obstet. Gynecol.* **59**:33–39, 1982.
31. Jeanty, P., Cantraine, F., Cousaert, E., Romero, R., and Hobbins, J.C.: The binocular distance. A new way to estimate fetal age. *J. Ultrasound Med.* **3**:241–243, 1984.
32. Jeanty, P., Rodesch, F., Delbeke, D., and Dumont, J. E.: Estimation of gestational age from measurements of fetal long bones. *J. Ultrasound Med.* **3**:75–79, 1984.
33. Johnson, M. L., Dunne, M. G., Mack, L. A., and Rashbaum, C. L.: Evaluation of fetal intracranial anatomy by static and real time ultrasound. *J. Clin. Ultrasound* **8**:311–318, 1980.
34. Lewis, P. J., Trudinger, B. J., and Mangez, J.: Effect of maternal glucose ingestion on fetal breathing and body movements in late pregnancy. *Br. J. Obstet. Gynaecol.* **85**:86–89, 1978.
35. Manning, F. A., Hill, L. M., and Platt, L. D.: Qualitative amniotic fluid volume determination by ultrasound-antepartum detection of intrauterine growth retardation. *Am. J. Obstet. Gynecol.* **139**:254–258, 1981.
36. Manning, F. A., Morrison, I., Lange, M. B., Harman, C. R., and Chamberlain P. F.: Fetal assessment based on fetal biophysical scoring: Experience in 12,620 referred high-risk pregnancies; perinatal mortality by frequency and etiology. *Am. J. Obstet. Gynecol.* **151**:343–350, 1985.
37. Manning, F. A., WynPugh, E., and Boddy, K.: Effect of cigarette smoking on fetal breathing

movements in normal pregnancies. *Br. Med. J.* **1**:552–553, 1975.
38. McCallum, W. D., Williams, C. S., Napell, S., and Diagle, R. E.:. Fetal blood velocity wave forms. *Am. J. Obstet. Gynecol.* **132**:425–429, 1978.
39. Miller, M. M., Tamura, R. K., Vaisrub, N., and Sabbagha, R. E.: Methods for dating pregnancy. *J. Ultrasound Med.* **3**:138–142, 1984.
40. Natale, R., Patrick, J., and Richardson, B.: Effect of human maternal venous plasma glucose concentrations on fetal breathing movements. *Am. J. Obstet. Gynecol.* **132**:36–41, 1978.
41. Nelson, L. H., Clark, C. E., Fishburne, J. I., Urban, R. B., and Penry, R. F.: Value of serial sonography in the in utero detection of duodenal atresia. *Obstet. Gynecol.* **59**:657–660, 1982.
42. O'Brien, W., Coddington, C., and Cefalo, R.: Serial ultrasonographic biparietal diameters for prediction of estimated date of confinement. *Am. J. Obstet. Gynecol.* **138**:467–468, 1980.
43. O'Brien, G. D., Queenan, J. T., and Campbell, S.: Assessment of gestational age in the second trimester by real-time ultrasound measurement of the femur length. *Am. J. Obstet. Gynecol.* **139**:540–545, 1981.
44. O'Keeffe, D. F., Garite, T. J., Elliott, J. P., and Burns, P. E.: The accuracy of estimated gestational age based on ultrasound measurement of biparietal diameter in preterm premature rupture of the membranes. *Am. J. Obstet. Gynecol.* **151**:309–312, 1985.
45. Patrick, J., Natale, R., and Richardson, B.: Patterns of human fetal breathing activity at 34–35 weeks' gestational age. *Am. J. Obstet. Gynecol.* **132**:507–513, 1978.
46. Phelan, J. P., Platt, L. D., Yeh, S. Y., Broussard, P., and Paul, R. H.: The role of ultrasound assessment of amniotic fluid volume in the management of the postdate pregnancy. *Am. J. Obstet. Gynecol.* **151**:304–308, 1985.
47. Philipson, E. H., Sokol, R. J., and Williams, T.: Oligohydramnios: Clinical associations and predictive value for intrauterine growth retardation. *Am. J. Obstet. Gynecol.* **146**:271–278, 1983.
48. Robinson, H. P., Hood, V. D., Gibson, A. A. M., and Ferguson-Smith, M. A.: Diagnostic ultrasound: Early detection of fetal neural tube defects. *Obstet. Gynecol.* **56**:705–710, 1980.
49. Romero, R., Cullen, M., Grannum, P., Jeanty, P., Reece, E. A., Venus, I., and Hobbins, J. C.: Antenatal diagnosis of renal anomalies with ultrasound. III. Bilateral renal agenesis. *Am. J. Obstet. Gynecol.* **151**:38–43, 1985.
50. Sabbagha, R. E.: Intrauterine growth retardation: Antenatal diagnosis by ultrasound. *Obstet. Gynecol.* **52**:252–256, 1978.
51. Sabbagha, R. E.: Intrauterine growth retardation avenues of future research in diagnosis and management by ultrasound. *Semin. Perinatol.* **8**:31–36, 1984.
52. Sabbagha, R. E., Barton, B. A., Barton, F. B., Kingas, E., Orgill, J., and Turner, J. H.: Sonar biparietal diameter. II. Predictive of three fetal growth patterns leading to a closer assessment of gestational age and neonatal weight. *Am. J. Obstet. Gynecol.* **126**:485–490, 1976.
53. Sabbagha, R. E. and Hughey, M.: Standardization of sonar cephalometry and gestational age. *Obstet. Gynecol.* **52**:402–406, 1978.
54. Sabbagha, R. E., Hughey, M., and Depp, R.: Growth adjusted sonographic age (GASA): A simplifed method. *Obstet. Gynecol.* **51**:383–386, 1978.
55. Sabbagha, R. E., Sheikh, Z., Tamura, R. K., DalCompo, S., Simpson, J. L., Depp, R., and Gerbie, A. B.: The predictive value, sensitivity, and specificity of targeted imaging for fetal anomalies in gravidas at high risk for fetal anomalies. *Am. J. Obstet. Gynecol.*, in press.
56. Sabbagha, R. E., Tamura, R. K., Dalcompo, S., Salvino, C., Shkolnik, A., and Gerbie, R. E.: Fetal cranial and craniocervical masses: Ultrasound characteristics and differential diagnoses. *Am. J. Obstet. Gynecol.* **138**:511–517, 1980.
57. Schulman, H., Fleischer, A., Stern, W., Farmakides, G., Jagani, N., and Blattner, P.: Umbilical velocity wave ratios in human pregnancy. *Am. J. Obstet. Gynecol.* **148**:985–990, 1984.
58. Shepherd, B. L. and Bonnar, J.: An ultrasound study of uteroplacental spiral arteries in hypertensive and normotensive pregnancy and fetal growth retardation. *Br. J. Obstet. Gynaecol.* **88**:695–705, 1981.
59. Simoni, G., Brambabti, B., Danesono, C., Terzoli, G.L., Romitti, I., Roselle, F., and Fraccaro, M.: Diagnostic application of first trimester trophoblast sampling in 100 pregnancies. *Hum. Genet.* **66**:252–259, 1984.
60. Simpson, J. L., Sabbagha, R. E., Elias, S., Talbot, C., and Tamura, R. K.: Failure to detect polycystic kidneys in utero by second trimester ultrasonography. *Hum. Genet.* **60**:295–296, 1982.
61. Smazal, S. F., Weisman, L. E., Hopper, K. D., Ghaed, N., and Shirts, S.: Comparative analysis of ultrasonographic methods of gestational age assessment. *J. Ultrasound Med.* **2**:147–150, 1983.
62. Smeltzer, J. S., Normoyle, J., and Sabbagha, R. E.: Ultrasonic estimation of gestational age: Superiority of the BPD and fronto-occipital diameter over other parameters. Scientific Program and Abstracts of the 32nd Annual Meeting of the Society for Gynecologic Investigation, Phoenix, AZ, 1985, p. 246 (Abstract 437).
63. Tamura, R. K. and Sabbagha, R. E.: Percentile ranks of sonar fetal abdominal circumference measurements. *Am. J. Obstet. Gynecol.* **138**:475–479, 1980.
64. Tamura, R. K., Sabbagha, R. E., Depp, R., Dooley, S. L., and Socol, M. L.: Diabetic macrosomia:

Accuracy of third trimester ultrasound. *Obstet. Gynecol.*, in press.

65. Verp, M. S., Milunsky, A., Simpson, J. L., Graham, A., and Sabbagha, R. E.: Elevated alpha-fetoprotein and acetylcholinesterase associated with hydrocele. *Am. J. Med. Genet.* **19**:651–652, 1984.
66. Weiner, C. P., Sabbagha, R. E., Vaisrub, N., and Socol, M. L.: Ultrasonic fetal weight prediction: The role of head circumference and femur length. *Obstet. Gynecol.* **65**:812–817, 1985.

13

ANTENATAL DIAGNOSIS AND GENETIC SCREENING FOR GENETIC DISORDERS

Approximately 3% of liveborn infants have a major congenital anomaly. About one-half of these major congenital anomalies are evident at birth. The remainder become evident later in life. Since prenatal diagnosis of genetic disorders was first accomplished in 1968, enormous advances have been made. Application of molecular genetics for diagnostic purposes is proving especially helpful.[46]

In this chapter the surgical techniques necessary for prenatal diagnosis are presented first. Thereafter, disorders amenable to genetic sceening and prenatal diagnosis are discussed. The material inevitably reflects the author's previous reviews of this topic.[41,49]

SPECTRUM OF GENETIC DISEASE

Phenotypic variation—normal or abnormal—may be considered in terms of several etiologic categories: (1) chromosomal abnormalities, numerical or structural; (2) single-gene (mendelian) disorders; (3) polygenic/multifactorial disorders (polygenic inheritance implies etiology resulting from cumulative effects of more than one gene, whereas multifactorial implies interaction with environmental factors as well); or (4) teratogenic disorders, which are caused by exposure to exogenous factors (e.g., drugs) that deleteriously affect an embryo otherwise destined to develop normally. Principles of these mechanisms are discussed elsewhere.[46] The first two are especially familiar to most physicians.

From surveys of more than 50,000 liveborn neonates, it is established that the incidence of chromosomal aberrations is 1:160 (Table 13-1). In addition to the 0.6% liveborns who are phenotypically abnormal as a result of chromosomal aberrations, some 1% are abnormal as a result of a single-gene mutation. There exist at least 934 autosomal dominant, 588 autosomal recessive, and 115 X-linked disorders. Even the most common mendelian disorders (cystic fibrosis in Caucasians, sickle cell anemia in Blacks, β-thalassemia in Greeks and Italians, α-thalassemia in Southeast Asians, Tay–Sachs disease in Ashkenazi Jews) are individually rare. Only sickle cell anemia has an incidence greater than 1 per 1000 in any ethnic group. In aggregate, however, mendelian disorders result in 1% of liveborns having a congenital defect.

Another 1% of neonates are abnormal but show a normal chromosomal complement and have not apparently undergone mutation at a single genetic locus. Included in this group are most common anomalies limited to a single organ system—for example, hydrocephaly, anencephaly and spina bifida (neural tube defects), facial clefts (cleft lip and palate), cardiac defects, pyloric stenosis, omphalocele, hip dislocation, uterine fusion defects, and club foot (Table 13-2). After birth of one affected child, the recurrence risk in subsequent progeny is 1–5%.[46] This is less than would be expected if only a single gene were responsible, but greater than expected for the general population. Risks are also 1–5% for offspring of affected parents.

TABLE 13-1. CHROMOSOMAL ABNORMALITIES IN LIVEBORN INFANTS AT VARIOUS MATERNAL AGES

Maternal Age	Incidence of Down's Syndrome	Incidence of All Chromosome Abnormalities*
20	1/1667	1/526*
21	1/1667	1/526*
22	1/1429	1/500*
23	1/1429	1/500*
24	1/1250	1/476*
25	1/1250	1/476*
26	1/1176	1/476*
27	1/1111	1/455*
28	1/1053	1/435*
29	1/1000	1/417*
30	1/952	1/384*
31	1/909	1/384*
32	1/769	1/322*
33	1/625	1/317
34	1/500	1/260
35	1/385	1/204
36	1/294	1/164
37	1/227	1/130
38	1/175	1/103
39	1/137	1/82
40	1/106	1/65
41	1/82	1/51
42	1/64	1/40
43	1/50	1/32
44	1/38	1/25
45	1/30	1/20
46	1/23	1/15
47	1/18	1/12
48	1/14	1/10
49	1/11	1/7

* 47,XXX excluded for ages 20–32 (data not available). Data of Hook and colleagues.[22, 23]

That recurrence risks are similar for sibs and offspring almost eliminates environmental causes as the exclusive etiologic factor. It is unlikely that households in different generations would be exposed to the same teratogen. Also excluding environmental factors as sole etiologic agents is the observation that monozygotic twins are much more often similarly affected (concordant) than are dizygotic twins, despite both types of twin sharing a common uterus.

All the above observations are best explained on the basis of polygenic/multifactorial inheritance. Principles are reviewed elsewhere in detail.[46] It is relevant to reiterate that only a few genes are required to produce the number of genotypes necessary to explain recurrence risks of 1–5%. That is, large numbers of genes and complex mechanisms need not be involved. Polygenic/ multifactorial etiology can reasonably be held responsible for most abnormal liveborns who have normal chromosomes and who have no mendelian mutations. Of course, proved teratogens (about twenty) are known.

Only a few comments are needed to reinforce the notion that the burden of genetic diseases on society is high. Genetic disorders account for about 20% of pediatric hospital admissions, and for an even higher percentage of long-term admissions. This already high total does not even include many disorders (e.g., diabetes mellitus) known to be influenced by heritable tendencies. An additional example of the burden of genetic disease is that about 20% of heart attacks in men under 60 years occur in those with a mendelian disorder of lipid metabolism.

TABLE 13-2. FREQUENCY OF UNBALANCED OFFSPRING AT AMNIOCENTESIS OR CHORIONIC VILLUS SAMPLING

Sex of Heterozygote		Amniocentesis*		Chorionic Villus Sampling†	
Pooled reciprocal translocations (all types)					
	Father	27/231	(11.75%)		
	Mother	44/378	(11.6%)		
	Not stated			7/19	(38.9%)
Pooled Robertsonian translocations (all types)					
	Father	0/119		0/7	
	Mother	28/293	(9.6%)‡	5/17	(29.4%)
Specific Robertsonian translocations					
13*q*14*q*	Father	0.73			
	Mother	0/157			
13*q*21*q*	Father	0/11			
	Mother	2/20	(10%)		
14*q*21*q*	Father	0/51			
	Mother	21/137	(15.3%)		
21*q*22*q*	Father	0/3			
	Mother	3/19	(15.8%)		
Pooled inversions (all types)					
	Father	2/51	(4.0%)		
	Mother	5/67	(7.5%)		
	Not stated			0/3	

* Boué and Gallano.[5]
† Mikkelsen.[32]
‡ All except one unbalanced offspring occurred in a translocation involving No. 21. Risk can be calculated as 10–15% if translocation involves a No. 21, but much lower if this chromosome is not involved.

COUNSELING THE APPARENTLY NORMAL COUPLE

Eliciting Genetic Information

One first should determine whether the patient, her husband, or their families have a disorder that might prove heritable. Inquire about the health of first-degree relatives (sibs, parents, offspring), second-degree relatives (uncles, aunts, nephews, nieces, and grandparents), and third-degree relatives (first cousins). Elicit abnormal reproductive outcomes, specifically spontaneous abortions, stillborns, and anomalous liveborn infants. Record drug exposure by husband and wife, including not only agents currently being taken, but also noxious agents (e.g., chemotherapeutic agents) to which exposure occurred prior to pregnancy.

Parental ages should be recorded, for indeed the most common indication for prenatal diagnosis is advanced maternal age. Advanced maternal age warrants discussion irrespective of a patient's difficulties in achieving pregnancy or the physician's convictions regarding pregnancy termination. Fathers over 55 years may be at increased risk for aneuploid offspring, and beginning in the fifth decade are definitely at increased risk for new dominant mutations. Unfortunately, the latter are not amenable to prenatal diagnosis.

Ethnic origin should be recorded. Ashkenazi Jews are at increased risk for offspring with Tay–Sachs disease and should be screened to determine heterozygote status (frequency 1/27). Increasing availability of prenatal diagnostic techniques also makes advisable routine heterozygote screening for β-thalassemia in Italians and Greeks, sickle cell anemia in Blacks, and α-thalassemia in Southeast Asians.

Some individuals consider it useful to obtain genetic information through use of questionnaires or checklists, often constructed to require action only to positive responses.

Communication

In counseling, one should use terms readily comprehensible to patients yet avoid a patronizing attitude. This truism is obvious but actually is much easier said than done. It is useful to preface remarks with a few sentences recounting the major causes of genetic abnormalities: cytogenetic, single gene, polygenic/multifactorial (can be labeled "complex"), and environmental. Write out unfamiliar words and use tables or diagrams to reinforce important concepts. Repetition is essential. Allow time not only to answer questions but also to allow couples to talk with each other to formulate their concerns.

In complex cases, written information (letters) serves as a useful permanent record, allays misunderstanding, and is helpful in dealing with relatives. For more common problems—advanced maternal age, repetitive abortions, previous offspring with neural tube defects, previous trisomic offspring—brochures or preprinted forms not only suffice but have the advantage of emphasizing that a couple's problem is not unique.

Nondirective Counseling

Most geneticists subscribe to the thesis that a counselor should provide information but not dictate (direct) a particular course of action. Of course, completely nondirective counseling is probably a myth. Witness, for example, the impact of a counselor's unwitting facial expressions, from which unstated opinions can be deduced readily. Merely offering antenatal diagnostic services implies an element of approval. It is difficult to remain truly objective. Nonetheless, one should attempt to provide information and not dictate a specific course of action.

COUNSELING COUPLES AFTER AN ABNORMAL OUTCOME

The emotion engendered in counseling couples who have had an abnormal child differs from that elicited in couples at increased risk (e.g., advanced maternal age) but not yet actually having an abnormal child. For the latter, counseling is approached with substantial psychologic overtones. Great sensitivity and substantial investment of time is thus necessary. Such couples are generally best managed by a geneticist, the role of most obstetrician-gynecologists being that of recognizing the problem and reinforcing salient genetic facts.

Confirmation of Diagnosis

Although the diagnosis may seem obvious, confirmation is always obligatory. Accepting a patient's word may not suffice, nor would accepting a diagnosis made by a physician not highly knowledgeable about the condition. It is thus often necessary to verify a diagnosis to assure accurate counseling. If possible, the anomalous individual should be examined. Examining first-degree relatives may also be helpful if the possibility of an autosomal dominant disorder (e.g., neurofibromatosis) exists. Alternatively, one may need to rely on medical records or laboratory tests.

Family History

The family history should be verified. In complex cases, there is merit in a physician personally taking pedigrees, despite the temptation to delegate the responsibility. While the counselor is eliciting pedigree information, most couples visibly become more at ease. Interaction between husband and wife can also be observed.

The family history elicited after an abnormality has been detected may differ from that obtained in routine screening (see below). Record outcomes of all pregnancies by first-degree, second-degree, and third-degree relatives. Elicit names and birth dates of these relatives, not so much for the intrinsic value of that information, as to assure that the couple actually recalls each relative. Generalizations like "There are no other birth defects in the family" may be misleading. If other relatives are said to be abnormal, either obtain medical records or examine that individual.

Psychologic Considerations

Psychologic defenses underlie all genetic counseling. If not appreciated, these defenses can impede the counseling process. Anxiety is low in couples requesting genetic counseling because of age or because of an abnormality in a distant relative. As long as anxiety remains low, comprehension of information is usually not impeded. However, couples who have experienced a stillborn infant, an anomalous offspring, or multiple repetitive abortions are more anxious. Their ability to retain information may be impeded.

Couples experiencing abnormal pregnancy outcomes show the same grief reactions that occur following death of a loved one: denial, anger, guilt, bargaining, and resolution. One should defer to this sequence by not attempting definitive counseling immediately following birth of an abnormal neonate. Offer support to parents, but avoid discussing specific recurrence risks for fear of adding to the immediate burden. By 4–6 weeks, the couple has begun to cope and is receptive to counseling.

An additional psychologic consideration is that of parental blame. It is natural to search for exogenous factors that might have caused an abnormal outcome. In the process of such a search, unjustifiable guilt often arises. There may subconsciously arise a tendency to blame the spouse. Of course, occasionally the "blame" is realistic, for example, in autosomal dominant traits. Fortunately, most couples can be assured that nothing could have prevented the abnormal pregnancy.

Appreciating the various psychologic defenses described above helps one to understand the ostensible failure of some intelligent couples to comprehend genetic information.

Communication

Communicating advice in readily comprehensible terms is essential. The ultimate principle is to allow parents to make their own reproductive decisions.

PRINCIPLES UNDERLYING GENETIC SCREENING

Genetic screening implies that ostensibly normal individuals are routinely monitored for the presence or absence of some disorder. Examples include (1) prenatal cytogenetic analysis (chorionic villus sampling or amniocentesis) in women aged 35 years or older and (2) serum phenylalanine assays to detect phenyketonuria (PKU) in neonates. In theory, a very large number of genetic disorders could be screened. For example, all chromosomal abnormalities could be detected in the neonatal period, and almost all disorders of amino acid metabolism are amenable to screening. On the other hand, screening is actually recommended for relatively few disorders. The reason is that certain prerequisites essential for initiating screening programs are not always met. These prerequisites are especially relevant to maternal serum alpha-fetoprotein screening programs (MSAFP) and deserve some emphasis.

Capacity to Alter Clinical Management

Although screening to achieve research objectives (e.g., determining the incidence of a disorder) is sometimes appropriate, widespread screening is ordinarily performed only if an abnormal finding would alter clinical management. Thus, neonates might be screened for those metabolic disorders (e.g., PKU) amenable to dietary treatment; however, neonates would not be screened for disorders that are not treatable. Lack of treatment thus precludes neonatal screening for infants with chromosomal abnormalities, Tay–Sachs disease, Duchenne muscular dystrophy, and cystic fibrosis. Sickle cell anemia is arguable.

On the other hand, it is reasonable to screen adults to determine if they are at increased risk for offspring with nontreatable disorders. Heterozygote determinations could alter reproductive choices and thus alter clinical management. Screening adults to determine heterozygote status is especially applicable if prenatal diagnosis is available. Mendelian disorders for which heterozygote determinations are possible include Tay–Sachs in Ashkenazi Jews, β-thalassemia in Greeks and Italians, α-thalassemia in Southeast Asians, and sickle cell anemia in Blacks. Screening is especially applicable for pregnant patients. Offering amniocentesis to women aged 35 years is well accepted. Rapidly becoming the standard as well is maternal serum alpha-fetoprotein (MSAFP) screening for neural tube defects.

Cost Effectiveness

Merely having the ability to identify a heterozygote or to detect an affected individual does not warrant that screening should be undertaken. Technology exists to screen perhaps a hundred mendelian disorders, and additional disorders will surely be detectable through advances in molecular genetics. However, only a few disorders are recommended for neonatal screening, heterozygote detection, or prenatal monitoring.

For only these few disorders does the high cost of a screening program justify the monetary and emotional savings of detecting a few affected cases. Thus, neonatal screening is universally recommended for hypothyroidism and phenylketonuria in the United States. Screening for other disorders is not generally recommended, although in some states galactosemia, maple-syrup-urine disease, and adenosine deaminase deficiency are screened. Chromosomal analysis and alpha fetoprotein assays are routinely performed in fluid obtained at amniocentesis; however, assays for other detectable disorders are not performed.

Reliability of Assay

The requisite assay must have a high predictive value. Following this general axiom is especially necessary for genetic diseases, all of which are individually rare. Even very low false positive rates could result in a single abnormal value being more likely to represent a false positive than true positive value.

Capacity to Handle Problems

Fulfilling all the above prerequisites still does not mean that screening programs for a particular disorder should be initiated. One final prerequisite must be met—ability to handle problems that inevitably arise in screening programs. Sometimes the high frequency of ancillary problems and the relative unavailability of staff to handle these problems obviates a screening program that would otherwise be attractive.

An example of the necessity for solving unexpected problems can be cited in PKU screening programs. After screening programs were initiated, it developed that most elevated phenylalanine values were not the result of PKU, but rather other conditions that did not even require dietary treatment. Ability to separate the latter cases (false positives) from true (PKU) cases is crucial. Another example of the potential inability to handle problems lies with maternal serum alpha-fetoprotein programs. Approximately 25 women will have an elevated serum value for every woman shown to have a fetus with a neural tube defect; 24 of 25 women with a single elevated value will eventually prove to have a normal fetus. In heterozygote screening programs (sickle cell anemia, Tay-Sachs disease, β-thalassemia), one must assure that heterozygotes do not become stigmatized or develop erroneous impressions that their own health is threatened.

TECHNICAL CONSIDERATIONS

Amniocentesis

Technique. Amniocentesis is best performed at 16–17 weeks' gestation (menstrual weeks). At this stage of gestation, the amniotic fluid volume of 200–225 ml is sufficient to remove 30–35 ml, the uterus is accessible to a transabdominal approach, the ratio of viable to nonviable cells in the amniotic fluid is relatively high, and the time before fetal viability is adequate to complete diagnostic studies. An ultrasound examination (preferably dynamic imaging) should be performed immediately prior to amniocentesis in order to determine fetal biparietal diameter, placental position, amniotic fluid location, fetal cardiac movement, and number of fetuses. Alternatively, ultrasound can also be performed current with amniocentesis.[13]

Bloody amniotic fluid is not infrequently aspirated at amniocentesis. The blood is almost always maternal in origin, and does not adversely affect amniotic cell growth. On the other hand, brown or dark red (wine-colored) amniotic fluid is associated with increased likelihood of poor pregnancy outcome. The color is indicative of previous intra-amniotic bleeding. Hemoglobin breakdown products account for the pigment. Pregnancy loss eventually occurs in perhaps 20–30%[13] of such cases. If abnormally colored fluid also shows an elevated alpha-fetoprotein, the outcome is almost always unfavorable (fetal death, anencephaly, spontaneous abortion, or fetal abnormality). Greenish amniotic fluid, presumably due to meconium staining, is not associated with poor pregnancy outcome.[27]

In multiple gestations, amniocentesis can usually be performed on both (or all) fetuses. Following aspiration of amniotic fluid from the first sac, 2–3 ml of indigo carmine (diluted 1:10 in bacteriostatic water) is injected before the needle is withdrawn. A second amniocentesis is then performed in the location of the second fetus, preferably determined after visualizing the membranes separating the two sacs. Aspiration of clear fluid confirms that the second sac has been entered. At large university centers, amniocentesis is successfully performed in more than 95% of twin pregnancies, with ostensibly no increased risks.[12,13] Triplets and other multiple gestations can be managed similarly by sequentially injecting dye into successive sacs.

Following amniocentesis, the patient may resume all normal activities. Common sense dictates that strenuous exercise (jogging, "aerobic" exercise) should be deferred for a day or so, and perhaps intercourse as well. Persistent uterine cramping, vaginal bleeding, leakage of amniotic fluid, or fever should be reported to the physician. Rh-immune globulin is usually administered, although absolute verification of its necessity is lacking.

If only one of the fetuses is abnormal, parents will ordinarily have to choose between terminating both (all) fetuses and continuing a pregnancy with one normal and one abnormal fetus. Selective termination of a single fetus has been achieved but must be viewed as an exception and possibly unreliable.

Safety. Amniocentesis potentially involves risks to both mother and fetus. Maternal risks are quite low, with symptomatic amnionitis occurring only very rarely. Minor maternal complications (e.g., transient vaginal spotting, minimal amniotic fluid leakage) occur more often, but still infrequently.

The frequency of increased fetal loss following amniocentesis has been addressed by several large collaborative studies, which are the only studies with appropriate controls. In the major U.S. study, 3.5% of pregnant women who underwent amniocentesis experienced fetal loss subsequent to the procedure compared to 3.2% of controls.[35] The small difference was not statistically significant and disappeared completely when corrected for maternal age. However, a later British collaborative study[53] found that the rate of fetal loss following amniocentesis was significantly increased. Neither collaborative study was conducted with high-quality ultrasound, and some participating obstetricians were relatively inexperienced in amniocentesis. Most centers now counsel that the risk of abortion secondary to amniocentesis is 1/200 or less. At our center, we mention that serious maternal complications and fetal injuries are "reported but very rare."

Chorionic Villus Sampling

Amniocentesis has the disadvantage of being performed in the second trimester. First-trimester methods are highly desirable, not only to allow pregnancy termination early in gestation but also to protect patient privacy. Eventually it should prove possible to analyze fetal cells circulating in maternal blood. At present, attention is focusing on chorionic villus sampling.

Historical Aspects. First-trimester sampling of fetal tissues was first attempted more than a decade ago. In 1973, Kullander and Sandahl[29] studied 39 Swedish women undergoing pregnancy termination. Subjects between 8 and 20 weeks' gestation underwent transcervical chorionic biopsy utilizing a 5 mm endoscope. Chromosomal studies were completed in 20 cases, all of which were consistent with sex of the abortus. In 19 cases, pregnancy termination was delayed between 7 and 43 days; the only complications observed were two infections. The study was stopped after the demonstration that amniocentesis was relatively safe and highly reliable.

In 1975, Chinese workers transcervically aspirated chorionic villi for X-chromatin studies.[10] Although ultrasound was not employed, only 4 of 100 subjects aborted following the procedure. Thirty other pregnancies were terminated after the sex became known, but the remaining 66 pregnancies continued uneventfully. Fetal sex was accurately predicted in 94% of the 66 cases. Other first-trimester techniques were attempted subsequently, but attempts became practical only after the advent of improved ultrasonographic techniques.

In 1982, Kazy et al.[28] obtained samples by either (1) transcervical fetoscopic biopsy immediately following ultrasound or (2) flexible biopsy forceps guided simultaneously by ultrasonography. All 13 patients continuing pregnancies were later delivered of normal infants. In 1982, Old, Ward, and their colleagues[37] described 63 patients in whom chorionic villus sampling was performed by transcervical aspiration with a 1.5 mm plastic cannula using ultrasonographically directed sampling. Continuing pregnancies were described. The first large sample was studied in Milan by Simoni, Brambati, and others.[38] The National Institutes of Health are now funding seven U.S. centers to investigate the safety and accuracy of CVS: Yale University, Mount Sinai Medical School, Jefferson Medical College, Michael Reese Medical Center, Baylor University, the University of California–San Francisco, my group (Northwestern University/University Tennessee). Results will be available in several years.

Technique. Chorionic villus sampling usually utilizes a hollow, malleable plastic catheter about 1.5 mm in diameter; a metal obturator extending just distal to the catheter tip is inserted.[14] The patient is placed in lithotomy position, her vagina cleansed, and the catheter/obturator introduced transcervically under simultaneous ultrasonographic visualization (Fig. 13-1). The catheter is directed toward the main portion of placenta (trophoblastic tissue). The obturator is then removed, and, by negative pressure, 10–25 mg of chorionic villi are aspirated into a 20–30 cc syringe. Optimal time for sampling is 9–11 weeks. Transabdominal CVS can also be performed.

Safety. The complication rate for CVS is yet to be established. Worldwide tabulations of the first 4000 cases indicate an absolute fetal loss rate of 4–5%.[25] In our hands, no immediate losses occurred in the first 80 cases. This loss rate must be compared to the background loss rate, which unfortunately is not well established. The appropriate comparison group would be a matched sample of women showing an ultrasonographically normal fetus at a comparable gestational stage. Data available from an NICHD-sponsored study, "Diabetes in Early Pregnancy,' are instructive in this regard.[43] In this collaborative study, pregnancies were diagnosed by β-hCG radioimmunoassay within 21

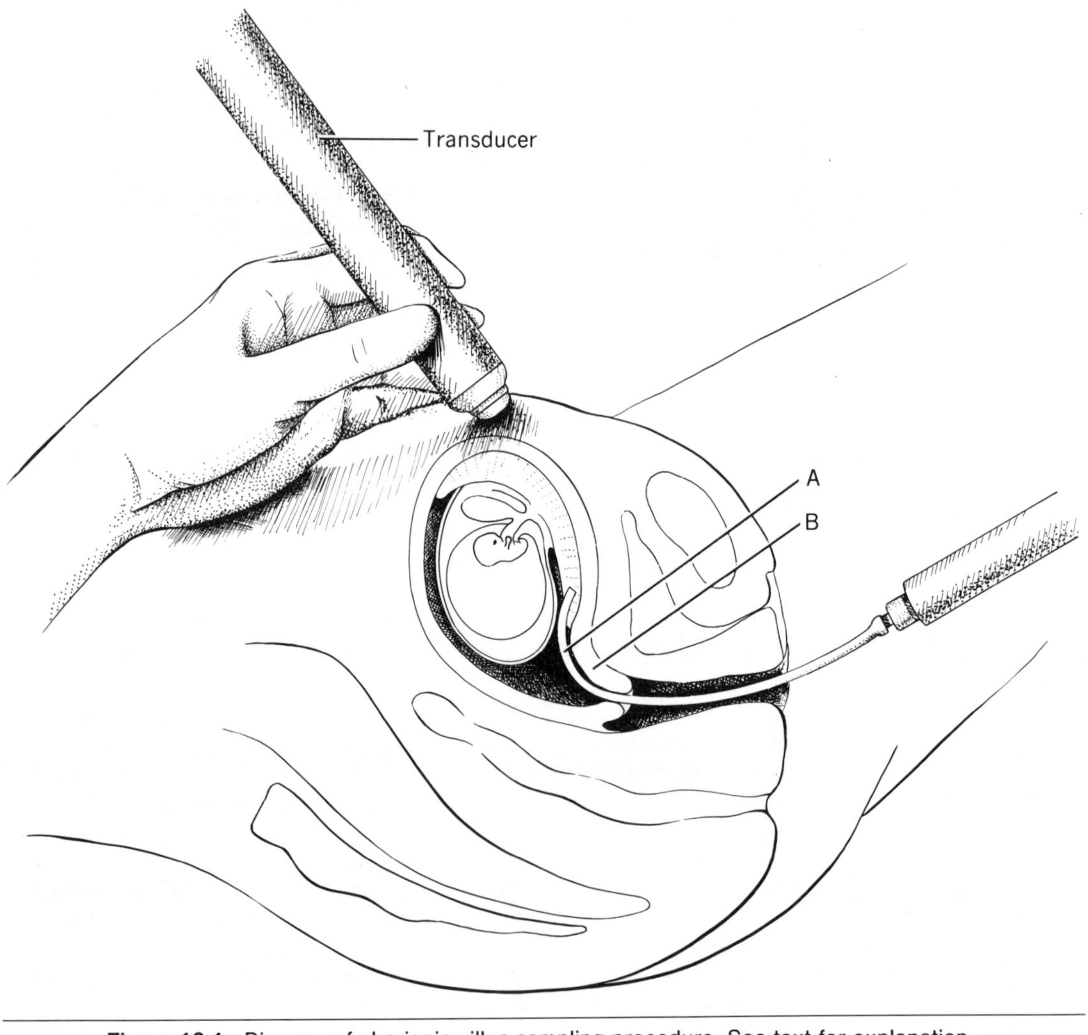

Figure 13-1. Diagram of chorionic villus sampling procedure. See text for explanation.

days of conception. Of 220 women having a normal ultrasound (crown-rump length, cardiac motion) eight weeks after their last menstrual period, only seven (3.2%) later experienced a fetal loss. Comparable data derived in other ways can be cited.[8,52] These low fetal loss rates indicate that ultrasonographically normal pregnancies are lost relatively infrequently. It follows that most losses that become clinically evident in the 8-12 week interval actually represent fetal demises that occurred weeks previously (missed abortions). Thus, the relatively low absolute loss rates observed after CVS are still compatible with increased risks of 1-2%.[14]

Diagnostic Limitations for CVS. Both chorionic villi and amniotic fluid cells offer information concerning chromosomal status, enzyme levels, and DNA patterns. The only major difference is that assays requiring amniotic fluid liquor, namely, alpha-fetoprotein, cannot be performed in CVS.

Fetal Cells in Maternal Blood

Ideally, fetal abnormalities would be detected without amniocentesis or CVS, both invasive procedures. If noninvasive techniques became available, one could justify screening all pregnant women, irrespective of age or previous obstetric history.

One attractive possibility involves recovering fetal cells from maternal blood. Fetal cells are present in the maternal blood during pregnancy. Unfortunately, these cells seem reluctant to undergo mitogen-stimulated transformation.[25] Without transformation, metaphases necessary for chromosomal analysis cannot be obtained.

If a reliable method of isolating and culturing fetal cells from maternal blood does become available, however, one could envision a screening program analogous to that utilized for neural tube defects. A blood sample could be obtained from all pregnant patients, with confirmatory amniocentesis or CVS performed in women whose blood reveals abnormalities. Identification of new mitogens that facilitate transformation or use of chromosome-specific (e.g., Nos. 13, 18, 21) DNA probes should eventually make this approach feasible.

Analysis of Amniotic Fluid Cells or Chorionic Villi

Analysis of either chorionic villi or amniotic fluid cells carries many pitfalls, some of which every obstetrician-gynecologist should recognize. First, cells may not grow, or growth may be insufficient for proper analysis. Failures of amniotic fluid cultures are now relatively uncommon, but still occur. Chorionic villi divide more rapidly than amniotic fluid cells. In fact, a few chorionic cells can be accumulated in metaphase within hours after sampling. This so-called direct analysis can provide rapid answers; however, these rapid ("direct") preparations sometimes yield metaphases of relatively poor quality. Initiation of cultures addresses this problem.

A second source of error involves analysis of maternal rather than fetal cells, a special fear in CVS. The frequency with which this error occurs in CVS is still being determined, but microscopic inspection of CVS aspirates is necessary to exclude maternal decidua. Utilization of both direct methods and culture techniques should minimize this error, since maternal decidual cells will ordinarily not divide as rapidly as chorionic villi. In amniocentesis, maternal cell contamination can be minimized by discarding the first few drops of aspirated amniotic fluid. Incidentally, cross-contamination in multiple gestations appears to be rare in amniocentesis. In our unit, we have never observed cross-contamination in unlike-sexed twins.

A third potential source of error involves aberrations that do not reflect fetal status. One reason for this is the occurrence of in vitro aberrations, aberrations which arise in culture. They should be suspected whenever an abnormality is restricted to only one of the several cultures (flasks) or clones initiated from a single amniotic fluid or CVS specimen. In fact, cells containing at least one additional structurally normal chromosome are detected in 1-2% of all amniotic fluid specimens.[24,47] If cells are confined to a single culture or clone, the phenomenon is termed pseudomosaicism. Clinically significant fetal mosaicism is assumed to exist only if cells with an abnormal complement are detected in more than one flask or clone (true mosaicism). True fetal mosaicism occurs in 0.25% of amniotic fluid samples and is usually (70-80%) confirmed by studies of the abortus or liveborn.[24] A second reason is that certain fetal tissues sampled may not always reflect embryonic status. Tetraploidy occurs in human amnion but not in fetal tissue. It may also be necessary to confirm (amniocentesis) certain monosomies (e.g., 45,X) and trisomies (e.g., No. 15) that are detected in chorionic villi.

A fourth dilemma is that some phenotypes are difficult to predict. This is true when a de novo translocation, inversion, or small supernumerary chromosome is identified. If a phenotypically normal parent has the same abnormality (e.g., balanced translocation) as that in the fetus, reassurance is usually appropriate. On the other hand, if a balanced translocation or inversion is present in the fetus but not in either parent (de novo origin), some 10% of fetuses are phenotypically abnormal.[51] Phenotypic abnormalities in such fetuses could reflect mutation or hemizygosity at one of the break points, a position effect, or a rearrangement not actually balanced. Similar information applies for de novo supernumerary chromosomes, about 10% of which are associated with phenotypic abnormalities.[51]

Sex chromosome abnormalities may also create quandries. A mildly abnormal phenotype, often with slow mental development, may be associated with the complements 47,XXX; 47,-XXY; and 47,XYY. However, most individuals with these complements are neither severely retarded nor grossly malformed. Couples thus may or may not choose to abort fetuses wih such complements.

INDICATIONS FOR PRENATAL CYTOGENETIC STUDIES

Virtually all chromosomal disorders could be detectable in utero. However, it is not appropriate to perform amniocentesis or chorionic villus sampling (CVS) in every pregnancy because, for many couples, the risk of these procedures outweighs the diagnostic benefits. This section considers current indications for cytogenetic studies.

Advanced Maternal Age

The most common indication for antenatal cytogenetic studies is increased maternal age. The overall incidence of trisomy 21 (1 per 800 liveborn births in the United States) increases with age (Table 13-1). Above age 30, the rate increases exponentially. The likelihood of a 35-year-old mother having a child with trisomy 21 is 1 in 385; at age 39 the risk is 1 in 137; at age 45 the risk is 1 in 30.[22] Trisomy 21 is not the only chromosomal abnormality that increases with maternal age. Trisomy 13, trisomy 18, 47,XXX, and 47,XXY also increase.[23] There is no accepted biologic explanation for the relationship between aneuploidy and advanced maternal age.

Based on the above data, it is standard medical practice to offer prenatal diagnosis to all women who will be 35 years or older when their infant is born (EDC). Because the choice of a particular age is largely arbitrary, however, flexibility is desirable when answering inquiries from women less than 35 years old.

It is worth emphasizing that these risk figures are applicable for liveborns. The prevalence of abnormalities in antenatal studies at 16–18 weeks' gestation is about 30% higher than in liveborn infants.[21] The prevalence at 9–11 weeks (time for CVS) is higher yet. The discrepancy between frequencies in liveborn infants and frequencies in fetuses is probably accounted for by the disproportionate number of chromosomally abnormal fetuses aborting spontaneously later in gestation. That is, some fetuses therapeutically aborted after antenatal studies would have spontaneously aborted.

Previous Child with Chromosome Abnormality

Following the birth of one child with trisomy 21, the likelihood that subsequent progeny will have a similar chromosomal abnormality is traditionally considered to be increased, even if the parental chromosomal complements are normal. However, the risk is actually not greatly increased. This relative increase is greatest if the mother is relatively young when the trisomic proband was born.[48] Parental anxiety alone dictates, however, that antenatal chromosomal studies should be discussed for couples who previously had a trisomic child.

Recurrence risks following births of liveborns with chromosomal abnormalities other than trisomy 21 are less well defined. The risk seems to be approximately 1% for either the same or for a different chromosomal abnormality. Thus, antenatal studies should also be offered to such couples. Whether risks are similar following the delivery of a trisomic stillborn or trisomic abortus remains uncertain.

Parental Translocation, Inversion, or Aneuploidy

Another indication for prenatal cytogenetic studies is presence of a parental chromosomal abnormality. Balanced translocations are the usual indication, but inversions and other abnormalities also occur.

Translocations. The clinical significance of translocations can be illustrated by recalling Robertsonian translocations, those involving centromeric fusion of the acrocentric chromosomes (13, 14, 15, 21, or 22). If a child has Down's syndrome resulting from such a Robertsonian translocation [eg., 46,XX,−14, +(14q;21q)], the rearrangement will have originated de novo in 50–75% of cases (i.e., it is present in neither parent). The likelihood of Down's syndrome recurring in progeny of parents whose offspring had a de novo translocation is minimal. On the other hand, the risk is significant in the 25–50% of families in which individuals have Down's syndrome as a result of a balanced parental translocation [e.g., parental complement 45,XX,-14,-21,+(14q;21q). The theoretical risk that a parent carrying a t(14q;21q) chromosome will have a child with Down's syndrome is 33% (Fig. 13-2). However, empiric risks may be considerably less in amniotic fluid studies. The likelihood is about 2% or less if the father carries translocation, and 10–15% if the mother carries the translocation (Table 13-2).[5] The risks are much higher in chorionic villi sampling,[32] presumably because spontaneous abortion of some abnormal fetuses has not yet occurred (Table 13-2). For other Robertsonian translocations, risks are lower. For example, in t(13q;14q), there is a low (1% or less) risk for unbalanced liveborns (trisomy 13) (Table 13-2).

Reciprocal translocations do not involve centromeric fusion and, hence, usually do not involve acrocentric chromosomes. Empiric data for specific translocations are rarely available, but generalizations can be made on the basis of pooled data derived from many different translocations. Again, theoretical risks for abnormal (unbalanced) offspring are greater than empiric risks. Based on limited data in amniocentesis registries, risks are 11% for offspring of female heterozygotes and 11% for offspring of male heterozygotes (Table 13-2).[5] In chorionic villus sampling, risks approximate 40% (Table 13-2).[32]

Inversions. In chromosomal inversions, the normal sequence of genes is altered. In paracentric inversions, the rearrangement results from reinsertion of a chromosomal segment in which break points occur on the same side of the centromere. In pericentric inversions, breaks occur on opposite sides. Individuals with inversions are phenotypically normal. However, they may produce unbalanced gametes if, during meiosis, crossing-over (recombination) occurs within the inverted sequence. For example, crossing-over within a pericentric inversion gives rise to two duplication-deficiency products and two normal products (Fig. 13-3).

Empiric risk data for specific pericentric inversions are rarely available, although pooled

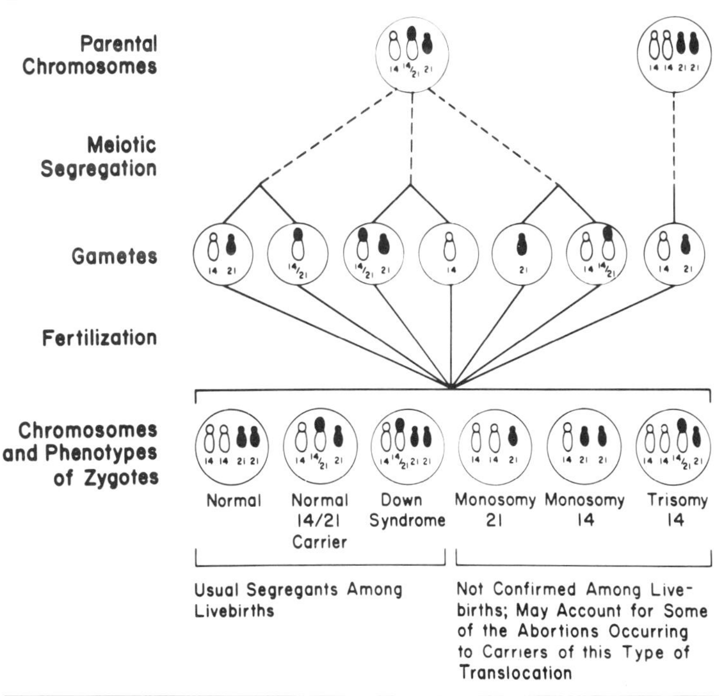

Figure 13-2. Diagram of possible gametes and progeny of a phenotypically normal individual heterozygous for a Robertsonian translocation between chromosomes 14 and 21 (a form of D/G translocation). Three of the six possible gametes are incompatible with life. The likelihood that an individual with such a translocation would have a child with Down syndrome is thus theoretically 33%. However, the empirical risk is considerably less. From Gerbie, A. and Simpson, J. L.: Antenatal detection of genetic disorders. *Postgrad. Med.* **59**(6):129–136, 1976.

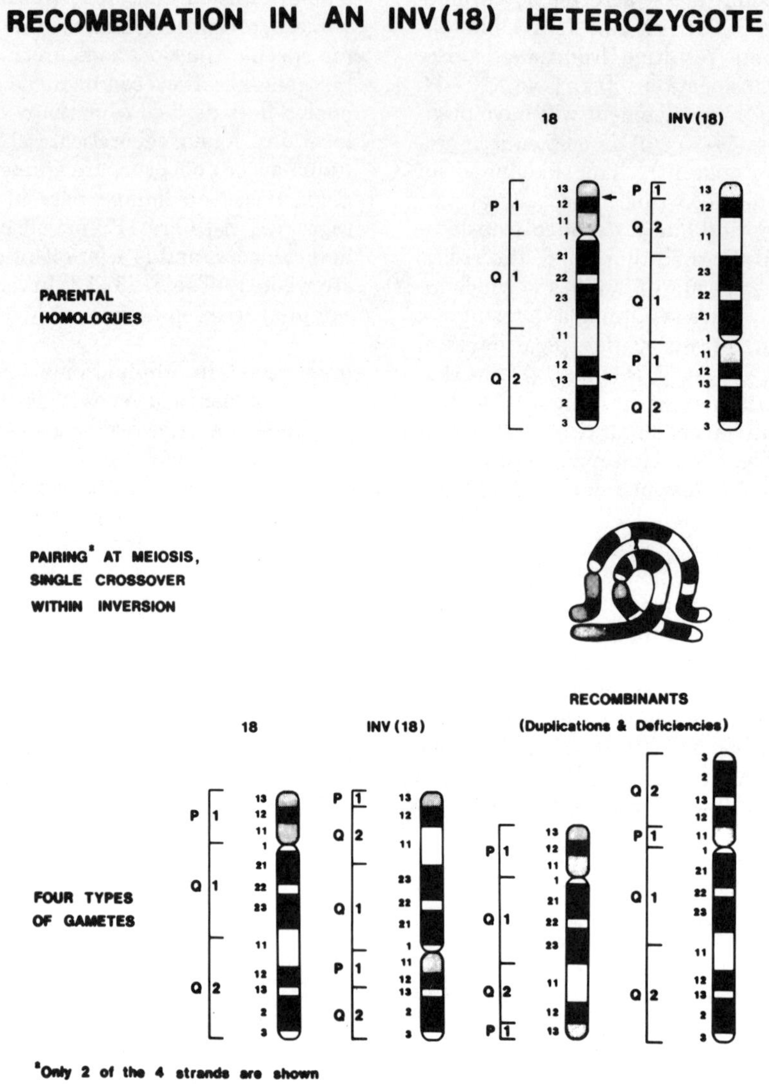

Figure 13-3. Diagram illustrating the break points leading to an inversion in chromosomes 18. The inversion loop resulting from pairing during meiosis is shown. As a result, crossing-over at meiosis I would be expected to produce the four types of gamete shown. Two of the four would be genetically balanced, although one would show the same inversion present in the parent. In addition, two types of gamete would be genetically unbalanced, showing complementary duplications and deficiencies. It is the chromosomal region outside the inverted segment that appears as duplications or deficiencies. From Martin, A. O., Simpson, J. L., Deddish, R., and Elias, S.: Clinical implications of chromosomal inversions. A pericentric inversion in No. 18 segregating in a family ascertained through an abnormal proband. *Am. J. Perinatol.* **1**:81–88, 1984.[30]

data indicate not inconsequential risks to progeny. Females with an inversion are at greater risk (8%) for abnormal unbalanced progeny than are males (4%). Paradoxically, inversions involving relatively longer segments (30–60% total chromosomal length) are more likely to produce anomalous offspring than pericentric inversion involving shorter segments. A relatively short pericentric inversion segment is apparently associated with decreased likelihood of recombination within the segment. The argument is discussed in detail elsewhere.[30,44]

Crossing-over within a paracentric inversion leads to one dicentric, one acentric, and two normal products. The acentric and dicentric products would be lost. Since all aberrant products are lethal, abnormal liveborns will rarely be the result of paracentric inversions. However, repeated abortions can occur.

Previous Stillborn or Abortuses Not Subjected to Chromosomal Analysis

Couples experiencing repetitive abortions should undergo cytogenetic studies to exclude the presence of an inversion or translocation, either of which clearly justifies antenatal chromosomal studies. Approximately 2–5% of couples with such histories will show a rearrangement.[30,45] Antenatal diagnosis is also not unreasonable for couples who have no chromosomal rearrangements but have had one or more spontaneous abortions or stillborn infants. The rationale is based on observations that 50–60% of all first-trimester abortuses show numerical chromosomal abnormalities. Of abortuses with chromosomal abnormalities, 50% are trisomic; thus, 25% of all first-trimester abortuses are trisomic. Furthermore, in successive abortuses, the chromosomal complements are usually either consistently normal or consistently abnormal (recurrent aneuploidy).[20] Thus, certain couples must be predisposed to aneuploid conceptuses.

If abortuses or stillborn infants were known to be trisomic, it would certainly be reasonable to offer antenatal cytogenetic studies in subsequent pregnancies, because another trisomic conceptus might not abort, but rather survive to be liveborn. Of course, chromosomal studies are not often performed on abortuses or stillborn infants. Therefore, one usually does not know whether a couple experiencing multiple abortuses or stillborns did or did not have recurrent aneuploid conceptions. Whether in these couples the theoretic risks for aneuploid liveborns outweigh the small yet finite risks of amniocentesis or CVS is arguable.

Advanced Paternal Age

Down's syndrome may also be associated with advanced paternal age. Originally it was suggested that the risk of siring offspring with trisomy 21 is increased by paternal age 55, and perhaps as early as age 41. However, the latest tabulations are revealing little if any paternal effect.[16] If advanced paternal age increases the risk, it would be particularly applicable when the mother is aged 30–34 years.

Exposure to Irradiation or Chemotherapeutic Agents

A common clinical query involves the propriety of antenatal chromosomal studies in individuals who received massive (therapeutic) doses of x-irradiation or chemotherapeutic agents prior to pregnancy. Fears of abnormal progeny generally prove unfounded, but several case-control studies have shown that women whose pregnancies terminated in liveborn offspring with Down's syndrome received significantly more x-irradiation prior to conception than did controls. On the other hand, increased anomalies were not observed in offspring of women treated with x-irradiation for Hodgkin's disease, nor did Japanese women exposed to x-irradiation through the atomic bomb explosions show an increased prevalence of Down's syndrome offspring.[49] Antenatal cytogenetic studies should be discussed but not encouraged for women or men who previously underwent radiotherapy. Of course, such individuals are also at theoretic risk for gene mutations, for which one cannot all be tested for.

Similar reasoning might also apply to individuals who have received chemotherapeutic agents. Such agents produce chromosomal damage and gene mutations. Fortunately, no increase in anomalous liveborns has been observed. Couples desiring antenatal diagnostic studies must realize that it is not possible to monitor gene mutations.

PRENATAL DIAGNOSIS FOR MENDELIAN AND POLYGENIC DISORDERS

Antenatal diagnosis for these genetic disorders was originally possible only for certain inborn errors of metabolism. Neural tube defects (NTDs) later became detectable on the basis of elevated amniotic fluid alpha-fetoprotein. Antenatal diagnosis of hemoglobinopathies, hemophilia, and other disorders thereafter became detectable, initially through assay of fetal sera (fetoscopy) and now through DNA analysis. Renal anomalies and other anatomic defects are also increasingly detectable by ultrasonographic visualization.

Despite these many advances, studies for mendelian and polygenic disorders continue to be performed less frequently than chromosomal studies.

Inborn Errors of Metabolism

Antenatal diagnosis is possible for at least 80 inborn errors of metabolism. Almost all are transmitted in autosomal recessive fashion, although a few are transmitted in X-linked recessive or autosomal dominant fashion. It is unreasonable to expect physicians who are not geneticists to be fully informed in all aspects of this complex topic. However, a few generalizations concerning metabolic disorders are appropriate.

First, couples will usually be identified as at risk for a child with a metabolic disorder because they previously had an affected child. Occasionally, screening programs identify heterozygotes at risk for a child with an autosomal recessive disorder, most commonly Tay-Sachs disease. Second, diagnosis of affected offspring (or two heterozygous parents) must always be verified in order for appropriate antenatal tests to be offered. Confirmation may not always be easy. If the affected child is no longer alive, the diagnosis may prove impossible to verify. Third, detection of metabolic errors requires that the enzyme be expressed in amniotic fluid cells or chorionic villus cells. This requirement is not fulfilled by all metabolic disorders, a prominent example being phenylketonuria (PKU). Fortunately, PKU now seems diagnosable by the molecular techniques described below. In general, enzymes present in amniotic fluid cell are also expressed in chorionic villi; however, this area is still undergoing investigation. Fourth, biochemical studies may require more cells than cytogenetic studies, at least in amniocentesis. Delays may also occur if the fluid or cultured cells must be transported to a referral laboratory.

Galjaard fully reviews metabolic disorders detectable in utero.[17] Two disorders deserve special comments.

Tay-Sachs Disease. Tay-Sachs disease (GM_2 gangliosidosis type 1) is an autosomal recessive disorder in which hexosaminidase A, the enzyme necessary for metabolizing sphingolipid, is virtually absent. Sphingolipids accumulate, interfere with neurologic development, and eventually result in death by 3–4 years of age. Routine screening programs for heterozygote detection are now standard clinical practice. Heterozygote frequency in the Gentile population is 1:300, but in Ashkenazi Jews it is 1:27. Intensive educational efforts directed at the Jewish population have resulted in widespread utilization of heterozygote detection tests. Pregnancies at risk can be monitored by assaying hexosamidase A levels in amniotic fluid fibroblasts or chorionic villus cells. At our university, we also recommend screening when only one partner is Ashkenazi.

Of importance to obstetricians is that serum hexosaminidase A decreases during pregnancy relative to total hexosaminidase (A,B). Therefore, pregnant women may erroneously be diagnosed as heterozygotes (false positive). Leukocyte assays should thus always be available whenever pregnant women are tested. However, a negative value (nonheterozygote) can be accepted as valid.

Cystic Fibrosis (CF). Cystic fibrosis is the most common mendelian disorder in the Caucasian population. Affected individuals show chronic dysfunction of exocrine and mucus-producing glands (pancreas, biliary tract, intestine, and bronchi). Life expectancy is 20–30 years, with deaths usually resulting from respiratory failure. The underlying defect has not been elucidated, despite years of study. Although CF is transmitted in autosomal recessive fashion, heterozygote detection is not yet reliably available. Thus, couples at risk are usually identified only after the birth of an affected child.

Many different methods have been attempted for antenatal diagnosis of this disorder. Unfortunately, early enthusiasm has repeatedly been replaced by disappointment. Current excitement centers around assays for various microvillar peptidases, such as the intestinal isozymes, amniotic fluid alkaline phosphatase, α-glutamyltranspeptidase, and amino peptidase. The strategy is that alkaline phosphatase and other microvillar enzymes are decreased in both normal as well as CF pregnancies, but in the latter the decrease is more marked and more consistently observed.[1,6] Thus, low amniotic fluid alkaline phosphatase in a couple having 25% risk for a CF child is quite likely (10:1 or so) to indicate an affected child. Even more recently, a host of studies describing informative restriction fragment-length polymorphisms (RFLPs) restriction fragment-length polymorphisms have been reported. At the time of this writing, the proportion of cases that can be detected by DNA analysis remains uncertain. Moreover, over 70% seem detectable, provided the index case in a given family is still available. Prenatal studies in families without an affected child must await further advances.

Neural Tube Defects

Failure of neural tube closure leads to anencephaly, spina bifida (myelomeningocele or meningocele), and encephalocele. These defects represent different manifestations of the same pathogenic process; thus, couples who have had a child with any type of neural tube defect (NTD) have approximately equal risks for subsequent offspring having either spina bifida or anencephaly. This holds true irrespective of the type of neural tube defect exhibited by the index case.

If the proband (index case) has a neural tube defect, the likelihood that a first-degree relative will have either anencephaly or spina bifida is 2% in the United States.[33] The risk is 5% in the United Kingdom. Second-degree relatives (nieces, nephews, grandchildren) and third-degree relatives (first cousins) are less likely to be affected. However, the risk of NTDs in first cousins of affected individuals remains increased over that of the general population. In particular, offspring of the sisters of women with an affected child have a 0.5–1.0% risk for offspring with NTD.

Antenatal diagnosis of neural tube defects can be accomplished readily by either ultrasound or amniotic fluid alpha-fetoprotein (AFP) assay. Ultrasonography performed by experienced investigators should readily exclude anencephaly, and spina bifida can be detected by serial views of the vertebral column. However, not all centers possess the necessary technical sophistication. Thus, AFP assays remain the preferable method for diagnosis of neural tube defects. Diagnosis of NTD is possible in all except the 5–10% of spina bifida cases in which skin covers the lesion. Whether Level II ultrasound examinations can detect closed lesions remains problematic.

Amniotic fluid AFP may be spuriously elevated if the amniotic fluid contains fetal blood (bloody tap). This error can be eliminated if amniotic fluid acetylcholinesterase is assayed simultaneously. Presence of acetylcholinesterase, an enzyme not detectable in maternal serum, verifies that elevated AFP is due to NTD or other fetal defects. On the other hand, fetal hemoglobin associated with absence of acetylcholinesterase suggests that the elevated AFP is due to fetal blood contamination (false positive).

Elevated AFP is sometimes associated with other anomalies: omphalocele, cystic hygroma, and congenital nephrosis. In these disorders, acetylcholinesterase may or may not be elevated. Ultrasonographic studies should thus always be undertaken to corroborate abnormal AFP results and to determine the precise nature of any defect present.

Maternal Serum AFP (MSAFP). Maternal serum AFP is elevated in 80–85% of pregnancies characterized by a fetus with a neural tube defect (NTD). This observation proves useful for reducing the incidence of NTD liveborns. Since relatively few of the total number of NTDs occur in families with previously affected offspring, a noninvasive screening method is needed to identify couples at increased likelihood for having a child with NTD. Maternal serum AFP elevations can serve such a purpose. Unfortunately, considerable overlap exists between MSAFP in normal pregnancies and MSAFP in pregnancies characterized by a fetus with NTD.[33,34] MSAFP values can ostensibly be elevated for other reasons: (1) underestimation of gestational age, inasmuch as values decrease as gestation progresses (Fig. 13-4); (2) multiple gestation, 60% of twins and almost all triplets showing elevations[50]; (3) threatened abortion, presumably due to fetal blood in maternal circulation; (4) Rh disease; and (5) anomalies other than neural tube defects. Maximum accuracy requires that the initial MSAFP assay be obtained at 15–17 weeks' gestation.

To minimize false positive values, MSAFP screening requires a second (confirmatory) MSAFP sample one week after the initial screen. If both values are elevated, ultrasound is necessary to exclude an overestimated gestational age, multiple gestations, or fetal demise. Increasingly, ultrasonography is being ordered after a single MSAFP elevation. If no explanation is found, amniocentesis for amniotic fluid AFP and acetylcholinesterase is necessary. Such a program identifies about 90% of anencephaly and 80% of spina bifida. Of some 25 women having a single elevated serum AFP, only one will eventually prove to have a child with neural tube defects (Table 13-3).[7] Women with one or certainly with more than one MSAFP elevation who have no NTD fetus are still at increased risk for other obstetric complications: intrauterine growth retardation, fetal demise, bleeding, and possibly placental abruption.[18]

Serum AFP screening programs are increasingly being initiated in the United States. It is prudent for obstetricians to inform their patients of MSAFP screening. Prior to initiating

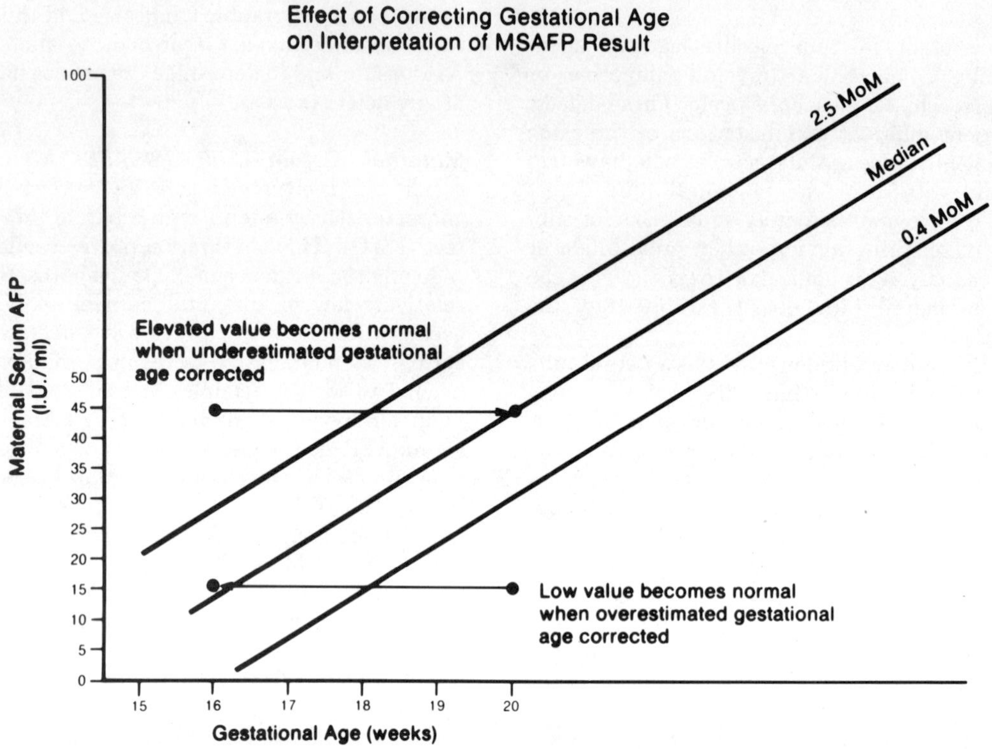

Figure 13-4. Media maternal serum alpha-fetoprotein (MSAFP) throughout gestation. That values increase with increasing gestational age requires accurate dating to interpret low or high MSAFP. From Simpson, J. L.: Genetic counseling and prenatal diagnosis. In: *Obstetrics: Normal and Problem Pregnancies.* S. G. Gabbe, J. F. Niebyl, and J. L. Simpson (Eds.). New York, Churchill-Livingstone, in press (by permission of the publisher).[41]

screening programs, however, one must assure availability of laboratory services, ultrasound, and counseling. All will be necessary to reassure women who have one or more elevated serum AFP levels but otherwise normal tests.

More recently, it is becoming clear that significance must be attached to low serum AFP values. An association with aneuploidy exists, although the magnitude of the increased risk is unknown. Serum values lower than 0.4 multiples of the median (MOM) value significantly increase the magnitude of the increased risk. The magnitude of the increased risk is still uncertain, but at least a three-fold increased risk of trisomy 21 over that expected on the basis of age alone seems to exist.[9] Various proposals have been made for resolving low MSAFP values, but no unanimity has been reached. It would seem best to allow each woman to make her own decision concerning propriety of amniocentesis, using revised risks for aneuploidy recalculated on serum AFP values. For example, a low (<0.4 MOM) value in a 33-year-old woman increases her risk from 1/625 to at least 1/222, approximately that of a 37-year-old woman with normal serum AFP.

Diagnosis by Fetal Visualization (Ultrasonography)

Defects inherited in polygenic/multifactorial fashion carry recurrence risks of 1–5% for first-degree relatives (sibs, offspring, parent). Included in this category are most common anatomic defects limited either to one organ system or to a single embryologically related system. Because the number of genes responsible for these defects is unknown, diagnosis by enzyme assays or even linkage analysis cannot seriously be considered. In utero visualization is also use-

TABLE 13-3. MATERNAL SERUM ALPHA-FETOPROTEIN SCREENING PROGRAM (MSAFP)

Initial sample				1000
Normal MSAFP* (no further testing)			950	
Elevated MSAFP			50	
Normal MSAFP (no further tests)		20		
Second elevated MSAFP		30		
Ultrasound (Level I) explanation:				
No further testing (erroneous dates greater than 2 weeks, twins, triplets, fetal demise)	15			
No ultrasound explanation	15			
Amniocentesis abnormal	1–2†			
Elevated amniotic fluid AFP: anencephaly, spina bifida, omphalocele, other defect				
Amniocentesis normal	13–14			

* Outcome of maternal serum AFP screening in population of 1000 pregnant women.
† 1 if anencephaly detected at Level I ultrasound, 2 if not.
Source: Simpson, J. L.: Genetic counseling and prenatal diagnosis. In: *Obstetrics: Normal and Abnormal.* S. G. Gabbe, J. F. Niebyl and J. L. Simpson (eds.). New York, Churchill-Livingstone, in press (by permission of the publisher).[41]

ful in mendelian disorders characterized by certain anatomic defects, for example, autosomal recessive (infantile) polycystic kidney disease, X-linked recessive aqueductal stenosis (hydrocephaly), various skeletal dysplasias, and other disorders.

Ultrasonography, fetoscopy, and roentgenography have all been utilized for fetal visualization. The latter two techniques are occasionally still utilized, but advances in ultrasonography now dictate its paramount use. The usual circumstance is that of a couple previously having a child with the defect, thus incurring a 1–5% risk for another affected child. In order to help alter clinical management, defects should be diagnosed by 20–24 weeks' gestation. This is sufficiently early for the alternative reproductive options of termination, fetal surgery, or intensive neonatal surgery.

Antenatal ultrasonography for anomaly detection should be performed only by physicians with great experience. Approximately 45 minutes must be devoted to the task, using the most modern equipment. Brief (Level I) exams by primary providers should not be used to derive information regarding anomaly detection. In fact, physicians scanning obstetric patients for fetal viability, presence or absence of twins, and placental location should explicitly inform their patients that no attempt at anomaly assessment is being made.

The predictive value of Level II ultrasonography for anomaly assessment is still uncertain, even in the best of hands. Some data are published, but even the definitions of "correct" and "incorrect" diagnosis are not uniform. How should one classify cases in which second-trimester exams reveal no anomalies, but the anomaly becomes evident in the third trimester? Such an occurrence is a diagnostic error so far as a couple's reproductive options are concerned, but it might merely have reflected normal developmental processes. Different sets of data have also been gathered using different equipment, reflecting continually improving technology. It follows that the only truly relevant data are those compiled by that ultrasonographer who will be performing a given examination.

Some generalizations can, nonetheless, be offered. First, it is worth emphasizing again that anomaly assessment should be eschewed by the casual ultrasonographer. Second, data from even the most experienced sonologists show predictive values of less than 100%, even when defining "correct" diagnosis in ways that maximize percentages of correct outcomes. For example, maximum favorable outcomes would be recorded if one considered a pregnancy to be monitored correctly whenever a corect diagnosis was achieved prior to delivery. Third, some diagnoses (hydrocephaly, neural tube defects, omphalocele, renal and bladder anomalies) are more readily achievable than others. By contrast, cardiac assessment is more hazardous, and gastrointestinal obstruction (e.g., duodenal atresia) probably cannot be detected prior to the third trimester. Although achieved, it also seems hazardous to render a diagnosis on the basis of decreased fetal motion (e.g., arthrogryposis or multiple flexion contractures). Finally, in some centers sex prediction is considered highly accurate late in pregnancy, but less accurate prior to 24 weeks. Fetal sex can be correctly predicted in about 80% of cases between 16 and 24 weeks' gestation, but cytogenetic methods should be utilized if fetal sexing is truly important (e.g., X-linked recessive traits).

Fetal Sex Determination for X-Linked Recessive Disorders

In X-linked recessive or male-limited autosomal dominant traits, ordinarily only males are affected. Lesch–Nyhan syndrome, Fabry's disease, glucose 6-phosphate dehydrogenase deficiency, Hunter's syndrome, the fragile X-syndrome, hemophilia, probably Duchenne's muscular dystrophy, and probably X-linked retinitis pigmentosam are X-linked traits for which a definitive diagnosis is or soon will be possible. As informative restriction fragment-length polymorphisms (RFLP) are identified along the X (see below), the list of detectable X-linked disorders should increase very rapidly. (See below for explanation of this approach.) For X-linked disorders that are not definitively diagnosable, one is currently restricted to avoiding misdiagnoses of an affected child by terminating all pregnancies in which the fetus is male. Unfortunately, 50% of males aborted from heterozygous females prove genetically normal.

Some investigators have suggested determining fetal sex on the basis of X-chromatin or Y-chromatin interphase nuclei. This approach has the theoretical advantage of speed. However, fetal sex is more accurately determined on the basis of chromosomal studies. One reason is that testicular determinants on the Y chromosome are located, not in the fluorescent portion of the Y long arm, but rather in the nonfluorescent region near the centromere.[39] The fluorescent region contains no important genes yet is responsible for Y-chromatin. Males lacking the entire fluorescent region would be Y-chromatin negative ("female"). Regions of autosomal fluorescence may also mimic Y-chromatin during interphase and lead to false positive diagnosis.

X-chromatin analysis may also be unreliable because slides containing a relatively high proportion of desiccated cells may lead to erroneous diagnoses. Alternatively, use of gene probes for Y-specific or X-specific regions might permit rapid sex determination with a few cells. Again, the probes need not necessarily correlate with chromosomal regions containing pivotal loci. Fetal sex determination is most reliably determined by chromosomal analysis.

Diagnosis Through Fetoscopic Tissue Sampling (Blood Skin, Liver)

If a gene is not expressed in amniotic fluid or chorionic villus cells, morphologic or biochemical evaluation of such cells will provide no information concerning presence or absence of the disorder. However, the gene might still be expressed in blood, skin, or liver. These tissues can be obtained by fetoscopy. Unfortunately, the likelihood of abortion following fetoscopy is about 1–3% over the background loss rate, or 5–6% absolute loss rate.[19] The severity of some disorders may justify this risk if no other method is available. Fetoscopic sampling is increasingly becoming obsolete in the United States because of the increasing availability of molecular techniques. On the other hand, fetoscopy is still used for diagnosis of β-thalassemia in certain Mediterranean countries.

As alluded to above, the initial experience in fetoscopy was gathered in the diagnosis of hemoglobinopathies. Until molecular techniques were developed, antenatal diagnosis of hemoglobinopathies was achievable, not with amniotic fluid cells, but only with fetal blood. Fetal cells obtained at fetoscopy were incubated with radioactive leucine, with the synthesis of the various globin chains assayed to determine the presence or absence of total globin (e.g., β-globin in β-thalassemia) or specific globin (e.g., presence or absence of β^S in sickle cell anemia). Fetoscopic hemoglobin assays are highly (99%) accurate.[2]

Other disorders potentially diagnosable by analysis of fetal serum include hemophilia A (Factor VIII deficiency), detectable on the basis of an increase in the ratio Factor VIII-related antigen/Factor VIII-coagulant antigen.[31] The latter, but not the former, is decreased in hemophiliac fetuses. Hemophilia B (Factor IX deficiency) can also be detected by similar methodology, as can homozygous von Willebrand's disease. Gene probes for both hemophilia A and B are now available. Molecular techniques should thus permit diagnosis to be achieved by less invasive means (amniocentesis or CVS).

Analysis of fetal liver permits diagnosis of other disorders, such as the urea cycle defects ornithine transcarbamylase (OTC) deficiencies.[19] (Again, gene probes for OTC are becoming available.) Fetal liver biopsies carry a fetal loss risk of 1–3% above background.

Mutant genes may also produce life-threatening dermatologic abnormalities. Examples include epidermolysis bullosa and congenital ichthyosis. Because the metabolic basis of these disorders is not known, antenatal diagnosis is possible only through fetal skin biopsy. The safety of skin biopsies is uncertain, but the risk of abortion is estimated at 1–3%. Diagnoses have been made for harlequin ichthyosis, epidermolysis bullosa dystrophica, the Sjögren–Larsson syndrome and several other disorders.[11]

Linkage Analysis

Each gene is located on a chromosome in definite linear relationship to other genes. A given gene is, therefore, closer to some genes than others. During meiosis I, recombination can occur between homologous chromosomes. Genes are said to be linked to one another if, after meiosis I, they remain together more often than expected by chance.[46] That is, genes are linked if they usually segregate to the same gamete rather than to complementary gametes. The distance between loci can be determined by calculating the frequency with which genes on the same chromosome become interchanged (recombine) during meiosis I. If genes at different loci remain on the same parental chromosome with a frequency of 90%, they are said to be 10 map units apart. When genes remain together in only 50% of segregants, one cannot distinguish loose linkage from absence of linkage (i.e., presence of genes on different chromosomes). However, a relationship between two loosely linked genes whose recombination frequency is greater than 50% can be recognized if both prove linked to a third gene located intermediate between the two.

Linkage analysis can be used to diagnose mendelian disorders in which there exist neither metabolic assays nor other techniques to measure the mutant gene. The principle involves testing for the presence or absence of a "marker" gene closely linked to the mutant gene that is of interest. Status of the mutant can be inferred by the status of the marker, even though the two are functionally independent.

Figure 13-5[40] illustrates a family in which one child had 21-hydroxylase adrenogenital syndrome (ag). This locus and the HLA locus are closely linked on chromosome 6. HLA typing was therefore performed on both parents and on the affected child. In both mother and father (coincidentally), HLA types of the affected child revealed that the No. 6 chromosome containing the mutant (ag) gene also contained HLA antigens A2 and B27. The homologous No. 6 chromosome must, therefore, code for the normal gene (+) at the ag locus and for either HLA-A26 B35 (maternal) or HLA-A1 B17 (paternal). Fetal status could then be deduced on the basis of HLA studies of amniotic fluid fibroblasts. The 46,XY fetus showed HLA antigens A1B17/A26 B35; thus, from both parents he received the normal allele (+) rather than the ag allele. He was unaffected. Incidentally, antenatal diagnosis of 21-hydroxylase deficiency can now be achieved more rapidly on the basis of elevated levels of 17α-hydroxyprogesterone in amniotic fluid. 11β-Hydroxylase deficiency is not linked to HLA.

An important caveat of linkage analysis is that the method is never 100% accurate. Recombination can occur even between closely linked loci. Nonetheless, linkage analysis is becoming increasingly more practical as a more complete map of the human genome is developed. Linkage analysis should prove especially useful for autosomal dominant traits, few of which are detectable by current techniques. A limitation in the past has been availability of only limited numbers of informative blood group and serum protein polymorphisms. However, innumerable DNA polymorphisms (restriction fragment-length polymorphisms, RFLP) now exist, as discussed below. Use of RFLPs should eventually allow almost all mendelian disorders to be detected by linkage analysis.

MOLECULAR GENETICS IN PRENATAL DIAGNOSIS

Although it is clinically convenient to discuss molecular genetic techniques at the end of this chapter, the converse will likely be true in the future. More and more disorders are proving detectable by molecular techniques. Initially, such techniques were applied to disorders heretofore diagnosed by fetoscopy. The hemoglobinopathies were the first to be studied, especially α-thalassemia[26] and sickle cell anemia.[4,36] Later, β-thalassemia[4] and hemophilia proved detectable, using the principles of link-

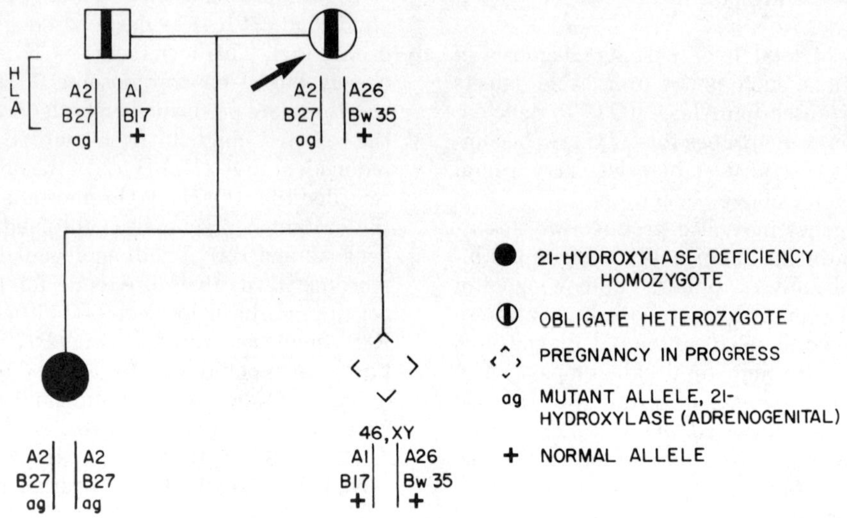

Figure 13-5. Linkage analysis. Antenatal studies of cultured fibroblasts excluded 21-hydroxylase deficiency in a fetus whose haplotypes differed from those of an affected liveborn sibling. The paternal chromosome 6 carrying the mutant allele for 21-hydroxylase contains A2B27; the maternal number 6 carrying the mutant also contains A2B27. The fetus is, however, homozygous for both normal alleles, assuming no recombination between the locus for ag and the locus for HLA 21-hydroxylase deficiency. In: *Genetic Issues in Pediatric and Obstetric Practice.* M. M. Kabach (Ed.). Chicago, Year Book Med. Publ., 1981, pp. 329–368 (by permission of the publisher).[40]

age analysis through RFLPs. More recently, it has proved possible to detect phenylketonuria, Duchenne's muscular dystrophy[3] and Huntington's chorea. In each case, linkage analysis is necessary. An inclusive list of currently detectable disorders is not practical, given the rapid advances. However, it is worthwhile to understand the rationale behind achieving diagnoses with molecular techniques.

Utilizing molecular genetics for prenatal diagnosis required the development of several analytical techniques. Each of the techniques can actually be used for a variety of different purposes, only a few of which need to be alluded to here. The principles are summarized in recent reviews.[15,42] After discussing the rationale, diagnostic approaches will be outlined.

Restriction Endonucleases and Restriction Fragment-Length Polymorphisms

A pivotal development in molecular genetics was the discovery of *restriction endonucleases*, bacterial enzymes that recognize and cut specific nucleotide sequences in double-stranded DNA molecules. The sites at which DNA are cut are called restriction sites. Approximately 200 different restriction enzymes are known, each recognizing a unique sequence of bases. Figure 13-6 illustrates the recognition sequence of one particular enzyme.

The availability of restriction enzymes allowed DNA to be cut into fragments whose lengths were consistent from experiment to experiment. DNA fragments resulting from restriction enzymes differ in length in direct proportion to the distance between recognition sites. The greater the distance between recognition sites, the longer the length of intervening DNA. Restriction fragments are specified according to numbers of bases (e.g., 10,000 bases = 10 kilobases = 10 kb). A single gene may or may not contain more than one restriction site for a given enzyme. Usually there is more than one site, but occasionally the sites might be situated in such a way that the entire gene lies between two sites. If a gene contains more than one restriction site, its DNA would ordinarily be subdivided into fragments of different lengths.

Of great diagnostic importance are observations that DNA from ostensibly normal individuals will not always show the same spectrum of

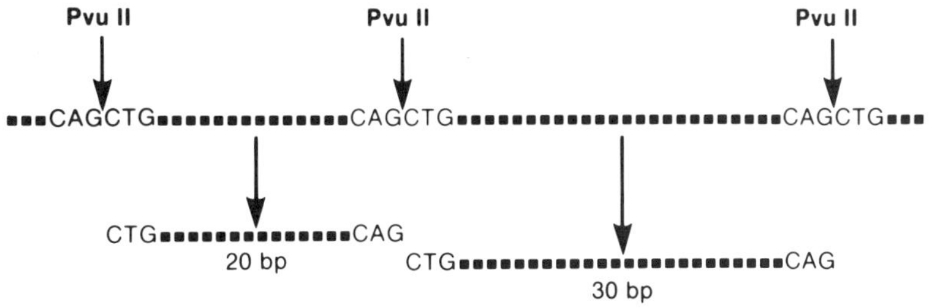

Figure 13-6. Simplified diagram illustrating the manner in which a restriction endonuclease cuts DNA at a specific nucleotide sequence. DNA nucleotide sequences shown as single-stranded. Pvu II recognizes the sequence CAGCTG and only that sequence. DNA is separated into fragments of different lengths on the basis of distances between restriction enzyme recognition sites. The further the distance between sites, the longer the length of intervening DNA. Shorter DNA fragments show greater mobility and migrate further in the agarose cell. From Simpson, J. L.: Genetic counseling and prenatal diagnosis. In: *Obstetrics: Normal and Problem Pregnancies.* S. G. Gabbe, J. F. Niebyl, and J. L. Simpson (Eds.). New York, Churchill-Livingstone, in press (by permission of the publisher).[41]

DNA fragments following exposure to a given restriction enzyme. The reason is that differences in DNA sequences exist among the population. Occasionally DNA differences are well known, producing diseases like sickle cell anemia. At other times, the differences confer no advantage or disadvantage. Thus, polymorphism exists with respect to the presence or absence of restriction sites. The term restriction fragment-length polymorphism (RFLP) has been coined to denote this phenomenon.

An RFLP is completely analogous to a blood group (e.g., ABO) or serum protein (e.g., G6PD) polymorphism. Individuals may or may not differ with respect to a given RFLP, as they may or may not differ with respect to a given protein polymorphism. The major difference is that RFLP polymorphisms need not involve coding DNA, whereas blood group polymorphisms always do. Innumerable RFLPs have been or will be in the human genome, greatly enhancing the number of polymorphic markers useful for linkage analysis. A given RFLP may be closely linked to a locus conferring a disease, allowing linkage analysis for presence or absence of a disorder. Since RFLPs exist every few centimorgans, linkage analysis will eventually permit prenatal diagnosis for almost all loci.

Southern Blotting and Hybridization

DNA digested by restriction endonucleases yields fragments of varying lengths. If allowed to migrate through an agarose gel, heavier DNA fragments prove less mobile. They remain near the origin of the gel. Lighter fragments migrate further (Fig. 13-7). The gel can be laid on a piece of nitrocellulose paper, and buffer allowed to flow through the gel onto the nitrocellulose filter. DNA fragments concomitantly migrate out of the gel and bind to the filter, creating a replica of the DNA fragment pattern.

If the nitrocellulose replicate is exposed to a specific *gene probe* (see below), the probe will hybridize only to that portion of the filter containing complementary DNA. To appreciate how a probe can be utilized, recall that DNA is double-stranded. If separated, the two strands will reapproximate themselves through complementary base pairing. If strands are disrupted (denatured), however, an interloping piece of DNA could compete and reaggregate with any existing complementary DNA sequences. The interloper could be cloned DNA (probe). If the probe consists of unique sequence DNA, it will locate its complementary DNA sequence, and only that sequence. If the probe is radioactive, autoradiographic techniques will signify the exact fragment in which the complementary sequence is located. That is, a gene (or, more specifically, a DNA sequence that is part of a gene) can be located among thousands of fragments, categorized according to length.

There are a variety of ways to make DNA probes. They can be synthesized from known human or animal genes, or from random (anonymous) DNA segments. Figure 13-8 illustrates

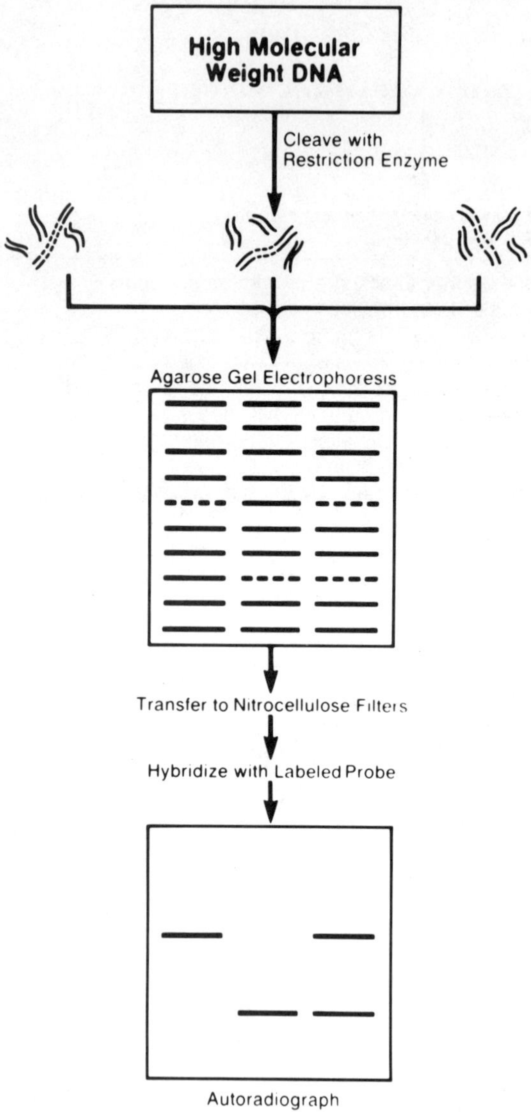

Figure 13-7. Southern blotting. DNA is cleaved with a restriction enzyme, and the cleaved DNA separated by size using agarose gel electrophoresis. The gel is then laid on a piece of nitrocellulose, and buffer is allowed to flow through the gel onto the nitrocellulose. DNA fragments migrate out of the gel and bind to the filter. A replica of the gel's DNA fragment pattern is thus made on the filter. The filter can then be hybridized with a suitable radioactively labeled probe; DNA fragments that hybridize to the probe are identified following autoradiography. From Simpson, J. L.: Genetic counseling and prenatal diagnosis. In: *Obstetrics: Normal and Problem Pregnancies.* S. G. Gabbe, J. F. Niebyl, and J. L. Simpson (Eds.). New York, Churchill-Livingstone, in press (by permission of the publisher).[41]

one way. This topic is considered in more detail elsewhere.[26,36,42]

Is the probe useful? To determine this, we need to ascertain if it is linked to the gene causing the disease of interest. This can be achieved by laborious techniques (and luck!). One hopes that the new probe will highlight an RFLP region that is linked to a known genetic locus or linked to a previously localized RFLP.

A natural extension of the techniques described above is the development of oligonucleotide probes. One can create DNA probes for sequences of any desired number of nucleotides. Technology exists that will create probes consisting of only a small number of nucleotides (oligonucleotides). These sensitive probes will hybridize only to sequences complementary for every single nucleotide. If only a single nucleotide is absent (or altered), the oligonucleotide probe will fail to hybridize. A variety of useful oligonucleotide probes are being developed, especially to diagnose hemoglobinopathies.

Diagnosis When the Molecular Basis Is Known

Let us now illustrate the value of the analytical techniques described above. Recall first that a gene mutation can result from any of several different mechanisms. Disorders may be caused by the complete absence of DNA (deletions) or by the presence of a single abnormal nucleotide (point mutation). An obvious way to detect a disorder characterized by absence of DNA would be to determine whether or not a DNA probe for the normal gene hybridizes DNA of an unknown individual. If the latter's DNA does not hybridize, he or she must lack the DNA sequence and thus must be affected. A related approach, utilized first for α-thalassemia, is to measure the rapidity with which complementary DNA (cDNA) hybridizes with DNA from an unknown individual. Since α-globin cDNA is complementary to α-globin structural genes, the rapidity of cDNA hybridization should reflect the number of α-globin genes (0,1,2,3,4) present. (Two genes code for α-globin; thus, each individual has four alleles. In homozygous α-thalassemia, all four α-globin alleles are deleted; in hemoglobin H disease, three of the four alleles are deleted.) Normal DNA (four alleles) will reanneal more quickly than DNA from hemoglobin H disease, which, in turn, reanneals more rapidly than homozygous α-thalassemia. DNA from the fetus in question could, of course, be derived from any available nucleated cell-

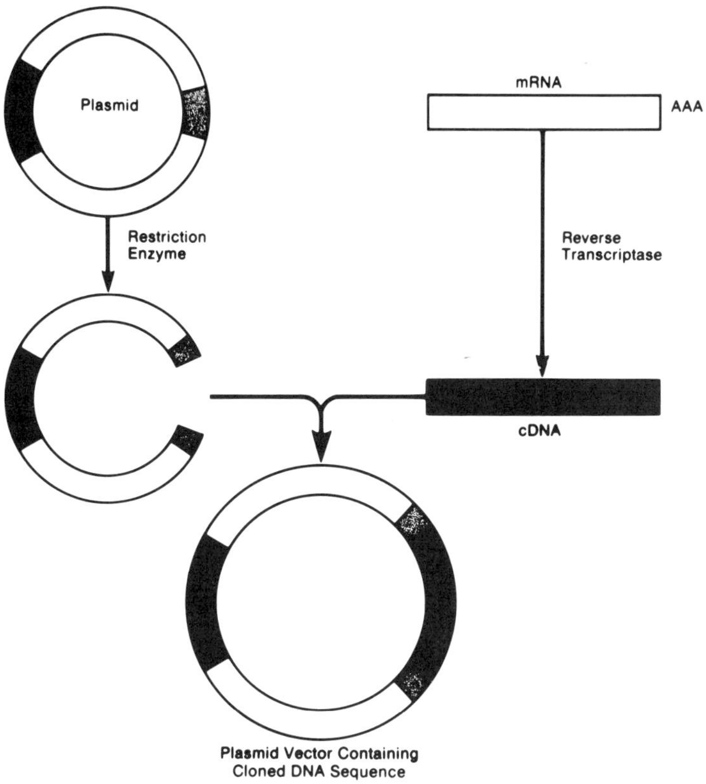

Figure 13-8. Diagram illustrating formation of a cloned DNA, from which a probe can be made. A DNA fragment is inserted in a plasmid vector, which can synthesize many copies of the inserted fragment. From Simpson, J. L.: Genetic counseling and prenatal diagnosis. In: *Obstetrics: Normal and Problem Pregnancies.* S. G. Gabbe, J. F. Niebyl, and J. L. Simpson (Eds.). New York, Churchill-Livingstone, in press (by permission of the publisher).[41]

chorionic villi, amniotic fluid cells, or perhaps trophoblasts in the maternal circulation.

A second general approach becomes applicable whenever the nucleotide sequence producing a mutation is known. Knowing the altered nucleotide sequence potentially allows one to select a restriction enzyme that acts at the specific site that has become altered. A useful restriction enzyme may or may not exist, but, if it does, prenatal diagnosis becomes possible. An example is sickle cell anemia, a disorder in which codon 6 (the triplet signifying the sixth amino acid) has undergone a mutation from adenine to thymine. Valine rather than glutamic acid is synthesized, this change alone being responsible for the altered hemoglobin structure. Restriction enzymes capable of recognizing the normal nucleotide sequence, but not capable of recognizing the mutant sequence, exist. For example, enzymes Mst II and Dde I require the normal nucleotide sequence at codon 6 (Fig. 13-9). Use of a β-globin DNA probe can differentiate DNA containing the mutant gene from DNA containing the normal gene. The probe

CTN*AG	Dde I cleavage site
C CTGAG GAG	Nucleotide sequence for Hgb A
C CTGTG GAG	Nucleotide sequence for Hgb S

* N = any nucleotide

Figure 13-9. Loss of Dde I restriction recognition site in βs (sickle cell anemia). Mutation of adenine to thymine results in a new nucleotide sequence, no longer recognized by Dde I. From Simpson, J. L.: Genetic counseling and prenatal diagnosis. In: *Obstetrics: Normal and Problem Pregnancies.* S. G. Gabbe, J. F. Niebyl, and J. L. Simpson (Eds.). New York, Churchill-Livingstone, in press (by permission of the publisher).[41]

highlights a longer fragment in the former as a result of the missing restriction site (Fig. 13-10). This approach is highly accurate for sickle cell anemia.

A third approach applicable when either a deletion or altered nucleotide sequence exists is to utilize an oligonucleotide probe. The probe will hybridize only to DNA containing each of a specified number of nucleotides. Alteration or absence of a single nucleotide results in failure of oligonucleotide hybridization. Oligonucleotide probes are available for many hemoglobinopathies.

Diagnosis When the Molecular Basis of a Disorder Is Not Known (Use of RFLP)

If the nucleotide sequence responsible for a given disorder is unknown, the approaches described above are not fruitful. Fortunately, one can still use molecular techniques if the mutant gene has been localized to a chromosome and if an RFLP is nearby. We have already noted that RFLPs exist throughout the genome. These RFLPs serve as markers, permitting linkage analysis by following segregation of mutant genes in a given family.

The difficulty lies in finding an RFLP closely linked to the mutant gene in question. Two general steps are required. First, one needs to screen a panel (library) of cloned DNA probes to locate one that identifies an RFLP near the gene in question. Various libraries have been created, and with effort one hopes to identify a clone located near the mutant. Prior knowledge helps, but trial-and-error is necessary, utilizing principles of linkage analysis.

Second, one must determine whether an in-

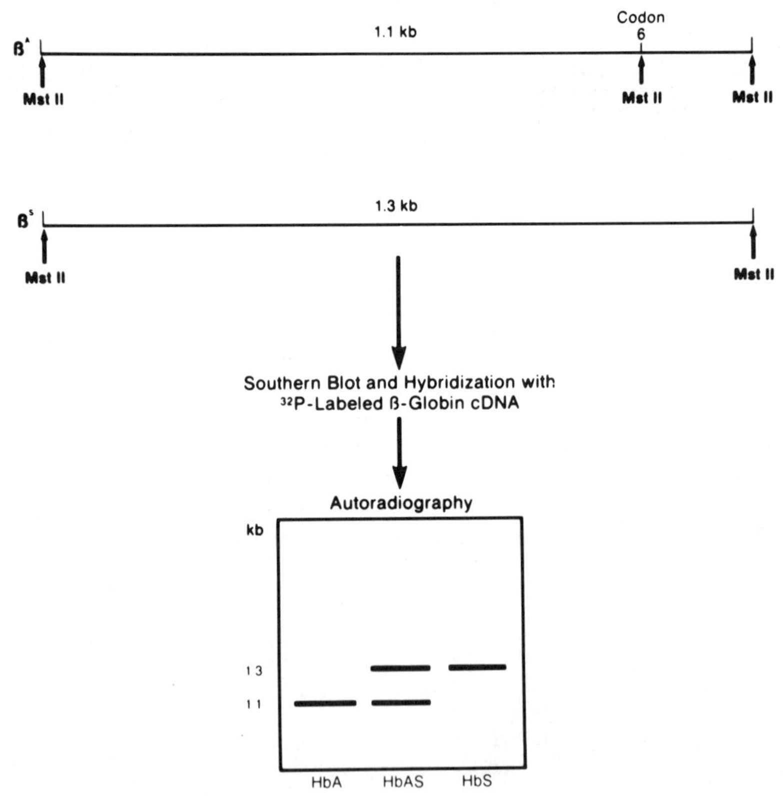

Figure 13-10. Using a radioactively labeled gene probe for β-globin to diagnose sickle cell anemia and those rare types of β-thalassemia in which the gene is deleted. In: *Obstetrics: Normal and Problem Pregnancies.* S. G. Gabbe, J. F. Niebyl, and J. L. Simpson (Eds.). New York, Churchill-Livingstone, in press (by permission of the publisher).[41]

formative situation exists in a given family, having identified a potentially informative probe. Suppose, for example, that a probe sometimes highlights a fragment of DNA 2000 bp long, whereas, at other times, it highlights a fragment 3000 bp long (Fig. 13-11). Still other individuals might show both a 2000 bp and a 3000 bp band, being heterozygous. Suppose further that this RFLP has already been proved to be closely linked to the locus corresponding to a given mutant. Analysis of RFLP patterns within a given family may then permit diagnosis. The approach is illustrated in Fig. 13-11. It is important to remember that the principles of linkage analysis apply whether the polymorphic locus is a blood group or an RFLP. That is, the RFLP pattern that will signal an affected fetus in one family (e.g., homozygous 2000 bp fragments in Fig. 13-11) may indicate just the opposite in another family. The RFLP merely serves as a marker, its presence or absence functionally independent from the disease. Moreover, DNA

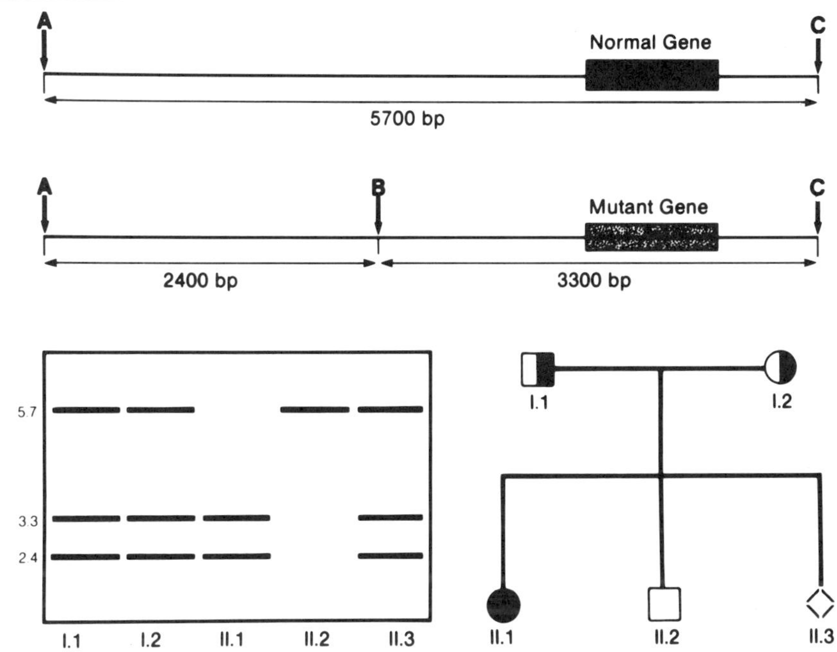

Figure 13-11. Prenatal diagnosis achieved by use of a restriction fragment-length polymorphism (RFLP), linked to the locus causing a disease. Suppose a restriction site, B, is closely linked to a gene. This restriction site is present in some individuals but not in others (i.e., polymorphism). A probe that hybridizes to DNA containing the polymorphic site will identify 2400 bp and 3300 bp fragments in individuals with the restriction site, but only a single 5700 bp fragment in those without the restriction site. On agarose gel electrophoresis, individuals heterozygous for the restriction site will display three bands (see individuals 1.1, 1.2, and 11.3), and individuals homozygous for the restriction site will display two bands (11.1). Homozygous individuals lacking the restriction site will display only one band (11.2).

In this family, parents (1.1, 1.2) are doubly heterozygous. They are each heterozygous for the mutant gene and are also heterozygous for the restriction site. DNA analysis of the affected child 11.1 shows only two bands (3.3 and 2.4 kb). We can conclude that in both parents the mutant gene is located on the chromosome characterized by the presence of restriction site B. Thus, DNA analysis reveals that their unaffected son (11.2) is not heterozygous but rather homozygous normal. DNA analysis from amniotic fluid cells or chorionic villi reveals that fetus (11.3) is normal but heterozygous. From Simpson, J. L.: Genetic counseling and prenatal diagnosis. In: *Obstetrics: Normal and Problem Pregnancies*. S. G. Gabbe, J. F. Niebyl, and J. L. Simpson (Eds.). New York, Churchill-Livingstone, in press (by permission of the publisher).[41]

patterns in a given family may not be informative. This circumstance would exist if, in Fig. 13-11, the mother, father, and affected fetus all showed only a 2000 bp fragment. It would be impossible to deduce disease status on the basis of this particular RFLP. However, another closely linked RFLP might be useful.

The beauty of RFLP linkage analysis is at least twofold. First, a limitless number of RFLPs exist throughout the human genome, eventually assuring prenatal diagnosis for any disorder whose chromosomal localization is known. Second, diagnosis can be accomplished without knowledge of the molecular basis of a disorder. This should especially prove advantageous for autosomal dominant disorders, about whose molecular basis we know very little.

REFERENCES

1. Aitken, D. A., Yaqoob, M., and Ferguson-Smith, M. A.: Microvillar enzyme analysis in amniotic fluid and the prenatal diagnosis of cystic fibrosis. *Prenat. Diagn.* **5**:119–127, 1985.
2. Alter, B .P.: Prenatal diagnosis of hemoglobinopathies and other hematologic disease. *J. Pediatr.* **95**:501–503, 1979.
3. Bakker, E., Hofker, M. H., Goor, N., Mandel, J. L., Wrogermann, K., Davies, K. E., Kunkel, L. M., Willard, H.F., Fenton, W.A., Sandkuyl, L., Majoor-Krakauer, D., v. Essen, A. J., Jahoda, M. G. J., Sachs, E. S., van Ommen, G. J. B., and Pearson, P. L.:. Prenatal diagnosis and carrier detection of Duchenne muscular dystrophy with closely linked RFLPs. *Lancet* **1**:655–658, 1985.
4. Boehm, C. D., Antonarakis, S. E., Phillips, J. A., III, Stetten, G., and Kazazian, H. H., Jr.: Prenatal diagnosis using DNA polymorphisms: Report on 95 pregnancies at risk for sickle cell disease and β-thalassemia. *N. Engl. J. Med.* **308**:1054–1058, 1983.
5. Boué, A. and Gallano, P.: A collaborative study of the segregation of inherited chromosome structural rearrangements in 1356 prenatal diagnoses. *Prenat. Diagn.* **4**(Spec. no.):45–67, 1984.
6. Brock, D. J.: A comparative study of microvillar enzyme activities in the prenatal detection of cystic fibrosis. Prenat. Diagn. **5**:129–134, 1985.
7. Brock, D. J. H.: *Early Diagnosis of Fetal Defects.* London, Churchill-Livingstone, 1982.
8. Christiaens, G. C. and Stoutenbeek, P.: Spontaneous abortion in proven intact pregnancies. (letter) *Lancet* **2**:571–572, 1984.
9. Cuckle, H. S., Wald, N. J., and Lindenbaum, R. H.: Maternal serum alpha-fetoprotein measurement: A screening test for Down syndrome. *Lancet* **1**:926–929, 1984.
10. Department of Obstetrics and Gynecology, Tietung Hospital of Anshan Iron and Steel Company, Anshan. Fetal sex prediction by sex chromatin of chorionic villi cells during early pregnancy. *Chin. Med. J.* **1**:117–126, 1975.
11. Elias, S., and Esterly, N. B.: Prenatal diagnosis of hereditary skin disorders. *Clin. Obstet. Gynecol.* **24**:1069–1087, 1981.
12. Elias, S. Gerbie, A. B., Simpson, J. L., Nadler, H. L., Sabbagha, R. E., and Shkolnik, A.: Genetic amniocentesis in twin gestations. *Am. J. Obstet. Gynecol.* **138**:169–174, 1980.
13. Elias, S. and Simpson, J. L.: Amniocentesis. In: *Genetic Disorders and the Fetus,* 2nd Edition. New York, Plenum Press, in press.
14. Bombard, A., Rosinsky, B. J., Baum, L. D. Chorionic villus sampling in continuous pregnancies. I. Low fetal loss rates in initial 109 cases. *Am. J. Obstet. Gynecol.* **154:**1349–1352, 1986.
15. Emery, E. H.: *An Introduction to Recombinant DNA.* Chichester, England, Wiley, 1984.
16. Ferguson-Smith, M. A. and Yates, J. R. W.: Maternal age specific rates for chromosome aberrations and factors influencing them: Report of a collaborative European study on 52,965 amniocenteses. *Prenat. Diagn.* **4**(Spec. no.):5–44, 1984.
17. Galjaard, H.: *Genetic Metabolic Diseases, Early Diagnosis and Prenatal Analysis.* Amsterdam, Elsevier, 1980.
18. Hamilton, M. P., Abdalla, H.I., and Whitfield, C. R.: Significance of raised maternal serum alpha-fetoprotein in singleton pregnancies with normally formed fetuses. *Obstet. Gynecol.* **65**:465–470, 1985.
19. Harrison, M. R., Golbus, M. S., and Filly, R. A.: *The Unborn Patient. Diagnosis and Treatment.* Orlando, FL, Grune & Stratton, 1984.
20. Hassold, T. J.: A cytogenetic study of repeated abortions. *Am. J. Hum. Genet.* **32**:723–730, 1980.
21. Hook, E. B.: Chromosome abnormalities and spontaneous fetal death following amniocentesis: Further data and association with maternal age. *Am. J. Hum. Genet.* **35**:110–116, 1983.
22. Hook, E. B.: Rates of chromosome abnormalities at different maternal ages. *Obstet. Gynecol.* **58**:282–285, 1981.
23. Hook, E. B., Cross, P. K., and Schreinemachers, D. M.: Chromosomal abnormality rates at amniocentesis and in liveborn infants. *JAMA* **249**:2034–2038, 1983.
24. Hsu, L. Y. F. and Perlis, T. E.: United States survey on chromosome mosaicism and pseudomosaicism in prenatal diagnosis. *Prenat. Diagn.* **4**(Spec. no.):97–130, 1984.
25. Jackson, L. G. and Wapner, R. J.: Chorionic biopsy. (letter) *N. Engl. J. Med.* **311**:539–540, 1984.
26. Kan, Y. W., Golbus, M. S., and Dozy, A. M.: Prenatal diagnosis of alpha-thalassemia. Clinical application of molecular hybridization. *N. Engl. J. Med.* **295**:1165–1167, 1976.

27. Karp, L. E. and Schiller, H. S.: Meconium staining of amniotic fluid at midtrimester amniocentesis. *Obstet. Gynecol.* **50**(Suppl.):47s–49s, 1977.
28. Kazy, Z., Rozovky, I. S., and Bakharev, V. A.: Chorion biopsy in early pregnancy: A method of early prenatal diagnosis for inherited disorders. *Prenat. Diagn.* **2**:39–45, 1982.
29. Kullander, S. and Sandahl, B.: Fetal chromosome analysis after transcervical placental biopsies during early pregnancy. *Acta Obstet. Gynecol. Scand.* **52**:355–359, 1973.
30. Martin, A. O., Simpson, J. L., Deddish, R. B., and Elias, S.: Clinical implications of chromosomal inversions. A pericentric inversion in No. 18 segregating in a family ascertained through an abnormal proband. *Am. J. Perinatol.* **1**:81–88, 1983.
31. Mibashan, R. S. and Rodeck, C. H.: Haemophilia and other genetic defects of haemostasis. In: *Prenatal Diagnosis.* C. H. Rodeck and K. H. Nicolaides (Eds.). Chichester, England, Wiley, 1984, pp. 179–194.
32. Mikkelsen, M.: Cytogenetic findings in first trimester chorionic villi biopsies: A collaborative study. In: *First Trimester Fetal Diagnosis* (M. Fraccaro, G. Simoni, B. Brambati) Berlin, Springer. Verlog, 1985, pp. 109–120.
33. Milunsky, A.: Prenatal diagnosis of neural tube defects. In:. *Genetic Disorders and the Fetus*, lst Edition. A. Milunsky (Ed.). New York, Plenum Press, 1979, pp. 379–430.
34. Milunsky, A., Alpert, E., Neff, R. K., and Frigoletto, F. D., Jr.: Prenatal diagnosis of neural tube defects. IV. Maternal serum alpha-fetoprotein screening. *Obstet. Gynecol.* **55**:60–66, 1980.
35. N.I.C.H.D. National Registry for Amniocentesis Study Group: Midtrimester amniocentesis for prenatal diagnosis. Safety and accuracy. *JAMA* **236**:1471–1476, 1976.
36. Old, J. M.: First trimester diagnosis of haemoglobinopathies by DNA analysis of chorionic villi. In: *Prenatal Diagnosis.* C. H. Rodeck and K. H. Nicolaides (Eds.). Chichester, England, Wiley, 1984, pp. 105–115.
37. Old, J. M., Ward, R. H., Petrou, M., Karagozlu, F., Modell, B., and Weatherall, D. J.: First trimester fetal diagnosis for haemoglobinopathies: Three cases. *Lancet* **2**:1413–1416, 1982.
38. Simoni, G., Brambati, B., Danesino, C., Rossella, F., Terzoli, G. L., Ferrari, M., and Fraccaro, M.: Efficient direct chromosome analyses and enzyme determinations from chorionic villi samples in the first trimester of pregnancy. *Hum. Genet.* **63**:349–357, 1983.
39. Simpson, J. L.: *Disorders of Sexual Differentiation. Etiology and Clinical Delineation.* New York, Academic Press, 1976.
40. Simpson, J. L.: Disorders of sexual differentiation resulting from mutant genes. In: *Genetic Issues in Pediatric and Obstetric Practice.* M. M. Kaback (Ed.). Chicago, Year Book, 1981, pp. 329–368.
41. Simpson, J. L.: Genetic counseling and prenatal diagnosis. In: *Obstetrics: Normal and Problem Pregrancies.* S. G. Gabbe, J. F. Niebyl, and J. L. Simpson (Eds.). New York, Churchill-Livingstone, 1986.
42. Simpson, J. L.: *Genetics.* CREOG Basic Science Monograph in Obstetrics and Gynecology. Washington, American College of Obstetricians and Gynecologists, 1986.
43. Simpson, J. L.: Low fetal loss rate after normal ultrasound at eight weeks gestation: Implications for chorionic villus sampling (CVS). (Abstract) *Am. J. Hum. Genet.* **36**(Suppl.):197s, 1984.
44. Simpson, J. L.: Pregnancies in women with chromosomal abnormalities. In: *Genetic Diseases in Pregnancy.* J. D. Schulman and J. L. Simpson (Eds.). New York, Academic Press, 1982, pp. 439–471.
45. Simpson, J. L.: Repetitive spontaneous abortion. In: *Perinatal Genetics.* I. H. Porter (Ed.). New York, Academic Press, in press.
46. Simpson, J. L., Golbus, M. S., Martin, A. O., and Sarto, G. E.: *Genetics in Obstetrics and Gynecology.* New York, Grune & Stratton, 1982.
47. Simpson, J. L., Martin, A. O., Verp, M. S., Elias, S., and Patel, V. A.: Hypermodal cells in amniotic fluid cultures: Frequency, interpretation, and clinical significance. *Am. J. Obstet. Gynecol.* **143**:250–258, 1982.
48. Stene, J., Stene, E., and Mikkelsen, M.: Risk for chromosome abnormality at amniocentesis following a child with a non-inherited chromosome aberration. A European collaborative study on prenatal diagnoses 1981. *Prenat. Diagn.* **4**(Spec. no.):81–95, 1984.
49. Verp, M. S. and Simpson, J. L.: Prenatal diagnosis of cytogenetic abnormalities. In: *Prenatal Diagnosis.* K. Filkins and J. F. Russo, eds. New York, Marcel Dekker, 1986, pp. 13–48.
50. Wald, N. J., Cuckle, H., Brock, J. H., Peto, R., Polani, P. E., and Woodford, F. P.: Maternal serum-alpha-fetoprotein measurement in antenatal screening for anencephaly and spina bifida in early pregnancy. Report of U.K. collaborative study on alpha-fetoprotein in relation to neural-tube defects. *Lancet* **1**:1323–1332, 1977.
51. Warburton, D.: Outcome of cases of de novo structural rearrangements diagnosed at amniocentesis. *Prenat. Diagn.* **4**(Spec. no.):69–80, 1984.
52. Wilson, R. D., Kendrick, V., Wittmann, B. K., and McGillivray, B. C.: Spontaneous abortion and pregnancy outcome after normal first-trimester ultrasound examination. *Obstet. Gynecol.* **67**:352–355, 1986.
53. Working Party on Amniocentesis. An assessment of the hazards of amniocentesis. Report to the Medical Research Council. *Br. J. Obstet. Gynaecol.* **85**(Suppl. 2):1–41, 1978.

14

CLINICAL TERATOLOGY

Teratology deals with the causes, mechanisms, and manifestations of developmental deviations of a structural or functional nature. Recently, emphasis in teratology has been placed on efforts to prevent such deviations. The word teratology, first used by Paré in the 16th century, is taken from the Greek word for wonderful or monstrous. In modern times, the term has taken on a broader meaning. It now includes a variety of aberrations of development such as intrauterine growth retardation, abortions, intrauterine death, and functional deficiencies, in addition to gross structural malformations. Thus, teratogenic effects include any abnormality of structure, function or metabolism, whether genetically determined or occurring as a result of an adverse influence during embryonic or fetal life. A teratogenic effect may cause disease from the time of conception through birth or even later in life. A teratogenic agent is a drug, chemical, virus, physical agent, or deficiency state that, if present during the embryonic or fetal period, alters morphology or subsequent function in the postnatal period.

The importance of teratology in biomedical science derives from the observation that between 2% and 4% of liveborn humans suffer from gross structural abnormalities. Given 3–4 million deliveries per year, some 60,000–120,000 grossly abnormal children are born each year in the United States alone. Approximately one-third to one-half of these individuals will require medical and/or surgical care. Life expectancy is significantly shorter than normal for many of them. The problem of birth defects is second only to the problem of prematurity in obstetrics. The costs of special education or institutionalization or the reduced productivity resulting from a flawed human life has drawn attention to this problem. The obstetrician plays a central role in prevention, prompt diagnosis, and development of technology for intrauterine therapy of birth defects.

PLACENTAL TRANSFER AND GENETIC SUSCEPTIBILITY TO ENVIRONMENTAL AGENTS

The preimplantation embryo may be exposed to therapeutic and environmental chemicals that reach tubal and uterine fluids. However, at this stage any damage to the conceptus either destroys it entirely or is adequately repaired such that no apparent adverse effects occur. This, then, appears to be an "all-or-nothing" period in embryonic life; chemicals potent enough to cause irreparable injury usually prevent survival of the affected embryo.[22]

After implantation, passage of drugs from mother to fetus occurs chiefly by placental transfer. The placenta does not represent a barrier to the passage of chemicals from the mother to the developing conceptus but should be considered a semipermeable membrane. Factors influencing the ease with which a molecule crosses the membrane include molecular weight and structure of the molecule, the degree of protein binding, the extent to which the compound is ionized, and the lipid solubility of the substance.

An unbound, un-ionized compound with a molecular weight less than 1000 daltons passes across such a membrane with ease. Because the molecular weight of most drugs is in the range of 250–500 daltons, placental transfer is readily accomplished.[56]

Whether or not a drug has any effect on the fetus depends on the ability of the drug to cross the placenta and on other factors. The dose that the fetus receives is of importance. In most cases, small or transient exposure to a chemical is unlikely to result in significant damage to the conceptus. The amount of any chemical that passes from mother to fetus is related to the concentration of the substance in maternal plasma and the length of time that a given concentration is maintained in the mother's blood. Most chemicals cross the placenta by simple diffusion. A higher concentration of the drug in the mother than in the fetus is required to expose the fetus to significant amounts of drug.

Concentration gradients across the placenta may be maintained in a number of ways. The most common are a continued high rate of ingestion of a drug by the mother or faster clearance of the drug by the fetus than by the mother. Our knowledge of how chemicals are distributed, metabolized, and cleared by the fetus is incomplete. The physiological distribution of drugs in the developing conceptus is likely to be different at different gestational ages.[55] For example at midpregnancy, total body water constitutes 95% of the weight of the fetus, whereas at term it constitutes 75% of the weight of the infant. Water-soluble drugs will therefore be proportionately more widely distributed in the younger fetus. Fat stores are limited in the fetus, even at term, and fat-soluble drugs (such as narcotics) may have greater access in the fetus than in the adult to the lipid-rich central nervous system.

The effectiveness of a potential teratogen depends on several factors. The dose reaching the fetus is important because there is likely to be a threshold dose below which no effect is seen.[36] However, duration of exposure and gestational age at which exposure occurs are also important. During the preimplantation stages of pregnancy (15–21 days from the beginning of the last menstrual period), a significant level of drug-induced damage which is not repaired is likely to destroy the embryo. During the period of major organogenesis (up to the end of the 10th menstrual week), morphologic damage is most likely. Therefore, during organ growth and development, drug effects are more likely to result in functional impairment.[77]

Another modifier of teratogenic drug action is the genetic predisposition of the fetus and/or mother. There are clear examples of genetically determined susceptibilities to the embryotoxic effects of drugs.[27] However, how genetic susceptibility and chemical exposure interact in determining abnormal intrauterine development is poorly understood.

Our knowledge of the causes and prevention of these problems is limited. About 15% of human congenital defects are associated with gene mutations and another 15% with chromosome aberrations. Between 3% and 5% of remaining anomalies can be attributed to chemical or physical agents or infections. For the remainder, the mechanism of teratogenesis is unknown.[20]

HUMAN TERATOGENS

Environmental agents that exert significant adverse effects during pregnancy include physical agents, maternal metabolic imbalances, infectious agents, and chemical agents. The list of teratogens has been modified over time as data and new knowledge have accumulated. For example, in 1973, thalidomide, steroid hormones and folic acid antagonists were considered "positively implicated" as teratogens,[78] whereas in 1979, cancer chemotherapeutic agents, DES, goitrogens/antithyroid drugs, hydantoins and trimethadione, Coumadin, and tetracycline were added to this group.[70] Table 14-1 lists agents that are currently considered teratogens, those that are possibly teratogens, and those unlikely to be teratogenic.

Physical Agents

Ionizing radiations have been implicated in poor pregnancy outcome for many years. Pregnant women exposed to atomic bomb explosions delivered children with microcephaly and low birth weight. An exposure of 50 rad or greater is associated with a significant probability of an observable embryopathic effect: increased incidence of death if exposure is during the preimplantation period; malformation if during the early organogenetic phase; or tissue hypoplasia with growth retardation if exposure is during the fetal stages. Risks of intermediate doses are more difficult to ascertain, particularly doses in the 10–15 rad range.[10] Exposure in the range utilized in usual diagnostic radiology (0.02–5 rad) presents low, if any, risks for poor pregnancy outcome.[52]

TABLE 14-1. TERATOGENIC AGENTS IN HUMANS

PHYSICAL AGENTS
- Radiation
  - Atomic weapons
  - Radioiodine
  - Therapeutic

INFECTIOUS AGENTS
- Cytomegalovirus
- Herpes simplex virus I and II
- Rubella virus
- Syphilis
- Toxoplasmosis
- Venezuelan equine encephalitis virus

MATERNAL METABOLIC IMBALANCE
- Alcoholism
- Diabetes
- Endemic cretinism
- Hyperthermia
- Phenylketonuria
- Rheumatic disease and congenital heart block
- Virilizing tumors

CHEMICAL AGENTS
- Androgenic hormones
- Aminopterin and methylaminopterin
- Busulfan
- Chlorobiphenyls
- Coumarin anticoagulants
- Cyclophosphamide
- Diethylstilbestrol
- Diphenylhydantoin
- Goitrogens and antithyroid drugs
- Lithium
- Mercury, organic
- Methimazole and scalp defects
- Streptomycin
- Tetracyclines
- Thalidomide
- 13-cis-retinoic acid
- Trimethadione and paramethadione
- Valproic acid

POSSIBLE TERATOGENS
- ? Binge drinking
- ? Cigarette smoking
- ? Diazepam (Valium)
- ? High Vitamin A
- ? Organic solvents (laboratory workers)
- ? Penicillamine
- ? Varicella
- ? Zinc deficiency

UNLIKELY TERATOGENS
- Agent Orange
- Anesthetics
- Aspartame
- Aspirin
- Bendectin (antinauseants)
- Birth control pills
- Illicit drugs (marihuana, LSD, cocaine)
- Metronidazole
- Rubella vaccine
- Spermicides
- Ultrasound
- Videodisplay terminals

? = Teratogenicity not fully established.
Source: Adapted and reproduced with permission from Shepard T. H.: Teratogenicity of therapeutic agents. In: Current Problems in Pediatrics. Gluck, L. et al. (Eds.) Copyright © 1979 by Yearbook Medical Publishers, Inc. Chicago.[70]

Concerns have been raised about the possibility that low-dose radiation exposure in utero is responsible for infertility, mutation, malignancy, behavioral alterations, and reduction of life span in the human. Some studies have suggested an increase in leukemia rates in children exposed to radiation in utero, even at low doses.[8,17] However, at present, no proof is available to support these concerns.

Infectious Agents

A number of infectious agents have been shown to exert teratogenic effects in the human. Maternal *Treponema pallidum* infection during pregnancy (congenital syphilis) is the oldest example of infectious teratogenic agents. Toxoplasmosis, herpes simplex, rubella, varicella, cytomegalovirus, and Venezuelan equine encephalitis virus are the important infectious agents known today as human teratogens.

Toxoplasmosis. An 11-month-old child with cysts due to parasites in the retina, congenital hydrocephalus, microphthalmos, and coloboma was reported by Janku in 1923.[37] A few years later, Levaditi recognized the cysts as being due to toxoplasma and proposed a possible association with congenital hydrocephalus.[45] More recently, a number of epidemiologic studies have determined the frequency of maternal and congenital toxoplasmosis and the risk for the fetus at various stages of pregnancy.[15,16,26,62]

Herpes Simplex. Batignani, in 1934, described a newborn who had herpes keratitis, and a case of hepatoadrenal necrosis with intranuclear inclusion bodies was reported by Hass in 1935.[33] With the availability of tissue culture techniques, specific immunological stains for herpes viruses, and electron microscopy, these newer methods were used to make the diagnosis and to expand information about the disease. The epidemiology of congenital herpes and the spectrum of clinical findings are now well described. (See Chapter 38.)

Rubella. Maternal infection with rubella and cataracts in children were first reported in 1941.[29] Epidemiological studies were later conducted to determine the full range of damage due to rubella and the importance of timing of the infection during gestation.[13,41,67]

Varicella. A child born to a mother who had had chicken pox during pregnancy and who suffered from hypoplasia of the right lower extremity, scarring of the left lower extremity, talipes equinovarus, cerebral cortical atrophy, cerebellar aplasia, and bilateral optic atrophy was reported in the late 1940s [42] Additional children with this syndrome have been described subsequently. The frequency of this association is low. A study of 190,000 pregnancies in New York City revealed only four malformations among babies of 135 mothers who had chicken pox during pregnancy, compared with five malformations among 146 matched controls.[72]

Cytomegalovirus. The description of large, inclusion-bearing cells in the kidneys of a stillborn infant who died of syphilis was reported in 1904. Inclusion-bearing cells in the kidneys and parotid glands of both stillborn and live infants have been reported since the beginning of the century.[28,59] Cytomegalovirus was recovered from infants with illnesses resembling cytomegalic inclusion disease in 1957.[75] Following this observation, epidemiological studies were carried out to determine the prevalence of CMV infections. The frequency and types of congenital disease which followed congenital CMV infection were later described.[35,58]

Venezuelan Equine Encephalitis. During the 1962 epidemic of Venezuelan equine encephalitis in Venezuela, pregnant women who contracted the disease had a high frequency of abortion and some delivered children with severe central nervous system damage. Children with microphthalmia, aplasia of the cerebellum, and only small nests of nervous tissue in the cranial cavities were described.[76] In other cases there was massive necrosis of the brain.

CHEMICAL AGENTS

Drugs. In the United States, about 45% of all pregnant women take one or more prescribed drugs. To this exposure, an additional unknown number of over-the-counter medications must be added. Analgesics, diuretics, antibiotics, antacids, and laxatives are the most frequently used drugs in pregnancy. If only the first trimester is considered, antiemetics, sedatives, antihistamines, hormones, analgesics, and laxatives/cathartics are used most frequently.[66]

Few human teratogens have been positively identified (Table 14-1) despite the fact that more than 600 drugs are teratogenic in animals. A detailed description of the teratogenic action of each drug is outside the scope of this chapter. Comments on selected agents are included. For a comprehensive description of human teratogens, the reader is referred to specialized publications (see next section of this chapter; sources of information on drugs in pregnancy).

Coumarin Anticoagulants. These drugs are among the most recently discovered human teratogens. The malformations elicited by treatment in the first trimester with warfarin, acenocoumarin, phenindione, or phenprocoumon include hypoplasia of the nasal structures and bone stippling reminiscent of the "chondrodysplasia punctata" lesion. Treatment with these drugs in the last trimester can cause fetal central nervous system malformations. Eighteen cases are now documented.

Ethanol. The defects produced in "fetal alcohol syndrome" (FAS) were described in France in 1967 by Lemoine et al.[44] and brought into sharper focus by Jones and Smith[38] in the United States. They include central nervous system dysfunction, growth deficiency, a cluster of facial abnormalities, and variable constellations of other malformations. About 618 cases have been reported,[73] but the actual risk of developing FAS is unknown.[36] It is not known if small doses of alcohol taken by the mother during pregnancy have harmful effects on the fetus.[61] (See Chapter 20.)

Diethylstilbestrol. Diethylstilbestrol (DES) is the first, and so far the only, example of a human transplacental carcinogen. The number of cases of vaginal adenocarcinoma in young women reported during a brief period exceeded the total number of such cases that had been reported in the world literature up to that time. Some 429 cases have been attributed to DES or possibly to the synthetic estrogens dienestrol or hexestrol given to women during gestation 7–30 years before.[34] However, no drug exposure could be documented in about one-third of reported cases. The risk of developing this abnormality is estimated at 1.4/1000 or less. Five-year survival is 80%. DES also exerts teratogenic effects. A number of vaginal and uterine abnormalities have been reported among these women.[39] Gonadal lesions have been described in the sons of women treated with DES during pregnancy.[7]

Antiepileptics. The anticonvulsants were first indicted in causing malformations in 1963. The association with increased congenital malformations is related to two different groups of these drugs: barbiturates and hydantoins, on the one hand, and oxazolidinedione compounds, on the other. Drugs of the former group are likely responsible for inducing about 6% abnormalities overall, or a two- to three-fold greater incidence than normal. The induced abnormalities are primarily cardiac defects, orofacial clefts, and skeletal defects, including the entity designated "fetal hydantoin syndrome."[32] Embryopathies attributed to phenobarbital [4,5] and primidone have also been reported. No real estimate exists for the number of cases of malformation due to anticonvulsant usage, but some features of the fetal hydantoin syndrome are said to occur in one-third of those exposed. The full expression of the syndrome is present in 11% of exposed fetuses.[31]

In the other group, the oxazolidinediones, trimethadione and paramethadione carry a much greater risk for malformations estimated as more than 80% upon exposure.[25] Speech impairment, heart disease, delayed mental development, malformed ears, urogenital malformations, facial clefts, and simian creases are features of the "fetal trimethadione syndrome" observed in the 36 cases reported to date.

Ototoxic Antibiotics. In 1950, deafness was noted in the child of a woman treated with streptomycin during the last month of pregnancy. To date, about 40 cases of deafness following use of the streptomycins and 10 cases due to kanamycin have been reported.[48] The effect is on the eighth cranial nerve with resulting hearing and/or vestibular defects. Exposure in early pregnancy seems to produce more adverse effects than exposure in late pregnancy. The risk of adverse effect is approximately 1 in 12 exposed infants.

Cancer Chemotherapeutic Drugs. (See Chapter 41.) The folic acid antagonists are teratogenic in humans. A number of antimetabolites and alkylating chemicals used as antineoplastic and/or immunosuppressive agents are also active teratogens. Since 1960, 23 cases have been reported in which cancer chemotherapeutic agents administered during pregnancy exerted teratogenic effects. Compounds reported to induce malformations include busulfan (multiple defects, 3 cases), chlorambucil (renal-urogenital defects, 2 cases), cyclophosphamide (digit defects, 2 cases), nitrogen mustard (digit and renal defects, 2 cases), cytarabine (digit defects, 2 cases), and fluorouracil (limb defects, 1 case). In addition, 11 embryos aborted after treatment with azauridine were described as abnormal.[63]

Lithium Carbonate. Lithium carbonate is likely to have teratogenic potential. This drug, used in the treatment of manic-depressive psychoses, is currently associated with 20 cases of malformation, 13 involving the heart and great vessels; 5 cases of the rare Ebstein's anomaly have been described.[49,54,64]

D-Penicillamine. D-penicillamine, the chelating drug used in the treatment of Wilson's disease, is probably a teratogen. Four cases of an identical defect, *cutis laxa*, a lesion characterized by extensive wrinkling and folding of the skin, have been reported following maternal exposure to D-penicillamine during pregnancy. The risk of this abnormality appears to be on the order of 4–5%, based on the ratio of affected : nonaffected cases.[63]

Ingestion of certain drugs during pregnancy clearly can induce adverse effects in the unborn child. However, few new teratogens or epidemics of birth defects have been identified since the thalidomide disaster, which attests both to effective laboratory testing of drugs in animals prior to clinical use and to extensive surveillance of use of therapeutic agents in women during pregnancy.

Other Environmental Chemicals. There is increasing concern not only that medications taken by the mother during pregnancy are potentially harmful to the developing conceptus, but that some occupations may also be harmful to human pregnancy. A few examples have already surfaced.

Organic mercury is associated with congenital encephalopathy in children exposed in utero subsequent to maternal ingestion of contaminated foodstuffs.[79] A widespread epidemic of methyl mercury poisoning occurred at Minamata Bay, Japan, in the early 1950s. Inorganic mercury compounds were discharged into the bay by a plastics factory. The metallic and inorganic mercury salts were converted by microorganisms to methyl mercury which entered the aquatic food chain, leading to high concentrations in fish. From 1953 to 1971, nearly 700 cases of poisoning were reported with a 38% mortality rate, and several infants were born with brain damage. Six percent of children born in the region between 1955 and 1959 developed cerebral palsy.[40,71]

In Iraq, massive poisoning occurred in individuals who consumed bread prepared from barley and wheat grain treated with methyl mercury fungicide.[2] From February to August of 1972, 6530 cases of poisoning were admitted to hospitals. There were 459 deaths. Of 31 hospitalized pregnant women, nearly half died. Several of the infants exposed in utero to methyl mercury developed severe brain damage.

Lead toxicity in pregnancy predisposes to fetal loss. High abortion and stillbirth rates have been noted in women working in British factories with elevated lead exposure.[30,60]

Concern has been expressed about a variety of environmental/occupational chemicals potentially harmful to the fetus. The number of chemicals included in this list is growing. However, the evidence for teratogenicity resulting from such exposures has been largely negative.

SOURCES OF INFORMATION ON DRUGS IN PREGNANCY

The introduction of thousands of new pharmaceutical and environmental chemicals each year places a special burden on the obstetrician who is relied on for accurate and up-to-date information regarding teratogens.

Although some information is available as to the relationship between certain chemicals and reproduction, interpretation of this information is often difficult. Our knowledge is incomplete and it is difficult to find clear-cut answers even when good data are available. There are thousands of chemicals for which data on reproductive toxicity are lacking entirely. On the other hand, the practical aspects of obstetrics demand that the most accurate answers be readily available. The need for practical information is well-recognized but so far only partially met. Some useful reference books are available.[6,11,47,68] A summary and guidelines for counseling have been published by the American College of Obstetricians and Gynecologists in a recent ACOG bulletin entitled *Teratology*.[1] References for detailed discussion of teratologic principles are available.[19,23,43,79]

A fairly complex literature search can be obtained through the National Library of Medicine or the Environmental Teratology Information Center (ETIC) which maintain a current listing of references on the reproductive effects of a large number of agents. Retrieval and reading of the literature may take several weeks and selection and interpretation of pertinent data can be difficult for the clinician. These disadvantages have been overcome by the Reproductive Toxicology Center in Washington, D.C., which offers an information system termed REPROTOX. By using REPROTOX, updated information on the effects of drugs and other chemicals on pregnancy and human reproduction can be obtained.[57]

METHODS TO ASSESS TERATOGENIC POTENTIAL

From the beginning of the 1960s, an intense search has been underway for a reliable system for evaluating the teratogenic potential of physical and chemical agents. We have not yet developed a perfect method and must rely on several approaches.[21]

It is helpful to have an idea of the methods being developed to test drugs for adverse reproductive effects.

Testing Methods in Experimental Systems

New drugs are usually given to laboratory animals to determine effects on reproduction. Rodents are commonly used because they are easily housed, relatively inexpensive, and reproduce rapidly. Test methods can become very elaborate, utilizing variations in dosing, in number of generations studied, and in timing of fetal exposure.[53] However, difficulties can arise when using animals to predict reproductive toxicity in humans. The chief problem is imperfect applicability of data from one species to predictions about other species. The classic example is thalidomide, which is not teratogenic in mice and rats but is highly teratogenic in rabbits, monkeys, and humans.

Testing chemicals in bacterial cultures and cell cultures is often less expensive, faster, and easier than using pregnant animals, but it is questionable whether these results can be extrapolated to the human.[18] Culture techniques utilizing whole embryos or organs may provide a more direct way to evaluate teratogenicity.[12]

Human Studies

Because teratogenicity in humans cannot be reliably inferred from experiments in laboratory animals, epidemiological surveillance of humans is necessary. Suspicion that a chemical or physical agent is a teratogen may be raised by the occurrence of a case or cluster of cases with an unusual abnormality or by the occurrence of an unusually high frequency of a fairly conmon abnormality. Questioning of the parents of anomalous children may suggest that exposure to a drug is associated with the anomaly. Hundreds of such associations are reported in the literature. lf a congenital abnormality is extremely rare in the general population, the collection of a handful of cases associated with use of a drug may be sufficient to establish causality. A typical example of this is the association of DES with clear-cell carcinoma of the vagina. However, in most cases, an association suggested by case reports needs to be tested in a controlled study. Of all the associations suggested by case reports, only a few will be confirmed by a controlled study.[14]

A prospective controlled study, called a cohort study, compares the outcome in a group of individuals exposed to the substance of interest with that in a suitable group of controls. One of the drawbacks of prospective studies is that a birth defect which occurs at low frequency requires a large study population in order to demonstrate an increase due to a given exposure. A common abnormality may be a practical starting point for such a study. Cohort studies yield a measurement called "relative risk" that represents the ratio of the incidence of the abnormality under study in the exposed versus the control population. A relative risk of 2.0 indicates that exposure to the drug is associated with a doubling of the incidence of the studied effect. If an adverse effect has a low baseline incidence, the absolute risk of the effect may still be small, even with a drug that imposes a high relative risk.

A retrospective study of drug effects is almost always easier to perform than a prospective study. The retrospective study, or case-control study, begins with a population of affected individuals. Suitable nonaffected controls are obtained and the putative cause of the effect is sought in both groups. Drug use may be ascertained by interview, review of medical records, or by looking for a laboratory marker of drug use (if one is available). From the difference between the history of drug use in the affected and nonaffected groups, an "odds ratio" is calculated. An odds ratio of 2.0, for example, indicates that affected individuals are twice as likely as the controls to have been exposed to a drug.

Case-control studies are subject to "recall bias." Parents with an affected child are likely to search for a reason for their misfortune. They may review events of the pregnancy in detail and are more likely to recall the use of medications than are the parents of normal babies. Recall bias can be neutralized by using as controls parents who have had abnormal babies in whom the abnormalities are clearly unrelated to the drug in question.

Any study of drug use in pregnancy may be influenced by confounding factors. For example, the use of marihuana and cocaine is often accompanied by the use of ethanol and tobacco. The effects of the latter two substances on reproduction may confound the measurement of an effect of the drug being studied.

Information generated by epidemiological studies must be interpreted with caution. Such data do not prove a cause and effect relationship between drugs and adverse pregnancy outcomes; rather, these data may show an association between drug use and adverse outcome. The statistical tests used in these studies give an estimate of the likelihood that any such association is due to chance.

PREVENTION OF TERATOGENIC EFFECTS DUE TO ENVIRONMENTAL CAUSES

Pregnancy should be ruled out in women of reproductive age before prescribing medications, vaccinations, or performing diagnostic procedures that may have potentially harmful effects for the conceptus. Clinically, this task is made easy by the accuracy and sensitivity of the hCG-beta-subunit assay. In spite of the availability of sensitive pregnancy tests, inadvertent administration of potentially harmful drugs or x-ray procedures to women unknowingly pregnant is not rare.

Concerning the use of drugs during gestation, the view that all medications should be avoided in pregnancy may be defensible, but is hardly practical. When the use of a therapeutic agent is necessary, the practitioner needs to know which of the available drugs is the safest. For most commonly used drugs, safety relies on a good track record after many years of clinical use in thousands of pregnancies. Ampicillin, for example, has not been associated with any pattern of abnormalities after use in large numbers of pregnant women, hence it is considered "probably safe." Newer and less frequently used medications cannot have developed such a record. Evaluation of these drugs must rely on indirect testing in animals and in in vitro systems and on whatever retrospective data are available.

The United States Food and Drug Administration regulations are designed to prevent a teratogen from being marketed for human use.[24] Each new drug is classified with regard to potential teratogenicity, based on the following characteristics:

Category A. Drugs for which well-controlled studies in women fail to demonstrate a risk to the fetus. The FDA issuance bulletin states, "Although such studies can never entirely exclude a risk, a reasonable presumption can be made that when such drugs are used during pregnancy, the possibility of fetal harm is remote. However, as with other drugs, they should be used during pregnancy only when clearly needed."

Category B. Indicates either that "animal studies have not demonstrated a fetal risk, but there are no adequate studies in women, or animal studies have uncovered some risk that has not been confirmed in controlled studies in women."

Category C. Means that "studies in animals have revealed adverse effects on the fetus and there are not adequate controlled studies in women, or studies in women and animals are not available."

Category D. Includes drugs whose potential benefits may be acceptable even though experience shows they are associated with birth defects (e.g., phenytoin for severe epilepsy). Such drugs are for use in life-threatening situations or serious diseases for which safer drugs cannot be used or are ineffective. "If a category D drug is given to a pregnant woman, or if the patient becomes pregnant while taking it, the physician should inform her of the potential risk to the fetus."

Category X. Includes drugs contraindicated for use during pregnancy because fetal abnormalities have been demonstrated in animal or human studies and potential risks clearly outweigh potential benefits. "FDA recommends that the physician advise the pregnant patient of the potential hazard if she intentionally or inadvertently used the drug."

Although a number of pitfalls are still present,[9] this classification is an improvement over the previous blanket disclaimer for new drugs.

Other preventive measures can be carried out. For example, fertile nonpregnant women, if candidates, should be vaccinated against diseases that, if contracted during pregnancy, present potential harm to the developing embryo or fetus. Postpartum rubella vaccination is an example of this type of prevention.

Women of child-bearing age treated with medications that are potentially harmful during pregnancy should be informed of the hazard and offered an effective birth control method. For example, pregnancy should not be initiated before one month passes after discontinuation of isotretinoin. Exposure to isotretinoin, a retinoid prescribed for the treatment of acne, during the first trimester of pregnancy, has been linked to a number of teratogenic effects, including increased abortion rate, microtia, craniofacial dysmorphism, and central nervous and cardiovascular system defects.

Women with diseases such as diabetes should have their diabetes controlled *before* they plan pregnancy.

Women on anti-epileptic medications who are planning to become pregnant should be evaluated before pregnancy for selection of the best medications to be taken.

A number of screening techniques should be carried out to identify subclinical diseases. An example is screening for syphilis so that treatment may be instituted.

Finally, women of child-bearing age should be educated about the risks to the offspring of infections such as rubella, syphilis, and toxoplasmosis and of practices such as alcohol consumption and tobacco smoking during pregnancy.

COUNSELING THE PREGNANT PATIENT EXPOSED TO POTENTIALLY HARMFUL AGENTS

Counseling regarding potentially harmful environmental exposures must be carried out in an atmosphere of openness in which the patient is encouraged to understand and to work out her problems. The counselor must be able to communicate with the patient. The counselor must realize that each woman facing a problem pregnancy must make a decision in a relatively short period of time. The decision-making process includes six major steps.[69] The woman should be helped to (1) define her problem fully, (2) explore and understand the implications of her present situation, (3) assess and understand her feelings about the situation, (4) accumulate information about all relevant aspects of her situation, (5) examine the positive and negative aspects of all choices available to her, and (6) make a decision and follow it through.

A quiet room and freedom from distraction are prerequisites for effective counseling. The participation of the father-to-be in the interview process is advisable because this increases the feeling of working out the problem as a team in which each participant has a role. Telephone conversations are not suitable for effective counseling.[69]

When a patient presents with a history of having taken a given medication in pregnancy, advice must be given cautiously. Most information is based on animal data of questionable applicability to humans. Most patient inquiries are related to exposures with low likelihood of causing harmful effects. The facts should be fully explained in a clear and simple manner to remove anxiety or guilt.

Some patients will have been exposed to agents known to be associated with increased risk for poor pregnancy outcomes, including birth defects. In these cases, the obstetrician must inform the parents of the risks and must be sure that the magnitude of the problem is understood by the patient. Sometimes it is useful to make literature available and to explain the significance of the printed information to her problem. These patients can be referred to specialized centers or to health professionals with special experience in teratology. The obstetrician should keep an accurate record of the source and type of information discussed with the patient.

REFERENCES

1. American College of Obstetricians and Gynecologists: *Teratology*. ACOG Technical Bulletin, No. 84, February 1985.
2. Bakir, F., Damluji, F., Amin-Zaki, L., Murtadha, M., Khalidi, A., Al-Rawi, N., Tikriti, S., Dhahir, H., Clarkson, T., Smith, J., and Doherty, R.: Methyl mercury poisoning in Iraq. *Science* **181**:230–240, 1973.
3. Batignani, A.: Conjunctivite da virus erpetico in neonato. *Boll. d'Ocul.* **13**:1217–1220, 1934.
4. Behtenod, M. and Frederich, A.: The children of drug-treated epileptics. *Pediatrics* **30**:227–248, 1975.
5. Berkowitz, F. E.: Fetal malformation due to phenobarbitone. A case report. *S. Afr. Med. J.* **55**:100–101, 1979.
6. Berkowitz, R. L., Coustan, D. R., and Mochizuki, T. K.: *Handbook for Prescribing Medications During Pregnancy*. Boston, MA, Little, Brown and Company, 1981.
7. Bibbo, M., Al-Naqeeb, M., Baccarini, I., Gill, W., Newton, M., Sleeper, K. M., Sonek, M., and Wied, G. L.: Follow-up study of male and female offspring of DES-treated mothers. A preliminary report. *J. Reprod. Med.* **15**:29–32, 1975.
8. Bithell, J. F. and Stewart, A. M.: Prenatal irradiation and childhood malignancy: A review of British data from the Oxford survey. *Br. J. Cancer* **31**:271–287, 1975.
9. Brent, R. L.: Methods of evaluating the alleged teratogenicity of environmental agents. In: *Prevention of Physical and Mental Congenital Defects, Part C: Basic and Medical Science, Education, and Future Strategies*. New York, Alan R. Liss, 1985, pp. 191–195.
10. Brent, R. L.: Radiation teratogenesis. *Teratology* **21**:281–298, 1980.
11. Briggs, G. C., Bodendorfer, T. W., Freeman, R. K., and Yaffe, S. J.: *Drugs in Pregnancy and Lactation, A Reference Guide to Fetal and Neonatal Risk*. Baltimore, MD, Williams & Wilkins, 1983.
12. Brown, N. and Fabro, S.: *The in Vitro Approach to Teratogenicity Testing. Developmental Toxicology*. London, Croom Helm Ltd., 1982.
13. Cooper, L. Z.: Rubella. A preventable cause of birth defects. In: *Birth Defects*. D. Bergsma (Ed.). Original Article Series, Vol. 4, No. 23. New York, National Foundation–March of Dimes, 1968.
14. Cordero, J. F. and Oakley, G. P.: Drug exposure during pregnancy: Some epidemiological considerations. *Clin. Obstet. Gynecol.* **26**:418–428, 1983.
15. Desmonts, G. and Couvreur, J.: Congenital toxoplasmosis. A prospective study of 378 pregnancies. N. Engl. J. Med. **290**:1110–1116, 1974.
16. Desmonts, G. and Couvreur, J.: Toxoplasmosis in pregnancy and transmission to the fetus. *Bull. N.Y. Acad. Med.* **50**:146–159, 1974.
17. Diamond, E. L., Schmerler, H., and Lilenfeld, A. M.: The relationship of intrauterine radiation to subsequent mortality and development of leukemia in children, a prospective study. *Am. J. Epidemiol.* **97**:282–313, 1973.
18. Fabro, S.: On predicting environmentally-induced human reproductive hazards: An overview and historical perspective. *Fundam. Appl. Toxicol.* 00:000, 1985.
19. Fabro, S.: Pharmacology and environmental toxicology of pregnancy. *Clin. Obstet. Gynecol.* **26**:377–378, 1983.

20. Fabro, S.: Reproductive toxicology: State of the art. *Am. J. Ind. Med.* 4:391–393, 1983.
21. Fabro, S., Brent, R. L., Clayson, D., Palmer, A. K., Jelinek, L. R., Krupp, P., Leonov, B., Lippman, A., Schardein, J. L., and Sever, J. L.: Workshop summary: Methods for judging human teratogenicity. *Prog. Clin. Biol. Res.* **163**:177–180, 1985.
22. Fabro, S., McLachlan, J., and Dames, N.: Chemical exposure of embryos during the preimplantation stages of pregnancy: Mortality rate and intrauterine development. *Am. J. Obstet. Gynecol.[1]* **148**:929–938, 1984.
23. Fabro, S. and Scialli, A.: *Principles of Drugs and Other Chemicals During Pregnancy.* New York, Marcel Dekker, 1986.
24. *Federal Register*: **44**:37434–37467, 1980.
25. Feldman, G. L., Weaver, D. D., and Lovrien, E. W.: The fetal trimethadione syndrome: Report of an additional family and further delineation of this syndrome. *Am. J. Dis. Child.* **131**:1389–1392, 1977.
26. Feldman, H. A. and Miller, L. T.: Congenital human toxoplasmosis. Ann. N.Y. Acad. Sci. **64**:180–184, 1956.
27. Genetic predisposition to chemically induced birth defects. S. Fabro (Ed.). *Reprod. Toxicol.* **2**:5–7, 1983.
28. Goodpasture, E. and Talbot, F. B.: Concerning the "protozoan-like" cells in certain lesions of infancy. *Am. J. Dis. Child.* **21**:415–425, 1921.
29. Gregg, N. M.: Congenital cataract following German measles in the mother. *Trans. Ophthalmol. Soc. Aust.* **3**:35–46, 1941.
30. Hamilton, A. and Hardy, H. L.: Hereditary lead poisoning. In: *lndustrial Toxicology.* Acton, MA, Publishing Sciences Group, 1974, pp. 119–121.
31. Hanson, J. W., Myrianthopoulos, N. C., Harvey, M. A. S., and Smith, D. W.: Risks to the offspring of women treated with hydantoin anticonvulsants, with emphasis on the fetal hydantoin syndrome. *J. Pediatr.* **89**:662–668, 1976.
32. Hanson, J. W. and Smith, D. W.: The fetal hydantoin syndrome. *J. Pediatr.* **87**:285–290, 1975.
33. Hass, M.: Hepato-adrenal necrosis with intranuclear inclusion bodies: Report of a case. *Am. J. Pathol.* **11**:127–142, 1935.
34. Herbst, A. L.: Clear cell adenocarcinoma and the current status of DES-exposed females. *Cancer* **48**:484–488, 1981.
35. Hildebrandt, R. J., Sever, J. L., Margeileth, A. M., and Callagen, D. A.: Cytomegalovirus in the normal pregnant woman. *Obstet. Gynecol.* **98**:1125–1128, 1967.
36. In utero alcohol exposure: Threshold for effects? S. Fabro (Ed.). *Reprod. Toxicol.* **1**:11–14, 1982.
37. Janku, J.: Pathogenesa a pathologika anatomie tak nazvaneho vrozencho kolobomu zlure skurny v oku normalue velikem a midrophtalmickem s nalezem parazitu v stinici. *Cas. Lek. Cesk.* **62**:1021–1027, 1923.
38. Jones, K. L. and Smith, D. W.: Recognition of the fetal alcohol syndrome in early infancy. *Lancet* **2**:999–1001, 1973.
39. Kaufman, R. H., Binder, G. L., Gray, P. M., Jr., and Adam, E.: Upper genital tract changes associated with exposure in utero to diethylstilbestrol. *Am. J. Obstet. Gynecol.* **128**:51–59, 1977.
40. Koos, B. J. and Longo, L. D.: Mercury toxicity in the pregnant woman, fetus and newborn infant. *Am. J. Obstet. Gynecol.* **126**:390–409, 1976.
41. Korones, S. B., Ainger, L. E., Monif, G. R. G., Roane, J., Sever, J. L., and Fuste, F.: Congenital rubella syndrome. Study of 22 infants. *Am. J. Dis. Child.* **110**:434–440, 1965.
42. La Foret, E. G. and Lynch, C. L., Jr.: Multiple congenital defects following maternal varicella. *N. Engl. J. Med.* **236**:534–537, 1947.
43. Larsen, J., Grossman, J., and Sever, J. L.: *Handbook of Perinatal lnfections.* Boston, MA, Little, Brown and Company, 1979.
44. Lemoine, P., Harousseau, H., Borteyru, J. P., and Menuet, J. C. Les enfants de parents alcooliques: Anomalies observees. A propos de 127 cas (Children of alcoholic parents: Anomalies observed in 127 cases). *Ouest. Med.* **21**:476–482 1968.
45. Levaditi, C.: Au sujet de certaines protozooses hereditaires humaines a localization oculaires et nerveuses. *C.R. Soc. Biol. (Paris)* **98**:297–299, 1928.
46. Nahmias, A., Alford, C., and Korowes, S.: Infection of the newborn with herpesvirus hominis. In: *Advances in Pediatrics.* I. Schulman (Ed.). Chicago, Year Book Medical Publishers, 1970, pp. 185–226.
47. Niebyl, J. R.: *Drugs in Pregnancy.* Philadelphia, Lea & Febiger, 1982.
48. Nishimura, H. and Tanimura, T.: *Clinical Aspects of the Teratogenicity of Drugs.* New York, Excerpta Medica, American Elsevier Company, 1976.
49. Nora, J. J., Nora, A. H., and Toews, W. H.: Lithium, Ebstein's anomaly, and other congenital heart defects. *Lancet* **2**:594–595, 1974.
50. Mace, D. R.: *Abortion: The Agonizing Decision.* New York, Abingdon Press, 1972.
51. Myrhe, S. A. and Williams, R.: Teratogenic effects associated with maternal primidone therapy. *J. Pediatr.* **99**:160–162, 1981.
52. Oppenheim, B. E., Griem, M. L., and Meier, P.: Effects of low-dose prenatal irradiation in humans: Analysis of Chicago-Lying-In data and comparison with other studies. *Radiat. Res.* **57**:508–554, 1974.
53. Palmer, A.K.: Regulatory requirements for reproductive toxicology: Theory and practice. In: *Developmental Toxicology.* New York, Raven Press, 1981, pp. 259–287.
54. Park, J. M., Sridaromont, S., Ledbetter, E. O., and Terry, W. M.: Ebstein's anomaly of the tricuspid valve associated with prenatal exposure to lith-

ium carbonate. *Am. J. Dis. Child.* **134**:703–704, 1980.

55. Philipson, A.: Persistence of ampicillin in the intrauterine content following single and multiple doses to pregnant women. *Acta Obstet. Gynecol. Scand.* **60**:121–123, 1981.
56. Rayburn, W. F. and Andresen, B. D.: Principles of perinatal pharmacology. In: *Drug Therapy in Obstetrics and Gynecology.* W. G. Rayburn and F. P. Zuspan (Eds.). Norwalk, CT, Appleton-Century-Crofts, 1982, pp. 1–8.
57. Reproductive Toxicology Center, Research Foundation of Columbia Hospital for Women, 2425 L Street, N.W., Washington, D.C. 20037 (202) 293-5137.
58. Reynolds, D. W., Stagno, S., Stubbs, K. G., Dahle, A. J., Livingston, M. M., Saxon, S. S., and Alford, C. A.: Congenital cytomegalovirus infection: Relation to auditory and mental deficiency. *N. Engl. J. Med.* **290**:291–296, 1974.
59. Rippert, H.: Uüber protozoenartigen Zellen in der Niereelines syphilitischem Neugeboren und in der Parotis von Kindern. *Zentralbl. Allg. Pathol.* **15**:945–948, 1904.
60. Rom, W. N.: Effects of lead on the female and reproduction: A review. *Mt. Sinai J. Med.* **43**:542–552, 1976.
61. Rosett, H. L. and Weiner, L.: *Alcohol and the Fetus: A Clinical Perspective.* New York, Oxford University Press, 1984.
62. Sabin, A. B., Eichenwald, H., Feldman, H., and Jacobs, L.: Present status of clinical manifestations of toxoplasmosis in man. Indications and provisions for routine serologic diagnosis. *JAMA* **150**:1063–1069, 1952.
63. Schardein, J.L.: *Current Status of Drugs as Teratogens in Man. Prevention of Physical and Mental Congenital Defects,* Part C: Basic and Medical Science, Education and Future Strategies. New York, Alan R. Liss, 1985, pp. 181–190.
64. Schou, M., Goldfield, M. D., Winstein, M. R., and Villeneuve, A.: Lithium and pregnancy. I. Report from the register of lithium babies. *Br. Med. J.* **2**:135–136, 1973.
65. Schroeder, H. A. and Balassa, J. J.: Abnormal trace elements in man: Cadmium. *J. Chronic Dis.* **14**:236–241, 1961.
66. Scialli, A. R.: Safe medications during pregnancy. *Contemp. Ob. Gyn.* **22**:40–66, 1983.
67. Sever, J. L., Hardy, J. B., Nelson, K. B., and Gilkeson, M. R.: Rubella in the collaborative perinatal research study. II. Clinical and laboratory findings in children through 3 years of age. *Am. J. Dis. Child.* **118**:123–132, 1969.
68. Shepard, T. H.: *Catalog of Teratogenic Agents.* Baltimore, MD, The Johns Hopkins University Press, 1980.
69. Shepard, T. H.: Counseling pregnant women exposed to potentially harmful agents during pregnancy. *Clin. Obstet. Gynecol.* **26**:478–483, 1983.
70. Shepard, T. H.: Teratogenicity of therapeutic agents. *Curr. Probl. Pediatr.* **10**:1–42, 1979.
71. Siedlecki, J. T.: Diagnosis of exposure to mercury-effect on pregnancy. *JAMA* **215**:648, 1971.
72. Siegel, M.: Congenital malformations following chicken pox, measles, mumps and hepatitis. Results of a cohort study. *JAMA* **226**:1521–1524, 1973.
73. Smith, D. W.: Alcohol effects on the fetus. In: *Drug and Chemical Risks to the Fetus and Newborn.* R. H. Schwarz and S. J. Yaffe (Eds.). New York, Alan R. Liss, 1980, pp. 73–82.
74. Warkany, J.: Antituberculous drugs. *Teratology* **20**:133–138, 1979.
75. Weller, T. H., Macauley, J. C., Craig, J. M., and Wirth, P.: Isolation of intranuclear inclusion-producing agents from infants with illnesses resembling cytomegalic inclusion disease. *Proc. Soc. Exp. Biol. Med.* **94**:4–12, 1957.
76. Wenger, F.: Massive cerebral necrosis of the fetus in cases of Venezuelan equine encephalitis. *Invest. Clinica* **21**:13–31, 1967.
77. Wilson, J. G.: *Environment and Birth Defects.* New York, Academic Press, 1973.
78. Wilson, J. G.: Present status of drugs as teratogens in man. *Teratology* **7**:3–16, 1973.
79. Wilson, J. G. and Fraser, F. C. (Eds.): *Handbook of Teratology,* Vols. 1–4. New York, Plenum Press, 1977-1978.

SECTION B
PROBLEMS SPECIFIC TO PREGNANCY AND LABOR

15

BLEEDING IN PREGNANCY

Vaginal bleeding during pregnancy can be caused by a variety of conditions. It is useful to categorize vaginal bleeding into bleeding originating as a consequence of pregnancy and bleeding that is not directly related to pregnancy. The latter category includes such entities as tumors of the genital tract, traumatic injuries of the genital tract, and cervical erosions and will not be discussed in this chapter. Bleeding directly related to pregnancy is best considered in relation to the time in pregnancy at which the bleeding presents. Although there is some overlap, separate consideration of the various causes of bleeding in the first and second halves of pregnancy is useful clinically.

BLEEDING DURING THE FIRST HALF OF PREGNANCY

The most common pregnancy-related causes of bleeding in the first half of pregnancy are spontaneous abortion, ectopic pregnancy, and, much less frequently, trophoblastic tumors.

About 20% of women report some bleeding during early pregnancy. Approximately half of these pregnancies continue to viability, although the incidence of low-birth-weight infants, prematurity, and perinatal morbidity and mortality is increased.

Abortion

Abortion, defined as the termination of pregnancy before the fetus is capable of extrauterine survival, is the most common cause of first-trimester bleeding. Although small fetuses now have the potential to survive, 20 weeks' gestation or 500 grams weight is the usual criterion used to separate abortions from immature or premature deliveries.

Classification. Abortions are classified as spontaneous or induced. Although there has been considerable debate about the true incidence of spontaneous abortion, the controversy centers around the definition of and methods of detection of pregnancy. If the definition is restricted to clinically apparent abortion, abortion occurs in about 10% of pregnancies. The incidence of abortion rises with maternal age, perhaps with parity, and is higher in women with a history of previous abortion. Spontaneous abortion is further subdivided into threatened, inevitable, incomplete, and missed abortion. When a woman experiences repeated spontaneous abortion, the designation habitual abortion is applied.

Threatened Abortion. A threatened abortion is defined by the occurrence of vaginal bleeding prior to the end of the 20th week of pregnancy. The bleeding may be scanty or moderate. The woman may experience no pain or may note pain over the lower back or crampy pain reminiscent of menstrual cramps. The likelihood that the pregnancy will continue is decreased if pain accompanies the bleeding.

Inevitable Abortion. If the cervix has begun to dilate and there is evidence that the membranes have ruptured, abortion is said to be inevitable.

Incomplete Abortion. If the fetus is expelled but the placenta (or a portion thereof) is retained in the uterus, the abortion is said to be incomplete.

Missed Abortion. A missed abortion is an abortion in which the fetus dies in utero before the 20th week of gestation, but the products of conception are retained in utero for a prolonged (but unspecified) period of time.[2] Missed abortion is suspected when the nausea and vomiting of early pregnancy diminish sharply or disappear, accompanied by a decrease in breast size and tenderness, and the uterus fails to grow, as judged by serial examinations. In cases of late missed abortion or fetal death in utero, the patient may note cessation of fetal movements.

Management of Abortion

Diagnosis. Patients who complain of bleeding in pregnancy should be examined. A speculum examination will confirm that the blood is coming from the external os of the cervix. In addition, visual inspection will reveal the presence of other causes of bleeding, such as polyps or erosions. Speculum examination is also useful to ascertain whether the cervix has begun to dilate, and whether any products of conception, including amniotic fluid, have already passed into the vagina.

Abdominal examination is useful to exclude tenderness to palpation and rebound tenderness. As discussed below, bleeding in early pregnancy is sometimes a symptom of extrauterine pregnancy.

Bimanual examination is useful to ascertain the presence of uterine tenderness and to search for adnexal tenderness and masses.

After the examination, if the diagnosis of threatened abortion is still entertained, ultrasonographic examination is a useful adjunct (see Chapter 5). If a well-defined sac, characterized by an echogenic circular or ovoid rim surrounding a transonic area, is identified by gray scale ultrasound, and if central echoes from the embryo are noted, the pregnancy is probably healthy. If the mean diameter of the gestational sac is appropriate for the age of the gestation, the impression of normality is reinforced. Finally, if the mean diameter of the gestational sac is 30 mm or more, fetal heart movements will be present if the pregnancy is normal. If the initial examination is inconclusive or suggests that the conceptus is dead, several sonographic examinations, done about one week apart, should be used to document failure of growth of the conceptus and uterus, or decreased size of the gestational mass.

If the fetal death occurs after the 13th week of gestation, gray scale ultrasonography may detect a coarsening and thickening of the outline of the fetal skull and thorax. This finding, which begins within 12 hours of fetal death, is due to movement of fluid into the dermis. Between 12 and 48 hours after fetal demise, this process, called "fluffing," progresses to the rest of the fetal body.[2]

Treatment. Threatened abortion should be treated by reassuring the patient. Bed rest, although of dubious therapeutic value in terms of the conception, is useful in that it makes the women a participant in her care. Inevitable abortion should be managed expeditiously. If uterine contractions do not begin spontaneously within a few hours of rupture of the membranes, uterine activity should be induced with an oxytocin infusion in order to expedite the expulsion of the products of conception and thus avoid intrauterine infection.

After the products of conception have been aborted, they should be examined to see if the fetus is grossly normal, and to attempt to ascertain whether or not the abortion is complete. If it is determined, from examining the aborted products of conception and/or from examining the patient, that the abortion is complete, no further therapy is necessary. If the abortion is not complete, the patient should be managed as an incomplete abortion. Incomplete abortions can be completed in an ambulatory setting. The patient should be given an analgesic. Paracervical block may be utilized if necessary. Retained products of conception, usually the placenta or placental fragments, can be grasped with an ovum forceps, which usually passes through the internal os quite easily. It is almost never necessary to dilate the cervix. After removing the retained products of conception with ovum forceps, gentle curettage can be performed with a sharp curette.

The management of missed abortion depends on the size of the uterus when the diagnosis is made. If the uterus is 12 weeks' size or smaller, we prefer to dilate the cervix and to evacuate the uterus by aspiration. When the uterus is 13–20 weeks' size, one may elect to observe the patient for spontaneous evacuation or uterine activity may be induced. For many reasons, including the desire to avoid the development of a coagulopathy, we prefer more aggressive intervention. One of two methods of intervention may be employed. Prostaglandin E_2

(PGE_2) vaginal suppositories, 20 mg, may be utilized. The frequency of administration is governed by the uterine response and by the presence of side effects of the medication. This is the preferred method, because it avoids amniocentesis. In this setting, the rendered amniotic fluid may be scanty, and amniocentesis may be difficult to perform. The second method employs amniocentesis. If amniotic fluid is obtained, 80 g of 59% urea and 5 mg of prostaglandin $F_{2\alpha}$ ($PGF_{2\alpha}$) are instilled into the amniotic sac. The risk of maternal side effects is increased because the $PGF_{2\alpha}$ may be rapidly absorbed via the necrotic fetal tissues.

Habitual Abortion. The classic definition of "habitual abortion" is applied to the woman who has experienced three or more consecutive abortions. This definition was based on the theoretical calculation of Malpas which assumed that (1) the spontaneous abortion rate is constant regardless of parity; (2) patients who abort fall into two groups, accidental and recurrent; and (3) the recurrent factors are unvarying from pregnancy to pregnancy. These assumptions are incorrect. In actuality, about three-fourths of women who have experienced three consecutive abortions will be successful in carrying the next pregnancy to term. Although the incidence of spontaneous abortion does increase slightly when the patient has experienced two or three previous abortions, it seems likely that the etiologic factors operative in patients who experience multiple abortions are not different from those operative in a single spontaneous abortion.[46]

Etiology of Abortion

Genetic Causes. Chromosomal abnormalities of the embryo are demonstrable in 50–60% of first-trimester spontaneous abortions. The abnormalities are usually in the number of chromosomes, rather than in the structure of chromosomes. Trisomy accounts for 50–60% of chromosomally abnormal fetuses, monosomy for 20%, and polyploidy for about 25%. If the first aborted fetus has chromosomal abnormalities, there is an 80% chance that a second abortus will have chromosomal abnormalities, as compared to a 50% chance if the first abortus had normal chromosomes.[9]

Anatomic Causes. The anatomic causes of habitual abortion include anomalies resulting from failures of fusion and canalization of the Müllerian duct, leiomyoma uteri, intrauterine synechiae, and cervical incompetence. Congenital malformations are the consequence of errors during embryogenesis. At six weeks of embryonic life, the Müllerian ducts appear as an invagination of the embryo's coelomic epithelium. They grow caudally and medially toward the urogenital sinus. The cephalad portions of the Müllerian ducts become the fallopian tubes, which open to the peritoneal cavity. The caudad portions fuse to form the uterus, cervix, and upper two-thirds of the vagina. Concomitantly, an invagination of the inferior part of the cloaca is converted into the lower third of the vagina. The uterus, cervix, and upper vagina are formed by fusion of the two Müllerian ducts. Fusion is followed by canalization or disappearance of the septum formed by the fused walls of the right and left ducts. The cervix is the first part of the genital system to lose its longitudinal septum, the vagina loses it next and, finally, at four to five months, the uterus does likewise.

Failures of development, of fusion or of the septa to disappear, result in genital tract anomalies. The most severe, such as congenital absence of the uterus and upper vagina, are caused by failure of the Müllerian system to develop. A number of malformations result from different degrees of failure of Müllerian duct fusion. They range from complete separation of the ducts, as in the case of a uterus didelphys with a septate vagina, to incomplete fusion of the two ducts (uterus duplex, bicornis) to failures of canalization (septate, or subseptate). Asymmetric development of the Müllerian ducts can lead to asymmetric uterus bicornis or arcuatus, uterus didelphys with unilateral obstruction, or uterus unicornis. Renal malformations commonly accompany this type of malformation because the mesonephric and paramesonephric ducts are closely related. Uterine anomalies are a significant cause of repetitive abortion. Patients with major uterine anomalies have an abortion rate of about 30%. With proper patient selection, uterine unification operations result in successful pregnancies in about 75% of patients.

Uterine myomas are found in association with repeated abortion. It is not certain that the relationship is causal. Some women with large multiple myomas are fertile, whereas other women with small myomas are infertile or abort repeatedly. When multiple myomectomy is performed in infertile women in whom no other cause of infertility can be demonstrated, about 50% will deliver living infants after the operation.

Intrauterine synechiae may or may not be a significant factor in habitual abortion. Most women with severe synechiae do not conceive. After lysis of adhesions, the incidence of abortion is still quite high.

The role of the incompetent cervical os in repetitive midtrimester pregnancy wastage is unquestioned. Uterine cerclage procedures are very effective in preventing pregnancy wastage secondary to incompetent os.

Hormonal Causes

Thyroid. Although subclinical thyroid dysfunction is usually included in discussions of putative etiologies of abortion, there is little or no evidence to implicate thyroid dysfunction in habitual abortion.

Luteal Phase Defects. In general, the literature supports the idea that some women who suffer repetitive abortion produce inadequate amounts of progesterone during the luteal phase of the menstrual cycle. However, there is no evidence that progesterone therapy, given after pregnancy is established, is of any value in the management of threatened or habitual abortion. Although it is possible that progesterone therapy administered during the luteal phase and continued into early pregnancy may improve pregnancy salvage in patients with luteal phase defects, controlled studies have not yet proved this efficacy of progesterone therapy.[22]

Immunologic Causes. Some authorities contend that the most common etiology of recurrent spontaneous abortion is an immunologic process.[48] This contention is based on four observations. (1) Women who suffer abortions do not produce the inhibitors of cell-mediated immunity found in maternal blood during normal pregnancy. (2) Couples who suffer repetitive abortions share more HLA antigens at the A and B loci than would be expected by chance. (3) Classical implantation antigens are absent on human trophoblast. Other alloantigens are present. (4) Some trophoblast allotypic determinants are shared with lymphocytes and are coded for in the HLA region. In couples in which HLA antigens are shared by husband and wife, it is likely that trophoblast-specific antigens (TLX antigens) would also be shared between the conceptus and the mother. If TLX-compatible embryos do not stimulate maternal protective (blocking) factors, the conceptus would be rejected as would any foreign tissue.[6] The theory of immunogenic abortion thus holds that, because HLA antigens are not present in pregnancy, the normal maternal response is to make antibodies to paternal HLA antigens expressed on the nontrophoblast embryonic cells. These antibodies function to suppress maternal cellular reactivity to paternal HLA antigens. This suppressor or antibody system fails in pregnancies in which the conceptus and the mother are TLX compatible. Failure of the protective effect or system results in spontaneous abortion. If further study validates this hypothesis, immunotherapy may become useful in the management of some couples who experience recurrent spontaneous abortions.

Infectious Causes. The infectious agents that have been implicated in repeated abortion are: Toxoplasma, Listeria, herpes virus, chlamydia, and mycoplasma.

Toxoplasma gondii. Although *Toxoplasma gondii* can invade the placenta and fetus and is a cause of stillbirth, there is no evidence that the organism causes repeated abortion. The prevalence of Toxoplasma antibodies is the same in women who have never aborted, who have had an occasional abortion, and in those with habitual abortion.

Listeria monocytogenes. There is no evidence that this agent causes abortion in women.

Chlamydia trachomatis. At this time, there is no firm evidence that chlamydia causes abortion in humans.

Mycoplasma. It is possible that mycoplasma may cause abortions, but this contention is not yet proved. Women with histories of habitual abortion have more colonies of T-mycoplasma in their endometria than do normal fertile women.

Systemic Illnesses. Cardiovascular disease and severe chronic renal disease may be associated with habitual abortion and other pregnancy wastage, probably because of inadequate uterine blood flow.

Diabetes Mellitus. In spite of a common conception that diabetes is associated with habitual abortion, there is no evidence to support this association.

Lupus Erythematosus. When lupus becomes clinically evident, the abortion rate rises dramatically, to over 40% in some studies. In addition, repetitive spontaneous abortions may occur while lupus is still in its subclinical stage.

Psychologic Factors. Some authors think that women who abort repeatedly either are basically immature and thus unwilling to accept the responsibility of motherhood, or are career-oriented, independent women who do not place maternity high in their system of values.[66] The evidence for these contentions remains nebulous. At this moment, the role of psychodynamics in repetitive abortion is incompletely defined.

Management of Habitual Abortion. Patients who experience two or more consecutive abortions should be given a diagnostic evaluation. In taking the history, the etiologic factors discussed above should be searched for. In addition to the physical examination, the adequacy of the luteal phase should be ascertained using a combination of hormonal measurements and ultrasonography to follow follicular development. Hysteroscopy and/or hysterosalpingography are utilized to search for uterine anomalies or other anatomic problems.

If a woman has three abortions, both members of the couple should be karyotyped. Karyotyping is also necessary if, in addition to one or two abortions, the couple has had a child with congenital malformations. Any time that a fetus or abortus is found to have a translocation, the parents should be karyotyped. If an abortus is trisomic, the risk of trisomy in future pregnancies is increased. Amniocentesis should be utilized for prenatal diagnosis.

Ectopic Pregnancy

Ectopic pregnancy is a common cause of bleeding in early pregnancy. Bleeding is often the initial symptom of ectopic pregnancy. However, many women who suffer ectopic pregnancy are not aware that they are pregnant. In the United States, the incidence of ectopic pregnancy is 10.1 per 1000 women per year. The case fatality is 9.5 per 1000 cases. Ectopic pregnancy now accounts for 10% of maternal deaths in the United States.

Etiology. Although many risk factors have been identified, the etiology of ectopic pregnancy remains enigmatic.

Diagnosis

Clinical Diagnosis. Many patients afflicted by eccyesis do not experience the classic symptom complex of amenorrhea, bleeding, fainting, and abdominal pain. The frequencies of symptoms documented in the literature are: abdominal pain, 96%; shoulder pain, 17%; amenorrhea, 76%; abnormal vaginal bleeding, 83%; fainting, 21% Most of this information comes from retrospective chart reviews. It is likely that careful questioning would reveal abnormal bleeding or delay of menses in a higher percentage. Vaginal bleeding may vary from spotting to hemorrhage. A common clinical error is to eliminate tubal pregnancy as a possibility because vaginal bleeding is profuse. It is likely that the distribution of reported symptoms will change during the next decade, because the diagnosis is now made earlier.

The physical findings in ectopic pregnancy are also variable. In some instances, the diagnosis is apparent, with obvious signs of intraperitoneal hemorrhage and vascular collapse. In others, the diagnosis is obscure. Physical examination is important. The temperature rarely rises above 101.5° F. The breasts may be engorged, or occasionally lactating. The patients are usually normotensive or slightly hypotensive. Tachycardia or bradycardia may be the only manifestations of decreased blood volume. Inspection of the abdomen with the patient supine may reveal infraumbilical distention, with a relatively flat hypochondrium. Such distention is evidence of intraperitoneal hemorrhage. Auscultation of the abdomen reveals active peristaltic sounds, in contrast to the situation in pelvic inflammatory disease, in which diminished or absent peristalsis is the rule. Tenderness upon palpation of the abdomen is usually, but not invariably, present. Rebound tenderness may be noted secondary to the generalized peritoneal reaction in the pelvis. The uterus may or may not be enlarged. It is not uncommon to encounter a normal-sized uterus at operation for ectopic pregnancy. A uterus larger than the size of a 3 1/2 months' gestation is not compatible with the diagnosis of ectopic pregnancy.

A pelvic mass is present in a significant number of patients with ectopic pregnancy, especially of the "chronic" variety. The mass may be felt in either adnexal region or in the cul-de-sac. Adnexal tenderness to palpation is usually present and may be exquisite. Most patients with ectopic pregnancy complain of pain if the cervix is moved laterally. This is due to the tension on the involved tube resulting from displacement of the corpus to the opposite side. Unilateral adnexal pain upon cervical motion is a valuable sign if present; however, pain is commonly elicited by motion of the cervix to either side.

Ancillary Aids to Diagnosis. By maintaining a high index of suspicion and by properly utilizing diagnostic aids, the physician can hold the rate of erroneous diagnosis to less than 10%. The ancillary diagnostic procedures most commonly employed are culdocentesis, laparoscopy, and ultrasonography.

Culdocentesis is simple to perform and does not cause severe pain if properly done. The results of culdocentesis are classified as negative if clear peritoneal fluid is obtained, positive if nonclotting blood is obtained, and indeterminate if neither peritoneal fluid nor blood is obtained. False-negative culdocentesis results are obtained in less than 5% of patients with ectopic pregnancy, but 5%–10% of patients with positive results do not have ectopic pregnancy. The more experience a given physician gains in performing culdocentesis, the greater the accuracy of diagnosis.

Laparoscopy is useful in the diagnosis of eccyesis. The patient can be discharged quickly if ectopic gestation is not present. The false negative and positive rates are each about 3%. Complications of the procedure include hemorrhage into the abdominal wall, intestinal perforations, gas embolism, parietal and mediastinal emphysema, and pneumothorax.

The most useful aid to diagnosis in uncertain cases is a combination of quantitative serum β-hCG assays with gray scale ultrasonography. The concentration of hCG in serum doubles every 48–72 hours during the first six weeks of pregnancy. In normal pregnancy, a well-defined gestational sac can be measured at 28 days after ovulation. At this time, the β-hCG titer is between 6000 and 6500 mIU/ml. Thus, if the hCG titer is above 6000 mIU/ml and a well-defined intrauterine gestational sac is not identified with gray scale ultrasound, ectopic pregnancy is likely. If no sac is seen and the hCG titer is below 6000 mIU/ml, no diagnosis can be established.[40] In this eventuality, if the clinical diagnosis is still unclear, it is wise to repeat the hCG titer in two days. If the titer has not doubled or nearly doubled, an ectopic pregnancy or an abnormal intrauterine pregnancy is indicated. Conversely, if a well-defined intrauterine sac is present and the hCG titer is lower than 6000 mIU/ml, the intrauterine pregnancy is abnormal.

Treatment. The treatment of ectopic pregnancy is directed toward two goals: preserving life and preserving fertility. Few patients die after the abdomen has been opened. In the acute case, accompanied by hemoperitoneum and shock, immediate laparotomy is mandatory. Procrastination to await blood transfusion is futile. Hemostasis is superior to transfusion in the treatment of ruptured tubal pregnancy. If donor blood cannot be obtained, the patient's own blood can be recovered and administered during the operation.

The second goal is much more difficult to accomplish. A woman who suffers an ectopic pregnancy has only one chance in three of thereafter delivering a living child. Although pregnancy occurs more frequently than that, a disproportionate number end in repeat ectopic pregnancy or abortion. A woman who develops a tubal gestation has about a 10% chance of developing a second tubal pregnancy. Conversely, about 10% of ectopic pregnancies are repeat experiences.

The first consideration in preservation of fertility usually entails a decision at the time of surgery. Although many gynecologists now consider repair rather than excision of the involved tube, that course of action is not without cost. Most evidence suggests that, if the opposite tube appears normal, conservation of the tube containing the ectopic pregnancy improves the future pregnancy rate only slightly but raises the incidence of recurrent ectopic pregnancy significantly.

Upon opening the abdomen, the surgeon may encounter any of three situations: The ectopic pregnancy may be in the patient's sole remaining tube; the other tube may be present and apparently normal; or the other tube may be present but diseased. The therapeutic choices depend on the patient's wishes with regard to fertility and the surgeon's assessment of risks versus potential gain. For example, the tube containing the gestation may be excised and the condition of the contralateral tube ignored. Conversely, in the presence of an abnormal contralateral tube, the pregnant tube may be removed and a tuboplasty performed on the abnormal opposite tube; both tubes may be repaired; or the pregnant tube may be repaired.

An experienced gynecologic surgeon can usually make an accurate judgement concerning the patency of the opposite tube from its appearance. If uncertain, the patency of the opposite tube can be determined by injecting a warmed solution of methylene blue in sodium chloride into the uterus and observing fimbrial spill.

The surgeon may elect to preserve the pregnant tube if the patient desires more children and is willing to accept the risk of another tubal pregnancy. Sometimes the pregnancy can simply be 'milked out' of the abdominal ostium. In other unruptured tubes, linear salpingotomy is performed and the gestational sac is shelled out, or segmental resection and anastomosis are done. If the tube is ruptured, repair of the rupture or partial salpingectomy with anastomosis or reimplantation of the oviduct may be performed. If the opposite tube is present, but abnormal, and if fertility is important to the patient, many gynecologists preserve the pregnant tube and also repair the opposite tube. We believe that, in most cases, however, such patients would be better served by sterilization. Although reparative surgery allows the chance for future pregnancy, it also carries a greatly increased risk of recurrent eccyesis.

The recent resurgence of interest in tubal plastic surgery, stimulated greatly by the popularization of microsurgical repair of the tubes, has raised another pertinent question. Having made the decision that either or both tubes require surgical repair, the physician must determine whether or not it would be best to perform the least manipulation necessary to secure hemostasis and to close the abdomen. Reparative surgery could then be done electively under optimal conditions, with the full surgical team attending a healthy patient in an unhurried procedure. Some clinicians prefer to perform the reparative surgery at the time of initial laparotomy. The most appropriate timing and procedure to perform have not yet been determined by a careful study.

Gestational Trophoblastic Neoplasia

In the United States, gestational trophoblastic neoplasia (GTN) is seen once in about 1200 pregnancies. GTN is classified as benign or malignant. The benign group includes hydatidiform mole, molar degeneration of the placenta (transitional mole), and hydropic villi in a blighted ovum. The first of these is the one that usually first presents with bleeding during pregnancy. The malignant group, which is outside the scope of this chapter, includes metastatic and nonmetastatic malignant trophoblastic disease.[3] Although hydatidiform mole is an uncommon cause of bleeding in pregnancy, bleeding during the first trimester of pregnancy is the most common symptom of hydatidiform mole.

Diagnosis. The uterus is smaller than would be predicted from the menstrual dates in about 25% of patients with mole. In another 50%, the uterine size is significantly larger than predicted. In addition to bleeding and discordance between uterine size and dates, persistent hyperemesis gravidarum and the development of pregnancy-induced hypertension during the first half of pregnancy, or the development of hyperthyroidism should arouse the suspicion that a trophoblastic tumor is present.

About 90% of patients with trophoblastic neoplasia complain of bleeding. Other symptoms include nausea and vomiting in 15%, pregnancy-induced hypertension in 12%, and pain in 10%. Fewer than 1% develop symptoms of hyperthyroidism.

Most patients with GTN become symptomatic prior to the 17th week of pregnancy.[25] When a patient presents with bleeding in pregnancy and the fetal heart is not detectable although the uterus is larger than 12 weeks' gestational size, GTN should be suspected. The diagnosis of GTN is supported (but not proved) if the serum β-hCG level is above 40,000 mIU/ml, because such high values are uncommon (but not unknown) in normal pregnancy. The most useful aid to the diagnosis of GTN is ultrasonography. Sonograms demonstrate the characteristic appearance of GTN. However, multiple leiomyomas and multiple pregnancies can yield similar sonographic images. If sonography is not available, or the sonogram is not diagnostic, one of two courses can be followed, depending on the clinical setting. If the clinical setting is consistent with missed abortion, serial ultrasonography may be utilized. If the clinical picture is strongly suggestive of GTN, amniography may be done. This is rarely necessary.

To perform amniography, the abdomen is prepared and draped to provide a surgically clean field. A 22-gauge spinal needle is passed successively through the abdominal wall and the uterine wall to enter the uterine cavity. Twenty milliliters of water-soluble radio-opaque medium is then injected into the uterine cavity. About 10 minutes after injecting the radio-opaque medium, an x-ray of the abdomen is taken. The pattern of opacification associated with hydatidiform mole is quite typical.

Treatment. The treatment of choice for evacuating a hydatidiform mole is suction curettage. Although other methods have been utilized, such as intrauterine instillation of saline or prostaglandins, intravaginal prostaglandin suppositories, and oxytocin infusions, these methods increase blood loss and may increase the risk of deporting trophoblast to other locations, such as the lung, via the venous circulation.

Before the operative procedure is undertaken, the degree of anemia and hypovolemia should be ascertained. These patients undergo the same physiologic adjustments in plasma volume as those seen in normal pregnancy. Dilutional anemia should not be treated. Volume overload should be avoided. Transfusion is used only as required to stabilize vital functions.

Although paracervical block can be used for anesthesia, most clinicians prefer general anesthesia. The cervix is initially dilated sufficiently to allow passage of an 8 mm suction curette. Should a larger curette be required, the cervix is dilated further. The cervix dilates readily, therefore most authorities do not utilize laminaria for dilatation. When about two-thirds of the molar tissue has been evacuated, an oxytocin infusion (20 units of oxytocin in 1000 ml of physiologic saline) is begun. The oxytocin infusion should be continued for 24 hours. Some clinicians prefer to curette the uterus gently with a sharp curette after most of the molar tissue has been evacuated with the suction curette. This step is designed to remove any trophoblastic tissue that might have been missed, especially in the cornual regions.

During the immediate postoperative period, the patient should be closely observed for bleeding. Another complication, much less common, is pulmonary compromise. The latter is secondary to microembolization of the pulmonary vasculature by deported trophoblast. If the patient does not respond to conservative therapy, mechanical ventilation utilizing positive end expiratory pressure may be necessary.

After evacuation, the patient must be advised to delay pregnancy for at least six months. Contraceptives should be used. Serial quantitative hCG determinations are also necessary. For details of follow-up, appropriate monographs and review articles should be consulted.

BLEEDING IN THE SECOND HALF OF PREGNANCY

Vaginal bleeding is reported by 3–4% of pregnant women during the second half of pregnancy.[39] Such bleeding usually occurs in the third trimester. It differs etiologically from bleeding in the first half of pregnancy. The cause of the bleeding may have trivial impact on the pregnancy or it may represent a threat to the life of the mother and/or fetus.

Initial Evaluation

When a patient presents with a complaint of vaginal bleeding in the second half of pregnancy, the physician immediately thinks of a differential diagnosis and then proceeds to rule in or rule out disorders by taking a directed history and by performing a few simple procedures. Causes of bleeding are listed in Table 15-1.

The history gives the first clue to the etiology and severity of the bleeding episode. The physician needs to know the approximate volume of blood lost. The patient may estimate the volume of blood lost and may be asked whether or not the loss is more than that experienced with menses. Estimates of blood loss by the patient may be inaccurate, but bloody clothes, towels, lower extremities or bedding attest to heavy loss. The association of light bleeding mixed with mucus makes one think of "bloody show" that often precedes labor or coincides with early labor. A history of genital tract trauma points to an obvious etiology. Uterine contractions associated with vaginal bleeding are classically associated with abruptio placentae, but they may accompany bleeding from other causes. Painless vaginal bleeding implies that placenta previa is the cause, but painful contractions may be present with placenta previa and causes other than previa may present with painless bleeding. Bleeding initiated by intercourse or other cervical contact makes the physician think of cervical lesions and placenta previa. Bleeding after

TABLE 15-1. CAUSES OF BLEEDING IN THE SECOND HALF OF PREGNANCY

Cervical cancer
Cervicitis
Cervical ectropion
Cervical polyp
Trauma
"Heavy show"
Vasa previa
Placenta previa
Abruptio placentae
Circumvallate placenta
Unexplained

abdominal trauma suggests premature placental separation.

Vital signs remain normal during pregnancy despite significant blood loss. Hypotension, tachycardia, postural hypotension, and other signs of hypovolemia should be taken very seriously in pregnant women, because they develop relatively late in the course of blood loss and usually indicate heavy bleeding.

Speculum Examination. Speculum examination is safely performed in patients with vaginal bleeding and provides useful information regarding the etiology of the disorder.[31,43] Cervical cancer sufficiently extensive to cause bleeding should be readily visible on speculum examination. Likewise, bleeding from trauma, cervicitis, or cervical polyps can be seen coming from the cervix or the vagina. When blood is seen coming out of the cervical os, the source of bleeding is intrauterine. Estimation of the amount of bleeding can be done during speculum examination and blood can be taken for analysis for fetal hemoglobin at this time.

Sonography. When blood is coming through the cervical os, sonography is indicated to locate the placenta. Placenta previa can be diagnosed with a high degree of accuracy by sonography. Abruptio placentae may or may not be diagnosed with sonar. Sonar is not helpful for diagnosing other causes of bleeding. The main value of sonography is in locating the placenta. If the placenta is away from the region of the internal os, digital examination of the cervix can be done safely.

Differential Diagnosis. This rapid initial evaluation usually determines the most likely cause of bleeding in the second half of pregnancy. Cervical lesions such as cancer, cervicitis, ectropion, or polyp are usually not associated with pain or heavy bleeding. Bleeding from these entities may well be initiated by intercourse. They can be seen on speculum examination. A history of genital tract trauma reported by the patient is confirmed by speculum examination. In all these instances, the source of bleeding can be seen.

Bleeding that comes through the cervical os suggests vasa previa, placenta previa, or abruptio placentae. Vasa previa is confirmed by finding fetal hemoglobin in the blood. Placenta previa is diagnosed sonographically. Abruptio placentae is a clinical diagnosis which may be supported by sonographic findings, but which is confirmed after delivery. Circumvallate placenta may be presumed to be a mild abruption before delivery. The diagnosis is established after delivery. Formerly a large percentage of all cases of bleeding in the second half of pregnancy went unexplained. Since the advent of sonography, we have discovered that numerous patients who have placenta previa early in pregnancy do not manifest this condition at the time of delivery (see below). Presumably some cases of unexplained vaginal bleeding are represented in this group.

Vasa Previa

When the cord inserts into the fetal membranes rather than into the placenta or when there is a bilobed placenta with vessels running in the membranes between the lobes, the designation velamentous insertion of the umbilical cord is applied. Should these fetal vessels cross the region of the internal os, they are referred to as vasa previa. Vessels of vasa previa typically rupture at the same time that the membranes rupture. The mother is in no danger from this event, but the fetus is at great risk of exsanguination.

The incidence of vasa previa is estimated at 1 in 5000 deliveries and the perinatal mortality at 70%.[41] The best perinatal survival is obtained when the vasa previa is diagnosed before the vessels rupture. The vasa previa may be seen during amnioscopy or the vessels may be felt as a band running across the membranes. When vasa previa is diagnosed prior to rupture, delivery should be by cesarean section.

Painless vaginal bleeding from vasa previa prior to rupture of the membranes has been reported,[12] but the clue to the diagnosis of vasa previa usually is bleeding that begins when the membranes rupture. Whenever vasa previa is suspected as the cause of bleeding, the fetus should be monitored carefully for indications of fetal distress and a rapid test for fetal hemoglobin should be performed on the blood. Depending on the facilities available, this test might be a hemoglobin electrophoresis, an acid elution stain of a blood film (Kleihauer–Betke), or a modification of the Apt test, which originally was designed to differentiate adult from fetal hemoglobin in bloody stools of newborns.[4] The modified Apt test (Table 15-2) is rapid, accurate, easy to perform, and inexpensive. If fetal blood is detected and the fetus is viable, deliv-

TABLE 15-2. APT TEST FOR FETAL HEMOGLOBIN

Step 1.	Mix blood with tap water to cause hemolysis.
Step 2.	Centrifuge the solution for several minutes at 2000 rpm to separate debris from a pink supernatant containing the hemoglobin.
Step 3.	Add 1 ml of 0.25 normal (1%) NaOH with each 5 ml of supernatant solution.
Step 4.	Read the results in 2 minutes. Adult hemoglobin will change color to a yellowish brown; fetal hemoglobin will remain pink.

If desired, controls of maternal and/or fetal blood can be run at the same time to confirm the results.

ery should be accomplished at once in the interest of the fetus. This usually means by cesarean section.

Placenta Previa

Definition, Incidence, and Etiology. Placenta previa is defined as implantation of the placenta low in the uterus, either overlying or reaching the vicinity of the internal cervical os. Placentas previa are subdivided into central or total placenta previa, in which the os is completely covered by placenta; partial placenta previa, in which the os at complete cervical dilatation would be partially covered by placenta; and low-lying or marginal placenta previa, in which the os is not covered, but the edge of the placenta extends close to the region of the internal os. The frequency of each type of placenta previa reported in the literature varies. Some authors do not include low-lying placentas in their data on placenta previa. Low-lying placentas account for approximately half the cases of placenta previa. The other half of cases are approximately equally divided between total and partial previas. We manage low-lying placentas as previas because they present the same way and because their sonographic appearance cannot always be differentiated from that of partial previas. Indeed, some central and partial previas become low-lying placentas as pregnancy progresses.

The reported total incidence of placenta previa is approximately 0.5%. This figure is remarkably constant regardless of the definition used or of the source of the report.[7,13,31] In a referral hospital, the observed incidence of placenta previa is usually higher.

The etiology of placenta previa is unknown. Factors associated with a higher incidence of previa include increasing maternal age, increasing parity, multiple gestation, previous low-segment cesarean delivery, and male fetus.[7,10,15] The relationship between previous induced abortion and placenta previa has been explored. The results of these studies are inconclusive.[5,24]

Clinical Presentation. Painless vaginal bleeding is the chief complaint of 70–80% of women with placenta previa. Another 10–20% of patients complain of bleeding associated with labor pains and approximately 10% of patients have their previa diagnosed in the absence of vaginal bleeding.[15,47]

The bleeding associated with placenta previa may begin in the first half of pregnancy, but three reports have found the average duration of pregnancy at the time of the first bleed to be between 27 and 32 weeks.[45,47,70] Central placenta previas usually bleed earlier in pregnancy, bleed more heavily, and result in more premature deliveries and perinatal deaths than do other types of placenta previa.[54]

Malpresentations of the fetus are found in one-fourth to one-third of cases of placenta previa.[15,45] The bulk of the placenta low in the uterus probably interferes with the mechanisms that adapt the fetal head to the lower uterine segment. Breech presentation and transverse lie occur with almost equal frequency.[45]

Diagnosis. The definitive diagnosis of placenta previa depends on digital examination. Direct palpation of the placenta through the cervical os proves the diagnosis. Vaginal examination induces torrential hemorrhage in approximately 6% of patients with placenta previa.[31,47] Therefore, digital examination should not be performed unless the fetus is sufficiently mature to be delivered. The examination should be done in an operating room prepared for surgery. Blood should be available for transfusion.

Because manual examination is dangerous in women with suspected placenta previa, alternative diagnostic techniques have been developed to locate the placenta in order to make a presumptive diagnosis of placenta previa. All the techniques formerly employed have been replaced by ultrasonography. It is recommended that all labor and delivery suites have access to ultrasonography 24 hours a day. Sonography is highly accurate for placental localization. If the placenta is seen on the corpus or fundus of the uterus, one can exclude placenta previa. Likewise, if a central placenta previa is seen with ultrasonography, there is no need to perform a pelvic examination. Delivery can be accomplished by cesarean section at the appropriate time. Varieties of placenta previa may not always be differentiated sonographically. It is difficult to tell a partial previa from a low-lying placenta. In this instance, vaginal examination at term may be desirable to select the route of delivery.[13]

One of the most interesting developments in recent years is the sonographic demonstration that the placenta occupies different locations within the uterus at different gestational ages. At 16 weeks' gestation, the placenta occupies one-half the inner surface area of the uterus, whereas at term it occupies one-fourth to one-third of the area.[38] During pregnancy, the placenta migrates from the lower part of the uterus toward the fundus. At term, placenta previa may no longer be present in patients who had displayed the condition in early pregnancy.[14,59,67]

Although 5–50% of women may demonstrate a type of placenta previa in mid-pregnancy, few or none require intervention at term because of bleeding or placenta previa.[59,67] If placenta previa is present at 30 weeks' gestation, the incidence of clinical problems at the time of delivery may be as high as 24%.[14]

A prospective study of low implantation of the placenta in the midtrimester revealed that women with low implantation were significantly older than controls, were of significantly higher parity,and had a significant history of uterine operations. At term, only 3% of patients with a low placental implantation had a placenta previa. However, these women suffered a significantly increased incidence of third-trimester bleeding, abruptio placentae, cesarean delivery blood loss with vaginal delivery, low-birth-weight infants, and perinatal mortality. Sonography at 33 weeks' gestation revealed no evidence of a previa in almost all patients in whom placenta previa was demonstrated earlier in pregnancy.[50]

The precise significance of an asymptomatic placenta previa noted on a midtrimester sonographic examination is unknown. At best, it seems to be a normal form of placental implantation in early pregnancy. At worst, it persists as a placenta previa in up to 10% of patients. Women with low implantation of the placenta may be at higher risk for pregnancy complications as noted above. Most physicians agree that when an asymptomatic, midtrimester previa is noted on sonography, the patient should be informed and reassured that it is usually a benign, self-limited condition. Activities need not be limited, but repeat sonography is indicated.[59] If the previa persists past 30 weeks' gestation, it is likely to be present at the time of delivery. If the patient develops bleeding, she should, of course, be managed as any other patient with a placenta previa.

Management. With placenta previa, hemorrhage is unavoidable at the time of labor and vaginal delivery. Many devices and techniques were developed to minimize hemorrhage at delivery, but the maternal mortality associated with the condition remained 10% overall and 25% with central previas into the late 1920s.[8]

Modern management of placenta previa began in 1927 when the treatment of placenta previa with blood transfusion and cesarean section, two new and risky procedures, was initiated.[8] Prior to that time, the maternal mortality associated with previas had been unchanged for 20 years. Women usually died of hemorrhage after delivery and rarely died if they were undelivered or if they had no intrauterine manipulations. Maternal mortality was related to the condition of the patient at the time of delivery and to the method of delivery. Therapy was therefore aimed at replacing blood loss prior to delivery and at delivering the patient in a way that minimized the danger of trauma to the cervix and lower uterine segment. These aims were accomplished by blood transfusion if the red cell count dropped below 3 million per cu mm or if the blood pressure dropped below 90/60. Delivery was by cesarean section.[8]

Institutions that followed the above precepts noted a decline in maternal mortality to less than 1%. Cesarean section became the method of choice for delivery of women with placenta previa because it was safest for the mother.

Despite improved maternal mortality figures, the outlook for the fetus with a placenta previa remained dismal. Most authors reported perinatal mortality figures of 50% or higher.

The second step in the modern management of placenta previa came about because the condition was now no longer life-threatening to the mother and because prematurity was the chief cause of perinatal mortality. To improve perinatal mortality, the pregnancy should be allowed to continue while maintaining safety for the mother. In 1945, authors in Texas and Northern Ireland presented similar guidelines for the management of women suspected of having a previa.[37,43] They noted that placenta previa was not an obstetric emergency that required immediate delivery with the first bleeding episode. Indeed, the first bleed was rarely severe unless the patient had a vaginal examination. They advocated hospitalization when the diagnosis was suspected and vaginal examination only when delivery was contemplated. The examination was to prove or disprove the diagnosis of previa and, thereby, to choose the route of delivery. Johnson, who termed this "conservative management," stated that he knew of no woman with a placenta previa who bled to death in the absence of cervical or intrauterine manipulation or manual removal of the placenta.[37]

A series of 105 women with placenta previa was reported in 1948. Among women managed by immediate delivery, the perinatal mortality rate was 37.5%; women not delivered at once had a perinatal mortality rate of 12%.[69] There was only one maternal death in the series; it was from sepsis, not hemorrhage. The author designated this delay in delivery "expectant management," the term most physicians still use.

Expectant management of patients with placenta previa terminates when the fetus is mature, the mother is in labor, the blood loss is excessive, the fetus is dead, or there is evidence of intra-amniotic infection. Few of these criteria for terminating expectant management are rigidly defined. The issue of continued hospitalization for women undergoing expectant management has been debated. Both points of view (maintenance in the hospital versus observation at home) have merit. We are willing to manage patients at home when the bleeding has stopped for several days if the patient and her family understand her condition, if she will refrain from intercourse, if she is not anemic, if she has a telephone, if someone is always with her and transportation is available, and if she does not live more than 30 minutes away from the hospital. Whereas we have been satisfied with this approach, others assert that continued hospitalization is more cost-effective.[19]

In the 1960s and early 1970s, the results of expectant management were not as good as hoped for in terms of perinatal mortality.[16,31] Expectant management was often precluded because of uterine contractions and heavy bleeding. The main factor in the success of expectant management seemed to be the type of previa and the time in pregnancy when the first bleed occurred. The worst results were obtained when there was a central previa which bled for the first time prior to 32 weeks' gestation.[54]

Recently, several clinicians have advocated "conservative aggressive" or "aggressive expectant" management of patients with placenta previa.[15,63] These differ from traditional expectant management in the more liberal use of transfusions, the use of tocolytics for women who are having contractions, use of amniocentesis for fetal lung maturity studies, and bioelectronic fetal monitoring to assure fetal well-being. Perinatal mortality rates of 4–8% have been reported by institutions using this approach.[45,63]

The "double set up" examination is still occasionally necessary to help determine the route of delivery. Should sonography clearly demonstrate a central previa when it is time for delivery, there is nothing to be gained by vaginal examination. If, however, sonography is equivocal, vaginal examination may be helpful.[13] This examination is termed a "double set up" because it should take place in a fully equipped operating room set up for vaginal or cesarean delivery, with blood available, anesthesia present, and the attendants prepared for immediate cesarean delivery if hemorrhage is provoked. Under sterile conditions, a finger is inserted through the cervical canal. The relationships of the placenta and the fetal head to the pelvis are both important. Some physicians assert that the location of the placenta is not critical, as long as the head descends into the pelvis. Others attempt vaginal delivery when there is a low-lying placenta or partial previa of a minor degree. The posterior low-lying placenta has been termed "the dangerous placenta" because, in that location, the placenta covers the sacral promontory and obstructs the pelvic inlet to some degree.[64]

Complications in the Fetus and Newborn. Placenta previa has become a much safer condition for the mother because of blood transfusions and cesarean delivery in almost all cases. The well-being of the fetus and newborn has also been improved because of recent modifications in expectant management.

Repeated episodes of bleeding during pregnancy and low implantation of the placenta have been thought to have an adverse effect on fetal growth and survival. Such concerns seem to have no basis.[21,45] Repeated episodes of bleeding do not correlate with growth retardation or with perinatal mortality. The amount of blood lost does correlate with perinatal mortality. Severe hemorrhage was associated with intrauterine fetal loss in 9% of cases managed expectantly in one series.[54]

A study of the impact of placenta previa on newborns noted that such infants were more likely to die in the first month of life than were infants without placenta previa, regardless of duration of pregnancy and birth weight.[61] The study was not designed to identify a cause of the increased deaths.

Maternal Complications. Women with placenta previa are more likely to have placenta accreta than are women with a normally implanted placenta.[44] This is especially true if the woman has had a previous cesarean delivery. (Placenta accreta is discussed in Chapter 47.) Almost all cases of placenta previa accreta should be managed by hysterectomy.

Postpartum hemorrhage is also encountered commonly after delivery of a woman with placenta previa. This is because the implantation site is in the lower uterine segment which is composed mostly of collagen and cannot achieve hemostasis through the mechanism of uterine contraction. Ecbolic agents are, therefore, ineffective and surgical therapy is often necessary (see Chapter 47).

Abruptio Placentae

Abruptio placentae is a more difficult topic to discuss than is placenta previa. There is no uniform classification, the diagnosis is usually clinical with little help from sonography, and the interval from abruption to delivery is usually short. Despite advances in perinatal medicine, there is currently no way to predict abruptions, the etiology of abruptions is often obscure, and the attendant perinatal mortality remains high.

Definition and Incidence. Abruptio placentae is defined as the premature separation of a normally implanted placenta. This implies separation after the 20th week of pregnancy, but before delivery of the fetus. The pathophysiology involves maternal hemorrhage into the decidua basalis with formation of a clot which separates the placenta from its attachment. This process, in turn, can progress to further placental separation and hemorrhage.

The extravasated maternal blood and clot may remain totally within the uterus. In this instance, the abruption is termed "concealed;" there is no external bleeding. Alternatively, all or almost all the blood may exit from the uterus and appear as vaginal bleeding. The blood may find escape into the amniotic cavity and appear later as bloody amniotic fluid with or without external signs of bleeding. Combinations of the above findings are the rule rather than the exception. In contrast to the situation with placenta previa, the amount of blood apparently lost with a placental abruption bears no constant relationship with the amount of blood actually lost from the woman's circulation. This is a key point in the diagnosis and management of abruptio placentae.

The incidence of abruptio placentae varies more widely than does the incidence of previa. The definition used to confirm abruption and the nature of the reporting hospital influence the incidence figures. The overall incidence is reported to be from less than 1% to 2.5%.[20,35,39,62] Abruptions severe enough to kill the fetus occur in approximately 0.2% of pregnancies.[57] Abruptio placentae is one of the leading causes of perinatal mortality because of stillbirths and, to a much lesser extent, prematurity.

Etiology. There are several known etiologies and several associations with placental abruption. Pritchard, in 1970, gave a very complete description of the causes of abruption in 201 cases sufficiently severe to cause fetal death.[56] Among the possible causes of abruptio placentae, the following deserve note:

Sudden Decompression of a Distended Uterus. The reported incidence of abruption due to rupture of the membranes in women with polyhydramnios ranges from 0.5–2%.[29,56] The mechanism seems to be rapid adjustment of intrauterine area with subsequent shearing off of the placenta similar to the normal mechanism of placental separation in the third stage of labor. Similar mechanisms can cause problems for the second and subsequent fetuses in cases of multiple gestation. Strangely, in one series of abruptions, 2% of the abruptions occurred in cases of polyhydramnios prior to rupture of the membranes.[29]

Uterine Anomaly. This is a very rare cause of abruption occurring in only one of Pritchard's 201 patients.

Inferior Vena Cava Occlusion. In pregnant dogs, experimental occlusion of the inferior vena cava causes placental abruption.[49] The hypothesized mechanism involves a rapid rise in venous pressure in the placental bed that causes placental separation. The evidence for a similar mechanism in pregnant women is lacking.[65] There are ample benefits to the pregnant woman in avoiding the supine position without adding the avoidance of abruption.

Maternal Folate Deficiency. In the 1960s, investigators in England reported that 97% of abruptions were caused by maternal folate deficiency.[29] Supplemental folate administration to pregnant women was touted to prevent abruptions as well as spontaneous abortions, congenital anomalies, growth retardation, and premature delivery. Investigators in the United States and Ireland failed to find the same association between abruptions and maternal folate deficiency.[20,68] The addition of folate to prenatal vitamin supplements has certainly not prevented 97% of abruptions.[56]

Hypertensive Disorders. Maternal hypertensive disorders have been considered unimportant by some[28,30] and by others to be the most important factor in the genesis of placental abruptions. The bulk of the clinical evidence points to a definite relationship between maternal hypertension and placental abruption.[1,20,56]

Parity. There is a consistent association between increasing parity and abruption. Maternal age may or may not have an association with abruption separate from that of parity.

Past History. The incidence of abruption is higher in women who have had prior abruptions.[20,30,56] This is especially true if they are hypertensive and have a parity above three. Among Pritchard's 201 women with an abruption severe enough to kill the fetus, there was a 30-fold increase in severe abruptions in the subsequent pregnancy![56]

Trauma. Trauma is a well-documented but infrequent cause of abruptions. Abruptions secondary to trauma seem to account for approximately 1% of all abruptions. Automobile accidents and falls are the main causes of traumatic abruption.

Trauma is the leading cause of death in women aged 15–35. Half of these deaths are due to automobile accidents.[32] In at least one state, trauma is the most frequent nonobstetric cause of maternal death.[11] It has been estimated that 7% of pregnant women are involved in accidents during pregnancy.[11]

Blunt abdominal trauma causes 80% of abdominal injuries in pregnancy. Automobile accidents account for over half of the instances of blunt abdominal trauma.[11] In these cases, the most common cause of fetal death is maternal death and the best chance for fetal survival is to assure maternal survival.[60] Among women who survive abdominal trauma, abruptio placentae is the most frequent cause of fetal death.[32] In contrast to the situation with abortions, where trauma can rarely be proved as the cause of pregnancy loss,[27] a recent study of pregnant trauma patients revealed that more than one-fourth of them sustained placental abruption.[32] Most traumatic abruptions occur within 48 hours of the traumatic event, but abruption has been reported as late as five days after an automobile accident.[32]

The use of automobile seat belts by pregnant women has received attention. One study found that use of only lap belts made no significant difference in maternal or fetal loss. Lap belts were recommended because they prevented ejection of the accident victim from the automobile.[17] Subsequent studies utilizing pregnant baboons suggest that lap belts are inferior to lap belts with a shoulder restraint. The use of shoulder restraint prevents forward flexion and possible injury due to the lap belt itself.[18]

Maternal response to injury is altered by pregnancy. The diagnosis and treatment of injured women is often modified by the pregnancy. Necessary laboratory and roentgenographic studies should be obtained in the interest of both mother and fetus. Hemorrhagic shock should be treated vigorously (see Chapter 47). As many as 80% of women admitted in hemorrhagic shock may sustain an unsuccessful pregnancy outcome.[60] It has been suggested that the manner of treating trauma patients in the supine position adversely affects pregnancy outcome through the development of supine hypotension and possible fetal distress.[11]

Clinical Presentation. Although painless abruptio placentae may rarely occur,[51] abdominal pain and vaginal bleeding are the usual complaints of women with abruptio placentae. Both are highly variable in magnitude. The pain may be no more intense than menstrual cramps or normal labor or it may be severe abdominal pain associated with a penetrating sacral backache.

Uterine contractions are almost always associated with the pain. Formerly, it was believed that the uterus contracted in a tetanic fashion in cases of severe placental abruption. Abdominal palpation gives the examiner this impression. Monitoring of intrauterine pressure demonstrates that the resting pressure of the uterus is elevated to between 20 and 60 torr in many cases of abruption and that frequent contractions of low intensity occur. These contractions cannot be appreciated by the examining hand and the physician feels what seems to be a tetanic contraction (Fig. 15-1). At times, the contractions simulate those of normal labor; they may also be more frequent or more intense than normal labor. Uterine tenderness to palpation is also characteristic of abruptions.

The amount of blood apparently lost may not accurately reflect the amount actually lost. Concealed abruptions often have more complete placental separation than abruptions in which all blood finds egress. As more and more placenta separates, fetal distress and eventually fetal death ensue. Separation of approximately 50% of the placenta is sufficient to cause fetal demise.

When enough blood is lost, the woman develops hypovolemic shock. It was formerly taught that, in cases of abruptio placentae, the shock was out of proportion to the blood loss.[53] Several studies have now shown that to be inaccurate; the blood loss was usually grossly underestimated because of inability to estimate the size of the retroplacental hematoma. In abruptions severe enough to kill the fetus the average blood loss is 2500 ml![57] In Ireland, the amount of blood given to women with abruptions tripled when blood replacement was guided by central venous pressure monitoring instead of by estimated blood loss; the number of women with hypovolemic renal damage also decreased dramatically with the increase in volume of blood transfusion.[20,52]

Disseminated intravascular coagulation with resultant coagulopathy occurs almost exclusively in abruptions that are sufficiently severe to kill the fetus. The authors have seen only one

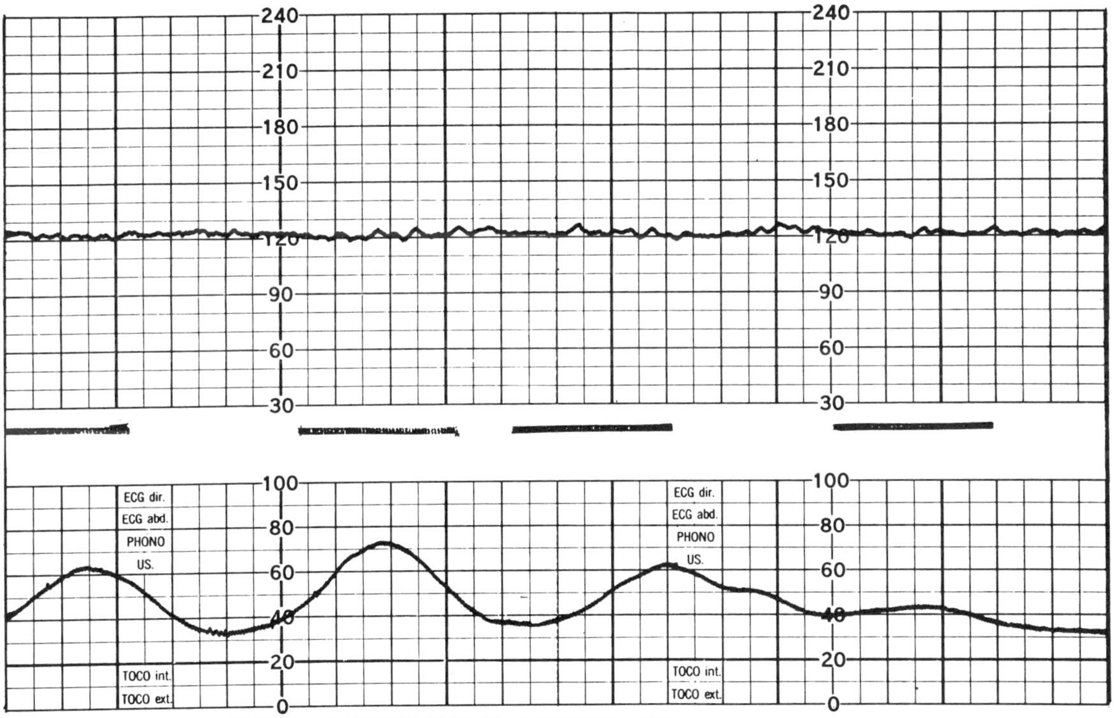

Figure 15-1. Characteristic pattern of uterine activity and fetal heart rate with abruptio placentae. This oscillograph record from a woman with a placental abruption shows elevation of the uterine resting pressure and frequent contractions of low intensity. The fetal heart rate tracing exhibits borderline bradycardia and decreased beat-to-beat variability.

significant coagulopathy associated with a live fetus. Coagulopathy occurs in 13–38% of abruptions associated with fetal demise.[20,30,57] To some extent, the incidence varies with the definition used to diagnose coagulopathy. Typically, fibrinogen and platelets are low and fibrin degradation products are elevated in peripheral blood. Observation of a tube of the patient's blood for the time it takes to clot is a highly effective way to diagnose coagulopathy. If no clot forms, the fibrinogen level is below 60 mg/dl; if a firm clot forms which does not lyse, the fibrinogen is above 150 mg/dl.[34] Bleeding from the gums and venipuncture sites correlates with a fibrinogen level below 60 mg/dl and a severe coagulopathy.

Diagnosis. The diagnosis of abruptio placentae is clinical. Finding a retroplacental blood clot after delivery confirms the diagnosis. The antepartum clinical diagnosis is based on the clinical presentation of pain and vaginal bleeding. The findings of uterine contractions, tenderness, and tetany make the diagnosis more secure. If there is associated fetal death, the diagnosis is even more certain.

Sonography, which is so helpful in cases of placenta previa, is not as reliable in cases of abruptio placentae.[23,33,51,71] The characteristic sonographic appearance of abruption includes a retroplacental or intraplacental sonolucent area, thickening or rounding of the placental edges, and a thicker placenta.[36] Exceptions to all these findings occur and some cases demonstrate none of them. It is thought that if most of the blood escapes the retroplacental location, there are no characteristic findings.[33] Retroplacental veins, which are sonolucent, can be mistaken for hematomas as can normal myometrium, especially if there is a contraction behind the placental area.[71]

Ultrasonography was used to identify abruptions in three women who presented with abdominal pain and no bleeding. In these instances, all blood remained behind the placenta and was correctly detected sonographically.[58] Nevertheless, the diagnosis remains clinical; sonography may or may not be helpful in an individual case.

One of the problems in discussing abruptions is the lack of a commonly accepted classification. Until there is an accepted antepartum classification, it is difficult to compare cases and forms of management. The simplest classification is to divide abruptions into those that do and those that do not kill the fetus.[57] Other classifications have been based on placental findings, estimated blood loss, and symptoms[39] or partly on fetal death, partly on the volume of concealed hemorrhage, and partly on maternal shock.[26] Page's grading of the severity of abruptions uses clinical factors and is very helpful. Perhaps the most useful classification of placental abruptions was that proposed by Sher[62] (Table 15-3).

A classification system is important to assess quickly the maternal and fetal prognosis, to plan management, and to compare results among institutions.

Management. Fetal life or death is the most important determinant of the management of abruptio placentae. By Sher's definition, Grade I abruptions are diagnosed only in retrospect so we are discussing Grade II and Grade III abruptions.

When the fetus is alive, major maternal complications are rare.[62] Patients in this group represent our only chance to improve perinatal outcome. It has been suggested that all women with an abruption and a live fetus be stabilized rapidly and delivered by cesarean if vaginal delivery is not imminent.[39] This management was suggested as part of a study to determine the best management for abruptions associated with a live fetus. To date, the results of the study have not been reported. This suggestion was based on the observation that 75% of fetal losses occurred more than an hour and a half after admission to the hospital with a diagnosis

TABLE 15-3. CLASSIFICATION SYSTEM FOR PLACENTAL ABRUPTIONS

Grade I	The mildest form of placental abruption. The cause of hemorrhage is uncertain until after delivery when a retroplacental clot is found.
Grade II	Antepartum hemorrhage with a tense, tender uterus and a live fetus.
Grade III	Classic features of abruptio placentae and a dead fetus. This grade is further subdivided according to the presence or absence of coagulopathy.
Grade III A	No coagulopathy
Grade III B	Coagulopathy present

Source: Sher.[62]

of abruption and a live fetus. Other clinicians do not share this experience.[30,35] At our institution, it is rare for a fetus alive on admission to die prior to delivery. A review of our abruptions led to the conclusion that cesarean delivery for all live fetuses would not change the perinatal mortality.

Fetal distress is a constant concern in patients with an abruption and a live fetus. The development of distress is based on the initial condition of the fetus, the amount of placental separation, the amount of blood lost, and the development of uterine hypertonus. Intrauterine pressure is the only one of these factors that can be measured accurately. Amniotomy and intrauterine pressure monitoring should begin as soon as possible after admission. A fetal electrode should be placed at once for constant monitoring of the fetal heart rate. Uterine hypertonus often precedes the development of fetal heart rate changes suggestive of fetal distress.

Intravenous fluids should be given and blood crossmatched. Immediate cesarean delivery should be accomplished when there is any evidence of fetal distress and the fetus is sufficiently mature to benefit from abdominal delivery.

Maternal clot observation and coagulation profile, as well as blood count, platelet count, urinalysis, and recording of urine output, should be performed. These are usually normal with Grade II abruptions. Table 15-4 summarizes management of placental abruptions with a live fetus.

Grade III abruptions, those with a dead fetus, pose a threat to the woman's life. Perinatal mortality is no longer a factor and prompt action is necessary in the maternal interest. With these severe abruptions, several facts are known: the average blood loss is 2500 ml and the chance of a coagulopathy developing is about 30%.[57]

Initial management involves crossmatch for six units of packed red cells and administration of two of the units as soon as they are available. Intravenous fluids should also be given. Amniotomy for intrauterine pressure monitoring should be done at once. Clot observation and clotting studies for fibrinogen, fibrin split products, platelet count, prothrombin time and partial thromboplastin time should be drawn on admission and every two hours thereafter. Blood count and urinalysis are performed also.

Fortunately, 30% of women with Grade III abruptions deliver within one hour of admission to the hospital,[57] but the other 70%, are a cause of great concern. Some method of evaluating the adequacy of initial treatment must be established. Vital signs are always recorded, but they are not always helpful if normal, as pregnant women can have normal vital signs despite heavy blood loss. The woman's urinary output is of great importance; a rate of 30 ml/hour is considered minimal evidence of adequate fluid replacement. Hourly hematocrit determinations above 30% are also reassuring. Central venous pressure monitoring is effective in the management of transfusion therapy for patients with

TABLE 15-4. MANAGEMENT OF PATIENTS WITH ABRUPTIO PLACENTAE AND A LIVE FETUS: GRADE II

Laboratory studies	Blood count, platelet count, urinalysis, clot observation, coagulation studies, crossmatch 2 units of packed red cells.
Fetal evaluation	Rupture membranes, insert pressure catheter and fetal electrode. Monitor fetal heart rate and uterine activity constantly.
Continuing evaluation	Intravenous fluid therapy monitored by hematocrit and urine output every hour until delivery. Keep hematocrit above 30% and urine output above 30 ml/hour. Repeat clot observation every 2 hours.
Delivery	Anticipate vaginal delivery if there is no contraindication. Use oxytocin if necessary to obtain adequate uterine activity. Watch carefully for fetal distress; if it appears, deliver the patient by cesarean section unless vaginal delivery is imminent or the fetus is too small to survive.

abruptions[52]; balloon flotation catheters may be of value in some women (see Chapters 47 and 49).

Coagulopathy, if it develops, need not be treated unless surgical therapy is planned. Fibrinogen was used successfully to treat coagulopathies in the past, but it is no longer available because of the high incidence of hepatitis associated with its use. Fresh frozen plasma and platelets are excellent therapy for the coagulopathy when therapy is indicated.

Delivery of women with Grade III abruptions should be by vagina unless there is some other reason for cesarean delivery. Delivery within 6–8 hours of admission has been advocated to decrease the maternal complications of abruptio placentae.[34,53] It is now believed, however, that the maternal complications can be prevented by adequate transfusion therapy, thus avoiding surgery on critically ill women in order to satisfy an arbitrary time limit.[52] The authors are not ready to totally abandon a time limit approach, having seen some women who would have benefitted from such an approach, but the weight of the evidence suggests that most women can be managed by careful clinical monitoring.

A summary of the management of women with Grade III abruptions is contained in Table 15-5.

TABLE 15-5. MANAGEMENT OF PATIENTS WITH ABRUPTIO PLACENTAE AND A DEAD FETUS: GRADE III

Laboratory studies	Blood count, platelet count, urinalysis, clot observation, coagulation studies, crossmatch 6 units of packed red cells.
Maternal therapy	Insert large intravenous infusion line and begin therapy with saline solution. Give 2 units of packed cells when available; if patient is in shock, you may have to give type-specific blood. Rupture membranes and insert intrauterine pressure monitor. Place indwelling catheter in urinary bladder. Consider placement of a central venous pressure line or balloon flotation catheter if necessary.
Continuing evaluation	Record vital signs, urine output, hematocrit, and clot observation every hour. Coagulation studies should be repeated every 2 hours. Expect rapid progress in labor; if it does not occur, base decision to use oxytocin on the uterine activity demonstrated by the pressure catheter. Be sure patient has had adequate blood and volume replacement as judged by hematocrit and urine output or by invasive monitoring techniques. The blood pressure and pulse rate are helpful guides if they indicate hypovolemia.
Delivery	Anticipate vaginal delivery. Indications for cesarean delivery for a Grade III abruption include a contraindication to labor, excessive bleeding that cannot be replaced, and prolonged labor that is ineffective—this was formerly 6–8 hours; there is no definite limit now as long as the patient's condition is stable.
Watch for complications	Coagulopathy occurs in over one-fourth of cases. It merits treatment with fresh frozen plasma and possibly with platelets if surgical treatment is planned or occasionally if there is postpartum bleeding. Uterine rupture may occur as may postpartum hemorrhage due to uterine atony and amniotic fluid infusion.

Fetal and Newborn Complications. Perinatal mortality has been essentially unchanged over the years. Reports of perinatal mortality rates of 30–36% are still seen.[35,62] In a recent report, over 15% of all perinatal deaths in one institution were from abruptions.[35] There is no test to predict abruptions and most of the perinatal mortality occurs before the patient arrives for medical attention. The immediate hope for improving perinatal mortality is to adopt a liberal cesarean delivery policy for women with Grade II abruptions. Any suspicion of fetal distress should prompt immediate delivery.

Most nursery deaths are a result of premature delivery and its complications. Unfortunately, there is no real equivalent of the expectant management used in women with placenta previa that can be applied to women with placental abruptions. Clinically evident abruptions are rarely amenable to an expectant approach to management.

Maternal Complications. Maternal death is virtually limited to Grade III abruptions. The most common mechanism of death reported in the past was renal failure from renal cortical necrosis as a result of prolonged hypotension. The second most common cause was hypovolemic shock.[20,42] Both these entities have a common cause—blood loss, and a common treatment—transfusion. In the last 20 years, with better knowledge of the amount of blood actually lost and with better techniques for evaluating the adequacy of transfusion therapy, deaths and renal compromise associated with abruptions have become unusual. Vigorous transfusion therapy is of the utmost importance in treating severe abruptions.

Coagulopathy contributes to maternal morbidity by increasing blood loss. At one time, effort was directed at different forms of management for the coagulopathy. Arguments raged over the relative merits of epsilon amino caproic acid and heparin in the therapy of coagulation problems. It is now generally recognized that the best therapy is to deliver the baby and let the woman correct her own coagulopathy after delivery. The coagulopathy will not correct until after delivery and then it does so promptly. Specific therapy with fresh frozen plasma and platelets is generally not necessary unless the patient is to have surgical treatment.

Uterine rupture is a complication of abruptio placentae that is not often discussed. We have seen three women spontaneously rupture their uteri in association with the hypertonic contractions of placental abruption.

Postpartum hemorrhage due to uterine atony is specifically associated with abruptio placentae. A uterus which becomes suffused with blood to the extent that it does not contract after delivery is termed a Couvelaire uterus and may require surgical therapy.[34] A uterus which is suffused with blood, but contracts, requires no treatment.

The number of women who sustain an amniotic fluid embolus is quite small, but 45% of fatal cases reviewed in one year were associated with placental abruptions.[55] Amniotic fluid embolus is discussed in Chapter 39.

REFERENCES

1. Abdella, T. N., Sibai, B. M., Hays, J. M., Jr., and Anderson, G. D.: Relationship of hypertensive disease to abruptio placentae. *Obstet. Gynecol.* **63**:365–370, 1984.
2. A.C.O.G. Technical Bulletin: Diagnosis and management of missed abortion and antepartum fetal death. No. 55, November 1979.
3. A.C.O.G. Technical Bulletin: Management of gestational trophoblastic neoplasia. No. 59, December 1980.
4. Apt, L. and Downey, W. S., Jr.: "Melena" neonatorum: The swallowed blood syndrome. A simple test for the differentiation of adult and fetal hemoglobin in bloody stools. *J. Pediatr.* **47**:6–12, 1955.
5. Barrett, J. M., Boehm, F. H., and Killam, A. P.: Induced abortion: A risk factor for placenta previa. *Am. J. Obstet. Gynecol.* **141**:769–772, 1981.
6. Beer, A. E., Billingham, R. E., and Yang, S. L.: Further evidence concerning the antigenic status of the trophoblast. *J. Exp. Med.* 135:1177–1184, 1972.
7. Bender, S.: Placenta previa and previous lower segment cesarean section. *Surg. Gynecol. Obstet.* **98**:625–628, 1954.
8. Bill, A. H.: The treatment of placenta previa by prophylactic blood transfusion and cesarean section. *Am. J. Obstet. Gynecol.* **14**:523–529, 1927.
9. Boué, J. and Boué, A.: Chromosomal analysis of two consecutive abortuses in each of 43 women. *Humangenetik* **19**:275–280, 1973.
10. Brenner, W. E., Edelman, D. A., and Hendricks, C. H.: Characteristics of patients with placenta previa and results of "expectant management." *Am. J. Obstet. Gynecol.* **132**:180–191, 1978.
11. Buchsbaum, H. J.: Accidental injury complicating pregnancy. *Am. J. Obstet. Gynecol.* **102**:752–769, 1968.
12. Carp, H. J. A., Mashiach, S., and Serr, D. M.: Vasa praevia: A major complication and its management. *Obstet. Gynecol.* **53**:273–275, 1979.
13. Chervenak, F. A., Lee, Y., Hendler, M. A., Monoson, R. F., and Berkowitz, R. L.: Role of at-

tempted vaginal delivery in the management of placenta previa. *Obstet. Gynecol.* **64**:798–801, 1984.

14. Comeau, J., Shaw, L., Marcell, C. C., and Lavery, J. P.: Early placenta previa and delivery outcome. *Obstet. Gynecol.* **61**:577–580, 1983.
15. Cotton, D. B., Read, J. A., Paul, R. H., and Quilligan, E. J.: The conservative aggressive management of placenta previa. *Am. J. Obstet. Gynecol.* **137**:687–695, 1980.
16. Crenshaw, C., Jr., Jones, D. E. D., and Parker, R. T.: Placenta previa: A survey of twenty years experience with improved perinatal survival by expectant therapy and cesarean delivery. *Obstet. Gynecol. Surv.* **28**:461–469, 1973.
17. Crosby, W. M. and Costiloe, J. P.: Safety of lap-belt restraint for pregnant victims of automobile collisions. *N. Engl. J. Med.* **284**:632–636, 1971.
18. Crosby, W. M., King, A. I., and Stout, L. C.: Fetal survival following impact: Improvement with shoulder harness restraint. *Am. J. Obstet. Gynecol.* **112**:1101–1106, 1972.
19. D'Angelo, L. J. and Irwin, L. F.: Conservative management of placenta previa: A cost benefit analysis. *Am. J. Obstet. Gynecol.* **149**:320–326, 1984.
20. de Valera, E.: Abruptio placentae. *Am. J. Obstet. Gynecol.* **100**:599–606, 1968.
21. Gabert, H. A.: Placenta previa and fetal growth. *Obstet. Gynecol.* **38**:403–406, 1971.
22. Glass, R. H. and Golbus, M. S.: Habitual abortion. *Fertil. Steril.* **29**:257–265, 1978.
23. Grannum, P. A. and Hobbins, J. C.: The placenta. *Radiol. Clin. North Am.* **20**:353–365, 1982.
24. Grimes, D. A. and Techman, T.: Legal abortion and placenta previa. *Am. J. Obstet. Gynecol.* **149**:501–504, 1984.
25. Hammond, C. B. and Surwit, E. A.: Achieving a high cure rate for GTN. *Contemp. OB/GYN* **17**:163–174, 1981.
26. Hendelman, M. and Fraser, W. D.: A clinical analysis of abruptio placentae. *Am. J. Obstet. Gynecol.* **80**:17–20, 1960.
27. Hertig, A. T. and Sheldon, W. H.: Minimal criteria required to prove prima facie case of traumatic abortion or miscarriage. *Ann. Surg.* **117**:596–606, 1943.
28. Hibbard, B. M.: Abruptio placentae, pre-eclampsia, and essential hypertension. *J. Obstet. Gynaecol. Br. Commonw.* **69**:282–287, 1962.
29. Hibbard, B. M. and Hibbard, E. D.: Aetiological factors in abruptio placentae. *Br. Med. J.* **2**:1430–1436, 1963.
30. Hibbard, B. M. and Jeffcoate, T. N. A.: Abruptio placentae. *Obstet. Gynecol.* **27**:155–167, 1966.
31. Hibbard, L. T.: Placenta previa. *Am. J. Obstet. Gynecol.* **104**:172–182, 1969.
32. Higgins, S. D. and Garite, T. J.: Late abruptio placenta in trauma patients: Implications for monitoring. *Obstet. Gynecol.* **63**:10S–12S, 1984.
33. Hill, L. M., Breckle, R., and Gehrking, W.: Abruptio placentae: An unusual ultrasonic presentation. *Am. J. Obstet. Gynecol.* **148**:1144–1145, 1984.
34. Hodgkinson, C. P. and Neuffeld, J.: Premature separation of the normally implanted placenta. *Clin. Obstet. Gynecol.* **3**:585–598, 1960.
35. Hurd, W. W., Miodovnik, M., Hertzberg, V., and Lavin, J. P.: Selective management of abruptio placentae: A prospective study. *Obstet. Gynecol.* **61**:467–473, 1983.
36. Jaffe, M. H., Schoen, W. C., Silver, T. M., Bowerman, R. A., and Stuck, K. J.: Sonography of abruptio placentae. *Am. J. Roentgenol.* **137**:-1049–1054, 1981.
37. Johnson, H. W.: The conservative management of some varieties of placenta previa. *Am. J. Obstet. Gynecol.* **50**:248–254, 1945.
38. King, D. L.: Placental migration demonstrated by ultrasonography. *Radiology* **109**:167–170, 1973.
39. Knab, D. R.: Abruptio placentae: An assessment of the time and method of delivery. *Obstet. Gynecol.* **52**:625–629, 1978.
40. Kodar, N., De Vore, G., and Romero, R.: Discriminatory hCG zone: Its use in the sonographic evaluation for ectopic pregnancy. *Obstet. Gynecol.* **58**:156–161, 1981.
41. Kouyoumdjian, A.: Velamentous insertion of the umbilical cord. *Obstet. Gynecol.* **56**:737–742, 1980.
42. Krupp, P. J., Barclay, D. L., Roeling, W. M., and Wegener, G.: Maternal mortality: A 20 year study of Tulane Department of Obstetrics and Gynecology at Charity Hospital. *Obstet. Gynecol.* **35**:823–829, 1970.
43. Macafee, C. H. G.: Placenta previa—A study of 174 cases. *J. Obstet. Gynaecol. Br. Emp.* **52**:313–324, 1945.
44. McHattie, T. J.: Placenta previa accreta. *Obstet. Gynecol.* **40**:795–798, 1972.
45. McShane, P. M., Heyl, P. S., and Epstein, M. F.: Maternal and perinatal morbidity resulting from placenta previa. *Obstet. Gynecol.* **65**:176–182, 1985.
46. Moghissi, K. S.: What causes habitual abortion? *Contemp. OB/GYN* **20**:45–64, 1982.
47. Morgan, J.: Placenta previa: Report on a series of 538 cases. *J. Obstet. Gynaecol. Br. Commonw.* **72**:700–705, 1965.
48. Mowbray, J. F. and Underwood, J. L.: Immunology of abortion. *Clin. Exp. Immunol.* **60**:1–7, 1985.
49. Nesbitt, R. E. L., Jr., Powers, S. R., Jr., Boba, A., and Stein, A.: Experimental abruptio placentae: Histologic and physiologic studies. *Obstet. Gynecol.* **12**:359–368, 1958.
50. Newton, E. R., Barss, V., and Cetrulo, C. L.: The epidemiology and clinical history of asymptomatic midtrimester placenta previa. *Am. J. Obstet. Gynecol.* **148**:743–748, 1984.
51. Notelovitz, M., Bottoms, S. F., Dase, D. F., and Leichter, P. J.: Painless abruptio placentae. *Obstet. Gynecol.* **53**:270–272, 1979.
52. O'Driscoll, K. and McCarthy, J. R.: Abruptio

placentae and central venous pressure. *J. Obstet. Gynaecol. Br. Commonw.* **73**:923–929, 1966.
53. Page, E. W., King, E. B., and Merrill, J. A.: Abruptio placentae: Dangers of delay in delivery. *Obstet. Gynecol.* **3**:385–393, 1954.
54. Pedowitz, P.: Placenta previa: An evaluation of expectant management and the factors responsible for fetal wastage. *Am. J. Obstet. Gynecol.* **93**:16–25, 1965.
55. Peterson, E. P. and Taylor, H. B.: Amniotic fluid embolism:. An analysis of 40 cases. *Obstet. Gynecol.* **35**:787–793, 1970.
56. Pritchard, J. A.: Genesis of severe placental abruption. *Am. J. Obstet. Gynecol.* **108**:22–27, 1970.
57. Pritchard, J. A. and Brekken, A. L.: Clinical and laboratory studies on severe abruptio placentae. *Am. J. Obstet. Gynecol.* **97**:681–695, 1967.
58. Rivera-Alsina, M. E., Saldana, L. R., Maklad, N., and Korp, S.: The case of ultrasound in the expectant management of abruptio placentae. *Am. J. Obstet. Gynecol.* **146**:924–927, 1983.
59. Rizos, N., Doran, T. A., Miskin, M., Benzie, R. J., and Ford, J. A.: Natural history of placenta previa ascertained by diagnostic ultrasound. *Am. J. Obstet. Gynecol.* **133**:287–291, 1979.
60. Rothenberger, D., Quattlebaum, F. W., Perry, J. F., Jr., Zabel, J., and Fischer, R. P.: Blunt maternal trauma: A review of 103 cases. *J. Trauma* **18**:173–179, 1978.
61. Schlesinger, E. R., Mazundar, S. M., and Logrillo, V. M.: The impact of placenta previa on survivorship of offspring to four years of age. *Am. J. Obstet. Gynecol.* **116**:657–660, 1973.
62. Sher, G.: A rational basis for the management of abruptio placentae. *J. Reprod. Med.* **21**:123–129, 1978.
63. Silver, R., Depp, R., Sabbagha, R. E., Dooley, S. L., Socol, M. L., and Tamura, R. K.: Placenta previa: Aggressive expectant management. *Am. J. Obstet. Gynecol.* **150**: 15–22, 1984.
64. Stallworthy, J.: The dangerous placenta. *Am. J. Obstet. Gynecol.* **61**:720–737, 1951.
65. Stone, S. R., Whalley, P. J., and Pritchard, J. A.: Inferior vena cava and ovarian vein ligation during late pregnancy. *Obstet. Gynecol.* **32**:267–273, 1968.
66. Tupper, C. and Weil, R. J.: The problem of spontaneous abortion. IX. The treatment of habitual aborters by psychotherapy. *Am. J. Obstet. Gynecol.* **83**:421–424, 1962.
67. Wexler, P. and Gottesfeld, K. R.: Second trimester placenta previa: An apparently normal placentation. *Obstet. Gynecol.* **50**:706–709, 1977.
68. Whalley, P. J., Scott, D. E., and Pritchard, J. A.: Maternal folate deficiency and pregnancy. 1. Placental abruption. *Am. J. Obstet. Gynecol.* **105**:670–677, 1969.
69. Williams, T. J.: The expectant management of placenta previa. *Am. J. Obstet. Gynecol.* **55**:169–173, 1948.
70. Yepes, L. G. and Eastman, N. J.: The management of placenta previa. *South. Med J.* **39**:291–296, 1946.
71. Yiu-Chiu, V. and Chiu, L.: Sonographic features of placental complications in pregnancy. *Am. J. Roentgenol.* **138**:879–885, 1982.

16

SECOND TRIMESTER PREGNANCY LOSS

The least well studied and therefore least understood contributor to reproductive failure is that group of entities together designated 'midtrimester loss." The availability of accurate karyotyping and sophisticated hormone assays has now helped to delineate principal factors operating both in first trimester spontaneous abortion and in recurrent first trimester loss. The advanced technologies of perinatal and neonatal medicine have offered enormous insight into the normal physiology and maturation of the developing fetus and maternal milieu in late pregnancy. In turn, new knowledge has helped to better define pathologic states at the end of gestation and opportunities for third trimester preventative intervention.

Reproductive failure during the first and last trimesters of gestation has become the focus of attention because first trimester loss is most common and third trimester complications are the most dramatic and traumatic to the childbearing couple. Traditional teaching has been facilitated by an arbitrary division of the normal nine-month pregnancy into three presumably equal trimesters. For a long time, viability conveniently coincided only with birth after the 28th week of gestation, the traditionally accepted onset of the third trimester. Legal definitions relating to abortion, stillbirth, and neonatal death were also tied to this concept, although great variations have always existed among nations and even among states within the United States. By default, the second trimester was defined as that period greater than 12 but less than 28 weeks' gestation, a span covering 16 of the 40 weeks of pregnancy. Today, the second trimester can no longer be viewed as a fixed period isolated from the other two. It is now recognized that reproductive losses do not simply segregate along traditional trimester periods. For example, chromosomal defects result in fetal loss both before and after the 12th week, whereas placental causes of bleeding in pregnancy usually commence much earlier than the 28th week of gestation. Medical diseases complicate pregnancy throughout gestation. Most importantly, the premature birth of a 26-week fetus can now result in a normal healthy surviving infant. Why then give special consideration to the intermediate stage of fetal development? Because of the realization that the most difficult clinical judgments and ethical decisions confronting the modern obstetrician are those related to threatened loss during this critical period of time. Additionally, the concept of a continuum of reproductive failure implies that the clustering of pathologic events by trimester is not fixed and often varies from pregnancy to pregnancy, even in an individual woman. Sound prevention programs must take cognizance of this concept in developing prospective strategies from a well-documented historical data base.

INCIDENCE

Because of inconsistencies in definition and reporting, it is difficult to find reliable estimates of the overall scope of the midpregnancy problem.

Although multiple interactive causes of second trimester reproductive failure are acknowledged, quantitative discussions have traditionally focused on individual etiologies. These are provided independent of one another and, except perhaps for the problem of habitual wastage, there has been little or no effort to summate etiologies. Prior to 20 weeks' gestation, all losses are categorized as abortion, a definition which meets both legal and clinical criteria because fetuses are not viable prior to this point in gestation. Beyond 20 weeks' gestation, categorization becomes more complicated. The 20–24-week period is also considered previable, but some jurisdictions require that the birth of infants of this age be reported. The 24 to 28-week gestational period now constitutes a composite of stillbirths, neonatal deaths, and surviving premature infants.[51] The subject of this chapter revolves around pregnancies which terminate either spontaneously, or by design, between the 13th and 28th week from the last recalled menstrual period. Elective second trimester abortions are carefully excluded from this group.

To shed light on this group of infants, it is useful to review the life-table data assembled with respect to human reproduction. It is now believed, based on sensitive β-hCG pregnancy testing data, that only about 30% of all human conceptions survive to birth.[67] As many as 55% of conceptions are lost prior to the first missed menstrual period. Approximately 15% of clinically recognized pregnancies abort spontaneously during the first 12 weeks.[100] Second trimester losses account for less than 10% of all spontaneous abortions, but among these are included a disproportionate contribution from women who evidence a tendency to abort repeatedly.[30,39,56] For example, current data suggest that, after two preceding losses, the risk for a repeat abortion is approximately one in four pregnancies, whereas after three preceding losses it approaches one in three.[88,89] (See also Chapter 15.)

Although the term "habitual aborter" has been restricted to women who have experienced three consecutive miscarriages, it is preferable to think in an etiologic rather than quantitative manner, even after a single second trimester event.[22] In this manner, potentially recurrent causes of reproductive failure may be identified earlier and thus become amenable to appropriate interconception treatments or to early intervention in a subsequent pregnancy.

ETIOLOGY

The data concerning etiology of second trimester losses have largely been derived from studies of couples with prior recurrent loss.[45] Most of these studies have been retrospective and have been marked by inclusion criteria which vary among investigators. One exception was a recent prospective study which was, however, restricted to women with three consecutive prior second trimester losses.[73] No prospective epidemiologic information with respect to all second trimester occurrences currently exists. Therefore, loss at this stage of pregnancy cannot be placed in true perspective. Furthermore, even with couples studied because of so-called 'habitual abortion," etiologic diagnosis has been achieved in only approximately 60% (Table 16-1).

GENETIC FACTORS

It is well established that the frequency of chromosomally abnormal fetuses decreases progressively from early first trimester pregnancies to surviving infants at birth. Whereas as much as 50% of first trimester abortus material reveals chromosomal abnormalities, only approximately 0.6% of newborns demonstrate them at term. Natural selection appears to explain such a discrepancy. At midpregnancy, 5–10% of stillborn infants are chromosomally abnormal. This incidence is approximately doubled among second trimester abortion specimens.[30,39,55]

The single most common chromosomal abnormality in the first trimester is 45X (Turner's syndrome), which has been documented in approximately 18% of spontaneous abortion material. (See Chapter 13.) The most common autosomal aneuploidies are trisomy 16, trisomy 21, trisomy 13, and trisomy 18. Various polyploidies and sex chromosome abnormalities, for example, 47XXY (Klinefelter's syndrome) are also much more common in abortuses than among newborns. Although translocations are

TABLE 16-1. KNOWN CAUSES OF SECOND TRIMESTER REPRODUCTIVE FAILURE

Genetic	Endocrinopathies
Diabetes mellitus	Autoimmune diseases
Cervical incompetence	Infections
Uterine abnormalities	Psychological factors
Medical conditions	Other miscellaneous

documented in only a small percentage of cases, they play an important role in repetitive miscarriages. It is principally for this etiology that genetic studies are advocated. It has been estimated that one parent will show a balanced translocation in about 2–5% of couples experiencing recurrent early loss.[89]

Unfortunately, no comparable direct data on the distribution of chromosomal abnormalities in the midtrimester are available. Indirect data, however, have been extrapolated from women undergoing amniocentesis for advanced maternal age or because of a prior history of genetic defects. In this highly selected high-risk group, the incidence of aneuploidy is significantly higher than that encountered at term in comparable women. Although the exact proportion of Down's syndrome zygotes that end in intrauterine demise is unknown, it appears to be as high as 65% or greater. A significant fraction of this loss apparently occurs in the second trimester. It has been estimated that perhaps as many as half of trisomy 21 fetuses diagnosed at amniocentesis would undergo spontaneous fetal demise if left undisturbed.[41] Similarly, less than 1% of Turners (45X) conceptuses result in a liveborn infant. Higher rates of diagnosis from amniocentesis than among live births is also noted in other cytogenetic abnormalities such as trisomy 18, trisomy 13, and 47XXY. A high fetal death rate after the 16th week of gestation appears to contribute to the disparity. The relative ratios of increased risk for these abnormalities as compared with Down's syndrome are shown in Table 16-2.[42] These data suggest that

TABLE 16-2. RATES OF MAJOR ANEUPLOIDIES FOUND AT AMNIOCENTESIS COMPARED WITH RATES IN LIVE BIRTHS

	Trisomy			
	21	19	13	45X
Rates in live births per 1000	1.26	0.12	0.05	1.2
Rates in prenatal diagnosis* per 1000	17.3	2.7	1.1	5.4
Ratio	13.7	22.0	20.4	4.4
Relative rate†	1.0	1.6	1.5	0.3

* Studied prenatally because of advanced maternal age.
† Normalized to a value of 1.0 per Down's syndrome.
Source: Adapted from Hook, E. B., Cross, P. K., and Schreinemachers, D. M.: Chromosomal abnormality rates at amniocentesis and in live-born infants. *JAMA* **249**:2034–2038, 1983 (copyright 1983, American Medical Association).

relatively more 47+18 and 47+13 fetuses and relatively fewer 47XXY and 47XXX fetuses are lost in the second trimester as compared with 47+21 fetuses. Recurrence risks for trisomies due to nondisjunction are estimated to be 1–2%. Thus, in the absence of a balanced translocation in one of the parents, genetic studies of the couple contribute little toward solving the problem of second trimester reproductive failure.

Recently, Merkatz et al.[64] described an association between fetal autosomal trisomies and low maternal serum alpha-fetoprotein values (MSAFP). Because most children with Down's syndrome and other aneuploidies are born to younger mothers who would not otherwise have been candidates for genetic amniocentesis, the possibility of identifying an at-risk group through MSAFP testing was suggested. Cuckle et al.[19] confirmed this finding in Great Britain, where MSAFP screening is routinely practiced, and developed an algorithm for incorporating maternal age and MSAFP values into the decision of whether or not to recommend genetic amniocentesis. The sensitivity, specificity, and cost-benefit consideration of such a proposal is still to be adequately demonstrated. However, the potential implication for patients with prior second trimester loss is clear, since this screening could readily be incorporated into the prenatal care of this high-risk population.

DIABETES MELLITUS

The association between diabetes mellitus and second trimester reproductive loss remains unclear and highly controversial. Despite an acknowledged relationship between uncontrolled or undetected maternal diabetes and an increased incidence of fetal anomalies,[26] there is as yet no proof of an increased early spontaneous abortion rate among diabetic women or of a unique role for maternal diabetes in repetitive pregnancy loss during the first trimester. The consensus is that the spontaneous abortion rate among diabetic women is approximately 12.5%, similar to that recognized in the population as a whole.[18,27,52] The frequency of repetitive miscarriage is also similar to that in the population at large. Diabetes mellitus is not a frequent cause of recurrent first trimester pregnancy wastage.

On the other hand, a recent prospective analysis provided evidence that the overall risk of spontaneous abortion among insulin-dependent diabetic women may indeed be substantially higher than that of the general population.[69]

The spontaneous abortion rate for the diabetic group was 30%, with only 70% of pregnancies progressing beyond 20 weeks. Twenty-seven percent of the abortions occurred in the interval between 13 and 20 weeks, yielding a markedly increased overall second trimester abortion rate of approximately 8%. No data were provided for pregnancy outcome in the interval between 20 and 28 weeks. It is presumed, however, that there were additional reproductive failures during this period. An additional 25% of the abortions apparently occurred during the 12th week of gestation, the gateway to the second trimester. These data agree with previous studies demonstrating that the early spontaneous abortion rate among diabetic women is comparable to that among the nondiabetic population. However, the rate of second trimester reproductive failure appears to be markedly increased. The clinical conclusion to be derived from these findings is that, although first trimester aborters need not have special screening for occult diabetes mellitus, a woman with a documented second trimester loss of unknown etiology must be considered at risk for occult diabetes mellitus. Glucose tolerance testing may or may not prove positive in the interconceptional period but must be repeated periodically in a subsequent pregnancy. There are as yet no good data linking the tightness of diabetes control to the likelihood of second trimester loss, but, in view of a clear relationship between control and perinatal mortality and morbidity, it is not unreasonable to presume that such a relationship may ultimately be documented. Known insulin-dependent diabetics require careful preconceptional counseling. Preconceptional control has been advocated as a means to reduce congenital malformations.[66] It may eventually be established that good metabolic control early in gestation will also minimize the risk of second trimester reproductive failure.

INCOMPETENT CERVIX

There is as yet no universally accepted definition of the term "incompetent cervix" because there has been poor correlation of anatomic and physiologic testing with subsequent cervical function. The condition has, therefore, always been defined by clinical rather than objective methods. The cervix is said to be characterized by an "inability to contain the products of normal conception in the second trimester." However, current insight recognizes that an incompetent cervix may contribute to preterm births in the third trimester. The outcome of subsequent pregnancies may vary widely with or without therapeutic intervention. The published incidences differ greatly from report to report because different criteria are utilized for clinical diagnosis (Table 16-3). Best estimate is that 0.05–1% of all pregnancies are affected by cervical incompetence and that the condition is etiologic in as many as 15% of all second trimester reproductive failures.[4,33]

In the absence of effective treatment, the same sequence of events may be expected to repeat itself in each successive pregnancy. A history of repeated painless dilatation of the cervix during the second trimester of pregnancy is therefore sought. It is assumed that the membranes then prolapse through the cervix and balloon into the vagina without associated bleeding or contractions. Eventually, the membranes may rupture with subsequent rapid expulsion of the immature fetus, or the fetus may be expelled within an intact sac.

A more subtle expression of the same condition may present as very early premature rupture of the membranes without associated labor. In this circumstance, a variety of clinical events may eventually ensue, including spontaneous labor and preterm delivery, as well as the development of chorioamnionitis. Bleeding or mild uterine contractions may develop, confounding the search for the classic history. Thus, when looking in retrospect for etiologic factors for midpregnancy loss, the expectation that a woman with cervical incompetence should not have experienced the usual discom-

TABLE 16-3. THE REPORTED UTILIZATION OF CERCLAGE PROCEDURES

Author	Year	Number of Procedures	Rate per Deliveries
Barter	1958	110	1:1842
Crocker	1958–61	34	1:1000
Goldstein	1959–62	36	1:714
Hofmeister	1958–66	72	1:266
Kuhn	1969–74	242	1:182
Toaff	1966–72	410	1:54
Harger	1971–78	251	1:222
Barford	1973–82	147	1:152

Incidence modified from Harger, J. H.: Comparison of success and morbidity in cervical cerclage procedures. *Obstet. Gynecol.* **56**:543–548, 1980. Reprinted with permission from the American College of Obstetricians and Gynecologists.

forts of labor may be met in only the most obvious cases of incompetent cervix. The astute obstetrician must be aware of the multiple presentations of this clinical entity and must increase sensitivity to its presence if multiple pregnancy losses are to be prevented. On the other hand, a more common tendency has been for physicians to be nonspecific in their diagnostic criteria and therefore to overutilize surgical intervention. For this reason, many questions have been raised regarding both the existence of the condition and the value of the procedures for its correction.[35] In Great Britain, for example, the Medical Research Council and the Royal College of Obstetricians and Gynecologists have recently noted that only a large randomized controlled clinical trial will define the value of the cerclage procedure.[59]

The cervix is a predominantly fibrous rather than a muscular structure. Recognition of the collagenous nature of the cervical stroma has led to improved understanding of the changing function, structure, and biochemistry of the cervix throughout gestation.[20] At the end of pregnancy, the cervix undergoes a process that leads to the progressive ripening, dilatation, and effacement associated with normal parturition. During most of gestation, the cervix is presumed to play a role in retaining the conceptus within the uterus.[21] The implication of this assumption is that damage to the cervix might predispose to late abortion or to preterm birth. In the 1950s, the clinical concept of cervical incompetence was introduced and methods to deal with the problem were suggested.[54]

At present, traumatic, congenital, and dysfunctional categories of cervical incompetence are recognized.[43] Traumatic causes occur in at least one-third of patients and are associated with clearly identifiable structural damage to the cervical integrity. In this group, damage most frequently has been attributed to a prior dilatation and curettage either for the treatment of dysmenorrhea and other gynecological complaints or for elective pregnancy termination. Second trimester pregnancy termination via vaginal methods or intra-amniotic instillations may also cause cervical damage. Laceration of the collagenous fibers within the internal os of the cervix is assumed to be present, even though this disruption may not be obvious to the examiner. Other causes of trauma include cervical amputation and conization for gynecological indications, obstetrical lacerations associated with instrumental delivery, precipitous labor, malpresentation, infants of excessive size, and cesarean section with lower segmental tears.

The pathogenesis of cervical incompetence among women who lack a history of cervical damage is less well understood. Some congenital conditions undoubtedly are operative, since the classic painless midpregnancy loss has been documented in nulliparous women. This category of incompetence has recently been extended to include women who are the offspring of mothers treated with diethylstilbestrol (DES) during pregnancy. Exposure to DES in utero may produce not only a primary uterine abnormality, but also a distinct cervical defect. Both malformations are seen in some women.[5]

As many as one-third of women with congenital anomalies of the uterus, in particular those with a bicornuate uterus, have functional cervical incompetence.[8] It is not clear how much of this incompetence is due to the fundal abnormality and how much is due directly to a less visible congenital alteration of the cervix itself. In many instances, cerclage is effective with or without correction of the fundal anomaly. Some women may have a congenitally shortened cervix without any other obvious associated uterine anomalies. They are at risk for both second trimester reproductive failure and otherwise unexplained preterm births.

There remains a small group of women without structural or traumatic alteration of the cervix, who possess a dysfunction in which the changes in the cervix normally expected at term occur much earlier in gestation. This dysfunction of the cervix leading to clinical cervical incompetence has been thought to relate to an alteration of cervical composition characterized by an abnormally high ratio of muscle to collagen with associated loss of the fibrous capacity to retain the conceptus.[21]

In order to diagnose these various categories of cervical incompetence, a thorough history and physical examination, preferably prior to pregnancy, but at least during the initial prenatal visit, are required. This applies to primigravidas as well as to multiparous women. To await an utward pregnancy history is to expose the patient to the potential of considerable anguish, suffering, and unnecessary cost. Likewise, patient education to pregnancy risk factors should take place within the context of any suggestive historical or physical findings. Education should include specific information about preterm labor and about third trimester pregnancy danger signs such as bleeding. A patient who presents with a prior history of preterm birth or midtrimester loss requires even greater attention to detail in both diagnosis and education. These patients must be taught to recognize the vague clinical symptoms such as lower abdominal discomfort, sensation of heaviness, lower back pain, vaginal discharge, and fullness which have been retrospectively associated with the earliest protrusion of the amniotic membranes into the internal os.

All too frequently, a pregnancy terminates under circumstances suggestive of an incompetent cervix, but in the absence of interconceptional evaluation and counseling. In an ideal reproductive health care system, the risk identification process will automatically be initiated in preparation for a subsequent pregnancy. Most of the recommended diagnostic procedures can be applied only in the nonpregnant state. All efforts should be extended to conduct a thorough interconceptional evaluation in the woman at risk in order to minimize subsequent losses.

A wide assortment of biophysical tests havc been employed in an effort to predict the functional competence of the cervix. The measurement of cervical canal dilatation by the ability of the cervix to resist the passage of a number 8 Hegar dilator has been the most frequently utilized technique, but the end-point is too subjective.[2,46] Hysterosalpingography may reveal an anatomical defect in the fundus, cavity, or cervix itself, but the shape and width of the lower uterine segment may vary with the menstrual cycle. Hysterosalpingography has proved to be a relatively nonspecific diagnostic tool. Embellishments of mechanical measurement techniques utilizing radio-opaque dyes, Foley catheters, and intracervical balloons have also yielded differing rates of success. None of these techniques has withstood the test of time.[47,76]

Most recently, studies of cervical compliance by generating pressure volume curves by controlled inflation of intracervical balloons have offered some promise.[71] The advantage of this relatively noninvasive technology is that reproducible quantitative data can be obtained at various points in the menstrual cycle and in repetitive cycles of the nonpregnant woman. Such quantitative data may be utilized to evaluate the sensitivity and specificity of diagnoses and the efficacy of therapy.

During a pregnancy at risk, the use of ultrasonography to visualize the amniotic sac at the level of the internal os has been advocated.[83,97] With this tool, the very earliest encroachment of the membranes into the cervical canal may be recognizable. In theory, such a diagnostic regimen offers a considerable advantage over the more traditional approach of frequent vaginal examination for digital detection of occult cervical effacement and dilatation.[17] The ability of such examinations reliably to discriminate early cervical incompetence has long been in question.[25,72,84] Cervical dilatation of as much as 1–2 cm exists during the midtrimester in a significant percentage of nulliparous and multiparous patients. The cervices of as many as 16% of gravidas demonstrate such change. Furthermore, the rate of premature labor is not significantly different in women with or without 1–2 cm of dilatation.[25,74] When a strong clinical suspicion of incompetent cervix exists, the examiner is more likely to detect occult progression of cervical effacement or dilation. However, in the absence of such a level of concern, by the time objective changes are recognized, it may already be too late to salvage the pregnancy. An early decision as to whether or not an incompetent cervix is the presumed basis for prior pregnancy loss is critical. All treatments yield greater efficacy when applied on a timely basis. On the other hand, overdiagnosis and overtreatment should be avoided.

Bed rest, hormones, and pessaries have been utilized to treat patients with cervical incompetence, but none have proved consistently effective. If the diagnosis is correct, the accepted effective therapy is surgical reinforcement of the weakened cervix. A wide assortment of surgical procedures has been suggested (Table 16-4). Two main categories of operation are most widely utilized (Fig. 16-1).[62,87] The first, initially described by Shirodkar, utilizes encerclage of the cervix with a nonabsorbable material placed submucosally after advancing the bladder. Presently, a 5 mm wide mersilene band is employed and is placed by utilizing a large, curved atraumatic needle.[87] The major theoretical advantages of this operation are that (1) with the bladder advanced, the suture can be located high at the level of the internal os; and (2) it can be left in situ for subsequent pregnancies. The procedure requires a high level of expertise and entails risks of bleeding, bladder trauma, infection, rupture of the membranes, and uterine artery or ureteral injury.

McDonald[61,62] suggested a much simpler procedure that employed a purse string suture of braided silk or mersilene. This suture is placed at the level of the junction of the smooth mucosa of the portio vaginalis and the rugose mucosa of the vagina. It does not necessitate a

TABLE 16-4. HISTORICAL APPROACH TO REPAIR OF THE INCOMPETENT CERVIX

Author	Year	Procedure
Lash, A. F. and Lash, S. R.	1950	Repair in nonpregnant state
Shirodkar, V. V.	1955	Fascia lata cerclage
Baden, F. and Baden, E.	1957	Trachelorrhaphy in pregnancy
Barter, R. H.	1958	Dacron mesh
Page, E. M.	1958	Oxycel gauze impregnated with talc
Johnson, J. W.	1959	Stainless steel wire
Lewis, G. C. and Reid, T. B.	1959	Nylon through polythene tube
Barnes, A. C.	1961	Electrocautery to produce stenosis
Hefner, J. D.	1961	Two mattress sutures (Wurm)
Hunter, R. G.	1961	Skin graft from thigh
Ritter, H. A. and Ritter, P. J.	1961	Dacron ribbon
McDonald, I.	1963	Purse string suture with mersiline tape
Benson, R. and Durfee, J.	1965	Transabdominal uterocervical cerclage
Yosowitz, E.	1972	"Baylor balloon"
Novy, M. O.	1982	Transabdominal cervicoisthmic cerclage

large midline incision nor reflection of the bladder. The cervical wall and the endocervical canal are avoided. A minimum of four needle bites are utilized at 10, 7, 5, and 2 o'clock, respectively. The suture is tied on the anterior surface of the cervix in the midline. The recommended timing for placement of either cerclage is in the early second trimester, in order to avoid the likelihood of a coincidental first trimester spontaneous miscarriage. With the availability of contemporary ultrasound technology for confirming fetal viability, earlier placement may be employed in selected cases.

Reported success rates with both surgical procedures are quite similar. Postcerclage survival rates vary from 50-90%.[34] Thus, many investigators have become advocates of the simpler operation. However, no good randomized prospective comparison of the two operations has yet been reported. The wide variation in clinical diagnosis of the incompetent cervix and indications for cerclage make noncontemporaneous comparisons between different centers difficult. It may be presumed that both operations are overutilized and therefore many "successes" are not directly attributable to the surgical intervention. A standardized method for evaluation of patients and a randomized approach to treatment, utilizing both surgical and nonsurgical modalities, are mandated to answer finally this serious and important question.

Neither the Shirodkar nor McDonald procedure is optimal when satisfactory placement of the sutures is difficult. Examples of such circumstances include the congenitally short or extensively amputated cervix, marked cervical or vaginal scarring from repeated prior cerclage attempts, multiple deep or high lacerations, chronic or subacute infection, and the markedly effaced or dilated cervix.

Transabdominal cervicouterine cerclage may be utilized to treat such conditions.[7] In this operation, the peritoneal cavity is approached abdominally, the vesicocervical fold of peritoneum opened, and the bladder displaced inferiorly to provide access to the avascular space at the level of the anatomic internal os. The cerclage suture is placed by puncturing the posterior leaf of the broad ligament just above the corpocervical junction. This procedure may yield a high success rate in high-risk patients, including those with previous transvaginal cerclage failure.[73] It is also possible to perform a similar procedure via a transvaginal approach.[62,79] This type of surgical procedure may increase complications such as intraoperative bleeding, premature labor and intrauterine fetal hypoxia or death because of the potential for compromise of the uterine circulation. The risk of inadvertent puncture of the amniotic membranes or of ureteral injury is also present. Thus, the method should be reserved for highly selected indications and should be performed only by experienced and competent operators.

An alternative method of dealing with the dilated and effaced cervix, particularly after 20 weeks' gestation, is to utilize the Wurm procedure,[38] which entails less extensive surgery. In this operation, two crossing mattress sutures are placed transvaginally at the level of the internal os, utilizing a heavy, nonabsorbable suture material. One suture extends across the

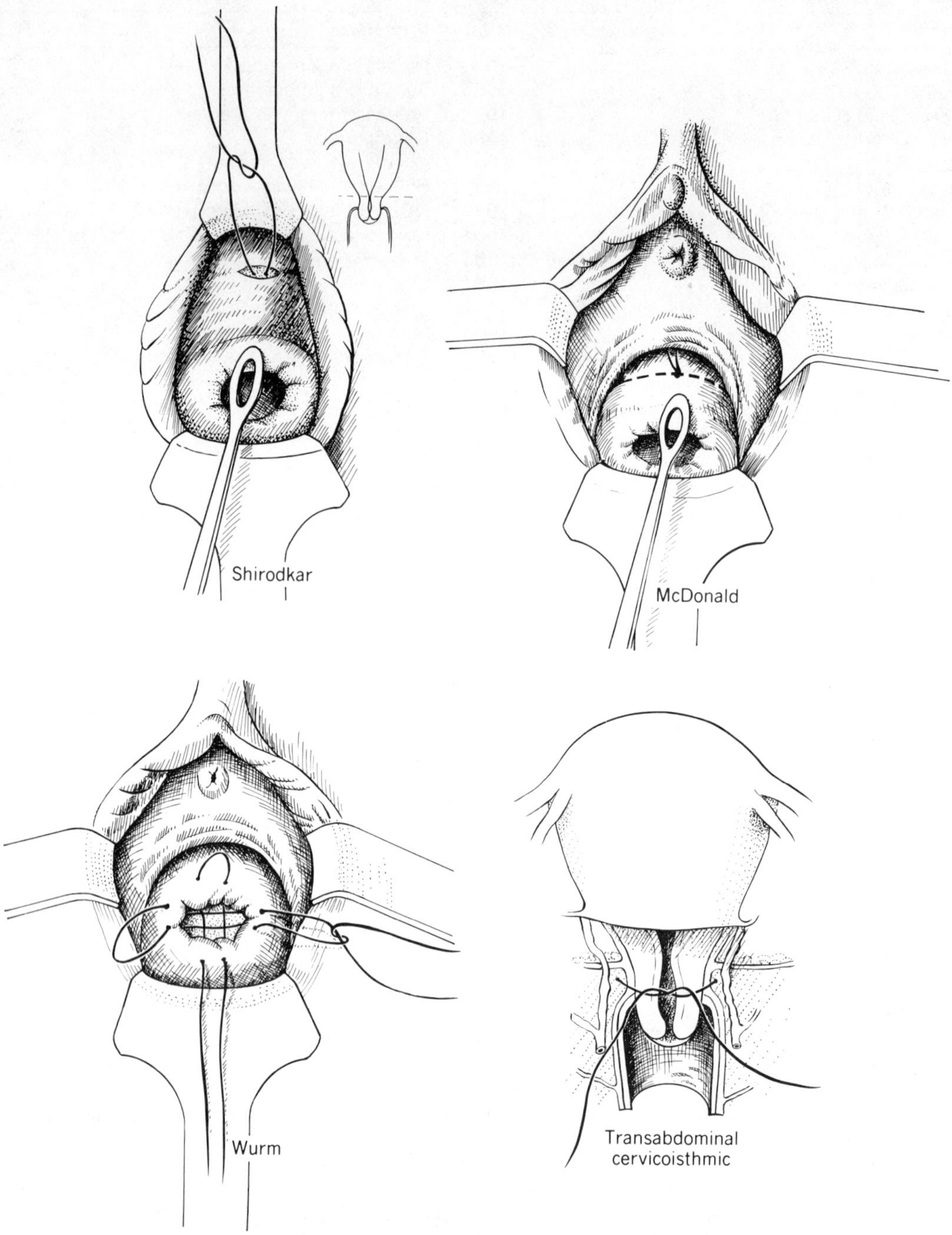

Figure 16-1. Panel (a) depicts the Shirodkar procedure. The bladder is reflected upward in order to expose the cervix at the level of the internal os. A submucosal permanent suture is then placed to encircle the cervix. Panel (b) depicts the McDonald procedure. The bladder is left undisturbed. A purse string suture is placed through the mucosa of the cervix. Panel (c) depicts the Wurm technique in which mattress sutures are placed perpendicular to each other. Panel (d) depicts the transabdominal approach to the uterine cervicoisthmic junction. The suture is placed at the level of the internal os, piercing the parametria to encircle the cervix.

cervical canal from 12 to 6 o'clock and back again, and the second is placed perpendicularly from 3 to 9 o'clock and back, 1 centimeter inferior to the first ligature. The two sutures are then tied, closing the dilated cervix at two distinct points. Since the suture material traverses the cervical canal, the risk of subsequent infection must be considered.

An additional circumstance necessitating individualization of corrective surgery is that in which the amniotic membranes have already prolapsed through the incompetent cervix. The likelihood of chorioamnionitis is then greatly enhanced and this risk must be carefully weighed prior to operative intervention. Some clinicians believe that any suturing of the cervix in this state is contraindicated, whereas others attempt initial conservative management with bed rest in deep Trendelenberg position to await spontaneous reduction of the membranes prior to considering surgery. A third group ascertains whether any evidence of infection exists at the time. If no signs of infection are evident, they move rapidly to surgery to minimize further exposure of the sac to the environment and flora of the vagina.

Operating under such conditions requires maintaining an active reduction of the herniated amniotic membranes to facilitate suture placement. This may be technically difficult to accomplish, particularly since trauma to the membranes must be avoided. With the patient in Trendelenberg position, downward traction is applied to the anterior and posterior lips of the cervix, while upward reduction of the membranes is performed with a moistened sponge held either manually or by ovum forceps (Fig. 16-2). An alternative approach utilizes an inflated Foley catheter bulb to effect reduction.[40] This technique provides a smooth, rounded, atraumatic surface with which to progressively push and hold the membranes back into the uterine cavity. Once the membranes have been reposited into the uterus, the bulb is further inflated and left in position while the cerclage suture is inserted. While the suture is being tied down, the catheter is deflated and removed.

Cervical cerclage is not without hazards (Table 16-5). In addition to the immediate surgical complications previously described, subsequent difficulties encountered include severe infection aggravated by the foreign body, premature labor, cervical or vaginal laceration, and rupture of the uterus in the face of active uterine contractions.[16,23,77,81] Anesthetic risks during pregnancy increase with each surgical proce-

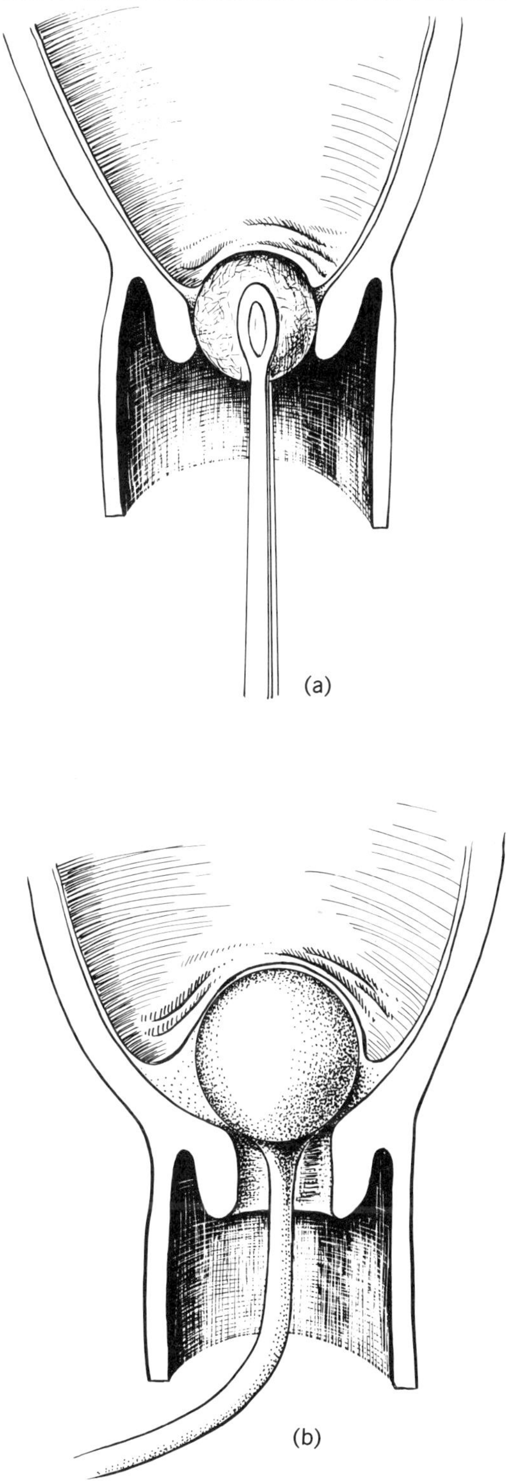

Figure 16-2. The membranes may be reduced either by pressing upward with a sponge held in a uterine forceps (a) or by making pressure with the balloon of a Foley catheter (b).

TABLE 16-5. ILLUSTRATIVE REPORTED RATES OF LATE POSTOPERATIVE CERCLAGE COMPLICATIONS

Event	Frequency (%)
Premature rupture of membranes	9.0–11.0
Chorioamnionitis	0.8– 7.7
Suture displacement	3.0–13.0
Cervical laceration	0.7–13.2
Elective cesarean section	0.7–67.0
Cervical dystocia	1.4– 5.0

dure, and choosing cerclage may eventually mandate several. Maternal deaths from each of these severe complications have been recorded. Therefore, in addition to avoiding unwarranted use of the procedure, the clinician must remain alert to the need for prompt removal of the suture in the presence of ruptured membranes, signs of infection, or early onset of labor.

CONGENITAL UTERINE ANOMALIES

Most women with uterine malformations enjoy normal reproductive function. The diagnosis may be established only coincidentally or at postmortem examination. The majority of women with uterine malformations are able to have successful term gestations.[28] Reproductive failure is seen in 25–50% of patients with a unicornous or didelphic uterus.[50,82]

On the other hand, some women with uterine malformations experience a high rate of late first trimester and midpregnancy fetal wastage and others undergo preterm labor and delivery, often complicated by malpresentations of the fetus.[70] The etiology of reproductive failure among such patients is unclear. Cervical incompetence, reduced uterine volume, poor vascularization, and increased uterine contractions secondary to altered myometrial physiology have all been implicated.[12,86]

Women with bicornuate and septate uteri appear to be more at risk for poor outcome (see Chapter 15). Increased incidence of spontaneous abortion, repeated or habitual abortion, preterm labor, and breech presentation are all associated with these uterine anomalies.[50,86]

Confusion arises because many reports of the potential benefits of surgical procedures for correcting uterine malformations deal with series of women identified because of significant prior reproductive wastage.[31] These series often provide an excessively pessimistic view of the likelihood of a viable pregnancy in the absence of surgical correction and probably overestimate the success rate attributable to the operation itself. Randomized controlled studies are lacking. Data from large series indicate that only about 20% of patients with Müllerian fusion defects experience related reproductive failure. Corrective surgery is to be employed in selected patients. For example, complete fusion failure (uterus didelphys) is a comparatively benign condition. It should not necessitate surgical correction except to excise a vaginal septum if dyspareunia exists.[82]

A bicornuate uterus, with two externally visible horns, but a single cervix and vagina, is more common. The condition, when associated with pregnancy wastage, may require surgical correction. The Strassman procedure was originally designed for this type of anomaly (Fig. 16-3). The two uterine horns are opened with a transverse incision and then rejoined in an anteroposterior closure perpendicular to the incision in order to create the maximum uterine cavity.[93]

It is generally agreed that the one type of anomaly associated with reproductive problems which does require surgical correction is the septate uterus.[49] The uterus is usually characterized by an essentially normal external appearance. Internally, there is a vertical septum running from the fundus either partially or completely to the cervical os. It is believed that high fetal wastage occurs either through interference with normal uterine distension or because of the poor vascularity of the septum.[13] The fibrous, avascular septum fails to provide an adequate site for nidation and placental development.[49]

Two principal surgical approaches have been recommended. Jones and Jones first popularized a technique of converging anteroposterior incisions from fundus to internal os, wedging the uterine septum from the rest of the uterus and then repairing the defect.[14,48] Excessive blood loss may be associated with the procedure. Various methods for achieving hemostasis have been suggested. These include techniques of parametrial clamping as well as the use of various pharmacologic agents. Tompkins described a simpler procedure in which the septum is incised via a sagittal midline incision in the uterus directly through the septum. The myometrium is then sutured to unify the cavities.[92] The relative avascularity of the septum reduces concern about potential blood loss. The success rate with the procedure is very high.

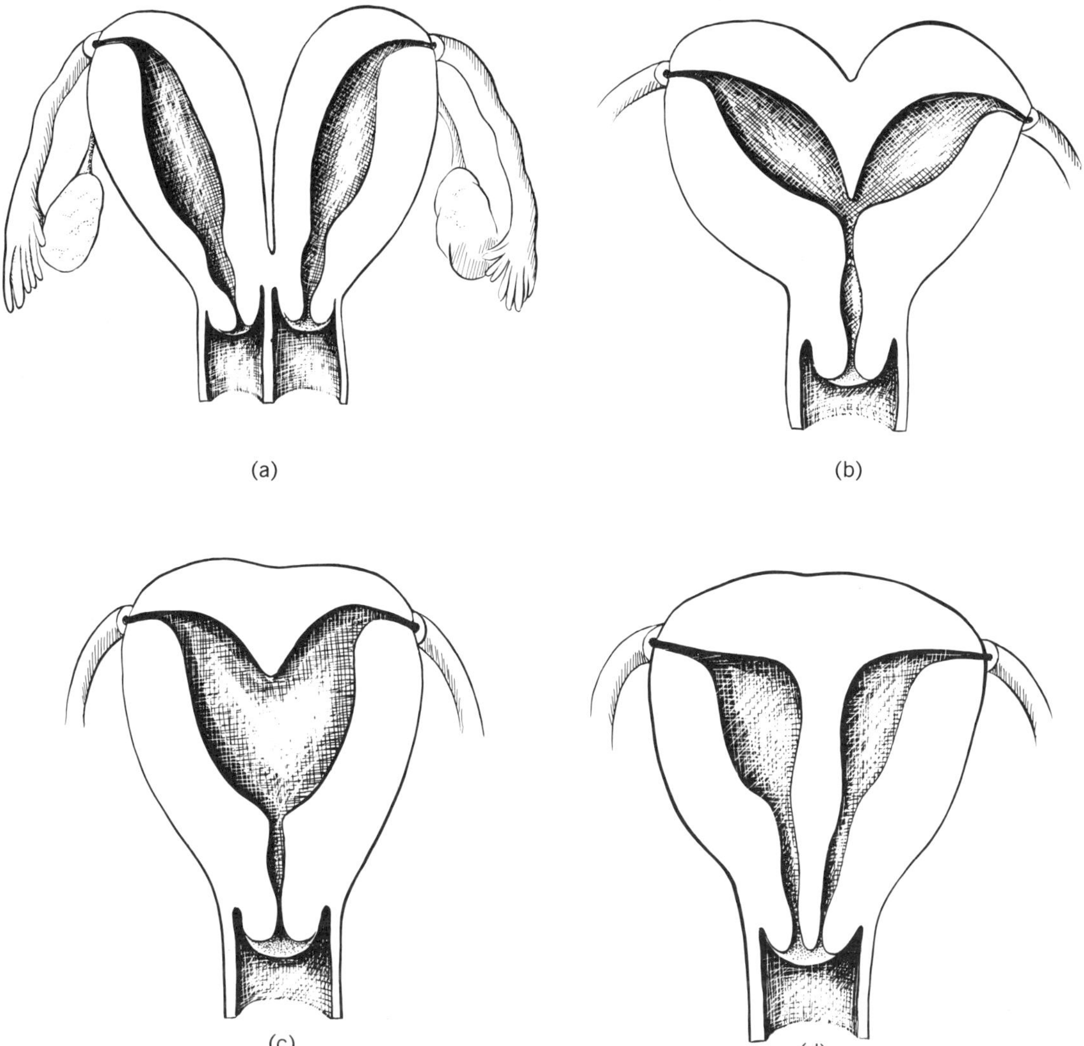

Figure 16-3. The uterus didelphys is shown in panel (a). This anomaly generally does not require surgical therapy. Uterus bicornis unicollis is depicted in panel (b). The authors prefer to utilize the Strassman technique where surgical therapy of this anomaly is required. Panels (c) and (d) depict uterus subseptate and uterus septate, respectively. The Tompkins procedure is the procedure of choice when reconstruction is necessary, but the Jones procedure also gives good results.

Under rare circumstances, the uterine septum is complete and extends to the level of the internal os. When it is totally removed, the possibility of incompetent cervix is extant. Cerclage may be required to restore normal anatomic function.[12,60]

An adequate evaluation must precede any consideration of corrective surgery. It is more important to individualize decision-making than it is to insist that a specified number of midtrimester pregnancy losses first occur. Women suspected to be at risk because of a history of a second trimester loss, repeated abortion, premature labor, and/or fetal malpresentation should undergo a work-up that includes hysterosalpingography and, at times, laparoscopy and hysteroscopy. Bicornuate and subseptate uteri may present similar shadows on hysterosalpingography. The distinction between them is made through direct visualization. Uterine malformations are associated with a 9% incidence of coexisting renal malformations. Intravenous pyelography should be performed.[68] Hysterosalpingography also reveals symptomatic submucous myomata as well as the "T" shaped anomaly caused by exposure in utero to maternal diethylstilbestrol (DES) ingestion. Unfavorable pregnancy outcome has been associated with the latter malformation, but no specific therapy has been established.

MISCELLANEOUS

After all potential genetic, metabolic, and anatomic etiologies of second trimester reproductive failure have been considered, the clinician is still confronted with many patients in whom a pathophysiologic diagnosis is difficult to establish. In the final analysis, the etiology will remain unknown in many. In a significant percentage of couples with a prior history of habitual abortion, the etiology remains obscure after thorough evaluation. It is possible that psychologic factors are important in the etiology of recurrent abortion in some of these women.[60,73]

In other women, reproductive function is complicated by systemic medical illnesses such as chronic renal failure, autoimmune diseases, endocrinopathies, and infection. Most of these conditions are discussed in considerable detail elsewhere in this book, but it is worthwhile briefly to reiterate some of the highlights of their individual contributions to the problem of midpregnancy loss. Women with untreated hypothyroidism who become pregnant have increased rates of both abortion and stillbirth.[96] Pregnant women with hyperthyroidism may demonstrate increased rates of late fetal loss if the mother is inadequately treated.[65]

Chronic renal diseases are associated with high rates of fetal midpregnancy loss, especially when hypertension exists. Treatment by chronic dialysis has yielded few pregnancy successes, but renal transplantation has generally proved effective in leading to satisfactory subsequent reproductive performance.[63]

The collagen–vascular diseases may provide a natural experiment in immunologically mediated reproductive failure. Recently, a number of studies acknowledge the repeated midgestational fetal loss experienced by women with these conditions.[1,11,24,90] Systemic lupus erythematosus (SLE) is the most common of the collagen–vascular diseases affecting women in the childbearing years. Scleroderma is the second most common. Total pregnancy loss from the first trimester onward experienced by women with SLE may approximate 50%. Research points to the importance of the lupus anticoagulant as a specific risk marker.[15,72,78] Antibodies to cardiolipin, a phospholipid antigen, are common in patients with SLE. These antibodies have been implicated in causing coagulation abnormalities predisposing to placental thrombosis and infarction.[6,37,44] The presence of this antibody in pregnant women with SLE apparently correlates better with the occurrence of midpregnancy fetal distress and fetal death than does the lupus anticoagulant.[57] Other immunologic phenomena associated with transplacental passage of antibodies are providing additional clues for future study of the perinatal implications of this disease. In particular, the presence of anti-ribonucleoprotein antigen, that is, Anti-Ro (SS-A), has been implicated in the pathogenesis of the congenital complete heart block seen in offspring of mothers with collagen–vascular diseases.[85] Prospective pregnancy studies of known lupus patients are clearly indicated for elucidating the true risk of untoward outcome. At present, it appears that careful control of the disease process for at least six months prior to embarking on a pregnancy offers the best opportunity for a successful live birth.[95] The work-up of patients with unexplained fetal demise should also include a search for occult autoimmune disease.

Numerous investigators have attempted to establish a causal relationship between various low-grade chronic endometrial infections and midtrimester reproductive failure (Table 16-6). In general, the bacterial and viral organisms which have been implicated are of low virulence and often exist as facultative intracellular parasites. They include *Mycoplasma hominis, Ureaplasma urealyticum, Chlamydia tracho-*

TABLE 16-6. SOME OF THE GENITAL TRACT PATHOGENS SUGGESTED AS ETIOLOGIC IN SECOND TRIMESTER PREGNANCY LOSS

Chlamydia trachomatis	*Toxoplasma gondii*
Herpes simplex virus	*Treponema pallidum*
Listeria monocytogenes	*Ureaplasma urealyticum*
Mycoplasma hominis	

matis, Listeria monocytogenes, Toxoplasma gondii, herpes simplex virus, and *Treponema pallidum*.[32] The difficulty in all these associations has been a lack of specificity in correlating the finding of the infectious agent with poor pregnancy outcome (see Chapter 15). When controlled studies have been attempted, the frequency of positive cultures for most of these low-grade pathogens has usually been as high in normal controls as in patients with repeated midpregnancy loss.[91] This generic statement applies to ureaplasma[73] (although a link between ureaplasma infection and excessive stillbirth is possible[53]) and *T. gondii*[94] (although it is speculated that the toxoplasma parasite can both invade and cross the placenta during a primary infection and that chronic endometrial infections may be responsible for poor placentation[75]).

Listeria monocytogenes is a gram positive facultative anaerobe eliminated from affected hosts by mechanisms generally dependent on cell-mediated immunity.[29] It is therefore more commonly encountered among patients with chronic diseases or immune suppression. The infection is associated with pregnancy wastage in various animal species, particularly cattle and sheep. However, prospective attempts to establish a similar relationship in humans have revealed no evidence that this type agent contributes to unexplained midpregnancy loss.[3,9,58] No evidence of *L. monocytogenes* has been found in cultures from more than 700 repeated aborters.[55,77]

Low-grade infection of the amniotic membranes has been suggested as a major causative factor of preterm labor and of premature rupture of the membranes early in pregnancy. Considerable debate exists as to whether the increased bacterial colonization found in amniotic fluid cultures or upon pathologic examination of the placenta and membranes is etiologically primary or is secondary to a dilated cervix, decreased host resistance, and continued uterine activity.[68] For this reason, the National Institutes of Health recently initiated a large prospective, multicentric study designed to obtain vaginal-cervical cultures in midgestation and to undertake a controlled trial of prophylactic antibiotic therapy.[98] It is hoped that the results of this study may clarify the relationships among chronic low-grade genital tract infection, prematurity, and midpregnancy reproductive failure. In the interim, there seems little justification to assume that either cultures or antibiotic treatment should be incorporated as a routine component of care for the woman who has experienced a second trimester loss.

REFERENCES

1. Abramowsky, C. R.: Lupus erythematosus, the placenta and pregnancy: A natural experiment in immunologically mediated reproductive failure. *Prog. Clin. Biol. Res.* **70**:309–320, 1981.
2. Anthony, G. S., Calder, A. A., and MacNaughton, M. C.: Cervical resistance in patients with previous spontaneous mid-trimester abortion. *Br. J. Obstet. Gynaecol.* **89**:1046–1049, 1982.
3. Ansbacher, R., Borchardt, K. A., Hannegan, M. W., and Boyson, W. A.: Clinical investigation of *Listeria monocytogenes* as a possible cause of human fetal wastage. *Am. J. Obstet. Gynecol.* **94**:386–390, 1966.
4. Barford, D. A. and Rosen, M. G.: Cervical incompetence:. Diagnosis and outcome. *Obstet. Gynecol.* **64**:159–163, 1984.
5. Barnes, A. B., Colton, T., Gundersen, J., Noller, K. L., Tilley, B. C., Strama, T., Townsend, D. E., Hatab, P., and O'Brien, P. C.: Fertility and outcome of pregnancy in women exposed in utero to diethylstilbestrol. *N. Engl. J. Med.* **302**:609–613, 1980.
6. Bell, D. A., Komar, R., Chodirker, W. B., Bloch, J., and Cairns, E.: A comparison of serologic reactivity among SLE patients with or without anti-Ro (SS-A) antibodies. *J. Rheumatol.* **11**:315–317, 1984.
7. Benson, R. C. and Durfee, R. B.: Transabdominal cervicouterine cerclage during pregnancy for the treatment of cervical incompetence. *J. Obstet. Gynecol.* **25**:145–155, 1965.
8. Berger, M. I. and Goldstein, D. P.: Impaired reproductive performance in DES-exposed women. *Obstet. Gynecol.* **55**:25–27, 1980.
9. Bottone, E. J. and Sierra, M. F.: *Listeria monocytogenes*: Another look at the "Cinderella among pathogenic bacteria." *Mt. Sinai J. Med. (N.Y.)* **44**:42–59, 1977.
10. Boue, J., Boue, A., and Lazar, P.: Retrospective and prospective epidemiological studies of 1500 karyotyped spontaneous human abortions. *Teratology* **12**:11–26, 1975.
11. Bulmash, J. M.: Systemic lupus erythematosus and pregnancy. *Obstet. Gynecol. Annu.* **7**:153–194, 1978.
12. Burchell, R. C., Creed, F., Rosoulpour, M., and Whitcomb, M.: Vascular anatomy of the human uterus and pregnancy wastage. *Br. J. Obstet. Gynaecol.* **85**:698–706, 1978.
13. Buttram, V. C., Jr., and Gibbsons, W. E.: Mullerian anomalies: A proposed classification (an analysis of 144 cases). *Fertil. Steril.* **32**:40–46, 1979.
14. Buttram, V. C., Zanotti, L., Acosta, A. A., Vanderheyden, J.S., Besch, P. K., and Franklin, R. R.:

Surgical correction of the septate uterus. *Fertil. Steril.* **25**:373–379, 1974.

15. Carreras, L. O., Defreyn, G., Machin, S. J., Vermylen, J., Deman, R., Spitz, B., and Van Assche, A.: Arterial thrombosis, intrauterine death and "lupus" anticoagulant: Detection of immunoglobulin interfering with prostacyclin formation. *Lancet* **1**:244–246, 1981.
16. Charles, D. and Edwards, W. R.: Infectious complications of cervical cerclage. *Am. J. Obstet. Gynecoly.* **141**:1065–1070, 1981.
17. Cousins, L. M.: Cervical incompetence. In: *Maternal Fetal Medicine: Principles and Practice.* R. K. Creasy and R. Resnik (Eds.). Philadelphia, W. B. Saunders, 1984, pp. 394–399.
18. Crane, J. P. and Wahl, N.: The role of maternal diabetes in repetitive spontaneous abortion. *Fertil. Steril.* **36**:477–479, 1981.
19. Cuckle, H. S., Wald, N. J., and Lindenbaum, R. H.: Maternal serum alpha-fetoprotein measurement: A screening test for Down syndrome. *Lancet* **1**:926–929, 1984.
20. Danforth, D. N.: Cervical incompetency as a cause of spontaneous abortion. *Clin. Obstet. (N.Y.)* **2**:45–56, 1959.
21. Danforth, D. N.: Early studies of the anatomy and physiology of the human cervix and implications for the future. In: Dilatation of the Uterine Cervix. F. Naftolin and P. G. Stubblefield (Eds.). New York, Raven Press, 1980, pp. 3–15.
22. DeCherney, A. H. and Polan, M. L.: Helping habitual aborters. *Contemp. Ob. Gyn.* **20**:241–248, 1982.
23. Dunn, L. J., Robinson, J. C., and Steer, C. M.: Maternal death following suture of incompetent cervix during pregancy. *Am. J. Obstet.* **78**:335–339, 1959.
24. Firkin, B. G., Howard, M. A., and Radford, N.: Possible relationship between lupus inhibitor and recurrent abortion in young women. (Letter) *Lancet* **2**:366, 1980.
25. Floyd, W. S.: Cervical dilatation in the mid-trimester of pregnancy. *Obstet. Gynecol.* **18**:380–381, 1961.
26. Gabbe, S. G.: Congenital malformations in infants of diabetic mothers. *Obstet Gynecol. Surv.* **32**:125–132, 1977.
27. Gellis, S. S. and Hsia, D. Y. Y.: The infant of the diabetic mother. *Am. J. Dis. Child.* **97**:1–41, 1959.
28. Green, L. K. and Harris, R. E.: Uterine anomalies. Frequency of diagnosis and associated obstetric complications. *Obstet. Gynecol.* **47**:427–429, 1976.
29. Grieco, M. H.: Humoral and cellular responses to infection. In: *Infections in the Abnormal Host.* M. H. Grieco (Ed.). New York, Yorke Medical Books, 1980, pp. 231–304.
30. Grobstein, C.: External human fertilization. *Sci. Am.* **240**:57–67, 1979.
31. Gros, A., David, A., and Serr, D. M.: Management of congenital malformations of the uterus: Fetal salvage. *Acta Eur. Fertil.* **5**:301–304, 1974.
32. Hammer, G. S. and Hirschman, S. Z.: Infections in pregnancy. In: *Medical, Surgical, and Gynecologic Complications of Pregnancy,* 3rd Edition. S. Cherry, R. Berkowitz, and N. Kase (Eds.). Baltimore, Williams & Wilkins, 1985, pp. 2–28.
33. Harger, J. H.: Cervical cerclage: Patient selection, morbidity, and success rates. *Clin. Perinatol.* **10**:321–341, 1983.
34. Harger, J. H.: Comparison of success and morbidity in cervical cerclage procedures. *Obstet Gynecol.* **56**:543–548, 1980.
35. Harger, J. H.: Effectiveness of cervical cerclage. (Letter) *Am. J. Obstet. Gynecol.* **148**:834, 1984.
36. Harger, J. H., Archer, D. F., Marchese, S. G., Muracca-Clemens, M., and Garver, K. L.: Etiology of recurrent pregnancy losses and outcome of subsequent pregnancies. *Obstet Gynecol.* **62**:574–581, 1983.
37. Harris, E. N., Gharavi, A. E., Boey, M. L., Patel, B. M., Mackworth-Young, C. G., Loizou, S., and Hughes, G.R.:. Anticardiolipin antibodies: Detection by radioimmunoassay and association with thrombosis in systemic lupus erythematosus. *Lancet* **2**:1211–1214, 1983.
38. Hefner, J. D., Patow, W. E., and Ludwig, J. M.: A new surgical procedure for the correction of the incompetent cervix during pregnancy. *Obstet Gynecol.* **18**:617–620, 1961.
39. Hertig, A. T., Rock, J., Adams, E. C., and Menkin, M. C.: Thirty-four fertilized human ova, good, bad and indifferent, recovered from 210 women of known fertility; a study of biologic wastage in early human pregnancy. *Pediatrics* **23** (Part 2):202–211, 1959.
40. Holman, M. R : An aid for cervical cerclage. *Obstet Gynecol.* **42**:468–469, 1973.
41. Hook, E. B.: Differences between rates of trisomy 21 (Down syndrome) and other chromosomal abnormalities diagnosed in livebirths and in cells cultured after second-trimester amniocentesis—suggested explanations and implications for genetic counseling and program planning. *Birth Defects* **14**:249–267, 1978.
42. Hook, E. B., Cross, P. K., and Schreinemachers, D. M.: Chromosomal abnormality rates at amniocentesis and in live-born infants. *JAMA* **249**:2034–2038, 1983.
43. Hunter, R. G., Henry, G. W., and Judd, C. S., Jr.: Physiologic or dysfunctional incompetence of the cervix. Diagnosis and surgical treatment in the nonpregnant woman. *Am. J. Obstet. Gynecol.* **81**:1183–1190, 1961.
44. Isenberg, D. A. Shoenfield, Y., and Schwartz, R. S.: Multiple serologic reactions and their relationship to clinical activity in systemic lupus erythematosus. *Arthritis Rheum.* **27**:132–138, 1984.
45. Jarvinen, P. A. and Kokkonen, J.: Etiology and treatment of failed pregnancies. *Int. J. Fertil.* **17**:81–85, 1972.

46. Jennings, C. L., Jr.: Temporary submucosal cerclage for cervical incompetence: Report of forty-eight cases. *Am. J. Obstet. Gynecol.* **113**:1097–1102, 1972.
47. Johnstone, F. D., Beard, R. J., Boyd, I. E., and McCarthy, T. G.: Cervical diameter after suction termination of pregnancy. *Br. Med. J.* **1**:68–69, 1976.
48. Jones, H. W., Jr.: Operations for congenital anomalies of the uterus and vagina. *Clin. Obstet. Gynecol.* **2**:1053–1066, 1959.
49. Jones, H. W., Jr.: Reproductive impairment and the malformed uterus. *Fertil. Steril.* **36**:137–148, 1981.
50. Jones, W. S.: Obstetric significance of female genital anomalies. *Obstet Gynecol.* **10**:113–127, 1957.
51. Kissane, J. M.: Reproductive failure. A survey of pathogenic mechanisms with emphasis on mechnisms for repeated failures. In: *Perinatal Medicine*. R. L. Naeye, J. M. Kissane, and N. Kaufman (Eds.). Baltimore, Williams & Wilkins, 1981, pp. 369–380.
52. Kitzmiller, J. L., Cloherty, J. P., Younger, M. D., Tabatabaii, A., Rothchild, S. B., Sosenko, I., Epstein, M. F., Singh, S., and Neff, R. K.: Diabetic pregnancy and perinatal morbidity. *Am. J. Obstet. Gynecol.* **131**:560–580, 1978.
53. Kundsin, R. B. and Driscoll, S. G.: Mycoplasmas and human reproductive failure. *Surg. Gynecol. Obstet.* **131**:89–92, 1970.
54. Lash, A. F. and Lash, S. R.: Habitual abortion: The incompetent internal os of the cervix. *Am. J. Obstet. Gynecol.* **59**:68–76, 1950.
55. Lawler, F. C., Wood, W. S., King, S., and Metzger, W. I.: *Listeria monocytogenes* as a cause of fetal loss. *Am. J. Obstet. Gynecol.* **89**:915–923, 1964.
56. Lindley, M.: Life and death before birth. *Nature* **280**:635–636, 1979.
57. Lockshin, M. D., Druzin, M. L., Goei, S., Qamar, T., Magid, M. S., Jovanovic, L., and Ferenc, M.: Antibody to cardiolipin as a predictor of fetal distress or death in pregnant patients with systemic lupus erythematosus. *N. Engl. J. Med.* **313**:152–156, 1985.
58. MacNaughton, M. C.: Listeria monocytogenes in abortion. *Lancet* **2**:484, 1962.
59. MacNaughton, M. C.: M.R.C./R.C.O.G. cervical cerclage trial. (Letter) *Lancet* **1**:1320, 1981.
60. Mann, E. D.: Habitual abortion. *Am. J. Obstet. Gynecol.* **77**:706–718, 1959.
61. McDonald, I. A.: Incompetent cervix as a cause of recurrent miscarriage. *J. Obstet. Gynaecol. Br. Emp.* **64**:346–350, 1957.
62. McDonald, I. A.: Incompetence of the cervix. *Aust. N.Z. J. Obstet. Gynaecol.* **18**:34–37, 1978.
63. Merkatz, I. R. and Goldfarb, J. M.: The renal transplant recipient. In: *Management of High-Risk Pregnancy*, 2nd Edition. J. T. Queenan (Ed.). New Jersey, Medical Economics Books, 1985, pp. 333–339.
64. Merkatz, I. R., Nitowsky, H. M., Macri, J. N., and Johnson, W. E.:. An association between low maternal serum alpha-fetoprotein and fetal chromosomal abnormalities. *Am. J. Obstet. Gynecol.* **148**:886–894, 1984.
65. Mestman, J. H.: Hyperthyroidism. In: *Management of High-Risk Pregnancy*, 2nd Edition. J. T. Queenan (Ed.). New Jersey, Medical Economics Books, 1985, pp. 361–369.
66. Miller, E., Hare, J. W., Cloherty, J. P., Dunn, P. J., Gleason, R. E., Soeldner, J. S., and Kitzmiller, J. L.: Elevated maternal hemoglobin A/c in early pregnancy and major congenital anomalies in infants of diabetic mothers. *N. Engl. J. Med.* **304**:1331–1334, 1981.
67. Miller, J. F., Williamson, E., Glue, J., Gordon, Y. B., Grudzinskas, J. G., and Sykes, A.: Fetal loss after implementation. A prospective study. *Lancet* **2**:554–556, 1980.
68. Minkoff, H.: Prematurity: Infection as an etiologic factor. *Obstet Gynecol.* **62**:137–144, 1983.
69. Miodovnik, M., Lavin, J. P., Knowles, H. C., Holroyde, J., and Stys, S. J.: Spontaneous abortion among insulin-dependent women. *Am. J. Obstet. Gynecol.* **150**:372–376, 1984.
70. Musich, J. R. and Behrman, S. J.: Obstetric outcome before and after metroplasty in women with uterine anomalies. *Obstet Gynecol.* **52**:63–66, 1978.
71. Newman, M. R., Merkatz, I. R., Selim, M. A., Zador, I. E., and Roux, J. F.: Continuous monitoring of cervical dilatation during labor and measurement of cervical compliance in the human. In: *Dilatation of the Uterine Cervix*. F. Naftolin and P. G. Stubblefield (Eds.). New York, Raven Press, 1980, pp. 233–246.
72. Nilsson, I. M., Astedt, B., Hedner, U., and Berezin, D.: Intrauterine death and circulating anticoagulant ("antithromboplastin"). *Acta Med. Scand.* **197**:153–159, 1975.
73. Novy, M. J.: Transabdominal cervicoisthmic cerclage for the management of repetitive abortion and premature delivery. *Am. J. Obstet. Gynecol.* **143**:44–54, 1982.
74. Parikh, M. N. and Mehta, J. C.: Internal cervical os during the second half of pregnancy. *J. Obstet. Gynaecol. Br. Commonw.* **68**:818–821, 1961.
75. Pedersen, B.S.: A prospective study of acquired toxoplasmosis among 8,043 pregnant women in the Oslo area. *Am. J. Obstet. Gynecol.* **136**:399–406, 1980.
76. Peterson, P. G. and Keifer, W. S., Jr.: Diagnosis of an incompetent internal cervical os. *Am. J. Obstet. Gynecol.* **116**:498–504, 1973.
77. Ranney, B.: Congenital cervical incompetence in primigravidas. *Am. J. Obstet. Gynecol.* **86**:52–65, 1963.
78. Recce, E. A., Romero, R., Clyne, L. P., Kriz, N. S., and Hobbins, J. C.: Lupus-like anticoagulant in pregnancy. (Letter) *Lancet* **1**:344–345, 1984.
79. Ritter, H. A.: Surgical closure of the incompetent

cervix:. 15 years' experience. *Int. J. Gynaecol. Obstet.* **16**:194–196, 1978-1979.

80. Robau, E. and David, A.: *Listeria monocytogenes* in abortion. *J. Obstet. Gynaecol. Br. Commonw.* **70**:481–482, 1963.
81. Robboy, M. S.: The management of cervical incompetence. U.C.L.A. experience with cerclage procedures. *Obstet Gynecol.* **41**:108–112, 1973.
82. Rock, J. A. and Jones, H. W., Jr.: The clinical management of the double uterus. *Fertil. Steril.* **28**:798–806, 1977.
83. Sarti, D. A., Sample, W. F., Hobel, C. J., and Staisch, K. J.: Ultrasonic visualization of a dilated cervix during pregnancy. *Radiology* **130**:417–420, 1979.
84. Schaffner, F. and Schanzer, S. N.: Cervical dilatation in the early third trimester. *Obstet Gynecol.* **27**:130–133, 1966.
85. Scott, J. S., Maddison, P. J., Taylor, P. V., Esscher, E., Scott, 0., and Skinner, R. P.: Connective tissue disease, antibodies to ribonucleoprotein, ad congenital heart block. *N. Engl. J. Med.* **309**:209–212, 1983.
86. Semmens, J. P.: Congenital anomalies of the female genital tract. *Obstet Gynecol.* **19**:328–350, 1962.
87. Shirodkar, V. N.: *Surgical Treatment of Habitual Abortion, Tendances Actuelles en Gynecologie et Obstetrique.* Librairie de L'Universite, S.A. Geneve, Georg. O. Cie, 1955.
88. Simpson, J. L.: Antenatal diagnosis of chromosomal abnormalities. In: *Management of High-Risk Pregnancy,* 2nd Edition. J.T. Queenan (Ed.). New Jersey, Medical Economics Books, 1985, pp. 29–39.
89. Simpson, J. L.: Genes, chromosomes and reproductive failure. *Fertil. Steril.* **33**:107–116, 1980.
90. Slat, W. G. and Graham; A. R.: Scleroderma and pregnancy. *Am. J. Obstet. Gynecol.* **101**:335–341, 1968.
91. Southern, P. M., Jr.: Habitual abortion and toxoplasmosis. Is there a relationship? *Obstet Gynecol.* **39**:45–47, 1972.
92. Speert, H.: Pregnancy prognosis following repeated abortion. *Am. J. Obstet. Gynecol.* **68**:665–673, 1954.
93. Strassman, E. O.: Fertility and unification of double uterus. *Fertil. Steril.* **17**:165–176, 1966.
94. Stray-Pedersen, B. and Stray-Pedersen, S.: Etiologic factors and subsequent reproductive performance in 195 couples with a prior history of habitual abortion. *Am. J. Obstet. Gynecol.* **148**:140–146, 1984.
95. Thurman, G. R.: Systemic lupus erythematosus. *Curr. Prob. Obstet. Gynecol. Infertil.* **8**:12–30, 1985.
96. Tompkins, P.: Comments on the bicornuate uterus and twinning. Surg. Clin. N. Am. 42:1049–1062, 1962.
97. Vaalamo, P. and Kivikoski, A.: The incompetent cervix during pregnancy diagnosed by ultrasound. *Acta Obstet. Gynecol. Scand.* **62**:19–21, 1983.
98. Vaginal Infection and Pregnancy Study. 1983-6: National Institute of Child Health and Human Development, U.S. Department of Health and Human Services, Public Health Service.
99. Warburton, D. and Fraser, F. C.: Spontaneous abortion risks in man: Data from reproductive histories collected in a medical genetics unit. *Am. J. Hum. Genet.* **16**:1–25, 1964.
100. Witski, E.: Teratogenic effect from overripeness of the egg. In: *Congenital Malformations.* F.C. Fraser and V.A. McKusick (Eds.). Amsterdam, Excerpta Medica, 1976, pp. 157–160.

17

PREMATURE RUPTURE OF THE MEMBRANES

Premature rupture of the membranes (PROM) is a common but poorly understood problem. There is little understanding of its basic pathophysiology, and much controversy surrounds its management. Indeed, the problem is intricate. Gestational age and demographic factors influence the outcome of PROM. Therapeutic modalities added within the last 10 years include corticosteroids, tocolytics, and more potent antibiotics. Of major importance is the marked improvement in survival of low-birth-weight infants. This chapter emphasizes works published since 1970. Earlier literature has been extensively reviewed.[37]

Lack of standard and specific terminology has hindered our understanding of PROM. We define PROM as rupture at any time before the onset of contractions. Regrettably, "premature" also carries the connotation of preterm pregnancy. To avoid confusion, we shall use the word "preterm" to refer to gestational age <37 weeks. Terminology is further confused because others have used the expression "prolonged rupture of the membranes" and have used the same acronym, PROM.[82,86]

The latent period is defined as the time from membrane rupture to onset of contractions, and is to be distinguished from the "latent phase," designating the phase of labor that precedes the active phase (see Chapter 7).

Respiratory distress syndrome (RDS) requires careful definition. Most studies used the following criteria: early onset after birth, tachypnea, expiratory grunting, retractions, cyanosis and hypoxia, and a chest radiograph showing a reticulogranular pattern with air bronchograms. However, some studies do not define RDS. One defined RDS as "any breathing difficulty" and reserved "hyaline membrane disease" for the more specific findings, noted above.[65]

Terms recently used to describe maternal or perinatal infections durng labor include: "fever in labor," "intrapartum fever," "chorioamnionitis," "amnionitis," and "intrauterine infection." Whereas the first two terms are objective, they are also nonspecific, and the degree of temperature used to define "fever" is selected arbitrarily. The latter three terms are usually presumptive, based on combinations of maternal fever, uterine irritability or tenderness, leukocytosis, or purulent cervical discharge. After delivery, maternal infection is referred to as "endometritis" or "postpartum infection." In few studies, though, were presumed maternal infections confirmed by blood or genital tract cultures. Rather, these clinical diagnoses are usually based on fever, uterine tenderness, and exclusion of other sources of fever.

In neonates, the most common term used to report infection was neonatal sepsis, but some authors mean strictly a positive blood or cerebrospinal fluid culture, whereas others mean simply clinical signs or symptoms of sepsis.

INCIDENCE

In several recent reports, the incidence of PROM has ranged from 4.5% to 7.6% of total deliveries,[5,19,28] whereas PROM in preterm patients occurred in approximately 1% of all pregnancies.[12,25,36] In 1970, Gunn and colleagues noted that the incidence ranged from 2.7% to 17% with an average of about 10%.[37]

ETIOLOGY

Clinical Variables

Clinical variables, including cervical incompetence, cervical operations and lacerations, multiple pregnancies, polyhydramnios, antepartum hemorrhage, and heavy smoking have been associated with PROM.[23,25] However, in the majority of instances, none of these clinical variables is present. No association has been found between the frequency of PROM and maternal age, parity, maternal weight, fetal weight and position, trauma, or type of work.[37,59]

Physical Properties of the Membranes. There has been continued interest in the physical properties of membranes which rupture prematurely. The collagen content of amnion normally decreases in late pregnancy, even in patients without PROM, but these changes have been reported to occur earlier in gestation in patients with PROM.[75] However, others found no significant difference in the collagen content of fetal membranes among patient groups with term spontaneous ROM, with term artificial ROM, and with preterm PROM.[1] Differences in methodology may underlie these divergent conclusions.

Other reports have shown that membranes from cases with PROM are thinner.[3,64] Using in vitro techniques to measure rupturing pressure, three groups of investigators have found that the membranes from patients with PROM withstand either the same or higher pressure before bursting than do membranes from those without PROM.[1,3,50] Such observations have suggested a local defect at the site of rupture, rather than a diffuse weakening, in membranes that rupture before labor. These studies of physical properties should be interpreted cautiously because of differences in measuring techniques, possible deterioration of membrane preparations, and need for proper controls.

Infection. Subclinical infection may be a cause rather than a mere result of PROM. Acute inflammation of the placental membranes is twice as common when membranes rupture within 4 hours before labor than when they rupture after the onset of labor, suggesting that this "infection" may be the cause of PROM.[59] An additional analysis considered two successive singleton pregnancies in each of 5230 women (10,460 pregnancies). Preterm PROM occurred in only 2% of 773 pregnancies when recent coitus and histologic chorioamnionitis were absent, but in 23% of 96 pregnancies when both of these features were present.[58] Although this study shows an impressive increase in preterm PROM associated with these two factors, a causal role is not established because there may be other factors which were not considered. Evaluation of successive pregnancies would not necessarily eliminate these confounding variables.

In South African Blacks, histologic chorioamnionitis and PROM were increased when coitus had occurred within the last 7 days. Use of a condom during coitus resulted in less placental inflammation. In addition, PROM was more frequent ($p < 0.01$) when there had been orgasm during coitus.[60]

Cederqvist and colleagues investigated cord blood immunoglobulins and noted two patterns of onset of infection after PROM.[11] In one, there was clinical and immunologic evidence of infection within 12 hours of PROM. This observation suggests that infection occurred before rupture and may have been the cause.

Further evidence is provided by bacteriologic studies. Patients with PROM prior to term are more likely to have anaerobes in endocervical cultures than are women without PROM at term.[16] This observation may be interpreted to show that subclinical anaerobic "infection" leads to PROM. However, the increased presence of anaerobes in cervical cultures may reflect hormonal or other influences at different stages of gestation or perhaps an inhibitory effect of leaking amniotic fluid on aerobes at term. This latter possibility is supported by the observation that anaerobes are found more commonly in the cervices of women with ROM longer than 12 hours.[20]

DIAGNOSIS

PROM is generally readily diagnosed by history, physical findings, and simple laboratory tests. These diagnostic tests have been summarized recently.[29,76] Standard tests are based on determination of pH (nitrazene test) or detection of a "ferning" pattern or of fetal cells.

Although these tests are accurate in approximately 90% of cases, they each yield false-positive and false-negative results, especially in cases with small amounts of amniotic fluid in the vagina. Other approaches to diagnosing PROM in equivocal cases include biochemical and histochemical tests[24,35,55,69,78,85] and intra-amniotic injection of various dyes.[4,15,57,66] However, these newer tests have not gained wide use, and the dye-injections seem fraught with potential problems. Ultrasound examination has also been mentioned as a diagnostic technique, since a finding of oligohydramnios might suggest PROM,[49] but oligohydramnios is hardly specific and perhaps not sufficiently sensitive for diagnosis of PROM.

LABOR

Onset

The onset of labor occurs within 24 hours after membrane rupture in 80–90% of term patients.[37] The latent period exceeds 24 hours in 19% of patients at term and exceeds 48 hours in 12.5%.[45,46] Only 3.6% of term patients do not go into labor within 7 days.[45]

Latent periods are longer among patients with PROM prior to term. Confirming older studies, more recent investigations have shown latent periods 24 hours in 57–83%,[46,62] 72 hours in 15–26%,[28,43,53] and 7 days in 19–41%.[12,23,46] There is an inverse relationship between gestational age and the proportion of patients with latent periods 3 days.[43] One-third of pregnancies between 25 and 32 weeks had latent periods >3 days, whereas for pregnancies 33–34 and 35–36 weeks, the corresponding values were 16% and 4.5%, respectively. In 1984, Taylor and Garite reported the outcome in 53 cases of PROM at 16–25 weeks (mean, 22.6 weeks). The median length of time from PROM to delivery was 6 days (range 1–87 days; mean 17).[81] Thus, the natural history of PROM reveals that labor usually develops within a few days. Accordingly, tocolytics have been given to patients with PROM in order to prolong the pregnancy.

Tocolysis

In a few studies, investigators have given tocolytic agents either with or without steroids to patients with PROM before term.[6,13,23,48,52,62,77,79] In some, tocolytics were used to delay delivery for approximately 48 hours after steroid administration; in others, no limit was placed on duration of tocolytic therapy. With PROM, tocolytics delay delivery for a period of 1–3 days in most cases. However, nearly all patients deliver within a week as tocolytics are less effective with PROM than with intact membranes.[13,2,79]

Cesarean Delivery

In recent reports, the percentage of patients delivered by cesarean ranges from 7% to 48% (Table 17-1), markedly higher than the range of 1–7% reported before 1970.[37] This increase is important, as cesarean birth is the major risk factor for puerperal infection and a significant risk factor for RDS. Two recent studies have reported a significantly higher rate of cesarean delivery when induction was attempted, compared to when an expectant policy was followed (39% vs. 12%, respectively) in patients at term with PROM and unfavorable cervices.[22,45] The prospective, randomized study by Duff and colleagues found the rate of cesarean delivery to be 8% in the expectant group and 20% in the induction group ($p < 0.05$).[22] In patients managed by induction, 58% of cesarean sections were the result of failed induction (see Fig. 17-1). Management schemes which urge induction in either term or preterm pregnancies with unfavorable cervices are likely to yield higher cesarean delivery rates.

COMPLICATIONS

Analysis of complications from recent studies is difficult because of the complexity of these studies and the differences in study design.[5,8,10,14,31,36,43,45,46,48,54,62,65,73,82–84] Table 17-1 summarizes studies each of which contained more than 100 infants. Direct comparisons of data from one study to another require extreme caution. The wide-ranging differences may be attributed to major differences from study to study in population at risk, gestational age, definitions employed, and management.

The risks of PROM generally are those of infection versus those of prematurity. The most common complication among pregnancies with PROM before 37 Weeks is RDS, which is found in 10–40% of neonates. (A small number of studies have reported RDS in as high as 60–80% of newborns.) Bona fide neonatal sepsis was documented in less than 10%, whereas amnionitis

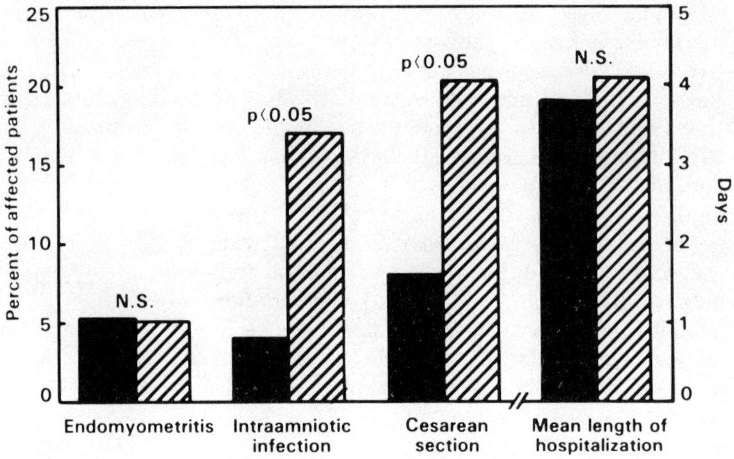

Figure 17-1. Maternal outcome in term patients who have premature rupture of membranes and a cervix unfavorable for induction of labor. Solid bars indicate expectant management. Hatched bars indicate intervention. (Reprinted with permission from the American College of Obstetricians and Gynecologists [*Obstet. Gynecol.* **63**(5):697–702, 1984].)

(based on clinical criteria only) occurred in approximately 4–33%. Endometritis developed in 3–29% of patients in most reports, but it is not clear whether patients with amnionitis are also included in the endometritis category. In selected groups, such as patients with cesarean section after PROM, endometritis occurs in up to 70% of patients.

Causes of perinatal death may be determined by examining data from four large series (Table 17-2). Two of these studies included stillbirths; two others excluded stillbirths. Overall, RDS was the leading cause of death. Deaths were presumed to be due to anoxia when there was an ante- or intrapartum death of a very small infant. Congenital anomalies and infection were each responsible for a clear minority of deaths. In terms of both frequency and severity, RDS was a greater threat than infection to the preterm fetus.

When PROM occurred prior to 26 weeks and with long intervals (e.g., more than 5 weeks) between rupture and delivery, Nimrod and colleagues noted a 27% incidence of fetal pulmonary hypoplasia.[61]

Asphyxia, defined as an Apgar score of <7 at 5 minutes of life, is noted in 15–64% of live born infants.[25,28,65,72] This complication is most common among the very low birth weight infants. Other complications of PROM, especially in the preterm pregnancy, are malpresentation, cord prolapse, and congenital anomalies. In view of the long list of potential hazards, it is not surprising that premature infants surviving after PROM are subject to prolonged hospitalization.

INTERACTION OF TREATMENT AND OUTCOME

Effect of Treatment on Infection

A number of treatment plans potentially affect maternal and fetal infection.

Corticosteroids and Infection. A number of workers have used steroids in at least some patients with PROM. A summary of recent prospective, randomized studies is provided in Table 17-3.[6,9,14,31,51,56,63,80] In three studies, the investigators found evidence for an increased rate of maternal postpartum infection after administration of steroids. The infections occurred mainly after vaginal delivery and were mild.[31] Maternal infection may increase significantly when the duration of PROM is longer than 48 hours.[80] In patients with PROM and a cervical suture, a higher rate of fetal infection was noted when steroids were used.[48] The results of other nonrandomized studies were variable.

Latent Period and Incidence of Amnionitis. Some recent reports have found an increased rate of amnionitis with increasing length of the latent period,[5,28,82] but other investigators have found no increase in the incidence of amnionitis among preterm pregnancies with increasing latent periods.[72,83] Still others found a variable effect, depending on weight groups.[54] In patients with preterm PROM, vaginal examination should be avoided until labor develops.[73]

TABLE 17-1. MATERNAL–FETAL OUTCOME IN RECENT, LARGER STUDIES (>100 INFANTS) OF PREMATURE RUPTURE OF MEMBRANES (PROM)

Author, Year, Location	Gestational Age or Birth Weight	Number of Patients	Cesarean Delivery	Complications: PNM†	Complications: RDS‡	Complications: Infection§	
Schutte,[73] 1983, Amsterdam, Netherlands	16 weeks to term	321 Mothers 334 Infants	N.R.*	10% for 28–38 weeks; 2.6% for ≧37 weeks	N.R.	Neonates: Preterm Term Maternal fever on day of delivery	 16% 3% 15%
Brame,[10] 1983, North Carolina	26–35 weeks	214	7%	7%	23%	Maternal Neonatal	3% 4%
Wilson,[84] 1982, Virginia	<37 weeks	143 Mothers 145 Infants	22%	15%	85% (used ventilator therapy)	Maternal NN	10% 7%
Kuhn,[48] 1982, Melbourne	25–33 weeks	216	N.R.	N.R. for group with PROM	"Severe" 18.6%	Maternal NN	18% 20%
Graham,[36] 1982, Texas	<34 weeks	109	N.R.*	21–41%	41–76%	NNS (includes clinical diagnosis)	15–28%
Kappy,[45] 1982 Massachusetts	>36 weeks	150	12–100%	0	—	Overall, "febrile morbidity" NNS	13% 0
Perkins,[65] 1982, New Mexico	<2001 g	133 Infants 125 Mothers	29%	10%	20%	"Fever" NNS	23% 0
Garite,[31] 1981, California	28–34 weeks	160 Mothers	25–35%	2–6%	17–21%	Amn. Endo. NNS	14% 14–29% 0–5%
Varner,[83] 1981, Iowa	28–36 weeks	127 Infants 116 Mothers	7%	3%	25%	Amn. Endo. NNS	9% 7% 7%
Daikoku,[19] 1981, Maryland	≧37 weeks	454	Approx. 8%	0.2%	N.R.	"Mat. Fever" NNS	2.0% 0.5%
	<37weeks	203	Approx. 13%	<32 weeks, 33% 33–36 weeks, 4%	N.R.	"Mat. Fever" NNS	6.9% 0.5%

TABLE 17-1. Continued

Author, Year, Location	Gestational Age or Birth Weight	Number of Patients	Cesarean Delivery	Complications: PNM†	Complications: RDS‡	Complications: Infection§	
Johnson,[43] 1981, Maryland	25–36 weeks	447	N.R.	25–28 weeks, 43.5% 29–32 weeks, 11.3%	N. R.	N.R.	
Collaborative Group,[14] 1981	26–37 weeks	288	N.R. for these subgroups	N.R. for these subgroups	10–12%	N.R. for these subgroups	
Nochimson,[62] 1980, Connecticut; New York	27–34 weeks	42 (1977–1979) 61 (1974–1977)	17% 10%	5% 10%	12% 31%	"Mat. Fever" "Mat. Fever"	7% 25%
Kappy,[46] 1979, Massachusetts	24–40 weeks	78 ≧ 37 weeks 110 < 37 weeks	36% 31%	1% 10%	— 10%	Mat. infection at delivery NNS	2.3% 0.5%
Miller,[54] 1978, North Carolina	1000–2500 g	151	7%	1000–1500 g, 29% 1501–2500 g 2%	1000–1500 g, 42% 1500–2500 g 7%	Amn. Endo. NNS	8% 7% 2%
Fayez,[28] 1978, Missouri	>34 weeks	59 observed 53 induced	0 6%	0 0	0 0	Amn. NNS Amn.	12% 4% 4%
Berkowitz,[8] 1977, Connecticut	<36 weeks	340	N.R.	21%	41%	NN deaths related to sepsis	1.7%
Bada,[5] 1977, Kentucky	All	963 total 270, <38 weeks	N.R.	Term, 0.1% Preterm, 13%	13% of preterm	Amn. NNS (Clinical diagnosis)	11% 5%
Thibeault,[82] 1977, California	25–34 weeks	153	N.R.	19–34%	ROM <24 h, 60% ROM >72 h, 0%	Amn. NNS	4–33% 3%

* NR—Not reported.
† PNM—Perinatal mortality.
‡ RDS—Respiratory distress syndrome (see text).
§ Infection: NNS—Neonatal sepsis (positive blood culture unless otherwise noted); Amn.—Amnionitis; Endo.—Endometritis.

TABLE 17-2. PRIMARY CAUSES OF DEATH AMONG INFANTS BORN WITH PREMATURE RUPTURE OF THE MEMBRANES BEFORE TERM*

Cause	Percentage of Perinatal Deaths
RDS	29–70%
Infection	3–19%
Congenital anomaly	9–27%
Asphyxia–anoxia	5–46%†
Others‡	9–27%

* Data are from four studies with more than 20 perinatal deaths and with causes of death indicated.[5,8,18,23] Overall perinatal mortality was 13–24%.
† Includes stillbirths with birth weight between 500 and 1000 grams.
‡ Includes "atelectasis," erythroblastosis fetalis, intracranial hemorrhage, and necrotizing enterocolitis.

Prophylactic Antibiotics. Many studies have employed prophylactic antibiotics for either mothers or newborns, but rarely in standardized fashion. There is no agreement regarding the value of prophylaxis among infants born after membranes have been ruptured for 24 hours or more.[38,86] Prophylaxis for mothers with PROM has usually been reserved for patients undergoing cesarean delivery. Others have favored use of prophylaxis in women receiving steroids.[53]

Many favor the use of intrapartum antibiotics (e.g., penicillin or ampicillin) in patients with PROM and a positive genital culture for group B streptococci. Although this approach decreases intrapartum transmission of group B streptococci when membranes are intact, its efficacy with PROM is unclear, as infection may be established before onset of labor.

Accordingly, we favor a short course of antibiotics as soon as the culture is identified. However, many patients will deliver before the results are available, and use of such therapy may increase infection due to penicillin-resistant bacteria.

Diagnosis of Infection. Several authors have evaluated use of amniocentesis and microscopic examination of amniotic fluid for presence of bacteria.[32,91] This approach is limited, however, as amniotic fluid was available in only half the patients. Clinical chorioamnionitis was more common in women with positive smears or cultures, but approximately 20–30% of such women had no clinical evidence of infection. In addition, amniocentesis may potentially be accompanied by trauma, bleeding, initiation of labor, or introduction of infection, although Yeast and co-authors reported no increase in onset of labor and no trauma in their retrospective series.[88]

The clinical usefulness of amniocentesis in preterm patients with PROM has not been determined. Most patients with PROM and positive amniotic fluid cultures are in labor within 48 hours, and, because of delays in reporting cultures, results are often available after the fact. Since at least some patients have positive cultures with no clinical evidence of infection, there is concern regarding unnecessary delivery of preterm infants. Finally, it has not been demonstrated that delivery before chorioamnionitis is clinically evident leads to an improved perinatal outcome.

Others have evaluated C-reactive protein as a predictor of infection (Table 17-4).[26,27,39,70] In sum, elevated serum CRP in patients with premature rupture of the membranes has good predictive value for histologic amnionitis, but its predictive value for clinically evident infection is poor (30–45%). The predictive value of a normal CRP for predicting absence of clinical chorioamnionitis is better (80–97%). The role of CRP in management remains unresolved. In view of the low predictive value of a positive test, it does not appear wise to deliver solely on the basis of an elevated CRP.

Course of Amnionitis. Perinatal outcome in the face of clinically diagnosed amnionitis has been improving.[30,33,47,89] In contrast to earlier studies which had reported high perinatal mortality rates (as high as 32–50%) in cases of amnionitis,[37] these recent studies showed lower PNM with few deaths being attributable to infection per se. Rather, the deaths were more commonly due to problems accompanying prematurity. Maternal outcome was excellent in all studies, although an approximately threefold increase in cesarean delivery rates has been noted. (Further data on outcome are presented in Chapter. 38)

Effect of Treatment on Respiratory Distress Syndrome

Use of Steroids and Development of RDS in Patients with PROM. A summary of prospective, randomized studies is provided in Table 17-3. Two studies reported significant (or nearly significant) decreases in RDS,[51,63] but others

TABLE 17-3. EFFECT OF CORTICOSTEROID ADMINISTRATION ON RESPIRATORY DISTRESS SYNDROME AND ON INFECTION IN PATIENTS WITH PREMATURE RUPTURE OF THE MEMBRANES, AS OBSERVED IN PROSPECTIVE, RANDOMIZED STUDIES

Author, Year	Design of Study; Agent	Gestational Age Range	Number of Patients with PROM		Effect of Steroids on	
			With Steroids	Without Steroids	Respiratory Distress Syndrome	Infection
Iams,[40] 1985	Prospective; randomized use of hydrocortisone	28–34 weeks	38	35	None	Increased endometritis
Schmidt,[71] 1984	Double-blind administration of betamethasone, methylprednisolone, hydrocortisone, or placebo	26–32 weeks	45	17	None	Increased endometritis after vaginal delivery in hydrocortisone-treated women
Barrett,[6] 1982	Prospective; betamethasone use if L/S immature and Gram stain of AF was negative	26–34 weeks	36	53	No significant decrease, but 14% in steroid group vs. 29% in no steroid group	No increase
Garite,[31] 1981	Prospective; randomized use of betamethasone	28–34 weeks	80	80	None	Increased endometritis mainly after vaginal delivery ($p < 0.05$)
Collaborative study,[14] 1981	Double-blind administration of dexamethasone or placebo	26–37 weeks	153	135	No significant decrease	Not reported for subgroup with PROM, but no increase overall

TABLE 17-3. Continued

Author, Year	Design of Study; Agent	Gestational Age Range	Number of Patients with PROM: With Steroids	Number of Patients with PROM: Without Steroids	Effect of Steroids on: Respiratory Distress Syndrome	Effect of Steroids on: Infection
Papageorgiou,[63] 1979	Double-blind administration of betametha-sone or placebo	25–34 weeks	17*	19*	Decreased ($p < 0.039$)	No increase
Taeusch,[80] 1979	Double-blind administration of dexametha-sone or placebo	<33 weeks	17*	24*	Not significantly decreased	Increase in maternal infection when ROM >48 hours $p < 0.008$)
Morrison,[56] 1978	Double-blind administration of hydrocorti-sone or placebo	<34 weeks	24	23	No comment about subgroup with PROM	No increase
Block,[9] 1977	Double-blind administration of betametha-sone, methyl-prednisolone, or placebo	32–37 weeks	43	26	No significant difference	None apparent
Liggins,[51] 1976	Double-blind administration of betametha-sone or cortisone acetate (''relatively inactive'' steroid)	<37 weeks	118*	94*	Decreased ($p = 0.07$)	No increase in ''deaths with pneumonia''

* In these reports, the number of patients with PROM is not published. Numbers listed are patients with rupture of membranes >24 hours; these patients probably all had PROM.

TABLE 17-4. C-REACTIVE PROTEIN AND PREDICTION OF CHORIOAMNIONITIS IN PATIENTS WITH PREMATURE RUPTURE OF THE MEMBRANES

Author, Year	N	Endpoint Measured	Predictive Value Negative	Predictive Value Positive
Evans, 1980	119	"Inf. morbidity"	86%	100%
Farb, 1983	31	Clin. amnionitis	80%	45%
Hawrylyshyn, 1983	52	Hist. amnionitis	88%	96%
		Clin. amnionitis	—	29%
Romem, 1984	51	Clin. amnionitis	97%	43%
		Clin. amnionitis*	97%	86%

* Detection of clinical amnionitis after excluding patients with other alleged causes for elevated CRP (including labor >6 hours, urinary tract infection, endocarditis, and superficial thrombophlebitis in a drug addict).

found no significant decrease when steroids were used in patients with PROM.[6,9,14,31,40,71,80] Data from the large, blinded, collaborative study on antenatal dexamethasone administration showed no significant effect of steroids in reducing RDS among patients with PROM.[14] Yet, there are major difficulties in interpreting these studies. In some of the more rigorously designed studies of steroid use, the numbers of patients with PROM are small. Thus, real differences may have been missed (a beta error). Indeed, in most studies, there are at least small decreases in RDS in the steroid group. A relatively wide range of gestational ages were studied. The minimum number of weeks gestation for entry into a study varied from 25 to 32, and the maximum varied from 32 to 37. Since it is unlikely that an equal effect of steroids on RDS will be seen at all gestational age intervals, real differences may have been missed in some gestational age intervals because of combining them with infants of other gestational ages. Finally, experiments measuring the surfactant-inducing potency of steroids suggest differences in the efficacy of the various steroid preparations and differences in efficacy with varying doses.[2] Although this is a highly controversial area, our interpretation is that the bulk of the data does not favor use of steroids with PROM.

Latent Period on Development of RDS. Many studies have addressed this question, but results are conflicting. Some studies noted that prolonged ROM decreased the incidence of RDS.[7, 8,68,74,82,90] others noted no significant effect,[5, 12,21,23,44,51,67,72,80,87] and two noted a variable effect depending on weight groups.[54,65] These discrepancies may be explained by differences in experimental design (such as grouping of varying gestational ages and using varying sample sizes) or differences in definitions of clinical complications.

Tocolytics on Development of RDS. This is another confusing area. Some studies suggested a decrease in RDS with use of β-adrenergics, but in the National Collaborative Study, use of tocolytics in patients with ruptured membranes increased the odds of RDS by about 350%.[17] This is an unexpected and unexplained finding, that urges caution in the use of tocolytics in patients with PROM.

Determination of Fetal Lung Maturity. Because RDS is the single greatest threat to infants with PROM, some clinicians determine the status of fetal pulmonary maturity and proceeded with delivery if the lungs are mature. Amniotic fluid may be collected by amniocentesis[32,91] or by collection from the posterior vagina. [34,41,77] Presence of either phosphatidylglycerol or an L/S 2 in amniotic fluid collected vaginally has been reported to be a good predictor of pulmonary maturity. In a series of patients with PROM before 36 weeks, the authors determined whether phosphotidyl glycerol (PG) was present in the vaginal pool and delivered patients when there was presence of PG, or spontaneous labor, or evidence of sepsis. Of 214 patients, 47 had PG present initially and were delivered. Of the remaining 167, 36 (21%) developed PG and were induced or delivered by cesarean section. Evidence of maternal infection developed in 8 (5%); spontaneous labor developed in 123 (74%) of the 167 patients. PG in amniotic fluid from the vagina reliably predicted fetal lung maturity. However, absence of PG did not necessarily mean that RDS would develop. Of the 131 patients who did not show

PG in the vaginal pool in any sample, 82 (62%) were delivered of infants who had no RDS.[10]

Even with PROM, delivery of a premature infant simply because its lungs show biochemical maturity may be questioned in view of other potential hazards of prematurity and the potential difficulties of the induction.

PERINATAL MORTALITY

In the past decade, perinatal mortality (PNM) rates have decreased considerably among low-birth-weight infants, with and without PROM. In any given study, factors affecting outcome are exclusion or inclusion of stillbirths, range of gestational ages studied, size of the study, and the span of years studied as well as calendar years in which the study was performed. Thus, it is not surprising to find PNM ranging from 2.5% to 50% of all births. Most series have few perinatal deaths, and others do not specify the primary causes of death. Table 17-2 summarizes large, recent studies.

MATERNAL MORTALITY

Recent studies document only one maternal death (due to chorioamnionitis, severe toxemia, and cardiorespiratory arrest) in over 3000 women with PROM.[18] From the same institution, reports from the early 1950s document four other maternal deaths from longstanding infection.[43] Citations of maternal death from sepsis complicating PROM appear sporadically.[42]

MANAGEMENT

As shown in Table 17-5, there are numerous proposals for management, but there have been few prospective, randomized, comparative studies of management of preterm PROM. Because of differences in populations, studies are largely noncomparable and unconvincing. No plan has become the accepted standard.

In general, physicians following a policy of intervention (such as for fetal pulmonary maturity) must consider the risks of diagnostic procedures (e.g., amniocentesis), of difficult inductions and ensuing high cesarean section rates, and of hazards of prematurity other than RDS. Those following a policy of expectancy must acknowledge that, in the majority of instances, labor or infection will ensue within 3–7 days.

TABLE 17-5. MANAGEMENT OPTIONS PROPOSED FOR PATIENTS WITH PROM

TERM PREGNANCY

- Induction if spontaneous labor does not ensue in approximately 12 hours or if there are other complications (e.g., toxemia).
- Expectant management for women with uncomplicated pregnancies and a cervix unfavorable for induction.

PRETERM PREGNANCY

- Expectant management. Delivery if labor or signs of infection ensue.
- Determine fetal pulmonary status by amniocentesis or from vaginal pool. Delivery if mature.
- Determine risk of infection by amniotic fluid stains or by C-reactive protein. Delivery if evidence of infection develops.
- Administer corticosteroids, with or without delivery in 24–28 hours. Tocolytics as needed.
- Delivery after an arbitrary latent period, for example, 16–72 hours.
- Combinations of the above.

On our service, we follow an expectant policy for PROM before term. We use neither tocolytic agents nor steroids, but penicillin is used when a patient has group B streptococci. Delivery is effected when clinical evidence of amnionitis becomes evident, but not solely for positive cultures, elevated WBCs, or elevated CRPs. For patients with PROM at term, we induce labor if the cervix is ripe (2 cm dilated and 80% effaced) or if there are pregnancy complications. We follow expectant management if the cervix is unripe and the pregnancy is uncomplicated.

We lack a clear understanding of the pathophysiology of PROM and thus a scientifically sound basis for its management. Conclusions about management of PROM must be regarded as tentative, at least in part, but a number of shifts have become evident in the last decade.

First, although maternal death is extremely rare, there has been a marked rise in the cesarean delivery rate in cases with PROM and very probably an increase in postpartum infection. Second, RDS is a greater threat to the neonate than is sepsis in PROM before term. Third, caution must be raised regarding use of tocolytics in cases of PROM. Although these agents appear to delay delivery, it is for a limited time only. Subclinical infection may be the cause of the uterine activity, and tocolytics may increase

RDS in preterm PROM. Fourth, use of amniocentesis to predict pulmonary maturity and infection is an unproved approach. Reliable information regarding fetal pulmonary status may often be obtained from amniotic fluid collected in the vagina, but Gram staining or culturing of this specimen to demonstrate infection is not reliable. The fluid is likely to be heavily contaminated with lower genital tract bacteria. Evidence of pulmonary maturity may not in itself warrant delivery in view of the other hazards of prematurity and of difficult inductions. We don't know whether or not there is any real advantage to delivery before infection is clinically evident (i.e., when there is only a positive Gram stain or a positive culture of the amniotic fluid). Fifth, despite numerous investigations, there is still no agreement regarding the effect of prolonged latent periods on the incidence of RDS. Sixth, the value of corticosteroids in decreasing RDS in preterm infants born after PROM is debatable.

In view of the present confusion regarding management of preterm pregnancies where PROM is present, we believe that caution should be exercised to avoid use of unproved therapeutic modalities, and complete perinatal care should be provided in tertiary centers.

REFERENCES

1. Al-Zaid, N. S.: Bursting pressure and collagen content of fetal membranes and their relation to premature rupture of the membranes. *Br. J. Obstet. Gynaecol.* **87**:227–229, 1980.
2. Anderson, G. C., Lamden, M. P., Cidlowski, J. A., and Ashikaga, T.: Comparative pulmonary surfactant-inducing effect of three corticosteroids in the near-term rat. *Am. J. Obstet. Gynecol.* **139**:562–564, 1981.
3. Artal, R., Sokol, R. J., Neuman, M., Burstein, A. H., and Stojkov, J.: The mechanical properties of prematurely and non-prematurely ruptured membranes, methods, and preliminary results. *Am. J. Obstet. Gynecol.* **125**:655–659, 1976.
4. Atlay, R. D. and Sutherst, J. R.: Premature rupture of the fetal membranes confirmed by intraamniotic injection of dye (Evans blue T-1824). *Am. J. Obstet. Gynecol.* **108**:993–994, 1970.
5. Bada, H. S., Alojipan, L. C., and Andrews, B. F.: Premature rupture of membranes and its effect on the newborn. *Pediatr. Clin. North Am.* **24**:491–500, 1977.
6. Barrett, J. M. and Boehm, F. H.: Comparison of aggressive and conservative management of premature rupture of fetal membranes. *Am. J. Obstet. Gynecol.* **144**:12–16, 1982.
7. Bauer, C. R., Stern, L., and Colle, E.: Prolonged rupture of membranes associated with a decreased incidence of respiratory distress syndrome. *Pediatrics* **53**:7–12, 1974.
8. Berkowitz, R. L., Kantor, R. D., Beck, G. J., and Warshaw, J. B.: The relationship between premature rupture of the membranes and the respiratory distress syndrome. An update and plan of management. *Am. J. Obstet. Gynecol.* **131**:-503-508, 1978.
9. Block, M. F., Klin, O. R., and Crosby, W. M.: Antenatal glucocorticoid therapy for the prevention of respiratory distress syndrome in the premature infant. *Obstet. Gynecol.* **50**:186–190, 1977.
10. Brame, R. G. and MacKenna, J.: Vaginal pool phospholipids in management of premature rupture of membranes. *Am. J. Obstet. Gynecol.* **145**:992–1000, 1983.
11. Cederqvist, L. L., Zervoudakis, I. A., Ewool, L. C., and Litwin, S. D.: The relationship between prematurely ruptured membranes and fetal immunoglobulin production. *Am. J. Obstet. Gynecol.* **134**:784–788, 1979.
12. Christensen, K. K., Christensen, P., Ingemarsson, I., Mardh, P.-A., Nordenfelt, E., Ripa, T., Solum, T., and Svenningsen, N.: A study of complications in preterm deliveries after prolonged premature rupture of the membranes. *Obstet. Gynecol.* **48**:670–677, 1976.
13. Christensen, K. K., Ingemarsson, I., Leideman, T., Solum, T., and Svenningsen, N.: Effect of ritodrine on labor after premature rupture of the membranes. *Obstet. Gynecol.* **55**:187–190, 1980.
14. Collaborative group on antenatal steroid therapy: Effect of antenatal dexamethasone administration on the prevention of respiratory distress syndrome. *Am. J. Obstet. Gynecol.* **141**:276–287, 1981.
15. Cowett, R. M., Hakanson, D. O., Kocon, R. W., and Oh, W.: Untoward neonatal effect of intraamniotic administration of methylene blue. *Obstet. Gynecol.* **48**:74S–75S, 1976.
16. Creatsas, G., Pavlatos, M., Lolis, D., Aravantino, D., and Kaskarelis, D.: Bacterial contamination of the cervix and premature rupture of membranes. *Am. J. Obstet. Gynecol.* **139**:522–525, 1981.
17. Curet, L. B., Rao, A. V., Zachman, R. D., Morrison, J. C., Burkett, G, Poole, W. K., and Bauer, C.: Association between ruptured membranes, tocolytic therapy, and respiratory distress syndrome. *Am. J. Obstet. Gynecol.* **148**:263–268, 1984.
18. Daikoku, N. H., Kaltreider, F., Khouzami, V. A., Spence, M., and Johnson, J. W.: Premature rupture of membranes and spontaneous preterm labor: Maternal endometritis risks. *Obstet. Gynecol.* **59**:13–20, 1982.
19. Daikoku, N. H., Kaltreider, F., Johnson, T. R., Jr., Johnson, J. W., and Simmons, M. A.: Premature rupture of membranes and preterm labor: Neonatal infection and perinatal mortality risks. *Obstet. Gynecol.* **58**:417–425, 1981.

20. DelBene, V. E., Moore, E., Rogers, M., and Kreutner, A. K.: Bacterial flora of patients with prematurely ruptured membranes. *South. Med. J.* **70**:950–954, 1977.
21. Dluholucky, S., Babic, J., and Taufer, I.: Reduction of incidence and mortality of respiratory distress syndrome by administration of hydrocortisone to mother. *Arch. Dis. Child.* **51**:420–423, 1976.
22. Duff, W. P., Huff, R. W., and Gibbs, R. S.: Management of the term patient who has premature rupture of the membranes and a cervix unfavorable for induction. *Obstet. Gynecol.* **63**:697–702, 1984.
23. Eggers, T. R., Doyle, L. W., and Pepperell, R. J.: Premature rupture of the membranes. *Med. J. Aust.* **1**:209–213, 1979.
24. Elmfors, B., Tryding, N., and Tufvesson, G.: The diagnosis of ruptured fetal membranes by measurement of diamine oxidase (DAO) activity in vaginal fluid. *J. Obstet. Gynaecol. Br. Commonw.* **81**:361–362, 1974.
25. Evaldson, G., Lagrelius, A., and Winiarski, J.: Premature rupture of the membranes. *Acta Obstet. Gynecol. Scand.* **59**:385–393, 1980.
26. Evans, M. I., Hajj, S. N., Devoe, L. D., Angerman, N. S., and Moawad, A. H.: C-reactive protein as a predictor of infectious morbidity with premature rupture of membranes. *Am. J. Obstet. Gynecol.* **138**:648–652, 1980.
27. Farb, H. F., Arnesen M., Geistler, P., and Knox, G. E.: C-reactive protein with premature rupture of membranes and premature labor. *Obstet. Gynecol.* **62**:49–51, 1983.
28. Fayez, J. A., Hasan, A. A., Jonas, H. S., and Miller, G. L.: Management of premature rupture of the membranes. *Obstet. Gynecol.* **52**:17–21, 1978.
29. Friedman, M. L. and McElin, T. W.: Diagnosis of ruptured fetal membranes. Clinical study and review of the literature. *Am. J. Obstet. Gynecol.* **104**:544–550, 1969.
30. Garite, T. J. and Freeman, R. K.: Chorioamnionitis in the preterm gestation. *Obstet. Gynecol.* **59**:539–545, 1982.
31. Garite, T. J., Freeman, R. K., Linzey, E. M., Braly, P. S., and Dorchester, W. L.: Prospective randomized study of corticosteroids in the management of premature rupture of the membranes and the premature gestation. *Am. J. Obstet. Gynecol.* **141**:508–515, 1981.
32. Garite, T. J., Freeman, R. K., Linzey, E. M., and Braly, P.: The use of amniocentesis in patients with premature rupture of membranes. *Obstet. Gynecol.* **54**:226–230, 1979.
33. Gibbs, R. S., Castillo, M. S., and Rodgers, P. J.: Management of acute chorioamnionitis. *Am. J. Obstet. Gynecol.* **136**:709–713, 1980.
34. Goldstein, A. S., Mangurten, H. H., Libretti, J. V., and Berman, A. M.: Lecithin/sphingomyelin ratio in amniotic fluid obtained vaginally. *Am. J. Obstet. Gynecol.* **138**:232–233, 1980.
35. Gorodeski, I. G., Paz, M., Insler, V., and Fishel, J.: Diagnosis of rupture of the fetal membranes by glucose and fructose measurements. *Obstet. Gynecol.* **53**:611–616, 1979.
36. Graham, R. J., Gilstrap, L. C., III, Lauth, J. C., Kodack-Garza, S., and Conaster, D. G.: Conservative management of patients with premature rupture of fetal membranes. *Obstet. Gynecol.* **59**:607–610, 1982.
37. Gunn, G. C., Mishell, D. R., and Morton, D. G.: Premature rupture of the fetal membranes: A review. *Am. J. Obstet. Gynecol.* **106**:469–483, 1970.
38. Habel, A. H., Sandor, G. S., Conn, N. K., and McCrae, W. M.: Premature rupture of membranes and effects of prophylactic antibiotics. *Arch. Dis. Child.* **47**:401–404, 1972.
39. Hawrylyshyn, P., Bernstein, P., Milligan, J. E., Soldin, S., Pollard, A., and Papsin, F. R.: Premature rupture of membranes: The role of C-reactive protein in the prediction of chorioamnionitis. *Am. J. Obstet. Gynecol.* **147**:240–246, 1983.
40. Iams, J. D., Talbert, M. L., Barrows, H., and Sachs, L.: Management of preterm preaturely ruptured membranes: A prospective randomized comparison of observation versus use of steroids and timed delivery. *Am. J. Obstet. Gynecol.* **151**:32–38, 1985.
41. Isherwood, D. M., McMurray, J. A., Campbell, C., and Jenkins, D. M.: Prediction of fetal pulmonary maturity from amniotic fluid obtained from the vagina after premature rupture of the membranes. A patient treated with dexamethasone. *Acta Obstet. Gynecol. Scand.* **60**:83–85, 1981.
42. Jewett, J. F.: Committee on maternal welfare. Prolonged rupture of the membranes. *N. Engl. J. Med.* **292**:752–753, 1975.
43. Johnson, J. W., Daikoku, N. H., Niebyl, J. R., Johnson, T. R., Jr., Khouzami, V. A., and Witter, F. R.: Premature rupture of the membranes andprolonged latency. *Obstet. Gynecol.* **57**:547–556, 1981.
44. Jones, M. D., Jr., Burd, L. I., Bowes, W. A., Jr., Battaglia, F. C., and Lubchenco, L. O.: Failure of association of premature rupture of membranes with respiratory-distress syndrome. *N. Engl. J. Med.* **292**:1253–1257, 1975.
45. Kappy, K. A., Cetrulo, C. L., Knuppel, R. A., Ingardia, C. J., Sbarra, A. J., Scerbo, J. C., and Mitchell, G. W.: Premature rupture of the membranes at term. A comparison of induced and spontaneous labors. *J. Reprod. Med.* **27**:29–33, 1982.
46. Kappy, K. A., Cetrulo, C. L., Knuppel, R. A., Ingardia, C. J., Sbarra, A. J., Scerbo, J. C., and Mitchell, G. W.: Premature rupture of the membranes: A conservative approach. *Am. J. Obstet. Gynecol.* **134**:655–661, 1979.
47. Koh, K. S., Chan, F. H., Manfared, A. H., Ledger,

W. J., and Paul, R. H.: The changing perinatal and maternal outcome in chorioamnionitis. *Obstet. Gynecol.* **53**:730–734, 1979.

48. Kuhn, R. J., Speirs, A. L., Pepperell, R. J., Eggers, T. R., Doyle, L. W., and Hutchison, A.: Betamethasone, albuterol, and threatened premature delivery: Benefits and risks. Study of 469 pregnancies. *Obstet. Gynecol.* **60**:403–408, 1982.
49. Larsen, J. W.: Premature amniorrhexis. *Obstet. Gynecol. Annu.* **8**:203–221, 1979.
50. Lavery, J. P. and Miller, C. E.: Deformation and creep in the human chorioamniotic sac. *Am. J. Obstet. Gynecol.* **134**:366–375, 1979.
51. Liggins, G. C.: Prenatal glucocorticoid treatment: Prevention of respiratory distress syndrome. Lung maturation and the prevention of hyaline membrane disease. Report of the 70th Ross Conference on pediatric research, Columbus, OH, 1976, pp. 97–105.
52. Mead, P. B. and Clapp, J. F.: The use of betamethasone and timed delivery in management of premature rupture of the membranes in preterm pregnancy. *J. Reprod. Med.* **19**:3–7, 1977.
53. Miller, J. M., Jr., Brazy, J. E., Gall, S. A., Crenshaw, M. C., Jr., and Jelovsek, F. R.: Premature rupture of the membranes: Maternal and neonatal infectious morbidity related to betamethasone and antibiotic therapy. *J. Reprod. Med.* **25**:173–177, 1980.
54. Miller, J. M., Pupkin, M. J., and Crenshaw, C.: Premature labor and premature rupture of the membranes. *Am. J. Obstet. Gynecol.* **132**:1–6, 1978.
55. Montanari, G. D., Grismondi, G. L., and Zonoio, L.: 3:4 benzpyriene-induced *in vitro* flourescence of fetal lipids in the diagnosis of ruptured membranes. *J. Obstet. Gynaecol. Br. Commonw.* **77**:148–150, 1970.
56. Morrison, J. C., Whybrew, W. D., Bucovaz, E. T., and Schneider, J. M.: Injection of corticosteroids into mother to prevent neonatal respiratory distress syndrome. *Am. J. Obstet. Gynecol.* **131**:358–366, 1978.
57. Morrison, L. and Wiseman, H. J.: Intra-amniotic injection of Evans blue dye (Letter) *Am. J. Obstet. Gynecol.* **113**:1147, 1972.
58. Naeye, R. L.: Factors that predispose to premature rupture of the fetal membranes. *Obstet. Gynecol.* **60**:93–98, 1982.
59. Naeye, R. L. and Peters, E. C.: Causes and consequences of premature rupture of fetal membranes. *Lancet* **1**:192–194, 1980.
60. Naeye, R. L. and Ross, S.: Coitus and chorioamnionitis: A prospective study. *Early Hum. Dev.* **6**:91–97, 1982.
61. Nimrod, C., Varela-Gittings, F., Machin, G., Campbell, D., and Wesenberg, R.: The effect of very prolonged membrane rupture on fetal development. *Am. J. Obstet. Gynecol.* **148**:540–543, 1984.
62. Nochimson, D. J., Petrie, R. H., Shah, B. L., Pampati, N., and Brunelle, D.: Comparison of conservative and dynamic management of premature rupture of membranes/premature labor syndrome. New approaches to the delivery of infants which may minimize the need for intensive care. *Clin. Perinatol.* **7**:17–31, 1979.
63. Papageorgiou, A. N., Desgranges, M. F., Masson, M., Colle, Shatz, R., and Gelfand, M. M.: The antenatal use of betamethasone in the prevention of respiratory distress syndrome: A controlled double-blind study. *Pediatrics* **63**:73–79, 1979.
64. Parry-Jones, E and Priya, S.: A study of the elasticity and tension of fetal membranes and of the relation of the area of the gestational sac to the area of the uterine cavity. *Br. J. Obstet. Gynaecol.* **83**:205–212, 1976.
65. Perkins, R. P.: The neonatal significance of selected perinatal events among infants of low birth weight. II. The infuence of ruptured membranes. *Am. J. Obstet. Gynecol.* **142**:7–16, 1982.
66. Plunkett, G. D.: Neonatal complications. *Obstet. Gynecol.* **41**:476–477, 1973.
67. Quirk, J. G., Raker, R. K., Petrie, R. H., and Williams, A. M.: The role of glucocorticoids, unstressful labor, and atraumatic delivery in the prevention of respiratory distress syndrome. *Am. J. Obstet. Gynecol.* **134**:768–771, 1979.
68. Richardson, C. J., Pomerance, J. J., Cunningham, M. D., and Gluck, L.: Acceleration of fetal lung maturation following prolonged rupture of the membranes. *Am. J. Obstet. Gynecol.* **118**:1115–1118, 1974.
69. Rochelson, B. L., Richardson, D. A., and Macri, J. N.: Rapid assay—possible application in the diagnosis of premature rupture of the membranes. *Obstet. Gynecol.* **62**:414–418, 1983.
70. Romem, Y. and Artal, R.: C-reactive protein as a predictor for chorioamnionitis in cases of premature rupture of the membranes. *Am. J. Obstet. Gynecol.* **150**:546–550, 1984.
71. Schmidt, P. L., Sims, M. E., Strassner, H. T., Paul, R. H., Mueller, E., and McCart, D.: Effect of antepartum glucocorticoid administration upon neonatal respiratory distress syndrome and perinatal infection. *Am. J. Obstet. Gynecol.* **148**:178–186, 1984.
72. Schreiber, J. and Benedetti, T.: Conservative management of preterm premature rupture of the fetal membranes in a low socioeconomic population. *Am. J. Obstet. Gynecol.* **136**:92–96, 1980.
73. Schutte, M. F., Treffess, P. E., Kloostrerman, G. J., and Soepatmi, S.: Management of premature rupture of membranes: The risk of vaginal examination to the infant. *Am. J. Obstet. Gynecol.* **146**:395–400, 1983.
74. Sell, E. J. and Harris, T. R.: Association of premature rupture of membranes with idiopathic respiratory distress syndrome. *Obstet. Gynecol.* **49**:167–169, 1977.
75. Skinner, S. J., Campos, G. A., and Liggins, G. C.: Collagen content of human amniotic membranes:

Effect of gestation length and premature rupture. *Obstet. Gynecol.* **57**:487–489, 1981.

76. Smith, R. P.: A technique for the detection of rupture of the membranes. A review and preliminary report. *Obstet. Gynecol.* **48**:172–176, 1976.
77. Stedman, C. M., Crawford, S., Staten, E., and Cherny, W. B.: Management of preterm premature rupture of membranes: Assessing amniotic fluid in the vagina for phosphatidyl- glycerol. *Am. J. Obstet. Gynecol.* **140**:34–38, 1981.
78. Steinman, G., Kleiner, G. J., and Greston, W. M.: Spontaneous rupture of membranes. Rapid strip tests for detection. *N.Y. State J. Med.* **79**:1849–1851, 1979.
79. Stubblefield, P. G. and Heyl, P. S.: Treatment of premature labor with subcutaneous terbutaline. *Obstet. Gynecol.* **59**:457–462, 1982.
80. Taeusch, H. W., Frigoletto, F., Kitzmiller, J., Avery, M. E., Hehre, A., Fromm, B., Lawson, E., and Neff, R. K.: Risk of respiratory distress syndrome after prenatal dexamethasone treatment. *Pediatrics* **63**:64–72, 1979.
81. Taylor, J. and Garite, T. J.: Premature rupture of membranes before fetal viability. *Obstet. Gynecol.* **64**:615–620, 1984.
82. Thibeault, D. W. and Emmanouilides, G. C.: Prolonged rupture of fetal membranes and decreased frequency of respiratory distress syndrome and patent ductus arteriosus in preterm infants. *Am. J. Obstet. Gynecol.* **129**:43–46, 1977.
83. Varner, M. W. and Galask, R. P.: Conservative management of premature rupture of the membranes. *Am. J. Obstet. Gynecol.* **140**:39–45, 1981.
84. Wilson, J. C., Levy, D. L., and Wilds, P. L.: Premature rupture of membranes prior to term—consequences of nonintervention. *Obstet. Gynecol.* **60**:601-606, 1982.
85. Wishart, M. M., Jenkins, D. T., and Knott, M. L.: Measuement of diamine oxidase activity in vaginal fluid—an aid to diagnosis of ruptured fetal membranes. *Aust. N.Z. J. Obstet. Gynaecol.* **19**:23–24, 1979.
86. Wolf, R. L. and Olinsky, A.: Prolonged rupture of fetal membranes and neonatal infections. *S. Afr. Med. J.* **50**:574–576, 1976.
87. Worthington, D., Maloney, A. H., and Smith, B. T.: Fetal lung maturity. I. Mode of onset of premature labor. Influence of premature rupture of the membranes. *Obstet Gynecol* **49**:275–279, 1977.
88. Yeast, J. D., Garite, T. J., and Dorchester, W.: The risks of amniocentesis in the management of premature rupture of the membranes. *Am. J. Obstet. Gynecol.* **149**:505–508, 1984.
89. Yoder, P. R., Gibbs, R. S., Blanco, J. D., Castaneda, Y. S., and St. Clair, P. J.: A prospective, controlled study of maternal and perinatal outcome after intra-amniotic infection at term. *Am. J. Obstet. Gynecol.* **145**:695–701, 1983.
90. Yoon, J. J. and Harper, R. G.: Observations on the relationship between duration of rupture of the membranes and the development of idiopathic respiratory distress syndrome. *Pediatrics* **52**:161–168, 1973.
91. Zlatnik, F. J., Cruikshank, D. P., Petzold, C. R., and Galask, R. P.: Amniocentesis in the identification of inapparent infection in preterm patients with premature rupture of the membranes. *J. Reprod. Med.* **29**:656–660, 1984.

18

PRETERM LABOR

ETIOLOGY

In the absence of a complication of gestation, preterm labor is most probably initiated by precocious activation of the system normally initiating parturition at term. Many of the complications of pregnancy may also induce premature stimulation of the same system. Central to our current understanding is the concept that the fetus and fetal tissues such as the placenta and membranes play a major role in the initiation of parturition. Although the exact mechanism of parturition is yet to be clearly defined, it should be viewed as a paracrine event involving interactions between mother and fetus, between different cells, and between different hormones and enzymes within the uterus. To explain parturition, one must consider not only the onset of uterine contractions, but also the complex changes in the connective tissue of the cervix which permit it to become distensible and to respond to the uterine activity.

Parturition in Animal Models

As with many enigmas in medicine, it has been extremely useful to study various animal species in order to gain insight into the human situation. The mechanisms of parturition have been most clearly defined in the sheep model, wherein an enhanced responsiveness of the fetal adrenal to fetal corticotropin results, near the end of gestation, in increased fetal cortisol secretion, which then leads to a series of events initiating labor.

Progesterone is essential for maintenance of pregnancy in various animal species. In some species, such as the rabbit, the corpus luteum is the source of progesterone throughout gestation, whereas in others such as the sheep and humans, the placenta takes over progesterone production after the first part of pregnancy. In sheep, the placenta synthesizes mainly progesterone throughout gestation with little estrogen being formed. However, the increased fetal cortisol secretion results in stimulation and activation of placental 17α-hydroxylase, 17-20-desmolase, and aromatase enzyme activities. These placental enzymatic changes lead to an increase in estrogen production and secretion and a decrease in progesterone formation and secretion. The resulting abrupt and marked alteration in the estrogen:progesterone ratio is followed by stimulation of prostaglandin synthesis by intrauterine tissues and parturition.[68,69,110]

Parturition in Women

The series of events leading to parturition in the sheep cannot be directly applied to an understanding of the onset of labor in humans. There are no significant changes in circulating concentrations of maternal estrogens or progesterone prior to parturition. Although some controversy exists concerning changes in maternal and fetal concentrations of cortisol prior to term which may affect maturation of various fetal tissues, the lack of significant 17α-hydroxylase in the human placenta prevents this mechanism from causing an abrupt change in the estrogen: progesterone ratio. However, the human placenta has an abundant supply of aromatizing enzymes to convert androgens to estrogen. Fetal adrenal dehydroisoandrosterone from the fetal zone of the adrenal may be converted to estrogen in the placenta.[104] Estrogen concentrations in maternal plasma rise throughout gestation without apparent abrupt change prior to the onset of labor. Thus, lack of a demonstrable change in the estrogen:progesterone ratio or withdrawal of progesterone, as reflected by peripheral plasma concentrations, has led to a consideration of local changes in steroid production or action within the uterus as a stimulus to parturition. In addition, prostaglandins are currently thought to play a pivotal role in most, if not all, mammalian species, including the human. Again, local changes in prostaglandin metabolism may be operative without being reflected in changes in peripheral plasma concentration.

Prostaglandins and Parturition

Prostaglandin (PG) synthesis and release are necessary for the initiation of parturition.[17,19,66] Both exogenously administered PGF_{2a} (PGF) and PGE_2 (PGE) stimulate uterine contractions at any stage of pregnancy. This stimulatory activity follows their administration by the intravenous, oral, intra-amniotic, or extraovular routes. Drugs such as aspirin or indomethacin, which inhibit the enzyme cyclooxygenase necessary for synthesis of prostaglandins, suppress preterm and term labor and prolong induction to abortion intervals. During labor, the concentrations of PGE and PGF and their metabolites are elevated in maternal plasma and amniotic fluid. Their obligatory precursor, arachidonic acid, is also elevated in amniotic fluid during labor and has been used successfully as an intra-amniotic abortifacient.

Mechanism of Action. It is likely that various prostaglandins affect all the tissues of the uterus and not just the myometrium. There is evidence to support prostaglandin action on other sites such as the blood vessels, the decidua, and the cervix.

The mechanisms of smooth muscle contractility and relaxation have been recently reviewed.[47] In essence, myosin light-chain kinase is the key regulatory enzyme which phosphorylates inactive myosin to permit its interaction with the active site of actin to form actomyosin and thus to induce smooth muscle contraction. The activity of myosin light-chain kinase is dependent on the protein calmodulin. Calmodulin is a calcium-sensitive enzyme which, upon binding with calcium, activates myosin light-chain kinase. Therefore, the intracellular concentration of free calcium is central to the myosin and actin interaction. Prostaglandins are thought to promote release of calcium from the sarcoplasmic reticulum and/or to enhance calcium ion transport across the cell membrane.

An important aspect of uterine contractility during labor is the integration of all the uterine muscle cells by cell-to-cell communications known as gap junctions.[34] Such cell-to-cell communication can permit the propagation of an electrical signal to synchronize the individual myometrial cells. The number of these gap junctions increases significantly at the time of parturition, both preterm and term, in various animal species and in humans. Formation of gap junctions is stimulated by estrogen and inhibited by progesterone. The role of PG in gap junction formation is currently not well defined. In the rat, progesterone levels begin to decrease a few days before parturition as estrogens and PGF begin to rise, followed by an increase in the number of gap junctions and then by parturition. However, simultaneous combined estrogen and indomethacin treatment, the latter inhibiting prostaglandin synthesis, increases gap junction formation in the rat. Inhibition of prostaglandin synthesis may decrease prostacyclin (PGI_2) which causes uterine relaxation, or may alter binding of steroids to their receptors, such as by decreasing the numbers or the binding affinity of progesterone receptors.

Prostaglandin Synthesis. The biochemistry and metabolism of the various prostaglandins have been well established. Interest with regard to parturition currently centers on prostaglandins of the two double-bond series. Prostaglandins are synthesized and metabolized quite rapidly, the initial step being the release of arachidonic acid from stored phospholipids by the action of phospholipases such as phospholipase A_2 and phospholipase C. Once there is a release of the substrate arachidonic acid, it is converted to prostaglandins of the two series by cyclooxygenase, an enzyme that appears to be activated by the presence of the substrate.

The Site of Prostaglandin Synthesis. The site of prostaglandin synthesis involved in parturition is an interaction of the amnion, chorion, and decidua. There is a significant decrease in the arachidonic acid content of phosphatidylethanolamine and phosphatidylinositol in amnion obtained during early labor as compared to before labor. The principal prostaglandin produced by amnion, with its very high concentration of cyclooxygenase activity, is PGE. PGE is not metabolized further by the amnion. In chorion, PGE is also formed, and in decidua approximately equal amounts of PGE and PGF are formed. In the chorion, there is significant activity of 15 hydroxyprostaglandin dehydrogenase which catalyzes conversion of prostaglandin to their metabolites.[17]

Control of Prostaglandin Synthesis. The inhibition of, or stimulus to, prostaglandin synthesis during gestation in humans is unknown. It is probable that specific substances of fetal origin inhibit prostaglandin synthesis during gestation until term approaches, when their activity decreases, and/or specific stimulators may increase at term.

Inhibition. Amniotic fluid contains an endogenous inhibitor of prostaglandin synthesis, the activity of which decreases at term. This activity inhibits the synthesis of prostaglandin from arachidonic acid.[100] More recently, two proteins which inhibit the release of arachidonic acid and PGF synthesis from dispersed endometrial cells have been found in amniotic fluid.[116] These proteins do not inhibit cyclooxygenase activity, but rather the release of arachidonic acid, the rate-limiting step in prostaglandin synthesis. The source and control of these proteins remains to be determined.

Stimulation. Enzymatic activities of phospholipases A_2 and C are increased in amnion as term approaches. Both enzymes are calcium-ion dependent.[10] Calcium may have a direct effect or may act indirectly by altering other enzymatic systems.

As amniotic fluid is in part composed of fetal urine and the fetus is involved with the onset of parturition, it is possible that the stimulant of prostaglandin synthesis is derived from the fetal kidney. Fetal urine significantly stimulates PGE production from dispersed human amnion cells, but not from myometrial, endometrial, or adipose dispersed cells in monolayer culture.[17]

Although there is still controversy as to whether oxytocin synthesis and release are increased prior to parturition, the increase in myometrial sensitivity to oxytocin can be explained by the increase in numbers of myometrial oxytocin receptors as term approaches in animals and humans.[32] Oxytocin also stimulates prostaglandin production by the myometrium and decidua. There would appear to be significant potential interaction between oxytocin, oxytocin receptors, and prostaglandins, in paracrine fashion.

The Cervix

Any consideration of parturition must include the cervix. Uterine contractions will not cause dilatation of the cervix unless the connective tissue of the cervix has undergone biochemical changes which increase its compliance or distensibility (see Chapter 7). The cervix remains unyielding throughout gestation so that the fetus may be retained in utero, yet, with parturition, it is suddenly changed to permit birth. The decrease in cervical resistance is independent of uterine activity at term in experimental animals.[108] In addition, oxytocin is a poor cervical ripening agent.

Estrogen, relaxin, and prostaglandins have all been implicated in the biochemical changes in the cervix prior to parturition, and all have been used clinically prior to induction of labor,[106] but the endogenous mechanisms responsible for these changes in the human remain to be identified. The fact that prostaglandin release from fibroblasts has been observed in inflammatory reactions, which are, in some ways, similar to that of cervical ripening, suggests a major role for prostaglandin in cervical ripening.[66]

DEFINITION OF PRETERM LABOR

The World Health Organization defines the upper limit of preterm birth as any delivery that occurs before 37 completed weeks of gestation, as calculated from the first day of the last menstrual period. The lower limit of a preterm birth has not been adequately addressed. However, as pregnancies that end before 20 completed weeks of gestation are classified as abortions, it is appropriate to define preterm birth as any birth occurring between 20 and 37 completed weeks, or between 114 and 259 days of gestation.

INCIDENCE–MORTALITY–MORBIDITY

The incidence of preterm birth varies widely, depending on the population that is being investigated. Since conception occurs in some patients with irregular menses, or who have recently used oral contraception, resulting in an overestimation of gestational age, the incidence of preterm delivery is probably underestimated. However, intrauterine growth retardation is a contributor to low-birth-weight infants. Failure to differentiate preterm births from growth-retarded low-birth-weight infants born after 37 completed weeks may lead to overestimation of the incidence of preterm birth.

The preterm delivery rate in New York was reported to be 7.6%, in one center in England as 5.1%, and in all of New Zealand as 6.7%.[33,83,98] A recent report for the United States, using birth registration data and excluding 20% of births from analysis, reported the preterm birth rate to be 3.55% in 1980, 2.97% in the white population, and 6.77% in the black population.[57] Unpublished information from five university centers currently studying preterm birth, with careful attention to the determination of gestational age using a number of criteria, reveals the preterm birth rate in their varied populations to range from 5% to 11% (Creasy, R. K.: Unpublished observations). The incidence of reported preterm birth has been relatively stable over the past two decades, with a few rare exceptions.

Preterm births now account for the majority of perinatal deaths in nonanomalous newborns. In England, 62% of perinatal deaths, and 85% of neonatal deaths not due to major anomalies, occurred in infants delivered between 22 and 37 weeks of gestation,[98] and in one report from the United States, 75% of perinatal deaths were associated with preterm delivery[33] Advances in neonatal care over the past 20 years have led to improved survival of preterm births. Many tertiary centers report close to 100% survival if delivery occurs after 32 completed weeks of gestation (Table 18-1). Most of the mortality associated with preterm birth occurs in newborns delivered between 20 and 32 completed weeks of gestation, who comprise approximately 30% of preterm births. It is important to stress that these survival rates are for babies born in centers with available neonatal intensive care and, therefore, are likely to be higher than the survival attained under all circumstances nationwide.

Due to increased survival rates for preterm infants, attention must also be focused on morbidity associated with preterm birth. Surprisingly, the actual incidence of anticipated

TABLE 18-1. SURVIVAL RATES OF PRETERM LIVEBIRTHS PER GESTATIONAL AGE (GA) AT BIRTH*

GA	Liveborns per GA Category	Birth weight† per GA Category	Survivors n	Survivors %
≦25	5	575 ± 170 g	0	0
26–27	16	884 ± 164 g	9	56
28–29	32	1211 ± 247 g	29	91
30–31	33	1468 ± 310 g	32	97
32–33	44	1831 ± 323 g	44	100
34	40	2157 ± 356 g	40	100
35	36	2420 ± 293 g	36	100

* Excluding maternal and fetal complications other than those related to preterm birth.

† Mean ± S. D.

Source: Konte, J. M., Holbrook, R. H., Jr., Laros, R. K., Jr., and Creasy, R. K.: Short-term neonatal morbidity associated with preterm birth and effect of a preterm birth prevention program on expected incidence of morbidity. *Am. J. Perinatol.* **3**:283–288, 1986.

TABLE 18-2. MORBIDITY RATES PER GESTATIONAL AGE (GA) AT BIRTH*

GA	26–27	28–29	30–31	32–33	34	35
n	16	32	33	34	40	36
ICN						
n	16	32	31	40	29	8
%	100%	100%	94%	91%	73%	22%
RDS						
n	13	19	10	13	9	1
%	81%	59%	30%	30%	23%	3%
PDA						
n	8	16	7	6	5	—
%	50%	50%	21%	14%	13%	—
Sepsis						
n	5	8	5	3	2	2
%	31%	25%	15%	7%	5%	6%
NEC						
n	4	2	2	1	—	—
%	25%	6%	6%	2%	—	—

GA = Completed weeks of gestation; ICN = Intensive care nursery admission; RDS = Respiratory distress syndrome; PDA = Patent ductus arteriosus; NEC = Necrotizing enterocolitis.

* Excluding maternal and fetal complications other than those related to preterm birth.

Source: Konte, J. M., Holbrook, R. H., Jr., Laros, R. K., Jr., and Creasy, R. K.: Short-term neonatal morbidity associated with preterm birth and effect of a preterm birth prevention program on expected incidence of morbidity. *Am. J. Perinatol.* **3**:283–288, 1986.

morbidity at a particular gestational age is not well established for two reasons. The first reason is that there has been a continuum of improving neonatal care and survival, and the second is that few reports have focused on morbidity associated only with preterm delivery, excluding other complications of pregnancy. One recent report of 206 inborn preterm infants, without any detectable maternal or fetal complications, is summarized in Tables 18-1 and 18-2.[60]

EPIDEMIOLOGY-ETIOLOGY

The various factors associated with preterm birth may be considered under the following categories.[4,45,86,107]

Medical History

The past reproductive performance correlates strongly with preterm birth. One of the major risk factors for preterm birth is a previous preterm birth. A history of the first birth being preterm is associated with a risk of recurrence of between 15% and 30%. The incidence rises significantly with two or more previous preterm births. The risk of repeating a preterm birth, depending on the previous outcomes of pregnancy, in more than 20,000 women having three births in a 10-year period in Norway, is summarized in Table 18-3. A number of previous reports have indicated an increased incidence of subsequent preterm delivery following one first trimester abortion, but when proper controls are introduced, there does not appear to be a significant risk. It is still uncertain whether or not multiple first trimester abortions are associated wih subsequent preterm labor and delivery. However, second trimester abortion is associated with subsequent preterm birth.

Three to 16% of preterm births are asso-

TABLE 18-3. THE RISK OF PRETERM BIRTH IN SUBSEQUENT BIRTHS

First Birth	Second Birth	Subsequent Preterm Birth (%)
Not preterm		4.4
Preterm		17.2
Not preterm	Not preterm	2.6
Preterm	Not preterm	5.7
Not preterm	Preterm	11.1
Preterm	Preterm	28.4

Source: Bakketeig, L. S. and Hoffman, H. J.: Epidemiology of preterm birth: Results from a longitudinal study of births in Norway. In: *Preterm Labor.* M. G. Elder and C. H. Hendricks (Eds.). London, Butterworths, 1981, pp. 17–46.

ciated with uterine anomalies, but the association of spontaneous preterm labor with a specific anomaly is unknown, because the incidence of pregnancy in women with uterine anomalies is not established. The incidence varies from 4% to 17% with a septate uterus to between 20% and 80% with other proven anomalies.[41] The T-shaped uterus that may be present in women exposed in utero to diethylstilbestrol is frequently associated with preterm birth, as is the uterus with postoperative synechiae.

Incompetence of the cervix due to an inherent defect or secondary to dilatation or cone biopsy can occur, but its incidence and its effect on preterm births are uncertain. Preterm delivery rates between 0 and 33% have been reported after cone biopsy of the cervix.

Spontaneous preterm birth is more likely to occur in women who have a history of previous renal disease such as pyelonephritis or recurrent urinary tract infections.

Socioeconomic Status

A strong correlation exists between preterm newborns and low socioeconomic status when the latter is defined on the basis of education or income. The components of low socioeconomic status that predispose to the increased incidence of preterm birth are poorly defined. The incidence of preterm birth is higher in women less than 20 years of age for both initial and subsequent pregnancies. The age group at highest risk is women over 35 years of age having their first pregnancy. The woman over 35 is not at increased risk if she had a previous pregnancy before age 35.

Nutritional status at the onset of gestation appears to influence the incidence of preterm delivery. Preterm deliveries are three times as frequent in women weighing less than 50 kg as compared to those weighing 57 kg or more at the start of pregnancy.[2] Nutritional status during gestation in women whose preconceptional status is normal appears to affect fetal growth more than gestational age.[61]

Behavior During Pregnancy

An increasing body of evidence from Europe demonstrates a relationship between type of occupation, work status, and spontaneous preterm labor.[45,72,86] Women at particular risk are those involved in service and manufacturing work or jobs likely to produce fatigue or high psychological stress (Table 18-4).

Cigarette smoking increases the risk of both poor fetal growth and spontaneous preterm births. The risk increases with the amount of smoking.[75] Alcohol and narcotic addiction are associated with low-birth-weight infants, but it is not clear whether this effect is on fetal growth or gestational age.

Numerous anecdotal reports suggest that psychosocial trauma may trigger spontaneous preterm labor. Prospective studies have also shown an association between adverse major life events in the third trimester and preterm labor and delivery.[82]

Complications of Pregnancy

One of the major contributors to spontaneous preterm birth is the multiple gestation. Thirty

TABLE 18-4. PERCENT DISTRIBUTION AND RELATIVE RISK OF ONE OR MORE PRETERM BIRTHS BY MOTHER'S OCCUPATION. (BASED ON 30,979 MOTHERS WITH THEIR FIRST THREE SINGLETON BIRTHS IN NORWAY, 1967–1976.)

Mother's Occupation	Percentage of Mothers	Relative Risk of 1 Preterm Birth	Relative Risk of 2 or 3 Preterm Births
Housewife or unemployed	60.3%	0.78	0.59
Agriculture/fishing	3.3%	0.85	0.62
Technical/professional	12.1%	1.04	0.99
Clerical/sales	13.9%	1.21	1.29
Services	6.7%	1.43	2.15
Manufacturing	3.8%	1.38	2.47
TOTAL	100.0%	1.00	1.00

Source: Hoffman, H. J. and Bakketeig, L. G.: Risk factors associated with the occurrence of preterm birth. *Clin. Obstet. Gynecol.* **27**:539–552, 1984.

to 50% of twin gestations deliver before 36 completed weeks of gestation.

Gross fetal anomalies, particularly multiple anomalies involving the central nervous system, are accompanied by an increased possibility of preterm labor. This is particularly true of those anomalies that are accompanied by polyhydramnios (30–40% risk of preterm labor) or oligohydramnios. Renal agenesis is associated with a 60% preterm delivery rate. Anencephaly may prolong pregnancy, but if associated with polyhydramnios, preterm labor is likely.

Antepartum hemorrhage, whether from placenta previa or abruption of the placenta, carries the highest association with preterm delivery in some reports. First trimester bleeding also increases the risk of preterm labor in that pregnancy.[45] The association of advancing parity and preterm labor noted in cross-sectional data is not confirmed in longitudinal analyses. Although hypertensive disease and preeclampsia may lead to an increased incidence of indicated preterm delivery, the risk of spontaneous preterm labor is not increased. Diabetes mellitus does not predispose to preterm labor unless polyhydramnios is present. Hyperthyroidism, hepatitis, and obstetrical cholestasis have been suggested as additional risk factors for preterm labor, but the exact risk with these factors is currently poorly defined. Abdominal surgery during the latter half of gestation is usually associated with excessive uterine activity, which in some patients may progress to preterm labor. Inadvertent elective preterm delivery still occurs.

There appears to be little question that some cases of preterm labor with intact membranes are caused by intrauterine infection, but the incidence, specific high-risk organisms, and pathogenesis are relatively undefined. Colonization of the vagina with such organisms as group B streptococcus, *Chlamydia trachomatis*, mycoplasmas, or various anaerobes may be associated with preterm labor. However, a statistically significant correlation between bacterial colonization of the vagina, placenta, and amniotic fluid and subsequent preterm labor remains to be defined.[91] Infectious organisms may also enter the intrauterine environment from transplacental passage from the maternal bloodstream. Examples of this etiology of preterm labor are infections with *Listeria monocytogenes*, mycobacteria, and *Treponema pallidum*. Viruses such as cytomegalovirus, herpes, rubella, hepatitis, and smallpox, and protozoans such as *Toxoplasma gondii* and *Plasmodium falciparum* have also been indicted.[91,93]

Asymptomatic bacteriuria associated with underlying renal disease, or progressing to pyelonephritis, is associated with an increased preterm delivery rate, but the mechanism by which premature labor is stimulated is unknown. Maternal systemic disease such as untreated bacterial pneumonia and acute appendicitis with sepsis or peritonitis also increases the possibility of preterm labor.

PREDICTION OF PRETERM LABOR

Ideally, with preterm labor and delivery, as with any major public health problem, it is preferable to prevent the problem rather than to try to treat the problem. It is necessary to be able to predict with a high degree of discrimination whether preterm labor will occur in a given pregnancy so that some prevention modality, such as behavior modification (i.e., decrease in physical activity) or administration of a prophylactic tocolytic agent, may be instituted. The early signs of preterm labor may be so subtle that the process is not recognized until the cervix is widely dilated or the membranes are ruptured (an occurrence in 30–40% of patients at the time of diagnosis of preterm labor). The result is that only 10–20% of patients are candidates for the use of tocolytic drugs.[74,107] One other potential way of achieving a reduction in preterm births would therefore be to increase the number of patients who are candidates for treatment by improving the early diagnosis. The ideal group to observe closely would be those at increased risk of preterm labor.

Prediction Systems

Risk Scoring. Risk-scoring systems have developed with the goal of predicting whether spontaneous preterm labor will occur in a specific individual. Unfortunately, many of the reports have not differentiated between indicated and spontaneous preterm births in their analyses, or they have included premature rupture of the membranes as a risk factor. Few investigators have evaluated the systems prospectively in a population that has not been exposed to some prevention modality.

One of the first attempts to predict preterm labor using a large number of factors, such as socioeconomic factors, reproductive performance, and the status of the current pregnancy, was published in 1969.[85] This approach could predict up to 75% of preterm births, but approximately 40% of the population at large was placed in the at-risk category. The accuracy of prediction was improved by rescoring later in pregnancy. A modification of this system has been studied prospectively in a population that was not treated with any prevention methods (Table 18-5).[23] Approximately 9% of patients were identified as high risk at their initial visit. The number increased to 13% at the repeat screening. The system identified 44% (sensitivity) of all subsequent spontaneous preterm births by initial screening and 64% by using a repeat screening. However, only 30% of high-risk patients delivered preterm. The importance of the past reproductive history in predicting preterm labor was clearly demonstrated. The high-risk group contributed to only 31% of primigravid spontaneous preterm births, but to 77% of multigravid spontaneous preterm births. These results are generally similar to other reports. It is unlikely that further refinements in using epidemiologic factors will improve prediction. It is necessary to determine whether or not biochemical or biophysical means of predicting preterm labor can improve the discrimination of the risk-scoring indices.

Biochemical Predictors. Biochemical predictors of preterm labor have been suggested by numerous authors. Particular attention has been focused on maternal serum estradiol or progesterone concentrations. However, weekly measurement of estradiol and progesterone has proved to be of no value.[11] Although there is evidence of a central role of prostaglandins in the initiation of parturition, there are, at present, no reports documenting an increase in serum prostaglandins or in their metabolites prior to the onset of preterm labor. There has been a suggestion that maternal serum alpha-

TABLE 18-5. SYSTEM FOR DETERMINING RISK OF SPONTANEOUS PRETERM DELIVERY*

Points Assigned	Socioeconomic Factors	Previous Medical History	Daily Habits	Aspects of Current Pregnancy
1	Two children at home Low socioeconomic status	Abortion x 1 Less than 1 year	Works outside home	Unusual fatigue
2	Maternal age 20 years or 40 years Single parent	Abortion x 2	Smokes more than 10 cigarettes per day	Gain of less than 5 kg by 32 weeks
3	Very low socioeconomic status Height 150 cm Weight 45 kg	Abortion x 3	Heavy or stressful work Long, tiring trip	Breech at 32 weeks Weight loss of 2 kg Head engaged at 32 weeks Febrile illness
4	Maternal age 18 years	Pyelonephritis		Bleeding after 12 weeks Effacement Dilation Uterine irritability
5		Uterine anomaly Second trimester abortion DES exposure Cone biopsy		Placenta previa Hydramnios
10		Preterm delivery Repeated second trimester abortion		Twins Abdominal surgery

*Score is computed by adding the number of points given any item. The score is computed at the first visit and again at 22–26 weeks' gestation. A total score of 10 or more places patient at high risk for spontaneous preterm delivery.

Source: Adapted from Creasy, R. K., Gummer, B. A., and Liggins, G. C.: A system for predicting spontaneous preterm birth. *Obstet. Gynecol.* **55**:692–695, 1980. Reprinted with permission from the American College of Obstetricians and Gynecologists.

fetoprotein measurements are abnormally high at 16–18 weeks of gestation in women destined to enter preterm labor, but further confirmation is necessary.

Biophysical Predictors. Biophysical predictors of preterm labor such as alterations in the cervix or patterns of uterine activity have also been used in attempts to predict preterm labor. If effacement occurs before 35 weeks of gestation, up to 30% of patients will deliver before term.[117] Although the degree of cervical dilatation may be related to the onset of labor, its usefulness in predicting preterm labor has been questioned.[3] Early engagement of the presenting part may also be a predictive sign.[114] It appears that early cervical effacement or dilatation, or engagement of the presenting part may help predict preterm labor in selected patients, but the usefulness of these evaluations to predict preterm labor on a population basis remains to be determined. These evaluations in regard to the early diagnosis of preterm labor are discussed later.

The total amount of uterine activity increases as gestation advances. Two specific types of uterine contraction pattern are encountered. The first is a high-frequency, low-amplitude pattern. The second is characterized by high-amplitude contractions which become more frequent as pregnancy progresses. Diurnal rhythmicity observed in the primate has yet to be fully evaluated in the human. An alteration in baseline uterine activity days to weeks before the onset of established preterm labor has been described.[7,53] In ambulatory patients using a portable tocodynamometer, the frequency of contractions was significantly greater in women who subsequently developed preterm labor than in women who later delivered at term (Fig. 18-1a). This difference was apparent in many patients several weeks before the onset of labor. There also appears to be a difference in baseline uterine activity between singleton and multiple gestations. Twin gestations display significantly more uterine activity than singletons do; the activity increases as term approaches (Fig. 18-1b).[54] Further characterization of uterine activity is necessary before it can be determined whether monitoring of uterine activity can predict preterm labor with sufficient specificity and sensitivity to warrant prophylaxis in a given patient.

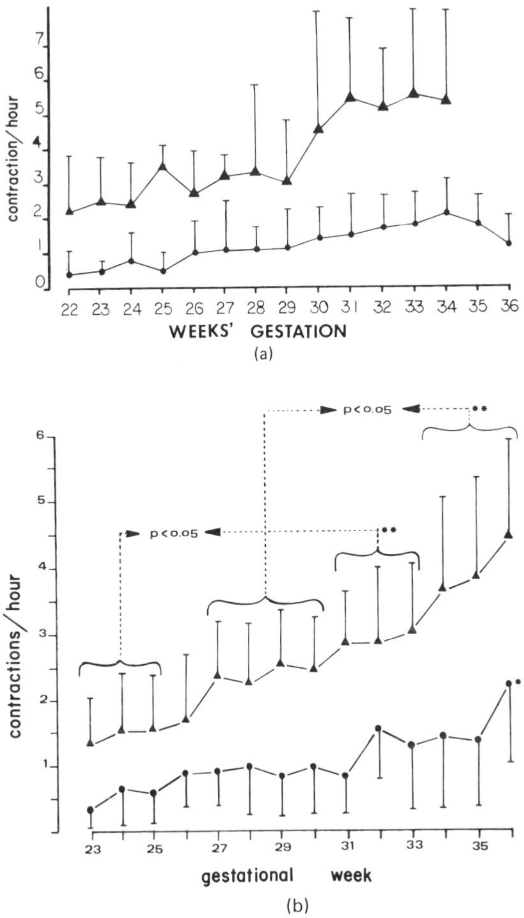

Figure 18-1. (a) Frequency of contractions during pregnancy in patients having preterm labor (▲) and patients having term labor (•). Mean ± S.D. From: Katz, M., Newman, R. B., and Gill, P. J.: Assessment of uterine activity in ambulatory patients at high risk of preterm labor and delivery. *Am. J. Obstet. Gynecol.*, **154**:44–47, 1986. (b) Frequency of contractions in ambulatory single ton (•) and twin (▲) gestations, delivery at term. Mean ± S.D. From: Newman, R. B., Gill, P. J., and Katz, M.: Uterine activity during pregnancy in ambulatory patients. comparison of singleton and twin gestations. *Am. J. Obstet. Gynecol.*, **154**:530–531, 1986.

PREVENTION OF PRETERM LABOR

The difficulty in accurately predicting preterm labor has resulted in difficulty in evaluating methods of preventing spontaneous preterm labor. The majority of prevention modalities have been assessed in multiple gestations, and studies in twin gestations are not necessarily applicable to the singleton gestation.

Bed Rest

One of the most widely held views is that bed rest prevents the initiation of preterm labor. Although several reports have suggested that bed rest is effective in preventing preterm labor in twin pregnancies,[59,89] its value has yet to be validated in prospective controlled twin pregnancy trials[77,114] or in singleton gestations. If bed rest is to be of value in decreasing mortality, it should be instituted by 24–25 weeks of gestation. Surprisingly, bed rest has even been shown to increase the incidence of preterm delivery in a recent prospective trial of twin gestations.[101]

Cervical Cerclage

The placement of an encircling suture around the proximal cervix is accepted by most obstetricians as appropriate treatment for the patient with a classical history of incompetent cervix. Cerclage is of no value as prophylaxis against preterm labor in singleton [64,99] or in multiple[114] gestations (Table 18-6). If anything, controlled trials show a trend of an increase in preterm labor, use of tocolytics, and painful contractions in patients with a cerclage. If a cerclage is placed, prostaglandins are elevated at least during the time that the surgery is performed.[9]

Tocolytics–Steroids

As beta-adrenergics are utilized for inhibiting established preterm labor, it is appropriate to consider their use in prophylaxis against preterm labor. Prospective studies using low-dose beta-adrenergic drugs in twin gestations have shown no beneficial effect.[84] However, a retrospective trial in which the beta-adrenergic was administered in higher doses (doses resulting in maternal tachycardia) demonstrated a decrease in preterm births. Beta-adrenergic agonists also decrease the incidence of recurrent preterm labor.[15,22] The role of beta-adrenergics as prophylactic agents needs further clarification. If they are used, the dosage should be titrated against maternal pulse rate as well as against uterine activity.

The previously held idea that parturition is preceded by withdrawal of progesterone naturally led to trials to test the possibility that treatment with exogenous progesterone could prevent preterm labor. Patients at risk of preterm delivery on the basis of a history of two abortions, two preterm births, or a combination of abortion and preterm birth were given either weekly injections of 17α-hydroxyprogesterone caproate or no treatment. The preliminary results showed no births before 36 weeks in the treatment group versus an incidence of 41% in the no-treatment group. When the study was continued in a noncontrolled manner, 24% of patients receiving treatment delivered preterm.[49,50] This incidence of preterm birth is that expected in the population selected. A more recent study of women chosen and treated in a similar fashion reported that preterm birth occurred in 14 of 37 (38%) controls versus 5 of 31 (16%) patients in the treatment group.[118] Other studies have not been encouraging. A prospective double-blind study in 168 high-risk patients showed no benefit,[39] and no benefit was shown when the study was conducted on twin pregnancies.[38] In addition, no benefit has been shown when progesterone is used as prophylaxis against preterm labor in women undergoing abdominal surgery during pregnancy.[44] The use of progesterone to inhibit established preterm labor is of no benefit, nor does progesterone treatment affect the duration of gestation when used after 36 weeks. Thus, the use of these agents as prophylaxis against preterm labor is still very questionable at best.

Antibiotics

The relation between infection and preterm labor, although poorly defined, is well estab-

TABLE 18-6. RESULTS OF TRIAL TO EVALUATE CERCLAGE AS MEANS OF PREVENTING PRETERM BIRTH

	Cerclage (%)	No Cerclage (%)
Admission to hospital (excluding cerclage or birth)	32	17
Oral tocolytics	47	30
Preterm birth	6.7	5.5

Source: Lazar, P., Guegun, S., Dreyfus, F., Pontonnier, G., and Papiernik, E.: Multicentered controlled trial of cervical cerclage in women at moderate risk of preterm delivery. *Br. J. Obstet. Gynaecol.* **91**:731–735, 1984.

lished in some patients. The demonstration that certain organisms in the vaginal flora exhibit high phospholipase A_2 activity,[6] which could theoretically lead to prostaglandin synthesis by the membranes and trigger labor, led to the suggestion that antibiotic treatment could reverse this potential pathogenesis. Random treatment of nonbacteriuric patients with tetracycline daily, as part of a study of bacteriuria in pregnancy, resulted in fewer preterm births and more completed weeks of gestation in the treatment group.[28] These results are compatible with the theory that antibiotic therapy may have an effect against organisms in the vaginal flora that might trigger preterm labor. However, prospective trials will be necessary before any conclusions concerning this possibility can be established.

Coitus

There are several suggestions of an association between coitus and preterm labor. It is also possible that coitus may contribute to the pathogenesis of intrauterine infection. It is known that the uterus contracts with orgasmic activity and that semen contains prostaglandins, with the suggestion that these mechanisms may lead to preterm labor. Since the majority of pregnant women continue to have coitus and only 5–10% experience preterm labor, the association needs clarification before cessation of coitus in pregnancy should be recommended. Cessation of coitus may be recommended between 20 and 36 weeks in patients at very high risk, such as women with two or three previous preterm births, but such routine advice is not warranted. Another approach would be to have patients monitor themselves for regular uterine contractions some 2–3 hours after coitus and to seek prompt medical advice if regular contractions are present at that time.

EARLY DETECTION OF PRETERM LABOR

As the status of preventing preterm labor is not encouraging at the present time, attention must also be directed at preventing preterm birth by the inhibition and arrest of preterm labor by the use of tocolytic drugs. The efficacy of these drugs is minimal if the cervix is completely effaced or more than 3–4 cm dilated, or if the membranes are not intact when therapy is begun. In addition, a significant reduction in the incidence of preterm birth is unlikely if only 10–20% of patients are candidates for treatment.[21] Therefore, every attempt must be made to detect preterm labor early in its course.

Symptoms

Symptoms of preterm labor are often so subtle that they are not recognized by the patient or physician until labor and cervical dilatation are far advanced. In a recent questionnaire evaluation of 100 women in established preterm labor, with uterine contractions occurring at least every 4–5 minutes, only 45 of the patients recognized that they were having contractions at least once every 10 minutes and only 55% of these described the contractions as painful.[36] The early symptoms of labor are listed in Table 18-7. Uterine contractions or menstrual-like cramps are the most frequently reported symptoms, but they may not be reported or may be reported as occurring only once or twice per hour. Constant rather than intermittent backache or pelvic pressure is reported by one-fourth of patients. Increased vaginal discharge, frequently mucoid in nature, changed in color, or pink- or red-stained, is reported by one-third to one-half of patients. Urinary frequency is also significantly increased. The frequency of symptoms does not appear to be different between primigravid and multigravid women. The presence of these symptoms indicates the need for close observation of the patient.

Preterm Birth Prevention Programs

Preterm birth prevention programs have been developed with initial encouraging results.[23,43,86] In general, these programs include special education of the patient, increased awareness by the health care team of the insidious symptoms of preterm labor, and prompt treatment once a diagnosis of preterm labor is made. It is important for patients to receive antenatal care by

TABLE 18-7. EARLY SYMPTOMS OF PRETERM LABOR

- Uterine contractions
- Menstrual/intestinal-like cramps
- Constant backache
- Constant pelvic pressure
- Increased vaginal discharge
- Blood-stained vaginal discharge

midgestation if these programs are to be effective.

The specific components of one program[43] involve (1) weekly visits for patients at high risk of preterm labor after 20 weeks of gestation or as soon as the increased risk is recognized; (2) education of the patient concerning the problems and symptoms of preterm labor; (3) education in self-detection of regular but usually painless contractions by uterine palpation twice a day, or if symptoms occur, or after coitus (the portable home tocodynamometer recorder may be used in the future); (4) weekly evaluation of the cervix to detect any significant change in consistency, position, effacement, or dilatation, or a change in the station of the presenting part; (5) a liberal policy of direct patient observation and brief uterine monitoring for any regular uterine activity or increased vaginal mucoid or pink discharge; and (6) prompt treatment of preterm labor. Preliminary results of this approach include an increased number of patients who are candidates for treatment, a reduction of more than 50% in preterm births, and a reduction of approximately 70% in perinatal morbidity and mortality.[21,60] The ability to decrease preterm birth in other obstetrical populations is currently being assessed in multicenter trials in order to determine the limitations of this approach in different obstetrical populations.

There has been concern that repeated digital evaluation of the cervix may stimulate uterine activity and preterm labor because vaginal examination in pregnancy has been reported to increase prostaglandin metabolite concentrations in the maternal circulation shortly after examination.[78] In addition, there is a concern that the cervical examination may increase the incidence of infection or bleeding. These issues have been studied in 133 preterm labor patients who had received regular cervical examinations as part of a preterm birth prevention program.[46] The incidence of chorioamnionitis, postpartum endometritis, and ruptured membranes was not increased as compared to other patients experiencing preterm labor but not receiving cervical evaluations. The onset of preterm labor which occurred within 7 days of a cervical examination was not temporally associated with the preceding examination (Fig. 18-2). Preterm labor was diagnosed initially in approximately 18% of patients by the weekly cervical evaluation.

DIAGNOSIS OF PRETERM LABOR

Clinical trials of various tocolytic drugs in patients diagnosed, on the basis of regular uterine

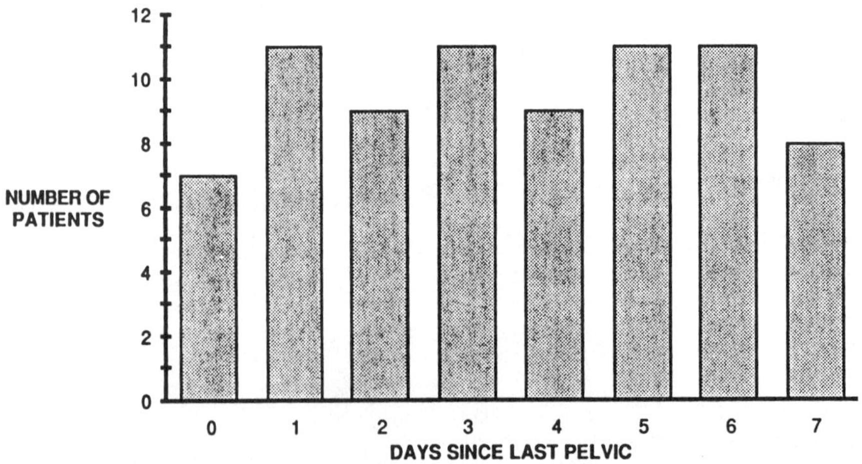

Figure 18-2. Histogram of the number of preterm labor patients experiencing the onset of preterm labor on each of seven days following the last weekly cervical examination prior to preterm labor. The distribution is not significantly different from a random distribution, indicating that the cervical examination did not stimulate preterm labor. From: Holbrook, R. H., Jr., Falcon, J., Herron, M., Lirette, M., Laros, R. L., and Creasy, R. K.: Evaluation of the weekly cervical examination in a preterm birth prevention program. Submitted for publication.

TABLE 18-8. SUGGESTED CRITERIA FOR A DIAGNOSIS OF PRETERM LABOR

Gestational age—20–36 weeks
AND
Regular uterine contractions
AND either
- Ruptured membranes
- Cervical change
- Dilatation ≧2 cm
- Effacement 80%
- Absence of fetal breathing movements

contractions, as being in preterm labor demonstrated the value of placebo treatment in 30–50% of patients. In patients admitted with a diagnosis of preterm labor based only on uterine activity, who were initially treated with only hydration and morphine, only 45% had persistent uterine activity which necessitated treatment with a tocolytic agent.[112] It is doubtful that transient hydration and sedation would stop established preterm labor. If regular uterine contractions are associated with cervical change,the placebo effect is minimized. The suggested criteria for a diagnosis of preterm labor are listed in Table 18-8. Because elevations in prostaglandins in the fetal circulation inhibit fetal breathing movements, the absence of fetal breathing movements as detected by ultrasound examination may help to diagnose preterm labor.[18] Nineteen of 20 patients admitted with suspected preterm labor, in whom fetal breathing movements were not detected, delivered within 48 hours. Twenty-five of 34 patients in whom fetal breathing movements were present delivered at least more than one week later, but seven patients developed spontaneous rupture of the membranes. These initial results are encouraging in regard to finding a more accurate method of diagnosing preterm labor, particularly because the absence of fetal breathing movements seemed to indicate true preterm labor. Ultrasonic evaluation of the cervix to evaluate cervical length, thickness of the anterior lower uterine segment, and dilatation of the endocervical may also be of assistance.[5]

MANAGEMENT OF PRETERM LABOR

Initial Evaluation

The first step in evaluating the patient at risk for possible preterm delivery is to place the patient at bed rest and to initiate continuous fetal heart and uterine activity monitoring. If the membranes are intact, the cervix should be evaluated digitally to establish a baseline. The history and physical examination are then completed in an effort to identify any conditions present which may have initiated the preterm labor or any fetal or maternal conditions that would contraindicate tocolytic therapy or that would affect the type of tocolytic to be chosen.

A urinary analysis and culture should be obtained because of the frequent association of asymptomatic urinary tract infection. Some have advocated that cultures of the vaginal and cervical flora be obtained, but the value of this procedure is unproven. A positive herpes or beta hemolytic streptococcus culture might affect future obstetrical or neonatal management should the membranes rupture or the preterm labor progress (see Chapter 17). If a fever of unknown origin is present, amniocentesis should be done and a gram stain and culture of the amniotic fluid performed. The presence of bacteria on the gram stain is highly correlated with a positive culture. Although preterm labor may be caused by chorioamnionitis, in an otherwise asymptomatic patient, routine amniocentesis in all preterm labor patients is not indicated.[113]

If the cervix is uneffaced and not dilated, tocolytic treatment is not indicated. Hydration with 500 cc of intravenous fluids, sedation, and bed rest are frequently associated with cessation of uterine activity. If uterine contractions persist, but the cervix remains unchanged, frequent cervical evaluation is warranted so that occult advanced cervical change does not occur. Treatment is indicated once the diagnosis is established according to the guidelines noted above.

Contraindications to tocolytic pharmacologic treatment are either absolute or relative. Absolute contraindications include chorioamnionitis, severe fetal growth retardation, fetal anomaly incompatible with life, fetal death, severe pregnancy-induced hypertension, and severe hemorrhage. Relative contraindications, in which tocolytic treatment might be used with very close patient observation, include mild hypertensive disorders, mild abruptio placentae with normal uterine tonus and normal fetal heart rate, placenta previa without significant hemorrhage, fetal anomaly compatible with life, mild fetal growth retardation depending on gestational age, and fetal distress as indicated by variable decelerations in the presence of normal amniotic fluid volume. Maternal heart disease, hyperthyroidism, and diabetes mellitus may affect selection of the tocolytic drug, because the beta-adrenergics are relatively contraindicated in these conditions.

Tocolytic treatment is usually not indicated if the cervix is more than 4 cm dilated. Successful tocolysis is not likely under these conditions.[97] However, if the gestation is at the critical juncture of 24–26 weeks of gestation, delay of delivery for 1–2 weeks significantly improves perinatal results.[60] Tocolytic treatment may occasionally arrest cervical dilatation even when the cervix is 4 cm dilated, particularly in twin pregnancies. A careful analysis of the potential costs and benefits in an individual patient may thus make tocolytic attempts prudent.

Pharmacologic Tocolysis

The agents currently in use clinically include the beta-adrenergic drugs and magnesium sulfate. Ethanol, previously used extensively, has fallen from favor due to the necessity for maternal inebriation. Also, retrospective studies comparing a beta-adrenergic drug with intravenous ethanol demonstrated a higher incidence of low Apgar scores, respiratory distress syndrome, and neonatal demise in infants of ethanol-treated mothers. The adverse outcomes were mainly confined to newborns delivered within 12 hours of maternal treatment.[120] There are only minimal results published in regard to prostaglandin synthetase inhibitors and calcium antagonists, which should be considered experimental at this time. There is no sound evidence to support the use of narcotics or sedatives in the treatment of established preterm labor, even though they may be used to differentiate true from false preterm labor.[112] They may also be useful in dealing with the anxiety generated by the possibility of preterm delivery, but ideally should not be used if preterm delivery is likely to occur within hours after their use because of potential neonatal depression.

The efficacy of tocolytic drugs in delaying delivery for 1–3 days appears well established, but their efficacy in preventing preterm births is still controversial.[42,58] Lack of consistent definitions of tocolytic success, different definitions of preterm labor, lack of randomization, and variations in dosage make comparison and evaluation of tocolytic drugs difficult.

Beta-Adrenergic Agonists. A number of beta-adrenergic agents are in clinical use. This class of tocolytic drugs is the most widely used to inhibit preterm labor. The beta-adrenergic compounds used for tocolysis include isoxsuprine, hexoprenaline, fenoterol, orciprenaline, ritodrine, salbutamol, and terbutaline.[24,115]

Mechanism of Action. The beta-adrenergic agents which are used clinically are derivatives of epinephrine that have been formulated in attempts to maximize the beta$_2$-adrenergic effects on the uterus, although they all have some beta$_1$-adrenergic activity. The beta-adrenergic agonists used for tocolysis interact with receptors located on the cell membrane, resulting in activation of the enzyme adenylate cyclase. This enzyme catalyzes the conversion of adenosine triphosphate (ATP) to cyclic adenosine monophosphate (cAMP) within the cell.[109] The increase in intracellular cAMP results in activation of a cAMP-dependent protein kinase that phosphorylates several proteins. Relaxation of smooth muscle is achieved by (1) the protein kinase activation, resulting in phosphorylation of membrane proteins which may be responsible for decreasing intracellular free calcium, and (2) the protein kinase phosphorylating myosin light-chain kinase, thus reducing the phosphorylation of myosin and preventing its interaction with action that is necessary for smooth muscle shortening.[47,95]

Pharmacology. The metabolism of the clinically available beta-adrenergic tocolytics is probably different from that of endogenous catecholamines, because the former are not substrates for catecholamine-0-methyl transferase. Minimal information is available about their binding to proteins. Available information indicates that clinical beta-adrenergic tocolytics are excreted unaltered or as conjugates by the kidneys. The degree of substitution on the amino group of the side chain as well as the presence of hydroxy groups in the three and five positions increases beta$_2$ activity. Placental transfer depends on protein binding, fat solubility, and equilibrium constants. Minimal information is available concerning these issues, except that available data indicate that some agents such as ritodrine and terbutaline cross into the fetus, whereas fenoterol and hexoprenaline probably cross the placenta to a lesser degree.

The concentration of ritodrine in maternal blood increases linearly with increasing infusion rates, with the concentrations varying to some degree from patient to patient, at least at low infusion rates.[16] At the end of an infusion, there is an initial rapid half-life of 5–10 minutes, followed by a second-phase half-life of 1.5–2.5 hours, followed by a more protracted third phase. Oral administration of ritodrine or salbutamol produces maximal serum concentrations in 30–60 minutes. Following oral administration, there is an initial half-life of 1–2 hours followed by a 10–12 hour decay, with wide variability. The bioavailability after oral administration is approximately 30% of that following intravenous usage.[24]

The increase in maternal heart rate following ritodrine infusion is reported to be linearly related to the log of the ritodrine concentration, but considerable variability is present. Tachyphylaxis of the heart rate response with continued beta-adrenergic infusions has been reported.[16] This could simply be a reflection of initially high endogenous catecholamine release due to patient anxiety or could be due to desensitization or down-regulation of receptors secondary to continuous agonist exposure such as that which has been noted in other systems.[65] Continuous exposure of perfused human myometrial strips to beta agonists in vitro results in initial inhibition of contractions which gradually return, whereas intermittent exposure maintains relative relaxation.[55] Because none of the beta-adrenergic tocolytics are pure beta$_2$ agonists, there is usually some component of beta$_1$ stimulation as well as beta$_2$ stimulation in sites other than the uterus (Table 18-9).

Efficacy. The efficacies of the different beta-adrenergic tocolytics are quite comparable. Little evidence supports the superiority of one versus another. There is little question that these drugs can delay delivery for 1–3 days, but the evidence for their ability to decrease preterm births is still inconclusive. Some studies show definite benefit and others do not.[58,112] With these drugs, delay of delivery at a critical time in gestation is likely to improve perinatal outcome.

Clinical Use. Prior to initiation of intravenous beta-adrenergic tocolysis, the usual method of initial treatment consists of the patient being weighed, placed on bed rest in the lateral decubitus position, and an intravenous infusion established with a solution of 5% dextrose in water. Fetal heart rate and uterine activity are recorded continuously. Baseline determinations of hematocrit, glucose, potassium, and colloid osmotic pressure are obtained and repeated every 6–12 hours while intravenous therapy is being used. Intake and output should be recorded. Total fluid intake should be between 1500 and 2500 cc per 24 hours. The lungs should be auscultated every 8–12 hours, searching for any evidence of early pulmonary edema. The beta-adrenergic drug is usually diluted in normal saline and infused into the main intravenous infusion line near its entry into the skin.

The initial intravenous dose utilized is the lowest recommended by the manufacturer. The infusion rate is increased every 10–30 minutes, depending on the uterine response and any adverse maternal side effects. The infusion rate should not be elevated further if maternal pulse rate reaches 130 beats per minute or there is significant maternal hypotension. Once tocolysis is achieved, the infusion is usually continued for 12–24 hours.

Intramuscular or subcutaneous injections may occasionally be used as initial treatment. The injections are given every 2–4 hours for 24 hours.

Oral medication is used after intravenous, intramuscular, or subcutaneous use of the drug has achieved satisfactory tocolysis (uterine contractions absent or at least every 10–15 minutes

TABLE 18-9. BETA-ADRENERGIC RECEPTOR RESPONSES

Beta$_1$-Adrenergic Responses	Beta$_2$-Adrenergic Responses
Cardiac	Smooth Muscle
↑ Heart rate	↓ Uterine activity
↑ Stroke volume	↓ Vascular tone
Intestine	↓ Bronchial tone
↓ Motility	Renal
Fat	↑ Renin release
↑ Lipolysis	↓ Urinary output
	Metabolic
	↑ Glycogenolysis
	↑ Insulin release

apart). Oral medication is initiated 30 minutes before stopping intravenous treatment and repeated at 2–4 hour intervals in most patients. Oral medication decreases the incidence of recurrence of preterm labor.[15,22] After 24 hours of successful oral tocolysis, limited ambulation is begun. If contractions do not recur, the patient is discharged to continue oral treatment at home until 36–37 weeks of gestation. If uterine contractions are absent on oral medication, it is difficult to know what dose and frequency should be used. As there is a correlation between maternal pulse rate and serum concentrations of beta-adrenergic tocolytics, and there is a close correlation between the onset of uterine inhibitory effects and the onset of an increase in pulse rate,[71] one can use the maternal pulse rate to determine oral medication usage. A sustained mild tachycardia indicates the probability of a uterine effect.

Maternal Side Effects. As indicated earlier, beta-adrenergic tocolytics affect beta receptors in many different tissues, thereby eliciting a number of effects other than the desired uterine relaxation. Some of these may be minor, but potential serious side effects may occur.[24,115] The most serious maternal cardiovascular side effects include hypotension, myocardial ischemia, severe arrhythmias, and pulmonary edema. The reported incidence of these serious complications varies between 1% and 5%.

The major changes in normal cardiovascular physiology during pregnancy (see Chapter 3), such as increased plasma volume, increased cardiac output, and hyperdynamic function, are altered even further by beta-adrenergic treatment. These drugs raise cardiac output an additional 50%. This increase in cardiac output does help to compensate for the drug-induced vasodilatation, preventing significant hypotension in most patients. There is a widening of pulse pressure. Systolic pressures rise and diastolic pressures fall. Mild palpitations and flushing are common.

Myocardial ischemia has been reported with several of the tocolytics. Although not necessarily dose-related, ischemia does occur at high heart rates. Active maternal cardiac disease is a definite contraindication to the use of these agents. Cardiac arrhythmias are usually asymptomatic, include premature ventricular and nodal contractions, and usually respond quickly to cessation of treatment.

Pulmonary edema is the most common serious adverse side effect and usually responds quickly to cessation of the beta-adrenergic infusion and institution of appropriate treatment. However, if this condition is not acted on quickly, it can lead to adult respiratory distress syndrome. Predisposing factors are twin gestations (approximately half of the reported cases) in which plasma volume is greater than in singletons, anemia below 9 gram% hemoglobin, iatrogenic fluid overload, and a persistent heart rate over 130 beats per minute. The beta-adrenergics increase water imbibition in animals, stimulate the renin–aldosterone system, and decrease urinary output.[24,62] Experimental studies in the baboon over 24 hours revealed that these agents cause an increase in extracellular fluid and retention of sodium and a slow, progressive rise in pulmonary capillary wedge pressure.[40] All these actions tend to predispose the patient to fluid overload over time. Most of the reported cases reveal pulmonary edema occurring approximately 36–48 hours after initiation of treatment, whether or not intravenous treatment is continuing. The concomitant use of corticosteroids (to induce fetal lung maturity) and beta-adrenergic tocolytics in patients developing pulmonary edema has suggested that corticosteroids may be a predisposing factor. However, the incidence of corticosteroid therapy in patients who develop pulmonary edema is similar to that in the overall preterm labor population who receive tocolytics, indicating that corticosteroids are not a factor in the pathogenesis of beta-adrenergic-induced pulmonary edema.[96]

Significant metabolic changes occur with beta-adrenergic therapy. There is a rapid increase in blood glucose secondary to increased hepatic glycogenolysis. The elevations begin to decrease after 3 hours, but glucose levels remain elevated at 24 hours.[119] Prolonged oral administration does not appear to be associated with hyperglycemia. Insulin secretion is increased secondary to maternal hyperglycemia and stimulation of the pancreatic islet cells. These alterations in carbohydrate metabolism may lead to ketoacidosis in the insulin-dependent pregnant diabetic. Coincident with the hyperglycemia is the presence of hypokalemia.[119] Urinary excretion of potassium is not increased. Although advocated by some, there is no evidence at present to indicate that exogenous potassium should be administered. There are no known changes in serum calcium or magnesium. With increased lipolysis and glycogenolysis, there is an increase in free fatty acids, beta-hydroxybutyrate and lactate, but maternal acidosis is rare.

Fetal-neonatal effects. It is probable that most of the beta-adrenergic drugs cross the placenta, but detailed information is minimal. At low maternal infusion rates, there is no change in fetal heart rate. A mild elevation occurs at high infusion rates. Studies in experimental animals reveal a redistribution of fetal cardiac output favoring vital organs.[103] Suggestions that maternal beta-adrenergic treatment results in increased fetal weight and a decreased incidence of respiratory distress syndrome are still unproven. Neonatal hypoglycemia, hypocalcemia, ileus, and hypotension have been reported in observational reviews,[14] but prospective trials have not routinely substantiated these findings. If adverse neonatal effects do occur secondary to maternal tocolytic treatment, they are probably more likely to occur if delivery occurs within 8 hours of tocolytic treatment. Follow-up studies of newborns exposed in utero to beta-adrenergic agonists show normal growth and development at 2 years of age.[31]

Magnesium Sulfate. Although magnesium sulfate has been used extensively in obstetrics for the treatment of preeclampsia, it has only been used, to any degree, for the inhibition of preterm labor over the past 5–10 years.

Mechanism of Action. The mechanism responsible for magnesium sulfate tocolysis remains unknown at present. Magnesium decreases the frequency of depolarization and uncouples depolarization from the contraction. It may act by competing with calcium for entry into the cell.

Pharmacology. Magnesium concentrations in maternal serum of 4–7 mg/100 ml are necessary for inhibition of human myometrial contractions.[37,90] Magnesium concentrations of this magnitude are reached only with intravenous or intramuscular treatment. Excretion is almost entirely by the kidney, with at least 90% being excreted within 24 hours. As magnesium is reabsorbed by a transport-limited mechanism, the glomerular filtration rate significantly affects excretion. Magnesium crosses the placenta rapidly.

Efficacy. There has been only one placebo-controlled tocolytic trial reported. Most studies have been retrospective and observational, or magnesium sulfate has been compared with a beta-adrenergic compound. Success in delaying delivery for at least 24 hours appears nearly comparable to that reported for the beta-adrenergic agents.[20,29,105] Magnesium sulfate appears to be less efficacious if the cervix is more than 1 cm dilated.

Clinical Use. Prior to beginning therapy, the patient should be evaluated as outlined earlier for the clinical use of beta-adrenergics. Serum magnesium concentrations are obtained as a baseline and every 6 hours subsequently. A loading dose of 4–6 grams is administered intravenously over 20 minutes, followed by a maintenance dose of 1–3 grams per hour for 12–24 hours if uterine relaxation is achieved. Continued treatment with oral beta-adrenergic tocolytics as outlined earlier is then advised. Magnesium sulfate has been suggested to be the therapy of choice when treating the insulin-dependent diabetic for preterm labor.

There have been preliminary trials of combining magnesium sulfate with beta-adrenergic tocolytics, particularly if response to the beta-adrenergic treatment is less than desired. The benefits and risks of this combined therapy remain to be delineated.

Maternal Side Effects. The most serious potential side effects are respiratory depression and cardiac conduction defects which may occur at serum concentrations above 12 mg/100 ml. Deep tendon reflexes may be lost at 8–10 mg/100 ml. Vasodilatation results in flushing and a sense of warmth, with potential minor and usually transient decreases in blood pressure. A mild increase in heart rate and cardiac output is seen in nonpregnant patients.[79] Pulmonary edema has also been reported. It is therefore necessary to pay careful attention to intake and output. Paralytic ileus has been reported. Maternal hypocalcemia is associated with increases in magnesium concentrations, the total calcium concentrations falling by approximately 25%.[25] Levels of parathyroid hormone are increased. The hypocalcemia results from increased urinary excretion. Calcium gluconate should be available to reverse any serious toxic effect.

Fetal–Neonatal Effects. Magnesium concentrations in the newborn are similar to those in maternal serum.[25] The mean half-life of the elevated magnesium levels is more than 40 hours. Total calcium levels are minimally reduced. Neurobehavioral changes have been reported in a group of newborns whose mean magnesium concentration was 4.15 mEq/liter.[92] Decreased Dubowitz scores, decreased muscle tone, and poor suckling necessitating intravenous fluids were observed with increased frequency. These differences from a control group disappeared by 48 hours of age.

Prostaglandin Synthesis Inhibitors. Since prostaglandins are thought to play a significant stimulatory role in labor, there has been interest in the possibility that inhibitors of prostaglandin synthesis might arrest preterm labor.

Mechanism of Action. Nonsteroidal anti-inflammatory agents such as indomethacin decrease prostaglandin synthesis by inhibiting the enzyme cyclooxygenase which is necessary for the conversion of arachidonic acid to various prostaglandins.

Pharmacology. Indomethacin is absorbed after rectal or oral administration, reaching peak concentrations within 2 hours of oral intake.[1] It is extensively protein bound and is eliminated largely unchanged. It readily passes across the placenta. Fetal serum concentrations reach equilibration with maternal concentrations. The half-life is approximately 20–25 hours in preterm neonates.[8]

Efficacy. A small prospective, randomized, controlled trial of 24 hours of indomethacin treatment reported that preterm delivery occurred within 24 hours in 1 of 15 patients receiving treatment, versus 9 of 15 controls.[80] In a noncontrolled trial in which patients usually were treated for only 24–48 hours, the preterm delivery rate was 41%, but delivery was delayed for more than 72 hours in 79% of patients.[26]

Maternal Side Effects. Indomethacin and other cyclooxygenase inhibitors, probably due to inhibition of platelet aggregation, are associated with an increase in maternal bleeding during labor and postpartum, but the incidence is not well defined.

Fetal–Neonatal Effects. A number of case reports have suggested that these drugs may cause constriction of the ductus arteriosus in the fetus and cause pulmonary hypertension in the newborn. Acetylsalicylic acid given to fetal lambs in the last fifth of gestation causes constriction of the ductus arteriosus,[94] and indomethacin is used clinically to cause closure of the patent ductus in preterm newborns. A large collaborative trial demonstrated ductal closure in 77% of preterm newborns. The closure was not dependent on gestational age.[35] However, in at least two studies concerned with tocolytic effect, no adverse drug-related side effects could be detected.[26,80] It may be that normal fetuses can tolerate partial ductal closure, but some fetuses, such as the growth retarded fetus which is critically dependent on ductal flow, cannot. When indomethacin is given to newborns, there is a decrease in glomerular filtration and urinary output. Oligohydramnios develops when indomethacin is given for a number of days antenatally.[48]

Calcium Antagonists. Because free intracellular calcium plays a pivotal role in uterine muscle contraction, interest has arisen in the use of these agents as tocolytic drugs. Minimal knowledge concerning this approach is available at present.

Tocolysis and Gestational Age

In view of risks of neonatal mortality before 30–32 weeks of gestational age, it is advisable to attempt to stop preterm labor if it occurs prior to 32 weeks and there are no maternal or fetal contraindications. After 32 weeks neonatal morbidity becomes the determining factor in deciding whether or not to attempt tocolysis. A recent study of more than 200 newborns delivered on a tertiary high-risk service has examined the morbidity associated with preterm birth, excluding complications that could be ascribed to factors other than preterm delivery such as maternal diabetes, anomalies, congenital infection, and growth retardation.[60] The incidence of six major morbidity events is listed in Table 18-2. Note that intraventricular hemorrhage was diagnosed only after clinical findings suggested that radiologic examination was indicated. Significant decreases in admissions to intensive care (70%), respiratory distress syndrome (87%), patent ductus arteriosus (100%), and mean number of hospital days (39%) were observed by delaying delivery from 34 to 35 completed weeks (35 days prior to term), and extension of pregnancy from 35 to 36 completed weeks reduced admissions to neonatal special care by 75% and length of hospitalization by 42%.

MANAGEMENT OF PROGRESSIVE PRETERM LABOR

Ample accumulated evidence shows that delivery of small preterm newborns is best accomplished in a specialized perinatal center. Preterm infants have less chance of mortality and both short- and long-term morbidity if born in an intensive care setting than if they are transferred after birth for specialized care.[111] Short-term tocolytic therapy can delay delivery sufficiently to permit transfer of the mother and fetus to a center with specialized perinatal and neonatal facilities and personnel. The regionalization of perinatal care can make available the appropriate level of care necessary for all patients through cost-effective utilization of resources.[102]

Survival of Very Low-Birth-Weight Infants

Over the past 25–30 years, survival of low-birth-weight preterm infants has increased progressively. Currently, the critical birth weight appears to be approximately 800 grams or a gestational age of 26 weeks, at which time survival is approximately 60%.[60] Below this weight or gestational age, survival falls rapidly. As survival rates of these small infants have improved, the frequency of major handicaps in survivors has remained stable.[51] It is therefore important to estimate fetal weight accurately. The use of ultrasonic estimations of fetal weight of large infants has a considerable error, but this error is minimized at smaller fetal sizes, being in the range of ±50–75 grams in infants under 900 grams.[56] Therefore, ultrasonic determination of fetal size may aid significantly in obstetrical management. The tendency clinically to underestimate fetal weight may result in a nonintervention approach with resultant worse neonatal outcome.[88]

Fetal Monitoring

Perinatal asphyxia is a major risk factor for short- and long-term neurological abnormalities in both preterm and term infants. Survival in the asphyxiated preterm baby appears to be much lower than in the term baby, whereas severe long-term disabilities are the same, or less frequent, in the preterm as compared to the term infant.[76,81] If neonatal seizures follow the perinatal asphyxia, the risk of major disability in later life rises significantly. Birth asphyxia also predisposes the preterm newborn to the development of respiratory distress syndrome.[30] The inverse relationship between gestational age and intraventricular hemorrhage in infants between 26 and 34 weeks of gestation appears to be higher in asphyxiated infants, but this is not well established.

Continuous fetal heart rate monitoring is valuable when dealing with progressive preterm labor. Monitoring of fetuses of less than 1500 grams can aid in significantly reducing neonatal mortality.[87] Fetal heart rate recordings that are normal or reassuring are rarely associated with fetal acidosis. In infants under 1500 grams, ominous periodic deceleration patterns, such as late decelerations or severe variable decelerations, are associated with increased fetal acidosis, and increased morbidity and mortality.[12,73,87] If there is a prompt response to ominous patterns, these babies may still evidence perinatal asphyxia at birth but need not suffer increased neonatal morbidity and mortality.[12] Thus, intensive obstetrical and neonatal observation and management can improve outcome.

Fetal Lung Maturation

At least seven controlled trials have now been performed establishing the potential value of the use of maternal corticosteroid therapy to induce lung maturation and to reduce respiratory distress syndrome in the preterm neonate of less than 34 weeks of gestation when membranes are intact. There is a significant reduction in the incidence of neonatal respiratory distress syndrome in fetuses less than 34 weeks if betamethasone or dexamethasone is given to the mother and delivery is delayed for at least 24 hours from the first injection.[67,70] The percentage reduction in respiratory distress syndrome is not as pronounced in infants of less than 30 weeks' gestational age but may be improved if delivery can be delayed for 48–72 hours. The corticosteroid treatment is not as well established when the clinical association also includes rupture of the membranes. Some studies did not show a benefit under these circumstances.

Method of Delivery

At the present time, there is no convincing evidence to suggest that vaginal delivery should not be the mode of delivery when (1) the presentation is vertex, (2) labor is progressing in normal fashion, and (3) the fetal heart rate tracing is essentially normal. This approach assumes the capability to respond quickly to an ominous fetal heart rate tracing by immediate cesarean section and the availability of neonatal intensive care. In general, an episiotomy is recommended to help effect controlled delivery of the fetal head and to reduce the length of the second stage. However, no significant data on this issue are available. The recommendation that low forceps delivery should be employed in order to protect the less-well-calcified vertex from maternal soft tissue resistance has not been substantiated.

A large number of observational studies strongly support the concept that cesarean section is the optimal method of delivery when the fetus is in the breech presentation and below 1500–1750 grams or below 33 weeks of gestation. Cesarean delivery of the breech weighing between 500 and 1500 grams, when compared to vaginal delivery, is associated with significantly decreased mortality, birth asphyxia, and intraventricular hemorrhage.[13,63] Similar findings have been reported in a paired retrospective study.[27] Prospective studies have not yet confirmed this approach. It has been reported that vaginal delivery is appropriate if the preterm breech is presenting as a complete breech or frank breech.[52] However, if the breech presents as a footling, with the associated increase in cord prolapse, and entrapment of the aftercoming head, cesarean section is indicated. The incidence of incomplete breech presentation is much higher in small preterm fetuses than at term. The incidence of congenital anomalies may be nearly 20% when the preterm fetus presents as a breech.[52] Thus, there is a need for careful ultrasonic evaluation of the preterm breech in an attempt to make certain that a lethal congenital anomaly is not present before proceeding with abdominal delivery.

REFERENCES

1. Alvan, G., Orme, M., Bertilsson, L., Ekstrand, R., and Palmer, L.: Pharmacokinetics of indomethacin. *Clin. Pharmacol. Ther.* **18**:364–373, 1975.
2. Anderson, A. B.: Factors associated with spontaneous pre-term birth. *Br. J. Obstet. Gynaecol.* **83**:342–350, 1976.
3. Anderson, A. B. M. and Turnbull, A. C.: Relationship between length of gestation and cervical dilatation, uterine contractility, and other factors during pregnancy. *Am. J. Obstet. Gynecol.* **105**:1207–1214, 1969.
4. Bakketeig, L. S. and Hoffman, H. J.: Epidemiology of preterm birth: Results from a longitudinal study of births in Norway. In: *Preterm Labor.* M. G. Elder and C. H. Hendricks (Eds.). London, Butterworths, 1981, pp. 17–46.
5. Bartolucci, L., Hill, W. C., Katz, M., Gill, P. J., and Kitzmiller, J. L.: Ultrasonography in preterm labor. *Am. J. Obstet. Gynecol.* **149**:52–56, 1984.
6. Bejar, R., Curbelo, V., Davis, C. and Gluck, L.: Premature labor. II. Bacterial sources of phospholipase. *Obstet. Gynecol.* **57**:479–482, 1981.
7. Bell, R.: The prediction of preterm labour by recording spontaneous antenatal uterine activity. *Br. J. Obstet. Gynaecol.* **90**:884–887, 1983.
8. Bhat, R., Vidyasagar, D., Vadapalli, M., Whalley, C., Fisher, E., Hastreiter, A., and Evans, M.: Disposition of indomethacin in preterm infants. *J. Pediatr.* **95**:313–316, 1979.
9. Bibby J. G., Brunt J., Mitchell, M. D., Anderson, A. B., and Turnbull, A.C.: The effect of cervical encerclage on plasma prostaglandin concentrations during early human pregnancy. *Br. J. Obstet. Gynaecol.* **86**:19–22, 1979.
10. Bleasdale, J. E., Okasaki, T., Sagawa, N., et al.: The mobilization of arachidonic acid for prostaglandin production during parturition. In: *Initiation of Parturition: Prevention of Prematurity: Report of The Fourth Ross Conference on Obstetric Research.* P. C. MacDonald and J. Porter (Eds.). Columbus, OH, Ross Laboratories, 1983, pp. 129–137.
11. Block, B. S., Liggins, G. C., and Creasy, R. K.: Preterm delivery is not predicted by serial plasma estradiol or progesterone concentration measurements. *Am. J. Obstet. Gynecol.* **150**:716–722, 1984.
12. Bowes, W. A., Jr., Halgrimson, M., and Simmons, M. A.: Results of intensive perinatal management of very low birth weight infants (501 to 1500 grams). *J. Reprod. Med.* **23**:245–250, 1979.
13. Bowes, W. A., Jr., Taylor, E. S., O'Brien, M., and Bowes, C.: Breech delivery: Evaluation of the method of delivery on perinatal results and maternal morbidity. *Am. J. Obstet. Gynecol.* **135**:965–973, 1979.
14. Brazy, J. E. and Pupkin, M. J.: Effects of maternal isoxsuprine administration on preterm infants. *J. Pediatr.* **94**:444–448, 1979.
15. Brown, S. M. and Tejani, N. A.: Terbutaline sulfate in the prevention of recurrence of premature labor. *Obstet. Gynecol.* **57**:22–25 1981.
16. Caritis, S. N., Lin, L. S., Toig, G., and Wong, L. K.: Pharmacodynamics of ritodrine in pregnant women during preterm labor. *Am. J. Obstet. Gynecol.* **147**:752–759, 1983.
17. Casey, M. L. and MacDonald, P. C.: Endocrinology of preterm birth. *Clin. Obstet. Gynecol.* **27**:562–571, 1984.
18. Castle, B. M. and Turnbull, A. C.: The presence or absence of fetal breathing movements predicts the outcome of preterm labour. *Lancet* **2**:471–473, 1983.
19. Challis, J. R. G.: Factors responsible for parturition. In: *Preterm Labour and Its Consequences.* R. W. Beard and F. Sharp (Eds.). London, Royal College of Obstetricians and Gynaecologists, 1985, pp. 61–69.

20. Cotton, D. B., Strassner, H. T., Hill, L. M., Schifrin, B. S., and Paul, R. H.: Comparison of magnesium sulfate terbutaline and a placebo for inhibition of preterm labor. A randomized study. *J. Reprod. Med.* **29**:92–97, 1984.
21. Creasy, R. K.: Prevention of preterm birth. *Birth Defects* **19**:97–102, 1983.
22. Creasy, R. K., Golbus, M. S., Laros, R. K., Jr., Parker, J. T., and Roberts, J. M.: Oral ritodrine maintenance in the treatment of preterm labor. *Am. J. Obstet. Gynecol.* **137**:212–219, 1980.
23. Creasy, R. K., Gummer, B. A., and Liggins, G. C.: A system for predicting spontaneous preterm birth. *Obstet. Gynecol.* **55**:692–695, 1980.
24. Creasy, R. K. and Katz, M.: Basic research and clinical experience with β-adrenergic tocolytics in the United States. In: *Preterm Birth: Causes, Prevention and Management*, Chapter 10. F. Fuchs and P. G. Stubblefield (Eds.). New York, Macmillan Publishing Co., 1984, pp. 150–170.
25. Cruikshank, D. P., Pitkin, R. M., Reynolds, W. A., Williams, G. A., and Hargis, G. K.: Effects of magnesium sulfate treatment on perinatal calcium metabolism. I. Maternal and fetal responses. *Am. J. Obstet. Gynecol.* **134**:243–249, 1979.
26. Dudley, D. K. and Hardie, M. J.: Fetal and neonatal effects of indomethacin used as a tocolytic agent. *Am. J. Obstet. Gynecol.* **151**:181–184, 1985.
27. Duenhoelter, J. H., Wells, C. E., Reisch, J. S., Santos-Ramos, R., and Jimenez, J. M.: A paired controlled study of vaginal and abdominal delivery of the low birth weight breech fetus. *Obstet. Gynecol.* **54**:310–313, 1979.
28. Elder, H. A., Santamarina, B. A., Smith, S., and Kass, E. H.: The natural history of asymptomatic bacteriuria during pregnancy: The effect of tetracycline on the clinical course and outcome of pregnancy. *Am. J. Obstet. Gynecol.* **111**:441–462, 1971.
29. Elliott, J. P.: Magnesium sulfate as a tocolytic agent. *Am. J. Obstet. Gynecol.* **147**:277–284, 1983.
30. Farrell, P. M. and Avery, M. E.: Hyaline membrane disease. *Am. Rev. Respir. Dis.* **111**:657–688, 1975.
31. Freysz, H., Willard, D., Lehr, A., Messer, J., and Boog, G.: A long term evaluation of infants who receive a beta-mimetic drug while in utero. *J. Perinat. Med.* **5**:94–99, 1977.
32. Fuchs, A. R., Fuchs, F., Husslein, P., Soloff, M. S., and Fernstrom, M.J.: Oxytocin receptors and human parturition. A dual role for oxytocin in the initiation of labor. *Science* **215**:1396–1398, 1982.
33. Fuchs, F.: Prevention of prematurity. *Am. J. Obstet. Gynecol.* **126**:809–820, 1976.
34. Garfield, R. E.: Control of myometrial function in preterm versus term labor. *Clin. Obstet. Gynecol.* **27**:572–591, 1984.
35. Gersony, W. M., Peckham, G. J., Ellison, R. C., Miettinen, O. S., and Nadas, A. S.: Effects of indomethacin in premature infants with patent ductus arteriosus. Results of a national collaborative study. *J. Pediatr.* **102**:895–906, 1983.
36. Goodyear, K., Katz, M., and Creasy, R. K.: Signs and symptoms of preterm labor. Submitted for publication.
37. Harbert, G. M., Jr., Cornell, G. W., and Thornton, W. N., Jr.: Effect of toxemia therapy on uterine dynamics. *Am. J. Obstet. Gynecol.* **105**:94–104, 1969.
38. Hartikainen-Sorri, A. L., Kauppila, A., and Tuimala, R.: Inefficacy of 17α-hydroxyprogesterone caproate in the prevention of prematurity in twin pregnancy. *Obstet. Gynecol.* **56**:692–695, 1980.
39. Hauth, J. C., Gilstrap, L. C., 3d, Brekken, A. L., and Hauth, J. M.: The effect of 17α-hydroxyprogesterone caproate on pregnancy outcome in an active-duty military population. *Am. J. Obstet. Gynecol.* **146**:187–190, 1983.
40. Hauth, J. C., Hankins, G. D., Kuell, T. J., and Pierson, W. P.: Ritodrine hydrochloride infusion in pregnant baboons. I. Biophysical effects. *Am. J. Obstet. Gynecol.* **146**:916–924, 1983.
41. Heinonen, P. K., Saarikoski, S., and Pystynen, P.: Reproductive performance of women with uterine anomalies. An evaluation of 182 cases. *Acta Obstet. Gynecol. Scand.* **61**:157–162, 1982.
42. Hemminki, E. and Starfield, B.: Prevention and treatment of premature labour by drugs: Review of controlled clinical trials. *Br. J. Obstet. Gynaecol.* **85**:411–417, 1978.
43. Herron, M. A., Katz, M., and Creasy, R. K.: Evaluation of a preterm birth prevention program: Preliminary report. *Obstet. Gynecol.* **59**:452–456, 1982.
44. Hill, L. M., Johnson, C. E., and Lee, R. A.: Prophylactic use of hydroxyprogesterone caproate in abdominal surgery during pregnancy. A retrospective evaluation. *Obstet. Gynecol.* **46**:287–290, 1975.
45. Hoffman, H. J. and Bakketeig, L. S.: Risk factors associated with the occurrence of preterm birth. *Clin. Obstet. Gynecol.* **27**:539–552, 1984.
46. Holbrook, R. H., Jr., Falcon, J., Herron, M., Lirette, M., Laros, R. L., and Creasy, R. K.: Evaluation of the weekly cervical examination in a preterm birth prevention program. Submitted for publication.
47. Huszar, G. and Naftolin, F.: The myometrium and uterine cervix in normal and preterm labor. *N. Engl. J. Med.* **311**:571–581, 1984.
48. Itskovitz, J., Abramovici, H., and Brandes, J. M.: Oligohydramnion, meconium and perinatal death concurrent with indomethacin treatment in human pregnancy. *J. Reprod. Med.* **24**:137–140, 1980.
49. Johnson, J. W., Austin, K. L., Jones, G. S., Davis, G. H., and King, T. M.: Efficacy of 17α-hydroxyprogesterone caproate in the prevention of premature labor. *N. Engl. J. Med.* **293**:675–680, 1975.
50. Johnon, J. W., Lee, P. A., Zachary, A. S., Calhoun, S., and Migeon, C. J.: High-risk prematurity—

progestin treatment and steroid studies. *Obstet. Gynecol.* **54**:412–418, 1979.

51. Jones, R. A. and Davies, P. A.: The outcome for preterm infants. In: *Preterm Labor.* M.G. Elder and C.H. Hendricks (Eds.). London, Butterworths, 1981, pp. 289–316.
52. Karp, L. E., Doney, J. R., McCarthy, T., Meis, P. J., and Hall, M.: The premature breech. Trial of labor or cesarean section? *Obstet. Gynecol.* **53**:88–92, 1979.
53. Katz, M., Newman, R. B., and Gill, P. J.: Assessment of uterine activity in ambulatory patients at high risk of preterm labor and delivery. *Am. J. Obstet. Gynecol.*, **154**:44–47, 1986.
54. Newman, R. B., Gill, P. J., and Katz, M.: Uterine activity during pregnancy in ambulatory patients. Comparison of singleton and twin gestations. *Am. J. Obstet. Gynecol.* **154**:530–531, 1986.
55. Ke, R., Vohra, M., and Casper, R.: Prolonged inhibition of human myometrial contractility by intermittent isoproterenol. *Am. J. Obstet. Gynecol.* **149**:841–844, 1984.
56. Key, T. C., Dattel, B. J., and Resnik, R.: The ultrasonographic estimation of fetal weight in the very low-birth-weight infant. *Am. J. Obstet. Gynecol.* **145**:574–578, 1983.
57. Kessel, S. S., Villar, J., Berendes, H. W., and Nugent, R. P.: The changing pattern of low birth weight in the United States, 1970 to 1980. *JAMA* **251**:1978–1982, 1984.
58. King, J. F., Keirse, J. N. C., Grant, A., and Chalmers, I.: Tocolysis—The case for and against. In: *Preterm Labour and Its Consequences.* R. W. Beard and F. Sharp (Eds.). London, Royal College of Obstetricians and Gynaecologists, 1985, pp. 199–208.
59. Komaromy, B. and Lampe, L.: The value of bed rest in twin pregnancies. *Int. J. Gynaecol. Obstet.* **15**:262–266, 1977.
60. Konte, J. M., Holbrook, R. H., Jr., Laros, R. K., Jr., and Creasy, R. K.: Short-term neonatal morbidity associated with preterm birth and effect of a preterm birth prevention program on expected incidence of morbidity. *Am. J. Perinatol.* **3**:283–288, 1986.
61. Kristal, A. R. and Rush, D.: Maternal nutrition and duration of gestation: A review. *Clin. Obstet. Gynecol.* **27**:553–561, 1984.
62. Lammintausta, R. and Erkkola, R.: Renin-angiotensin-aldosterone system and sodium in normal pregnancy: A longitudinal study. *Acta Obstet. Gynecol. Scand.* **56**:221–225, 1977.
63. Lamont, R. F., Dunlop, P. D., Crowley, P., and Elder, M. G.: Spontaneous preterm labour and delivery at under 34 weeks' gestation. *Br. Med. J.* **286**:454–457, 1983.
64. Lazar, P., Gueguen, S., Dreyfus, F., Reynaud, R., Pontonnier, G., and Papiernik, E.: Multicentered controlled trial of cervical cerclage in women at moderate risk of preterm delivery. *Br. J. Obstet. Gynaecol.* **91**:731–735, 1984.
65. Lefkowitz, R. J. and Williams, L. T.: Molecular mechanisms of activation and desensitization of adenylate cyclase coupled beta-adrenergic receptors. *Adv. Cyclic Nucleotide Res.* **9**:1–17, 1978.
66. Liggins, G. C.: Initiation of spontaneous labor. *Clin. Obstet. Gynecol.* **26**:47–55, 1983.
67. Liggins, G. C.: Prenatal glucocorticoid treatment: Prevention of respiratory distress syndrome. In: *Report of the 70th Ross Conference on Pediatric Research.* T. D. Moore (Ed.). Columbus, OH, Ross Laboratories, 1977, pp. 97–103.
68. Liggins, G. C., Fairclough, R. J., Grieves, S. A. Kendall, J. Z., and Knox, B. S.: The mechanism of initiation of parturition in the ewe. *Recent Prog. Horm. Res.* **29**:111–159, 1973.
69. Liggins, G. C., Fairclough, R. J., Grieves, S. A., Forster, C. S., and Knox, B. S.: Parturition in the sheep. In: *The Fetus and Birth.* Ciba Foundation Symposium (new series; vol. 47), Amsterdam, Elsevier, 1977, pp. 5–30.
70. Liggins, G. C. and Howie, R. N.: A controlled trial of antepartum glucocorticoid treatment of the respiratory distress syndrome in premature infants. *Pediatrics* **50**:515–525, 1972.
71. Lipshitz, J.: The uterine and cardiovascular effects of oral fenoterol hydrobromide. *Br. J. Obstet. Gynaecol.* **84**:737–739, 1977.
72. Mamelle, N., Laumon, B., and Lazar, P.: Prematurity and occupational activity during pregnancy. *Am. J. Epidemiol.* **119**:309–322, 1984.
73. Martin, C. B., Jr., Siassi, B., and Hon, E. H.: Fetal heart rate patterns and neonatal death in low birthweight infants. *Obstet. Gynecol.* **44**:503–510, 1974.
74. Merkatz, I. R., Peter, J. B., and Barden, T. P.: Ritodrine hydrochloride. A betamimetic agent for use in preterm labor. II. Evidence of efficacy. *Obstet. Gynecol.* **56**:7–12, 1980.
75. Meyer, M. B. and Tonascia, J. A.: Maternal smoking, pregnancy complications and perinatal mortality. *Am. J. Obstet. Gynecol.* **128**:494–502, 1977.
76. Milligan, J. C., Painter, M. J., O'Donoghue, P. A., MacDonald, H. M., Allen, A. C., and Taylor, P. M.: Neonatal asphyxia. II. Neonatal mortality and long-term sequelae. *J. Pediatr.* **96**:903–907, 1980.
77. Misenhimer, H. R. and Kaltreider, D. F.: Effects of decreased prenatal activity in patients with twin pregnancy. *Obstet. Gynecol.* **51**:692–694, 1978.
78. Mitchell, M. D., Flint, A. P. F., Bibby, J., Brunt, J., Arnold, J. M., Anderson, A. B., and Turnbull, A. C.: Rapid increases in plasma prostaglandin concentrations after vaginal examination and amniotomy. *Br. Med. J.* **2**:1183–1185, 1977.
79. Mroczek, W. J., Lee, W. R., and Davidov, M. E.: Effect of magnesium sulfate on cardiovascular hemodynamics. *Angiology* **28**:720–724, 1977.
80. Niebyl, J. R., Blake, D. A., White, R. D., Kumor, K. M., Dubin, N. H., Robinson, J. C., and Egner,

P. G.: The inhibition of premature labor with indomethacin. *Am. J. Obstet. Gynecol.* **136**:1014-1019, 1980.

81. Nelson, K. B. and Ellenberg, J. H.: Apgar scores as predictors of chronic neurologic disability. *Pediatrics* **68**:36-44, 1981.
82. Newton, R. W. and Hunt, L. P.: Psychosocial stress in pregnancy and its relation to low birth weight. *Br. Med. J. 288*:1191-1194, 1984.
83. New Zealand Health Statistics Report, 1978. New Zealand Dept. of Health, Wellington, New Zealand.
84. O'Connor, M. C., Murphy, H., and Dalrymple, I. J.: Double blind trial of ritodrine and placebo in twin pregnancy. *Br. J. Obstet. Gynaecol.* **86**:706-709, 1979.
85. Papiernik, E.: Coefficient de risque d'accouchement premature. *Presse Med.* **77**:793-794, 1969.
86. Papiernik, E.: Proposals for a programmed prevention policy of preterm birth. *Clin. Obstet. Gynecol.* **27**:614-635, 1984.
87. Paul, R. H. and Hon, E. H.: Clinical fetal monitoring. V. Effect on perinatal outcome. *Am. J. Obstet. Gynecol.* **118**:529-533, 1974.
88. Paul, R. H., Koh, K. S., and Monfared, A. H.: Obstetric factors influencing outcome in infants weighing from 1001 to 1500 grams. *Am. J. Obstet. Gynecol.* **133**:503-508, 1979.
89. Persson, P. H., Grennert, L., Gennser, G., and Kullander, S.: On improved outcome in twin pregnancies. *Acta Obstet. Gynecol. Scand.* **58**:3-7, 1979.
90. Petrie, R. H.: Preterm parturition. Tocolysis using magnesium sulfate. *Semin. Perinatol.* **5**:266-273, 1981.
91. Polk, B. F.: Infectious processes and preterm labor. In: *Preterm Birth: Causes, Prevention and Management.* F. Fuchs and P. G. Stubblefield (Eds.). New York, Macmillan Publishing Co., 1984, pp. 86-97.
92. Rasch, D. K., Huber, P. A., Richardson, C. J., L'Hommedieu, C. S., Nelson, T. E., and Reddi, R.: Neurobehavioral effects of neonatal hypermagnesemia. *J. Pediatr.* **100**:272-276, 1982.
93. Remington J. S. and Klein J. O.: *Infectious Disease of the Fetus and Newborn Infant*, 2nd Edition. Philadelphia, W. B. Saunders, 1983.
94. Rudolph, A. M. and Heymann, M. A.: Hemodynamic changes induced by blockers of prostaglandin synthesis in the fetal lamb in utero. *Adv. Prostaglandin Thromboxane Res.* **4**:231-237, 1978.
95. Roberts, J. M.: Current understanding of pharmacologic mechanisms in the prevention of preterm birth. *Clin. Obstet. Gynecol.* **27**:592-605, 1984.
96. Robertson, P. A., Herron, M., Katz, M., and Creasy, R. K.: Maternal morbidity associated with isoxsuprine and terbutaline tocolysis. *Eur. J. Obstet. Gynaecol. Reprod. Biol.* **11**:317-318, 1981.
97. Renaud, R., Irrmann, M., Gandar, R., and Flynn, M. G.: The use of ritodrine in the treatment of premature labour. *J. Obstet. Gynaecol. Br. Commonw.* **81**:182-186, 1974.
98. Rush, R. W., Keirse, M. J., Howat, P., Baum, J. D., Anderson, A. B., and Turnbull, A. C.: Contribution of preterm delivery to perinatal mortality. *Br. Med. J.* **2**:965-968, 1976.
99. Rush, R. W., Isaacs, S., McPherson, K., Jones, L., Chalmers, I., and Grant, A.: A randomized controlled trial of cervical cerclage in women at high risk of spontaneous preterm delivery. *Br. J. Obstet. Gynaecol.* **91**:724-730, 1984.
100. Saeed, S. A., Strickland, D. M., Young, D. C., Dang, A., and Mitchell, M. D.: Inhibition of prostaglandin synthesis by human amniotic fluid: Acute reduction in inhibitory activity of amniotic fluid obtained during labor. *J. Clin. Endocrinol. Metab.* **55**:801-803, 1982.
101. Saunders, M. C., Dick, J. S., Brown I. M., McPherson, K., and Chalmers, I.: The effects of hospitalization for bed rest on the duration of twin pregnancy: A randomized trial. *Lancet* **2**:793-795, 1985.
102. Scott, K. E., Peddle, L. J., and Rees, E. P.: Impact of regional organization and planned services to reduce perinatal mortality. In: *Preterm Birth: Causes, Prevention and Management*, Chapter 22. F. Fuchs and P. G. Stubblefield (Eds.). New York, Macmillan Publishing Co., 1984, pp. 348-376.
103. Siimes, A. S., Creasy, R. K., Heymann, M. A., and Rudolph, A. M.: Cardiac output and its distribution and organ blood flow in the fetal lamb during ritodrine administration. *Am. J. Obstet. Gynecol.* **132**:42-48, 1978.
104. Siiteri, P. K. and Seron-Ferre, M.: Some new thoughts on the fetoplacental unit and parturition in primates. In: *Fetal Endocrinology.* M. J. Novy and J. A. Resko (Eds.). New York, Academic Press, 1981, pp. 1-34.
105. Spisso, K. R., Harbert, G. M., Jr., and Thiagarajah, S.: The use of magnesium sulfate as the primary tocolytic agent to prevent premature delivery. *Am. J. Obstet. Gynecol.* **142**:840-845, 1982.
106. Steiner, A. L. and Creasy, R. K.: Methods of cervical priming. *Clin. Obstet. Gynecol.* **26**:37-46, 1983.
107. Stubblefield, P. G.: Causes and prevention of preterm birth. An overview. In: *Preterm Birth: Causes, Prevention and Management.* F. Fuchs and P. G. Stubblefield (Eds.). New York, Macmillan Publishing Co., 1984, pp. 3-20.
108. Stys, S. J., Clewell, W. H., and Meschia, G.: Changes in cervical compliance at parturition independent of uterine activity. *Am. J. Obstet. Gynecol.* **130**:414-418, 1978.
109. Sutherland, E. W., Robinson, G. A., and Butcher, R. W.: Some aspects of the biological role of adenosine 3,5-monophosphate (cyclic AMP). *Circulation* **37**:279-306, 1968.
110. Thorburn, G. D. and Challis, J. R.: Endo-

crine control of parturition. *Physiol. Rev.* **59**:863–918, 1979.

111. Usher, R.: Changing mortality rates with perinatal intensive care and regionalization. *Semin. Perinatol.* **1**:309–319, 1977.
112. Valenzuela, G., Cline, S., and Hayashi, R. H.: Follow up of hydration and sedation in the pretherapy of premature labor. *Am. J. Obstet. Gynecol.* **147**:396–398, 1983.
113. Wallace, R. L. and Herrick, C. N.: Amniocentesis in the evaluation of premature labor. *Obstet. Gynecol.* **57**:483–486, 1981.
114. Weeks, A. R., Menzies, D. N., and de Boer, C. H.: The relative efficacy of bed rest, cervical suture, and no treatment in the management of twin pregnancy. *Br. J. Obstet. Gynaecol.* **84**:161–164, 1977.
115. Weidinger H.: The European experience with β-mimetic agents. In: *Preterm Birth: Causes, Prevention and Management,* Chapter 9. F. Fuchs and P. G. Stubblefield (Eds.). New York, Macmillan Publishing Co., 1984, pp. 131–149.
116. Wilson, T., Liggins, G. C., Aimer, G. P., and Skinner, S. J. M.:. Partial purification and characterization of two compounds from amniotic fluid which inhibit phospholipase activity in human endometrial cells. *Biochem. Biophys. Res. Commun.* **131**:22–29, 1985.
117. Wood, C., Bannerman, R. H. O., Booth, R. T., and Pinkerton, J. H. M.: The prediction of premature labor by observation of the cervix and external tocography. *Am. J. Obstet. Gynecol.* **91**:396–402, 1965.
118. Yemini, M., Borenstein, R., Dreazen, E., Apelman, Z., Mogilner, B. M., Kessler, I., and Lancet, M.: Prevention of premature labor by 17α-hydroxyprogesterone caproate. *Am. J. Obstet. Gynecol.* **151**:574–577, 1985.
119. Young, D. C., Toofanian, A., and Leveno, K. J.: Potassium and glucose concentrations without treatment during ritodrine tocolysis. *Am. J. Obstet. Gynecol.* **145**:105–106, 1983.
120. Zervoudakis, I. A., Krauss, A., and Fuchs, F.: Infants of mothers treated with ethanol for premature labor. *Am. J. Obstet. Gynecol.* **137**:713–718, 1980.

19

THE MANAGEMENT OF POSTDATE PREGNANCY

More than 100 years ago, Oliver Wendell Holmes questioned whether the placenta as an organ of transfer kept pace with the developing fetus or whether it fell behind at some point in time. Just as a definitive answer to the question continues to elude us, so do definitive programs of clinical management for this condition. Although a risk of increased fetal morbidity and mortality is clearly associated with continued intrauterine existence beyond term, the risk is small. Problems are presented if one undertakes a policy of routine termination of all pregnancies that go beyond term. Management strategies in vogue today reflect different perceptions of the maternal and fetal risks involved and, we believe, an unfortunate misunderstanding of the pathogenesis of injury in the postdate pregnancy. The current medical-legal climate adds another dimension to the debate and, in so doing, distracts from the medical issues.

DEFINITIONS

We consider a pregnancy postdate or prolonged when it exceeds 294 days (42 weeks) from the first day of the last menstrual period or 280 days (40 weeks) from the day of ovulation. Thus, the terms postdate pregnancy and prolonged pregnancy represent obstetrical diagnoses based on the clinical estimation of the length of gestation.

The terms postmature, postmaturity syndrome, and dysmaturity describe the neonate with manifestations of intrauterine nutritional deprivation—who also happens to be postdate (see below). These features, originally described by Ballantine in 1922[3] and then by Clifford,[17] include long fingernails, absent lanugo and vernix, abundant scalp hair, desquamation of the skin with reddish color absent. These features are associated with decreased amniotic fluid volume and passage of meconium. The dysmaturity of prolonged pregnancy is not unique. It is common to nutritional failure from any cause at any gestational age near term or beyond.

ETIOLOGY OF POSTDATE PREGNANCY

Many theories of the etiology of post-term pregnancy have been proposed.[1,57,81] In attempting to elucidate the mechanisms of postdate pregnancy, investigators have concentrated on two separate lines of inquiry. The first investigates the reasons for the delay in onset of parturition; the second deals with the mechanisms of placental insufficiency leading to evidence of dysmaturity/postmaturity syndrome. Etiology remains elusive in both areas.

ONSET OF LABOR

The past several years have witnessed great strides in understanding the manifold processes resulting in labor. We have come to understand that the fetal pituitary–adrenal axis appears necessary for the timely initiation of labor. Malformations of the fetal hypothalamus, pituitary (anencephaly), or adrenal gland (hypoplasia) generally result in post-term pregnancy if uncomplicated by hydramnios.[60] Normally, fetal plasma corticosteroid levels rise prior to the onset of labor. Indeed, recent evidence suggests that failure to elevate plasma cortisol in the fetus contributes to prolonged pregnancy, whereas intra-amniotic administration of steroids in post-term pregnancy induces labor.[62-64,82] Other theories suggest that prolongation of pregnancy may be secondary to failure of regulatory hormonal factors, which either stimulate uterine activity (prostaglandins) or suppress activity (progesterone). Diminished production of progesterone by the placenta promotes labor,[20] as does administration of prostaglandins E_2 and $F_{2\alpha}$. Progesterone inhibits spontaneous uterine contractions by blocking the activity of endogenous prostaglandin $F_{2\alpha}$. A retrospective survey suggested that taking aspirin (a prostaglandin inhibitor) during the last six months of pregnancy prolongs the duration of pregnancy.

This theory is supported in animals and humans by the decrease in level of progesterone and rise in 17β-estradiol in maternal plasma prior to the onset of labor.[87] This finding is denied by others, but since the effect need be only a local one, systemic levels may not truly reflect local hormonal dynamics.

Post-term pregnancy is associated with congenital anomalies of the fetus, including anencephaly, trisomies 16 and 18, and Seckel's dwarfism. Lastly, placental sulfatase deficiency and extrauterine pregnancy are associated with post-term gestation.

FETAL DEPRIVATION—THE PLACENTA

Dysmaturity occurs in 20–30% of post-term pregnancies.[81] Patients with isolated placental sulfatase deficiency manifest prolonged pregnancy, but generally without signs of fetal deprivation. The placenta is an obvious place to search for the etiology of nutritional insufficiency in the postmature infant. A number of studies suggest decreased placental function after 40 weeks of gestation. Indeed, placental transfer of water, electrolytes, and glucose diminishes after this time, accompanied by a rapid decline in amniotic fluid volume. The diminution of amniotic fluid volume may be the most reliable sign of impending or established placental insufficiency.[77] Abundant amniotic fluid seems to preclude significant nutritional compromise. On the other hand, most babies with decreased amniotic fluid volume are not obviously compromised.

Most placentas from postdate pregnancies do not show characteristic lesions other than those of aging. These include an increased incidence of infarcts, calcification, intervillous thrombosis, perivillous fibrin, retroplacental hematomas, fetal arterial thrombosis, obliterative endarteritis, and compensatory villous growth.[89] A profusion of syncytial knots and an increase in stromal fibrosis, accompanied by decreased vascularization of villi, suggest reduced fetal blood flow and placental ischemia. Accompanying ultrastructural changes include decreased syncytial microvilli, decreased size and number of mitochondria, sparse Golgi apparatus, and decreased syncytial pinocytosis.[86] These changes are similar to those found in preeclampsia, suggesting a common pathogenesis of decreased uterine blood flow. A review of 4205 post-term placentas revealed no characteristic lesion.[30] Placental weight correlates with outcome in postdate pregnancy. In one study, the average placental weight in survivors was about 580 g, whereas the average placental weight in nonsurvivors was 452 g.[44] Placentas weighing more than 700 g were not associated with increased mortality.

Antepartum and intrapartum fetal monitoring data do not support a role for impaired uteroplacental blood flow and fetal asphyxia early in the pathogenesis of the postmaturity syndrome. The majority of post-term pregnancies terminated by cesarean section because of fetal distress reveal variable decelerations (thought to reflect umbilical cord compression) rather than late decelerations. Even infants destined to suffer neurological handicaps rarely manifest late decelerations.

At least two features of postdate pregnancy appear to predispose the post-term fetus to variable decelerations. Oligohydramnios diminishes the fluid buffer around the cord and predisposes to variable decelerations.[32] Indeed, instillation of water via an intrauterine catheter into the uterus of patients with variable decelerations and oligohydramnios ameliorates the deceleration pattern in a high percentage. Oligohydramnios is not an isolated feature in postmature pregnancy. The elevated hematocrit, parched skin, diminished size and turgor of the umbilical cord, and diminished placental weight all reflect generalized fluid deprivation and increase the risk of umbilical cord compression and perhaps other sequelae. Thus, in contrast to the usual explanation of postmaturity syndrome, which indicts global placental insufficiency, we prefer to separate two placental functions—respiratory and nutritional. The respiratory function maintains blood-gas homeostasis, whereas the nutritional function affords foodstuffs and water to the developing fetus. There is little doubt that the designation postmaturity syndrome describes fetal wasting, with evidence of fetal weight loss. However, there is little evidence for concurrent impaired respiratory function of the placenta in the majority of fetuses with postmaturity syndrome. One might argue that, if the respiratory function of the placenta were as severely affected as the nutritional, the fetus would not survive. Although insufficient placental blood flow accounts for 25% of perinatal mortality in post-term gestation,[60] it seems unreasonable to equate nutritional with respiratory placental insufficiency except late in the syndrome.

The postmature infant is of normal length and head circumference but shows evidence of weight loss and nutritional deprivation. Three stages of postmaturity are recognized, according to the degree of fetal nutritional deprivation (Table 19-1).[16,17] There is a direct correlation among the appearance of the neonate, the severity of fetal distress, and perinatal morbidity and mortality. Biochemically, the affected neonate manifests dehydration, polycythemia, increased hemoglobin concentration,[60,89] elevated plasma levels of bilirubin, pentoses, and nitrogen, and glycosuria, albuminuria,[81] and hypoglycemia.

The majority of babies who deliver post-term do not suffer from dysmaturity. In many of these fetuses, growth continues apace. These infants thus may reach macrosomic weights (see below).

TABLE 19-1. CLIFFORD CLASSIFICATION OF POSTMATURITY[53]

Stage 1
- Dry, cracked, peeling, loose, wrinkled skin
- Long nails, abundant hair
- Loss of vernix
- Malnourished appearance, recent weight loss
- Decreased subcutaneous tissue
- Open-eyed and alert infant

Stage 2
- All features of Stage 1
- Meconium staining (greenish)
- Fetal distress or anoxia, birth asphyxia in some cases

Stage 3
- All features of Stages 1 and 2
- Meconium staining (yellow) of cord and nails
- Perinatal mortality

DIAGNOSIS

The diagnosis of post-term gestation requires careful review of menstrual history and early clinical examination. Ultrasound evaluation should be performed early if dates are uncertain or if uterine size and dates are discordant. As many as 22% of pregnancies cannot be assigned reliable dates.[23] The menstrual history should include questions about the period, the previous period, and use of contraceptive pills. Although some clinicians classify and manage patients based on the presumed accuracy of the menstrual history (Table 19-2),[90] this strategy seems to be of little value and belies the element of uncertainty in all such estimates of gestational age. Definitive dates must be assigned early in pregnancy. Once a due date has been assigned, it must never be revised. The accuracy of the assignment of gestational age by any technique decreases with advancing age. We believe it inappropriate to attempt to use amniotic fluid volume or cervical ripeness late in pregnancy to determine the accuracy of the due date. The cervix tends to be unfavorable in post-term gestation,[40,45] refuting the notion that, if the cervix is not favorable near the estimated delivery

TABLE 19-2. CLASSIFICATION OF DATING HISTORY AT 42 WEEKS OF GESTATION

Good dates

The presence of one of the following:
- Positive pregnancy test documented by 6 weeks from the last menstrual period
- First examination performed by the 10th week of gestation with bimanual examination
- Fetal heart tones heard with a DeLee stethoscope at 20 weeks' gestation and/or 22 weeks or longer since fetal heart tones were first heard
- Gestational age confirmed with ultrasound examination before 28 weeks

Poor dates

Failure to substantiate the menstrual dates by the above criteria date, dating must have been incorrect.[10] On an average, amniotic fluid volume decreases to less than 300 ml at 42 weeks' gestation.[89] Some suggest that normal amounts of amniotic fluid require thorough reexamination of the historically determined dates.[72]

IMPLICATIONS OF POSTDATE PREGNANCY

Perinatal mortality in prolonged pregnancy exceeds that of term pregnancies by twofold.[1,30,44] A variety of reasons account for the increase[60]:

Congenital anomaly	26%
adrenal hypoplasia	
anencephaly	
Infection	19%
Abruptio placentae	10%
Rh	8%
Growth failure	8%
Placental infarcts	7%
Miscellaneous	22%

Anoxia is prominent in about one-third of deaths.[28,53,60] Modern management has done much to reduce perinatal mortality, but a residual morbidity that requires attention remains. The majority of postdate babies continue to grow. The incidence of macrosomia increases with advancing gestational age. Macrosomia, in turn, predisposes to dysfunctional labor, traumatic delivery, shoulder dystocia, and brachial plexus injury. If placental insufficiency is present, there is a high incidence of fetal distress during labor, accompanied by meconium staining and acidosis.[31] Neonatal problems include asphyxia, meconium aspiration syndrome, persistent fetal circulation, respiratory distress, and metabolic disturbances which include hypoglycemia, hypothermia, and hypocalcemia.[17,50,51,57,89,91] The consequences of intrauterine deprivation and compromised neonatal adaptation continue to be reflected in later morbidity. Such babies reflect an increased early mortality, increased frequency of illness, feeding and sleep disturbances, and low developmental and mental scores.[91]

INCIDENCE

Post-term gestations occur more frequently in young and elderly primigravidas and tend to recur in successive pregnancies. Prolonged gestation also occurs more frequently when the fetus is male.[89]

The exact incidence of post-term gestation is uncertain but has been estimated to be between 3.5% and 15.0%.[1,10,50] Approximately 4.0–7.3% of pregnancies deliver after 43 weeks.[91] The duration of pregnancy calculated from Naegle's rule assumes a 28-day cycle with conception at midcycle. For menstrual cycles longer than 28 days, the estimated date of confinement (EDC) must be advanced by the duration of the cycle in excess of 28 days. Such "delayed ovulation" is the major cause of prolonged pregnancy when the EDC is calculated from the last menstrual period. When adjusted for cycle length, the true incidence of post-term gestation varies between 5% and 8%.[77] When accurate and consistent with early physical exam, menstrual data are the most reliable criteria for dating pregnancy. Pelvic examination before 10 weeks' gestation is optimal. If the uterus is retroverted or the patient is obese, confirmation of dates by uterine size may be difficult. Fetal heart tones are usually heard with a conventional stethoscope by the 19th to 20th week of gestation but may be audible as early as 17 weeks. If heart tones have been documented for 20 weeks, the pregnancy may be considered to be at term. If ultrasonic doppler probes are used, fetal cardiac activity will usually be documented no later than 12 weeks.

Urine pregnancy tests can detect hCG between 4 and 7 days after the first missed period (see Chapter 5). The β-hCG test becomes positive one week after conception. We emphasize that, despite the limitations and pitfalls of early examination, fetal auscultation, and detection of hCG in urine, the earlier in pregnancy that the examination is performed, the more accurate is assessment of gestational age.

Ultrasound is useful for dating pregnancy in both the first and second trimesters. In the first trimester, before 12 weeks' gestation, evaluation of the crown–rump length (CRL) is accurate to within 3 days.[13,73] Beyond 14 weeks, the biparietal diameter (BPD) is widely used, but, increasingly, gestational age is computed from composite information including cephalic index, femur length, and head and abdominal circumferences. The BPD should be obtained between 14 and 28 weeks. If the LMP is known, a single examination at 20 weeks is sufficient. If the dates are uncertain or the examination between 14 and 20 weeks is inconsistent, then a repeat examination done before 30 weeks is indicated. The interval between examinations should be at least 3–4 weeks. The growth rate between the

16th and 24th weeks is 3–3.5 mm per week.[13]

A significant portion (40–70%) of apparently prolonged pregnancies result from poor assignment of gestational age.[9,22] Careful attention to history and physical examination and liberal ultrasound scanning prior to 24 weeks' gestation should decrease the incidence of post-term pregnancy by eliminating inappropriate assignments of gestational age.

In our institutions, we do not allow reassignment of gestational age. At the initial visit, an EDC is assigned if the periods are regular and the examination before 10 weeks is consistent. If these factors are not present or the patient has recently used birth control pills, we do not assign a date until we have obtained an ultrasound examination. Once the date is assigned, it is never changed, because, as discussed above, the accuracy of the estimation of gestational age diminishes as pregnancy advances.

Although the primary concern in postdate pregnancy is for the safety of the fetus, reassurance of the mother is important and should begin long before 42 weeks. Mothers should be informed of the variation in duration of pregnancy and of the consequences of going beyond term.

MANAGEMENT OF PROLONGED PREGNANCY

The management of the uncomplicated, prolonged pregnancy remains controversial. One must weigh the risk of increased fetal morbidity and mortality associated with continued intrauterine existence beyond 42 weeks' gestation against problems associated with routine induction of labor. Those advocating conservative management rely on one or more antepartum tests of fetal well-being, including the nonstress test (NST),[74] the oxytocin challenge test (OCT), also designated the contraction stress test (CST),[28] amniocentesis or amnioscopy for detection of meconium,[89] determination of estriol levels,[7] measurement of human placental lactogen (hPL),[41] and real-time ultrasound scanning for analysis of fetal breathing movements (FBM), fetal movements (FM), and amniotic fluid volume (AFV).[56,69,78] In general, the various parameters predict normal outcome well but are less accurate in predicting poor outcome; none is a good predictor of postmaturity.

Advocates of routine intervention at 42 weeks' gestation cite multiple factors to support their philosophy of aggressive management. These factors include increasing maternal and physician anxiety over fetal well-being and the potential of perinatal morbidity and mortality. Increasing fetal size and weight (macrosomia) make the course of labor potentially more difficult and longer with birth trauma more likely with vaginal delivery. Cesarean delivery for failure to progress during labor is more frequent in the presence of macrosomia. Continued intrauterine existence increases the likelihood of meconium passage in utero and the potential for meconium aspiration or postmaturity syndrome. The development of oligohydramnios increases the likelihood of cord compression, significant fetal heart rate decelerations antepartum and intrapartum, thereby increasing the likelihood of cesarean delivery for fetal distress. Although routine induction of labor is associated with an increased rate of cesarean delivery,[33,61,89] more reliable techniques of induction or cervical ripening may decrease this risk. Breast self-stimulation successfully ripens the cervix in term pregnancies and can decrease the incidence of unfavorable cervices at 42 weeks gestation and facilitate induction of labor.[26,27]

Advocates of conservative or expectant management cite several problems associated with elective induction, including inappropriate gestational age assignment, universally acceptable perinatal outcome in the majority of fetuses left in utero, and the high rate of failure of elective induction necessitating cesarean intervention. Cesarean delivery is associated with increased maternal and fetal morbidity in subsequent pregnancies.[70] Despite philosophical differences, most authors agree that, when the cervix is favorable and no contraindications to induction exist, induction of labor at 42 weeks' gestation is appropriate[22,31,72,89,90]

A recent survey of the management of post-term pregnancy revealed that the approach to management among institutions training fellows in maternal–fetal medicine varies considerably.[36] A minority routinely terminate the pregnancy regardless of cervical examination at 42 weeks' gestation. The majority of institutions favor regular assessment of fetal well-being when expectant management is followed.

ASSESSMENT OF FETAL WELL-BEING

Biochemical Assessment

As a result of conflicting reports on their usefulness, the use of estriol (E_3) determinations to assess fetal well-being in post-term pregnancy has declined drastically in recent years.[41,56,69,70,78,79] During pregnancy, the production of E_3 by the mother results from a complex process involving the maternal liver and kidneys, the placenta and the fetal adrenal and liver (see Chapter 3). Estriol derives from placental bioconversion of fetal 16-α-hydroxydehydroepiandrosterone sulfate.[75] Falsely low estriol values, in the absence of placental dysfunction, are found in certain conditions (Table 19-3).[49] Measurement of urinary E_3 has the theoretical advantage over serum E_3 measurement of sampling the steroid over a longer period of time. The 24-hour urine estriol method eliminates diurnal variation. The estriol to creatinine ratio can be used to assure proper collection technique. However, the collection methodology is inconvenient, is associated with delay in obtaining results, masks acute changes, often requires repetition, and is associated with falsely low levels when renal disease is present.[49] Plasma E_3 measurement allows for ease of obtaining the sample and rapid results but fails to account for diurnal variation and false elevation in the presence of renal disease. To be effective, serial 24-hour urinary E_3 measurement should be initiated at 41.5 weeks for baseline excretion determination and repeated three times weekly.[7,83] A 35% decrease in urinary E_3 excretion is regarded as critical, prompting further evaluation or delivery.[34] The estrogen:creatinine ratio from single-voided and 24-hour urine collections is highly predictive of fetal dysmaturity and may ultimately prove useful in management of post-term pregnancy.[42,71]

Amniocentesis

Meconium is present in 20–40% of postdate pregnancies. Given the high correlation, the search for meconium by amniocentesis or amnioscopy enjoyed considerable vogue for a time but has since fallen out of fashion. Though meconium passage is associated with fetal distress, it is more reasonably a function of gestational age, representing maturity of the gastrointestinal system of the postdate fetus. The presence of meconium at amniocentesis does not correlate with perinatal outcome unless co-associated with abnormal fetal heart rate pattern.[2,37,79] Since amniocentesis is not without risk, especially with diminished amniotic fluid, we find little to support its utilization in the post-term patient.

TABLE 19-3. ETIOLOGY OF LOW ESTRIOL DETERMINATIONS

1. Placental dysfunction
2. Fetal anencephaly
3. Fetal adrenal disorders
   (a) Primary congenital adrenal hypoplasia
   (b) Secondary adrenal hypoplasia secondary to maternal steroid administration
4. Fetal liver cirrhosis
5. Placental sulfatase deficiency
6. Maternal renal disease (urinary measurement)
7. Maternal antibiotic administration and interruption of hepatointestinal circulation

Maternal Perception of Fetal Activity

Maternal monitoring of fetal activity has been a helpful adjunct to standard evaluation techniques. Active fetal movements are an expression of fetal well-being.[76] Decreased fetal movements are associated with chronic uteroplacental insufficiency and may herald the onset of hypoxia or asphyxia. Monitoring of fetal activity has been suggested as a screening test to be utilized prior to traditional fetal monitoring techniques.[35] Nevertheless, total reliance on such testing seems inappropriate in light of variable patient compliance and reliability and of the proven ability of traditional monitoring techniques.[22]

Antepartum Electronic Fetal Monitoring

Antepartum fetal heart rate monitoring in the form of the NST or the OCT is the most efficient, reliable technique of monitoring the progression of prolonged pregnancy.[22,39]

Regardless of testing and management philosophy, the major inconvenience of the OCT is that it is time consuming. The reliability and predictive abilities of the OCT are less than ideal. When the OCT was utilized as the primary means of surveillance in post-term pregnancy, patients experienced low perinatal morbidity and high cesarean delivery rates.[31] However, FHR decelerations were noted in 38.5% of tests. The last test prior to delivery was normal in only 57.9% of tests. Furthermore, pregnancy termination was performed in 25.4% of patients, although only 5.5% of tests demonstrated repetitive late decelerations (positive OCT). There was clearly a therapeutic benefit of early intervention in postdate pregnancies irrespective of OCT test result. Unfortunately, this good outcome associated with OCT testing has not been duplicated by others who found a significant risk of morbidity in patients so managed.[45,70,79] Further experience with the OCT should clarify these discrepancies.

The restriction of the analysis of the NST to the presence (reactive) or absence (nonreactive) of FHR accelerations has been viewed as an extremely simplified method of interpretation of the NST.[47] "Full visual analysis" of the NST is a less rigid and more individualized method that allows evaluation of FHR decelerations and baseline heart rate and variability.[48,88] The controversy concerning NST evaluation criteria stems from testing philosophy and use of the OCT when the NST is nonreactive. Complete visual analysis of the NST appears to make OCT performance unnecessary, because of occasional spontaneous uterine contractions during NST testing. Because spontaneous contractions are invariably present during NST testing during the post-term period, attention to spontaneous contractions and FHR decelerations appears appropriate.[47] A direct comparison between approaches is lacking.

The use of the NST as a primary means of surveillance in post-term pregnancy has its advocates.[48,66,74,78,88] However, recent reports of poor perinatal outcome following NST testing in post-term pregnancies have reheated the NST versus the OCT controversy.[4,59,68] Recent data support the concept that the reactive NST is a reliable sign of fetal well-being in post-term pregnancy.[25] When delivery is effected immediately after a reactive NST is found, there is virtually no serious morbidity. However, we must be more circumspect about findings other than reactivity in antepartum test results. With normal AFV (by ultrasound) and absent decelerations, the reactive NST suffices. When AFV is diminished or episodic decelerations are seen on the reactive NST, delivery must be considered irrespective of the reactive NST. The frequency of testing may also be of crucial importance because semi-weekly testing may also contribute to improved perinatal outcome when compared to weekly testing.[25]

Real-Time Ultrasound Assessment

An alternate technique for fetal surveillance is the biophysical profile (RTBS), which includes evaluation of the NST, FBM, gross fetal body movements (FM), flexion (tone), and AFV.[56] Evaluation of AFV is crucial to the assessment of fetal well-being in post-term gestations.[25,50] The association between decreased AFV and FHR decelerations in antepartum and intrapartum testing in postdate pregnancies has been clearly demonstrated.[24,25,32,50,65,80] No infant was found to have the postmaturity syndrome when normal amniotic fluid was found by real-time ultrasound scanning.[25]

Assessment of Fetal Well-Being Protocol

The evidence suggests that the reactive NST is at least as good a predictor of immediate normal outcome as is the negative OCT and that prolongation of pregnancy in post-term gestation increases the risk of abnormal outcome.[25] Thus, there is clearly a therapeutic benefit of early intervention in post-term pregnancies, irrespective of test results or test schemas. The testing scheme presented in Fig. 19-1 employs routine semi-weekly NST and ultrasound AFV scanning for the assessment of fetal well-being in post-term gestations.[25] The scheme assumes that the NST is a suitable screening test provided FHR decelerations are absent during testing and amniotic fluid is normal. When FHR decelerations occur during the NST or decreased AFV is seen, the post-term patient should be hospitalized and pregnancy terminated, irrespective of the underlying FHR pattern.

This scheme produces results comparable to those of the OCT, including low morbidity rates and high cesarean section rates.[25,66] On the basis of the outcome results, there seems little to choose between the OCT and the NST/ultrasound scheme for management of post-term pregnancy. However, the NST/ultrasound scheme is faster, more simple and less subject to equivocal results, poses no danger, and carries only minimal inconvenience. In addition, ultrasound scanning provides information concerning placental location, fetal presentation, and the presence or absence of fetal anomalies.

INTRAPARTUM MANAGEMENT

General Considerations

Although statistics generally point to a rise in mortality and morbidity after 42 weeks, it is unreasonable to believe either that (1) the rise is a step function or (2) that the antecedents of fetal embarrassment are not already present at 42 weeks' gestation. Only about 10–20% of postdate pregnancies are in fact compromised, but the

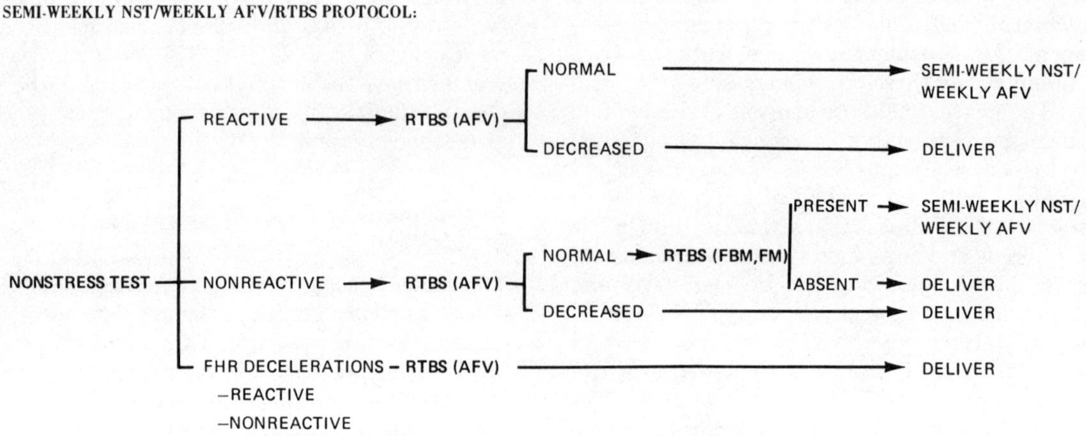

Figure 19-1. This scheme outlines the use of the nonstress test utilized in conjunction with weekly evaluation of amniotic fluid volume by real-time B-scan [RTBS (AFV)] combined with use of real-time B-scan to determine fetal breathing movements and fetal movements (FBM, FM). (Reprinted from Eden, R. D., Gergely, R. Z., Schifrin, B. S. and Wade, M. E.: Comparison of antepartum testing schemes for the management of the postdate pregnancy. Am. J. Obstet. Gynecol. **144:**683–692, 1985, with permission of the C. V. Mosby Co.)

majority of those are found to be compromised at the time of initial examination after 42 weeks. We believe that it is not possible to expect optimal outcome in postdate pregnancy if testing begins after the 42nd week of pregnancy (294 days). Accordingly, it has been our policy to begin testing in the 41st week, that is, on or before the 287th day of pregnancy as calculated from the last menstrual period.

The goals of intrapartum management are prevention and early detection of intrapartum asphyxia, prevention of meconium aspiration, and prevention of traumatic delivery. For these purposes, we require electronic fetal monitoring in spontaneous or induced labor. We prefer direct electrode monitoring, but this may not be possible early in labor, especially with an unfavorable cervix. If the external tracing is adequate, surveillance may be continued by this technique. We believe that inability to obtain adequate electronic surveillance of the post-term fetus during labor mandates cesarean section.

Every attempt is made to avoid difficult delivery. We recommend careful assessment of fetal size and attention to the course of labor, with particular attention to the risks of shoulder dystocia with protracted descent in the second stage[8] (see Chapter 45).

Irrespective of methodology of antepartum assessment or timing of delivery, labor is dangerous for the post-term fetus. Patients should be encouraged to come to the hospital in early labor and the fetus should be monitored as soon as possible. Careful attention to fetal heart rate patterns, liberal use of fetal scalp blood pH sampling, and close attention to progress of labor are warranted in these patients.

The incidence of the passage of meconium is increased in post-term pregnancies.[45,58] Meconium staining of the amniotic fluid is noted at the time of rupture of the membranes in approximately 20% of such patients and its incidence doubles by the time of delivery. If no fluid is obtained at amniotomy or at spontaneous rupture of the membranes, meconium must be anticipated. The consistency of the meconium in the amniotic fluid is inversely related to the amount of fluid. With severe oligohydramnios, meconium may be so inspissated that it may not flow and may not appear at the cervix if the head is well engaged. Meconium appears in about 50% of babies with oligohydramnios. Irrespective of the passage of meconium, cesarean intervention for fetal distress should be reserved for those fetuses demonstrating fetal heart rate patterns and acidosis, because the majority of post-term infants tolerate labor well.[58] In the absence of abnormal heart rate patterns, meconium per se is not considered an indication for delivery. However, the presence of meconium does demand the availability of adequate personnel at delivery to manage fetal resuscitation. Timely aspiration of the oral pharynx during delivery is mandatory to minimize the risk of meconium aspiration. The infant's nose and oropharynx should be cleared by suction with a bulb syringe and a DeLee trap prior to delivery of the chest.[14]

The neonatal management of the meconium-covered baby by trained and experienced personnel requires repeated emphasis (see Chapter 10). A pediatrician/neonatologist trained in neonatal resuscitation should be present at every post-term delivery when fetal distress or meconium is present. The degree of resuscitation is governed by the degree of birth asphyxia and the presence of meconium.

Meconium aspiration resulting from fetal or infant gasping may obstruct the airway, interfere with gas exchange, and cause severe respiratory distress. Tracheal meconium is visualized in approximately 50% of infants if the amniotic fluid is meconium stained. Tracheal meconium may be present without evidence of meconium in the mouth or larynx. The amount and texture of the meconium is related to the severity of respiratory distress. Tracheal suction should be accomplished under direct vision when meconium is present in the hypopharynx. Direct visualization and proper suctioning of meconium favorably affect neonatal outcome.[14,38] Positive pressure respiration should be delayed until adequate tracheal suction has been accomplished. Intubation is accomplished under direct laryngoscopy before inspiration. Suction is performed until the trachea is cleared. This should be accomplished rapidly before significant bradycardia occurs.

Depressed infants having tracheal meconium at birth are at risk for meconium aspiration pneumonia and should be observed for respiratory distress. When pulmonary parenchymal changes are noted on x-ray, chest physiotherapy and oropharyngeal suctioning with positional change should be performed frequently.[18] Broad-spectrum antibiotics should be initiated following culture, since meconium promotes the growth of bacteria.[11]

Significant meconium aspiration leads to mechanical obstruction of both large and small airways and a chemical pneumonitis often resulting in severe hypoxemia and pulmonary artery hypertension.[18] A 10–20% incidence of pneumothorax or pneumomediastinum is associated with meconium aspiration. This incidence is increased when mechanical ventilation is required.[11,43]

Management of Polycythemia in the Neonate

Increased viscosity and decreased blood flow diminish oxygen transport when the central hematocrit rises above 60%.[6,85] Since infant erythrocytes are less deformable than adult erythrocytes, there is an impairment of tissue oxygenation and formation of microthrombi with increasing blood viscosity. Polycythemia in post-term infants results from placental insufficiency and chronic hypoxia. Infants are plethoric in appearance and may experience respiratory distress, congestive heart failure, renal vein thrombosis, priapism, hypoglycemia, and hyperbilirubinemia. Volume expansion is the preferred method of treatment, but partial exchange transfusion should be performed when the hematocrit is greater than 65% or when symptoms appear.[19]

PROGNOSIS

Interpretation of perinatal morbidity and mortality statistics associated with prolonged pregnancy is controversial.[10,17,21,25,54,55,57,66,67,81,90] Early reports suggested an increase in perinatal mortality with post-term pregnancy with a rate twice that of term gestations at 43 weeks, tripled at 44 weeks, and quintupled at 45 weeks.[10,17] Furthermore, perinatal mortality increases with maternal age and decreases with increasing gravidity. Recent evidence suggests that the risk of antepartum and intrapartum death resides in the small, growth-retarded fetus.[21,55,81] A review of stillbirths following nonstress testing revealed a stillbirth rate of 2.8 per 1000.[5] The OCT and NST/ultrasound testing schemes have reduced that rate even further.[25,66]

An increased incidence of neonatal illness, sleep and feeding disturbances, delayed social development, difficult temperament, and hospitalizations occurs in post-term infants.[12,15,46,52,84] The increase in mortality of these infants extends to up to two years of age.[91] The most controlled investigation of postmature infants revealed that Brazelton interaction and motor and Denver Developmental Scale scores were lower than in term controls at four months.

However, at eight months only the mental scores were lower.[29]

CONTROVERSIES

The management of previous cesarean delivery patients in the post-term period is also controversial. Currently most patients are electively delivered by repeat cesarean section at 42 weeks. Further experience with vaginal delivery following previous cesarean may allow selected patients to await spontaneous onset of labor in the post-term period.

SUMMARY

Prolonged pregnancies represent difficulties in clinical management. There is increased anxiety on the part of the patient, increased concern on the part of the physician, and no universally satisfying solution to these problems. We believe that much anxiety can be reduced if the problem of postdate pregnancy is anticipated and discussed early in pregnancy, when the most accurate dating of pregnancy takes place. Timely fetal testing, including amniotic fluid measurement, should be initiated soon after the due date, and prompt intervention should occur if fetal testing or amniotic fluid volume is abnormal. During labor, attention to fetal condition and the progress of labor can do much to optimize outcome.

REFERENCES

1. Abdul-Karim, R. W. and Rizk, P. T.: Prolonged pregnancy and postmaturity. In: *Perinatology Case Studies*. A. Langer and L. Iffy (Eds.). Garden City, New York, Medical Examination Publishing Co., 1978.
2. Abramovici, H. and Brandes, J. M.: Meconium during delivery: A sign of compensated fetal distress. *Am. J. Obstet. Gynecol.* **118**:251–255, 1974.
3. Ballantine, J. W. and Browne, F. J.: The problems of foetal post-maturity and prolongation of pregnancy. *J. Obstet. Gynaecol. Br. Emp.* **29**:177–238, 1922.
4. Barrett, J. M., Salyer, S. L., and Boehm, F. H.: The nonstress test: An evaluation of 1,000 patients. *Am. J. Obstet. Gynecol.* **141**:153–157, 1981.
5. Barss, V. A., Frigoletto, F. D., and Diamond, F.: Stillbirth after nonstress testing. *Obstet. Gynecol.* **65**:541-544, 1985.
6. Baum, R. S.: Viscous forces in neonatal polycythemia. (Abstract) *J. Pediatr.* **69**:975, 1966.
7. Beischer, N. A., Brown, J. B., Smith, M. A., and Townsend, L.: Studies in prolonged pregnancy. II. Clinical results and urinary excretion in prolonged pregnancy. *Am. J. Obstet. Gynecol.* **103**:483–495, 1969.
8. Benedetti, T. J. and Gabbe, S. G.: Shoulder dystocia, a complication of fetal macrosomia and prolonged second stage of labor with midpelvic delivery. *Obstet. Gynecol.* **52**:526–529, 1978.
9. Boyce, A., Mayaux, M. J., and Schwartz, D.: Classical and "true" gestational postmaturity. *Am. J. Obstet. Gynecol.* **125**:911–917, 1976.
10. Browne, J. C.: Postmaturity. *JAMA* **186**:1047–1052, 1963.
11. Bryan, C. S.: Enhancement of bacterial infection by meconium. *Johns Hopkins Med. J.* **121**:9–14, 1967.
12. Callenbach, J. C. and Hall, R. T.: Morbidity and mortality of advanced gestational age: Post-term or postmature. Obstet. Gynecol. **53**:721–724, 1979.
13. Campbell, S. and Neumann, G. B.: Growth of the fetal biparietal diameter during normal pregnancy. *J. Obstet. Gynaecol. Br. Commonw.* **78**:513–519, 1971.
14. Carson, B. S., Losey, R. W., Bower, W. A., and Simmons, M. A.: Combined obstetric and pediatric approach prevents meconium aspiration syndrome. *Am. J. Obstet. Gynecol.* **126**:712–715, 1976.
15. Chamberlain, R. N. and Simpson, R. N.: Cross-sectional studies of physical growth in twins. Postmature and small-for-dates children. *Acta Paediatr. Scand.* **66**:457–463, 1977.
16. Clifford, S. H.: Clinical significance of yellow staining of the vernix caseosa, skin, nails and umbilical cord of the newborn. (Abstract) *Am. J. Dis. Child.* **69**:327, 1945.
17. Clifford, S. H.: Postmaturity—with placental dysfunction: Clinical syndrome and pathologic findings. *J. Pediatr.* **44**:1–13, 1954.
18. Cloherty, J. P : Meconium aspiration. In: *Manual of Neonatal Care*. J. P. Cloherty and A R. Stark (Eds.). Boston, Little, Brown and Company, 1980, pp. 163–167.
19. Cloherty, J. P.: Polycythemia. In: *Manual of Neonatal Care*. J. P. Cloherty and A. R. Stark (Eds.). Boston, Little Brown and Company, 1980, pp. 231–233.
20. Csapo, A. I.: Dr. Csapo's "Seesaw" theory of pregnancy. *Contemp. OB/GYN* **8**:51–55, 1976.
21. Dawkins, M. J.: Perinatal mortality survey under auspices of National Birthday Trust Fund (Preliminary Communication). Associations of intrauterine asphyxia. *Proc. R. Soc. Med.* **54**:1090–1091, 1961.
22. Depp, R.: Postmaturity. In: *Management of High-Risk* Pregnancy. J. Queenan (Ed.). Oradell, NJ, Medical Economics, 1981, pp. 531–547.
23. Dewhurst, C. J., Beazley, J. J., and Campbell, S.:

Assessment of fetal maturity and dysmaturity. *Am. J. Obstet. Gynecol.* **113**:141–149, 1972.

24. Druzin, M. L., Gratacos, H., Keegan, K. A., and Paul, R. H.: Antepartum fetal heart rate testing. VII. The significance of fetal bradycardia. *Am. J. Obstet. Gynecol.* **139**:194–198, 1981.
25. Eden, R. D., Gergely, R. Z., Schifrin, B. S., and Wade, M. E.: Comparison of antepartum testing schemes for the management of the postdate pregnancy. *Am. J. Obstet. Gynecol.* **144**:683–692, 1982.
26. Elliot, J. P. and Flaherty, J. F.: The use of breast stimulation to prevent postdate pregnancy. *Am. J. Obstet. Gynecol.* **149**:628–632, 1984.
27. Elliot, J. P. and Flaherty, J. F.: The use of breast stimulation to ripen the cervix in term pregnancies. *Am. J. Obstet. Gynecol.* **145**:553–556, 1983.
28. Evans, T. N., Koeff, S. T., and Morley, G. W.: Fetal effects of prolonged pregnancy. *Am. J. Obstet. Gynecol.* **85**:701–709, 1963.
29. Field, T. M., Dabiri, C., Hallock, N., and Schumann, H. H.: Developmental effects of prolonged pregnancy and the postmaturity syndrome. *J. Pediatr.* **90**:836–839, 1977.
30. Fox, H.: The placenta in pregnancies of abnormal duration. In: *Pathology of the Placenta (Major Problems in Pathology*, Vol. 7). H. Fox (Ed.). London, W. B. Saunders, 1978.
31. Freeman, R. K., Garite, T. J., Modanlow, H., Dorchester, W., Rommal, C., and Devaney, M.: Post-date pregnancy: Utilization of contraction stress testing for primary fetal surveillance. *Am. J. Obstet. Gynecol.* **140**:128–135, 1981.
32. Gabbe, S. A., Ettinger, B. B., Freeman, R. K., and Martin, C. B.:. Umbilical cord compression associated with amniotomy: Laboratory observations. *Am. J. Obstet. Gynecol.* **126**:353–355, 1976.
33. Gibb, D. M. F., Cardozo, L. D., Studd, J. W. W., and Cooper, D. J.: Prolonged pregnancy: Is induction of labour indicated? A prospective study. *Br. J. Obstet. Gynaecol.* **89**:292–295, 1982.
34. Goebelsmann, V., Freeman, R. K., Mestman, J. H., Nakamura, R. M., and Woodling, B. A.: Estriol in pregnancy. *Am. J. Obstet. Gynecol.* **115**:795–802, 1973.
35. Goodlin, R. C. and Haesslein, H. C.: When is it fetal distress? *Am. J. Obstet. Gynecol.* **128**:440–445, 1977.
36. Granados, J. L.: Survey of the management of postterm pregnancy. *Obstet. Gynecol.* **63**:651–653, 1984.
37. Green, J. N. and Paul, R. H.: The value of amniocentesis in prolonged pregnancy. *Obstet. Gynecol.* **51**:293–298, 1978.
38. Gregory, G. A., Goodling, C. A., Phibbs, R. H., and Tooley, W. H.: Meconium aspiration in infants—a prospective study. *J. Pediatr.* **85**:848–852, 1974.
39. Hammacher, K.: Früherkennung intrauterine Gefahrenzustande durch Elektrophonokardiographie und Tokographie. In: *Die Prophylaxe Frühkindlicher Hirnschaden*. R. Elert, and K. A. Huter (Eds.). Stuttgart, Georg Thieme, 1966.
40. Harris, B. A., Huddleston, J. F., Sutliff, G., and Perlis, H. W.: The unfavorable cervix in prolonged pregnancy. *Obstet. Gynecol.* **62**:171–174, 1983.
41. Josimovich, J. B., Soffonoff, P., Starkovsky, N., and Mueller-Heubach, E.: Evaluation of postterm pregnancy with maternal serum placental lactogen and alpha fetoprotein concentrations. *Obstet. Gynecol.* **50**:445–449, 1977.
42. Khouzami, V. A., Johnson, J. C., Hernandez, E., Rotmensch, J., Frye, R., and Daihohu, N.: Urinary estrogens in post-term pregnancy. *Am. J. Obstet. Gynecol.* **141**:205–211, 1981.
43. Klaus, M.: Cleansing the neonatal trachea. *J. Pediatr.* **85**:853, 1974.
44. Kloosterman, G. J.: The obstetrician and dysmaturity. In: *Nutricia Symposium of Prematurity and Dysmaturity, Groningen, 1967.* Aspects of prematurity and dysmaturity. H. E. Leiden, and K. N. V. Stensert (Eds.). Springfield, IL, Thomas, 1968, pp. 263–280.
45. Knox, G. E., Huddleston, J. F., and Flowers, C. E.: Management of prolonged pregnancy: Results of a prospective randomized trial. *Am. J. Obstet. Gynecol.* **134**:376–381, 1979.
46. Krebs, H. B., Peters, R. E., Dunn, L. J., Jordan, H. V. F., and Segretti, A.: Intrapartum fetal heart rate monitoring. III. Association of meconium with abnormal fetal heart rate patterns. *Am. J. Obstet. Gynecol.* **137**:936–943, 1980.
47. Kubli, F.: Antepartum monitoring of fetal heart rate. In: *Fetal Physiology and Medicine, The Basis of Perinatology*, 2nd Edition. R. N. Beard, and P. W. Nathanielsz (Eds.). New York, Marcel Dekker, 1984.
48. Kubli, F., Boos, R., Ruttgers, H., Hagens, C., and Vanselow, H.: Antepartum FHR-monitoring. In: *Current Status of* FHR Monitoring and Ultrasound in Obstetrics. Proceedings of the Scientific Meeting of the Royal College of Obstetricians and Gynaecologists, December 2, 1977. R. W. Beard, and S. Campbell (Eds.). London, The College, 1977.
49. Laros, R. K.: Evaluation of the fetus. In: *Anesthesia for Obstetrics.* S. M. Shnider and G. Levinson (Eds.). Baltimore, William & Wilkins, 1979, pp. 343–356.
50. Leveno, J. J., Quirk, J. G., Cunningham, F. G., Nelson, S. D., Rigoberto, S.-R., Toofanian, A., and DePalma, R. T.: Prolonged pregnancy. I. Observations concerning the causes of fetal distress. *Am. J. Obstet. Gynecol.* **150**:465–473, 1984.
51. Lindell, A.: Prolonged pregnancy. *Acta Obstet. Gynecol. Scand.* **35**:136–163, 1956.
52. Lovell, K. E.: The effect of postmaturity on the developing child. *Med. J. Aust.* **1**:13–17, 1973.
53. Lucas, W. E., Anctil, A. O., and Callagan, D. A.: The problem of post-term pregnancy. *Am. J. Obstet. Gynecol.* **91**:241–250, 1965.

54. Macafee, C. H. and Bancroft-Livingston, G.: Studies in prolonged pregnancy. IV. Clinical assessment. *J. Obstet. Gynaecol. Br. Commonw.* **65**:7–15, 1958.

55. Magram, H. M. and Cavanagh, W. V.: Problem of postmaturty: Statistical analysis. *Am. J. Obstet. Gynecol.* **79**:216–223, 1960.

56. Manning, F. A., Platt, L. D., and Sipos, L.: Antepartum fetal evaluation: Development of a fetal biophysical profile. *Am. J. Obstet. Gynecol.* **136**:787–795, 1980.

57. Mead, P. B. and Marcus, S. L.: Prolonged pregnancy. *Am. J. Obstet. Gynecol.* **89**:495–502, 1964.

58. Miller, F. C. and Read, J. A.: Intrapartum assessment of the postdate fetus. *Am. J. Obstet. Gynecol.* **141**:516–520, 1981.

59. Miyazaki, F. S . and Myazaki, B. A.: False reactive nonstress tests in post-term pregnancies. *Am. J. Obstet. Gynecol.* **140**:269–276, 1981.

60. Naeye, R. L.: Causes of perinatal mortality excess in prolonged gestations. *Am. J. Epidemiol.* **108**:429–433, 1978.

61. Nakano, R.: Post-term pregnancy. A five-year review from Osaka National Hospital. *Acta Obstet. Gynecol. Sand.* **51**:217–222, 1972.

62. Nwosu, U. C., Wallach, E. E., Boggs, T. R., and Bongiovanni, A. M.: Possible adrenocortical insufficiency in postmature neonates. *Am. J. Obstet. Gynecol.* **122**:969–974, 1975.

63. Nwosu, U. C., Wallach, E. E., Boggs, T. R., Nemiroff, R. L., and Bongiovanni, A. M.: Possible role of the fetal adrenal glands in the etiology of postmaturity. *Am. J. Obstet. Gynecol.* **121**:366–370, 1975.

64. Nwosu, U. C., Wallach, E. E., and Bolognese, R. J.: Initiation of labor by intraamniotic cortisol instillation in prolonged human pregnancy. *Obstet. Gynecol.* **47**:137–142, 1976.

65. O'Leary, J., Andrinopoulos, G., and Giordano, P.: Variable decelerations and the nonstress test: An indication of cord compromise. *Am. J. Obstet. Gynecol.* **137**:704–706, 1980.

66. Paul, R. H. and Miller, F.: Antepartum FHR monitoring. *Clin. Obstet. Gynecol.* **21**:375–396, 1978.

67. Perlin, I. A.: Postmaturity. *Am. J. Obstet. Gynecol.* **80**:1–5, 1960.

68. Phelan, J. P., Platt, L. D., Yeh, S. Y., Trujillo, M., and Paul, R.H.: Continuing role of the nonstress test in the management of postdates pregnancy. *Obstet. Gynecol.* **64**:624–628, 1984.

69. Platt, L. D., Egligton, G. S., Sipos, L., Broussard, P., and Paul, R. H.: Further experience with the fetal biophysical profile. *Obstet. Gynecol.* **61**:480–485, 193.

70. Pritchard, J. A., MacDonald, P. C., and Gant, N. F. (Eds.): *Williams Obstetrics*, 17th Edition. Norwalk, Appleton-Century-Crofts, 1985, pp. 745–768.

71. Rayburn, W. F., Motley, M. E., Stempel, L. F., and Gendreau, R. M.: Antepartum prediction of the postmature infant. *Obstet. Gynecol.* **60**:148–153, 1982.

72. Resnik, R.: Post-term pregnancy. In: *Maternal Fetal Medicine*. R. Creasy and R. Resnik (Eds.). Philadelphia, Saunders, 1985, pp. 443–448.

73. Robinson, H. P.: Sonar measurement of fetal crown-rump length as means of assessing maturity in the first trimester of pregnancy. *Br. Med. J.* **4**:28–31, 1973.

74. Rochard, F., Schifrin, B. S., and Sureau C.: Nonstressed fetal heart rate monitoring in the antepartum period. *Am. J. Obstet. Gynecol.* **126**:699–706, 1976.

75. Ryan, K. J.: Placental synthesis of steroid hormones. In: *Maternal-Fetal Endocrinology*. D. Tulchinsky and K. J. Ryan (Eds.). Philadelphia, W. B. Saunders, 1980, pp. 3–16.

76. Sadovsky, E. and Polishuk, W. Z.: Fetal movements in utero: Nature, assessment, prognostic value, timing of delivery. *Obstet. Gynecol.* **50**:49–55, 1977.

77. Saito, M., Yazawa, K., Hashiguchi, A., Kumasaka, T., Nishi, N., and Kato, K.: Time of ovulation and prolonged pregnancy. *Am. J. Obstet. Gynecol.* **112**:31–38, 1972.

78. Schifrin, B. S., Guntes, V., Gergely, R. Z., Eden, R. D., Roll, K., and Jacobs, J.: The role of real-time scanning in antenatal fetal surveillance. *Am. J. Obstet. Gynecol.* **140**:525–530, 1981.

79. Schneider, J. M., Olsen, R. W., and Curet, L. B.: Screening for fetal and neonatal risk in the postdate pregnancy. *Am. J. Obstet. Gynecol.* **131**:473–478, 1978.

80. Shime, J., Gare, D. J., Andrews, J., Bertrand, M., Salgado, J., and Whillans, G.: Prolonged pregnancy: Surveillance of the fetus and the neonate and the course of labor and delivery. *Am. J. Obstet. Gynecol.* **148**:547–552, 1984.

81. Sjostedt, S., Engleson, G., and Rooth, G.: Dysmaturity. *Arch. Dis. Child.* **33**:123–130, 1958.

82. Smith, I. D. and Shearman, R. P.: Fetal plasma steroids in relation to parturition: I. The effect of gestational age upon umbilical plasma corticosteroid levels following vaginal delivery. *J. Obstet. Gynaecol. Br. Commonw.* **81**:11–15, 1974.

83. Smith, K., Greene, J. W., Jr., and Touchstone, J. C.: Urinary estriol determination in the management of prolonged pregnancy. *Am. J. Obstet. Gynecol.* **96**:901–906, 1966.

84. Starks, G. C.: Correlation of meconium-stained amniotic fluid, early intrapartum fetal pH and Apgar scores as predictors of perinatal outcome. *Obstet. Gynecol.* **56**:604–609, 1980.

85. Stone, H. O., Thompson, H. K., Jr., and Schmidt-Nielsen, K.: Influence of erythrocytes on blood viscosity. *Am. J. Physiol.* **214**:913–918, 1968.

86. Thliveris, J. A. and Baskett, T. F.: Fine structure of the human placenta in prolonged pregnancy: Preliminary report. *Gynecol. Obstet. Invest.* **9**:40–48, 1978.

87. Turnbull, A. C., Patten, P. T., Flint, A. P. E.,

Keirse, M. J. N., Jeremy, J. Y., and Anderson, A. B. M.: Significant fall in progesterone and rise in oestradiol levels in human peripheral plasma before onset of labour. *Lancet* **1**:101–104, 1974.

88. Visser, G. H. A., Redman, C. W. G., Huisjes, H. J., and Turnbull, A. C.: Nonstressed antepartum heart rate monitoring: Implication of decelerations after spontaneous contractions. *Am. J. Obstet. Gynecol.* **138**:429–435, 1980.
89. Vorherr, H.: Placental insufficiency in relation to post-term pregnancy and fetal postmaturity: Evaluation of fetoplacental function; management of the postterm gravida. *Am. J. Obstet. Gynecol.* **123**:67–103, 1975.
90. Yeh, S-Y. and Read, J. A.: Management of post-term pregnancy in a large obstetric population. *Obstet. Gynecol.* **60**:282–287, 1982.
91. Zwerdling, M. A.: Factors pertaining to prolonged pregnancy and its outcome. *Pediatrics* **40**:202–212, 1967.

20

POOR OBSTETRICAL OUTCOME

"Poor obstetric outcome" connotes failure of normal ante- or intrapartum mechanisms sufficient to prevent the delivery of a healthy infant. The etiologies of suboptimal outcome are myriad and range from acute intrapartum insults to those occurring at the time of conception. The conditions addressed in this chapter represent disorders that commonly confront the obstetrician. They are frequently associated with intra- as well as extrauterine deficits that compromise fetal well-being. Knowledge of their pathogenesis, diagnosis, and management will maximize the potential for effective intervention and optimal outcome. The disorders discussed include intrauterine growth retardation, congenital malformations, fetal wastage, fetal macrosomia and nonimmune hydrops fetalis.

INTRAUTERINE GROWTH RETARDATION (IUGR)

Disturbances of intrauterine growth frequently portend a variety of fetal and neonatal complications capable of inducing physical and intellectual deficits. Intrauterine growth retardation (IUGR) broadly refers to suboptimal fetal growth and development occurring secondary to a variety of mechanisms. Although IUGR does not universally presage poor outcome, infants so affected are at increased risk for a variety of complications, including hypoglycemia, polycythemia, hypocalcemia, and intrapartum asphyxia.[17,37] Perinatal mortality is from 4 to 8 times greater for these infants.[82]

Depending on the parameters chosen, disorders of fetal growth complicate from 3% to 10% of all gestations.[82] A variety of criteria are used to define IUGR, including birth weights below the 3rd,[17,18] 5th,[9,86] 10th,[20,28,82], and 25th[14] percentiles for gestational age and birth weight more than two standard deviations below the mean for a particular gestational age.[76,88] Birth weight below the 10th percentile for gestational age is the criterion most often employed and most generally applicable to the identification of fetuses with impaired growth and its potential attendant complications.

Depending on the pattern of growth inhibition and coexisting maternal conditions, IUGR is classified as either symmetric or asymmetric.

Symmetric IUGR refers to uniform reduction in head circumference, abdominal circumference, and body length. This category encompasses two-thirds of infants whose birth weights are less than the 10th percentile.[78] In general, symmetric IUGR is associated with exogenous factors to which the fetus is exposed early in gestation or with inherent conditions restricting growth potential. However, not all newborns whose birth weights fall below the 10th percentile are victims of a pathologic insult in utero. Infants whose parents are below average in height and weight may have similarly reduced growth potential manifest as a birth weight which is below average but appropriate for gestational age.

A variety of drugs have been associated with increased risk of IUGR. Two of the most ubiquitous are alcohol and tobacco. Although many of the studies that explore the relationship of maternal alcohol consumption to pejorative fetal effects are flawed to some extent, evidence to date suggests that maternal alcohol abuse can produce the Fetal Alcohol Syndrome (FAS). The key features of this syndrome include IUGR, characteristic facial configuration, and mental retardation. The exact risk to the progeny of heavy drinkers is not known, nor is it clear exactly how heavy the drinking must be to induce these abnormalities. Furthermore, the syndrome does not uniformly occur with known maternal alcohol abuse. There is also evidence suggesting that the defects associated with maternal alcohol consumption do not represent a unique and consistent collection of abnormalities. Thus, there apparently are individual differences in susceptibility to the effects of alcohol. FAS may represent a distinctive form of IUGR. Typically, these infants fail to demonstrate the "catch-up" growth generally characteristic of asymmetric IUGR and exhibit long-term growth retardation and neurobehavioral delay. In summary, the evidence suggests that women ingesting relatively large quantities of alcohol or those who are genetically more susceptible to its effects are at increased risk of having children with growth retardation and an increased frequency of various major and minor congenital defects often forming no unique pattern, although there may be some (e.g., midfacial anomalies) suggesting an alcoholic etiology.

In developed countries, cigarette smoking is one of the most powerful determinants of IUGR. The decrease in birth weight in the infants born to smokers averages 150–250 g. The correlation between smoking and low birth weight is consistent and is independent of maternal age, gravidity, socioeconomic class, or geographic region. The effect of smoking is dose and time dependent; growth retardation is most pronounced in the fetuses of mothers smoking more than ten cigarettes per day and in those exposed during the third trimester. Infants of mothers smoking less than seven to ten cigarettes per day or those whose mothers discontinue smoking in the first trimester seem to be spared growth deficiencies.[7,89]

Other drugs suspected of impairing fetal growth in utero include phenytoin, heroin, methadone, propranolol, warfarin, and steroids.[82]

Approximately 10% of all IUGR is attributed to infection.[52] Rubella, cytomegalovirus, and toxoplasmosis have all been associated with symmetrically impaired fetal growth in addition to a variety of organ specific malformations. Neonatal, as well as intrauterine, growth is retarded in infants infected in utero. As a rule, long-term prognosis is inversely proportional to the timing and duration of exposure; the earlier the infection and the longer the duration, the more pronounced the organ and general growth deficits.

Symmetrically retarded intrauterine growth is also an integral component of a number of congenital syndromes. In addition to decreasing neonatal survival, trisomy 13 and 18 and Potter's syndrome (renal agenesis)[54] also impair fetal growth. Cytogenetic defects can be demonstrated in approximately 10% of growth-retarded infants with mental impairment.[41] Typically, growth retardation occurring in association with nonlethal genetic conditions tends to persist into postnatal life.

Maternal undernutrition is commonly assumed to be a significant environmental cause of IUGR, but the data are inconsistent. Despite severe starvation in pregnant women during the famine of 1945 in Western Holland, the average decrease in birth weight was only 240 g. There was no increase in the number of infants with birth weights below 2250 g. Low birth weight has been associated with poor maternal weight gain and prepregnancy maternal weight of less than 50 kg, although this may represent the birth of a constitutionally small infant to a constitutionally small mother. Severe caloric restriction in pregnant subhuman primates is not invariably associated with reduced intrauterine growth.[41] The total metabolic requirements of the term fetus are served by 90–100 kcal/kg per day. Therefore, it is probable that only excessive maternal dietary restriction interferes with the minimum fetal requirements for growth.

As reviewed above, symmetric IUGR results from a variety of perinatal insults, the prognosis depending on the etiology. Regardless of the cause and associated defects, however, these infants are at increased risk for peripartum asphyxia, long-term disability, and perinatal mortality.

Asymmetric IUGR denotes a pattern of intrauterine growth that is normal until the late second or early third trimester, at which time the abdominal circumference, reflecting fetal trunk growth, fails to enlarge at the expected rate. In contrast, head growth, as manifested by the biparietal diameter (BPD), generally remains within normal limits or demonstrates only a later growth deficit. As opposed to symmetric IUGR, in which the fetus is affected early by either extrinsic or intrinsic insults that produce general stunting of growth, asymmetric IUGR results from incremental deprivation secondary to gradually worsening uteroplacental insufficiency. This pattern of "head (brain) sparing" may represent a fetal attempt to adapt to a progressively compromised nutrient supply by reapportioning cardiac output to maintain central nervous system growth and development at the expense of the carcass. Animal experiments lend credence to this supposition. Fetal hypoxia in sheep results in increased blood flow to the brain and the heart with a corresponding decrease in flow to the muscle and viscera.[64]

Unlike symmetric IUGR, which usually results from specific insults, asymmetric IUGR may accompany any condition that causes progressive impairment of uteroplacental blood flow. Placental vascular insufficiencies are generally secondary to suboptimal perfusion or to decreased placental surface area available for exchange. Disorders associated with the former include maternal hypertensive disease, cyanotic heart disease, and decreased prepregnancy blood volume. Conditions limiting placental membrane area include various placental pathologies such as circumvallate placenta. Indirect measures of uteroplacental blood flow in humans indicate a reduction in placental perfusion in pregnancies complicated by IUGR.[92] Additionally, experimentally induced reductions in placental blood flow in sheep result in substantial fetal growth retardation.[23]

Considering that the pathogenesis of asymmetric IUGR involves chronic uteroplacental insufficiency resulting in an intrauterine environment not conducive to optimal growth of an otherwise normal fetus, it is not surprising that infants so affected demonstrate exaggerated postnatal "catch up," growth during the first six months of extrauterine life. This is in contradistinction to infants born after symmetric IUGR. Although many asymmetrically growth-retarded infants remain shorter than controls, and their weights remain below the 10th percentile, neurobehavioral and motor development is typically close to normal.[40,41] In general, long-term outcome for infants with asymmetric IUGR is improved over that for infants with symmetric IUGR of nonconstitutional etiology.[24]

In addition to the factors already discussed, IUGR is associated with multiple gestation, prepregnancy weight of less than 50 kg, weight gain less than 0.9 kg/wk, and a poor past obstetric history. A 25% risk of recurrence has been demonstrated in mothers with a history of a previously growth-retarded infant and with no other risk factors. The prior birth of a growth-retarded infant may well be the most important single risk factor for recurrence.[81]

A high index of suspicion is essential to the diagnosis of IUGR. Clinical and laboratory aids reputedly useful in diagnosis of IUGR include serial fundal height measurements, glucose tolerance determinations, a variety of hormonal assays, and ultrasonographic evaluation. These will be separately considered.

Serial measurement of fundal height, which usually reflects an increase in the size or growth of intrauterine contents, could logically be expected to provide an index of growth, or lack thereof. Clinically, this has been demonstrated to offer varying accuracy. Utilizing serial fundal height measurements in a group of 298 normal pregnant women who subsequently delivered infants with birth weights appropriate for gestational age, the 10th, 50th, and 90th percentiles of uterine height have been determined.[6] The 10th percentile corresponds to a fundal height of 4 cm or more less than the gestational age in weeks. The predictive value of this parameter has been evaluated in women delivering low-birth-weight neonates and those with infants appropriate for gestational age. Of 44 women delivering neonates with birth weights less than the 10th percentile, 38 had fundal heights less than the 10th percentile (86% sensitivity). Of 95 women delivering neonates with birth weights appropriate for gestational age, 85 had uterine heights above the 10th percentile (90% specificity). The 14% false negative rate and 10% false positive rate suggest that systematic and accurate determination of fundal height is of value in detecting pregnancies with suboptimal fetal growth. Any patient in whom the fundal height lags 4 cm or more behind the gestational age in weeks is a candidate for further evaluation.

Maternal glucose tolerance testing has been recommended as an effective early screening test for pregnancies at risk of fetal growth retardation based on the supposition that maternal hypoglycemia results in fetal hypoglycemia and hypoinsulinemia.

The resultant decreased substrate availability allegedly causes diminished fetal growth and possibly growth retardation. A number of investigators have found a correlation between maternal hypoglycemia during glucose tolerance testing and subsequent births of infants small for gestational age.[51,85]

A variety of biochemical tests of fetoplacental function have been advocated for the detection and evaluation of growth retardation and other complications of pregnancy. Serial determinations of maternal urinary estriols, estriol:creatinine ratios, serum estrogens, and human placental lactogen are variably prognostic for IUGR.[82] These assays are infrequently employed in the diagnosis and management of pregnancies at risk for IUGR, due to technical and logistical disadvantages, wide overlap with normal values, the interference of other maternal diseases and therapies with their determinations, and lack of superiority over other diagnostic techniques.

Ultrasound, which is commonly used to determine gestational age and serial growth, is especially suited to the diagnosis of fetal growth abnormalities. Although the BPD is the most reproducible and readily obtained fetal dimension, its use as the sole parameter to evaluate fetal growth is limited by the fact that fetal weight and BPD are not directly related. Dolichocephaly, or flattening of the BPD, results in an artifically small measurement. In asymmetric IUGR, there is relative brain sparing precluding use of the BPD in diagnosis. Consequently, the accuracy of the BPD alone in the diagnosis of IUGR ranges from 50% to 60%.[78,82] Measurement of fetal abdominal circumference (AC), obtained from a plane perpendicular to the fetal spine at a point where the umbilical vein can be visualized coursing through the liver, is of additional value. The AC reflects liver mass and subcutaneous tissue, both of which are reduced in IUGR. Reductions in AC occur in symmetric and asymmetric IUGR and represent overall growth impairment. Since brain growth often continues at the expense of body growth under conditions of intrauterine deprivation, the ratio of head:body disproportion, reflected by the head circumference (HC) to AC ratio, frequently reflects the degree of compromise. Use of AC alone or in combination with the HC in a head:body ratio correctly predicts impaired fetal growth in 71–96% of cases of IUGR.[11,38,55] Normally, the ratio of HC to AC is greater than one until approximately 36 weeks, after which the ratio reverses. Characteristic changes occur in the HC to AC ratio, depending on the pattern of growth delay, symmetric or asymmetric. In symmetric growth retardation, the ratio is often unaffected, although absolute values are less than expected. Asymmetric growth retardation, characterized by head sparing, results in substantial alterations in HC to AC ratios.

Additional ultrasound parameters potentially useful in diagnosis of IUGR include estimations of total intrauterine volume, placental maturity, amniotic fluid volume, fetal weight, and lung maturity. Determinations of total intrauterine volume are of limited value due to technical imprecision as well as associated confounding variables, including bladder volume, localized contractions, and uterine shape.[15] Placental maturity studies, based on characteristic changes in placental density and architecture with advancing gestational age, have recently been utilized in the diagnosis of IUGR. Placentas are assigned a grade, 0, I, II, or III, with 0 representing the least mature and III the most mature placental morphology. A prospective study of placental grade and fetal maturity reported that 62% of infants with birth weights less than the 10th percentile could be correctly predicted by the prior finding of a Grade III placenta.[49] If the fetus is smaller than predicted by gestational dates, Grade III placenta is associated with a definite increase in risk of low birth weight as compared with pregnancies with a placental grade of less than III. Although promising, the utility of this parameter remains to be determined.

Oligohydramnios, usually defined as absence of at least one amniotic fluid pocket greater than 1 cm in its greatest diameter, may result from diminished fetal urine production secondary to hypoxemia-stimulated redistribution of cardiac output. Despite conflicting reports regarding the absolute predictive value of decreased amniotic fluid, it is generally agreed that finding oligohydramnios on ultrasound examination should raise the suspicion of IUGR and stimulate further evaluation.[15]

Evidence of pulmonary maturity, as demonstrated by a mature lecithin/sphingomyelin (L/S) ratio, Foam Stability lndex, or the presence of phosphatidyglycerol (PG) in association with a BPD of less than 87 mm or an estimated fetal weight of less than 1500 g, suggests IUGR and may be useful in discriminating between a stunted fetus and an appropriately grown premature fetus.[30]

Antepartum management of the patient with impaired fetal growth includes treatment of contributing maternal factors, fetal testing, appropriately timed delivery, and intrapartum surveillance.

Although it is unclear to what degree, if any, fetal growth impairment is reversible,[5] treatment of associated maternal conditions is advocated. Such conditions include chronic hypertension, malnutrition, renal disease, anemia, and substance abuse. The cornerstone of antenatal testing is electronic fetal monitoring. The nonstress test (NST) is frequently the initial testing procedure of choice in evaluation of at-risk pregnancies. In pregnancies complicated by IUGR, the loss of variability and lack of fetal heart rate (FHR) accelerations with fetal movements often presage a poor outcome.[26] Such abnormal tests dictate follow-up stress testing, traditionally performed with oxytocin, although encouraging preliminary results have been reported with the use of breast nipple stimulation to induce uterine contractions. IUGR is frequently associated with a positive stress test which predicts increased likelihood of fetal distress during labor and perinatal mortality.[59,69]

A combination of the two most useful techniques for fetal evaluation, electronic monitoring and ultrasound, has resulted in the development of the biophysical profile, which includes assessment of fetal movement, tone, breathing movements, qualitative amniotic fluid volume, and fetal heart rate responses. Determinations of amniotic fluid volume and fetal heart rate reactivity are especially relevant to the growth-retarded fetus. Decreased amniotic fluid volume and fetal heart rate reactivity should heighten suspicion of IUGR and chronic stress in utero. The biophysical profile has a higher positive predictive value than the NST of low Apgar scores. [62] Use of the biophysical profile also rules out major anomalies.

Timing of delivery should be guided by antepartum testing, rate of fetal growth in utero, and fetal maturity. In the absence of fetal compromise or maternal deterioration, IUGR is not an indication for preterm delivery. The combination of prematurity and growth retardation poses a greater threat than either condition alone. Therefore, provided there is evidence of fetal well-being, pregnancy should be allowed to continue until maturity is established.

The growth-retarded fetus has a decreased tolerance for hypoxia and is at increased risk for birth asphyxia.[60,61] Approximately one-third of all infants with IUGR develop late decelerations when allowed a trial of labor.[48,60] The ability to monitor the fetus electronically is essential. Fetal scalp pH determinations are necessary in cases of apparent distress. The attendant risks of meconium aspiration, neonatal hypoglycemia, hypocalcemia, and sepsis mandate that ante-intrapartum preparations include prior notification of a pediatrician to attend the delivery. Cesarean section solely for IUGR does not necessarily improve outcome.[42,69] Mode of delivery should be determined by the condition of the cervix and by the ability to monitor the fetus. Patients with an unfavorable cervix or those in whom continuous intrapartum monitoring is not feasible are candidates for cesarean section.[59]

CONGENITAL MALFORMATIONS

Major congenital malformations are structural defects that occur antenatally and are capable of causing death or severe functional impairment. Such abnormalities affect about 3% of newborns. These disorders are classified on the basis of known or suspected etiology and include (in decreasing order of frequency) those of unknown cause; those presumed due to a combination of genetic and nongenetic factors (commonly referred to as multifactorial); those occurring secondary to single mutant genes; those attributed to chromosomal anomalies; and those resulting from exogenous influences such as maternal disease or teratogen exposure.

Despite the relative frequency of malformations, an estimated 60%[27] are unrelated to known intrinsic or extrinsic insults, therefore limiting attempts at diagnosis, prevention, and counseling.

Malformations resulting from combined environmental and genetic factors are classified as multifactorial and constitute approximately 20%[27] of congenital malformations. In most cases, the defect involves a single structure and the infant is otherwise normal. Common malformations of presumed multifactorial origin include neural tube defects (anencephaly, encephalocele, and spina bifida); certain forms of hydrocephaly; facial clefts; cardiac anomalies; tracheoesophageal fistula; esophageal atresia; duodenal atresia; Meckel's diverticulum; diaphragmatic, umbilical, and inguinal hernias; omphalocele, renal, ureteral, and bladder anomalies; imperforate anus; and clubfoot. Counseling for multifactorial disorders requires exclusion of mendelian single gene factors and specific teratogenic factors that carry different risks and different potential for prenatal diagnosis. This category contains a heterogenous collection of abnormalities for which empiric or average recurrence risks are used rather than the precise probabilities that can be calculated for single-gene disorders. The fact that a structural defect represents a single primary developmental anomaly in most cases allows the obstetrician to give recurrence risk estimates of 2–5% to unaffected parents with one affected child.

Single-gene (mendelian) disorders include autosomal and sex chromosomal traits which collectively account for 7.5%[46] of congenital malformations. These mutant gene disorders are inherited according to the laws Mendel described in 1866.

Features of autosomal dominant transmission include multiple generation involvement, male-to-male transmission, spontaneous mutations, and marked variability in clinical expression. A carrier of a mutant gene has a 50% chance of transmitting it to each offspring if the other parent is normal. Autosomal recessive disorders occur when both alleles at a particular locus are mutant, because of a mutant contribution from each parent. As opposed to autosomal dominant disorders, both sexes are affected with the risks of recurrence 1 in 4 for an affected child, 2 in 4 for a carrier (heterozygote) child, and 1 in 4 for a homozygous normal child. Unaffected siblings of an affected person have a 2 in 3 risk of being a carrier and a 1 in 3 chance of being homozygous normal. Such traits are often associated with consanguinity. X-linked recessive disorders are expressed by all males who possess the mutant gene, because males have only one X chromosome. Females possessing a single X-linked mutant gene are carriers because they also have a second, normal, X chromosome. Under these conditions, half of their sons receive the X chromosome bearing the mutant gene and are affected, whereas half of their daughters also receive the abnormal X chromosome and are carriers. The other half of a carrier's sons and daughters do not receive the mutant gene and are not at risk of transmitting the X-linked condition to their progeny. An affected male passes his abnormal X chromosome to all his female offspring. Therefore they will all be carriers. Males receive only the Y chromosome from their father; therefore, no male-to-male transmission is possible for X-linked diseases.

Currently, more than 3000 disorders are thought to be inherited in mendelian fashion in humans. Those having an impact on reproductive function include: the hemoglobinopathies (most often sickle cell disease, α- and β-thalassemia, and HgbSC disease); hemolytic anemias (hereditary spherocytosis, glucose-6-phosphate dehydrogenase deficiency); coagulation factor deficiencies (hemophilia A and B, von Willebrand's disease); metabolic disorders (phenylketonuria, homocystinuria, the porphyrias); endocrine disorders (hypogonadism syndromes, adrenal, thyroid, and parathyroid abnormalities); renal disorders (polycystic kidney disease); skeletal and connective tissue disorders (Ehlers–Danlos syndrome, Marfan's syndrome, osteogenesis imperfecta, achondroplasia); neurologic disorders (myotonic dystrophy, neurofibromatosis); cardiovascular disorders (idiopathic hypertrophic subaortic stenosis, autosomal recessive hypoplastic left heart syndrome, X-linked aortic and mitral insufficiency); and respiratory disorders (cystic fibrosis).

In 1956, the diploid number of human chromosomes was determined to be 46.[93] The first abnormality of chromosome number was described in 1959 when Lejeune[58] demonstrated the extra chromosome associated with Down's syndrome. Abnormalities of chromosome number or structure have subsequently been reported involving each of the 23 pairs of chromosomes. Either a portion or an entire chromosome may be present in triplicate (e.g., trisomy 21) or singly (e.g., monosomy X). In general, monosomy results in more severely affected offspring than does trisomy. In contrast to the single-gene disorders previously discussed, chromosome abnormalities involve thousands of genes, thus often affecting multiple organ systems. Chromosome anomalies affect approximately one of every 160 newborns and, as a group, account for 6%[46] of all congenital malformations. Clinically important autosomal abnormalities include trisomy 21, 18, and 13; other trisomies; mosaicisms; monosomies; deletions; and inversions. Common sex chromosome anomalies include Turner's syndrome (45,X), Kleinfelter's syndrome (XXY), and X-linked mental retardation (fragile X syndrome). As a rule, the sex chromosome aberrations produce less severe physical and/or mental impairment than do the autosomal disorders.

Diverse but less common causes of congenital defects involve extrinsic and intrinsic insults, including maternal disease, environmental agents, and drug exposure. Maternal disorders known to cause congenital abnormalities include infections, diabetes mellitus, and phenylketonuria. Of the host of maternal infections putatively associated with malformations in the infant, only the rubella virus, cytomegalovirus, and *Toxoplasma gondii* are unquestionably associated with specific congenital defects.[46] Primary maternal rubella infection in pregnancy carries a risk of fetal involvement ranging from

50% in the first month to 10% by the third month.[65] Abnormalities consistently associated with rubella infection in utero include cataracts, patent ductus arteriosus, and deafness. Since the advent of rubella vaccination, the incidence of congenital rubella has decreased from 28 cases per 100,000 births in 1966 to one case per 100,000 births in 1982.[12] Cytomegalovirus is the most common cause of intrauterine infection.[33] About 50,000 infants are born each year in the United States with some evidence of infection. Clinical manifestations are quite broad. Ninety to 95% of congenitally infected infants are asymptomatic at birth. In infants with clinically apparent infection at birth, characteristic findings include mental retardation, chorioretinitis, cerebral calcifications, and micro- or hydrocephaly. *Toxoplasma gondii* is an intracellular parasite acquired by consuming raw or undercooked meat or by contact with oocysts from infected cat feces. Congenital infection with toxoplasmosis is an uncommon event. The incidence in this country has decreased over the last decade from 1/1000 to 1/8500.[75] Most infants with congenitally acquired toxoplasmosis demonstrate only serologic abnormalities. Clinical disease is associated primarily with acute infection. As with congenital cytomegalovirus, a broad spectrum of signs and symptoms have been associated with toxoplasmosis. The classic triad of malformations includes intracerebral calcifications, chorioretinitis, and hydrocephaly. Other agents (herpes simplex virus Type 2, *Treponema pallidum*, varicella, and coxsackie virus) have been implicated in the genesis of fetal malformation. None is consistently associated with specific characteristic abnormalities in the newborn. Collectively, these three infectious diseases account for 2% of congenital malformations.[46]

A multitude of noninfectious systemic maternal disorders have the potential to cause congenital malformations. Of these, only diabetes mellitus is implicated consistently enough to present a quantifiable risk for fetal maldevelopment in infants of insulin-requiring diabetic mothers (but not in gestational diabetics). Defects commonly associated with clinical diabetes mellitus include cardiovascular, neural-tube, and sacral malformations. The frequency of malformed children born to insulin-requiring diabetic mothers ranges from 6.6% to 13.0% with a mean rate of 9.1%,[46] or three times the incidence of malformations in the general population. Taken together, diabetes-related defects represent 1.4% of all congenital malformations.[46]

Phenylketonuria, fetal virilizing diseases (functional lesions of the ovary and adrenal gland), and endemic cretinism produce defects in utero, but their contribution to the total number of congenital malformations is so slight as to be unquantifiable. Only about 3.5% of all congenital defects can be attributed to maternal illness (2% due to infections, 1.4% due to diabetes, and less than 1% to the other diseases described above).

Exogenous causes of congenital malformations include various chemicals: environmental agents (e.g., additives, contaminants, and pollutants), drugs, and agents prescribed as treatment for illness.

Of all major environmental agents suspected of causing congenital malformations (lead, hexachlorophene, dioxin, organic solvents, and anesthetic gases), for only one, organic mercury, is there conclusive evidence of interference with prenatal development. Neurologic damage secondary to maternal ingestion of fish contaminated with methylmercury from industrial wastes was first recognized in 1953 in Minamata City in Southwest Japan.[94] Similar cases were subsequently reported from Niigata,[94] another Japanese coastal town, and Iraq,[3] where exposure occurred due to consumption of grain treated with a fungicide containing methylmercury. Prolonged intrauterine exposure to organic mercury disturbs brain development, resulting in neurologic damage. Such disturbances are primarily related to exposures during late gestation. First trimester exposure is unrelated to major malformations.

Chemicals suspected of interfering with intrauterine development include caffeine, tobacco, alcohol, and various addictive drugs. Heroin, methadone, lysergic acid diethylamide (LSD), cocaine, amphetamines, and tranquilizers are not convincingly associated with fetal structural abnormalities, although heroin and methadone are associated with an increased risk of intrauterine demise, decreased birth weight, and neonatal withdrawal symptoms.[47] Heavy caffeine consumption (4–8 cups per day or more) has been associated with reduced birth weight.[39] Smoking more than 10 cigarettes daily has been correlated with increased risk of spontaneous abortion and perinatal mortality as well as intrauterine growth retardation.[1,63] Neither has been shown to be a true teratogen.

Drug use is common among women of reproductive age and is little affected by pregnancy. Fifteen percent of women surveyed take systemic medication at some time during the six months prior to conception, and nearly 20% are exposed during the second and third months of pregnancy.[10] Pregnant women may inadvertently take drugs prior to confirmation of pregnancy, may require therapy for a preexisting medical condition, or may use over-the-counter preparations with the misconception that nonprescription drugs are inherently safer than their prescription counterparts. Although many such agents have, at one time or another, been suspected of causing congenital malformations, none of the most frequently self-prescribed medications has been clearly demonstrated to be teratogenic.

Fortunately, only one class of drugs, the anti-epileptics, is known to have consistent adverse effects on the fetus.

Infants born to women taking anticonvulsants have a two- to three-fold increase in congenital anomalies,[16] especially cleft lip and palate, digital hypoplasia, and congenital heart disease. Nonetheless, the exact etiology of these defects is not easily established. Epilepsy itself may be genetically linked to congenital anomalies as suggested from the higher than expected incidence of anomalies among epileptics and their relatives,[91] and from the observation that offspring of epileptic fathers may also be at increased risk for malformations.[83] The hypoxia and acidosis that frequently accompany epileptic convulsions may result in metabolic disturbances with teratogenic potential.[87]

Despite these reservations, the bulk of evidence suggests that some anticonvulsants are teratogenic and are primarily responsible for the increased incidence of malformations among the children of epileptics. The agents considered to have the highest teratogenic potential are phenytoin, trimethadione, and valproic acid. Phenytoin and trimethadione have been associated with syndromes including pre- and postnatal growth retardation, microcephaly, mental retardation, and facial dysmorphisms.[25,34] Distal digital hypoplasia is reported to be specific to phenytoin.[34] Valproic acid has been associated with lumbrosacral spina bifida.[13] When feasible, other anticonvulsants should be administered during pregnancy. It is estimated that anticonvulsant exposure is responsible for 1.26% of all malformed children.[47]

Anticoagulation with warfarin derivatives during the first trimester has been associated with multiple abnormalities, the most characteristic being epiphyseal stippling, nasal skeletal hypoplasia, and optic atrophy. A survey of women taking oral anticoagulants during at least the first trimester revealed a 14.7% incidence of spontaneous abortion, a 6.8% incidence of stillbirth, and a 9.0% incidence of drug-related embryopathy among liveborn infants.[32] Maternal therapy initiated beyond the first trimester is mainly associated with fetal hemorrhage and its sequellae. (See Chapter 30.)

Among cancer chemotherapeutic agents in pregnancy, only the folate antagonists, aminopterin and methotrexate, are known teratogens.[44] However, any drug designed to kill growing cells could be expected to have pejorative effects on the developing embryo. (See Chapter 41.)

Defects associated with the intentional or inadvertent administration of female sex hormones may be divided into two classes: genital and nongenital. Despite an alleged association between exposure to those agents early in gestation and a syndrome of multiple congenital anomalies (vertebral, anal, tracheoesophageal, renal, and limb [VACTERL]), recent evidence indicates that when used as oral contraceptives or for pregnancy testing, these substances have little if any potential for inducing nongenital defects.[47] In contrast, genital development may be disturbed following exposure to sex hormones during pregnancy. Androgenic steroids are clearly associated with masculinization of female external genitalia, and intrauterine exposure to DES can cause clear-cell adenocarcinoma of the female genital tract, although the incidence of both these abnormalities is quite low. [47] Structural anomalies of the female reproductive system may also occur secondary to intrauterine exposure to DES,[8] although their relation to subsequent carcinogenesis and fertility is uncertain. Current evidence indicates that most women exposed to DES in utero have had normal pregnancies and deliveries.[80]

In summary, an estimated 3% of all newborns will be affected with a structural abnormality severe enough to impair viability or function. As other causes of neonatal morbidity and mortality have become amenable to diagnosis and therapy, the impact of congenital malformations has grown proportionately. Such abnormalities are responsible for over 21% of infant mortality.[96] Attempts at prevention must take into account the diverse etiologies of these defects. Unfortunately, there are no known causes in an estimated 60% of cases. An additional 20% are attributed to interaction between multiple and poorly defined genetic and environmental factors. Efforts to reduce the frequency of such malformations are limited and will depend on efforts to define their underlying cause. The next largest group of congenital malformations are those with a genetic basis. Together, single-gene disorders and major chromosomal anomalies account for approximately 13.5% of all congenital defects. Attempts to influence the incidence of these disorders are limited to genetic counseling and selective pregnancy termination. Most couples are not known to be at risk until the birth of an affected child, and prenatal diagnosis is not available for all disorders. Therefore, preventive measures cannot at present be expected to impact significantly on the occurrence of congenital malformations. The remaining causes of congenital anomalies can be attributed to diabetes mellitus, anticonvulsant agents, rubella, toxoplasmosis, and cytomegalovirus. These disorders combined account for approximately 5% of all major anomalies. The contribution of other diseases, such as phenylketonuria and fetal virilizing diseases, is minimal (less than 1%). Although responsible for a limited number of all malformations, the contributions from these disorders can be decreased by aggressive management and control of diabetes mellitus, use of nonteratogenic anticonvulsants, and conscientious infection control and surveillance.

FETAL WASTAGE

Fetal loss has been associated with a myriad of conditions including maternal overexertion, exposure to drugs and viruses, trauma, and hormonal deprivation. More recent data suggest that a characteristic pattern of genetic selection occurs during the antepartum period that can be divided into three phases defined by the fetal mortality rate and the type of associated chromosomal abnormality.

The first, and probably most intensive, phase of selection includes gametogenesis, conception, preimplantation, and early implantation. Failure of development in the earliest stages of gestation is probably frequent. The true incidence is difficult to estimate because such losses are often clinically inapparent. Available data indicate that the rate of morphologic aberrations among preimplantation and early implanted embryos is quite high. The uteri and fallopian tubes of women undergoing elective hysterectomy during preimplantation and early implantation revealed gross abnormalities sufficient to preclude further development in 4 of 8 preimplanted embryos and 9 of 26 implanted embryos.[37] Many of these abnormalities, which included necrotic blastomeres, multinucleate blastomeres, and decreased numbers of blastomeres, were considered to result from chromosomal anomalies. The genetic aberrations characteristic of these inapparent pregnancies are thought to be autosomal monosomies, trisomies of the larger autosomes (groups A, B, and C), or structural abnormalities of the chromosomes (translocations, inversions, etc.) severe enough to result in defective embryogenesis.[77] Nongenetic causes for preclinical pregnancy loss include, among others (see below), luteal phase deficiency. The underlying pathology is presumed to involve a luteal phase too abbreviated to permit the timely transfer of progesterone production from the corpus luteum to the trophoblast.

Embryonic demise occurring more than 6 weeks after the last menstrual period is usually clinically apparent as a spontaneous abortion. Approximately 15% of all documented pregnancies abort spontaneously. The peak incidence of abortion is between the 10th and the 12th weeks of pregnancy. Most cases reported in the literature fall into this category. An estimated 50–60% of first-trimester losses are associated with abnormalities of chromosome number or structure.[57] In general, an inverse relationship between gestational age and frequency of chromosomal abnormalities exists, suggesting that the more severe the anomaly, the less likely is survival. In the first trimester, the most common cytogenetic aberrations include trisomies, polyploidies, and monosomies. Of these, the trisomies are most frequently implicated in early fetal loss, especially trisomy 13, 16, 18, 21, and 22. Many trisomies occurring in spontaneous abortions are thought to be incompatible with life, having never been observed in liveborns. Twenty to 25% of chromosomally defective early abortuses and fetal losses represent polyploidies (both triploidy, $3n = 69$ and tetraploidy, $4n = 92$). Monosomy X (45,X) is observed in 20–25% of genetically abnormal abortuses, making it the single most common chromosomal disorder associated with first-trimester losses. Although the majority of chromosomal abnormalities occurring at this stage are lethal for the fetus and differ in distribution from chromosomally abnormal viable fetuses, some anomalies do occur that are similar to those observed in liveborns. For example, X monosomies are found in both abortuses and liveborns, albeit the incidence is much higher in the former than in the latter.

In contrast to first-trimester abortions, the majority of second-trimester losses are nongenetic in origin. Chromosomal abnormalities are associated with only about 10–34% of second-trimester abortuses.[77] The distribution of chromosome anomalies in midtrimester abortuses more closely approximates that found in newborn infants than that found in first-trimester losses. Autosomal trisomies, X-monosomies and gonosomal aneuploids, and mosaicism are the genetic aberrations most frequently found in second-trimester abortuses.

A number of other disorders have also been implicated in early pregnancy losses. Progesterone deficiency and luteal phase defects, accepted causes of infertility, have a poorly defined role in preclinical and early-pregnancy wastage. Although there is some evidence that luteal phase defects may be a cause of repetitive abortions, the studies are flawed by small sample size, lack of matched controls, and inconclusive evidence of the efficacy of treatment. Uterine defects potentially interfering with either conception, implantation, embryonic–fetal development, or retention include intrauterine adhesions, Müllerian fusion or canalization defects, leiomyomas, and cervical incompetence. Depending on circumstance, surgical correction of these defects may or may not improve reproductive capacity. The immunogenetics of early fetal loss is not yet clearly defined. Abnormalities of "blocking antibodies," which modify maternal cellular immune reactivity and thus protect the fetus, have been implicated in recurrent pregnancy loss. However, studies controlled for endocrinologic and cytogenetic variables are lacking. Intrauterine infection, more commonly associated with late fetal loss, can also result in early pregnancy loss due to overwhelming fetal infection or to derangement of organogenesis sufficient to impair differentiation. Variables affecting fetal morbidity and mortality include the size of the inoculum, virulence of the organisms, severity of maternal infection, and stage of gestation. It is often difficult to separate the direct effects of infection on the fetus from the indirect effects of compromised maternal health, fever, associated conditions, and therapies.

The following organisms have been associated with early fetal loss: brucella, candida, chlamydia, cytomegalovirus, malaria, mycoplasma, *Salmonella typhi*, smallpox, toxoplasmosis, and vaccinia. Certain environmental agents are well-known abortifacients when administered in sufficient doses during critical periods of embryogenesis. Irradiation and certain drugs (e.g., folate antagonists) are among the most common. Other agents (especially alcohol, tobacco, and environmental pollutants) are also implicated in fetal loss, although definitive cause-and-effect relationships have not been established in most cases. Contrary to the common wisdom, maternal medical illness is seldom responsible for first- and second-trimester pregnancy loss unless significant deterioration occurs after the initiation of pregnancy. Such maternal disorders more commonly result in growth retardation and late fetal demise.

Chromosomal abnormalities become progressively less important causes of fetal death as gestation advances. In contrast to the frequency of genetic aberrations in first- and second-trimester losses, only 5–10% of stillborns are secondary to chromosomal abnormalities. The majority are trisomies of the smaller autosomes, especially trisomy 18. Stillbirths more commonly result from major congenital anomalies, uteroplacental pathology (including fetoplacental insufficiency, placenta previa and abruptio placenta), maternal systemic illnesses (especially hypertension), trauma, and isoimmunization. From 5–20% of all late pregnancy losses are of unknown etiology.[31,53]

A history of repetitive abortions was historically thought to confer an even greater risk of loss with subsequent pregnancies.[84] More recent studies have demonstrated some principles regarding recurrent spontaneous abortions. The risk of recurrence following one or more abortions is 25–30%.[97] This risk is influenced by the presence or absence of a prior liveborn infant and by the chromosomal constitution of previous abortuses. A prior abortus with a normal chromosome complement confers a slightly greater risk of subsequent pregnancy loss, as does the lack of any liveborn offspring.

Evaluation of patients with a previous abortion or stillborn is warranted for the psychological relief that it may provide the parents and for the value of such information in determining the possible risk of recurrence with subsequent pregnancies.

Initial investigation of patients with pregnancy loss should include a medical, occupational, and obstetric history to identify any maternal systemic disorders, exposure to infections, drugs, or other potential abortifacients, or prior reproductive difficulties. A family history is also important to identify potentially heritable disorders capable of affecting reproductive capacity.

Medical evaluation of the patient with recurrent first- or second-trimester losses should be guided by clinical circumstance. Glucose tolerance testing, antinuclear antibody studies, and thyroid function tests are of greatest value in patients with a suggestive history or clinical symptoms. Repetitive first-trimester losses unassociated with chromosomal defects warrant evaluation for luteal phase defects. In the absence of endocrine or genetic factors, cervical cultures for genital mycoplasmas (*M. hominis* and *U. urealyticum*) may be of value. If positive, treatment of the patient and her spouse with doxycycline has been advocated, although the efficacy of this therapy in reducing the pregnancy loss rate is unproven.[36] Patients with second-trimester losses should also be investigated for reproductive tract defects, including cervical incompetence, leiomyomas, and uterine anomalies. Isoimmunization should be ruled out in Rh-negative women. Patients with two or more first-trimester losses or one or more losses beyond the first trimester should undergo chromosome analysis to rule out parental translocations that could increase the risk of unbalanced gametes and chromosomally abnormal or nonviable offspring. The identification of a parental chromosomal disorder or of a previous abortus with an autosomal trisomy are indications for prenatal diagnostic studies in subsequent pregnancies.

A prospective evaluation of 155 couples with two or more consecutive first- or second-trimester losses found that in 68% of women with three or more losses, at least one diagnostic test suggested a possible cause for their repetitive losses. The studies included thyroid function profiles, antinuclear antibody tests, endocervical cultures for *M. hominis* and *U. urealyticum*, hysterosalpingograms, and peripheral leukocyte karyotypes. The hysterosalpingogram, peripheral lymphocyte karyotype, and cervical culture for *U. urealyticum* were of greatest value. The prognosis for future pregnancy was favorable regardless of whether the diagnostic tests were normal (77% subsequent live births) or abnormal (71% live births).[35]

Gross and microscopic autopsy of the infant and placenta, photographs, x-ray studies, bacterial cultures, and fetal tissue karyotyping are useful in the evaluation of the stillborn infant. The single most useful examination allowing a specific diagnosis is the gross autopsy.[68] Photography, radiography and bacterial cultures are useful to establish the diagnosis when the autopsy is abnormal. In contrast, routine karyotyping and histopathological examination are often not essential to the diagnosis. Indications for karyotype and histopathological analysis should be based on the other studies, especially the gross autopsy. Karyotyping may be of value in multiple congenital anomalies, nonimmunologic hydrops, a family history of abnormal children, or a history of recurrent pregnancy loss. Histopathology should be performed in cases of Potter's syndrome, polycystic kidneys, unilateral renal agenesis, or other renal abnormalities. In summary, gross autopsy, bacterial cultures, photography, and radiography should be performed on all stillbirths. Tissue samples suitable for karyotype and histopathologic analysis may be obtained at the time of autopsy and held to be either utilized or discarded pending the results of the above studies. For most pregnancy losses in which a specific anomaly is diagnosed, the risk of recurrence is increased only for that disorder; there is no generalized increase in risk of a subsequent abnormal outcome. This approach maximizes the likelihood of identifying disorders that have an increased risk of recurrence.

In addition to the aforementioned studies of the stillborn infant, Kleihauer–Betke staining of maternal blood in cases of unexplained fetal death allows the diagnosis of fetomaternal hemorrhage, a significant, but often undetected, cause of fetal mortality. In a series of 119 fetal deaths, 29 were without apparent cause. Kleihauer–Betke stains were positive in 4 of these cases, implicating massive transplacental hemorrhage as the presumed etiology in 13.8% of unexplained fetal deaths and 3.4% of all fetal deaths. These results suggest that fetomaternal hemorrhage occurring without apparent cause or precipitating factors is a significant cause of fetal death which should be ruled out in cases of unexplained intrauterine demise.[56]

MACROSOMIA

Disorders of fetal growth also include fetal growth acceleration. Although often receiving less attention than their growth-retarded counterparts, pregnancies complicated by fetal macrosomia are subject to a variety of maternal, fetal, and neonatal problems.

Fetal macrosomia has been variously defined as a birth weight greater than 4000 g,[67] 4100 g,[29] or 4500 g,[72] and greater than the 90th percentile for gestational age.[98] Infants with birth weights in excess of 4000 g are considered to be of excessive size because perinatal mortality increases above this level [4]; 8–10% of infants weigh more than 4000 g at birth.[90]

Early, or primary, growth acceleration accompanied by other defects is characteristic of a number of identifiable syndromes including transposition of the great vessels, Sotos' syndrome (cerebral gigantism), Weaver's syndrome (accelerated skeletal maturation, camptodactyly, macrosomia, unusual facies), Marshall–Smith syndrome (accelerated growth and maturation, broad middle phalanges, shallow orbits), and Beckwith–Wiedemann syndrome (exomphalos, gigantism, macroglossia).

Secondary fetal growth acceleration resulting from extrinsic maternal or fetal conditions is much more common and more is known about its pathophysiology. Abnormal glucose metabolism, especially insulin-dependent diabetes, is among the most frequent causes of secondary growth excess. Glucose, the energy substrate for the fetus, crosses the placenta by facilitated diffusion. Fetal concentrations reach approximately 75% of maternal concentrations. With maternal diabetes the fetus is subjected to a carbohydrate surplus which, in turn, stimulates increased secretion of insulin from the fetal pancreas. This relative hyperinsulinemia results in increased fetal anabolism with accumulation of glycogen in the liver and increased triglyceride synthesis in adipose tissue. The net effect is an increase in fetal subcutaneous fat and overall body size. Because the increased size is not accompanied by a similar acceleration in maturity, these large infants are often less mature than their size suggests. In spite of increased glycogen and fat stores, these infants tolerate the transient hypocaloric stress of the immediate neonatal period poorly. They are subject to hyperinsulinemia, hypoglucagonemia, and impaired glycogenolysis, all of which predispose to neonatal hypoglycemia. Other complications occurring with increased frequency in the infants of diabetic mothers include respiratory distress syndrome, hypocalcemia, jaundice, polycythemia, and cardiac dysfunction. Because such complications are presumably secondary to gestational hyperglycemia, maternal glucose should be rigidly controlled throughout pregnancy.

Maternal factors, other than diabetes, that are associated with fetal macrosomia include multiparity, previous delivery of an infant weighing greater than 4000 g at birth, obesity (15-25% above normal weight), a prepregnancy weight of more than 90 kg, and weight gain in excess of 35 pounds during gestation. Of these, maternal obesity and previous delivery of a macrosomic infant are probably the two most common and significant factors in the genesis of fetal macrosomia.[66]

Other intrauterine conditions frequently resulting in fetal macrosomia include immune and nonimmune hydrops fetalis, fetal congestive heart failure, asphyxia, and chorioangiomas of the placenta.

Pregnancies complicated by macrosomia are more likely to require augmentation of labor with oxytocin than are controls.[66] The incidence of cesarean delivery is higher, primarily as a result of cephalopelvic disproportion and failure to progress. The risk of shoulder dystocia relates directly to increasing birth weight. For fetuses weighing more than 4000 g, the incidence of shoulder dystocia is reported to range from 1.7–8.4%.[67] Such dystocia is not infrequently accompanied by skeletal and/or nerve damage, leading many authors to recommend the liberal use of cesarean section if macrosomia is diagnosed antenatally. (See Chapter 45.) Excessive fetal size has also been associated with a prolonged second stage of labor and increased postpartum blood loss.[72] Maternal mortality among mothers delivering macrosomic infants is rare. An incidence of 0.17% was reported in an older series,[79] but no maternal deaths were noted in more recent reviews.[29,66]

In addition to increased perinatal and neonatal mortality, macrosomic infants are at risk for hematologic and metabolic abnormalities, including polycythemia, hyperbilirubinemia and hypoglycemia. The incidence of hypoglycemia among all infants of insulin-dependent diabetic mothers is estimated to be as high as 75% and among infants of gestational diabetics as high as 25%. The incidence of this complication involving macrosomic infants of mothers without apparent gestational hyperglycemia is more difficult to determine, occurring with an estimated frequency of up to 12%.[90]

Nearly half of the serious morbidity associated with macrosomia results from complications occurring at delivery, including Erb's palsy, meconium aspiration, and perinatal asphyxia.[66] Other birth injuries seen in macrosomic fetuses result from trauma to the head and neck. Cranial injury may result in cephalohematomas with secondary hyperbilirubinemia or intraventricular hemorrhage. Peripheral nerve injuries include cervical or brachial plexus damage which may be life threatening, as in the case of phrenic nerve paralysis requiring ventilatory support. Lesser injuries may also result in permanent functional impairment. Only about 7% of patients with Erb–Duchenne palsy completely recover.[2]

Delivery is the most dangerous time for the large infant. Obstetric trauma and attendant morbidity frequently result from ante- or intrapartum failure to recognize the excessively large infant, precluding possible prevention by cesarean delivery.

The macrosomic infant is subject to a greater risk of perinatal mortality than its normally grown counterpart. Older series comparing neonates weighing 4500 g or more at birth with term-size controls reported perinatal mortality rates at least five times higher for the macrosomic group.[90] A more recent investigation demonstrated a perinatal mortality rate of 13.9/1000 births for macrosomic infants versus 7.0/1000 births for their control group. This difference was not statistically significant.[66]

A five-year follow-up of 200 infants weighing 4536 g or more at birth revealed 30.9% with significant medical problems (including, in descending order, asthma, Erb's palsy, convulsive disorders, cerebral palsy, mental retardation, congenital heart disease, and clubfoot) and 11.4% with severe neurologic disability. Twenty percent of those whose deliveries were complicated by shoulder dystocia had permanent Erb's palsy.[79] A more recent study involved serial developmental examinations of 212 infants with birth weights more than two standard deviations above the mean for gestational age over a four-year period. No differences were noted in the prevalence of handicaps, health problems, or speech and hearing defects; abnormalities of gross and fine motor movements were equally low in both groups.[71]

The suboptimal outcome in such pregnancies is due in large measure to lack of antepartum recognition. Thus, prenatal diagnosis of fetal macrosomia is the most effective means of prevention. Although ultrasound has been more commonly applied to the diagnosis and evaluation of the growth-retarded fetus, its utility in diagnosis of the macrosomic fetus has been explored on a limited basis. A comparison of various ultrasound parameters from 30 infants with birth weights greater than the 90th percentile to 42 infants with birth weights between the 10th and 90th percentiles found the BPD of little value in identification of the large-for-dates infant. The BPD was greater than the 90th percentile only 7% of the time. Measurement of fetal chest area correctly predicted 80% of large fetuses.[98] Determination of fetal chest area is the preferred method for detection of macrosomic fetuses and can be utilized in cases of fundal height discrepancies and maternal diabetes. Ogata et al.[70] performed serial ultrasonographic measurements of fetal BPD and AC in 23 diabetic women, Class A through C, in an attempt to detect evolving macrosomia. In all cases, the BPD remained within normal limits for nondiabetic controls. However, the AC demonstrated "accelerated somatic growth" exceeding the upper limits of normal from weeks 28 to 32 onward in 44%. These infants demonstrated increased weight and subcutaneous fat at birth. Differential ultrasonography may be useful for diagnosing accelerated intrauterine growth in fetuses of diabetic mothers. Ultrasonic measurements of BPD and chest diameter may be used to predict diabetes-induced macrosomia. A "macrosomia index" can be calculated by subtracting the BPD from the chest diameter. A transthoracic diameter 1.4 cm or more greater than the BPD correctly identified 87% of those fetuses weighing more than 4000 g and served as a predictor of significant disproportions signaling the possibility of shoulder dystocia.[21]

In summary, macrosomia often increases the risk of operative delivery, perinatal asphyxia, and trauma to skeletal and nerve tissue. This is primarily due to trauma at delivery and not to intrapartum hypoxia, as evidenced by the fact that the incidence of abnormal FHR tracings in labor is not increased. Efforts to improve outcome should be directed toward antepartum identification of the macrosomic fetus, avoidance of intrapartum complications, and use of cesarean delivery.

NONIMMUNE HYDROPS FETALIS

Nonimmune fetal hydrops refers to generalized soft tissue edema (anasarca), fluid accumulation in fetal serous cavities (such as the pleural, pericardial, and peritoneal spaces), in the absence of hemotologic evidence of isoimmunization. Potter, in 1943,[74] was the first to distinguish this entity from immune hydrops, also known as erythroblastosis fetalis (hydropic changes secondary to Rh or other blood group incompatibility). (See Chapter 21.) Distinctive features of nonimmune hydrops are lack of hepatosplenomegaly, the frequency of Rh-positive primigravid mothers, the absence of abnormal erythropoiesis, and the decreased likelihood of recurrence. Prior to the advent of Rh-immune globulin prophylaxis, more than 80% of cases of fetal hydrops were attributable to Rh isoimmunization. Testimony to its effectiveness is the fact that, currently, the majority of cases of fetal hydrops are considered to be nonimmunologic in orgin.[45] The incidence of nonimmune hydrops is reported to range from 1/1600 to 1/7000,[45] with antepartum diagnosis occurring more frequently as a result of the expanded use of ultrasound during pregnancy.

The edema and serous effusions may be the result of any or all of the following factors: increased intravascular hydrostatic pressure caused by hemodynamic disturbances (e.g., primary myocardial failure, high-output failure, obstruction of venous return); decreased plasma oncotic pressure (as with decreased albumin formation, e.g., congenital cirrhosis, or increased albumin excretion, e.g., congenital nephrotic syndrome); increased capillary permeability (secondary to anoxia, congenital infection); and obstruction to lymphatic flow (e.g., Turner's syndrome).

Fetal hydrops is a nonspecific finding that occurs in association with an array of maternal and fetal disorders. Frequently, failure to identify an obvious mechanism for the intrauterine fluid accumulation precludes assignment of a definite cause-and-effect relationship.

Cardiovascular disorders are the single largest group of causes associated with nonimmune hydrops. Regardless of the underlying pathology, if heart function is sufficiently compromised in utero, fetal hydrops develops. A variety of congenital heart lesions, especially anomalies of the tricuspid and pulmonic valves, have been associated with intrauterine heart failure. Fetal cardiac arrhythmias are now increasingly recognized as important causes of fetal hydrops. Many cases of so-called "idiopathic hydrops" may actually be secondary to undiagnosed intrauterine arrhythmias. Supraventricular tachycardias, familial congenital heart block, other types of complete heart block, and parasystole have all been diagnosed in utero and following delivery in association with hydrops fetalis.[95] Disorders interfering with myocardial contractility (e.g., subendocardial fibroelastosis), congenital myocarditis, and intracardiac neoplasms can all lead to intrauterine heart failure and subsequent hydrops fetalis.

Various pulmonary disorders are also frequently associated with nonimmune hydrops, presumably secondary to obstruction of blood return to the heart. The most common pulmonary lesion is congenital cystic adenomatoid malformation, although diaphragmatic hernia and pulmonary hypoplasia have also been associated with hydrops fetalis.

Fetal anemia may result from a variety of causes other than hematologic incompatibility, and, if severe enough, results in heart failure and hydrops fetalis. Homozygous α-thalassemia is a frequent cause of hydrops in some parts of the world. Glucose-6-phosphate dehydrogenase deficiency may induce hydropic changes after maternal ingestion of agents precipitating hemolysis. Intrauterine fetal transfusion, from both fetus to mother and twin to twin can precipitate hydrops, secondary to anemia, hypovolemia and heart failure.

Renal, gastrointestinal, and hepatic disorders are uncommonly associated with nonimmune hydrops. Hydrops occasionally accompanies urinary obstruction, although ascites is a more common sequella than is generalized edema. Congenital hepatitis, cirrhosis, and hepatic infection with rubella and syphilis may result in hypoproteinemia and hydrops.

A number of chromosomal abnormalities are frequently associated with hydrops fetalis. The most common of these is Turner's syndrome (45,X), although trisomy 21 (Down's syndrome), trisomy 13 (Patau's syndrome), and triploidy have also been found in association with hydrops, even in the absence of cardiac or renal anomalies.

A variety of inherited disorders, most commonly inborn errors of metabolism, are associated with nonimmune hydrops fetalis. Infantile Gaucher's disease, gangliosidosis GM_1, sialidosis, Hurler's syndrome, and Salla disease may all be associated with hydrops fetalis. Tuberous sclerosis, a rare autosomal recessive disorder, may present with nonimmune hydrops, apparently secondary to cirrhosis. Achondroplastic and thanatophoric dwarfism and osteogenesis imperfecta are other genetic conditions associated with hydrops fetalis.

The oldest recognized cause of nonimmune hydrops is transplacental infection. The prototype of this group, syphilis, may affect the fetal heart and liver, contributing to heart failure, hypoproteinemia, and edema. Toxoplasmosis, cytomegalic inclusion disease, and rubella are other transplacental infections associated with nonimmune hydrops.

Tumors of the placenta and umbilical cord may induce high-output cardiac failure, relative hypovolemia, and hypoproteinemia, contributing to hydrops fetalis. Chorioangioma of the placenta is the most common neoplasm of the placenta and umbilical cord.

Fetal hydrops unrelated to specific disorders is designated idiopathic. Approximately 25%[45] of cases fall into this category. An associated potential etiology should be demonstrable in the majority of cases by appropriate antepartum evaluation.

The perinatal mortality rate for nonimmune fetal hydrops ranges from 50–98%.[19] The incidence of major congenital anomalies ranges from 25%[45] to 64%.[19] Efforts to improve on these rather dismal statistics rest largely on early intrauterine diagnosis and aggressive management. Maternal conditions that mandate further evaluation for nonimmunologic hydrops fetalis include polyhydramnios, anemia, and pregnancy-induced hypertension. If the above complications are considered indications for ultrasonography, approximately 80% of infants with nonimmune hydrops and a gestational age greater than 28 weeks will be detected.[43]

Patients at risk deserve a thorough ultrasound examination. Early determinations of gestational age avoid the distortion of HC and AC by hydrops fetalis and aid in timing delivery. The greatest vertical diameter of the placenta should be measured to identify placentomegaly (placental thickness >6 cm), a frequent finding in patients with hydrops fetalis. Estimation of amniotic fluid volume is useful, because of the association with polyhydramnios. A systematic evaluation of the fetus should then be performed, beginning with the fetal skull. Edematous separation of the scalp and cranium manifests itself as two concentric rings. The scalp edema appears as a halo around the parietal bones.

Cardiac evaluation should be directed toward determination of fetal heart rate and rhythm, and the presence or absence of pericardial effusion. The limited potential space of the pericardium renders it an especially useful landmark in the diagnosis of early fluid accumulation. Accumulation of fluid separates the pericardial and epicardial membranes, which is detectable with real-time or M-mode ultrasound. Pericardial effusions precede the development of obvious fetal hydrops in fetuses at risk for nonimmune hydrops, thus serial examinations of the pericardial sac at 1–2 week intervals are useful.[73]

Measurements of abdominal diameter and circumference at the level of the umbilical vein are useful in assessing fetal age, growth, and weight. Ascites presents as an echolucent separation between the liver and inner abdominal wall. Abdominal circumference normally enlarges about 1 cm per week. More rapid rates of growth should raise suspicion of hepatosplenomegaly and developing hydrops fetalis.

Once fetal hydrops is identified, management should be directed toward determining the underlying cause and associated pathology. Differentiation of isoimmune from immune hydrops can be accomplished by maternal blood typing and an antibody screen. Additional antepartum studies should include serology, TORCH titers, a Kleihauer–Betke test (to rule out fetomaternal hemorrhage), glucose tolerance testing, maternal glucose-6-phosphate dehydrogenase activity, tests for α-thalassemia in South Asian populations, and evaluation for maternal collagen vascular diseases in cases of known or suspected fetal heart block. The addition of fetal echocardiography may allow diagnosis of structural abnormalities and arrhythmias predisposing to fetal congestive heart failure.

Subsequent management depends on the stage of gestation and the etiology. If the diagnosis is made prior to viability, action should be taken to reverse hydropic changes when feasible. Fetal tachyarrhythmias are a common and potentially treatable cause of nonimmune hydrops. An immature fetus with a supraventricular tachycardia may respond to transplacental therapy. Although reported experience is limited, cardioversion in utero has been accomplished after maternal digoxin administration.[50]

Fetuses with nonimmune hydrops that is not amenable to therapy in utero should undergo frequent antepartum evaluation. Serial ultrasonography allows early detection of worsening effusions and heart failure. Nonstress testing, contraction stress testing, and the biophysical profile should be employed to assess fetal wellbeing.

The primary factors affecting survival are prematurity, associated major congenital anomalies, and the severity of the hydropic changes. Fetuses are generally best served by early delivery, prior to development of gross serous cavity effusions. Delivery should be planned and controlled. Vaginal delivery is often complicated by the inability of the edematous placenta to sustain the fetus during labor. Difficulty with placental delivery and postpartum hemorrhage occur in a significant percentage of mothers after vaginal delivery of hydropic infants.[43] In deference to the potential for perinatal asphyxia and trauma, the liberal use of cesarean section for potentially viable fetuses is considered appropriate.

Initial neonatal management should focus on ventilation and fluid management. Respiratory embarrassment may occur secondary to pleural effusions, pulmonary or airway edema, or pulmonary hypoplasia resulting from external thoracic compression in utero. Artificial ventilation, often with high peak and endexpiratory pressures, is frequently required. Peripheral perfusion may be compromised by decreased intravascular volume, anemia, hypoxemia, and decreased cardiac output. Therapy should be directed toward maintenance of perfusion, mobilization of edema fluid, and avoidance of fluid overload. Many infants undergo spontaneous diuresis with resolution of edema if fluids are managed conservatively and the underlying process effectively treated. Complications frequently associated with prematurity (hypoglycemia, hypocalcemia, hyperbilirubinemia) and asphyxia (seizures, necrotizing enterocolitis, acute tubular necrosis, and disseminated intravascular coagulation) should be anticipated and promptly corrected.

If the etiology of the hydrops remains unclear after delivery, neonatal studies of potential value include a complete blood count, blood type and Coombs' test, serology, IgM and TORCH titers, liver and renal function tests, bacterial and viral cultures, x-rays, chromosomal analysis, and evaluation of placental anatomy and histology.

In contrast to immune hydrops, recurrence of nonimmune hydrops is very unusual and is most often due to genetically determined diseases such as glucose-6-phosphate dehydrogenase deficiency, homozygous α-thalassemia, Gaucher's disease, congenital nephrosis, tuberous sclerosis, and familial heart block. In such cases, the risk of recurrence depends on the genetics of the particular condition. Parents with an affected child should be offered prenatal genetic counseling and diagnostic studies with any subsequent pregnancies.

In summary, optimum obstetric management of nonimmune hydrops fetalis depends on early recognition, delivery prior to the development of obvious serous cavity effusions, and availability of a perinatal intensive care unit experienced in the management of neonatal prematurity and asphyxia and their complications.

REFERENCES

1. Abel, E. L.: Smoking during pregnancy: A review of effects on growth and development of offspring. *Hum. Biol.* **52**:593–625, 1980.
2. Adler, J. B. and Patterson, R. L., Jr.: Erb's palsy: Long-term results of treatment in eighty-eight cases. *J. Bone Joint Surg. (Am.)* **49**:1052–1064, 1967.
3. Bakir, F., Damluji, S. F., Amin-Zaki, L., Murtadha, M., Khalidi, A., Al-Rawi, N. Y., Tikriti, S., Dhahir, H. I., Clarkson, T. W., Smith, J. C., and Doherty, R. A.: Methylmercury poisoning in Iraq: An interuniversity report. *Science* **181**:230–241, 1973.
4. Battaglia, F. C., Frazier, T. M., and Hellegers, A. E.: Birth weight, gestational age, and pregnancy outcome, with special reference to high birth weight-low gestational age infant. *Pediatrics* **37**:417–422, 1966.
5. Beischer, N. A., Abell, D. A., and Drew, J. H.: Management of fetal growth retardation. *Med. J. Aust.* **2**:64 -646 977
6. Belizán, J. M., Villar, J., Nardin, J. C., Malamud, J., and DeVicuña, L. S.: Diagnosis of intrauterine growth retardation by a simple clinical method: Measurement of uterine height. *Am. J. Obstet. Gynecol.* **131**:643–646, 1978.
7. Berkowitz, R. L., Coustan, D. R., and Mochizuki, T. K.: *Handbook for Prescribing Medications During Pregnancy*, 1st Edition. Boston, Little, Brown, and Company, 1981.
8. Bibbo, M., Gill, W. B., Azizi, F., Blouth, R., Fang, V. S., Rosenfield, R. L., Schumacher, G. F. B., Sleeer, K., Sonek, M. G., and Weid, G. I.: Follow-up study of male and female offspring of DES-exposed mothers. *Obstet. Gynecol.* **49**:1–8, 1977.
9. Breart, G., Rabarison Y., Plouin, P. F., Sureau, C., and Rumeau-Rouqette, C.: Risk of fetal growth reardation as a result of maternal hypertension. Preparation to a trial on antihypertensive drugs. *Dev. Pharmacol. Ther.* **4**:116–123, 1982.
10. Brocklebank, J. C., Ray, W. A., Federspiel, C. F., and Schaffner, W.: Drug prescribing during pregnancy. A controlled study of Tennessee Medicaid recipients. *Am. J. Obstet. Gynecol.* **132**:235–244, 1978.
11. Campbell, S. and Thomas, A.: Ultrasound measurement of the fetal head to abdomen circumference ratio in the assessment of growth retardation. *Br. J. Gynaecol.* **84**:165–174, 1977.
12. Centers for Disease Control. Rubella and congenital rubella—United States. 1980–1983. *Morb. Mortal. Wkly. Rpt.* **32**:505–510, 1983.
13. Centers for Disease Control. Valproic acid and spina bifida: A preliminary report—France. *Morb. Mortal. Wkly. Rpt.* **31**:565–566, 1982.
14. Chamberlain, R. and Davey, A.: Physical growth in twins, postmature, and small-for-dates children. *Arch. Dis. Child.* **50**:437–442, 1975.
15. Chervenak F. A., Jeanty P., and Hobbins J. C.:

Current status of fetal age and growth assessment. *Clin. Obstet. Gynecol.* **10**:423–444, 1983.

16. Committee on Drugs, American Academy of Pediatrics: Anticonvulsants and pregnancy. *Pediatrics* **63**:331–333, 1979.
17. Daikoku, N. H., Johnson, J. W. C., Graf, C., Kearney, K., Tyson, J. E., and King, T. M.: Patterns of intrauterine growth retardation. *Obstet. Gynecol.* **54**:211–219, 1979.
18. Daikoku, N. H., Tyson, J. E., Graf, C., Scott, R., Smith, B. Johnson, J. W., and King, T. M.: The relative significance of human placental lactogen in the diagnosis of retarded fetal growth. *Am. J. Obstet. Gynecol.* **135**:516–521, 1979.
19. Davis, C. L.: Diagnosis and management of nonimmune hydrops fetalis. *J. Reprod. Med.* **27**:594–600, 1982.
20. Dobson, P. C., Abell, D. A., and Beischer, N. A.: Mortality and morbidity of fetal growth retardation. *Aust. N.Z. J. Obstet. Gynaecol.* **21**:69–72, 1981.
21. Elliott, J. P., Garite, T. J., Freeman, R. K., McQuown, D. S., and Patel, J. M.: Ultrasonic prediction of fetal macrosomia in diabetic patients. *Obstet. Gynecol.* **60**:159–162, 1982.
22. Etches, P. C. and Lemons, J. A.: Non-immune hydrops fetalis: Report of 22 cases including 3 siblings. *Pediatrics* **64**:326–332, 1979.
23. Evans, M. I., Mukherjee, A. B., and Schulman, J. D.: Animal models of intrauterine growth retardation. *Obstet. Gynaecol. Surv.* **38**:183–192, 1983.
24. Fancourt, R., Campbell, S., Harvey, D. R., and Norman, A. P.: Follow-up study of small-for-dates babies. *Br. Med. J.* **1**:1435–1437, 1976.
25. Feldman, G. L., Weaver, D. D., and Lorrien, E. W.: The fetal trimethadione syndrome: Report of an additional family and further delineation of this syndrome. *Am. J. Dis. Child.* **131**:1389–1392, 1977.
26. Flynn, A. M., Kelly, J. and O'Connor, M.: Unstressed antepartum cardiotocography in the management of the fetus suspected of growth retardation. *Br. J. Obstet. Gynaecol.* **86**:106–110, 1979.
27. Fraser, F. C.: Relation of animal studies to the problem in man. In: *Handbook of Teratology*, Vol. 1. J. G. Wilson and F. C. Fraser (Eds.). New York, Plenum, 1977, pp. 75–96.
28. Galbraith, R. S., Karchmar, E. J., Piercy, W. N., and Low, J. A.: The clinical prediction of intrauterine growth retardation. *Am. J. Obstet. Gynecol.* **133**:281–286, 1979.
29. Golditch, I. M. and Kirkman, K.: The large fetus management and outcome. *Obstet. Gynecol.* **52**:26–30, 1978.
30. Gross, T. L., Sokol, R. J., Wilson, M. V., and Zador, I. E.: Using ultrasound and amniotic fluid determinations to diagnose intrauterine growth retardation before birth: A clinical model. *Am. J. Obstet. Gynecol.* **143**:265–269, 1982.
31. Gruenberger, W. and Gerstner, G. J.: The causes of antepartum fetal death: A clinical-pathological study. *Clin. Exp. Obstet. Gyn.* **VII**:210–214, 1980.
32. Hall, J. G., Pauli, R. M., and Wilson, K. M.: Maternal and fetal sequelae of anticoagulation during pregnancy. *Am. J. Med.* **68**:122–140, 1980.
33. Hanshaw, J. B.: Cytomegalovirus. In: *Infectious Diseases of the Fetus and Newborn Infant.* J. S. Remington and J. O. Klein (Eds.). Philadelphia, W. B. Saunders, 1983, pp. 104–142.
34. Hanson, J. W. and Smith, D. W.: The fetal hydantoin syndrome. *J. Pediatr.* **87**:285–290, 1975.
35. Harger, A. H., Archer, D. F., Marchese, S. G., Muracca-Clemens, M., and Garver, K. L.: Etiology of recurrent pregnancy losses and outcome of subsequent pregnancies. *Obstet. Gynecol.* **62**:574–581, 1983.
36. Harrison, R. F., Hurley, R., and deLouvois, J.: Genital mycoplasmas and birth weight in offspring of primigravid women. *Am. J. Obstet. Gynecol.* **133**:201–203, 1979.
37. Hertig, A. T., Rock, J., Adams, E. C., and Menkin, M. C.: Thirty-four fertilized human ova, good, bad, and indifferent, recovered from 210 women of known fertility. A study of biologic wastage in early human pregnancy. *Pediatrics* **23**:202–211, 1959.
38. Hobbins, J. C., Berkowitz, R. L., and Grannum, P. A. T.: Diagnosis and management of intrauterine growth retardation. *J. Reprod. Med.* **21**:319–325, 1978.
39. Hogue, C. J.: Coffee in pregnancy. *Lancet* **1**:554, 1981.
40. Holmes, G. E., Miller, H. C., Hassanein, K., Lansky, S. B., and Groggin, J. E.: Postnatal somatic growth in infants with atypical fetal growth patterns. *Am. J. Dis. Child.* **131**:1078–1083, 1977.
41. Hill, D. F.: Physical growth and development after intrauterine growth retardation. *J. Reprod. Med.* **21**:335–342, 1978.
42. Hutchins, C. J.: Delivery of the growth retarded infant. *Obstet. Gynecol.* **56**:683–686, 1980.
43. Hutchison, A. A., Drew, J. H., Uy, V. Y. H., Williams, M. L., Fortune, D. W., and Beischer, N. A.: Nonimmunologic hydrops fetalis: A review of 61 cases. *Obstet. Gynecol.* **59**:347–352, 1982.
44. Iams, J. D. and Rayburn, W. F.: Drug effects on the fetus. In: *Drug Therapy in Obstetrics and Gynecology.* W. F. Rayburn and F. P. Zuspan (Eds.). Norwalk, Appleton-Century-Crofts, 1982, pp. 9–17.
45. Im, S. S., Rizos, N., Joutsi, P., Shime, J., and Benzie, R. J.: Nonimmunologic hydrops fetalis. *Am. J. Obstet. Gynecol.* **148**:566–569, 1984.
46. Kalter, H. and Warkany, J.: Congenital malformations—etiologic factors and their role in prevention (First of two parts). *N. Engl. J. Med.* **308**:424–431, 1983.
47. Kalter, H. and Warkany, J.: Congenital malformations (Second of two parts). *N. Engl. J. Med.* **308**:491–497, 1983.
48. Kariniemi, V. and Ammala, P.: Short-term vari-

ability of fetal heart rate during pregnancies with normal and insufficient placental function. *Am. J. Obstet. Gynecol.* **139**:33–37, 1981.

49. Kazzi, G. M., Gross, T. L., Sokol, R. J., and Kazzi, N. J.: Detection of intrauterine growth retardation: A new use for sonographic placental grading. *Am. J. Obstet. Gynecol.* **145**:733–737, 1983.
50. Kerenyi, T. D., Gleicher, N., Meller, J., Brown, E., Steinfield, L., Chitkara, U., and Raucher, H.: Transplacental cardioversion of intrauterine supraventricular tachycardia with digitalis. *Lancet* **2**:393–394, 1980.
51. Khouzami, V. A., Ginsburg, D. S., Daikoku, N. H., and Johnson, J. W. C.: The glucose tolerance test as a means of identifying intrauterine growth retardation. *Am. J. Obstet. Gynecol.* **139**:423–426, 1981.
52. Knox, G. E.: Influence of infection on fetal growth and development. *J. Reprod. Med.* **21**:352–358, 1978.
53. Knutzen, V. K. and Sher, G.: The major determinants of perinatal mortality in a large metropolitan hospital—results of a retrospective study. *J. Reprod. Med.* **27**:395–400, 1982.
54. Kurjak, A. and Kirkinen, P.: Ultrasonic growth pattern of fetuses with chromosomal aberrations. *Acta. Obstet. Gynecol. Scand.* **61**:223–225, 1982.
55. Kurjak, A., Kirkinen, P., and Latin, V.: Biometric and dynamic ultrasound assessment of small-for-dates infants: Report of 260 cases. *Obstet. Gynecol.* **56**:281–284, 1980.
56. Laube, D. W. and Scauberger, C. W.: Fetomaternal bleeding as a cause for "unexplained" fetal death. *Obstet. Gynecol.* **60**:649-651, 1982.
57. Lauritsen, J. G.: Aetiology of spontaneous abortion: A cytogenetic and epidemiological study of 288 abortuses and their parents. *Acta Obstet. Gynecol. Scand.* [Suppl.] **52**:1–29, 1976.
58. Lejeune, J.: Le mongolisme. Premiere exemple d'aberration autosomique humaine. *Ann. Genet.* **1**:41–49, 1959.
59. Lin, C. C., Devoe, L. D., River, P., and Moawad, A. H.: Oxytocin challenge test and intrauterine growth retardation. *Am. J. Obstet. Gynecol.* **140**:282–288, 1981.
60. Lin, C. C., Moawad, A. H., Rosenow, P. J., and River, P.: Acid-base characteristics of fetuses with intrauterine growth retardation during labor and delivery. *Am. J. Obstet. Gynecol.* **137**:553–559, 1980.
61. Low, J. A., Karchmar, J., Broekhoven, L., Leonard, T., McGrath, M. J., Pancham, S. R., and Piercy, W. N.: The probability of fetal metabolic acidosis during labor in a population at risk as determined by clinical factors. *Am. J. Obstet. Gynecol.* **141**:941–951, 1981.
62. Manning, F. A., Lange, I. R., Morrison I., and Harman, C. R.: Fetal biophysical profile score and the nonstress test: A comparative trial. *Obstet. Gynecol.* **64**:326–331, 1984.
63. Martin, J. C.: An overview: Maternal nicotine and caffeine consumption and offspring outcome. *Neurobehav. Toxicol. Teratol.* **4**:421–428, 1982.
64. Meschia, G.: Supply of oxygen to the fetus. *J. Reprod. Med.* **23**:160–165, 1979.
65. Miller, E., Cradock-Watson, J. E., and Pollock, T. M.: Consequences of confirmed maternal rubella at successive stages of pregnancy. *Lancet* **2**:781–784, 1982.
66. Modanlou, H. D., Dorchester, W. L., Thorosian, A., and Freeman, R. K.: Macrosomia—maternal, fetal and neonatal implications. *Obstet. Gynecol.* **55**:420–424, 1980.
67. Modanlou, H. D., Komatsu, G., Dorchester, W., Freeman, R. K., and Bosu, S. K.: Large-for-gestational age neonates. Anthropometric reasons for shoulder dystocia. *Obstet. Gynecol.* **60**:417–423, 1982.
68. Mueller, R. F., Sybert, V. P., Johnson, J., Brown, Z. A., and Chen, W. J.: Evaluation of a protocol for post-mortem examination of stillbirths. *N. Engl. J. Med.* **309**:586–590, 1983.
69. Odendaal, H. A.: The fetal and labor outcome of 102 positive contraction stress tests. *Obstet. Gynecol.* **54**:591–596, 1979.
70. Ogata, E. S., Sabbagha, R., Metzger, B. E., Phelps, R. L., Depp, R., Boehm, J. J., and Dooley, S. L.: Serial ultrasonography to assess evolving fetal macrosomia: Studies in 23 pregnant diabetic women. *JAMA* **243**:2405–2408, 1980.
71. Ounsted, M. K., Moar, V. A., and Scott, A.: Large-for-dates babies at the age of four years: Health, handicap, and developmental status. *Early Hum. Dev.* **9**:9–19, 1983.
72. Parks, D. G. and Ziel, H. K.: Macrosomia—a proposed indication for primary cesarean section. *Obstet. Gynecol.* **52**:407–409, 1978.
73. Platt, L. D. and DeVore, G. R.: In utero diagnosis of hydrops fetalis: Ultrasound methods. *Clin. Perinatol.* **9**:627–636, 1982.
74. Potter, E. L.: Universal edema of the fetus unassociated with erythroblastosis. *Am. J. Obstet. Gynecol.* **46**:130–134, 1943.
75. Remington, J. S. and Desmonts, G.: Toxoplasmosis. In: *Infectious Diseases of the Fetus and Newborn Infant.* J. S. Remington and J. O. Klein (Eds.). Philadelphia, W. B. Saunders, 1983, pp. 143-263.
76. Rolschau, J.: Circumvallate placenta and intrauterine growth retardation. *Acta. Obstet. Gynecol. Scand.* [Suppl]. **72**:11–14, 1978.
77. Ruzicska, P. and Czeizel, A.: Cytogenetic studies on mid-trimester abortuses. *Humangenetik* **10**:273–297, 1970.
78. Sabbagha, R. E.: Intrauterine growth retardation antenatal diagnosis by ultrasound. *Obstet. Gynecol.* **52**:252–256, 1978.
79. Sack, R. A.: The large infant. *Am. J. Obstet. Gynecol.* **104**:195–204, 1969.
80. Sandberg, E. C., Riffle, N. L., Higdon, J. V., and Getman, C. E.: Pregnancy outcome in women ex-

posed to diethylstilbestrol in utero. *Am. J. Obstet. Gynecol.* **140**:194-205, 1981.

81. Scott, A., Moar, V., and Ounsted, M.: The relative contributions of different maternal factors in small-for-gestational-age pregnancies. *Eur. J. Obstet. Gynecol. Reprod. Biol.* **12**:157-165, 1981.
82. Seeds, J. W.: Impaired fetal growth: Definition and clinical diagnosis. *Obstet. Gynecol.* **64**:303-310, 1984.
83. Shapiro, S., Hartz, S. C., Siskund, V., Mitchell, A. A., Slone, D., Rosenberg, L., Monson, R. R., and Heinonen, O. P.: Anticonvulsants and parental epilepsy in the development of birth defects. *Lancet* **1**:272-275, 1976.
84. Simpson, J. L., Golbus, M. S., Martin, A. O., and Sarto, G. E.: *Genetics in Obstetrics and Gynecology*, 1st Edition. New York, Grune & Stratton, 1982.
85. Sokol, R. J., Kazzi, G. M., Kalhan, S. C., and Pillay, S. K.: Identifying the pregnancy at risk for intrauterine growth retardation: Possible usefulness of the intravenous glucose tolerance test. *Am. J. Obstet. Gynecol.* **143**:220-223, 1982.
86. Sparks, J. W., Girard, J. R., and Battaglia, F. C.: An estimate of the caloric requirements of the human fetus. *Biol. Neonate* **38**:113-119, 1980.
87. Speidel, B. D. and Meadow, S. R.: Epilepsy, anticonvulsants, and congenital malformations. *Drugs* **8**:354-365, 1974.
88. Starfield, B., Shapiro, S., McCormick, M., and Bross, D.: Mortality and morbidity in infants with intrauterine growth retardation. *J. Pediatr.* **101**:978-983, 1982.
89. Stein, Z. A. and Susser, M.: Intrauterine growth retardation: Epidemiological issues and public health significance. *Semin. Perinatol.* **8**:5-15, 1984.
90. Stevenson, D. K., Cohen, R. S., Kerner, J. A.: Macrosomia: Causes and consequences. *J. Pediatr.* **100**:515-520, 1982.
91. Stumpf, D. A. and Frost, M.: Seizures, anticonvulsants, and pregnancy. *Am. J. Dis. Child.* **132**:746-748, 1978.
92. Tanguy, G., Thoumsin, J. H., Zorn, J. R., and Cedard, L.: DHEA-S-loading in cases of intrauterine growth retardation—relationship between the pattern of the maternal plasma metabolites and the fetoplacental dysfunction. *Gynecol. Obstet. Invest.* **12**:305-316, 1981.
93. Tjio, J. H. and Levan, A.: The chromosome number of man. *Hereditas* **42**:1-6, 1956.
94. Tsubaki, T. and Irukayama, K.: *Minamata Disease: Methylmercury Poisoning in Minamata and Niigata, Japan.* New York, Elsevier, 1977.
95. Turkel, S. B.: Conditions associated with nonimmune hydrops fetalis. *Clin. Perinatol.* **9**:613-625, 1982.
96. United States National Center for Health Statistics. Monthly Vital Statistics Report, Vol. 31, No. 5. Birth, marriages, divorces, and deaths for May 1982. Hyattsville, Maryland: Public Health Service, August 1982:1-10 [DHHS publication no. (PHS) 82-1120].
97. Warburton, D. and Fraser, F. C.: Spontaneous abortion risks in man: Data from reproductive histories collected in a medical genetics unit. *Am. J. Hum. Genet.* **16**:1-25, 1964.
98. Wladimiroff, J. W., Bloemsia, C. A., and Wallenburg, H. C. S.: Ultrasonic diagnosis of the large-for-dates infant. *Obstet. Gynecol.* **52**:285-287, 1978.

21

ALLOIMMUNE DISEASE

The human red blood cell (RBC) membrane appears deceptively smooth and simple when examined under the light microscope. On the molecular level, however, it is studded with discrete lumps and bumps, which can be differentiated by their individual antigenic behavior and sorted into families of antigens, known as blood group systems. At present, there are 12 known blood group systems and a large number of solitary antigens of varying frequency. An individual bears two sets of genetic information (haplotypes) for each system, inherited independently in mendelian pattern. To further multiply the possible variations in RBC antigens, haplotypes in several systems include multiple determinants (e.g., D, C, and E in the Rhesus system) for which there may be multiple alleles (e.g., C, c, C^w, C^u, and C^x for the C antigen).

Genes code for the synthesis of enzymes which, in turn, produce the antigen entities. This "indirect" expression of the gene allows further variation in observed red blood cell antigens, by antigen modification or inhibition by other separate genes. When such factors are added to the array of RBC antigens possible in each individual, it is not difficult to understand pregnancies in which mother and fetus do not have identical blood types.

This potential for differing blood types and the consequences of maternal immune response to (foreign) fetal red blood cell antigens form the basis of the problems discussed in this chapter. The sequential processes of maternal exposure, sensitization, and competent immune response to fetal RBC antigens inherited from the father are collectively termed *alloimmunization*. In most obstetric practices, alloimmunization is confined to a small group of antigens, of which the Rh system remains the most significant. The principles of this discussion, however, can be extended to any maternal–fetal blood group incompatibility.

HISTORICAL PERSPECTIVE

Descriptions of hydrops fetalis have appeared since the time of Hippocrates, but only since the turn of the century has etiology been clarified. In 1900, Landsteiner showed that human erythrocyte membrane surfaces carried differing structures—the ABO blood group antigens—and in 1905 Dienst first suggested that fetal blood group incompatibility provoked maternal immune responses, noting a postpartum rise in anti-A or anti-B titers in Group O women delivering Group A or B infants, respectively.[30] Although these contributions were of significant importance later, attempts to correlate ABO incompatibility with fetal/neonatal disease were frustrated during the next 20 years. The frequent inability of ABO differences to cause significant disease, indeed the protective nature of this incompatibility in preventing other alloimmunization, is discussed in detail later.

Ottenberg suggested in 1923 that "accidental placental transfusion of incompatible blood" into maternal circulation was related to the development of neonatal jaundice.[63] Still in the dark about the exact nature of maternal-fetal incompatibility, Darrow suggested that hemolytic anemia of the fetus/newborn was due to transmission of "immune bodies from an actively immunized mother."[22] The absence of significant correlation between incompatibilities of the known blood groups and neonatal disease (the M-N and P systems having been discovered in 1927) likely assisted Darrow in concluding that differences in structure between maternal and fetal hemoglobins, rather than red blood cell membranes, were the antigenic factors in this immune process.[75]

Clinical studies advanced on a parallel time scale. In 1932, Diamond concluded that four disease forms—hydrops fetalis, fetal erythroblastosis, icterus gravis neonatorum, and anemia of the newborn—were manifestations of the same disease process.[25,28] That the underlying cause of this spectrum of disease was related to a previously unknown form of maternal–fetal incompatibility was proposed by Levine and Stetson in 1939. They suggested that immunizing properties of the fetus, inherited from the father, were responsible for sensitization of the Group O patient against the Group O blood of her husband, used for transfusion.[51] This was a landmark report because it documented intragroup sensitization between two Group O individuals, without prior blood transfusion. Furthermore, when Levine and Stetson paneled the blood of their patient against 104 other Group O individuals, only 21 were compatible.

The unifying steps followed rapidly. In 1940, Landsteiner and Wiener showed that antisera developed in rabbits against Rhesus monkey red blood cells reacted differentially with human blood—85% of individuals reacted positively (Rhesus- or Rh-positive), whereas 15% did not react and therefore did not carry the antigen on their red blood cells (Rhesus- or Rh-negative).[47] The antigen that Landsteiner and Weiner actually were testing was the Rhesus antigen LW, not, in fact, the determinant of Rh type; nevertheless, the nomenclature and clinical sense of this classic work persist.[37] In 1940, Wiener and Peters demonstrated the antigenic nature of the human Rh factor in its ability to provoke an agglutinating and hemolyzing response by Rh-negative individuals to Rh-positive blood.[93] By 1941, Levine and colleagues solidified the concept of transplacental Rh alloimmunization.[50] Their theory that Rh-negative mothers were sensitized by the fetus' (paternally) inherited Rh-positive red blood cells, and that fetal/neonatal disease was the consequence of the intrauterine action of maternal anti-Rh agglutinins on the fetus, forms the essence of our current understanding.

This classic report also proposed the first significant advances in treatment. Correct Rh typing was necessary in transfusing mothers and in transfusion of affected Rh-positive newborn with Rh-negative blood. The further observation that different antisera reacted in varying strengths with different individuals gave one of the first insights into the multiplicity of Rh antigens.

Effort was turned to diagnostic techniques. Detection of Rh antibodies in maternal serum had used saline dilution of Rh-positive blood and, as we now know, detected the presence of *IgM*. Race showed that a second type of antibody ("incomplete" antibody) that blocked agglutination in saline suspensions existed in many Rh-negative individuals.[68] Diamond's laboratory developed a slide test using heated, concentrated Rh-positive preparations that would detect this incomplete (*IgG*) antibody[26] and showed improved results using albumin suspension.[29] The detection of circulating anti-Rh antibody in neonatal blood was reported by Coombs et al., also in 1945.[19]

Thus, the serology of the immediate maternal response (IgM, 19S, "saline" or "complete" antibody), the maternally produced agent of disease (IgG, 7S, "albumin" or "incomplete" antibody), and transmission of that agent to the surface of fetal RBCs (direct Coombs test) could be quantified. These tests and the continued development of antisera against Rh subgroups in the population led to a proliferation of reports. These saw evolution from the Rh yes/no theory of Landsteiner and Wiener to our current concept of the Rh antigen system of three loci—C, D, and E—with multiple alleles available for each site. As newborn treatment progressed, mortality from Rh hemolytic disease of the fetus and newborn (HDFN) fell progressively (Fig. 21-1). Before 1940, perinatal death occurred in 80–90% of pregnancies affected by severe HDFN. Routine use of Rh-negative blood for transfusion reduced this to 50% by 1945.[23] The development of detailed serology by 1945 also demonstrated that maternal antibody remained in the neonatal circulation to cause continued hemolysis for some time after birth.[25] Exchange transfusion via umbilical vein catheter saw a drop in mortality to 20–25% by 1951.[27] The addition of irradiation with blue

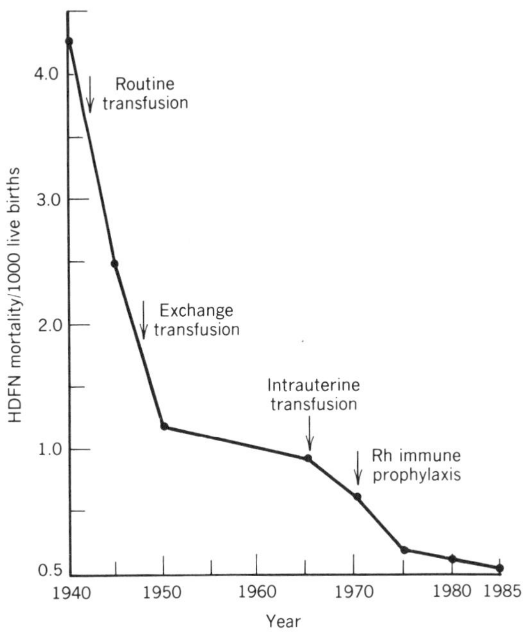

Figure 21-1. Graph of approximate mortality/1000 live births due to HDFN, showing treatment milestones (data from Diamond[25], Clark,[16] and Davey[23]).

light in the visual spectrum to accelerate breakdown of bilirubin (1958) was useful in reducing the requirement for exchange transfusion to prevent kernicterus.[20] Further reduction in the stillbirth rate was obtained with the introduction of intrauterine transfusion by Liley in 1963.[54]

At the same time as this last therapeutic innovation, definitive trials on *prevention* began. Using the acid-elution technique for identifying fetal RBCs in maternal blood (developed by Kleihauer, Braun, and Betke[46] in 1957), Zipursky and coworkers had shown that transplacental fetal-maternal hemorrhage was a common event at the time of delivery, and was the major probable source of antigen sensitization.[97] On the basis of this information, Clarke and colleagues in Liverpool attempted to eliminate Rh-positive cells injected to Rh-negative volunteers using 19S (IgM) anti-D plasma fractions. This trial in 1961 showed elimination of foreign (Rh-positive) red blood cells but did not prevent Rh alloimmunization.[31] The same year, using volunteers at Joliet Prison, Stern et al. were able to show that coating of the Rh-positive cells with 7S (IgG) anti-D before injection

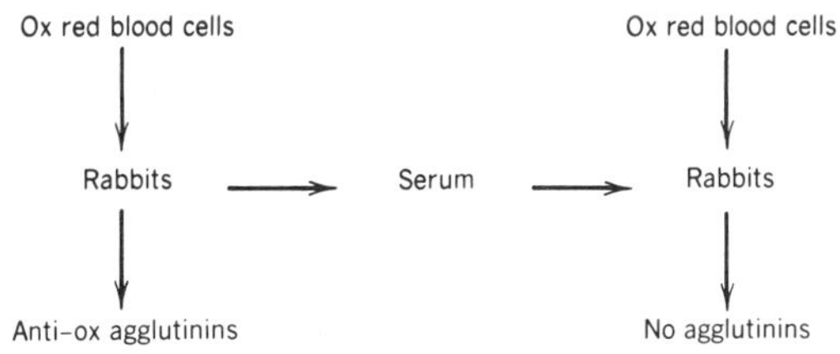

Figure 21-2. The investigations of Von Gungern (1900) were an early demonstration of the protective nature of passive immunity. Immune serum from the first group of rabbits immunized against ox red blood cells prevented immunization in the second group of rabbits.

did prevent antibody formation, regardless of the dose of coated cells.[82]

These important steps in prevention of Rh disease did not spring de novo from the 1960s. A summary of the conclusions of Von Dungern[88] (1900) is shown in Fig. 21-2. In 1909, Smith noted that excess antitoxin prevented diphtheria toxin from evoking immunity.[81] Finally, Race[68] and Wiener[92] showed that "incomplete" antibody (IgG) "blocked" agglutination of Rh-positive cells by saline agglutinin (IgM), demonstrating the ability of IgG to mask antigen sites.

Independent trials of Rh-immune prophylaxis were completed in the United States,[33] Britain,[17] and Canada[15] in the 1960s, establishing the ability to prevent most Rh disease. The sophistication of prevention and treatment continues to advance today, but our understanding is still incomplete, and Rh disease remains a significant clinical problem.

MECHANISMS OF ALLOIMMUNIZATION

Rh-antigen incompatibility is responsible for 90% of alloimmunization syndromes in pregnancy. In its complexity, the Rh system is second only to the HLA system. The ultimate outcome of pregnancy in Rh-negative women, therefore, is subject to varying influences of many factors (Fig. 21-3).

The Rh Antigens

Nomenclature. Rhesus blood type—positive or negative—is determined by the presence or absence, respectively, of an erythrocyte mem-

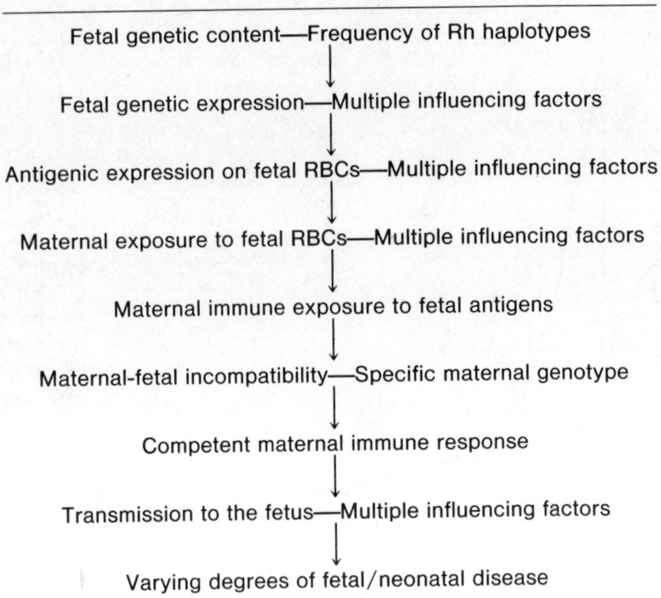

Figure 21-3. Generation of alloimmune disease in pregnant Rh-negative women depends on many complex interactions.

brane antigen called D. The Rhesus antigen, however, is more complicated than Rh typing suggests. In its ability to provoke antibodies, the complete Rh antigen behaves as if there were three antigenic sites; the designation CcDdEe summarizes the choice of alleles at these sites. The contribution from each parent (haplotype) is denoted CDE, Cde, and so on, and the format CDe/cDe specifies the Rh genotype of an individual. There are only five antigenic alleles—D, C, c, E, and e—all of which are expressed if present in the genetic complement ("codominant" genes). Lowercase d in this nomenclature signifies only the absence of D: there is no serologic evidence that an antigenic d exists.

This descriptive notation is that of Fisher and Race[69] and is focused on identifying each of the alleles borne by an individual. Inheritance of Rh antigens, however, does not conform to mendelian laws as would three separate pairs of alleles—certain triplets are much more common than others, and inheritance patterns are those of a single gene. For example, a child with parent Cde/cDE could inherit either Cde or cDE as one of its Rh haplotypes, but not cdE, cde, and so on. An alternate nomenclature devised by Wiener and Wexler[94] recognizes these patterns of inheritance and assigns a single character to designate the three-antigen unit (e.g., CDe is R^1 in this system). Finally, Rosenfeld et al.[73] proposed a system analogous to the HLA system, identifying each antigenic determinant (including the many variations to the five major antigens) by a number (e.g., CDe is Rh 1,2,5 in this system). Thus, a homozygous individual whose red blood cells agglutinate with anti-c and anti-E sera would be cDE/-cDE by the Fisher–Race system, R^2R^2 by the Wiener–Wexler system, and Rh 1,3,4 by the Rosenfeld system. Each system has its advantages; the descriptive ability of the Fisher–Race system has made it the most popular among obstetricians and neonatologists.

Antigen Distribution. The distribution of the common phenotypes and their most likely genotypes are shown in Table 21-1. The most common haplotypes are CDe (42% of the white population), cde (37%), cDE (14%), cDe (4%), Cde (2%), and cdE (1%). In blacks, cDe is the most common (44%) and CDe is found only 11% of the time. CDE and CdE are very rare.

Rhesus negativity is a Caucasian characteristic, but this varies throughout the world. In Finland, only 11% are Rh negative; in North America about 17% are Rh negative; and in Basque villages in Spain, the proportion may be as high as 37%. As seen in Table 21-1, about 44% of Rh-positive individuals are homozygous DD, 56% are Dd. These distribution statistics impact significantly on the likelihood of any Rh-negative women carrying an Rh-positive fetus.

Antigen Expression. The relative strength of Rh antigens is largely determined by the factors regulating the expression of genetic determi-

TABLE 21-1. Rh PHENOTYPES IN CAUCASIANS[74]

Antigens Expressed	Percentage of Population	Genotypes			
CcDe	35	CDe/cde	94%,	CDe/cDe	6%
CDe	20	CDe/CDe	95%,	CDe/Cde	5%
CcDEe	13	CDe/cDE	89%,	CDe/cdE	7%
cDEe	10	cDE/cde	93%,	cDE,cDe	6%
cDE	3	cDE/cDE	86%,	cDE/cdE	14%
cDe	2	cDe/cDe	97%,	cDe/cde	3%
ce	16	cde/cde	100%		
Cce	1	Cde/cde	100%		

Also: CDEe (0.3%), CcDE (0.1%), and cEe (0.2%). The remaining phenotypes are found in <0.1%: CcEe, CcE, Ce, cE, CDE, CEe, and CE.

nants. There are probably about 155,000 total antigenic sites available to the Rh antigens *per* red blood cell, and their distribution depends on the antigens coded for. For example, it has been suggested that, for genotype CDe/cDE, there are 37,000 D sites, 40,000 C sites, 40,000 c sites, 14,500 e sites, 8000 E sites and 12,500 G sites (G is a variant Rh antigen, C and/or D linked).[80]

The Rh antigen is probably a protein molecular weight 7000–10,000, dispersed in irregular clusters on the membrane. The antigen is likely anchored by concentrations of phospholipid in the membrane. It achieves full expression on RBCs by 4 weeks embryonic age, and anti-D agglutination of Rh-positive embryonic RBCs has been shown as early as 38 days.[45]

Rh Antigen Variants

D Variants

D^u/D Mosaic (Fig. 21-4). Variations in the expression of D antigen give rise to two paradoxical situations: (1) Rh-positive women who produce anti-D antibody and (2) Rh-negative women whose cells agglutinate with anti-D antibody. These observations have led to the "D-mosaic" theory: D antigen is composed of multiple epitopes.[83,84] The absolute number of components of the D antigen is unknown. "Normal" D expression may require all epitopes, and absence of a particular epitope (D-mosaic variant) or presence of one or more weaker epitopes (D^u variant) may give rise to the "incomplete" expression of Rh positivity. D antigenicity in D^u individuals (about 0.6% of the population) varies from readily detectable (appear Rh positive, although weakly) to minutely detectable (appear Rh negative on routine serotyping, detectable only indirectly by anti-anti-D binding). D-mosaic individuals always group as Rh positive but may alloimmunize to the D component(s) they lack. Although Bowman has rarely noted anti-D alloimmunization in such patients in more than 700,000 pregnancies,[5] there are several cases where this phenomenon has led to severe HDFN.[91] Issitt has reviewed these complexities in detail.[44]

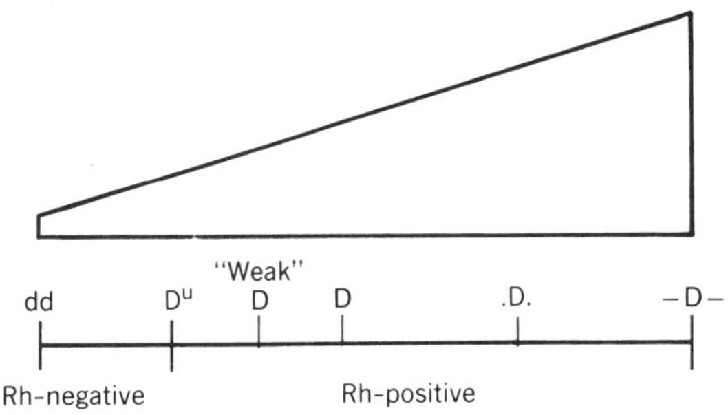

Figure 21-4. Variants of D antigenicity.

"Weak" D. As a result of the presence of C or E on the opposite chromosome ("trans" effect) D may be only weakly expressed. There is no evidence that the D antigen is unusual, only that it does not react as strongly with anti-D as does the "normal" Rh-positive population; such individuals are not at risk for anti-D alloimmunization.

-D- and .D.. In these rare individuals, no other epitopes (c, C, E, or e) are expressed. -D- individuals have *only* D antigen sites (Rh "superpositive"). .D. have an additional Rh antigen (Evans), and their expression of D is about half

that of -D- and twice that of normal Rh-positive homozygotes.[52]

dd. This, of course, is the designation for Rh-negative, or D-absent, individuals. Under special preparation, however, antigenic D can be extracted from Rh-negative cells.[64] Where these D antigens are concealed on the intact red blood cell is unknown.

C and E Variants. C^w is the most common of these and ranks ahead of the common antigens C and e in frequency of alloimmunization.[65] About 30 non-D variants exist, some of them of clinical significance in specific families or localities. In general, these antigens and their respective genes appear as paired alleles at the C or E sites; however, rare cases where more than two alleles are expressed have been reported.[52]

The possibility of incompatibility, therefore the potential for alloimmunization, even *within* Rh blood groups, emphasizes the need for accurate blood transfusion practices and for pregnancy surveillance. Regardless of blood type, all pregnant women should be screened with multiple antisera, on booking and again at 28–32 weeks, for red blood cell antibodies, many of which can cause disease as severe as that seen in anti-D alloimmunization (Table 21-2).

TABLE 21-2. MAJOR NON-D ANTIGENS ASSOCIATED WITH CLINICAL HDFN

Blood Group	Frequent	Uncommon
Rh	c, E, C^w	e, C, Ce, cE
Kell	K	Kp^a, Kp^b, k
Duffy		Fy^a
MNS		s
Private		Wr^a
ABO	A, B, H	AB

The Genes

Genetic information determining Rh phenotype is inherited in mendelian fashion and is located on the short arm of chromosome 1 (between 1p32 and the terminal point).[17] There may be a single locus on each chromosome, coding for production of an entire Rh-antigen complex (theory of Wiener[15]), or there may be three closely linked genes, coding separately for individual components—the Fisher–Race model.[69] If genes code for each antigenic type (epitope) of the complex Rh antigen, they must be at virtually adjacent loci. It has not been possible to separate the component genes in chromosome mapping, and the existence of any natural cross-over is limited.

Several factors may regulate the expression of Rh genes (Table 21-3). Although alleles are "codominant" (i.e., all alleles coded for are expressed), the extent of expression of each determinant may vary.

Maternal Exposure to Fetal Red Blood Cell Antigens

Trophoblast may express D antigen, but this remains doubtful.[36] Although other routes are theoretically possible, transplacental hemorrhage (TPH), bleeding from fetus to mother, is responsible for most pregnancy-related alloimmunization (Table 21-4). Mismatched transfusion was a leading cause of exposure before identification of the Rh group. Such instances

TABLE 21-3. REGULATION OF EXPRESSION OF Rh GENES

Mechanism	Illustration
Maximum expression limited to total available sites/RBCs	-D-/-D- individuals have 155,000 D antigenic sites, CDe/cDE have only 37,000
Gene dosage	c/c alleles = 80,000 c sites/cell c/C alleles = 40,000 c sites/cell
Presence of other alleles: cis (on same chromosome) or trans (on opposite chromosome)	cDE/cde produces less E than cdE/cde (cis); cdE/cDe produces less E than cdE/cde (trans)
"Incomplete" allele	D and D-mosaic variants
"Regulator" gene	Rh_{null} individuals express no Rh antigen–inhibition by separate gene

TABLE 21-4. MATERNAL EXPOSURE TO FOREIGN RBC ANTIGENS

Transplacental hemorrhage at delivery (previous pregnancy)
Antepartum TPH (current or previous pregnancy)
Blood transfusion
Grandmother theory*
Environmental, "naturally" occurring†

* Exposure in utero of the Rh-negative female fetus to Rh-positive maternal blood. Sensitization is "remembered" until the Rh-negative female reaches reproductive age and is reexposed.

† ABO antigens are ubiquitous and thorough sensitization is established early in life. "Natural" Rh antigens have not been proved but may include antigens in vaccines made from human sera.[96]

(including use of "emergency" O-positive blood) may account for 1–2% of modern alloimmunization. This factor is likely more important in alloimmune responses to non-D and non-Rh antigens. The roles of the "grandmother" mechanism and other environmental exposure to foreign RBC antigens remain largely theoretical.

Transplacental Hemorrhage (TPH). The role of TPH is central to alloimmunization in pregnancy. TPH increases near term and when the maternal-fetal interface is compromised (at delivery, with obstetric manipulation, manual removal of the placenta, abruptio placentae, etc.) (Table 21-5). Even in completely uncomplicated pregnancy, TPH may occur as often as 70% of the time.

Detection of TPH

Kleihauer Technique. Adult hemoglobin is eluted from red blood cells by exposure to acid buffer, pH 3.30, leaving maternal cells as "ghosts" and fetal cells intact.[46] Depending on laboratory expertise, light microscopy can provide quantitative assessment of TPH of volumes as low as 0.01 ml (Fig. 21-5). This is the most sensitive method of detecting TPH in current use.

TABLE 21-5. FREQUENCY OF TPH IN PREGNANCY

Event	Fetal Cells Present in Maternal Blood
Parturition	50%
Antepartum	20–30%
First trimester	5–8%
Second trimester	14–18%
Third trimester	25–30%
Spontaneous abortion	3–5%
Therapeutic abortion	6–20%
Ectopic pregnancy	5–8%
Molar pregnancy	Unknown
Amniocentesis	4–11%
Fetal death	Unknown

Antiglobulin Tests. Washed maternal blood is treated with anti-D and then with anti-immunoglobulin (Coombs) sera. Fetal (Rh-positive) cells, if present, bind the anti-D, which, in turn, binds the anti-Ig. In the *Rosette test*, the final step is addition of known Rh-positive cells pretreated with anti-D ("detector" cells) in a potentiating medium. The (anti-Ig)-(anti-D)-(D-positive fetal cell) complexes are bound by detector cells and rosettes are formed.[79] In the *enzyme-linked antiglobulin test* (ELAT), the antiglobulin serum is labeled with alkaline phosphatase, and the addition of an alkaline phosphatase substrate as a "developer" produces a color change that can be measured spectrophotometrically.[61] The *D^u screen* uses only the first two steps. The (anti-Ig)-(anti-D)-(D-positive) chains produce agglutination, observed microscopically.[66] These tests are shown in order of sensitivity.[78] Rosetting is a useful screen for TPH over 5 ml and ELAT for 30 ml or more; both should be followed by the definitive Kleihauer. The D^u screen is probably not sensitive enough for this application and is difficult to assess.

Alpha-Fetoprotein (AFP) Testing. This method has recently been suggested as a very sensitive indicator of TPH. Disruption of the maternal-fetal interface, by amniocentesis for instance, can be detected by rises in the post-tap maternal serum AFP.[13,48] Although AFP elevation may be a sensitive indicator of transplacental "leaks," it measures transplacental passage of fetal serum, not blood, and cannot be used to quantitate TPH.

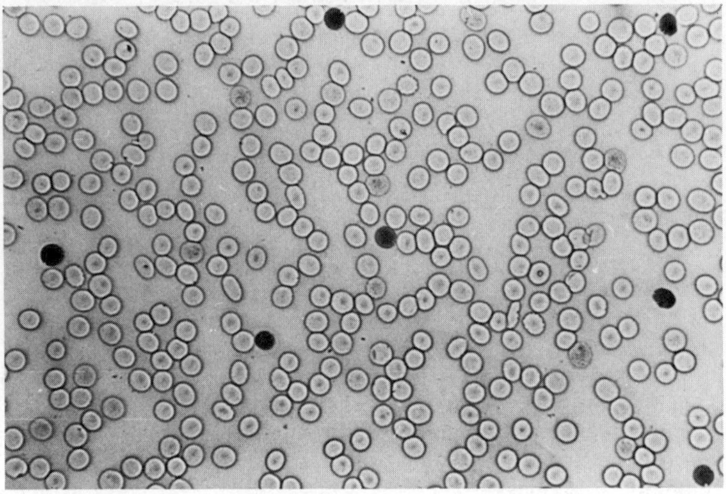

Figure 21-5. Kleihauer technique. Maternal cells are "ghosts," and intact fetal cells are dark. This illustration is from a patient who incurred a fetal–maternal hemorrhage of approximately 180 ml. (Courtesy Dr. J. M. Bowman, Rh Laboratory, Winnipeg, Canada.)

Maternal Immune Response to Fetal Red Blood Cell Antigens—Sensitization

The central elements determining the occurrence and extent of alloimmune disease—maternal immune exposure to fetal red blood cell antigens, recognition of these antigens as foreign, and generation of competent immune responses—comprise the process known as sensitization. Without sensitization, the secondary response which causes disease does not take place; once sensitization has occurred, there is little that will modify the secondary response and its resultant disease, although they may not take place until subsequent pregnancies.

Antibody evidence of sensitization appears slowly (2–6 months after primary exposure), in the form of rising maternal anti-D IgM and IgG. IgM, which does not cross the placenta, may be the principal antibody in the sensitizing response. Subsequent exposure to the antigen, however, causes a prompt (over a few days) "anamnestic" response in the form of IgG_1 and IgG_3 that readily cross the placenta.

Incidence of Sensitization. A primigravid Rh-negative woman delivering an Rh-positive, ABO-compatible fetus has a 16–17% risk of sensitization. Sensitization is detectable in 2% by the time of delivery (antepartum sensitization), in 7% by 6 months postpartum, and in the remainder by appearance of a secondary response with the next Rh-positive fetus. If the woman remains unsensitized, the same risk obtains with the next Rh-positive fetus. By delivery of the fifth Rh-positive, ABO-compatible fetus, 50–60% of women have become sensitized,[5] accounting for 90% of women who will ever become sensitized. Although new sensitization is unusual beyond this parity, Sacks[75] reported 8.4% being sensitized in pregnancies 6 through 8 and primary sensitization of two patients (0.3% of sensitized women) in their 12th pregnancy!

The secondary response, often in pregnancies subsequent to the sensitizing pregnancy, may be heightened by repetitive exposure and is more pronounced with longer re-exposure intervals. The factors affecting the magnitude of maternal secondary response are limited. Many factors, however, influence the occurrence of the primary sensitization response (Table 21-6).

Maternal Immune Exposure to Fetal Red Blood Cell Antigens. Distinction must be drawn between the simple presence of fetal red blood cells in maternal circulation and the generation of maternal immune responses to fetal red blood cell antigens: transplacental hemorrhage does not equal sensitization.

TABLE 21-6. FACTORS INFLUENCING RATE OF SENSITIZATION

Early transplacental hemorrhage
Large-volume TPH
Threshold effect
ABO incompatibility
Fetal antigen strength
Maternal nonresponder

TABLE 21-7. VOLUME OF Rh-POSITIVE BLOOD IN MATERNAL CIRCULATION

TPH volume	Percentage of All TPH[7,74]	Risk of Sensitization[5,98]
0–0.1 ml	75–80%	3%
>0.5 ml	10–15%	22%
>5.0 ml	1%	65%
>30 ml	0.1%	65%

Timing of TPH. About 90% of TPH occurs at delivery, substantiating the classic observations that first Rh-incompatible pregnancies are usually unaffected.[62] Early antepartum exposure, on the other hand, allows completion of the sensitization process, secondary response to repeated exposure, and the development of fetal/neonatal disease, even in first pregnancies.

Volume of TPH. Most fetal–maternal bleeds are of small volume and many very small TPHs may escape detection. Although risk of individual sensitization *does* rise with TPH volume, small-volume TPHs account for the large proportion of women who become sensitized (Table 21-7). The minimum volume of Rh-positive cells that can cause sensitization is unknown. In Rh-negative volunteers, repeated injections of only 0.1 ml caused sensitization 30% of the time.[98]

"Threshold" Effect. Pregnancy itself may have a protective effect against sensitization. At low levels of circulating Rh-positive cells, Rh-negative males and nonpregnant women sensitize more readily than do pregnant women with similar levels as a result of TPH.[45] Whether this is a biologically important effect is not known, and the mechanism is not defined.

ABO Incompatibility. The risk of sensitization falls from 16–1.5% when the Rh-incompatible mother and fetus are also ABO incompatible.[62] A similar decrease occurs in antepartum sensitization—2% versus 0.2%.

A brief digression into ABO-immune mechanisms will help to explain this protective effect. Preformed hemagglutinins are maintained in measurable concentrations to foreign ABO antigens (anti-B in type A individuals, anti-A and anti-B in type O individuals, etc.), likely on the basis of continued stimulation by naturally occurring A and B antigens in plants and food.[99] This "constant state of readiness" means rapid clearance of ABO-incompatible cells, by both IgM-activated complement-dependent *intravascular* hemolysis (with clearance of fragments by phagocytosis in the liver) and IgM-mediated hemagglutination (with microvascular trapping in many organs). Neither of these defense mechanisms allows much opportunity for antigen processing in the spleen or regional lymph nodes. As Rh antigens appear only on erythrocytes, this instant defense is not prepared, fetal cells are not rapidly cleared, and intact fetal cells are sequestered in the spleen and undergo *extravascular* hemolysis, allowing ample opportunity for antigen processing. Differential clearing of fetal cells is demonstrated by the data of Woodrow[95] (Table 21-8).

This protective effect is incomplete: large-volume TPH exceeds rapid clearance and Rh sensitization occurs.

Recognition of Fetal Antigens as Foreign. Two factors impact here: the likelihood of incompatibility and the nature of the incompatibility. The former is dependent on paternal Rh genotype and ABO type of both parents, whereas the latter is largely determined by antigen strength.

Predicting Sensitization in Rh-Negative Women. If the father is Rh negative, so too will all children be, and the risk of sensitization is zero. If the father is Rh positive, detailed blood typing of both parents will provide significant data for prediction. For instance, if the father is type O and expresses the phenotype CcDe (the most common Rh phenotype) and the mother is type O, the fetus will be ABO compatible but will have only a 50% chance of being Rh positive (94% of CcDe are Dd heterozygous), so the risk of sensitization is 8–9%. With detailed typing, prediction of paternal genotype becomes rea-

TABLE 21-8. WOMEN WITH FETAL RED CELLS IN THEIR CIRCULATION AFTER DELIVERY

	No cells	≦0.2 ml	0.2–1 ml	1–10 ml	>10 ml
ABO compatible	58%	31%	8%	2%	0.5%
ABO incompatible	83%	14%	2%	1.5%	0.2%

sonably accurate (Table 21-1). Other than such "educated guesses," however, there is no way at present of distinguishing DD from Dd among Rh-positive fathers (unless, of course, he has an Rh-negative parent or child, in which case he must be Dd). Although knowledge of exact phenotype may be helpful in some situations, and determination should always be performed for both parents, unless both are Rh negative the risk of sensitization is never zero and detailed management of the "Rh-negative gravida" must be performed diligently.

Antigen Strength. At its extreme, the D antigen is only moderately potent but still much stronger than the other Rh alleles.[74] This difference in immunogenic strength may explain the following differences between sensitization in Rh disease and c disease. When the mother is Rh negative (dd), approximately 83% of fathers will be Rh positive, of whom 54% will be Dd heterozygous and 46% will be DD homozygous, and the overall rate of sensitization is approximately 16%. This is contrasted with the much weaker c antigen, for when the mother is c negative (CC), 80% of fathers will be c positive, and of these 60% will be Cc heterozygotes, whereas the remaining 40% will be homozygotes, and sensitization occurs less than 1% of the time. Thus, despite similar likelihood of incompatibility, the antigen strength is directly associated with a lower frequency of sensitization. Anti-c disease, when it does occur, is just as serious as anti-D; hydrops is not uncommon.

Competent Maternal Immune Response. Many Rh-negative women will not develop anti-D antibody, regardless of the volume, number, or frequency of exposures. These "nonresponders" account for a full one-third of Rh-negative women but cannot be identified except by the absence of sensitization after several Rh-positive, ABO-compatible pregnancies. This character is probably genetically determined (HLA-A3 is more common among sensitized women; nonresponders may be A3 negative[21]); the site of action is not yet known.

Transmission of Immune Response to the Fetus

Once sensitization occurs, repeated exposure results in an immediate large-scale provocation of IgG, the agent of alloimmune disease. Anti-D IgG is actively transported across the placenta in endocytic vacuoles, released intact into the fetal circulation by exocytosis, and immediately begins the process of IgG-mediated extravascular hemolysis which leads to fetal disease. Activation is dependent only on antigen exposure—the volume of TPH, ABO-incompatibility, antigen strength, and so on have no ameliorating effect.

FETAL RESPONSES TO ALLOIMMUNIZATION

Variability in Rh disease does not end with maternal response. The extent of fetal disease depends on antibody level and its antigen affinity, but, in the face of similar antigenic attack, fetuses manifest all ranges of disease from hydropic stillbirth to moderate neonatal anemia. The factors determining individual fetal capacity for homeostatic compensation are poorly understood.

The strength of IgG binding on fetal RBCs varies with antigen density on RBCs, antibody concentration, and binding constant. Anti-D IgG is not complement activating but does cause immune identification (Fc receptor binding) by circulating macrophages and polymorphs. Using their multiple Fc receptors, these cells become surrounded by "rosettes" of antibody-coated fetal RBCs, develop pseudopods and digest portions of the RBC membranes. The red blood cells thus deformed are sequestered in the splenic reticuloendothelial system and cleared from the circulation by phagocytosis and extravascular hemolysis. The contribution to red blood cell destruction due to a second mechanism—antibody-dependent cellular toxicity (ADCC)—has not yet been determined.[85] (In the laboratory, lymphoid K cells and monocytes bind to the anti-D coated red blood cells, again via Fc receptors, and initiate lysis.) IgG has a serum half-life of 21 days in the neonate: the process of hemolysis is not interrupted by delivery.

Extravascular hemolysis has two consequences—generation of degradation products (stromal elements and hemoglobin) and anemia. Degradation products are cleared placentally and are not a factor in disease until after birth, when they participate in coagulation abnormalities and jaundice/kernicterus, respectively. The severity of anemia determines the compensatory efforts of the fetus and, in turn, the extent of intrauterine disease (Fig. 21-6). As anemia worsens, large numbers of immature red blood cells (normoblasts and erythroblasts) are

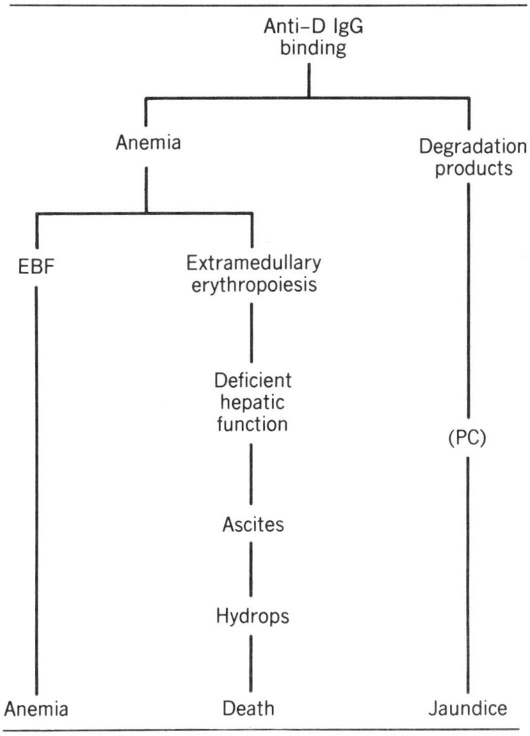

Figure 21-6. Pathophysiology of HDFN: EBF—erythroblastosis fetalis; PC—placental clearance.

released into the circulation (thus "erythroblastosis fetalis"). The second response is a return to extramedullary erythropoiesis, normally discontinued at 6 months' gestation. This affects primarily the liver, then the spleen, and other sites to a lesser extent. As anemia becomes progressively more severe, the islands of erythropoietic cells in the liver become larger and larger, distorting hepatic architecture and disrupting blood flow, with ensuing portal venous hypertension with ascites and umbilical venous hypertension with placental edema. The end point of this progression is hydrops fetalis: massive hepatomegaly, deficient liver function with hypoalbuminemia, anasarca with pleural and pericardial effusions, impaired placental circulation and intrauterine death (Fig. 21-7).

Range of Disease

IgG-mediated hemolysis continues after birth and, if untreated, leads to increasing disease (Table 21-9). Added to the excess bilirubin, hepatic impairment in severe disease further predisposes to kernicterus by delayed production of transport protein Y and hypoalbuminemia. Deposition of unconjugated bilirubin, lipid soluble, in the CNS results in neuronal death, yellow staining of dead areas (kernicterus), 80–90% mortality, and severely damaged survivors. With the advanced neonatal care now available, all infants with mild or moderate disease and 30–50% of those with severe disease should survive intact.

MANAGEMENT OF THE SENSITIZED GRAVIDA

The Manitoba Rh program has been active in alloimmune management since the first Canadian trials of Rh prophylaxis in the 1960s,[15] and it continues to be a model for centralized management of all Rh-negative women of reproductive age. Although the principles discussed are applicable to any obstetric practice, the availability of a broad range of clinical and laboratory experience is implicit, based on centralized referral and uniform application of standards. As will be noted, one of the current problems in management of Rh-negative women is failure to apply current knowledge in universal fashion. It is only through a highly motivated and diligent application of management principles by such programs that Rh disease can truly be eliminated.

Detection of Alloimmunization

All women should be screened in *all* pregnancies (Table 21-10). It is important not to omit the Rh-positive woman from this screening because 1.5–2% of all pregnant women show atypical blood group sensitization.[89]

Antibody Characterization. Antigenic specificity and concentration of the antibody are determined. The latter is done by (1) serial dilutions in albumin suspension that give the titer of IgG—for example, 1:4 and 1:16—and (2) quantitation by autoanalyzer technique that gives the specific antibody concentration in μ/ml.[59] Antibody titers are not perfect predictors of the severity of disease—they indicate the *range* of disease that is likely. Elevated ($\geqq$1:16) or rising (increase of 2 or more dilutions) titers detect only 60% of fetuses with severe disease.[9] Clinical use of autoanalyzer antibody levels suggests somewhat better correlation between antibody concentrations and likelihood of disease. When levels were always less than 0.8 μ/ml, no

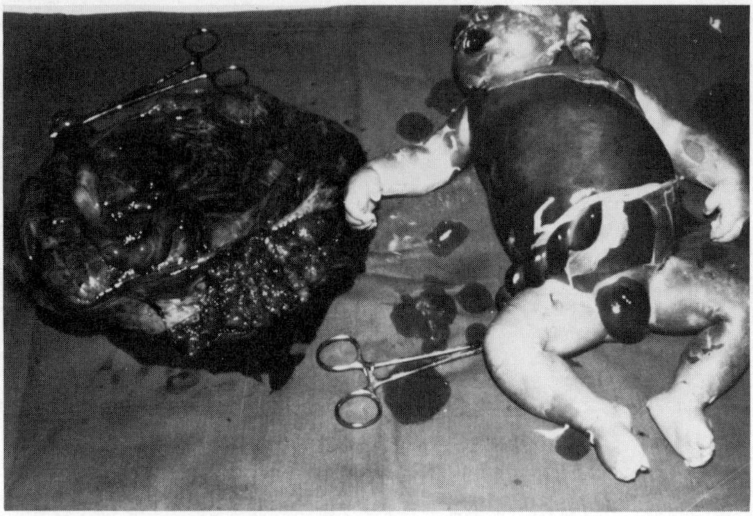

Figure 21-7. Severely hydropic stillborn infant. Massive hepatomegaly is evidenced by abdominal distension, marked peripheral edema (anasarca) and a hydropic placenta are also shown. (Reprinted from Bowman, J. M.: Rh-isoimmunization 1977. *Mod. Med. Can.* **32:**17, 1977 with permission of the publisher.)

newborns had hemoglobin less than 100 g/liter and the incidence of exchange transfusion was only 4%. Above 0.8 μ/ml, 22% had low hemoglobins and 78% required exchange at birth.[4] There is poor correlation among higher levels with severity of disease. The ADCC assay measures the strength of the maternal antibody in its ability to cause red blood cell lysis. It may become useful in selecting the antibody changes most likely to be associated with fetal disease.[85] For the present, however, *any* positive change in antibody status calls for more definitive *fetal* assessment.

"Suppression" of Sensitization

Promethazine Hydrochloride. This drug appears to interfere with several steps in the fetal immune response to IgG-coated red blood cells: Fc binding by macrophages, phagocytosis, and red blood cell membrane instability are all decreased in vitro.[37] In patients with previous serious Rh disease, administration of high doses (5 mg/kg maternal weight) was associated with improved outcome. Initial concerns about side effects of promethazine in reducing fetal T-cell populations[9] appear to be test-related rather than actual.[14] Properly formulated trials of this drug have not been conducted, and the improved outcome may well be related to better medical care, including very early delivery, rather than drug effect. Furthermore, better neonatal course may be due to drug-stimulated hepatic function rather than to amelioration of hemolysis.[86]

Oral Desensitization. Oral ingestion of material containing specific antigens produces antigen tolerance in animals, probably by

TABLE 21-9. NATURAL HISTORY OF HDFN

Percentage Affected		Extent of Disease
50–55%	"Mild"	Mild anemia, no treatment ± blue light
25–30%	"Moderate"	Alive, nonhydropic, severe jaundice, potential for kernicterus, severe anemia
20–25%	"Severe"	Stillbirth or neonatal death before term; 50% die at <34 weeks

TABLE 21-10. ANTIBODY SCREENING IN PREGNANCY[8]

Blood Groups	Maternal Samples at	Examined for
Rh positive	Booking, 32 weeks	Atypical antibodies*
Rh negative	Booking	All antibodies,† paternal blood typing
A. Not sensitized Rh-negative father	Repeat at 32 weeks and delivery; cord blood	All antibodies; cord antibodies typing
B. Not sensitized Rh-positive father	Repeat monthly to delivery,‡ 6 weeks, 6 months postpartum. Cord blood	Rh antibodies + atypical screen at 32 weeks and delivery; cord anti-bodies, typing
C. Sensitized (Incl. Rh+ atypical) stable or falling titers ≦8 albumin	Repeat monthly to 26 weeks. Every 2 weeks to delivery. Delivery, 6 weeks, 6 months postpartum. Cord blood	Specific antibody titers, screen all others; cord antibodies, typing.
D. Sensitized, changing titers or >16 albumin§	Central referral for management. Amniocentesis ± IUT, early delivery, exchange transfusions, photo-therapy, etc.	

* Multiple-cell screening, Lewis, Kell, Duffy, etc. may vary with population.
† Atypical screen plus routine Rh screen using Group O, CDe/cDE, Kell + cells.
‡ Includes quantitative Kleihauer for TPH.
§ Includes all patients with positive history, regardless of titer.

generation of antigen-specific T-suppressor cells.[59] Ingestion of capsules of Rh-positive red blood cell membranes (erythrocyte membrane oral therapy, EMOT) by Rh-negative women with poor previous outcomes was suggested as a means of suppressing maternal response.[3,5] Properly controlled trials have not been done. EMOT had no beneficial effect among a group of women selected for therapy on the basis of severe disease with previous hydropic stillbirths prior to 26 weeks' gestation.[34]

Intensive Plasma Exchange. In this automated procedure, large volumes of maternal plasma (anti-D IgG rich) are removed and replaced with a combination of plasma protein fraction, fresh frozen plasma, and albumin (antibody poor). Performed on a frequent basis, with removal of 2–5 liters or even as much as 20 liters per week, this procedure significantly lowers maternal antibody levels in about 50% of patients and may reduce overall mortality as well as the need for intrauterine transfusion.[7] Procedural complications occur approximately 17% of the time and include severe anaphylaxis to replacement products. In at least 50% of cases, plasma exchange produces only a temporary drop in antibody level, followed by a "rebound" which may raise anti-D IgG as much as 3.5 times the preexchange levels. No randomized trials evaluating this method have been performed. The institutions where this method is popular are those with the poorest experience with intrauterine transfusion.

These attempts at modifying established alloimmune disease point to dissatisfaction with present methods for antepartum management. Results with promethazine and/or EMOT are far from convincing. These agents do not form part of our approach to severe disease. Plasma exchange is not used as a primary means of suppression/treatment; the results are no better than IUT for moderately severe disease.[32,41] Plasma exchange *may* be useful, however, in postponing IUT from say 18 weeks to 22 weeks when IUT is technically much easier. This procedure is very expensive, time consuming, and has been associated with serious aggravation of fetal disease.[43]

Fc Receptor Blockade. The Fc receptors on immune cells can be saturated by incubation in vitro or intravenous infusion in vivo with hyperimmune serum. Lymphoid K cells ("killer" cells) and macrophages so treated will fail to bind with antigen–antibody complexes or structures (such as platelets or red blood cells) to which they would normally react strongly. Application of this principle in pregnancy has apparently prevented fetal/neonatal thrombocytopenia in women with immune-mediated thrombocytopenic purpura.[90] The nonspecific IgG (i.e., specific in small amounts to a multitude of antigens but no blood group antigens), administered intravenously to the mother, readily crosses the placenta and (theoretically) saturates the fetal immunocytes that would be active in anti-D IgG-mediated fetal hemolysis. The results of clinical trials in severely affected pregnancies are eagerly awaited.

EVALUATION OF THE ALLOIMMUNIZED FETUS

When maternal evidence indicates the possibility of disease, attention must be directed to the fetus. Amniotic fluid bilirubin measurement to predict the severity of disease was suggested by Bevis in 1956[2] and popularized by Liley in the 1960s.[55]

Bilirubin. The metabolic end product of the hemoglobin released by alloimmune hemolysis, bilirubin is cleared by the mother throughout pregnancy. Some is also excreted into the amniotic fluid, normally decreasing as term is approached. The primary route of excretion is probably via tracheopulmonary fluid, although a small amount may be excreted in the fetal urine. Bilirubin produces a characteristic absorption pattern on amniotic fluid spectrophotometry (Fig. 21-8). Plotted on semilog paper with a tangent drawn from 550 to 365 nm, the change in optical density (ΔOD) due to absorbance at the bilirubin peak (450 nm) measured vertically gives a value representative of the concentration of bilirubin (ΔOD 450; Fig. 21-9).

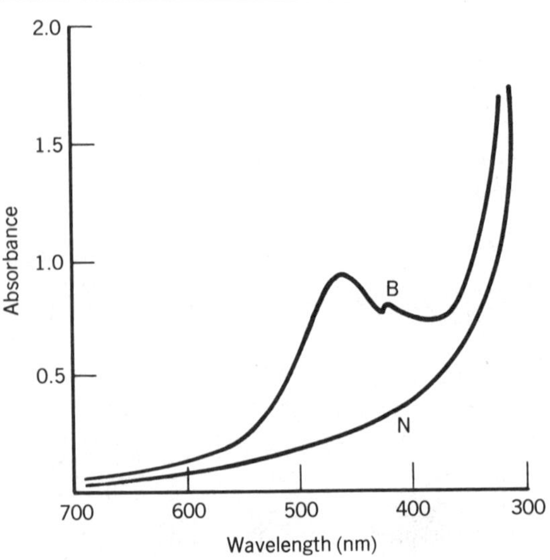

Figure 21-8. Absorption curves for normal amniotic fluid (N) and fluid stained with bilirubin (B).

Amniocentesis for ΔOD 450

This is the single most important means of evaluating severity of disease. Antibody levels and affinity are only rough predictors; maternal estriols have no value. The indications for this procedure are (1) previous loss or neonatal exchange transfusion due to alloimmune disease; (2) significant antibody titer (this must be standardized for each laboratory—at our institution, an albumin titer greater than 1:16 or autoanalyzer level greater than 1.0 μg/liter are critical levels); and (3) in unusual circumstances (e.g., recent large TPH, sudden hydramnios) where ultrasound findings suggest advancing disease before titers rise. About 50% of sensitized Rh-negative women meet one of these criteria.

The Procedure. Real-time ultrasound is now central to the safe and efficient performance of

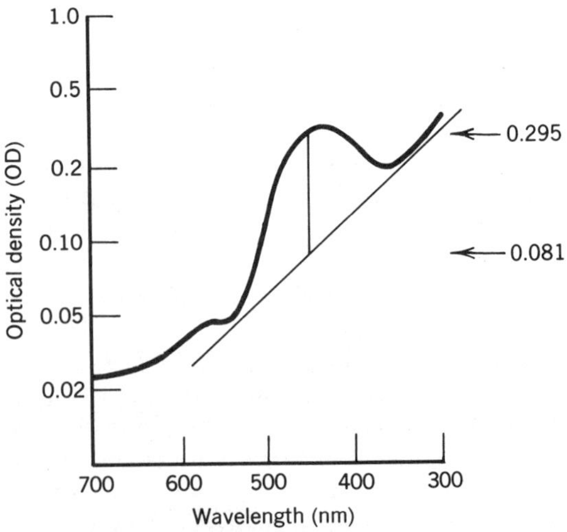

Figure 21-9. Semilog plot of optical density of amniotic fluid containing bilirubin at 29 weeks' gestation. A tangent (diagonal line) connects the OD at 550 and 365nm. At 450 nm (vertical line), the vertical distance from the tangent to the peak absorbance is the ΔOD 450, in this case the distance from 0.081 to 0.295, ΔOD 450 = 0.214.

amniocentesis. The aim of the procedure is to obtain an uncontaminated (by maternal blood) aliquot of amniotic fluid on the first attempt without provoking TPH and further aggravation of maternal response. To do this, particular care is taken to define a placenta-free site where fluid is accessible. If a completely anterior placenta offers no access to amniotic fluid at all, a transplacental tap is performed through a thin area of placenta far removed from the cord insertion.

Omitting amniocentesis in such cases may be an explanation for the partial success of plasma exchange: traumatic taps can seriously provoke maternal antibody production.[71] It is imperative, however, to define accurately the extent of disease in order to establish prognosis and a management plan. This *cannot* be done without ΔOD 450 measurement. In cases requiring a transplacental approach, subsequent amniocenteses may be spaced further apart if the titer is stable and there are no ultrasound signs of increasing disease.

As light causes prompt degradation of bilirubin, the samples should be wrapped immediately. The procedure is followed by a maternal Kleihauer determination (significant TPH at amniocentesis may require increased surveillance) and detailed ultrasound observation at the tap site.

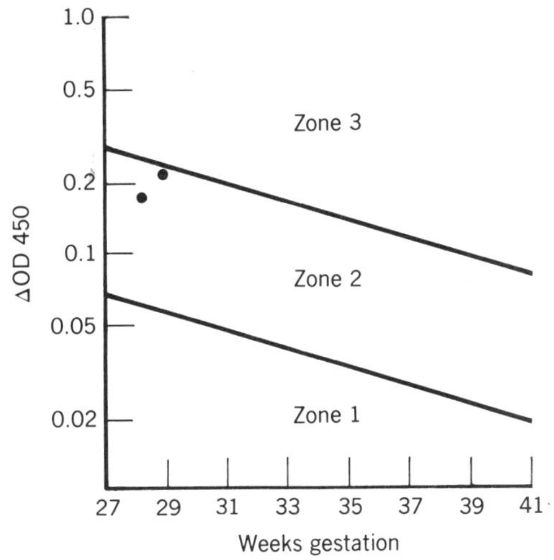

Figure 21-10. Liley zones correlating ΔOD with extent of disease and likely outcome. The ΔOD 450 from the fluid in Fig. 21-8, 0.214, when plotted at 29 weeks (upper dot) shows a rise from the value one week earlier, 0.178 (lower dot), and falls on the Zone 2–3 boundary, indicating severe disease, with 50–70% chance of stillbirth if untreated. IUT was performed the same day.

Interpretation of ΔOD 450. When performed and evaluated by experienced personnel, ΔOD 450 level is a very reliable indicator of fetal disease. On the basis of 101 Rh amniocenteses, Liley was able to establish "zones" of ΔOD 450 readings that correlated with severity of disease (Fig. 21-10).[53] Establishment of firm gestational age is critical to correct plotting of these values. The likelihood of significant disease increases within zones as well. For instance, ΔOD 450 in the top 80–90% of Zone 2 is associated with at least twice as many stillbirths as a Zone 2 reading near the Zone 1 boundary. In Liley's series, high Zone 3 readings usually meant hydropic stillbirth. The trend in serial ΔOD 450 readings is equally significant, since even a static ΔOD 450 may mean seriously increasing disease as gestation advances, whereas some Rh-negative (and therefore unaffected) fetuses may have high initial readings which fall progressively as pregnancy progresses. Rayburn et al. have documented normal ΔOD 450 levels for early pregnancy (16–24 weeks).[70]

Timing of Amniocentesis. Amniocentesis should begin as soon as a therapeutic response to serious disease is available. In centers with experienced intrauterine transfusion (IUT) teams, this is at 20–21 weeks. In some centers, direct fetal exchange transfusion by fetoscope-directed umbilical vessel catheterization[72] may make treatment possible (and therefore indicate amniocentesis) even earlier. The interval for serial repeat amniocenteses varies with severity of disease and the observed trend, from 4 days to 4 weeks; several ΔOD 450 measurements may be needed to establish a clear prognosis.

Sources of Error. Incorrect labeling, light exposure, and maternal or fetal urine or fetal ascites instead of amniotic fluid may all lead to inappropriate assessment. Ultrasound visualization markedly reduces the likelihood of the wrong fluid being obtained. Fetal urine is clear and has very low ΔOD 450, whereas ascitic fluid is bright amber and usually has a high protein content and low absorption above 575 nm, compared to amniotic fluid. Other pigments in amniotic fluid may prevent accurate spectrophotometry (Table 21-11). Finally, in a very small number of cases, a satisfactory specimen may yield a reading which does not correctly predict the severity of fetal disease.

TABLE 21-11. INTERFERENCE WITH ΔOD 450

Substance	Source	Absorbs (nm)	Result
Fetal serum	Traumatic amnio*	450	Falsely high
Oxyhemoglobin	Blood in a.f.	580, 540, 415	Obscures 450
Methemalbumin	Hemolysis in a.f.	405	Reduces 450
Meconium	Fetus	All, 420 peak	Obscures 450
76% Renografin	Amniography	All	Obscures 450
Bilirubin	GI obstruction†	450	Falsely high

* Also open neural tube defects, fetal nephrosis
† As in duodenal atresia, T-E fistula. N.B. Down's syndrome.

Ultrasound Assessment

Indications are identical to those for amniocentesis. Indeed, detailed real-time ultrasound evaluation should *always* accompany amniocentesis. This evaluation includes fetal morphology and measurement, fetal behavior, placental and cord morphology and measurement, and amniotic fluid volume assessment.

Fetus. Anomalies associated with elevated ΔOD 450 are excluded by detailed assessment of skull and spine, urinary, and GI tract structures. In the nonhydropic fetus, abdominal size, in particular liver size, gives valuable information on the extent of disease. Gross ascites is easily recognized (Fig. 21-11a), noting that a small rim less than 0.5 cm of peritoneal fluid may be a normal finding. In serial observations of the fetal abdomen during IUT, the first 15–30 ml of blood infused produces only an increase in contrast of the abdominal contents; 35–60 ml may be required before characteristic "ascites" appears.[40] Abdominal wall thickness (Fig. 21-11b) and scalp thickness (Fig. 21-11c) are indices of fetal edema. In its most severe form, hydrops may be associated with pericardial and pleural effusions (Fig. 21-12). Despite intrauterine treatment, this stage of disease is usually lethal. Detection of subclinical pericardial effusion in so-called "prehydrops" by specialized ultrasound techniques[24] has not proved significant in our experience.

Fetal behavior, as summarized by the Biophysical Profile Score (BPS), accurately determines fetal well-being.[58] A BPS of 4 or less indicates an increased risk of fetal loss. Appearance of a sinusoidal fetal heart rate pattern (Fig. 21-13) is an unreliable indicator of fetal disease; it should be followed immediately by ultrasound fetal assessment (BPS), in most cases repetition of maternal antibody titer, and, in many cases, amniocentesis for ΔOD 450. In some fetuses this pattern is an indicator of response to serious anemia,[87] but in many others it is a transient pattern not associated with poor outcome and is not an indication *by itself* for premature delivery.

Placenta and Umbilical Cord. As disease worsens, the placenta manifests increasing edema and may exceed 1.5 kg in weight. Increasing thickness and a diffuse "ground-glass" pattern become apparent (Fig. 21-14). Structural definition is lost, with disappearance of the chorionic plate and buckling of the fetal surface. Cord vein diameter may increase in severe disease.

Amniotic fluid volume is usually increased, often indicating overt hydramnios. Oligohydramnios indicates serious fetal compromise. As well as detailed evaluation of fetal disease, ultrasound provides fetal skeletal measurements important in confirming gestational age, demonstrating growth, and defining fetal and placental position for amniocentesis or IUT.

Overall Assessment

The combination of maternal antibody titers, ΔOD 450 measurement, and ultrasound evaluation provides an accurate description of fetal disease state in over 90% of cases. Maternal antibody levels usually err in overpredicting severe disease, but, on occasion, very rapid rises may not be detected soon enough to indicate accelerating fetal disease. ΔOD 450 measurement is subject to a number of confounding factors, and it may overpredict disease but seldom underestimates severity if performed serially. Ultrasound can unequivocally decide between hydrops/not hydrops but is limited in ability to quantify the extent of disease when hydrops is absent. *All* these modalities must be applied for accurate diagnosis and prognosis.

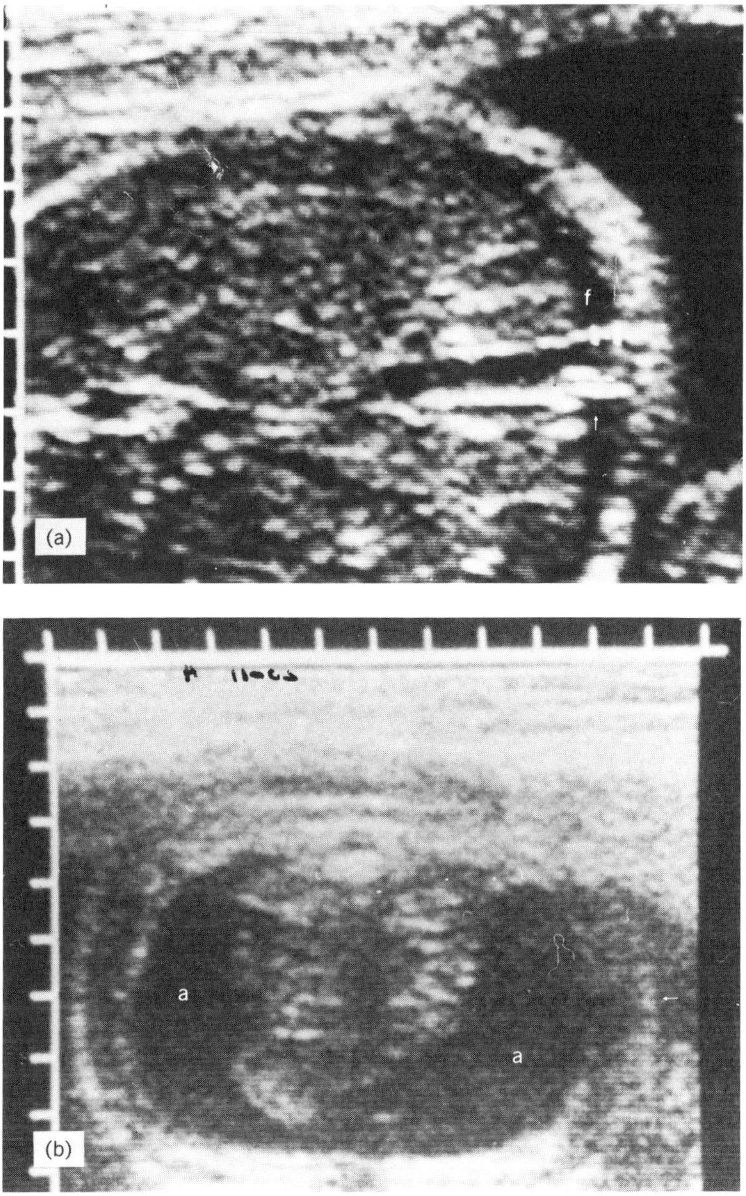

Figure 21-11. Ultrasound findings in hydrops fetalis. (a) Early ascites. Note fluid rim (f) and increased contrast of intra-abdominal contents, with umbilical vein outlined (arrow). (b) Fetal anasarca with markedly thickened abdominal wall (arrow) and gross ascites (a).

Continued on next page

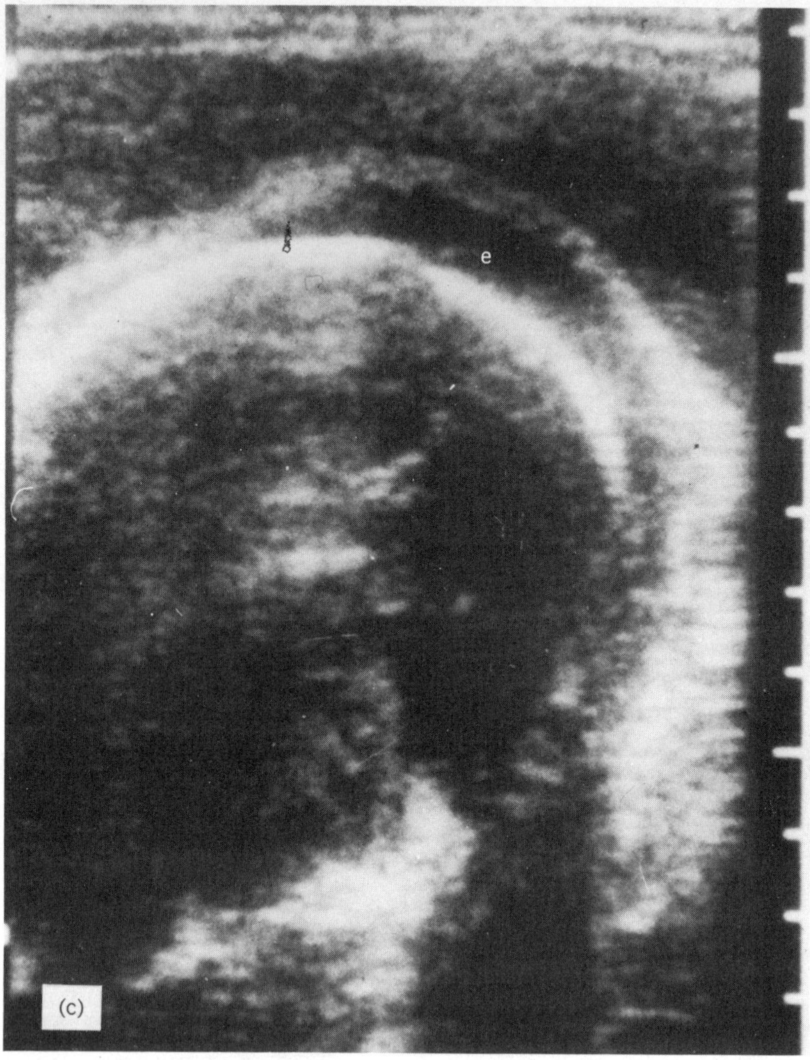

Figure 21-11 Continued. (c) Large "cuirasse" of scalp edema(e). Fetuses (a) and (c) survived with multiple IUT; (b) died in utero before transfusion.

Management of the Severely Affected Fetus

The combination of ΔOD 450 values and gestational age establishes the likelihood of severe disease, whereas ultrasound assessment determines the extent (hydrops or not) of this disease. Since intrauterine transfusion carries a definite risk of traumatic fetal death, it is undertaken only if fetal immaturity precludes early delivery (Table 21-12).

Early Delivery. After 34 weeks, early delivery and neonatal exchange transfusion are the rule. If a completely anterior placenta prevents ΔOD 450 determination, labor is induced rather than risk traumatic injury. Between 32 and 34 weeks, L:S ratio and phosphatidylglycerol are determined, with delivery if mature. The use of maternally administered dexamethasone or betamethasone may favorably influence fetal lung compliance at these gestational ages. In the nonhydropic fetus, full induction protocols are used. The hydropic fetus, however, is at considerable risk for intrapartum distress, and confirmation of fetal well-being with fetal pH is often prevented by massive scalp edema. Cesarean section is liberally employed in this group. De-

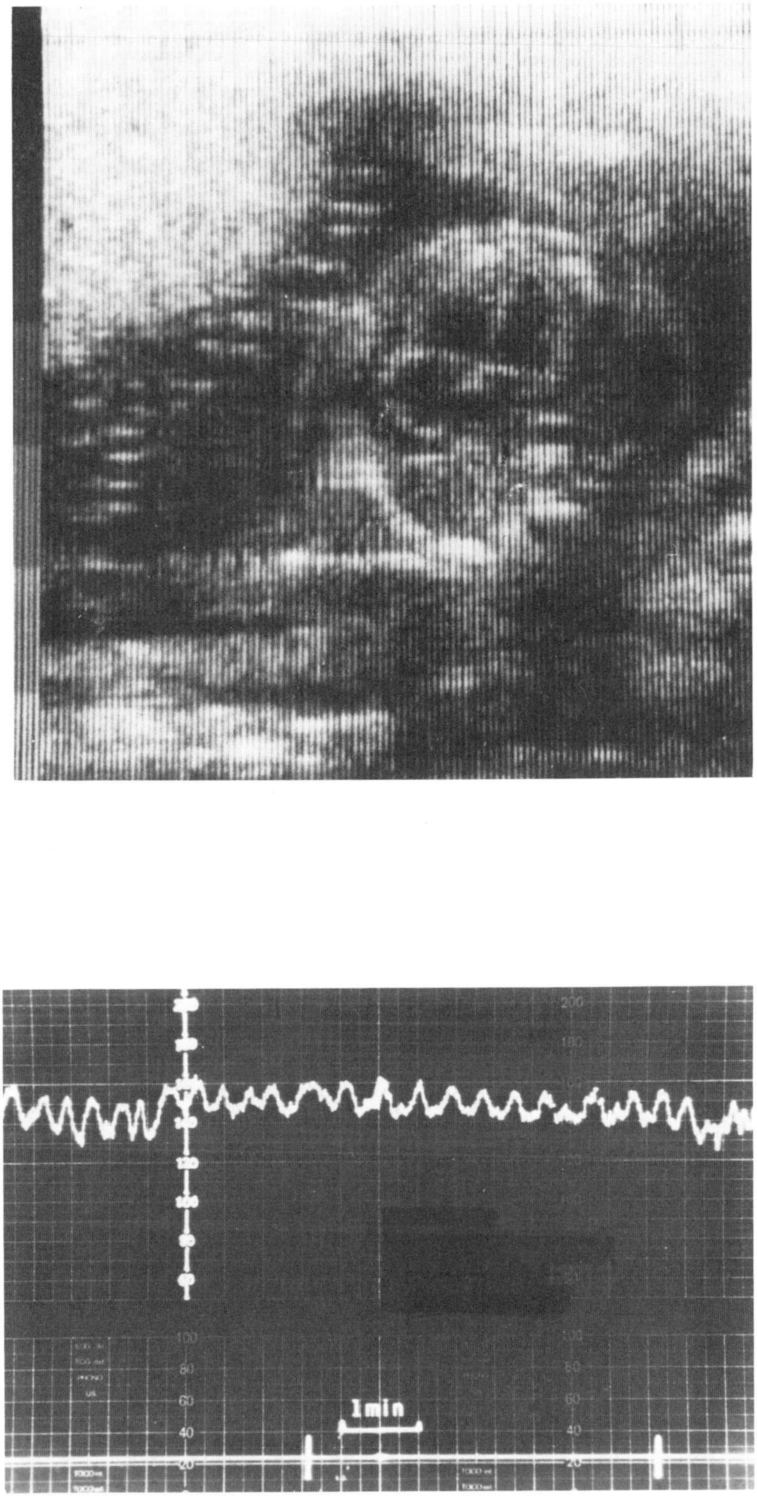

Figure 21-13. Sinusoidal heart rate pattern at 34 weeks' gestation, moderately severe (nonhydropic) disease. Pattern resolved spontaneously after 70 minutes. Serial ultrasound assessments showed no deterioration in fetal status; delivery at 35 5/7 weeks: cord hemoglobin 10.2, required two exchange transfusions and one simple transfusion.

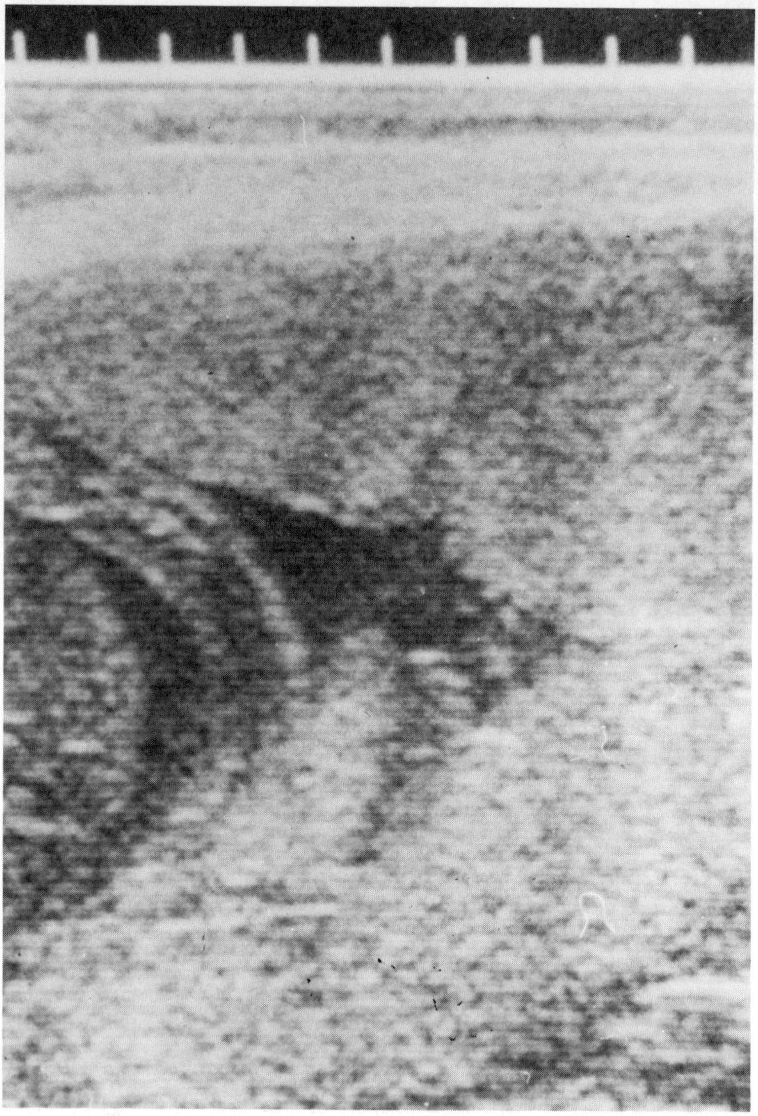

Figure 21-14. "Ground-glass" placenta, severe hydrops at 30 weeks. The chorionic plate is obscured and the placenta is "buckled" by edema.

livery of the fetus with severe disease should only be done where expert neonatal care, including immediate exchange transfusion in the resuscitation room, is available. Transfer of the mother with the baby in utero is preferred. Transfer of the severely affected neonate is dangerous and should not be planned.

Intrauterine Transfusion (IUT). In 10–12% of severely affected fetuses, intrauterine death will occur before pulmonary maturity is reached. In 1963, Liley published his classic description of intrauterine treatment of these fetuses,[54] utilizing intraperitoneal fetal transfusion to improve survival.

Criteria. Criteria for IUT are ΔOD 450 80–90% Zone 2 or in Zone 3, a very rapidly rising ΔOD 450 that has not quite reached these levels, or ultrasound evidence of hydrops at less than 32 weeks. IUT is rarely, if ever, undertaken beyond 32 weeks, delivery being the treatment of choice at that time, even if the L:S ratio is not fully mature. An anterior placenta is a relative contraindication: if the fetus is not hydropic and is nearing pulmonary maturity, IUT may be de-

TABLE 21-12. MANAGEMENT OF SEVERE FETAL DISEASE

ΔOD 450 ≧80% Zone 2, rapidly rising Zone 2, or ultrasound = Hydrops		
>34 weeks	**32–34 weeks**	**<32 weeks**
Delivery and neonatal treatment	L:S ratio, deliver if mature, or single IUT	Serial IUT delivery at 32–34 weeks

ferred if the ΔOD 450 is not rising rapidly. Transplacental amniocentesis is much less traumatic than transplacental IUT.

IUT Procedure. Centralized referral to a small, multidisciplinary "Intrauterine Transfusion Team" ensures continued technical competence. Ultrasound guidance is essential for correct positioning of the 16 gauge Tuohy needle in the fetal peritoneal cavity. Through this, a modified epidural catheter is threaded and the needle removed. Confirmation of free intraperitoneal placement by x-ray is essential, even in hydrops (Fig. 21-15), as placement within intra-abdominal fetal structures such as bladder, lesser sac, and retroperitoneal space

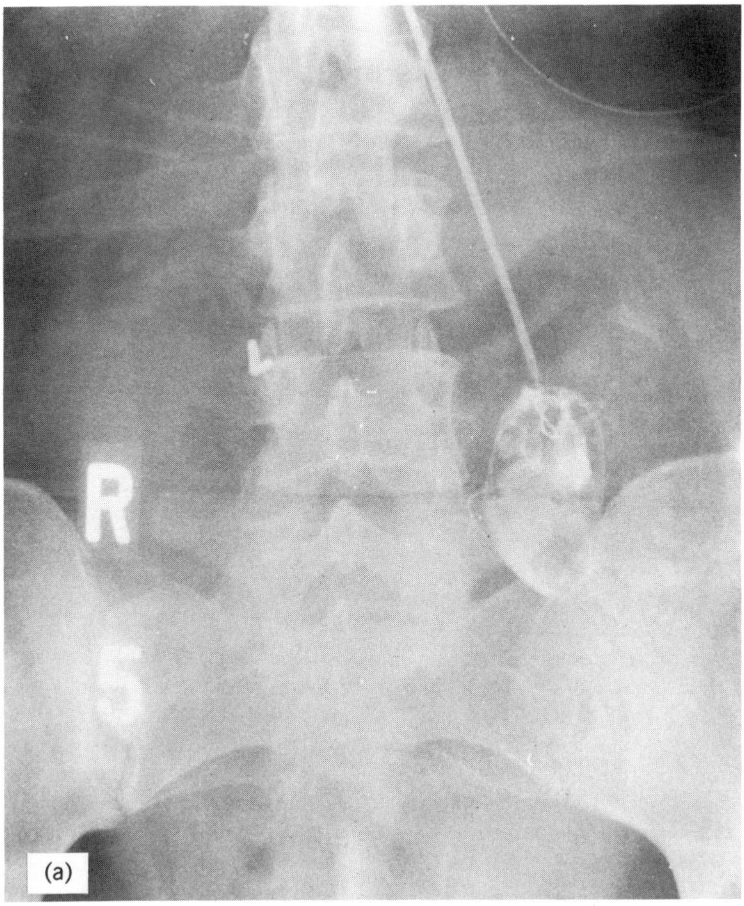

Figure 21-15. Dye-injection radiographs to confirm free intraperitoneal catheter placement. Part (a) demonstrates typical "semilunes," crescent-shaped negative shadows of small bowel loops.

Continued on next page

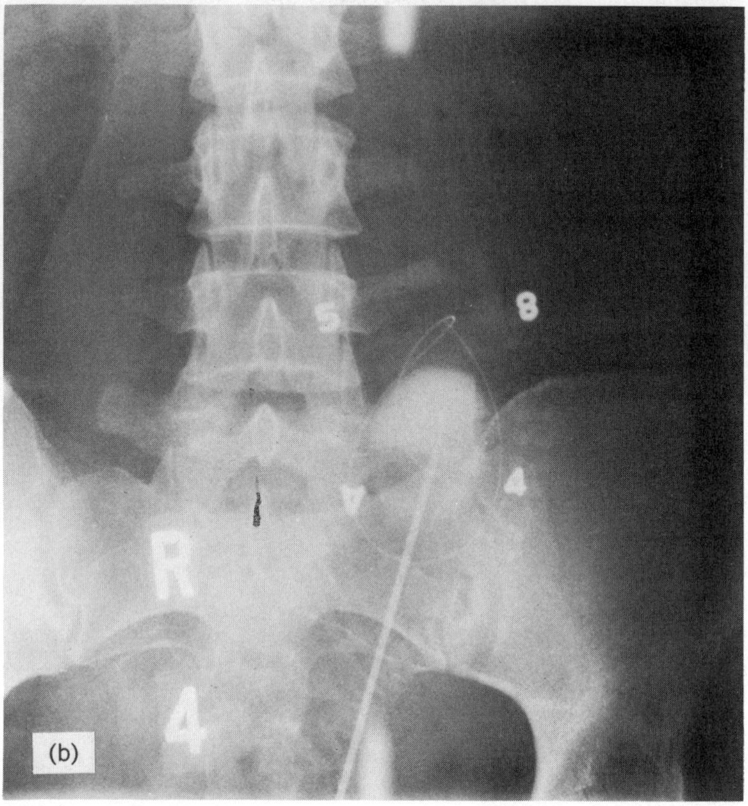

Figure 21-15 Continued. Part (b) shows the ''haze'' seen when dye is diffused by presence of ascites in hydrops at IUT.

markedly reduces absorption of the transfusion mass.

Fresh Type O, Kell-negative, D-negative red blood cells are carefully matched to the mother's serum. These RBCs, which bear no antigens foreign to the *mother*, are tightly packed (hematocrit above 85%), because plasma delays red blood cell absorption. The volume given is determined by gestational age, and the cells are administered slowly (35–50 minutes) with continuous fetal heart rate monitoring. FHR acceleration or tachycardia are normal responses, but sustained bradycardia may indicate overdistension of the fetal abdomen, and the transfusion should be stopped.

Absorption is via the subdiaphragmatic lymphatics, where small pores allow intermittent access in a "bellows-like" fashion, varying with diaphragm movement. Fetal "breathing movements" are well documented in the normal fetus; their absence may explain delayed absorption in some fetuses. Absorption is usually prompt and may be complete in as few as 3–4 days in the nonhydropic fetus.[39] Absorption in the hydropic fetus is much more variable. As fluid is absorbed preferentially to particles, ascites interferes with RBC uptake. For this reason, all ascitic fluid is removed at the time of IUT. Furosemide and digoxin are also given intraperitoneally to these fetuses.

Post-IUT Monitoring. In the viable premature fetus, post-IUT monitoring includes 2–4 hours of continuous FHR recording. Detailed ultrasound assessment is repeated, twice weekly for nonhydrops, daily for hydrops. Uptake of the transfusion mass is documented by serial measurements. The timing of the next IUT varies with the indices of disease. In general, IUT is repeated as follows: 2nd IUT 7–10 days; 3rd IUT 3–4 weeks later; 4th IUT 4 weeks later, until 32–34 weeks is reached. This schedule is flexible: lack of absorption or evidence of reaccumulation of ascites calls for more frequent

TABLE 21-13. IUT RESULTS AT WINNIPEG, 1980–1985

	IUT	Fetuses	Survivors	(%)
Hydrops	44	19	11	(58%)
Nonhydrops	64	33	29	(88%)
Total	108	52	40	(77%)

IUT. Fetal disease is not *treated* by a single transfusion in most cases; this usually arrests the progression of disease, but the appearance of hydrops between first and second IUT is not uncommon. If absorption is complete, the second IUT accomplishes the therapeutic aim: complete replacement with donor (nonantigenic) blood and inhibition of fetal hematopoiesis. Subsequent IUTs keep pace with the increasing blood volume of the growing fetus. The end result of successful intrauterine transfusion is a fetus with 100% donor (Rh-compatible) red blood cells, no fetal (Rh-incompatible) red blood cells, and no hematopoietic activity at any site.

The results of IUT at Winnipeg are shown in Table 21-13. These results reflect application of an ultrasound-directed management approach, a low rate of traumatic deaths at IUT (fewer than 2 deaths/100 IUT—tripled with anterior placenta), and expert neonatal management, all of which improve outcome. Increased centralization, however, may detract from previously published results[41] by concentrating very sick, very premature infants in one center. Nevertheless, the outlook for even the most severe disease is not hopeless: these results include many pregnancies where IUT began before 24 weeks' gestation, and twin pregnancy requiring up to 23 uterine punctures in the course of management[57] with successful outcome. Management in this fashion carries better prognosis than grossly premature delivery and attempts at neonatal management. Modern management of the hydropic fetus does not include pregnancy termination and voluntary sterilization on the basis of "hopeless" disease! Our management principles are summarized in Fig. 21-16.

PREVENTION OF ALLOIMMUNIZATION

As discussed previously, once a primary maternal response has been mounted, even as a purely IgM response, little can be done to modify IgG-mediated fetal hemolysis in subsequent Rh-incompatible pregnancies. This section, therefore, deals with the prevention of sensitization.

The laboratory and clinical experimental work leading to effective prophylaxis for Rh alloimmunization was completed by the late 1960s. It is clearly established that sensitization to D antigen can be prevented by administration of relatively small amounts of D-immune serum or purified preparations of anti-D IgG.[15-17,33] Two conditions apply: (1) the Rh-immune globulin (RhIg) must be given soon enough, and (2) it must be in sufficient concentration to prevent the process of sensitization from being completed. If these conditions are met, Rh-prophylaxis will always be successful.

Indications for Prophylaxis

Where prophylaxis has been previously given within 6–8 weeks, it may not be necessary to repeat it for a specific event (Table 21-14). For example, if a woman receiving RhIg at amniocentesis for L:S ratio is delivered a week later of an Rh-positive infant, postpartum prophylaxis is omitted, provided the maternal delivery Kleihauer excludes large-scale TPH (see below: Special Cases). The 72-hour period for postpartum prophylaxis allows for correct Rh typing of the infant. Two preparations are currently in use in North America: (1) alcohol-extracted RhIg (300 μg vial given i.m.), which may contain some IgM, IgA, and soluble protein as well as IgG, and 2) column-fractionated pure anti-D IgG (150 μg vial given i.v.). For spontaneous abortion, 150 μg RhIg is given;, otherwise, 300 μg is the standard dosage.

The debate on cost effectiveness of individual components of this approach continues. Despite some detractors[1,42] most analyses have shown benefit of both routine antenatal and event-specific prophylaxis, in addition to routine postpartum prophylaxis.[6,48,56,77]

Mechanism of Action of Prophylactic RhIg

Sufficient RhIg (about 20 micrograms RhIg per milliliter of Rh-positive RBCs) will prevent sensitization. Insufficient dosage (3–5 μg/ml) may augment and does not prevent sensitization. Therapeutic levels of RhIg prevent sensitization while binding only 10–30% of the D-antigen sites available. F(Ab) or $F(Ab)_2$ antibody fragments bind effectively to the D antigen, but

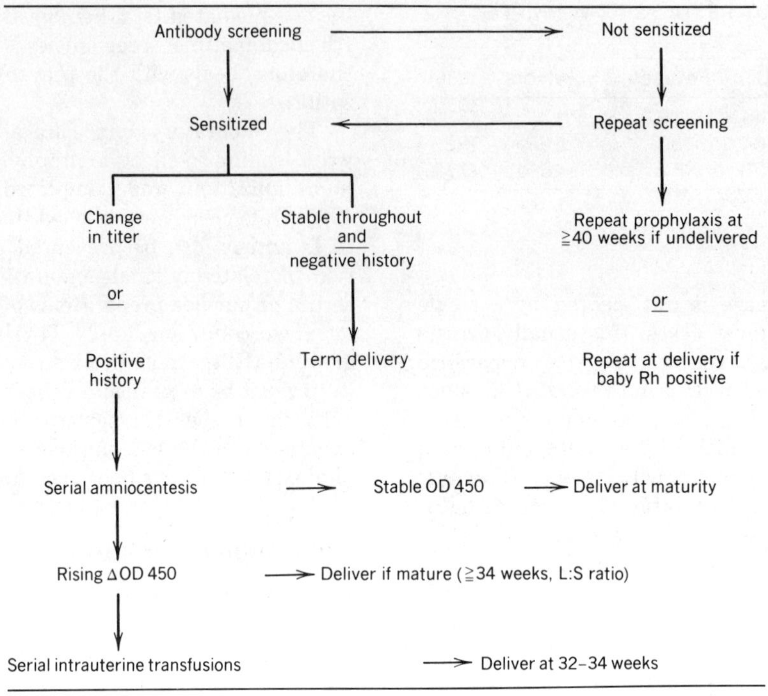

Figure 21-16. Summary of management of the Rh-negative gravida.

without the Fc portion of the antibody, prophylaxis does not occur. IgM anti-D and IgG anti-D bind equally well to Rh-positive RBCs, and both are associated with rapid clearance from maternal circulation; IgG anti-D effects prophylaxis, whereas IgM anti-D may aggravate antibody response and does not prevent it. These observations must be rationalized by any theory explaining the physiology of antibody-mediated immune suppression (AMIS).

The theory that most closely answers these questions is the "immunostat" theory of Gorman and Pollack.[35] This suggests central (i.e., cortex of regional lymph nodes, and white pulp of the spleen) immune inhibition. RhIg is bound to Rh-positive fetal cells, enabling efficient trapping of the foreign cells in immune-processing sites, but only a fraction of the antigen sites are covered. Therefore, immunocytes are presented simultaneously with the Fc portions of the bound antibody and with many unbound antigen sites. T-lymphocytes with Ig*G*-Fc receptor sites bind to the antigen–IgG complexes and function as suppressor cells, preventing B-lymphocyte responsiveness to the associated antigen. Conversely, T-lymphocytes with Ig*M*-Fc receptor sites augment B-cell response: the generation of plasma cell lines capable of

TABLE 21-14. PROPHYLAXIS IN UNSENSITIZED Rh-NEGATIVE WOMEN

Routine prophylaxis	28 weeks' gestation, *and* within 72 h of delivering an Rh-positive infant
Specific prophylaxis at the time of:	
	Amniocentesis (genetic or pulmonary maturity)
	Spontaneous or therapeutic abortion
	Antepartum hemorrhage
	Evacuation of molar or ectopic pregnancy
	Intrauterine fetal death

large-scale anti-D IgG production. It appears, therefore, that the role of "passive" anti-D IgG is to allow close approximation of suppressor T cells to the D antigen via Fc binding, provoking a chemical response ("soluble immune response suppressor") that prevents the translation of immune recognition into antibody response.[67]

Special Cases for Prophylaxis

Post-Term Pregnancy. Antepartum prophylaxis at 28 weeks may not be adequate for pregnancies extending beyond 40 weeks. Thus, Rh-negative women reaching their due date without delivery are re-treated (300 μg). Postpartum prophylaxis is omitted in these cases, provided the maternal Kleihauer test at delivery is negative.

Delayed/Omitted Prophylaxis. The 72-hour routine is based on procedural details of the original trials. Prophylaxis is at least partially effective 13 days after exposure to Rh-positive cells[76] and perhaps as late as 28 days.[5]

Spontaneous Abortion. In many cases, a single dose (150 μg) is sufficient coverage. However, if D&C is required or bleeding is heavy prior to passage of the conceptus, the standard dose is used. If there is doubt whether or not an early abortion has occurred, prophylaxis is given.

Amniocentesis. Despite improved safety of this procedure under ultrasound direction, the risk of TPH remains high: 3.3% for genetic amniocentesis and 3.9% for third-trimester taps.[11] Prophylaxis (300 μg) is used with all such procedures, and a maternal Kleihauer specimen is also drawn.

Large-Volume TPH. The standard 300 μg dose is estimated to offer full protection for TPH up to 30 ml, as determined by Kleihauer testing. When this test indicates TPH of ≧25 ml, an additional 300 μg is given for each 5 ml TPH increment. The Rosette test or the ELAT (discussed above) are adequate screening tests for this size of TPH.

Results of Prophylaxis

Before prophylaxis was introduced, the incidence of sensitization among Rh-negative Manitoba women was 118/1000 births, dropping to 18–20/1000 with the institution of postpartum prophylaxis. The rigorous application of the detailed approach to prophylaxis just described has produced the results shown in Table 21-15.

These data emphasize the impact of prophylaxis in reducing sensitization to 1.5/1000, but they also point out the most common current causes for prophylaxis failure. Serial values for 1979 through 1984 show progressive trends in the patterns of sensitization. The proportion of women who were sensitized prior to institution of prophylactic programs (1968 in Manitoba) has fallen from 35% in 1980 to only 8% in 1984. Furthermore, there has been a progressive increase in the relative number sensitized due to omission of appropriate treatment (22% in 1980–1981, 48% now).

Risks of Prophylaxis

Fetal risks are mainly theoretical. The small proportion of the IgG given to the mother that does cross the placenta occasionally results in a positive direct Coombs test but never causes HDFN. The theoretical possibility of immune deficiency due to AMIS in the fetus/newborn has never been proved clinically. Administering very large doses of RhIg (750 μg or more) in cases of large-volume antepartum TPH *may* result in some fetal hemolysis,[5] but Gorman suggests that it might take 50 maternal doses per day to create serious fetal effects.[35] Maternal risks such as anaphylaxis or anti-IgA sensitiza-

TABLE 21-15. Rh SENSITIZATION IN MANITOBA 1980–1985[12]

Total (including abortion)	129 women
Per 1000 births	1.57
Cause of alloimmunization	
Before prevention era	29 (22%)
Failure to receive treatment	42 (33%)
Antepartum—previous pregnancy	25 (19%)
Before 28 weeks—current pregnancy	15 (11%)
Unknown	18 (14%)

TABLE 21-16. ABO VERSUS Rh ALLOIMMUNIZATION

Factor	Rhesus	ABO
Incompatible pregnancy	9–11%	25–30%
Fetal antigen expressed	+++	±
Maternal antibody response	IgG	IgM>>IgG
Fetal targets	Red blood cells only	Multiple tissue sites
Placental targets	Uncertain	Definite
Antibody-antigen binding	Strong–very strong	Weak–moderate

tion are eliminated by the pure IgG RhIg now available.

Other Preventative Measures

Incorrect Transfusion. Through more detailed blood-banking practices, this type of error is becoming increasingly rare, both for D and for other less common antigens. Successful prevention of sensitization may be possible, even when whole units of Rh-positive blood are given, by a combination of exchange transfusion and high-dose Rhlg.

Genetic Amniocentesis in Rh-Negative Women. No cases of sensitization of Rh-negative women have occurred in Manitoba in over 1100 midtrimester amniocenteses. This is likely a result of prophylaxis (300 μg) in all patients and a policy of considering deferral of the procedure when the placenta is completely anterior. Furthermore, in the already-sensitized woman, transplacental amniocentesis for genetic reasons is only rarely carried out.

ALLOIMMUNIZATION TO "ATYPICAL ANTIGENS"

The preceding discussion of anti-D alloimmune disease can equally be applied to other Rhesus epitopes (C, E, etc.) and to most other blood group antigens (Kell, Duffy, Kidd, etc.). The relative importance of these "atypical" antibodies is displayed in Table 21-2. The low frequency of noncompatible pregnancies (or, more likely, incompletely matched blood transfusions) resulting in HDFN is such that preventative programs are not practical. Highly detailed crossmatching, however, is becoming more widespread, and this will undoubtedly continue to reduce the frequency of such maternal–fetal incompatibilities.

ABO Alloimmunization

ABO alloimmune disease is much more common than Rh disease. Between 20% and 30% of pregnancies are ABO incompatible, and about two-thirds of all HDFN is due to this incompatibility.[18] Most of this disease, however, appears as mild hyperbilirubinemia of the term newborn, without significant anemia. Mortality, hydrops, or even serious jaundice are extremely rare results of ABO incompatibility, and other reasons (other blood group immunization, drugs, breast-feeding, GI anomalies) should be carefully excluded in such cases.

Several protective mechanisms, different from Rh phenomena, account for this much milder form of alloimmunization (Table 21-16).

Most serious cases of neonatal jaundice from ABO incompatibility occur in Group O women with Group A_1 (as opposed to A_2) fetuses. These women are more likely to produce IgG than are Group A or B women. Immaturity of the antigen in the fetus (75% fewer antigens/red blood cell vs. adult blood), uptake of antibody by placental and non-RBC fetal tissue A/B determinants, and the lower binding constant relegate almost any ABO disease to a strictly neonatal disorder, with jaundice and its attendant risk of kernicterus being the significant problems. Less than 0.5% of ABO-incompatible newborns require exchange transfusion. In the rare woman with such a history, maternal testing for the level of IgG anti-A/B may help in planning delivery at a center with high-level neonatal care. Women who have only IgM anti-A/B will not have affected infants.

REFERENCES

1. Adams, M. M., Marks, J. S., and Ioplan, J. P.: Cost implications of routine antenatal administration of Rh immune globulin. *Am. J. Obstet. Gynecol.* **149**:633–638, 1984.

2. Bevis, D. C. A.: Composition of liquor amnii in haemolytic disease of the newborn. *Lancet* **2**:443, 1950.
3. Bierme S. J., Blanc, M., Abbal, M., and Fournie, A.: Oral Rh treatment for severely immunized mothers. *Lancet* **1**:604–605, 1979.
4. Bowell, P., Wainscoat, J. S., Peto, T. E. A., and Gunson, H. H.: Maternal anti-D concentrations in rhesus haemolytic disease of the newborn. *Br. Med. J.* **285**:327–329, 1982.
5. Bowman, J. M.: Blood group immunization in obstetric practice. *Curr. Probl. Obstet. Gynecol.* **7**:1–61, 1983.
6. Bowman, J. M.: Efficacy of antenatal Rh prophylaxis. In: *Rh Hemolytic Disease: New Strategy for Eradication.* F. D. Frigoletto, Jr., J. F. Jewett, and A. A. Konugres (Eds.). Boston, G. K. Hall, 1982, pp. 143–160.
7. Bowman, J. M.: The management of Rh-isoimmunization. *Obstet. Gynecol.* **52**:1–16, 1978.
8. Bowman, J. M.: The Manitoba Rh Programme. Protocol distributed to all practicing physicians. 1986.
9. Bowman, J. M.: Maternal blood group immunization. In: *Maternal-Fetal Medicine. Principles and Practice.* R. K. Creasy and R. Resnik (Eds.). Philadelphia, W. B. Saunders, 1984, pp. 1193–1239.
10. Bowman J. M.: Suppression of Rh-isoimmunization. A review. *Obstet. Gynecol.* **52**:385–393, 1978.
11. Bowman, J. M.: Transplacental hemorrhage associated with ultrasound-directed amniocentesis. *Obstet. Gynecol.* (in press, 1986).
12. Bowman, J. M., and Pollack, J. M.: Annual Report of the Rh Laboratory, Winnipeg, Canada, 1985.
13. Chamberlain, E. M., Scott, J. R., Wu, J. T., Rotens, N. S., Rote, N. S., and Egger, M. J.: A comparison of acid-elution techniques and alphafetoprotein levels for the detection of fetomaternal bleeding. *Am. J. Obstet. Gynecol.* **143**:912–917, 1982.
14. Charles, A. G. and Blumenthal, L. S.: Promethazine hydrochloride therapy in severely Rh-sensitized pregnancies. *Obstet. Gynecol.* **60**:627–630, 1982.
15. Chown, B., Duff, A. M., James, J., et al.: Prevention of primary Rh immunization: First report of the Western Canadian trial. *Can. Med. Assoc. J.* **100**:1021–1024, 1969.
16. Clark, C. A.: Prevention of Rh haemolytic disease by immunoglobulin anti-D. *Vox Sang.* **44**:396–399, 1983.
17. Clarke, C. A., Conohoe, W. T. A., McConnell, R. B., Woodrow, J. C., Finn, R., Krevans, J. R., Kulke, W., Lehane, D., and Sheppard, P. M.: Further experimental studies on the prevention of Rh haemolytic disease. *Br. Med. J.* **1**:979–984, 1963.
18. Cook, L. N.: ABO hemolytic disease. *Clin. Obstet. Gynecol.* **25**:333–339, 1982.
19. Coombs, R. R. A., Mourant, A. E., and Race, R. R.: Detection of weak and "incomplete" Rh agglutinins. new test. *Lancet* **2**:15–16, 1945.
20. Cremer, R. J., Perryman, P. W., and Richards, D. H.: Influence of light on the hyperbilirubinemia of infants. *Lancet* **1**:1094–1097, 1958.
21. Darke, C.: HLA types and the immune response to the Rh(D) antigen. *Tissue Antigens* **9**:171–173, 1977.
22. Darrow, R. R.: Icterus gravidus (erythroblastosis) neonatorum; examination of etiologic considerations. *Arch. Pathol.* **25**:378–417, 1938.
23. Davey, M.: The prevention of Rhesus isoimmunization. *Clin. Obstet. Gynaecol.* **6**:509–529, 1979.
24. DeVore, G. R., Donnerstein, R. L., Kleinman, C. S., Platt, L. D., and Hobbins, J. C.: Fetal echocardiography. II. The diagnosis and significance of a pericardial effusion in the fetus using real-time directed M-mode ultrasound. *Am. J. Obstet. Gynecol.* **144**:693–700, 1982.
25. Diamond, L. K.: Historic perspective on "exchange transfusion." *Vox Sang.* **45**:333–335, 1983.
26. Diamond, L. K., and Abelson, N. M.: Demonstration of anti-Rh agglutinins: An accurate and rapid slide test. *J. Lab. Clin. Med.* **30**:204–212, 1945.
27. Diamond L. K., Allen F. H., Jr., and Thomas, W. O., Jr.: Erythroblastosis fetalis. VII. Treatment with exchange transfusion. *N. Engl. J. Med.* **244**:39–49, 1951.
28. Diamond, L. K., Blackfan, K. D., and Baty, J. M.: Erythroblastosis fetalis and its association with universal edema of the fetus, icterus gravis neonatorum and anemia of the newborn. *J. Pediatr.* **1**:269–309, 1932.
29. Diamond, L. K. and Denton, R. L.: Rh agglutination in various media with particular reference to the value of albumin. *J. Lab. Clin. Med.* **30**:821–830, 1945.
30. Dienst, A.: Das Eklamsiegift. *Zentralbl. Gynakol.* **29**:353–364, 1905.
31. Finn, R., Clarke, C. A., Donohue, W. T. A., McConnell, R. B., Sheppard, P. M., Lehane, D., and Kulke, W.: Experimental studies on the prevention of Rh haemolytic disease. *Br. Med. J.* **1**:1486–1490, 1961.
32. Fraser, I. D., Bothamley, J. E., Bennett, M. O., and Airth, G. R.: Intensive antenatal plasmapheresis in severe Rhesus isoimmunization. *Lancet* **1**:6–9, 1976.
33. Freda, V. J., Gorman, J. G., and Pollack, W.: Successful prevention of experimental Rh sensitization in man with a anti-Rh gamma^2-globulin antibody preparation. *Transfusion* **4**:26–32, 1964.
34. Gold, W. R., Jr., Queenan, J. T., Woody, J., and Sacher, R. A.: Oral desensitization in Rh disease. *Am. J. Obstet. Gynecol.* **146**:980–981, 1982.
35. Gorman, J. G.: New applications of Rh immune globulin: Effect on protocols. In: *Rh Hemolytic Disease: New Strategy for Eradication.* F. D. Frigoletto, Jr., J. F. Jewett, and A. A. Konugres (Eds.). Boston, G. K. Hall, 1982, pp. 199–210.
36. Goto, S., Nishi, H., and Tomoda, Y.: Blood group

Rh-D factor in human trophoblast determined by the immunofluorescent method. *Am. J. Obstet. Gynecol.* **137**:707–712, 1980.

37. Greenwalt, T. J.: Rh isoimmunization—The importance of a critical case study. *JAMA* **251**: 1318–1320, 1984.
38. Gusdon, J. P.: The treatment of erythroblastosis with promethazine hydrochloride. *J. Reprod. Med.* **26**:454–458, 1981.
39. Harman, C. R., Biehl, D. R., Pollock, D. J., Bowman, J. M., and Manning, F. A.: Intrauterine transfusion: Kinetics of absorption donor cells in fetal lambs. *Am. J. Obstet. Gynecol.* **145**:830–836, 1983.
40. Harman, C. R., Manning, F. A., and Bowman, J. M.: Unpublished observations, Manitoba Intrauterine Transfusion Team, 1985.
41. Harman, C. R., Manning, F. A., Bowman, J. M., and Lange, I. R.: Severe Rh disease—poor outcome is not inevitable. *Am. J. Obstet. Gynecol.* **145**:823–829, 1983.
42. Hensleigh, P. A.: Preventing rhesus isoimmunization. Antepartum Rh-immune globulin prophylaxis versus a sensitive test for risk identification. *Am. J. Obstet. Gynecol.* **146**:749–755, 1983.
43. Isbister J. P., Ting, A., and Seeto K. M.: Development of Rh-specific maternal autoantibodies following intensive plasmapheresis for Rh immunization during pregnancy. *Vox Sang.* **33**:353–358, 1977.
44. Issitt, P. D.: *Serology and Genetics of the Rhesus Blood Group System.* Cincinnati, Montgomery Scientific Publications, 1979.
45. Keith, L., Danis, R. P., and Berger, G. S.: Clinical experience with the prevention of Rh-isoimmunization: A historical comparative analysis. *Am. J. Reprod. Immunol.* **5**:84–89, 1984.
46. Kleihauer, E., Braun, H., and Betke, K.: Demonstration von fetalem hämoglobin in den Erythrocytes eines Blutausstrichs. *Klin. Wochenschr.* **33**:637–638, 1957.
47. Landsteiner, K. and Wiener, A. S.: An agglutinable factor in human blood recognized by immune sera for Rhesus lood. *Proc. Soc. Exp. Biol. Med.* **43**:223, 1940.
48. Lavery, J. P.: Rh_0(D) immune globulin. When to use it in the Rh_0(D)-negative woman. *Postgrad. Med.* **75**:259–264, 1984.
49. Lele, A. S., Carmody, P. J., Hurd, M. E., and O'Leary, J. A.: Fetomaternal bleeding following diagnostic amniocentesis. *Obstet. Gynecol.* **60**:60–64, 1982.
50. Levine, P., Burnham, L., Katzin, E. M., and Vogel, P.: The role of isoimmunization in the pathogenesis of erythroblastosis fetalis. *Am. J. Obstet. Gynecol.* **42**:925–937, 1941.
51. Levine, P. and Stetson, R. E.: An unusual case of intra-group agglutination. *JAMA* **113**:126–127, 1939.
52. Lewis, M.: Recent advances in blood groups. *Clin. Lab. Med.* **2**:137–154, 1982.
53. Liley, A. W.: Errors in the assessment of hemolytic disease from amniotic fluid. *Am. Obstet. Gynecol.* **86**:485–494, 1963.
54. Liley, A. W.: Intrauterine transfusion of foetus in haemolytic disease. *Br. Med. J.* **2**:1107–1109, 1963.
55. Liley, A. W.: Liquor amnio analysis in management of pregnancy complicated by Rhesus isoimmunization. *Am. J. Obstet. Gynecol.* **82**:1359–1370, 1961.
56. Lim, O., Fleisher, A., and Ziel, H.: Reduction of Rh (D) sensitization: A cost-effective analysis. *Obstet. Gynecol.* **59**:477–480, 1982.
57. Manning, F. A., Bowman, J. M., Lange, I. R., and Chamberlain, P. F.: Intrauterine transfusion in an Rh-immunized twin pregnancy: A case report of successful outcome and a review of the literature. *Obstet. Gynecol.*, **65**:2S–6S, 1985.
58. Manning, F. A., Morrison, I., Lange, I. R., Harman, C. R., and Chamberlain, P. F.: Fetal assessment based upon fetal biophysical profile scoring: Experience in 12,620 referred high-risk pregnancies. 1. Perinatal mortality by frequency and etiology. *Am. J. Obstet. Gynecol.*, **151**:343–350, 1985.
59. Mattingly, J. A., and Waksman, B. H.: Immunologic suppression after oral administration of antigen. I. Specific suppressor cells formed in rat Peyer's patches after oral administration of sheep erythrocytes and their systemic migration. *J. Immunol.* **121**:1878–1883, 1978.
60. Moore, B. P. L.: Automation in the blood transfusion laboratory: 1. Antibody detection and quantitation in the Technicon AutoAnalyzer. *Can. Med. Assoc. J.* **100**:381–387, 1969.
61. Ness, P. M.: The assessment of fetal-maternal hemorrhage by enzyme-linked antiglobulin recipients. *Am. J. Obstet. Gynecol.* **143**:788–792, 1982.
62. Nevanlinna, H. R. and Vainio, T.: The influence of mother-child ABO incompatibility on Rh immunization. *Vox Sang.* **1**:26–36, 1956.
63. Ottenberg, R.: The etiology of eclampsia: Historical and critical notes. *JAMA* **81**:295–299, 1923.
64. Plapp, F. V., Kowalski, M. M., Tilzer, L., Brown, P. J., Evans, J., and Chiga, M.: Partial purification of Rh_0(D) antigen from Rh positive and negative erythrocytes. *Proc. Natl. Acad. Sci. USA* **76**:2964, 1979.
65. Polesky, H. F.: Diagnosis, prevention, and therapy in hemolytic disease of the newborn. *Clin. Lab. Med.* **2**:107–122, 1982.
66. Polesky, H. F. and Sebring, E. S.: Detection of fetal–maternal hemorrhage: An evaluation of serological tests related to Rh_0(D) immune globulin (human). *Transfusion* **11**:162–165, 1971.
67. Pollack, W.: Recent understanding for the mechanism by which passively administered Rh antibody suppresses the immune response to Rh antigen in unimmunized Rh-negative women. *Clin. Obstet. Gynecol.* **25**:255–265, 1982.
68. Race, R. R.: An "incomplete" antibody in human serum. *Nature* **153**:771–772, 1944.

69. Race, R. R.: The Rh genotype and Fisher's theory. *Blood* **3**:27–42, 1948.
70. Rayburn, W. F., Johnson, M. Z., and Menon, K. M. J.: Rh-isoimmunization: Normal amniotic fluid absorbance characteristics between 16 and 20 weeks. Proceedings of the 30th Annual Meeting of the Society for Gynecologic Investigation, Washington, DC, 1983, p. 26 (Abstract 44).
71. Robinson, A. E. A. and Tovey, L. A. D.: Intensive plasma exchange in the management of severe Rh disease. *Br. J. Haematol.* **45**:621–631, I980.
72. Rodeck, C. H., Holman, C. A., Karnicki, J., Kemp, J. R., Whitmore, D. N., and Austin, M. A.: Direct intravascular fetal blood transfusion by fetoscopy in severe rhesus isoimmunization. *Lancet* **1**:625–627, 1981.
73. Rosenfeld, R. E., Allen, F. H., Jr., and Rubenstein, P.: Genetic model for the Rh blood-group system. *Proc. Natl. Acad. Sci. USA* **70**:1303, 1973.
74. Rote, N. S.: Pathophysiology of Rh-isoimmunization. *Clin. Obstet. Gynecol.* **25**:243–253, 1982.
75. Sacks, M. S.: Hemolytic disease of the fetus and newborn. In: *Williams Obstetrics*, 10th Edition. N. J. Eastman (Ed.). New York, Appleton-Century-Crofts, 1950, pp. 1001–1025.
76. Samson, D. and Mollison, P. L.: Effect on primary Rh-immunization of delayed administration of anti-Rh. *Immunology* **28**:349–357, 1975.
77. Scott, J. R.: Antenatal prophylaxis: Experience at Utah. In: *Rh Hemolytic Disease: New Strategy for Eradication*. F. D. Frigoletto, Jr., J. F. Jewett and A. A. Konugres (Eds.). Boston, G. K. Hall, 1982, pp. 191–198.
78. Sebring, E. S.: Fetomaternal hemorrhage—lncidence and methods of detection and quantitation. In: *Hemolytic Disease of the Newborn*. G. Garratty (Ed.). Arlington, VA, American Association of Bloodbanks, 1984, pp. 87–117.
79. Sebring, E. S. and Polesky, H. F.: Detection of fetal-maternal hemorrhage with ficin-treated Rh positive indicator cells. *Transfusion* **20**:641, 1980.
80. Skov, F. and Hughes-Jones, N. C.: Observations on the number of available C antigen sites on red cells. *Vox Sang.* **33**:170–174, 1977.
81. Smith, T.: Active immunity produced by so-called balanced or neutral mixtures of diphtheria toxin and antitoxin. *J. Exp. Med.* **11**:241–256, 1909.
82. Stern, K., Goodman, H. S., and Berger, M.: Experimental isoimmunization to hemoantigens in man. *J. Immunol.* **87**:189–198, 1961.
83. Tippett, P. and Sanger, R.: Observations on subdivisions of the Rh antigen D. *Vox Sang.* **7**:9–13, 1962.
84. Unger, L. J., Wiener, A. S., and Katz, L.: Studies on blood group factors Rh^A, Rh^B and Rh^C. *J. Exp. Med.* **110**:495–510, 1959.
85. Urbaniak, S. J., Greiss, M. A., Crawford, R. J., and Fergusson, M. J. C.: Prediction of the outcome of Rhesus haemolytic disease of the newborn: Additional information using an ADCC assay. *Vox Sang.* **46**:323–329, 1984.
86. Vaisman, S. I., Lee, K. S., and Gardner, L. M.: The effect of promethazine hydrochloride on bilirubin metabolism in the rat. *Pediatr. Res.* **10**:788–791, 1976.
87. Visser, G. H. A.: Antepartum sinusoidal and decelerative heart rate patterns in Rh disease. *Am. J. Obstet. Gynecol.* **143**:538–544, 1982.
88. Von Dungern, F.: Beitrage zur Immunïttslehr. *Münch. Med. Wochenschr.* **47**:677, 1900.
89. Weinstein, L.: Irregular antibodies causing hemolytic disease of the newborn: A continuing problem. *Clin. Obstet. Gynecol.* **25**:321–332, 1982.
90. Wenske, C., Gaedicke, O., Kuenzlen, E., Heyes, H., Mueller-Eckhardt, C., Kleihauer, E., and Lauritzen, C.: Treatment of idiopathic thrombocytopenic purpura in pregnancy by high dose intravenous immunoglobulin. *Blut* **46**:347–353, 1983.
91. White, C. A., Stedman, C. M., and Frank, S.: Anti-D antibodies in D- and D^u-positive women: A cause of hemolytic disease of the newborn. *Am. J. Obstet. Gynecol.* **145**:1069–1075, 1983.
92. Wiener, A. S.: A new test (blocking test) for Rh sensitization. *Proc. Soc. Exp. Biol. Med.* **56**:173–176, 1944.
93. Wiener, A. S. and Peters, H. R.: Hemolytic reactions following transfusion of blood of the homologous group with three cases in which the same agglutinogen was responsible. *Ann. Intern. Med.* **13**:2306–2322, 1940.
94. Wiener, A. S. and Wexler, I. B.: *Heredity of the Blood Groups*. New York, Grune & Stratton, 1958.
95. Woodrow, J. C.: Rh immunization and its prevention. *Ser. Haematol.* **3**:1–151, 1970.
96. Zipursky, A.: Rh hemolytic disease of the newborn: The disease eradicated by immunology. *Clin. Obstet. Gynecol.* **20**:759–772, 1977.
97. Zipursky, A., Hull, A., White, F. D., and Israels, L. G.: Foetal erythrocytes in the maternal circulation. *Lancet* **1**:451–452, 1959.
98. Zipursky, A. and Israels, L. G.: The pathogenesis and prevention of Rh immunization. *Can. Med. Assoc. J.* **97**:1245–1257, 1967.
99. Zuelzer, W. W. and Cohen, F.: ABO hemolytic disease and heterospecific pregnancy. *Pediatr. Clin. North Am.* **4**:405–428, 1957.

22

ABNORMAL LABOR

Abnormal labor is a major problem in clinical obstetrics that most often is characterized by unusually slow progress or difficulty in accomplishing parturition. It is frequently referred to as dystocia, a term derived from the Greek roots "dys" meaning abnormal and "tokos" meaning labor or childbirth. From the viewpoint of its clinical consequences, abnormal labor consists not only of those conditions resulting in prolonged or arrested labor, but also of conditions leading to precipitous or tumultuous delivery.

The etiological factors resulting in abnormal labor have been divided (somewhat arbitrarily) into three categories which may exist singly but most often occur in combination.

Functional causes of abnormal labor are those attributable to dysfunction of the muscular forces that engender parturition. One functional form of abnormal labor may result from hypoactive uterine motility. In this form, myometrial contractions may be of insufficient intensity, duration, or frequency (hypotonic or hypocontractility) or inappropriately coordinated (hypertonic or hypercontractility) to generate the forces required for effacement and dilatation of the cervix. A second functional form of abnormal labor may result from hyperactive uterine motility which can compromise fetal status. This form of abnormal labor is manifested by uterine contractions of high frequency and intensity with or without increased baseline pressure. Dystocia may also result from inability of abdominal voluntary muscles to generate forces adequate to overcome the normal resistance of the maternal pelvic tissues for descent of the fetal presenting part to occur in a timely manner during the second stage of labor.

Fetal causes of abnormal labor are those attributable to size, shape, position, presentation, or attitude of the fetus or developmental abnormalities of such a character that they hinder or preclude extrusion of the fetus through the pelvis.

Maternal causes of abnormal labor are those attributable to some anatomical or positional abnormality of the pelvic organs that impedes or obstructs the descent of the fetal presenting part.

In some situations, inappropriate uterine contractility may be the sole cause for abnormal labor or dystocia, whereas in other cases the contractility may be relatively inadequate because of associated fetal or maternal causes. Factors that may directly influence muscle contractility include maternal fatigue, anxiety, fear, pain, and various drugs used during the course of labor. In cases where a fetal abnormality may be the predominant reason for abnormal labor, a dysfunctional pattern of uterine contractions and disadvantageous pelvic architecture may be associated factors. Maternal anatomic abnormalities may be severe enough to constitute the sole cause of abnormal labor, but, more often, they cause dysfunctional labor in conjunction with either a functional derangement of uterine contractility or with an abnormality of the fetus.

Once a particular labor aberration is recognized, the obstetrician must evaluate the conditions contributing to the specific abnormality and initiate the therapeutic regimen most appropriate to that individual patient. Even when the precise biochemical and hormonal facets of myometrial and cervical change associated with parturition have been fully elucidated (see Chapter 7), the diagnosis and management of abnormal labor will continue to require sound judgment and good obstetrical principles to determine the timing and best route of delivery for each pregnancy.

CHARACTERISTICS OF NORMAL LABOR

Labor uncomplicated by other factors displays characteristic patterns of uterine contraction and progresses in a predictable manner. Research performed in the 1950s and 1960s provided the foundation and many of the specific principles that comprise current knowledge of myometrial contractions and of the progress of cervical dilatation in normal and abnormal labor.

Myometrial Contractions

The principles of myometrial contractions at molecular and cellular levels are similar to those of skeletal muscle, but the kinetics of their reactions are different. Uterine contractions reflect the physiological interaction of a number of active compounds and are necessarily complex because the same organ must provide sequentially the optimal conditions for implantation, fetal growth and development and, finally, parturition. The uterine contractions of normal labor are characterized by a gradient of myometrial activity. Contraction intensity, duration, and total relative work per unit of time are greatest at the fundus and diminish toward the cervix.[91] "Fundal dominance" was confirmed by utilizing intramyometrial and intra-amniotic microballoons connected to strain-gauge transducers to measure local pressures in different regions of the uterine wall, as well as the total pressure generated within the fluid-filled sac of the amniochorionic membranes.[6] The duration and intensity of the myometrial contraction at a given site on the uterus are inversely proportional to the distance from the cornua. There is also a time difference in the onset of contractions in the fundus, midzone, and lower segments of the uterus. These triple descending gradients of propagation, duration, and intensity are essential to efficient cervical dilatation.

Early studies employing electrohysterography[63] described the exciting stimulus for each uterine contraction as starting in one cornu and then the other to join together and then to sweep over the fundus and down the uterus. Although no specific pacemaker areas or cells have been identified, later more sophisticated measurements of uterine electromyographic activity have confirmed that the electrical impulse propagates from the fundal portion of the uterus towards the cervix.[122]

The recorded pressure versus time curve of a uterine contraction is bell-shaped. The steep crescent slope leading to the peak of the curve represents the actual power of the uterine contraction and encompasses only one-third of the total duration of the contraction. The relaxation phase encompasses two-thirds of the contraction curve and is initially reflected by a rather steep decremental slope. This slope becomes more horizontal in the last one-third of the contraction, reflecting the gradual final relaxation process.

The intensity of a uterine contraction depends on the total myometrial mass and the number of excited myometrial cells. Contractions of the gravid uterus are perceptible by abdominal palpation when their intensity is approximately 10 mmHg above the level of baseline resting pressure or tonus. Elevation of uterine baseline pressure above the normal limits of 12–15 mmHg renders perception of the uterine contraction by abdominal palpation more difficult. The palpation perception threshold is influenced also by the thickness of the abdominal wall and the amount of amniotic fluid. Until the intensity of the contraction reaches 40 mmHg, the uterine wall can be readily depressed by abdominal palpation. Because the first and last part of each contraction is not perceived by abdominal palpation, the duration of the contraction as estimated clinically is shorter than that reflected on a polygraph recording.

Mechanical measurement of uterine contractions during labor most often employs either an external tocodynamometer placed on the abdominal wall over the uterine fundus or internal monitoring through an open-end, fluid-filled catheter inserted transcervically into the amniotic cavity (see Chapter 11). The contraction patterns, including moment-to-moment variations, are similar with both methods of measurement. External tocodynamometry, however, does not have units of measurement and cannot accurately reflect contraction intensity or the resting pressure during uterine diastole. Internal monitoring reflects the sum total effect of individual myometrial fiber contractions on intra-amniotic pressure (Pascal's principle). Contraction intensity and baseline pressure are usually recorded in millimeters of mercury. Inaccuracies may occur if the diaphragm of the pressure transducer is not placed at exactly the same level as the catheter tip or if these positional relationships vary with patient movement. Since 1 cm of water is the equivalent of 0.74 mmHg, a differential of 10 cm would alter the absolute value of the recorded pressure by 7.4 mmHg.

Six uterine contraction patterns recorded by internal monitoring of intra-amniotic pressure are depicted in Fig. 22-1. These patterns are representative of the changes that occur in prelabor and labor. Approximately 46–48 hours prior to delivery, contractions with intensities generally below 20 mmHg, but occasionally reaching 30–35 mmHg, occur every 5–10 minutes. Between these contractions, the small, focal, uncoordinated contractions typical of early gestation are recorded (Pattern 1). This is followed by a period of decreased contraction intensity (Pattern 2). The frequency of contractions is one every 8–15 minutes. The transition between prelabor and labor is gradual but progressive, and the small, focal, uncoordinated contractions tend to disappear as prelabor advances (Pattern 3). However, the configuration of the coordinated contractions remains unchanged. Waveform analyses indicate that the relationship of maximum amplitude to maximum and minimum slopes of the intra-amniotic pressure curve has no apparent differences between prelabor and active labor contractions.[111] During the prodromal or latent phase of labor, three to four uterine contractions with intensities of 20–30 mmHg occur in each 10 minute period (Pattern 4). In the active phase of labor with progressive cervical dilatation, contraction intensity increases from 30–40 mmHg to 50 mmHg or greater (Patterns 5 and 6). The intensity of contractions is greater in primiparous than in multiparous women.[113] Maternal expulsive efforts or Valsalva's maneuver may transiently increase intra-amniotic pressure to values of 100–150 mmHg. Throughout the active stage of labor, frequency of contractions progressively increases from approximately one contraction every 3–5 minutes to one every 2–3 minutes. During this stage, there is also a gradual but definite increase in baseline resting pressure.

Marked variations in repetition frequency, intensity, and apparent waveform may be noted during active labor, especially when the characteristics of large numbers of contractions are measured (Fig. 22-2). This irregular rhythmicity has been interpreted by some as further evidence to refute the concept of a uterine pacemaker.[96] It may be related, in part, to changes in maternal position. When a patient is positioned on her back, the average frequency of contractions is often higher, but the intensity lower than when she lies on her side. These alterations occur immediately after the change in po-

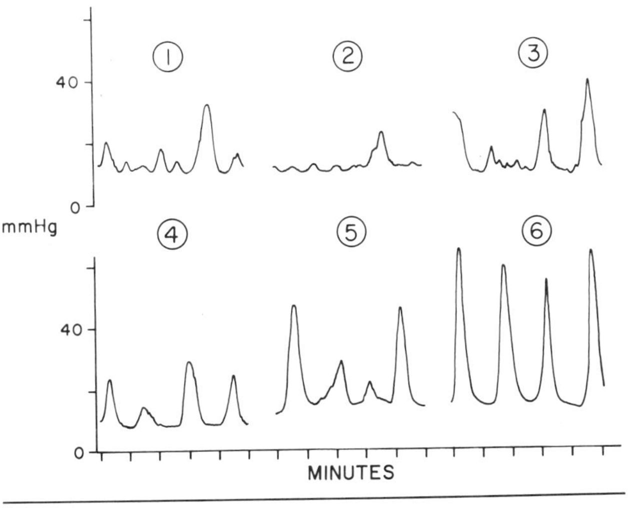

Figure 22-1. Representative patterns of changes in uterine contractions that occur in prelabor and labor. The recordings of intra-amniotic pressure were obtained at approximately 8 hour intervals over a 48 hour period ending at delivery.

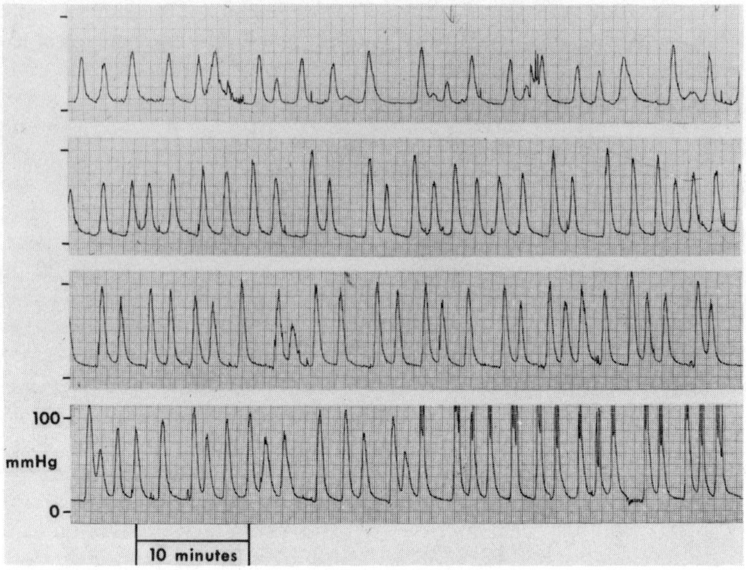

Figure 22-2. Polygraph tracing of intra-amniotic pressure illustrating the variations in repetition intensity, frequency, and waveform that occur during active spontaneous labor (recorded at a paper speed of 5 mm/min). During the four hours of recording depicted, the patient progressed from 4 cm to delivery of a 3060 g female infant with Apgar scores of 8 and 9.

sition and continue for as long as the new position is maintained.[9]

Cervicographic Analysis

Numerous authors have plotted the progress of cervical dilatation against the passage of time in an effort to apply more objective criteria to the course of labor than the intensity and frequency of uterine contractions or the total duration of labor. Among the names used to describe these plots have been labor graph, labor curve, cervimetry, parturograph, and partogram. Cervicographic analysis is a term applied to the use of these graphs or curves to define, characterize, and study labor. Based on these graphic studies, the first stage of labor has been divided somewhat artificially into two distinct phases: the prodromal or latent phase and the active phase[28] (see Chapter 7 for discussion). Others contend that the diagnosis of labor can be made only by observation of progress in cervical dilatation.[49,79] They use the term "labor" to refer to the active phase of labor only.

The latent phase or prodromal labor may last several hours or perhaps several days, during which time uterine contractions become organized and the cervix softens and effaces. Cervical dilatation is minimal. The duration of the latent phase is usually not influenced by maternal age, fetal size, or obstetrical abnormalities that may become apparent later in labor. However, the latent phase may be prolonged by exogenous factors including heavy sedation, analgesia, or conduction anesthesia. Another important factor affecting the duration of the latent phase is the initial status of the cervix. In general, the patient with a more favorable cervix at the onset of labor has a shorter latent phase.

The active phase of normal labor is characterized by progressive cervical dilatation and descent of the fetal presenting part through the pelvis (see Chapter 7).

CHARACTERISTICS OF ABNORMAL LABOR

Abnormal labor is defined by deviations from the limits set for the normal. Two major classifications of abnormalities of labor have evolved to replace less exact descriptions such as primary and secondary uterine inertia. One classification, devised primarily by South American and European investigators, is based on studies of the mechanical and electrical properties of the contracting uterus. It relies on alterations in the pattern of myometrial contractions to characterize abnormalities of labor. The second system was devised primarily by American investigators and relies on deviations from the temporal limits for normal progress in dilatation and descent for diagnosis and classification.

Myometrial Contractions

Abnormal patterns of uterine contraction are separated into those resulting from hypoactive uterine motility associated with insufficient generation of contractions (hypotonic uterine dysfunction), those resulting from ineffective contractility (hypertonic or uncoordinated uterine dysfunction), and those resulting from hyperactive uterine motility (Table 22-1).

Hypoactive Uterine Motility. Hypoactive disorders of uterine motility include hypotonic and hypertonic or uncoordinated uterine contractions.

Hypotonic Uterine Dysfunction or Hypocontractility. Hypotonic uterine dysfunction or hypocontractility reflects either a decrease in the frequency of electrical action potentials or a poor response to the signal. Since this distinction cannot be made without intramyometrial electrodes, hypotonic dysfunction is considered a single entity in clinical practice. Hypotonic dysfunction occurs in both nulliparous and multiparous women and may occur at any point in labor. Uterine contractions are infrequent and of low intensity. Baseline pressures are low or normal. Maternal discomfort is usually minimal.

Hypertonic or Uncoordinated Uterine Dysfunction (Hypercontractility). In this group of disorders, uterine contractions are generated either

TABLE 22-1. OUTLINE OF THE CLASSIFICATION AND CHARACTERISTICS OF ABNORMAL UTERINE CONTRACTIONS

Classification	Characteristics
I. HYPOACTIVE UTERINE MOTILITY	
A. Hypotonic uterine dysfunction (hypocontractility)	Infrequent, low intensity, low or normal baseline pressure. Nulliparous and multiparous women, slow progress
B. Hypertonic uterine dysfunction (hypercontractility)	Distortion of pattern, uncoordinated, elevated baseline pressure, primarily nulliparous women
1. Inversion of gradients	Appear normal in frequency and intensity. No progress
2. Uncoordinated contractions	
a. First-degree	Small contractions alternating with large ones having two or more peaks. Baseline pressure normal or slightly elevated. Slow or no progress
b. Second-degree (fibrillation)	Small, irregular, high-frequency contractions, slight elevation in baseline pressure. Usually little or no progress
II. HYPERACTIVE UTERINE MOTILITY	Intensities of 70 mmHg or greater, frequencies more than 5 per 10 min period, normal or increased baseline pressure. Progress varies, but usually increased
A. Tachysystole	Frequencies of more than 5 per 10 min period, progressive decrease of intensity and increase in baseline pressure. Progress usually increased

in the lower pole of the uterus or in multiple loci. In either circumstance, the contraction pattern interferes with the components necessary for normal labor, stretching of the lower uterine segment and descent of the presenting part. Hypertonic uterine dysfunction results in either an appreciable elevation in baseline pressure, a distortion of the pressure gradient by asynchronous contractions, or a combination of these abnormalities. Contractions become less frequent and the uterus is easily indentable even at the acme of a contraction. Hypertonic dysfunction is primarily observed in nulliparas and usually occurs early in labor. These contractions may produce significant, disproportionate maternal discomfort, often in the form of backache.

The qualitative abnormalities of hypertonic uterine contractions can be subdivided[7] into those resulting from inversion of the triple descending gradients (propagation, duration, intensity) and those resulting from varying degrees of incoordination. Inversion of the gradients may be total or partial, with the contraction wave starting in the lower part of the uterus and propagating upward. Because the tracings produced are almost identical in form to those recorded during normal labor, inversion gradients cannot be diagnosed from recordings made by external tocodynamometry or from intra-amniotic pressure measurements. If all three gradients are inverted, the contractions are totally ineffective in dilating the cervix, despite the fact that they may be as strong as those of normal labor. When only one or two of the components of the triple descending gradient are inverted, the contraction waves may dilate the cervix, but much more slowly than normal contraction waves do.

Hypertonic uterine activity resulting from uncoordinated uterine contractions is classified as first or second degree, depending on the number of areas within the uterus that are contracting independently or asynchronously. Because these conditions result in alterations of the contraction pattern, they can be detected by either external tocodynamometry or by internal monitoring of intra-amniotic pressure (Fig. 22-3).

First-degree incoordination is a fairly frequent deviation from the normal pattern of uterine activity. It is caused by interference with the normal interaction of the excitation centers of the uterus. If the excitation foci have different rhythms, their activity is asynchronous and produces a typical appearance on the intra-amniotic pressure tracing (Fig. 22-3a). Small contractions alternate with large ones. The large contractions tend to have two or more peaks and are lower and wider at the base than are normal contraction waves. Contractions localized to a very small area of the uterus are totally ineffective, whereas those covering a larger zone are capable of bringing about some dilatation of the cervix. The progress of labor is slower than normal. First-degree incoordination may present by itself or in combination with inverted gradients, hypotonia, or hyperactive uterine motility.

Second-degree incoordination or uterine fibrillation results when the uterus is divided functionally into numerous zones that contract independently and asynchronously. Two of the zones may obey the normal excitation foci, but the remaining ones are controlled by new foci that appear in other parts of the uterus. The records derived from external monitoring or from intra-amniotic pressure measurement show a characteristic pattern that makes the condition easy to recognize (Fig. 22-3b). There is a slight elevation of baseline pressure (15–18 mmHg) onto which is superimposed small, irregular contractions of high frequency. This is the most abnormal form of hypoactive uterine motility. Because only localized waves are produced, it is almost totally ineffective in promoting dilatation.

Hyperactive Uterine Motility. This condition is identified by myometrial contractions with intensities that raise intra-amniotic pressure to 70 mmHg or higher and occur more frequently than five per 10 minute period. The contractions are usually normal in contour. When manifested solely by the increased frequency of contractions, the condition is referred to as myometrial tachysystole. If the increased contraction frequency continues, it causes a progressive increase in baseline pressure and a decrease in contraction intensity. Total amplitude or intensity of the contraction complex usually remains the same.

Cervicographic Analysis

Abnormal labor has been divided into three categories based on the rates of cervical dilatation and descent of the fetal presenting part. These categories are (1) prolonged latent phase disorders,[37] (2) protraction disorders,[38] and (3) arrest disorders.[39] Because data generated for normal labor supported separation of nulliparous[31] from multiparous[29] patients, this distinction was

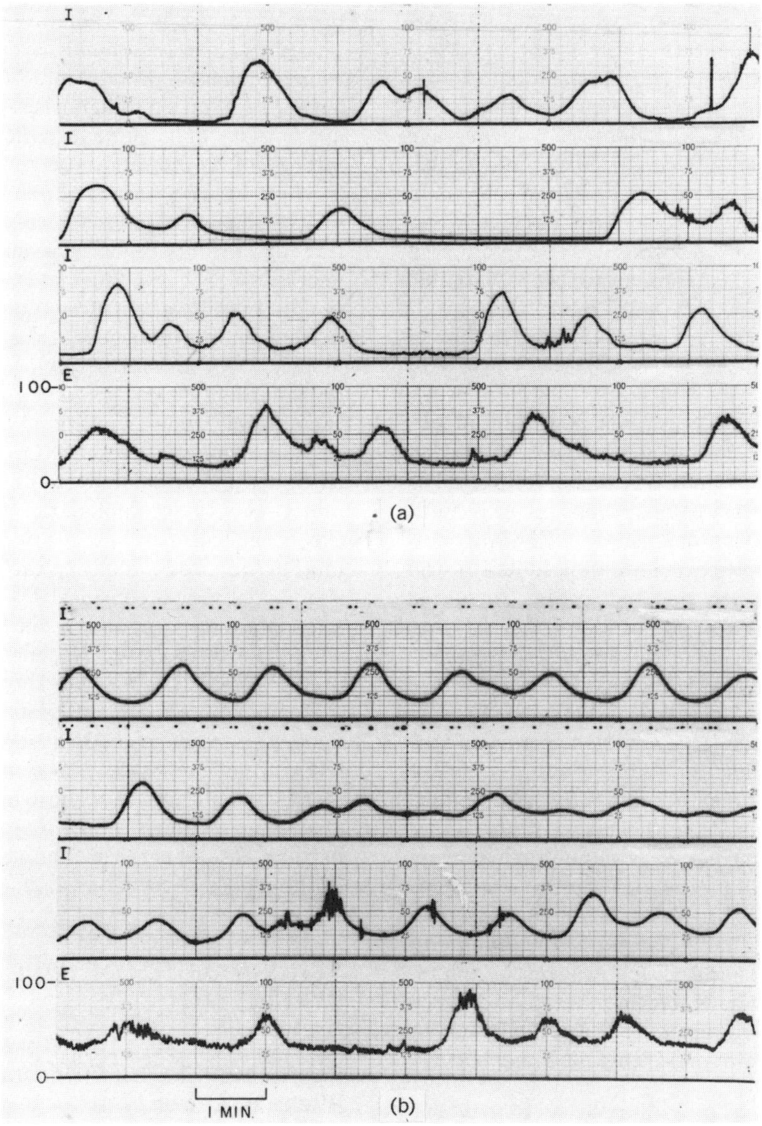

Figure 22-3. (a) Polygraph tracings of hypertonic uterine dysfunction showing the asynchronous patterns of first-degree incoordination. Contraction patterns were recorded by internal monitoring (I) in three patients and by external tocodynamometry (E) in one patient. (b) Three internal (I) and one external (E) monitor recordings illustrating the characteristics of second-degree incoordination.

also made for the diagnostic criteria of abnormal labor patterns.[35]

Prolonged Latent Phase Disorders. The diagnosis of prolonged latent phase is based on the passage of excessive time during which the cervix fails to dilate beyond 3–4 cm. In nulliparous women, the diagnosis is made if the latent phase is longer than 20 hours and, in multiparous patients, if it is longer than 14 hours.

Protraction Disorders. Protraction disorders consist of two subdivisions, (1) protracted active dilatation when the cervix fails to dilate at a rate considered to be normal and (2) protracted descent when the presenting part fails to descend at the normal rate but progress in cervical dilatation continues. Active phase dilatation is considered to be protracted in the nulliparous patient when the cervix dilates at an average rate of less than 1.2 cm/h and in the multiparous patient at a rate of less than 1.5 cm/h. Protracted descent is considered to occur when the presenting part descends less than 1 cm/h in nulliparous and 2 cm/h in multiparous patients.

Arrest Disorders. Arrest disorders are four in number and consist of (1) secondary arrest of dilatation, (2) arrest of descent, (3) failure of descent, and (4) prolonged deceleration phase. Two hours without change in cervical dilatation is considered the minimal criterion for diagnosis of secondary arrest of dilatation for both nulliparous and multiparous patients. For both nulliparous and multiparous women, failure of the presenting part to descend during a period greater than one hour is considered the criterion for arrested descent. The diagnostic criterion for failure of descent is absence of descent of the presenting part during late first stage or the second stage of labor. This criterion carries no specific time limits for either nulliparous or multiparous patients. In nulliparas, a prolonged deceleration phase is diagnosed when more than three hours passes without further progress in cervical dilatation. In multiparas, a prolonged deceleration phase is diagnosed when there is lack of change for more than one hour.

Combined disorders such as arrest of dilatation occurring when labor has already exhibited protraction disorders in cervical dilatation or descent of the fetal presenting part may occur.[36]

MANAGEMENT OF ABNORMAL LABOR

The management of abnormal labor begins with the ability to recognize and to characterize the abnormality. Since Friedman's work in the 1950s, American obstetrical management has relied heavily on the graphing and analysis of the cervical dilatation rate. However, use of the pattern of cervicographic changes for the diagnosis of abnormal labor requires the prior passage of some period of time without significant progress in order to establish the diagnosis. Evaluation of the frequency, duration, intensity, and configuration of myometrial contractions can indicate the presence of abnormal labor as it occurs. Consideration of the rate of cervical dilatation and the rate of descent of the fetal presenting part, in conjunction with the characteristics of the individual myometrial contractions, decreases procrastination and results in earlier recognition, diagnosis, and institution of appropriate management, which is in the best interest of mother and fetus.

Once it is established that labor is not progressing satisfactorily, evaluation of the patient and formulation of a management plan are necessary. Several questions should be answered initially and at frequent intervals as abnormal labor is managed: Is the patient in active labor? Are the contractions adequate? Is the fetus normally formed and in good condition? Is the mother in good condition? Is the pelvis adequate for the size, presentation, and position of the fetus? Is vaginal delivery or cesarean section more likely to accomplish the goal of obtaining the healthiest infant from the healthiest mother? If, after evaluating the abnormal labor, vaginal delivery is considered probable and safe, a flexible plan of management with time limits should be formulated. No one method can be used exclusively. The plan should be based on methods of management that are effective for managing the suspected cause of the abnormal labor. One can usually determine whether a method is effective in a short period of time by observing changes in myometrial contraction pattern, rate of cervical dilatation, and descent of the fetal presenting part.

ABNORMALITIES OF HYPOACTIVE UTERINE MOTILITY

Dysfunction in the Prodromal or Latent Phase of Labor

No matter what terminology is used, prodromal labor, prelabor, or latent phase, prolongation of early labor does occur and requires diagnosis and appropriate management.

O'Driscoll and associates have iterated[79] and reiterated[77] that painful uterine contractions alone are not sufficient evidence of labor and one cannot assume that a woman is in labor simply because she says so. In addition to painful uterine contractions, the diagnosis of labor requires either the passage of blood-stained mucus, spontaneous rupture of the membranes, or complete effacement of the cervix with or without dilatation. If the patient does not have at least one of these criteria in association with painful contractions, she is not kept in the active labor and delivery area.

The diagnosis of prolonged latent phase is most often made in retrospect. The disorder may be impossible to distinguish from false labor. If false labor can be ruled out, prolonged latent phase labor may be due to (1) injudicious use of analgesics or anesthetics, (2) hypoactive uterine motility, or (3) unknown reasons.

The early, inappropriate use of excessive narcotic or sedative analgesics and of regional epidural anesthesia is considered to be a frequent cause of this form of labor disorder. However, the literature relating to the effects of intrapartum medications on uterine activity is conflicting and often difficult to interpret. The investigative protocols are not uniform with regard to quantitation, time of administration, repetitive administration, drug dosage, stage of labor, whether the administration was carried out with one or more accompanying drugs, and consideration of the usual increase in uterine activity noted with the passage of time. Furthermore, drugs that alter uterine activity may or may not alter the progress of labor.

Meperidine is a popular medication used for analgesia during labor. The effect of meperidine on labor varies with the phase of labor at the time of administration. Prodromal labor may be inhibited by meperidine administration, whereas well-established active-phase labor is rarely affected by the usual dose of the drug.[19,85] Other investigators have reported a significant increase in uterine activity[102] or no effect[24] following meperidine administration in early labor.

Alphaprodine, hydroxyzine, and morphine demonstrate variability in suppression of labor similar to meperidine, but all reduce overall uterine activity below that expected in normal labor.[85] Promethazine, when used alone, inhibits amplitude and frequency of uterine contractions.[92] Pentazocine decreases intensity of contractions,[26] whereas diazepam reduces frequency of contraction during the postinjection interval.[123]

Studies on the effects of epidural anesthesia on uterine activity are also contradictory, but the controversy pertains more to active-phase than to latent-phase labor. Administration of epidural analgesia during the latent phase may readily inhibit the progress of labor. Administration of an epidural anesthetic in proper dosage (see Chapter 8) to a patient in well-established active-phase labor has little[25,94,95] or no effect.[56,86] However, a transient inhibition of uterine activity for 10–30 minutes following injection of anesthetic during all phases of labor has been reported by several investigators.[54,69,124,114] The addition of epinephrine to the anesthetic agent has been associated with a further decrease in the intensity of uterine activity,[71] although this decrease may be very transient.[18]

Treatment modalities available for management of a prolonged latent phase of labor are (1) therapeutic rest, (2) oxytocin stimulation of uterine contractions, and (3) amniotomy. Therapeutic rest and oxytocin infusion are equally effective in treatment of the prolonged latent phase. Amniotomy alone may not be an effective treatment for this labor disorder in nulliparous patients,[37] but it is often effective in multiparous patients.[35] However, even in the multiparous woman, amniotomy has the disadvantage of making an irreversible commitment to reasonably expeditious delivery because of the possibility of intra-amniotic infection or other complications. These circumstances may result in unnecessary operative intervention, especially if the cervix is unfavorable at the onset.

The regimen of therapeutic rest[35,37] involves the use of relatively large doses of narcotic analgesics. Depending on the physical size of the patient, 15–20 mg of morphine sulfate may be administered intramuscularly. This regimen generally results in 6–10 hours of moderate to deep narcosis. An additional dose of morphine may be required in rare instances if the first dose does not result in adequate rest. The vast majority of patients treated in this manner awaken in the active phase of labor without the likelihood of having subsequent abnormal labor patterns. Approximately 10% of patients awaken having no uterine contractions and a retrospective diagnosis of false labor will be made. A smaller number, approximately 5% of patients, awaken with persistence of the previous pattern. In these cases, the treatment has been unsuccessful, but the patient will be rested and better able to undergo other modes of management.

Oxytocin stimulation of uterine contractions in the latent phase of labor is advantageous in patients in whom delivery needs to be expedited or who are acceptable candidates for active management.[78,79,80] The patient will usually enter active-phase labor within three hours after initiation of oxytocin therapy. A disadvantage of oxytocin stimulation is that some of the patients are really in false labor and are actually undergoing induction, rather than stimulation of labor, sometimes under less than ideal circumstances. In addition, one may encounter the further disadvantage of initiating active labor in a woman who is already exhausted and frustrated.

Management. The dilemma of distinguishing between false and latent-phase labor may be resolved by external tocodynamometric monitoring. These polygraphic tracings may distinguish between the small, focally uncoordinated contractions that occur one to two days prior to labor (Fig. 22-1, Patterns 1 and 2) and the more coordinated contractions of advancing prelabor (Fig. 22-1, Patterns 3 and 4) or dysfunctional labor (Fig. 22-3). The passage of blood-stained mucus, complete effacement of the cervix, or spontaneous rupture of the membranes in a documented term gestation should be noted. Occurrence of any of these events associated with painful, regular, although perhaps infrequent, uterine contractions is a good indication that labor has begun.

Whenever the latent phase of labor is prolonged in the presence of sedative, analgesic, or anesthetic usage, the first step of management should be elimination of the exogenous factor. No additional treatment other than allowing the drug or drugs to be metabolized from the maternal circulation is needed unless the mother or the fetus is in specific danger from other causes such as intrauterine infection or evidence of fetal distress.

As with most obstetrical problems, a single approach applied to all patients results in overtreatment of some and undertreatment of others. This certainly applies to the management of prolonged latent-phase labor. The spectrum of patients extends from the exhausted, dehydrated nulliparous woman with a totally unfavorable cervix to the relaxed multiparous patient with a cervix that is 2–3 cm dilated and partially effaced. Therefore, for purposes of treatment, these patients are divided into two groups. The first group consists of all nulliparous patients and those multiparous patients with unfavorable cervices. All multiparous patients in whom the cervix is favorable should comprise the second group. These distinctions may not be clear-cut. Astute clinical judgment must be used, taking into consideration knowledge of the individual patient.

The first group of patients are the ones that will benefit most from the therapeutic rest regimen. In this group will be included most of the patients in whom evaluation of external tocodynamometric monitoring failed to reveal that they were actually in false labor. By therapeutic rest, these patients are saved an unnecessary and possibly unsuccessful elective induction of labor. Setting arbitrary time limits for the initiation of therapeutic rest is certainly not as important as is the clinical status of the patient. For example, if an exhausted, frustrated nulliparous woman has been having regular contractions for 16 hours or a multiparous woman for 10 hours, there is little justification for waiting four more hours to meet the definition of prolonged latent phse before treatment is initiated. Prior to drug administration, evaluations of the pelvis and of fetal parameters are mandatory. Because of the potential of neonatal depression, this regimen should not be used if there is any evidence that the patient is entering the active phase of labor.

The multiparous patient with a favorable cervix presents an entirely different situation. These women are usually calm, relaxed, and comfortable. There is little justification for allowing them to experience a prolonged latent phase. Management should consist of an observation period of two to four hours to confirm that no progress is occurring. This is followed by oxytocin stimulation. Prior to the use of oxytocin, the patient should be evaluated for disproportion and malpresentations that might make stimulation inadvisable. The obstetrician also must be assured of fetal maturity before oxytocin stimulation is instituted.

Oxytocin should be administered only by carefully controlled, continuous intravenous infusion, preferably using an infusion pump. Initial dosage should be very low with gradual increases until satisfactory labor is achieved (see Chapter 23). The success rate under these circumstances is very high, with few complications and a short interval between initiation of treatment and onset of active labor. This approach also may be used with caution for nulliparous women with very favorable cervices. Uterine activity and fetal heart rate patterns should be monitored continuously by external tocodynamometry. If for any reason the fetal heart rate cannot be monitored continuously, it is imperative that it be checked immediately following a contraction, rather than waiting a minute or more afterward. The membranes should not be ruptured artificially. Internal monitoring should not be used until progress in cervical dilatation is documented and a definite commitment to delivery is made.

Any choice of management of prolonged latent phase of labor should consider the thoughts and wishes of the patient, provided that they do not conflict with sound obstetrical judgment.

Regardless of whether or not the latent phase is recognized as a part of actual labor, there is agreement on one point: cesarean delivery is not indicated simply for failure to progress during this phase.

Dysfunction in the Active Phase of Labor

The foundation for any plan of management of abnormalities in the active phase of labor is recognition of the disorders. This usually requires continuous electronic monitoring of the uterine contraction pattern along with recording of the rate of cervical dilatation and descent of the fetal presenting part. When an abnormality of cervical dilatation occurs, distinction between hypoactive and hyperactive uterine dysfunction and between protracted labor and secondary arrest must be made.

The abnormalities of the active phase of labor allow for five methods of possible management: (1) observation with physiologic and emotional support, (2) maternal sedation or analgesia, (3) ambulation, (4) stimulation of myometrial contractions, and (5) cesarean delivery. The proper choice of these alternatives relies on the obstetrician's ability to recognize the type of abnormality, an understanding of its possible etiologies, and a thorough knowledge of procedures available for treatment.

Protraction Disorders. Protraction of cervical dilatation and descent of the fetal presenting part are closely related and are considered concurrently.

Myometrial contractions are characterized by hypoactive motility patterns. The contractions are either of inadequate intensity, too infrequent, uncoordinated, of too short duration, or combinations of these disorders. The obstetrician can usually identify the abnormal contraction patterns of hypotonic uterine dysfunction by abdominal palpation of the uterus, but either external or internal electronic measurement is helpful for documentation. Although hypotonic or hypocontractile contractions differ from the contractions of normal spontaneous labor in several respects in addition to maximal amplitude,[99] the differences most likely will not be appreciated by the clinician during the course of labor. When protraction disorders result from hypertonic or hypercontractility patterns of frequent, low-intensity, uncoordinated, short-duration contractions, electronic monitoring of uterine activity usually identifies the contraction abnormality (Fig. 22-3b).

The causes of these disorders are unknown but are undoubtedly related in part to abnormalities of the endocrinology of parturition. The concentrations of prostaglandins in amniotic fluid in normal labor differ from those in prolonged labor. Prostaglandin $F_{2\alpha}$ and 13,14-hydro-15-keto-prostaglandin $F_{2\alpha}$ are significantly lower in patients with prolonged labor.[90] Differences in oxytocin levels may also be involved in prolonged labor. The clearance rates and concentrations of oxytocin measured in plasma obtained from women during hypocontractile labor are similar to those recorded for nonpregnant individuals.[2] Although some investigators have found no difference in plasma oxytocin levels measured during active labor as compared to nonpregnant women,[65] others have reported plasma oxytocin levels during spontaneous labor to be consistently above levels observed one to two weeks before the onset of labor and higher than levels measured in control patients.[43]

Malpresentations and varying degrees of fetopelvic disproportion are associated with approximately one-third of cases of protracted labor. Heavy sedation also is considered to be a contributory factor. Rupture of the membranes prior to or early in the course of labor has been noted in a large number of these patients.[38] Overdistention of the uterus, as occurs with multiple gestation and hydramnios, also may contribute to primary uterine dysfunction. Protraction disorders occur more often in nulliparous women over the age of 30 years,[14,106] in post-term[106] or postmature pregnancies,[52] and in association with chorioamnionitis.[22] Hypotension can cause a decrease in frequency and intensity of uterine activity, as well as a decrease in baseline pressure. The fault seldom lies in a cervix that is too rigid to dilate. However, in elderly nulliparas and in women whose cervices are fibrosed from cervical conization, laser, or cryosurgery, excessive rigidity of the cervix may be a factor in the production of dystocia.

Treatment of protraction disorders is not universally established except in cases when absolute fetopelvic disproportion can be documented. Friedman and Sachtleben[35,38] recommend a regimen of passive supportive measures such as hydration, nutrition, rest, and psychological encouragement. They maintain that even with oxytocin stimulation, the rate of dilatation of the cervix and descent of the presenting part cannot be accelerated. This contention is supported by others,[48,53] especially in the presence of hypertonic or uncoordinated contractions. Artificial rupture of the membranes is considered by some to be of no value in the treatment of most instances of protracted labor.[34,53] Consequently, they believe that rupture of the membranes should be avoided.

The frequency and intensity of uterine contractions is affected by the patient's position and may be used to influence labor in protraction disorders. Frequency of contractions is increased when the patient assumes the sitting or standing position.[72] Contraction intensity and total uterine work also increase. The pressure on the uterine cervix is increased approximately 10 mmHg as a result of increased intrauterine pressure and an additional 20 mmHg from the weight exerted by the intrauterine contents transmitted to the lower uterine segment. There is an average increase of baseline pressure and contraction amplitude during labor of over 8 mmHg with walking as compared to bedrest. Ambulation may be as effective as oxytocin for the enhancement of labor.[89]

The regimen of passive support is opposed by other experienced clinicians who consider that active intervention is mandated if the rate of cervical dilatation does not exceed 1 cm each hour. [78-80] They recommend stimulation by artificial rupture of the amniochorionic membranes. After an interval of one hour, if progress is not satisfactory, oxytocin infusion is started. They and other authorities[8] believe that the uncoordinated contractions of hypertonic uterine dysfunction will respond to stimulation with oxytocic agents. They further advocate oxytocin stimulation as an essential prerequisite to the diagnosis of fetopelvic disproportion when the natural forces of labor are not adequate.

Management. The first step in the management of primary uterine dysfunction or protraction disorders in the active phase of labor requires clinical evaluation of the status of the patient and the course of labor. Factors such as sedation, conduction anesthesia, estimated fetal size, and maternal fatigue must be assessed. A careful vaginal examination should be performed to verify dilatation, station, presentation, and position and to reassess the pelvic structures. Vaginal examination performed during a contraction is helpful to determine the expelling force of the contraction, the response of the cervix to the contraction and to the pressure of the presenting part, and the response of the presenting part to the contraction and to the maternal pelvis. Unusual causes of dystocia such as obstruction from uterine, vaginal, or ovarian lesions, fetal malformation, and overdistention of the bladder must be excluded.

Next, a decision must be made whether to employ passive, supportive management, to stimulate labor with oxytocin, or to effect cesarean delivery. In the absence of absolute fetopelvic disproportion, resorting to abdominal delivery without a further trial of labor is not justified.

Once the diagnosis of hyoactive uterine dysfunction in the active phase of labor has been made and the fetal presenting part is engaged, or at least has descended through the pelvic inlet to near zero station, the membranes, if intact, should be ruptured. An intrauterine pressure catheter and a fetal scalp electrode should be applied. The visible presence of meconium in the amniotic fluid makes continuous monitoring of fetal heart activity in response to uterine contraction patterns critical (see Chapter 11). Following amniotomy, close observation should be employed for 30–60 minutes to see if the quality of labor improves. If it does not, oxytocin administration should be initiated. If the hypoactive uterine motility pattern being treated is uncoordinated, hypertonic contractions, internal monitoring of intra-amniotic pressure changes is mandatory to determine whether the abnormal contraction complexes convert to physiological patterns rather than become accentuated with an increase in baseline pressure.

The optimal period of time required for oxytocin stimulation prior to a decision as to success or failure is poorly defined. One characteristic of intravenous oxytocin is that, when successful, it acts promptly, leading to noticeable progress in cervical dilatation with little delay. For any given rate of infusion, the plasma level reaches a plateau after about 30 minutes as the rate of infusion and the rate of destruction of oxytocin achieve equilibrium. The drug, therefore, need not be used for an indefinite period, nor should it be used to force cervical dilatation at a rate that exceeds normal (Chapter 23). It should be employed for no more than a few hours. If by then the cervix has not changed appreciably and if a predictably easy vaginal delivery is not imminent, cesarean section should be performed.

Arrest Disorders. Management of the arrest disorders of labor centers on determining the adequacy of the maternal pelvis in order to select the most appropriate route of delivery. Relative or absolute fetopelvic disproportion and malpresentation are the most probable causes of these disorders. Excessive analgesic-sedative medication and improperly administered conduction anesthesia have also been implicated.

Myometrial contractions most often are of the hypoactive motility, hypotonic variety, but hypertonic abnormalities and hyperactive uterine motility may also be present. In hypotonic dysfunction, the usual forces of labor are replaced by myometrial contractions of lower amplitude and decreasing frequency with or without changes in duration. Development of hypotonic uterine dysfunction during the active phase of labor is often a protective mechanism against disproportion due to some degree of pelvic contracture or fetal abnormality. Typically, the uterus does not persist in spontaneous activity that would lead to its own destruction by rupture.

The coordinated contractions of hypotonic dysfunction may be replaced by uncoordinated contractions of higher frequency and elevated baseline pressure suggestive of hypertonic uterine dysfunction. These contractions must be differentiated from hyperactive uterine motility. This distinction between hypoactive, hypertonic dysfunction and hyperactive uterine motility, especially when associated with the arrest disorders of labor, is of considerable importance because of differing dangers imposed by these abnormalities and their response to therapy (see section entitled Abnormalities of Hyperactive Uterine Motility).

A comprehensive knowledge of pelvic anatomy is required for interpretation of clinical pelvimetry and determination of the presence of fetopelvic disproportion. In terms of objective measurements, only the diagonal conjugate and, to a lesser degree, the angle of the pubic arch and the bi-ischial diameter can be determined manually (see Chapter 7). Measurement of the diagonal conjugate is easily performed and accurately quantifiable. When the diagonal conjugate measures greater than 11.5 cm, the obstetrical conjugate is rarely less than 10 cm. This virtually excludes the possibility of contracture of the pelvic inlet in the anteroposterior diameter. Exceedingly narrow or wide measurements of the pubic arch and the bi-ischial diameter may suggest an unfavorable configuration of the mid or outlet portions of the maternal bony pelvis.

Accurate measurement of other pelvic dimensions can be ascertained only by x-ray pelvimetry. Measurements of the anteroposterior and transverse diameters of the pelvic inlet, midplane, and outlet are achievable by a number of radiological techniques. All systems of pelvimetry use these diameters either directly or in conjunction with measurements of the fetal skull. However, controversy exists about both the risks and the utility of x-ray pelvimetry in evaluating fetopelvic disproportion. Although x-ray pelvimetry must be considered as potentially hazardous to the fetus,[20,87,105] the existing evidence is contradictory.[17,51,82] Various investigators studying leukemia induction in children exposed to radiation in utero have found no statistically significant difference in relative risk compared to control populations.[1,45,59,67,74,81,120]

The utilization of x-ray pelvimetry in obstetrics has not changed substantially for many years,[5] but an increasing number of studies question the efficiency and value of the procedure. The conclusions of some of these studies have been that x-ray pelvic measurements obtained on patients with labor disorders did not differ from controls,[93] did not shorten the duration of labor or correlate with cesarean section rate,[60] were not related to the mode of delivery,[57] and did not improve neonatal mortality.[3] Other reports have held that the use of x-ray pelvimetry did correlate with the need for operative delivery[27,46,115] and with the incidence of perinatal mortality and morbidity.[44] Parsons and Spellacy[84] suggest that, in primigravida women, the elimination of x-ray pelvimetry does not lead to a compromise of infant outcome, provided electronic fetal monitoring is used. From these reports, one must conclude that x-ray pelvimetry may yield useful information in some patients, but it is seldom the pivotal point in patient management decisions.

Differences of opinion exist also in selection of those patients with the arrest disorders of labor, but without evidence of absolute fetopelvic disproportion, who are candidates for oxytocin stimulation. O'Driscoll and associates[77] make a very clear distinction between the management of primigravid and multiparous labor. They administer oxytocin to nulliparous women but feel that, because of the danger of uterine rupture, it should be avoided in the multiparous patient. Others believe that stimulation by oxytocin infusion is warranted in both nulliparous[97] and multiparous[98] patients. Similar views are held by Friedman and Sachtleben,[35,39] who consider the minimal time required to test the ability of oxytocin stimulation to produce additional cervical dilatation to be four hours.[40]

Management. The first step in treatment of arrest of active-phase labor is reevaluation of pelvic adequacy and of fetal presentation and attitude. Clinical pelvimetry is an integral part of the evaluation of all dysfunctional labor patterns but is of especial importance in arrest disorders. It should be ascertained that the pelvis is probably adequate for the size of the fetus and, if the presentation is vertex, that the fetal head is well-flexed so as to utilize the smallest (biparietal and suboccipitobregmatic) diameters to negotiate the pelvis. It is likely that the pelvis is adequate for a given fetus when (1) the diagonal conjugate is normal, (2) the pelvic sidewalls are nearly parallel, (3) the ischial spines are not prominent, (4) the sacrum is curved, (5) the pubic arch is wide, (6) the occiput is presenting, and (7) the fetal head descends further through the pelvic inlet with fundal pressure.

Abnormal fetal presentation and possible disproportion due to fetal macrosomia, congenital factors, or deflexion attitude of the presenting part must be excluded. Abdominal reexamination and performance of the maneuvers of Leopold (see Chapter 7) should be performed. Sonography may also aid in these determinations, but it is of limited value for evaluation of fetal factors below the brim of the mother's pelvis.

If the obstetrician cannot resolve these questions, a single standing lateral x-ray examination should be considered before subjecting mother and fetus to several hours of possible unsuccessful uterine stimulation or to abdominal delivery. Estimated exposure to the fetus from a single lateral x-ray of an average patient (15 inch lateral diameter) is 0.11 rads. The decision to use this procedure should rely on the probability of gaining information that will help to guide management. Reasons for obtaining x-ray pelvimetry should be individually established. The examination should be an aid to, not a requirement for, clinical decisions concerning obstetrical management.

The alternatives for management are cesarean section or oxytocin stimulation. Those mothers whose uterine contractions have been of normal quality and quantity, but who have failed to make normal progress, or whose fetus is exhibiting signs of distress, should be delivered by cesarean section. Patients in whom there is no evidence of serious disproportion or fetal distress should undergo a further trial of labor with oxytocin stimulation. When oxytocin is used, it is mandatory that the fetal heart rate and the uterine contraction pattern be monitored continuously.

A trial of labor requires a period of time to initiate the oxytocin infusion, additional time to adjust the dose to achieve the desired myometrial response, and a period of adequate contractility during which progress in effacement, dilatation, rotation, flexion, and descent of the presenting part can be observed. These procedures require a minimum of three to four hours, even when conducted most efficiently. Patients who respond to oxytocin augmentation with normal cervical dilatation and exhibit no signs of fetal distress should be allowed to continue labor. Vaginal delivery is anticipated. Supportive therapy with adequate hydration and appropriate analgesia should be initiated before maternal dehydration or exhaustion appear.

ABNORMALITIES OF MATERNAL EXPULSIVE FORCES

With descent of the presenting part toward the pelvic floor stimulating the perineal reflex, most women have an urge to push or bear down each time the uterus contracts. The combined forces created by the contractions of the uterus and by the abdominal musculature facilitate the propulsion of the fetus down the vagina and, in the case of spontaneous delivery, through the vaginal outlet. At times, the force created by voluntary contraction of the abdominal musculature is diminished sufficiently to retard, but seldom to prevent, spontaneous vaginal delivery.

Conduction anesthesia may reduce the reflex urge for the woman to push and may impair her ability to contract the abdominal muscles sufficiently to increase intra-abdominal pressure.[54-70,121] In some instances the reflex urge to push remains, but expulsive efforts are less effective because myometrial contractions have been depressed by the occurrence of maternal hypotension or aortocaval compression. Uterine activity has been shown to be decreased by postepidural hypotension[116] and by occlusion of the aorta [47,118] as may occur when the term pregnant woman is placed in the supine or dorsal lithotomy position.

In other instances, the reflex urge to push may be overridden by the intensification of the pain that is created by bearing down. Rarely, insufficient expulsive efforts may be the consequence of longstanding paralysis of the abdominal musculature, as after transsection of the spinal cord or poliomyelitis.

Management. Increased encouragement of the patient, oxytocin stimulation of weak contractions, and elective outlet forceps can be used to expedite delivery in the patient in whom expulsive efforts are ineffective.

Careful selection of the type and dosage of anesthesia and the timing of administration are important if compromise to voluntary expulsive efforts is to be avoided. With continuous epidural anesthesia, it may be necessary to allow the paralytic effects of the drug to wear off so that the mother, in response to coaching, can generate intra-abdominal pressures sufficient to accomplish spontaneous delivery or to move the fetal head into position appropriate for low forceps delivery. Oxytocin may also be employed to achieve these goals. In the absence of significant fetal distress or disproportion, the alternatives of a possibly difficult midforceps vaginal delivery or cesarean section are unsatisfactory choices.

For the woman who cannot bear down appropriately because of extreme discomfort, due either to the intensity of the contraction or to perineal pressure, analgesia is likely to be of benefit. Nitrous oxide mixed with an equal volume of oxygen and provided during each uterine contraction is safe for fetus and mother. At the same time, appropriate encouragement and instruction will be of benefit.

ABNORMALITIES OF HYPERACTIVE UTERINE MOTILITY

Hyperactive motility patterns are most commonly produced by the infusion of excessive amounts of oxytocic drugs. They also may occur spontaneously in obstructed labor, toxemia of pregnancy, with abruption of the placenta, and, in some cases, without evident cause. Maternal hyperthermia[73] and local application of heat to the maternal abdomen[61] may also provoke these patterns. Hyperactivity in the absence of mechanical obstruction usually produces precipitate or tumultuous labor.

Oxytocin Overdosage (Fig. 22-4). Oxytocin stimulates both electrical and contractile activity in uterine smooth muscle. It increases the intensity and frequency of uterine contractions, accelerates the spreading of the contractile waves through the uterus, and improves the coordination of the contractions.[10] Although usually both the intensity and the frequency of uterine contractions are increased, the relationship is inconsistent.[88] On occasion, infusion of oxytocin elicits a pronounced increase in intensity of contractions, but the frequency remains unchanged or, at times, slightly diminished. In other instances, an augmentation in the frequency of contractions may occur without significant effects on intensity. Change in baseline pressure or tonus of the uterus in response to oxytocin is independent of the changes in contraction frequency and intensity. Normally, the increase in baseline pressure is very slight, being most marked during the first 15 minutes after the start of the oxytocin infusion.

The rate of oxytocin infusion required to produce hyperactive uterine motility usually is related inversely to the preexisting degree of spontaneous uterine activity. With oxytocin overdosage, there may be a rapid, marked, and persistent rise in baseline pressure. Frequency of contractions may increase, but amplitude will decrease. This series of events may be incorrectly interpreted as a failure of response to oxytocin and, consequently, the rate of drug infusion increased. If the drug infusion is continued, the individual contractions may disappear and only a plateau of very high baseline pressure will be recorded. This condition is designated as "contracture" or "uterine tetany" and may signal impending uterine rupture. The elevated baseline pressure will remain as long as the oxytocin infusion is continued. When the oxytocin infusion is stopped, baseline pressure decreases progressively and individual contractions reappear, gradually increasing in amplitude and decreasing in frequency. If the baseline pressure exceeds 30 mmHg, the uterus becomes so firm during diastole that the contractions cannot be perceived by abdominal palpation, emphasizing the need for internal monitoring of intra-amniotic pressure in most instances of oxytocin stimulation.

Obstructed Labor. Mechanical factors such as a contracted pelvis and tumors located in the lower uterine segment or in the cul-de-sac and fetal causes such as macrosomia, congenital abnormalities, and malpresentations may prevent descent of the presenting part and engender hyperactive uterine motility. The patient may be restless and anxious and may have an increased body temperature and pulse rate.

At the beginning of labor, uterine contractions are normal in character and cause a progressive shortening of the upper uterine segments and stretching of the lower uterine segments, together with some effacement and

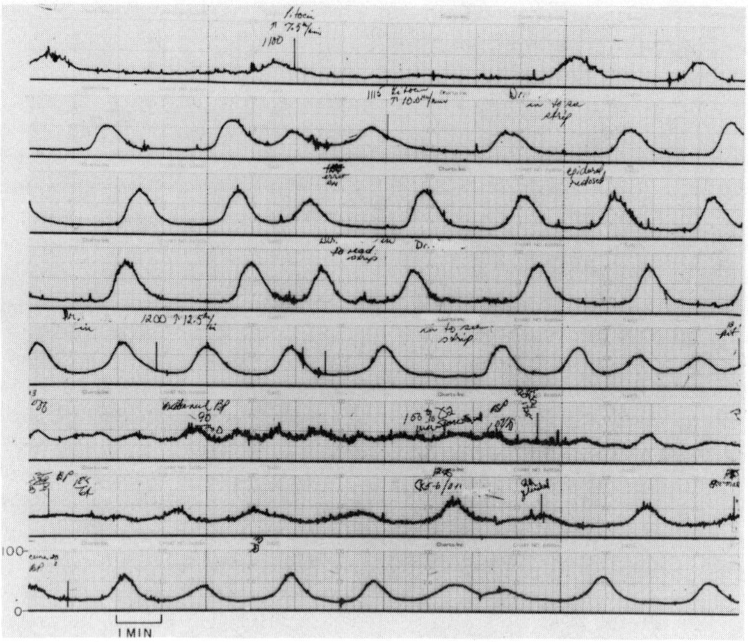

Figure 22-4. Polygraph tracing of 120 min of internal monitoring illustrating the effect of oxytocin overdosage. Oxytocin infusion rate was increased from 7.5 mU/min (segment 1) to 10 mU/min less than 20 minutes later (segment 2) and to 12.5 mU/min in segment 5. Oxytocin was discontinued at the beginning of segment 6. Approximately four hours later, the patient spontaneously delivered a 2900 g male infant with Apgar scores of 8 and 9.

dilatation of the cervix. In the presence of mechanical obstruction, the shortening of the upper uterine segment stretches the lower segment to a greater extent. After each contraction, the upper segment remains shorter and thicker and the lower segment becomes more distended and thinner. The physiological retraction ring discussed in Chapter 7 becomes more clearly defined and rises to an abnormally high position (Bandl's pathologic retraction ring). This elevation of the retraction ring is due to the extreme shortening of the upper uterine segment which is not counterbalanced by descent of the fetal presenting part. The round ligaments become very tense and easy to palpate abdominally (Frommel's sign) because their progressive retraction, which normally occurs simultaneously with that of the upper segment, has also been prevented.

The myometrial contractions progressively increase in amplitude and frequency, reaching and surpassing the maximal values recorded for normal labor. When the frequency of contractions surpasses five per 10 minute period, their amplitude progressively decreases and the baseline pressure increases because of incomplete relaxation, similar to the pattern observed with oxytocin overdosage. In some cases of obstructed labor, after a few hours of hyperactive uterine motility, myometrial contractions become progressively weaker and a contraction pattern consistent with hypoactive uterine motility develops.

Toxemia of Pregnancy and Abruption of the Placenta (Fig. 22-5). Uterine contractility is frequently much higher in intensity and frequency in patients with severe preeclampsia or eclampsia (Fig. 22-5a) than in patients of the same gestational age who do not have pregnancy-induced hypertension. [8,13,109,110] In some patients, only the intensity of contractions is abnormally high, whereas in others the frequency of the contractions and the baseline resting pressure of the myometrium are unusually high. The contractions may not be adequately coordinated to produce cervical dilatation. These patients often do not respond to rupture of the membranes, but the uterine response to oxytocin stimulation may be much greater than normal.

In placental abruption (Fig. 22-5b), the uter-

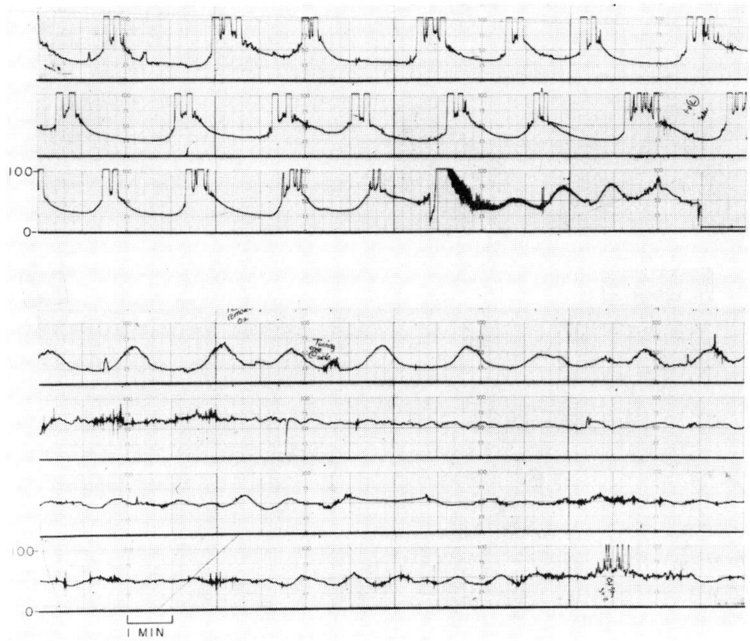

Figure 22-5. (a) Forty-eight minutes of intra-amniotic pressure recording obtained from a 16-year-old primigravida with pregnancy-induced hypertension. Near the end of segment 3, the patient experienced an eclamptic convulsion. Approximately one hour after the convulsion, she delivered a 3350 g male infant with Apgar scores of 4 and 8. (b) Polygraph tracing of intra-amniotic pressure recorded from a patient who experienced a 20% abruption of the placenta near the end of the first segment. This 18-year-old primigravida received four units of whole blood for stabilization and was delivered vaginally approximately two hours later of a 3990 g female infant with Apgar scores of 3 and 5.

ine baseline pressure may be two to four times greater than it is in normal labor.[8] Superimposed on the high baseline pressure, there may be rhythmic contractions of 20–30 mmHg intensity with a frequency similar to that of normal labor. In other cases, there may be tachysystole or incoordination, which add their hypertonic effects to the rise in baseline pressure. The combination of a rising baseline pressure and a high frequency of contractions is highly suggestive of severe placental abruption.[75] As in oxytocin overdosage and obstructed labor, the uterus may be so firm between contractions that individual increases in myometrial activity are not perceived by abdominal palpation or external tocodynamometry, giving the erroneous clinical impression that the uterus is not contracting.

Precipitate and Tumultuous Labor. In precipitate labor, the first and second stages of labor are usually less than three hours in duration. In some patients, the fetus may be delivered within only a few minutes after the onset of uterine contractions. Precipitate labor occurs predominantly in multiparous patients and may result from an abnormally low resistance of the pelvic structures or from abnormally strong uterine and abdominal muscle contractions. Precipitate labor should be distinguished from a precipitous delivery, which is the abrupt, frequently uncontrolled expulsion of the fetus at the end of the second stage of labor and unrelated to the total duration.

The rapid deliveries that follow precipitate labor may cause cervical, vaginal, and other pelvic lacerations. This is especially true when the etiology is related to hyperactive uterine motility rather than to decreased resistance of the pelvic tissues. The condition is frequently accompanied by hypoactive uterine contractility postpartum, with resultant hemorrhage from the placental site. The associated occurrence of amniotic fluid embolism, although very unusual, is more likely to occur when there is extensive maternal tissue damage.

Perinatal morbidity and mortality may be increased appreciably by precipitate or tumultuous labor. Due to the high intensity and frequency of myometrial contractions, shortening of the relaxation period takes place. The time for return of adequate uterine blood flow to allow oxygen equilibration between mother and fetus is decreased. This may cause progressive fetal hypoxia and hypercarbia. However, the incidence of abnormal fetal heart rate patterns is reportedly approximately one-half the frequency observed in patients with normal labor.[83] Physical injury to the fetus, including intracranial trauma, might also be expected, especially if the resistance of the pelvic tissues is great. Such fetal trauma is, however, rare. The literature on the effects of precipitate labor ranges from reports that the incidence of stillbirths and neonatal death are appreciably higher[112] to conclusions that precipitate labor need not be considered an intrapartum risk factor to the fetus[23] and statements that mother and baby react favorably to precipitate labor, which, in some respects, is more desirable than labor of normal length.[15] However, most of these reports did not utilize the diagnostic evaluation methods currently available to neonatologists.

Management. Treatment of hyperactive uterine motility depends on the etiological factors and the underlying pathophysiology.

The key to management of uterine hyperactivity secondary to oxytocin overdosage is prevention through an understanding of the pharmacodynamics of oxytocin and knowledge of its proper administration. If overstimulation does occur, stopping the intravenous infusion and instituting any supportive measures necessary for either mother or fetus are usually the only therapy required. Because the clearance rate of oxytocin is short during late pregnancy,[2,64] uterine contractions return to normal within minutes (Fig. 22-4). However, if the overdosage has been sufficient to produce uterine contracture or tetany, more than an hour may be needed before uterine activity returns to preinfusion values.[88]

Prolonged obstructed labor leading to localized constrictions of the uterus is not acceptable in current obstetrical practice but still occurs in rare neglected, unattended labors. In addition to the clinical signs and symptoms, diagnosis may be aided by sonographic examination to identify the thickened myometrium at the level of the retraction ring.[62] When the fetus is viable, delivery by cesarean section is usually performed because of the causative obstruction rather than because of the constriction ring itself.

Hyperactive uterine motility associated with severe preeclampsia, eclampsia, or abruption of the placenta usually responds to the procedures initiated for management of the primary condition. Specific therapy to decrease hyperactive uterine motility related to these or any other cause is seldom indicated. However, such therapy may be of benefit when acute, severe fetal distress occurs because of decreased placental perfusion due to hyperactivity of the uterus. Intervillous space blood flow in severe preeclamptics may improve significantly after lumbar epidural analgesia.[55] The improvement probably results from a decrease in maternal catecholamines that occurs after lumbar epidural anesthesia.[101] However, this approach is not generally used. Instead, magnesium sulfate given intravenously is utilized for its tocolytic effect. The usual dose is 4 g of magnesium sulfate administered as a 20% solution at a rate of approximately 1 g per minute. Ritodrine hydrochloride, 6 mg in 10 ml of normal saline given as an intravenous bolus infusion over 2–5 minutes, has also been used successfully.[125]

EFFECT OF ABNORMAL LABOR ON INFANT AND MOTHER

The normal fetus whose mother has no obstetrical or medical complication is usually capable of undergoing the stress of a normal labor without adverse effect. However, it is well recognized that even the normal fetus whose mother has an extremely prolonged or difficult labor or whose delivery is managed inappropriately may be overcome by the added stresses and be depressed, damaged, or die. Attempts at clarifying relationships between labor progress and infant condition are complicated both by the nonspecificity of the diagnosis "abnormal labor" and by the retrospective designs of the reports.

The physiological processes of labor can have varying effects on the fetus, depending on its initial status as labor begins. These effects can range from minimal to very significant. With each uterine contraction, there is a decrease or possible stoppage of blood flow into the intervillous space, which may result in fetal hypoxia or anoxia. Fetuses who are in good condition prior to onset of labor may show an increased incidence of abnormal heart rate patterns if they are subjected to abnormal labor. However, fetuses who are in poor condition when labor begins may have the same distribution of abnormal heart rate patterns regardless of the type of active labor.[83] In general, the relationship between labor patterns and fetal heart rate patterns is that, with increasing length of active first-stage labor, there is an increasing incidence of fetal heart rate patterns that reflect fetal stress, distress, or both.[68]

Adverse effects of labor on fetal heart rate patterns may be compounded by cephalopelvic disproportion. Patients with major disproportion have a significantly higher incidence of decreased baseline variability and of both late and variable decelerations.[107] The mean value of fetal scalp pH recorded just before delivery was 7.24 ± 0.40 SEM for the infants in the major cephalopelvic disproportion group as compared to 7.32 ± 0.53 SEM for the control group of infants.

Friedman and associates[33] have shown a direct relationship between increasing abnormal labor patterns and increasing perinatal mortality. Operative vaginal procedures, specifically midforceps, were felt to contribute heavily to this mortality, but even in spontaneous deliveries, there was a marked increase in perinatal loss when arrest of labor occurred as compared to normal labor.[30]

Vosburgh and colleagues[117] determined that the incidence of depressed infants, as well as perinatal mortality, was increased in association with uterine dysfunction and abnormal labor. Others have confirmed these findings and report that, even with the use of oxytocin there is a higher incidence of forceps deliveries and of infants with low Apgar scores,[108] even when the labor abnormality was a prolonged latent phase.[11]

Parallel relationships have been demonstrated between labor duration and development of neurological abnormalities.[4] A significantly higher incidence of abnormal neurological behavior, even in the absence of fetal asphyxia, is associated with the use of midforceps in prolonged labors.[12] Studies of the short- and long-term neurological sequelae demonstrated that infants delivered following dysfunctional labor tended to display a greater incidence of abnormal motor scores[32] and had lower IQ and hearing scores.[42]

Additional factors besides the abnormal labor pattern itself may affect fetal status and lead to fetal stress or distress. Oxytocin overstimulation can cause additional stress during labor because of increasing frequency, amplitude, and baseline pressure of the stimulated contractions[100,119] and increased frequency of abnormal contractions.[41]

Maternal anxiety and pain leading to elevated catecholamine levels can accentuate the effects of abnormal labor by interfering with coordinated uterine activity, diminishing uterine blood flow, and compounding the hypoxic effects of uterine contractions on the fetus.[16,66] Difficult labors and deliveries may also be more likely to leave psychological scars on the mothers. Two studies reported that difficult labor may exert a deleterious effect on future childbearing. Although more than two-thirds of their patients had further children after spontaneous delivery, only one-third did so after midforceps operations.[52,104] However, these findings are not supported by others.[58]

A major effect of abnormal labor on the mother is the morbidity that follows abdominal delivery performed because of "failure to progress" and "failure to progress with possible fetal distress." The incidence of primary cesarean sections done because of "failure to progress" or "uterine dysfunction" ranges from 14%[103] to 39%.[50] These figures exclude abdominal deliveries performed for cephalopelvic disproportion, malpresentation, and fetal distress. Thirty percent of the overall rise in the cesarean section rate from 1970 to 1978 was in the diagnostic category of "dystocia."[21]

O'Driscoll and associates[77] contend that maternal morbidity can be reduced by taking an active approach to the management of labor as an alternative to cesarean section for dystocia. In support of this contention, they cite their cesarean section rate of 4.8% in 1980. Primary cesarean section for dystocia was required in only 0.7% of all births. However, 13% of the 324 primary cesarean sections performed were done for the indication of dystocia, including persistent posterior position and cephalopelvic disproportion. Ineffective uterine activity, despite oxytocin therapy, accounted for 4.6%. The effects of their active management approach on the infant are uncertain. The authors used electronic fetal monitoring only when clinical criteria necessitated fetal scalp blood sampling for pH. They consider the perinatal morbidity data to be insufficient for valid comparison.[76] Uncorrected perinatal mortality for infants with a birth weight of 500 g or more was 16.8 per 1000.

Management. Any delay in cervical dilatation during the first stage or prolongation of the second stage of labor should alert the obstetrician to the possibility of abnormal labor. Undue procrastination often leads to an unfortunate outcome, whereas intervention too early results in needless cesarean deliveries. Appropriate obstetrical management of patients calls for repeated evaluation of fetal status throughout labor. Since even normal labor can produce stress or distress in the fetus, it is prudent to follow carefully all patients in labor. When abnormal labor is suspected or proved and when oxytocin is utilized in its treatment, continuous internal electronic monitoring of fetal heart rate and intra-amniotic pressure is essential (see Chapter 11).

Adverse effects of abnormal labor on infant and mother may be prevented, or at least reduced, by early recognition of dysfunction. Concurrent measurement of uterine activity and progression of cervical dilatation are complementary techniques to assess labor progress and to predict more quickly the course of labor. Both methods should be used to minimize delay in proper management of abnormal labor patterns and to avoid inappropriate therapy. No matter how much evaluation there may have been prior to the diagnosis of abnormal labor no decision as to treatment should be made without first performing a careful reexamination to search for the cause and to exclude the presence of absolute disproportion and malposition of the fetus.

As with all obstetrical patients, management of abnormal labor requires careful evaluation, sound judgment, and individualization of care. The primary objective of an obstetrician is to deliver a healthy mother of a healthy, intact infant. That failing, the next objective is to give the neonatologist an infant that has the best chance of responding favorably to neonatal management, if needed. It must be remembered that cesarean section always increases maternal morbidity, and the risk of maternal mortality in patients delivered by cesarean section is two to four times greater than that associated with vaginal delivery.[21]

REFERENCES

1. Ager, E. A., Schuman, L. M., Wallace, H. M., Rosenfield, A. B., and Gullen, W. H.: An epidemiological study of childhood leukemia. *J. Chronic Dis.* **18**:113–132, 1965.
2. Amico, J. A., Seitchik J., and Robinson, A. G.: Studies of oxytocin in plasma of women during hypocontractile labor. *J. Clin. Endocrinol. Metab.* **58**:274–279, 1984.
3. Barton, J. J., Garbaciak, J. A., and Ryan, G. M.: The efficacy of x-ray pelvimetry. *Am. J. Obstet. Gynecol.* **143**:304–311, 1982.
4. Bishop, E. H., Israel, S. L., and Briscoe, C. C.: Obstetric influences on the premature infant's first year of development. A report from the collaborative study of cerebral palsy. *Obstet. Gynecol.* **26**:628–635, 1965.
5. Brown, R. F.: The selection of patients for x-ray examinations. Public Health Service, Bureau of Radiological Health. DHEW publication (FDA) 80-8104. Rockville, MD, Government Printing Office, 1980.
6. Caldeyro, R., Alvarez, H., and Reynolds, S. R. M.: A better understanding of uterine contractility through simultaneous recording with an internal and a seven channel external method. *Surg. Gynecol. Obstet.* **91**:641–650, 1950.
7. Caldeyro-Barcia, R.: Uterine contractility in obstetrics. In: *Modern Trends in Gynaecology and Obstetrics: International Congress on Gynaecology and Obstetrics.* Montreal, Librairie Beauchemin, 1958, pp. 65–102.
8. Caldeyro-Barcia, R. and Alvarez, H.: Abnormal uterine action in labour. *J. Obstet. Gynaecol. Br. Emp.* **59**:646–662, 1952.
9. Caldeyro-Barcia, R., Noriega-Guerra, L., Cibils, L. A., Alvarez, H., Poseiro, J. J., Pose, S. V., Sica-Blanco, Y., Mendez-Bauer, C., Fielitz, C., and Gonzalez-Panizza, V. H.: Effect of position changes on the intensity and frequency of uterine contractions during labor. *Am. J. Obstet. Gynecol.* **80**:284–290, 1960.
10. Caldeyro-Barcia, R. and Poseiro, J. J.: Oxytocin and contractility of the pregnant human uterus. *Ann. N.Y. Acad. Sci.* **75**:813–830, 1959.
11. Cardozo, L. D., Gibb, D. M. F., Studd, J. W. W., Vasant, R.V., and Cooper, D. J.: Predictive value of cervimetric labour patterns in primigravidae. *Br. J. Obstet. Gynaecol.* **89**:33–38, 1982.
12. Chiswick, M. L. and James, D. K.: Kielland's forceps: Association with neonatal morbidity and mortality. *Br. Med. J.* **1**:7–9, 1979.
13. Cobo, E.: Uterine hypercontractility in toxemia of pregnancy. I. Its prolonged therapeutic control. *Am. J. Obstet. Gynecol.* **90**:505–510, 1964.
14. Cohen, W. R., Newman, L., and Friedman, E. A.: Risk of labor abnormalities with advancing maternal age. *Obstet. Gynecol.* **55**:414–416, 1980.
15. Conger, G. T. and Randall, J. H.: Precipitate labor. *Am. J. Obstet. Gynecol.* **73**:1321–1325, 1957.
16. Copher, D. E., and Huber, C. P.: Heart rate response of the human fetus to induced maternal hypoxia. *Am. J. Obstet. Gynecol.* **98**:320–335, 1967.
17. Court Brown, W. M., Doll, R., and Hill, A. B.: Incidence of leukaemia after exposure to diagnostic radiation in utero. *Br. Med. J.* **2**:1539–1545, 1960.
18. Craft, J. B., Jr., Epstein, B. S., and Coakley, C. S.:

Effect of lidocaine with epinephrine versus lidocaine (plain) on induced labor. *Anesth. Analg.* **51**:243–246, 1972.

19. DeVoe, S. J., DeVoe, K., Jr., Rigsby, W. C., and McDaniels, B. A.: Effect of meperidine on uterine contractility. *Am. J. Obstet. Gynecol.* **105**:1004–1007, 1969.
20. Diamond, E. L., Schmerler, H., and Lilienfeld, A. M.: The relationship of intra-uterine radiation to subsequent mortality and development of leukemia in children. *Am. J. Epidemiol.* **97**:283–313, 1973.
21. Draft Report of the Task Force on Cesarean Childbirth. U.S. Dept. of Health and Human Services, Public Health Service. Washington, DC, National Institutes of Health, 1980.
22. Duff, P., Sanders, R., and Gibbs, R. S.: The course of labor in term patients with chorioamnionitis. *Am. J. Obstet. Gynecol.* **147**:391–395, 1983.
23. Erkkola, R. and Nikkanen, V.: Precipitate labor. *Ann. Chir. Gynaecol.* [*Suppl.*] **97**:150–153, 1978.
24. Eskes, T. K. A. B.: Effect of morphine upon uterine contractility in late pregnancy. *Am. J. Obstet. Gynecol.* **84**:281–289, 1962.
25. Filler, W. W., Jr., Hall, W. C., and Filler, N. W.: Analgesia in obstetrics. The effect of analgesia on uterine contractility and fetal heart rate. *Am. J. Obstet. Gynecol.* **98**:832–846, 1967.
26. Filler, W. W., Jr. and Filler, N. W.: Effect of a potent non-narcotic analgesic agent (Pentazocine) on uterine contractility and fetal heart rate. *Obstet. Gynecol.* **28**:224–232, 1966.
27. Fine, E. A., Bracken, M., and Berkowitz, R. L.: An evaluation of the usefulness of x-ray pelvimetry: Comparison of the Thoms and modified Ball methods with manual pelvimetry. *Am. J. Obstet. Gynecol.* **137**:15–20, 1980.
28. Friedman, E. A.: The graphic analysis of labor. *Am. J. Obstet. Gynecol.* **68**:1568–1575, 1954.
29. Friedman, E. A.: Labor in multiparas: A graphicostatistical analysis. *Obstet. Gynecol.* **8**:691–703, 1956.
30. Friedman, E. A.: Patterns of labor as indicators of risk. *Clin. Obstet. Gynecol.* **16**:172–183, 1973.
31. Friedman, E. A.: Primigravid labor: A graphicostatistical analysis. *Obstet. Gynecol.* **6**:567–589, 1955.
32. Friedman, E. A., Niswander, K. R., and Sachtleben, M. R.: Dysfunctional labor. XI. Neurologic and developmental effects on surviving infants. *Obstet. Gynecol.* **33**:785–791, 1969.
33. Friedman, E. A. Niswander, K. R., Sachtleben, M. R., and Naftaly, N.: Dysfunctional labor. X. Immediate results to infant. *Obstet. Gynecol.* **33**:776–784, 1969.
34. Friedman, E. A., and Sachtleben, M. R.: Amniotomy and the course of labor. *Obstet. Gynecol.* **22**:755–770, 1963.
35. Friedman, E. A. and Sachtleben, M. R.: Dysfunctional labor: VI. Abnormal progress in the multipara. *Obstet. Gynecol.* **22**:478–494, 1963.
36. Friedman, E. A. and Sachtleben, M. R.: Dysfunctional labor: IV. Combined aberrant dilatation patterns in the nullipara. *Obstet. Gynecol.* **20**:761–773, 1962.
37. Friedman, E. A. and Sachtleben, M. R.: Dysfunctional labor: I. Prolonged latent phase in the nullipara. *Obstet. Gynecol.* **17**:135–148, 1961.
38. Friedman, E. A. and Sachtleben, M. R.: Dysfunctional labor: II. Protracted active phase dilatation in the nullipara. *Obstet. Gynecol.* **17**:566–578, 1961.
39. Friedman, E. A.. and Sachtleben, M. R.: Dysfunctional labor: III. Secondary arrest of dilatation in the nullipara. *Obstet. Gynecol.* **19**:576–591, 1962.
40. Friedman, E. A. and Sachtleben, M. R.: Dysfunctional labor: V. Therapeutic trial of oxytocin in secondary arrest. *Obstet. Gynecol.* **21**:13–21, 1963.
41. Friedman, E. A. and Sachtleben, M. R.: Effect of oxytocin and oral prostaglandin E_2 on uterine contractility and fetal heart rate patterns. *Am. J. Obstet. Gynecol.* **130**:403–407, 1978.
42. Friedman, E. A., Sachtleben, M. R., and Bresky, P. A.: Dysfunctional labor. XII. Long-term effects on infant. *Am. J. Obstet. Gynecol.* **127**:779–783, 1977.
43. Fuchs, A-R., Goeschen, K., Husslein, P., Rasmussen, A. B., and Fuchs, F.: Oxytocin and the initiation of human parturition. III. Plasma concentrations of oxytocin and 13,14-dihydro- 15-keto-prostaglandin F_2 alpha in spontaneous and oxytocin induced labor at term. *Am. J. Obstet. Gynecol.* **147**:497–502, 1983.
44. Goodwin, J. W. and Reid, D. E.: Risk to the fetus in prolonged and trial labor. *Am. J. Obstet. Gynecol.* **85**:209–222, 1963.
45. Gunz, F. W. and Atkinson, H. R.: Medical radiations and leukaemia. A retrospective survey. *Br. Med. J.* **1**:389–393, 1964.
46. Hannah, W. J.: X-ray pelvimetry—A critical appraisal. *Am. J. Obstet. Gynecol.* **91**:333–341, 1965.
47. Harbert, G. M., Brame, R. G., Wax, S. H., Cornell, G. W., McGaughey, H. S., and Thornton, W. N.: Uterine contractility response to blood flow in primates. *Surg. Forum* **17**:390–392, 1966.
48. Hellman, L. M.: Oxytocin in dysfunctional labor. *Clin. Obstet. Gynecol.* **2**:343–353, 1959.
49. Hendricks, C. H., Brenner, W. E., and Kraus, G.: Normal cervical dilatation pattern in late pregnancy and labor. *Am. J. Obstet. Gynecol.* **106**:1065–1082, 1970.
50. Hibbard, L. T.: Changing trends in cesarean section. *Am. J. Obstet. Gynecol.* **125**:798–804, 1976.
51. Jablon, S. and Kato, H.: Childhood cancer in relation to prenatal exposure to atomic-bomb radiation. *Lancet* **2**:1000–1003, 1970.
52. Jeffcoate, T. N. A.: Prolonged labour. *Lancet* **2**:61–67, 1961.
53. Jeffcoate, T. N. A., Baker, K., and Martin, R. H.: Inefficient uterine action. *Surg. Gynecol. Obstet.* **95**:257–273, 1952.
54. Johnson, W. L., Winter, W. W., Eng, M., Bonica,

J. J., and Hunter, C. A.: Effect of pudendal, spinal, and peridural block anesthesia on the second stage of labor. *Am. J. Obstet. Gynecol.* **113**:166–175, 1972.

55. Jouppila, P., Jouppila, R., Hollmen, A., and Koivula, A.: Lumbar epidural analgesia to improve intervillous blood flow during labor in severe preeclampsia. *Obstet. Gynecol.* **59**:158–161, 1982.
56. Jouppila, R., Jouppila, P., Karinen, J. M., and Hollmen, A.: Segmental epidural analgesia in labour: Related to the progress of labour, fetal malposition and instrumental delivery. *Acta Obstet. Gynecol. Scand.* **58**:135–139, 1979.
57. Joyce, D. N., Giwa-Osagie, F., and Stevenson, G. W.: Role of pelvimetry in active management of labour. *Br. Med. J.* **4**:505–507, 1975.
58. Kadar, N. and Romero, R.: Prognosis for future childbearing after midcavity instrumental deliveries in primigravidas. *Obstet. Gynecol.* **62**:166–170, 1983.
59. Kaplan, H. S.: An evaluation of the somatic and genetic hazards of the medical use of radiation. *Am. J. Roentgenol. Radium. Ther. Nucl. Med.* **80**:696–706, 1958.
60. Kelly, K. M., Madden, D. A., Arcarese, J. S., Barnett, M., and Brown, R. F.: The utilization and efficacy of pelvimetry. *Am. J. Roentgenol.* **125**:66–74, 1975.
61. Khamis, Y., Shaala, S., Damarawy, H., Romia, A., and Toppozada, M.: Effect of heat on uterine contractions during normal labor. *Int. J. Gynaecol. Obstet.* **21**:491–493, 1983.
62. Koontz, W. L., Seeds, J. W., and Cefalo, R. C.: Sonographic appearance of a pathologic retraction ring. *Am. J. Obstet. Gynecol.* **148**:823–825, 1984.
63. Larks, S. D.: *Electrohysterography, the Electrical Activity of the Human Uterus in Pregnancy and Labor.* Springfield, Thomas, 1960, pp. 46–94.
64. Leake, R. D., Weitzman, R. E., and Fisher, D. A.: Pharmacokinetics of oxytocin in the human subject. *Obstet. Gynecol.* **56**:701–704, 1980.
65. Leake, R. D., Weitzman, R. E., Glatz, T. H., and Fisher, D. A.: Plasma oxytocin concentrations in men, nonpregnant women, and pregnant women before and during spontaneous labor. *J. Clin. Endocrinol. Metab.* **53**:730–733, 1981.
66. Lederman, R. P., Lederman, E., Work, B. A., Jr., and McCann, D. S.: The relationship of maternal anxiety, plasma catecholamines, and plasma cortisol to progress in labor. *Am. J. Obstet. Gynecol.* **132**:495–500, 1978.
67. Lewis, T. L. T.: Leukaemia in childhood after antenatal exposure to x-rays (a survey at Queen Charlotte's Hospital). *Br. Med. J.* **2**:1551–1552, 1960.
68. Low, J. A., Cox, M. J., Karchmar, E. J., McGrath, M. J., Pancham, S. R., and Piercy, W. N.: The effect of maternal, labor, and fetal factors upon fetal heart rate during the intrapartum period. *Am. J. Obstet. Gynecol.* **139**:306–310, 1981.
69. Lowensohn, R. I., Paul, R. H., Fales, S., Yeh, S. Y., and Hon, E. H.: Intrapartum epidural anesthesia, an evaluation of effects on uterine activity. *Obstet. Gynecol.* **44**:388–393, 1974.
70. Maresh, M., Choong, K. H., and Beard, R. W.: Delayed pushing with lumbar epidural analgesia in labour. *Br. J. Obstet. Gynaecol.* **90**:623–627, 1983.
71. Matadial, L. and Cibils, L. A.: The effect of epidural anesthesia on uterine activity and blood pressure. *Am. J. Obstet. Gynecol.* **125**:846–854, 1976.
72. Mendez-Bauer, C., Arroyo, J., Garcia-Ramos, C., Menendez, A., Lavilla, M., Izquierdo, F., Villa-Elizaga, I., and Zamarriego, J.: Effects of standing position on spontaneous uterine contractility and other aspects of labor. *J. Perinat. Med.* **3**:89–100, 1975.
73. Morishima, H. O., Glaser, B., Niemann, W. H., and James, L. S.: Increased uterine activity and fetal deterioration during maternal hyperthermia. *Am. J. Obstet. Gynecol.* **121**:531–538, 1975.
74. Murray, R., Heckel, P., and Hempelmann, L. H.: Leukemia in children exposed to ionizing radiation. *N. Engl. J. Med.* **261**:585-589, 1959.
75. Odendaal, H. J.: Uterine contraction patterns in patients with severe abruptio placentae. *S. Afr. Med. J.* **57**:908–910, 1980.
76. O'Driscoll, K. and Foley, M.: Correlation of decrease in perinatal mortality and increase in cesarean section rates. *Am. J. Obstet. Gynecol.* **61**:1–5, 1983.
77. O'Driscoll, K., Foley, M., and MacDonald, D.: Active management of labor as an alternative to cesarean section for dystocia. *Obstet. Gynecol.* **63**:485–490, 1984.
78. O'Driscoll, K., Jackson, R. J. A., and Gallagher, J. T.: Active management of labour and cephalopelvic disproportion. *J. Obstet. Gynaecol. Br. Commonw.* **77**:385–389, 1970.
79. O'Driscoll, K., Jackson, R. J. A., and Gallagher, J. T.: Prevention of prolonged labour. *Br. Med. J.* **2**:477–480, 1969.
80. O'Driscoll, K., Stronge, J. M., and Minogue, M.: Active management of labour. *Br. Med. J.* **3**:135–137, 1973.
81. Oppenheim, B. E., Griem, M. L., and Meier, P.: The effects of diagnostic x-ray exposure on the human fetus. An examination of the evidence. *Radiology* **114**:529–534, 1975.
82. Oppenheim, B. E., Griem, M. L., and Meier, P.: Effects of low-dose prenatal irradiation in humans: Analysis of Chicago Lying-In data and comparison with other studies. *Radiat. Res.* **57**:508–544, 1974.
83. Ott, W. J.: Relationship of normal and abnormal late labor patterns to perinatal mortality. *Clin. Obstet. Gynecol.* **25**:105–109, 1982.
84. Parsons, M. T. and Spellacy, W. N.: Prospective randomized study of x-ray pelvimetry in the primigravida. *Obstet. Gynecol.* **66**:76–79, 1985.

85. Petrie, R. H., Wu, R., Miller, F. C., Sacks, D. A., Sugarman, R., Paul, R. H., and Hon, E. H.: The effect of drugs on uterine activity. *Obstet. Gynecol.* **48**:431–435, 1976.
86. Phillips, J. C., Hochberg, C. J., Petrakis, J. K., and Van Winkle, J. D.: Epidural analgesia and its effects on the "normal" progress of labor. *Am. J. Obstet. Gynecol.* **129**:316–323, 1977.
87. Polhemus, D. W. and Koch, R.: Leukemia and medical radiation. *Pediatrics* **23**:453–461, 1959.
88. Poseiro, J. J. and Noriega-Guerra, L.: Dose response relationships in uterine effects of oxytocin infusions. In: *Oxytocin.* R. Caldeyro-Barcia and H. Heller (Eds.). New York, Pergamon, 1961, pp. 158–173.
89. Read, J. A., Miller, F. C., and Paul, R. H.: Randomized trial of ambulation versus oxytocin for labor enhancement: A preliminary report. *Am. J. Obstet. Gynecol.* **139**:669–672, 1981.
90. Reddi, K., Kambaran, S. R., Norman, R. J., Joubert, S. M., and Philpott, R. H.: Abnormal concentrations of prostaglandins in amniotic fluid during delayed labour in multigravid patients. *Br. J. Obstet. Gynaecol.* **91**:781–787, 1984.
91. Reynolds, S. R. M., Heard, O. O., Bruns, P., and Hellman, L. M.: A multi-channel strain-gauge tokodynamometer: An instrument for studying patterns of uterine contractions in pregnant women. *Bull. Johns Hopkins Hosp.* **82**:446–469, 1948.
92. Riffel, H. D., Nochimson, D. J., Paul, R. H., and Hon, E. H. G.: Effects of meperidine and promethazine during labor. *Obstet. Gynecol.* **42**:738–745, 1973.
93. Russell, J. G. B. and Richards, B.: A review of pelvimetry data. *Br. J. Radiol.* **44**:780–784, 1971.
94. Schellenberg, J. C.: Uterine activity during lumbar epidural analgesia with bupivacaine. *Am. J. Obstet. Gynecol.* **127**:26–31, 1977.
95. Schifrin, B. S.: Fetal heart rate patterns following epidural anesthesia and oxytocin infusion during labour. *J. Obstet. Gynaecol. Br. Commonw.* **79**:332–339, 1972.
96. Schulman, H. and Romney, S. L.: Variability of uterine contractions in normal human parturition. *Obstet. Gynecol.* **36**:215–221, 1970.
97. Seitchik, J. and Castillo, M.: Oxytocin augmentation of dysfunctional labor. II. Uterine activity data. *Am. J. Obstet. Gynecol.* **145**:526–529, 1983.
98. Seitchik, J. and Castillo, M.: Oxytocin augmentation of dysfunctional labor. III. Multiparous patients. *Am. J. Obstet. Gynecol.* **145**:777–780, 1983.
99. Seitchik, J. and Chatkoff, M. L.: Intrauterine pressure wave form characteristics in hypocontractile labor before and after oxytocin administration. *Am. J. Obstet. Gynecol.* **123**:426–434, 1975.
100. Seitchik, J. and Chatkoff, M. L.: Oxytocin-induced uterine hypercontractility pressure wave forms. *Obstet. Gynecol.* **48**:436–441, 1976.
101. Shnider, S. M., Abboud, T. K., Artal, R., Henriksen, E. H., Stefani, S. J., and Levinson, G.: Maternal catecholamines decrease during labor after lumbar epidural anesthesia. *Am. J. Obstet. Gynecol.* **147**:13–15, 1983.
102. Sica-Blanco, Y., Rozada, H., and Remedio, M. R.: Effect of meperidine on uterine contractility during pregnancy and prelabor. *Am. J. Obstet. Gynecol.* **97**:1096–1100, 1967.
103. Sokol, R. J., Rosen, M. G., Bottoms, S. F., and Chik, L.: Risks preceding increased primary cesarean birth rates. *Obstet. Gynecol.* **59**:340–346, 1982.
104. Steer, C. M.: Effect of type of delivery on future childbearing. *Am. J. Obstet. Gynecol.* **60**:395–400, 1950.
105. Stewart, A., Webb, J., Giles, D., and Hewitt, D.: Malignant disease in childhood and diagnostic irradiation in utero. *Lancet* **2**:447, 1956.
106. Stewart, D. B.: Abnormal uterine action in labour. *J. Obstet. Gynaecol. Br. Emp.* **59**:641–643, 1952.
107. Stewart, K.S. and Philpott, R. H.: Fetal response to cephalopelvic disproportion. *Br. J. Obstet. Gynaecol.* **87**:641–649, 1980.
108. Studd, J. W. W., Crawford, J. S., Duignan, N. M., Rowbotham, C. J. F., and Hughes, A. O.: The effect of lumbar epidural analgesia on the rate of cervical dilatation and the outcome of labour of spontaneous onset. *Br. J. Obstet. Gynaecol.* **87**:1015–1021, 1980.
109. Talledo, O. E. and Zuspan, F. P.: Spontaneous uterine contractility in eclampsia. *Clin. Obstet. Gynecol.* **9**:910–921, 1966.
110. Taylor, E. S., Bruns, P. D., Anker, R. M., and Drose, V. E.: Correlation of urinary estrogen-pregnanediol excretion with uterine motility during pregnancy. *Am. J. Obstet. Gynecol.* **70**:894–909, 1955.
111. Thorne, D. O., Assadi, I., Fores, J., and Seitchik, J.: The relationship of the maximum amplitude and the maximum and minimum slope of the intrauterine pressure waveform in late pregnancy and labor. *IEEE Trans. Biomed. Eng.* **19**:388–390, 1972.
112. Tucker, B. E. and Benaron, H. B. W.: The immediate effects of prolonged labor with forceps delivery, precipitate labor with spontaneous delivery and natural labor with spontaneous delivery on the child. *Am. J. Obstet. Gynecol.* **66**:540–550, 1953.
113. Turnbull, A. C.: Uterine contractions in normal and abnormal labour. *J. Obstet. Gynaecol. Br. Emp.* **64**:321–333, 1957.
114. Tyack, A. J., Parsons, R. J., Millar, D. R., and Nicholas, A. D. G.: Uterine activity and plasma bupivacaine levels after caudal epidural analgesia. *J. Obstet. Gynaecol. Br. Commonw.* **80**:896–901, 1973.
115. Varner, M. W., Cruikshank, D. P., and Laube, D. W.: X-ray pelvimetry in clinical obstetrics. *Obstet. Gynecol.* **56**:296–300, 1980.
116. Vasicka, A., Hutchinson, H. T., Eng, M., and

Allen, C. R.: Spinal and epidural anesthesia, fetal and uterine response to acute hypo- and hypertension. *Am. J. Obstet. Gynecol.* **90**:800–810, 1964.

117. Vosburgh, G. J., Gates, M. J., Mackenzie, J., Deutschberger, J., Berendes, H., and Weiss, W.: The effects of uterine dysfunction and mechanical dystocia on pediatric outcome. *Bull. Sloane Hosp. Women Columbia Presbyt. Med.* **12**:72–76, 1966.
118. Weaver, J. B., Pearson, J. F., and Rosen, M.: Posture and epidural block in pregnant women at term. *Anaesthesia* **30**:752–756, 1975.
119. Weaver, J. B., Pearson, J. F., and Turnbull, A. C.: The effect upon the fetus of an oxytocin infusion in the absence of uterine hypertonus. *J. Obstet. Gynaecol. Br. Commonw.* **81**:297–302, 1974.
120. Wells, J. and Steer, C. M.: Relationship of leukemia in children to abdominal irradiation of mothers during pregnancy. *Am. J. Obstet. Gynecol.* **81**:1059–1063, 1961.
121. Willdeck-Lund, G., Lindmark, G., and Nilsson, B. A.: Effect of segmental epidural block on the course of labour and the condition of the infant during the neonatal period. *Acta. Anaesthesiol. Scand.* **23**:301–311, 1979.
122. Wolfs, G. M. J. A. and van Leeuwen, M.: Electromyographic observations on the human uterus during labour. *Acta Obstet. Gynecol. Scand.* [*Suppl.*] **90**:3–61, 1979.
123. Yeh, S. Y., Paul, R. H., Cordero, L., and Hon, E. H.: A study of diazepam during labor. *Obstet. Gynecol.* **43**:363–373, 1974.
124. Zador, G. and Nilsson, B. A.: Low dose intermittent epidural anaesthesia with lidocaine for vaginal delivery. II. Influence on labour and foetal acid-base status. *Acta Obstet. Gynecol. Scand. (Suppl.)* **34**:17–30, 1974.
125. Zentner, R.: Ritodrine in the management of a case of acute fetal distress. *Aust. N.Z. J. Obstet. Gynaecol.* **23**:250–252, 1983.

23

INDUCTION AND STIMULATION OF LABOR

Theobald, in an excellent review, described the history of the development of posterior pituitary extracts and oxytocin for the induction and augmentation of labor.[23] The first demonstration of the contractile effects of posterior pituitary extracts on the myometrium in vitro was reported by Dale in 1906. In vivo confirmation was provided by Frankl-Hochuart and Froöhlich in 1909. Hofbauer, in 1911, initiated the clinical application of oxytocin compounds, utilizing posterior pituitary extracts. Beginning in 1913, Watson systematically utilized such compounds to induce labor. Significant complications (ruptured uteri) resulted from the doses utilized in Watson's protocol.[24] The use of posterior pituitary extracts was discontinued until Theobald and associates described the administration of oxytocin via intravenous drip in 1948.[25] The initial dose utilized by Theobald and coworkers was 4–6 mU/min. This dosage was calculated by assuming that myometrial activity should be induced by a dose of oxytocin of the same magnitude as the dose of ADH required to inhibit water diuresis, a physiologic renal response.[25] Initial studies by Caldeyro-Barcia confirmed that the majority of patients responded to dosages of 5 mU/min or less.[24] Hendricks also found that 80% of patients undergoing induction of labor with pituitary extracts responded to 5 mU/min or less. Furthermore, infusions greater than 10 mU/min were required in only 3% of Hendricks' patients undergoing induction of labor.[24]

The Nobel prize-winning work of DuVigneaud and associates in the 1950s demonstrated the structure of oxytocin (Fig. 23-1).[3] Elucidation of the structure of the oxytocin molecule led to the production of synthetic oxytocin compounds. These compounds provide the obstetrician with a potent and effective but potentially harmful and often abused uterine stimulant.

This chapter is intended to provide the clinician with a rational, safe, and efficacious method of either initiating or augmenting labor in the term patient, utilizing oxytocin.

PHARMACOLOGY/PHYSIOLOGY OF ACTION

Oxytocin is an octapeptide with a chemical structure (Fig. 23-1) similar to antidiuretic hormone (ADH). Although both of these peptide hormones are released from the posterior pituitary by various reflex responses, they are synthesized in the supraoptic and paraventricular nuclei of the hypothalamus. From the site of synthesis, the peptides are transported to the posterior pituitary via the hypothalamic neurohypophyseal tract. In the pituitary gland they are stored at the perivascular nerve endings in neurosecretory granules. Stimulation of the paraventricular and/or supraoptic nuclei results in release of the active peptides into the vascular system.

The action of oxytocin on its target cells (myometrial cells of the uterus, myoepithelial

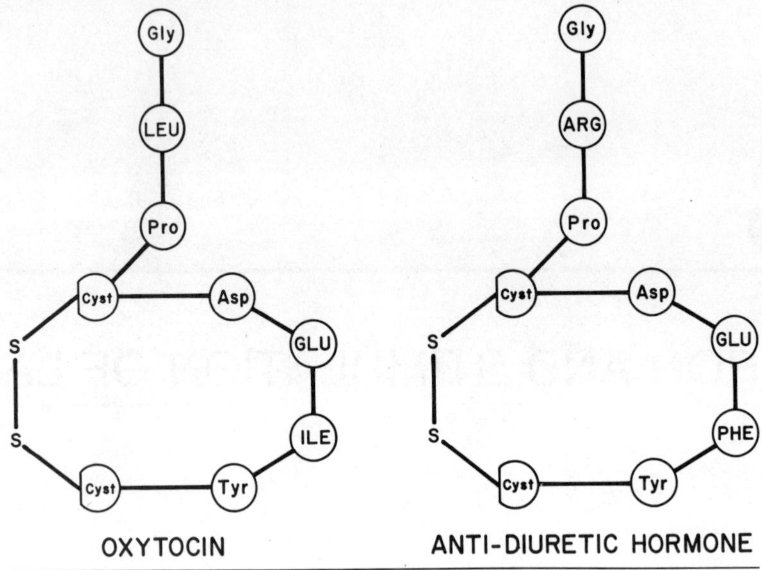

Figure 23-1. Chemical structure of oxytocin and antidiuretic hormone.

cells of the breast) is mediated by specific high-affinity membrane binding sites for oxytocin. Myometrial concentrations of oxytocin receptors increase approximately 12-fold between the early second trimester and the last four weeks of gestation.[7,8] Prior to the onset of spontaneous labor at term, there is a further twofold rise in oxytocin receptor concentration.[7,8] The increasing concentration of myometrial oxytocin receptors probably explains the increased uterine sensitivity to oxytocin with increasing gestational age. Myometrial oxytocin receptor concentrations have also been reported to be increased in patients with preterm labor.[8]

The intracellular mechanisms of oxytocin activation of receptor cells are not fully understood. Oxytocin may act through inhibition of the adenylate cyclase system, through alterations in intracellular calcium concentrations, through calcium "channel" action, or through some as-yet-undiscovered mechanism. Whatever its intracellular actions, oxytocin produces dose-dependent and receptor-concentration-dependent contractions of myometrial cells, in vivo and in vitro.

Plasma oxytocin levels of men, nonpregnant women, and nonlaboring pregnant women are all in the same ranges.[13] The absolute levels vary with the reporting laboratory. The oxytocin levels associated with spontaneous labor are still controversial.[9,14,17,25] The exact function of endogenous oxytocin in initiation and maintenance of labor is much debated. Maternal plasma levels of oxytocin have been described as increased or as unchanged during the active phase of spontaneous labor. Plasma oxytocin levels do increase during the expulsive phase of delivery.[14]

The function of oxytocin during parturition may not be totally determined by maternal plasma levels of oxytocin. Fetal production of oxytocin may play an important role. In the sheep[2] and the human,[16] fetal levels of oxytocin increase during active labor. A significant arteriovenous difference is measurable in cord blood. In addition, the changing milieu of oxytocin receptors preceding parturition may result in a significantly increased physiological response to relatively constant or slightly increased maternal oxytocin levels.

The syncytiotrophoblast produces a cysteine aminopeptidase (oxytocinase) which results in rapid in vitro degradation of oxytocin during pregnacy. Oxytocinase is released into the maternal circulation. In vitro incubation of oxytocin in plasma from pregnant women results in an 85% decrease in oxytocin concentration within an hour.[1,13] Plasma from men or nonpregnant women does not significantly degrade oxytocin.[13] Oxytocinase does not cross the placenta, as inferred from the fact that no degradation of oxytocin occurs in the plasma of cord blood.[13]

Despite the rapid degradation of oxytocin in

vitro, the increase in plasma oxytocinase during pregnancy is not reflected in increased metabolic clearance rates (MCRs) of infused oxytocin in pregnant women.[1,13,19] The MCRs for infused oxytocin are similar in men and nonpregnant and pregnant women. The mean MCR is 17-25 ml/kg/min. The in vivo half-life ($t_{1/2}$) of infused oxytocin is on the order of 1-3 minutes.

With a constant oxytocin infusion, plasma levels of oxytocin do not reach steady state in either pregnant or nonpregnant patients for 30-60 minutes.[19] Steady-state plasma oxytocin levels and the rates of oxytocin infusion show a positive linear correlation over a wide range of oxytocin infusion rates.[19]

These observations are consonant with the physiological responses demonstrated in pregnant patients at term.[23] At a given infusion rate, 14-60 minutes were required to obtain a maximum uterine response. Both the pharmacologic and physiologic responses to oxytocin infusion argue against increasing the rate of infusion at the 15-20 minute intervals often utilized by physicians.

Some patients undergoing induction of labor fail to demonstrate cervical dilatation despite apparently adequate uterine contractility.[11] Patients in whom induction is unsuccessful do not demonstrate increased plasma levels of prostaglandin F_2 metabolite in contrast to patients undergoing successful inductions with oxytocin. Therefore an important interaction may exist between oxytocin and prostaglandin. The initiation of uterine contractions by oxytocin does not appear to be prostaglandin dependent. However, cervical changes resulting from oxytocin infusions may be prostaglandin dependent through either changing biochemical or mechanical properties or increases in myometrial gap junctions with resultant synchronous, effective propagation of contractions.[9]

SIDE EFFECTS/COMPLICATIONS OF OXYTOCIN INFUSIONS

The known or presumed benefits of augmenting or inducing labor with oxytocin must be balanced against the potential complications. Uterine hypercontractility and fetal distress are commonly encountered complications of oxytocin infusion protocols that utilize high doses and short incremental time intervals for increasing dosages. Uterine hypercontractility is defined as a labor pattern of more than five contractions in 10 minutes or with baseline intrauterine pressures above 15 mmHg for longer than 15 minutes.[20] Management of uterine hypercontractility and/or fetal distress necessitates reducing the dose or discontinuing the oxytocin infusion. Tetanic contractions and/or severe fetal distress secondary to uteroplacental insufficiency may on occasion necessitate pharmacological or operative intervention. Terbutaline (0.125-0.250 mg intravenous [i.v.] bolus) can be utilized to relieve hyperstimulation and fetal distress, provided that no contraindications to beta sympathomimetic therapy exist.

A properly administered oxytocin infusion can significantly reduce the incidence of uterine hypercontractility and fetal distress.[20] The most important factor in reducing these complications is the interval between each incremental dose interval.[20] If infusion rates are increased before the maximum uterine response for a particular dose is evident (30-60 minutes), additive uterine stimulatory effects can occur, resulting in hyperstimulation and fetal distress. These complications often necessitate discontinuation of the oxytocin infusion. One of the criticisms of slowly increasing infusion rates has been that the induction/augmentation will require a longer time. Actually, the average time interval to delivery is decreased when augmentation is conducted utilizing an interval of 40 minutes between incremental doses, as compared to an interval of 20 minutes. The shortened average time is the result of a decreased incidence of oxytocin discontinuation.[20]

Oxytocin should never be given as an i.v. bolus, because premature ventricular contractions or hypotension can occur.

An increased incidence of neonatal jaundice has been reported in infants delivered after oxytocin-stimulated labors.[16] O'Driscoll states that such jaundice occurs only in induced labors. Other investigators note that jaundice results from traumatic deliveries that may be associated with oxytocin usage. At present, no definitive correlations have been shown.

High dosages of oxytocin may result in an antidiuretic effect. Urine output may begin to decrease at infusion rates greater than 20 mU/min. Water retention becomes a real possibility at rates greater than 40-50 mU/min. Fluid intake and output should be carefully monitored in any patient receiving an oxytocin infusion.

Judicious oxytocin administration and monitoring should make uterine rupture rare. As many as 50% of all uterine ruptures occur in patients receiving oxytocin infusions.[10] Administration of oxytocin infusions to patients with a transverse lower segment scar undergoing trial of labor appears to be safe and efficacious, provided that the infusion is properly administered and the patient is properly observed.[4] Although the risk of uterine rupture increases with advancing parity, oxytocin should not be reserved solely for nulliparous patients. Judicious use of oxytocin with close monitoring is safe in the multiparous patient. Grand multiparity (more than *seven* previous *deliveries*) is a relative contraindication to oxytocin infusion. In addition, conditions resulting in uterine overdistention (e.g., twins, macrosomia, polyhydramnios) should be viewed as relative contraindications to the use of oxytocin. Each patient's clinical status must be reviewed and the relative risks and benefits of an oxytocin infusion must be considered prior to beginning an infusion of this ecbolic agent.

MANAGEMENT OF OXYTOCIN INFUSION

Intrapartum management of oxytocin infusions require continuous uterine and fetal monitoring. Oxytocin infusions require qualified personnel in attendance at all times. Fluid intake and output must be carefully monitored. Vital signs should be obtained and documented every 15 minutes. Our requirements for intrapartum infusion of oxytocin are listed in Table 23-1.

TABLE 23-1. REQUIREMENTS FOR INTRAPARTUM INFUSION OF OXYTOCIN

A. Prior to the initiation of the induction/augmentation protocol the following must be documented on the chart:
   1. History and physical
   2. Presenting part/position/station
   3. Cervical status (effacement/dilatation)
   4. Estimated fetal weight (EFW)
   5. Clinical pelvimetry
   6. Evaluation of labor pattern
   7. Evaluation of fetal status (Fetal Heart Monitor pattern, meconium, etc.)
   8. Indication for oxytocin infusion (augmenation or induction and why)
   9. Specific order for oxytocin induction or augmentation
B. Responsible physician in close proximity.
C. All infusions shall be by continuous infusion pumps which are piggybacked into a main infusion line.
D. Oxytocin is commonly mixed in a concentration of 10 U in 500 cc D5W (20 mU/cc) and delivered via controlled infusion pump.
E. All infusions require the use of continuous electronic fetal and uterine monitoring.
F. All infusions require medical and/or nursing personnel in attendance at all times.

Oxytocin is utilized either to augment or to induce labor in selected patients. The responses of these two groups of patients to infused oxytocin can be quite different. For this reason, augmentation and induction must be managed as distinctly different clinical entities. Implicit to distinguishing between labor induction and augmentation is the obstetrician's ability to define and diagnose the onset of labor. Indeed, the diagnosis of labor is the single most important item in the management of labor and delivery.[16] It is critical to determine whether the patient is or is not in labor at the time of admission. Should uterine inertia occur in patients admitted to the labor and delivery suite with a diagnosis of labor based on bloody show, cervical effacement, and dilatation, accompanied by painful regular contractions, oxytocin infusion should be considered as an *augmentation* of labor. Patients admitted for delivery secondary to worsening maternal disease, fetal compromise, or abnormal fetal testing are to be considered for *induction* of labor, provided they do not evidence labor on admission. The physician should seldom be faced with a patient in whom one is unable to determine whether an oxytocin infusion would be for the purpose of induction or augmentation. Should this doubt exist, the patient should be managed as for augmentation.

Our recommended regimens for augmentation and induction are shown in Tables 23-2 and 23-3. The interval between doses remains 40 minutes in both groups.

Augmentation

Augmentation of labor occurs when a patient previously diagnosed as being in labor is given an oxytocin infusion because of a hypocontractile labor pattern. The decision to increase the dose is based on evaluation of uterine activity. Uterine activity may be evaluated by (1) clinical assessment of the frequency and quality of uterine contractions; (2) Montevideo units (MVUs), defined as the number of contractions in 10 minutes multiplied by the average amplitude of the contractions (requires internal monitors); or (3) the three-contraction score described by Seitchik (requires internal monitors and a programmed minicomputer).[18,21] Typically, 150 Montevideo units reflects adequate uterine activity, although many patients may demonstrate adequate progression with less than 150 MVUs.

TABLE 23-2. PROTOCOL FOR AUGMENTATION OF LABOR WITH OXYTOCIN

Augmentation Protocol

1. Begin at 1 mU/min.
2. Maintain each setting for a minimum of 40 minutes.
3. Evaluate uterine activity between 30 and 40 minutes after each setting:
   a. adequate activity/adequate fetal status—maintain dosage;
   b. inadequate uterine activity—increase dose by 1 mU/min.
4. No dosage (during augmentation) >9 mU/min unless the following is reevaluated and documented by the responsible physician:
   - labor pattern
   - fetal status
   - presenting part, position, station
   - EFW
   - clinical pelvimetry
   - evidence (or lack of) of chorioamnionitis.

Dysfunctional labor or hypocontractile labor requiring oxytocin augmentation is mainly a complication of first labors. O'Driscoll states that prolonged labor in a nullipara should be considered evidence of inefficient uterine activity, whereas prolonged labor in a multipara should be considered as evidence of cephalopelvic disproportion, malpresentation, or malformation.[16] The incidence of labor aberrations (excluding pure prolonged latent phase) is 6.22% in nulliparas in contrast to 0.5% in multiparas.[5] Prior to initiation of oxytocin augmentation, multiparas presenting with dysfunctional labor (evidenced by protracted active phase, secondary arrest of dilatation, or failure of descent) should be evaluated for complicating factors including chorioamnionitis, cephalopelvic disproportion, malpresentation, fetal malformation, multiple gestation, and macrosomia.

TABLE 23-3. PROTOCOL FOR THE INDUCTION OF LABOR WITH OXYTOCIN

Induction Protocol

1. Begin at 1–2 mU/min (depending on clinical evaluation).
2. Maintain each setting for a minimum of 40 minutes.
3. Evaluate the uterine activity between 30 and 40 minutes after each setting:
   a. activity adequate, fetal status stable—maintain infusion rate;
   b. inadequate uterine activity—double the preexisting oxytocin dosage.
4. No oxytocin dose greater than 20 mU/min may be given without the following additional documentation by the responsible physician:
   - evaluation of labor pattern (preferably internal pressure catheter)
   - evaluation of fetal status (fetal heart monitoring pattern, meconium)
   - clinical pelvimetry
   - presenting part, position, station
   - EFW
   - specific order for each dose >20 mU/min.

Both multiparous and nulliparous patients requiring augmentation respond to relatively low doses of oxytocin. Ninety percent of patients dilate their cervices on doses between 1 and 4 mU/min, and 15–20% respond to an infusion of 1 mU/min.[20,22]

The sensitivity to oxytocin of patients undergoing augmentation mandates initial dosages of 1 mU/min with increases (of 1 mU/min) at not less than 30–40 minutes. This schedule significantly decreases the incidence of uterine hyperstimulation and fetal distress, resulting in a decreased incidence of discontinuation or interruption of oxytocin infusion. The mean time interval from the beginning of augmentation to delivery is thus shortened when dosage increases are made every 30–40 minutes as compared to standard dosing intervals of 15–20 minutes.

Patients receiving oxytocin augmentation who require doses of greater than 8 mU/min should be carefully reevaluated for the presence of cephalopelvic disproportion (CPD), malpresentation, or chorioamnionitis.

Induction

Patients undergoing induction respond variably to infused oxytocin. Some of this variation may be related to the gestational age at which induction is initiated. Uterine sensitivity to oxytocin increases with increasing gestational age.[23] As noted above, this gestational age-related response may be explained by changes in uterine myometrial oxytocin receptor concentrations. The important interaction between oxytocin and prostaglandins in effecting cervical dilatation has also been discussed above.

The modified Bishop score (Table 23-4) remains a mainstay in predicting the success of oxytocin induction.[6,12] The modified Bishop score correlates with the success rate of induction and with the length of the latent phase.[6] Of the five factors included in the Bishop score, cervical dilatation is the most important determinant. Cervical position is the least important.[6] An "unripe" cervix should not necessarily

TABLE 23-4. MODIFIED BISHOP PELVIC SCORE

	Score			
Features	**0**	**1**	**2**	**3**
Station of head	−3	−2	−1–0	+1–+2
Cervical dilatation (cm)	0	1–2	3–4	>4
Cervical length (cm)	3	2	1	0
Cervical consistency	Firm	Medium	Soft	
Cervical position	Posterior	Mid	Anterior	

be considered as an indication for abdominal delivery. Vaginal delivery may be effected in a patient with an unfavorable cervix. Approximately 80% of patients with a Bishop score of ≧4 may be expected to undergo successful induction. The risks and benefits of prolonged induction versus operative delivery and the urgency of delivery must be considered in patients with "unfavorable" cervices.

Inductions should begin with infusion rates of 1-2 mU/min, depending on baseline uterine activity and clinical evaluation. Maximum uterine response to a given oxytocin infusion rate still requires 30–60 minutes; therefore, administration rates should not be increased at intervals of less than 30–40 minutes. Lack of uterine response or unsatisfactory uterine response after 30–40 minutes at a given infusion rate signals the need for a rate increase sufficient to double the previous dose (i.e., 1 mU/min, 2 mU/min, 4 mU/min, 8 mU/min etc.). Uterine response is evaluated as in augmentation of labor.

Unlike patients whose labors are augmented, it is not unusual for a patient undergoing induction to require more than 8 mU/min of oxytocin. Due to the risks associated with high infusion rates, clinical reassessment of all patients requiring more than 20 mU/min is required. Should infusion rates greater than 20 mU/min be necessary, the oxytocin should be administered in a more concentrated solution to minimize the volume of water given to the patient.

REFERENCES

1. Amico, J. A., Seitchik, J., and Robinson, A. G.: Studies of oxytocin in plasma of women during hypocontractile labor. *J. Clin. Endocrinol. Metab.* **58**:274–279, 1984.
2. Dawood, M. Y., Khan-Dawood, F. S., Ayromlooi, J., and Tobias, M.: Maternal and fetal oxytocin level during pregnancy and parturition in the sheep. *Am. J. Obstet. Gynecol.* **147**:584–588, 1983.
3. DuVigneaud, V., Nessler, C., and Trippett, S.: The sequence of amino acids in oxytocin, with a proposal for the structure of oxytocin. *J. Biol. Chem.* **205**:949–957, 1953.
4. Flamn, B. L., Dunnett, C., Fischerman, E., and Quilligan, E. J.: Vaginal delivery following cesarean section: Use of oxytocin augmentation and epidural anesthesia with internal tocodynamic and internal fetal monitoring. *Am. J. Obstet. Gynecol.* **148**:759–763, 1984.
5. Friedman, E. A.: *Labor: Clinical Evaluation and Management.* New York, Appleton-Century-Crofts, 1967.
6. Friedman, E. A., Niswander, K. R., Bayonet-Rivera, N. P., and Sachtleben, M. R.: Relation of prelabor evaluation to inducibility and the course of labor. *Obstet. Gynecol.* **28**:495–501, 1966.
7. Fuchs, A-R., Fuchs, F., Husslein, P., Soloff, M. S., and Fernstrom, M. J.: Oxytocin receptors and human parturition: A dual role for oxytocin in the initiation of labor. *Science* **215**:1396–1398, 1982.
8. Fuchs, A-R., Fuchs, F., Husslein, P., and Soloff, M. S.: Oxytocin receptors in the human uterus during pregnancy and parturition. *Am. J. Obstet. Gynecol.* **150**:734–741, 1984.
9. Fuchs, A-R., Goeschen, K., Husslein, P., Rasmussen, A. B., and Fuchs, F.: Oxytocin and the initiation of human parturition. III. Plasma concentrations of oxytocin and 13,14-dihydro-15-keto-prostaglandin $F_{2\alpha}$ in spontaneous and oxytocin induced labor at term. *Am. J. Obstet. Gynecol.* **147**:497–502, 1983.
10. Garnet, J. D.: Uterine rupture during pregnancy. An analysis of 133 patients. *Obstet. Gynecol.* **23**:898–905, 1964.
11. Husslein, P., Fuchs, A. R., and Fuchs, F.: Oxytocin and the initiation of human parturition. I. Prostaglandin release during induction of labor by oxytocin. *Am. J. Obstet. Gynecol.* **141**:688–693, 1981.
12. Lange, A. P., Secher, J. J., Westergaard, J. G., and Skovgard, I.: Prelabor evaluation of inducibility. *Obstet. Gynecol.* **60**:137–147, 1982.
13. Leake, R. D., Weitzman, R. E., and Fisher, D. A.: Pharmacokinetics of oxytocin in the human subject. *Obstet. Gynecol.* **56**:701–704, 1980.

14. Leake, R. P., Weitzman, R. E., Glatz, T. H., and Fisher, D. A.:. Plasma oxytocin concentrations in men, nonpregnant women, and pregnant women before and during spontaneous labor. *J. Clin. Endocrinol. Metab.* **53:**730–733, 1981.
15. Nagata, I., Kato, K., Makimura, N., Vesata, T., Seki, K., and Kikuchi, Y.: Comparison of plasma oxytocin levels during spontaneous labor and labor induced by amniotomy, prostaglandin $F_{2\alpha}$ and prostaglandin E_2. *Am. J. Obstet. Gynecol.* **147**:259–266, 1983.
16. O'Driscoll, K. and Meagher, D.: Diagnosis of labour. In: *Active Management of Labor*. Philadelphia, W. B. Saunders, 1980, pp. 23–30.
17. Sellers, S. M., Hodgson, H. T., Mountford, L. A., Mitchell, M. D., and Anderson, A. B.: Is oxytocin involved in parturition? *Br. J. Obstet. Gynaecol.* **88**:725–729, 1981.
18. Seitchik , J.: Measure of contraction strength in labor. *Am. J. Obstet. Gynecol.* **138**:727–730, 1980.
19. Seitchik, J., Amico, J., Robinson, A. G., and Castillo, M.: Oxytocin augmentation of dysfunctional labor. IV. Oxytocin pharmacokinetics. *Am. J. Obstet. Gynecol.* **150**:225–228, 1984.
20. Seitchik, J. and Castillo, M.: Oxytocin augmentation of dysfunctional labor. I. Clinical data. *Am. J. Obstet. Gynecol.* **144**:899–905, 1982.
21. Seitchik, J. and Castillo, M.: Oxytocin augmentation of dysfunctional labor. II. Uterine activity. *Am. J. Obstet. Gynecol.* **145**:526–529, 1983.
22. Seitchik, J. and Castillo, M.: Oxytocin augmentation of dysfunctional labor. III. Multiparous patients. *Am. J. Obstet. Gynecol.* **145**:777–780, 1983.
23. Sico-Blanco, Y. and Sala, N. L.: Uterine contractility at the beginning and end of any oxytocin infusion. In: *Oxytocin.* R. Caldeyro-Barcia R. and H. Heller (Eds.). New York, Pergamon Press, 1961, pp. 127–136.
24. Theobald, G. W.: Oxytocin reassessed. *Obstet. Gynecol. Surv.* **23**:109–131, 1968.
25. Theobald, G. W., Graham, A., Campbell, J., Gange, P. D., and Driscoll, W. J.: The use of post-pituitary extract in physiological amounts in obstetrics; a preliminary report. *Br. Med. J.* **2**:123–127, 1948.

24

BREECH PRESENTATION

Obstetricians have long recognized the excessive perinatal morbidity and mortality associated with breech presentation. Three to four percent of labors are complicated by breech presentation. Multiple factors are responsible for the three- to fourfold increase in poor outcome associated with breech presentation as compared to vertex presentation in labor.[5,12,34] The three major factors are congenital malformations, prematurity, and birth trauma. The incidence of prematurity and congenital anomalies is three to four times higher in breech as compared to cephalic presentation. In the past, severe birth trauma and stillbirth were common outcomes of breech labor and delivery.[48] Umbilical cord prolapse is increased as much as 20-fold, depending on gestational age and the type of breech.[20] Adverse obstetrical factors (placenta previa, abruptio placenta, multiple gestation) also play a role in the poor outcome noted for the breech fetus.

The majority of fetuses presenting in labor as breech are delivered by cesarean section.[42] This was not always the case. Before the development of blood banking, antibiotics, and safe anesthetic techniques, routine vaginal delivery was eminently reasonable. Maternal safety was the overwhelming concern of earlier practitioners. Because maternal morbidity and mortality associated with cesarean section were considered to be a greater threat than the adverse fetal and neonatal outcomes inherent to vaginal delivery, cesarean section was reserved for cases in which either the life of the mother or her child was clearly in jeopardy.

The liberalization of indications for cesarean section followed the development of increasingly safe operative procedures. As cesarean delivery became more acceptable, its application in breech presentation increased sharply, and rightfully so. In 1959, Wright[63] went so far as to state that any patient of more than 35 weeks gestation who entered labor with a living baby in breech presentation should be delivered by cesarean section, provided there was no maternal disease that contraindicated abdominal delivery. This conclusion was based on an earlier in-depth analysis of 1456 breech presentations delivered at seven hospitals in the early 1950s. This study concluded that cesarean delivery produced the lowest perinatal mortality but did not imply that it should be used in all breech deliveries. Perhaps the most important contribution of this study was the statement, "In discussing the perinatal mortality associated with breech presentation that it is not the same as breech delivery."[29]

Historic data did not usually separate perinatal morbidity and mortality by etiology. Thus, in the absence of neonatal intensive care facilities, cesarean section to save the premature infant was deemed unreasonable. In the past decade, the practice of obstetrics has changed markedly. The use of continuous electronic fetal monitoring, the ability to perform emergency cesarean delivery safely within minutes, and the support of neonatal intensive care units have made childbirth much safer. Obviously, these advances have had an impact on the outcome of breech delivery. The question may be asked as to how many infants may have formerly died as a direct result of problems that arose during labor and delivery. Such problems include fetal distress in labor, cord prolapse, placenta previa and placental abruption, and difficulties in delivery including entrapment of the aftercoming head. It is within this subgroup of fetuses that "routine" cesarean section might have made a difference in outcome.

Cesarean section has been extremely useful in decreasing the risk of birth trauma to the fetus presenting by the breech; however, other breech risk factors such as congenital anomalies (Table 24-1) and extreme prematurity are minimally altered by abdominal delivery.[10]

Review of several retrospective series during the 1940s and 1950s with only those deaths attributed to "breech factors" included demonstrated a definite relationship between the cesarean section rate and perinatal mortality for infants weighing more than 2500 grams (Fig. 24-1).[23] However, the maximum benefit achieved for term breech presentations occurred with a cesarean section rate of approximately 30%. Thus, the current section rate of 80–90% suggests that three cesarean sections are being performed for each one patient likely to benefit. Such observations have led to research designed to find criteria for selecting the route of delivery best suited to each individual.[3,24,43,60]

TABLE 24-1. CONGENITAL ABNORMALITIES MORE FREQUENTLY DIAGNOSED IN BREECH PRESENTATIONS THAN IN CEPHALIC PRESENTATIONS

Central nervous system
Hydrocephalus
Anencephaly
Meningomyelocele
Familial dysautonomia
Urinary system
Potter's syndrome
Cardiovascular system
Respiratory and gastrointestinal systems
Inguinal hernia
Skeletal system
Myotonic dystrophy
Dislocation of hips
Multiple abnormalities
Prader-Willi syndrome
Trisomy 13 syndrome
Trisomy 18 syndrome
Trisomy 21 syndrome
de Lange's syndrome
Werdnig-Hoffmann syndrome
Zollinger–Ellison syndrome
Smith–Lemli–Opitz syndrome
Fetal alcohol syndrome

Source: Brenner, W. E., Bruce, R. S. and Hendricks, C. H.: The characteristics and perils of breech presentation. *Am. J. Obstet. Gynecol.* **118**:700-712, 1974.

With the change from vaginal delivery to almost routine cesarean section, we have witnessed a shift from a predominant risk to the fetus at vaginal delivery to maternal risk at operative delivery. In the United States, cesarean section rates for the indication "breech" averaged 10% from the 1950s through the late 1960s. The section rate increased from approximately 10–12% in 1970 to more than 80% in 1980. It is estimated that approximately 9 of 10 breech-presenting infants were delivered by cesarean section in the United States in 1984. The cost of this policy stresses the health care system. One must ask whether or not all these operative procedures are necessary or whether there may be reasonable alternatives. Such alternatives include methods to select those breech presentations that may be allowed a trial of labor[8,25] as well as conversion of breech to a cephalic presentation prior to labor.[57]

To understand trends in breech management, it is necessary to delineate the main risks of vaginal delivery and of cesarean sections. Complications of labor and vaginal delivery are due to either umbilical cord prolapse and/or difficulty in delivering the extremities and the aftercoming head.[8,20,24,52] These hazards are disproportionately greater for the preterm breech infant.[21,26,35] With cesarean section, the major risks are operative risks imposed on the mother.[8] However, the risk of fetal injury is not eliminated by cesarean section, although it is minimized.[25]

Management of breech presentation challenges the clinician. Experience in the conduct of breech labor and delivery is crucial to good outcome. Skilled operators are necessary to maximize the safety of labor and vaginal delivery for breech-presenting infants. Many training programs have insufficient numbers of patients to allow residents in obstetrics and gynecology to develop the manual skills necessary to a safe vaginal breech delivery. However, safe delivery of the breech-presenting infant at cesarean section requires a total breech extraction, a fact that is often overlooked. This procedure itself carries an intrinsic risk that at times may equal or exceed assisted vaginal breech delivery. Since the mother is also exposed to surgical risk during cesarean section, a balanced approach should be sought. Although

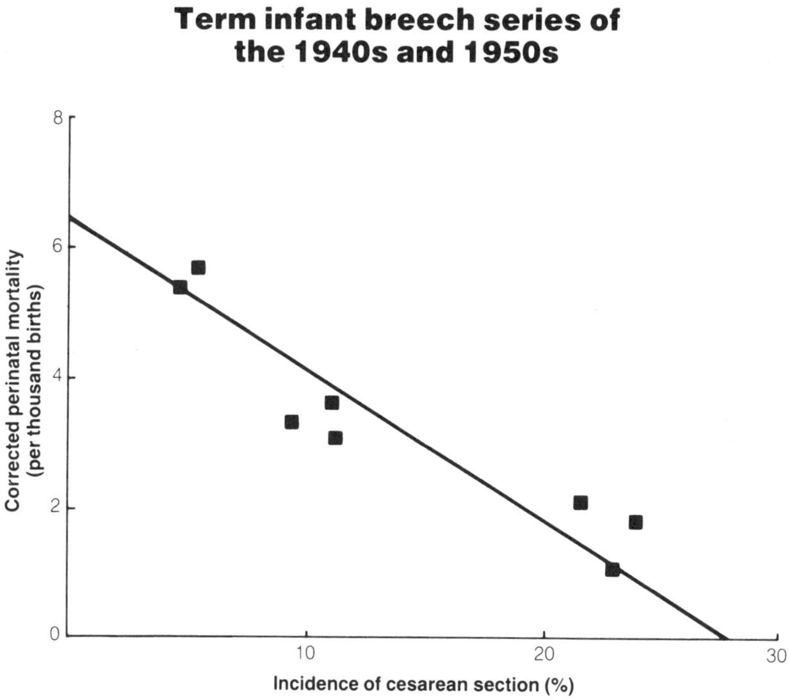

Figure 24-1. Relationship between death due to labor and delivery in breech presentation and cesarean section rate. (Reprinted from Gimovsky, M. L., and Petrie R. H.: Strategy for choosing the best delivery route for the breech baby. Contemp. OB/GYN **21** (April): 201–215, 1983, with permission of Medical Economics Company.)

many infants presenting by the breech are best delivered by cesarean section, safe cesarean delivery demands a clear understanding of the same mechanical techniques utilized in vaginal breech delivery. The breech-presenting fetus requires similar manipulations to effect delivery, regardless of route. Poorly performed breech extraction at cesarean section results in injuries similar to those sustained during vaginal delivery: branchial plexus injuries, bony fractures, spinal cord injury, and crush injuries to the viscera.[20,21,25]

To decide if a contemporary policy of routine section for breech is reasonable, we need to compare the results of cesarean and vaginal deliveries performed more recently and to reevaluate earlier advice and opinions. We must ask: Will cesarean section eliminate all preventable fetal morbidity and mortality? Are the maternal risks justified? Many report a corrected perinatal mortality rate of zero for term breech infant delivery by cesarean section. Infants who succumb following section for this indication invariably are either congenitally malformed or premature. The rare exception is a normal infant compromised by cord prolapse[20] or hyperextension.[11] Cesarean section results in far more maternal morbidity and mortality than does vaginal delivery. Cesarean section is therefore not cost effective unless it prevents a significant number of fetal injuries. Data that address these questions are available in recent studies[8,25,43] that allow liberal use of cesarean section for specific indications.

This chapter reviews clinical factors associated with breech presentation, an approach to labor and delivery of the breech-presenting infant, and selective use of cesarean section and of external cephalic version (ECV) in which the fetus, presenting as a breech, is converted to vertex. External cephalic version dramatically lessens the incidence of breech presentation and its attendant complications.[53,57,64]

Finally, we review protocols that attempt to minimize the need for cesarean section by selecting those breech fetuses in whom vaginal delivery can be safely attempted.[8,24,25,38,43,64] Selection of patients for trial of labor is complex and requires careful, thoughtful judgment and individualization. We believe that selected breech-presenting fetuses may safely be allowed a trial of labor and that the resulting decrease in cesarean sections maximizes the benefits to mother and infant, while minimizing the risks.[8,23,25]

DEFINITIONS

Breech Presentation

Breech presentation refers to the longitudinal lie of the fetus with the breech or buttocks as the presenting part. The position of a breech presentation is designated by the orientation of the sacrum with respect to the maternal pelvic outlet. Station in breech presentation refers to the lowermost portion of the buttocks in relationship to the level of the maternal ischial spines. It is often stated that, at a given point in labor, the breech is one station higher than its vertex counterpart.

There are several varieties of specific breech presentation (Fig. 24-2). These refer to conditions at the hip and knee joints. In *frank* breech presentation, both hip joints are flexed and both knee joints are extended. This is the most common type of breech presentation at term and is

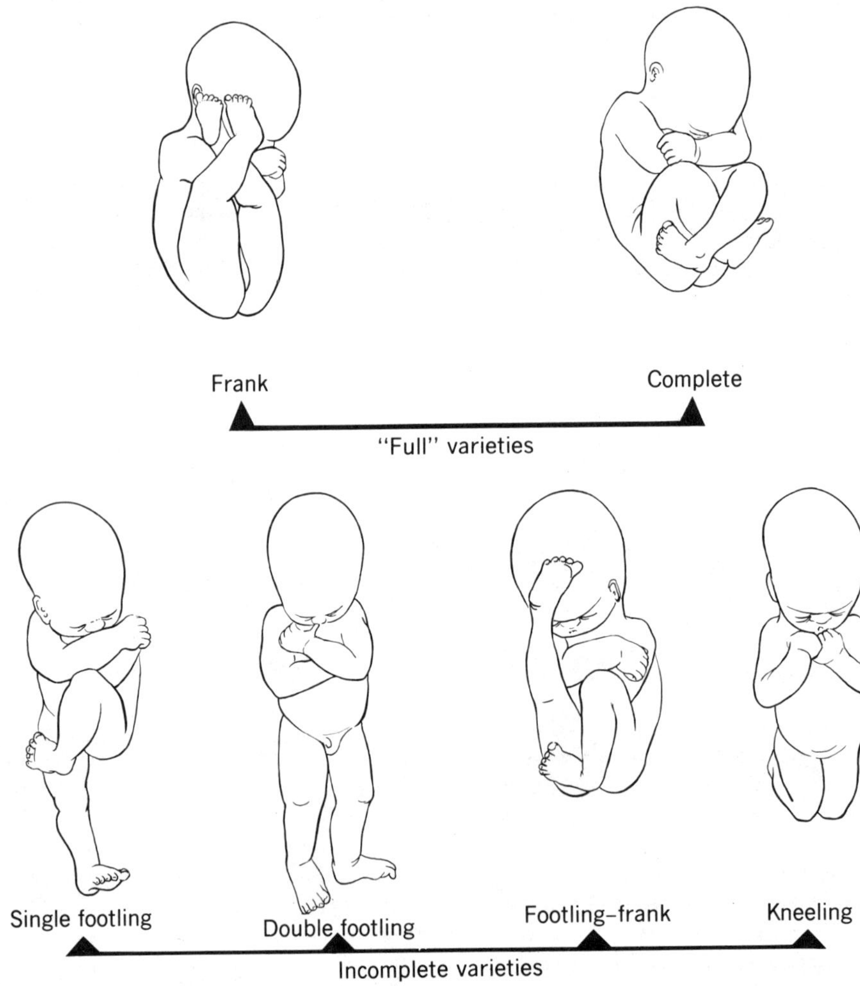

Figure 24-2. Types of breech presentation. Incomplete breech presentation refers to incomplete flexion of any hip or knee joint.

seen in more than 50% of breech fetuses during labor. In the *complete* breech presentation, both hip joints and both knee joints are flexed. In the *incomplete* breech, there may be "incomplete" flexion at either the hip or knee joints. Thus the incomplete breech may present as a single or double footling presentation. Although pelvic exam is helpful in deciding which type of breech presentation is present, confusion may occur (e.g., between double footling and complete breeches or between complete and incomplete breeches). Ultrasound may be helpful in clarifying the exact type of breech presentation, but an abdominal film is most useful in this regard. The x-ray exam also allows evaluation of the normalcy of the bony skull and of the relationship of the skull to the cervical spine (the degree of flexion or extension).

During the second stage of labor, the breech infant delivers successively larger diameters through the bony pelvis, culminating with the largest diameter, the aftercoming head. The vertex presentation may have hours to mould the head to allow adaptation to and safe navigation through the pelvis. The aftercoming head in breech presentation has only minutes to accomplish the same feat. Thus, any significant disproportion between the pelvis and the aftercoming head may result in significant fetal injury or even death.[24,48,56] Because the breech does not fill the birth canal as completely as the head and because the cord is physically closer to the breech than the head, there is an increased risk of umbilical cord prolapse during the first stage of labor[56] or umbilical cord compression during the expulsive maneuvers of the second stage and delivery. These are the major factors underlying the controversy regarding optimal management of breech presentation.

LABOR

Labor in breech presentation is influenced by the mechanical disadvantages caused by the breech. In comparison to the flexion that occurs at the cervical vertebrae in vertex deliveries, in breech presentation flexion occurs at the lumbar vertebrae. More significant usually is the lateral flexion of the trunk necessary for delivery. Flexion of the trunk is even more difficult in frank breech presentation than in nonfrank, because the legs tend to splint the body.

During labor, following lateral flexion of the trunk, the anterior hip is forced against and underneath the symphysis. The expulsive phase that follows delivers the anterior and then the posterior buttock. As the back rotates anteriorly, the shoulders enter the pelvic inlet transversely. The shoulders rotate 90° and deliver in the anterior/posterior diameter. As the anterior scapula is recognized at the introitus, the operator "sweeps" the infant's right humerus across the chest. Careful rotation of the body delivers the posterior scapula. The left humerus may then be delivered in a similar manner. It is important not to attempt to deliver the fetal arm until the scapula is visible. At this point, the aftercoming head usually enters the pelvic inlet obliquely. Internal rotation and flexion then occur. The back of the neck extends against the symphysis and the chin passes over the perineum.

Manual and operative procedures are utilized to assist in the delivery of the breech fetus.

Assisted Breech Delivery

This is a breech delivery in which the infant is supported and helped to deliver with minimal interference. The infant is allowed to deliver spontaneously to the umbilicus. In frank breech presentation, this may require slightly greater maternal expulsive efforts to allow the legs to be born. Several maneuvers may be used to assist breech delivery. The Lovset maneuver begins when the lower angle of the posterior scapula becomes visible. Rotation of the shoulder girdle with minimal resultant trauma is the goal of this technique (Fig. 24-3).[13] The fetal back is anterior and the trunk is encircled with both hands so that the thumbs lie against the infant's thighs. The fingers are applied to te baby's posterior pelvis with care to avoid excessive force in the area of the kidneys or adrenal glands. The trunk is guided downward with minimal traction. When the posterior scapula appears, rotation is employed to effect delivery of the upper extremities. The arms appear, followed by the head at the vulva. Manual pressure applied helps the fetal head to be born.

The Brandt maneuver is also commonly employed in assisted breech delivery. Once the infant has delivered spontaneously to the umbilicus, the obstetrician wraps the fetal body in a warm towel. Both hands are then applied to the posterior aspect of the fetal pelvis. One must avoid applying pressure over the fetal kidney and adrenal glands which are susceptible to crush injuries that may be fatal. Traction is then made in a downward direction. When the lower angle of the anterior scapula becomes vis-

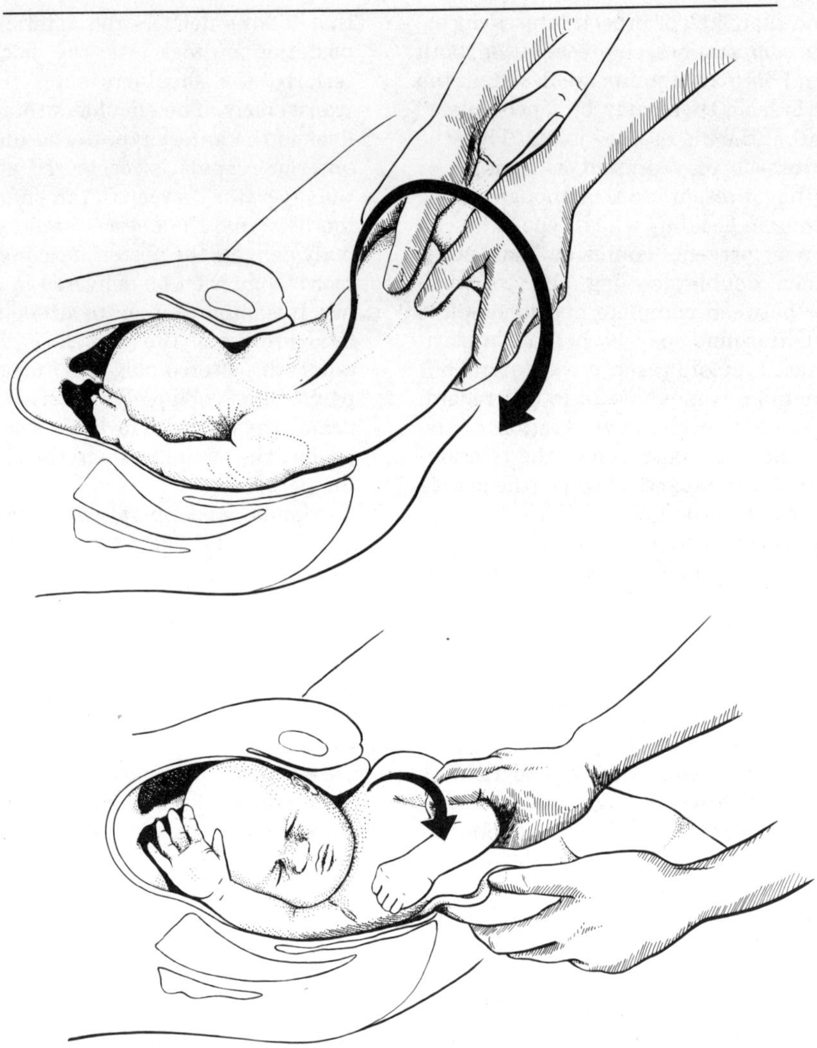

Figure 24-3. The Lovset maneuver for delivering a breech presentation. See text for detailed description.

ible, a finger is swept over the chest to release the arm. This having been accomplished, gentle rotation is used to bring the other scapula anteriorly. The second arm is released by gentle sweeping across the fetal chest. In performing the rotation at the cervical spine, the operator should remember that the vertebral arteries are susceptible to trauma at this point and that excessive rotation (past 105°) may result in either cervical spine injuries or trauma to the vertebral arteries. The head is next delivered by either manual or operative technique.

During delivery of the abdomen and chest, excessive haste may result in the loss of flexion of the aftercoming head or arms which are potentially serious problems. Delivery of nuchal arms may be managed by rotating the trunk. Most authors feel that deflexion of the aftercoming head is the single most difficult situation that may be encountered. Suprapubic pressure should be attempted to regain flexion.

Delivering the Aftercoming Head

As with other aspects of breech delivery, various techniques are available for effecting delivery of the aftercoming head. Maintaining flexion of the head and arms is cardinal to effecting safe breech delivery regardless of route. By placing one hand on the head abdominally, an assistant may "follow the head" into the pelvis to aid in maintaining this attitude (Naujok's maneuver, Fig. 24-4).

The Mauriceau–Smellie–Viet (MSV) maneuver (Fig. 24-5) is useful for effecting delivery when the head of the infant is in the occiput anterior position and the back turned toward the symphysis. The body of the infant, abdomen down, is supported on the operator's left arm and the index finger is inserted into the baby's mouth while two other fingers are applied to the face to maintain flexion. The head is then delivered by downward traction until the back of the neck extends under the pubic arch. A modification of the MSV maneuver encourages maintenance of flexion of the aftercoming head by pressure on the malar eminences and avoiding a finger in the mouth. Another modification of the MSV maneuver is the Wigand–Martin–Winkle maneuver. When the aftercoming head is higher than the operator had anticipated, the first tractive efforts made to accomplish delivery must complete flexion and internal rotation. Therefore, suprapubic pressure is made with one hand, while the other keeps the head flexed and helps to guide it out of the pelvis.[55]

Many times, the aftercoming head can be successfully delivered by the use of suprapubic pressure (Kristellar pressure). The principle here is the same: maintenance of flexion. This allows the smallest diameter of the aftercoming head to present. Loss of flexion substitutes a

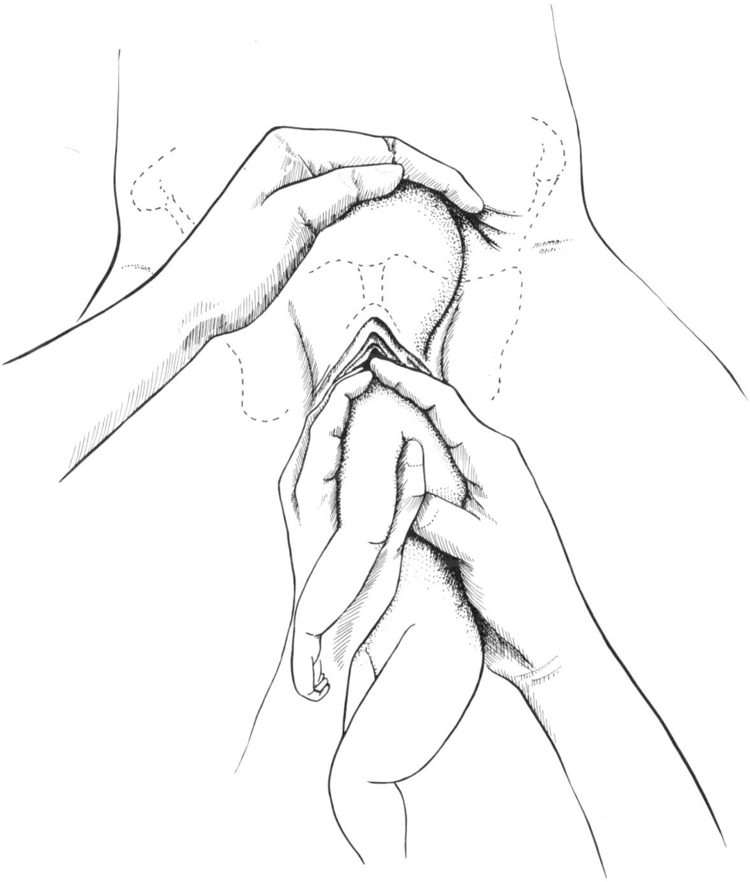

Figure 24-4. Naujok's maneuver is applied to the aftercoming head at high station. The attendant applies traction on the shoulders with both hands, while the assistant presses downward on the head to maintain flexion.

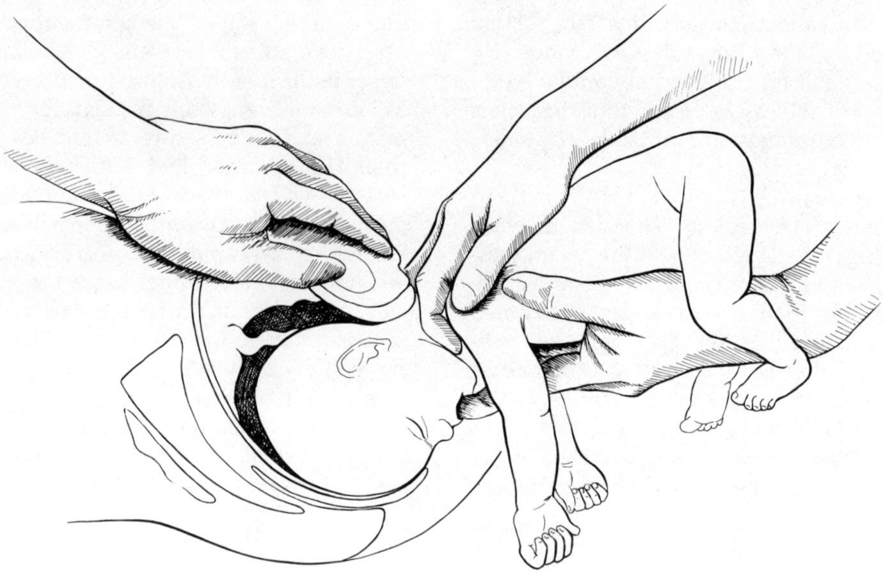

Figure 24-5. The Mauriceau–Smellie–Viet maneuver is useful in effecting delivery of the aftercoming head in occiput anterior position. See text for description.

longer diameter, thus making delivery more difficult.

Occasionally the occiput has turned posteriorly. The technique employed for delivery in this situation (modified Prague maneuver) describes the baby laid with his back on the operator's arm.[37] The index and middle fingers of the hand hook onto either side of the fetal neck from behind. An assistant inserts the index fingers of his hands into the child's mouth (or uses two fingers to maintain flexion on facial bones) and the infant is delivered maintaining flexion. Where the aftercoming head is directed posteriorly and is also complicated by deflexion, delivery may be effected as follows: The back of the baby is laid on the attendant's forearm, the other hand grasping the legs above the ankles. This results in the occiput passing forward over the sacral concavity and then over the perineum. The fetal larynx serves as a fulcrum in this type of delivery (Fig. 24-6).

Forceps in Breech Delivery

In 1924, Edmond Piper of Philadelphia introduced a special forcep for managing the aftercoming head in breech delivery.[9,47] Its main advantage is long shanks that allow a more suitable pelvic curve. This allows the handles to be at a lower level than the blade of the forcep, making these forceps relatively easy to apply to the aftercoming head (see Chapter 44). Very little traction is necessary in effecting delivery with Piper forceps. The aftercoming head must have descended to fill the pelvis and must be in the direct occiput anterior position. Delivery of the fetus using the forceps to elevate the aftercoming head about a point formed by the posterior aspect of the fetal neck where it meets the pubic symphysis allows delivery with maintenance of flexion. Kielland's forceps as well as Simpson's have also been applied successfully to the aftercoming head in breech delivery.

Spontaneous Breech Delivery

In spontaneous breech delivery, the patient effects delivery totally by her expulsive efforts. Whereas this may seem optimal, it is possible that the aftercoming head, subject to rapid and significant changes in external and internal pressure, may be subjected to greater trauma than that of the manual and operative techniques described above. In vaginal breech deliveries of multiparas and nulliparas, the lower five-minute Apgar scores seen with multiparous patients can be ascribed to this rapid change in pressure.[24]

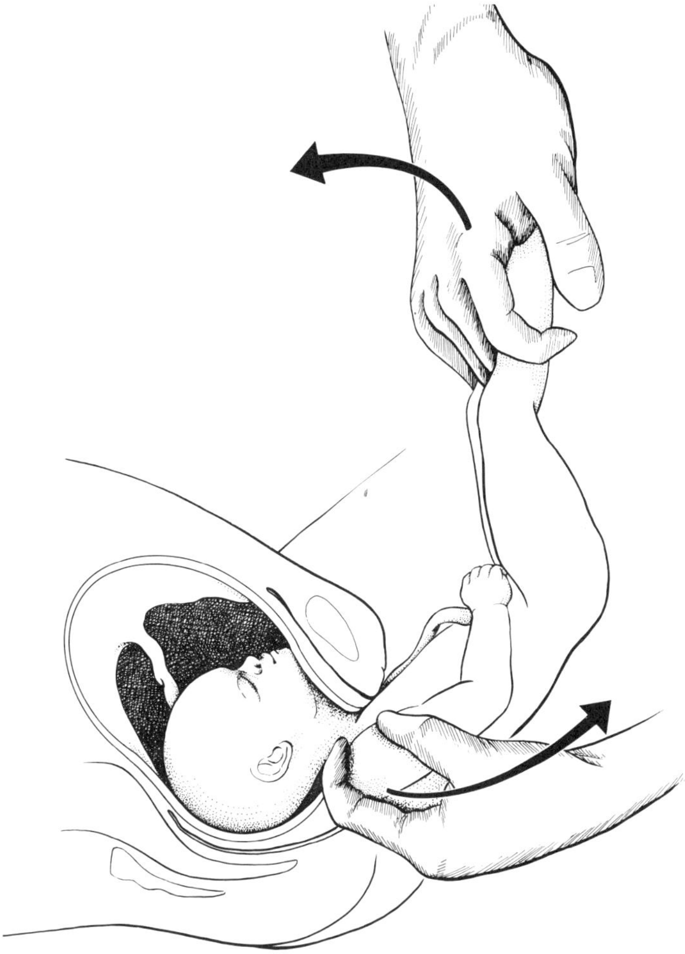

Figure 24-6. The Prague maneuver is utilized when the aftercoming head is in the occiput posterior position. The anterior larynx serves as a fulcrum point. See text for description.

The Breech Delivery Team

In effecting any vaginal breech delivery, it is important to stress the following. The obstetrician must have a gowned and gloved assistant. When feasible, the delivery room should be set up in advance and should include warm towels and Piper forceps in addition to the regular delivery instruments. The delivery room should be equipped with a fetal monitor to allow continuous monitoring of the fetus up to the point of delivery.

Expert anesthesia and pediatric support are crucial to the successful outcome of breech delivery, whether vaginally or by cesarean section. In about 10% of our vaginal breech deliveries, general anesthesia is employed during the delivery of the aftercoming head. By limiting maternal expulsive efforts, regional anesthesia may be very helpful in special situations associated with breech delivery, primarily premature breech infants and term nonfrank breech presentations.[9] In both instances, prolapse of either the umbilical cord or the fetal body through a partially dilated cervix is a major concern. By keeping the fetal membranes intact as long as possible and using regional anesthesia, these two difficult groups of breech presentations may be managed safely per vaginam.

The first few minutes after breech delivery are invariably associated with some degree of asphyxia.[15,28,62] This is evidenced by the high incidence of low one-minute Apgar scores seen at term breech delivery independent of delivery mode.[25,28] Umbilical cord gases frequently yield evidence of some degree of respiratory acidosis.

This probably results from partial cord compression as the body passes through the birth canal. A nuchal cord frequently accompanies breech presentation. Since breech infants are generally subjected to greater degrees of cord occlusion than are uncomplicated vertex deliveries, one may generally anticipate that the mild respiratory acidosis will resolve. Five-minute Apgar scores demonstrate no disadvantage for vaginal delivery in comparison to cesarean section when a conservative selective protocol has been employed.[20,25,62] The first few moments after birth represent a period in which many of these infants need some support, primarily supplemental oxygen. The short time available for moulding of the aftercoming head compared to that of cephalic deliveries increases the possibility of significant asphyxia and demands the presence of a skilled pediatrician at the delivery.

A great deal of anguish and haste has resulted from the dictum that once the cord appears, there are only "X" minutes available before severe neurologic sequelae occur to the infant. This misconception has yielded more traumatic injury than its putative benefits. This premise presupposes that the cord is totally occluded—the worst possible situation. The median time in our series for effecting delivery after the cord appears is 60 seconds.[25] Although this is a "long" minute or so for the attendants in the delivery room, it is vital that the obstetrician use only deliberate speed in effecting delivery. Acidosis (pH less than 7.20) is not frequent at vaginal breech delivery until six minutes or longer have passed.[19] It is rare (1/200) for delivery time to exceed six minutes when labor and vaginal delivery have been decided on by protocol selection.

If the appearance of umbilicus to delivery time is six minutes or less, the five-minute Apgar score is more than 7 virtually always.[8] We conclude that only partial cord occlusion generally occurs from the time that the umbilicus appears to the time of delivery. Thus, conclusions concerning *complete* cord occlusion and a critical "4 minute" time to delivery are not applicable to this situation.

A major current dilemma is that of obtaining sufficient experience at breech delivery. Little or minimal experience is gained in many training programs. Thus, many recently trained obstetricians may have great difficulty when faced with imminent delivery of a breech fetus in a facility unable to perform an emergency cesarean section. In our prospective series, 12% of patients randomized to cesarean section delivered vaginally before cesarean section could be performed. Thus, some breeches deliver per vaginam before they can be "saved" by a cesarean section. It behooves the obstetrician in training to learn as much as possible about the manual maneuvers required to safely effect and assist a breech delivery by practicing breech extraction techniques at cesarean section for breech presentation. The breech extraction performed at cesarean section should be conducted in a manner that maximizes experience.

To provide the best possible care for the parturient and her breech fetus, several other areas of concern should be considered, although not addressed in detail (Fig 24–7).

1. The question of standards of practice (medicolegal issues) (see Chapter 50).
2. Obtaining informed consent from the patient (see Chapter 50).
3. The desire and preference of the patient.

MANAGEMENT OPTIONS

Term Breech

External Cephalic Version. External cephalic version (ECV) refers to the conversion of a breech presentation to a cephalic presentation, usually prior to labor.[50,53] With use of tocolytic drugs to relax the uterus and appropriate surveillance methods (nonstress testing, ultrasound, and Kliehauer-Betke testing), ECV at 37–39 weeks of gestation is safe and effective.[57] A significant number of breech presentations diagnosed as late as 37–39 weeks may spontaneously convert from breech to vertex prior to labor. Thus the recognition of breech presentation at term but prior to labor is not a definitive indication for elective cesarean section. The physician must inform the patient of the option of attempted version with breech presentation. If her fetus remains in breech presentation, she should present herself for evaluation at the earliest suggestion of labor or rupture of membranes. At this point, in early labor or with rupture of membranes, the decision regarding cesarean section, trial of labor, or ECV must be made.

To perform ECV successfully, the breech must not be engaged and uterine activity must be abolished. There must be sufficient amniotic fluid to allow a safe attempt at rotation, and placentation must be normal. Anesthesia is contraindicated, since the necessity to avoid pain or

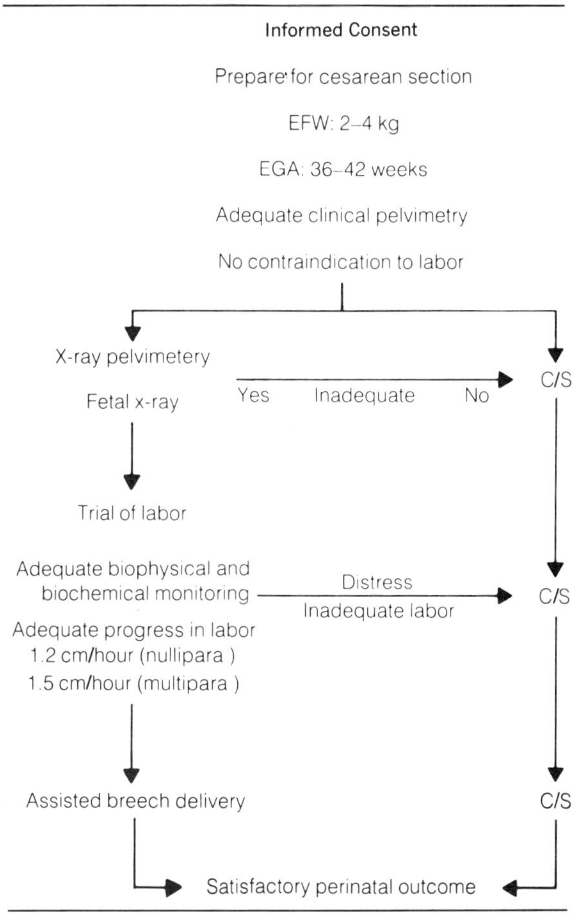

Figure 24-7. Evolving flow chart for management of breech presentation. (Reprinted from Gimovsky, M. L., and Petrie, R. H.: Strategy for choosing the best delivery route for the breech baby. Contemp. OB/GYN **21** (April): 201–215, 1983, with permission of Medical Economics Company.)

major discomfort during the procedure is a safeguard which limits the force applied.[53] External cephalic version should be performed in proximity to the laor and delivery suite, because it is possible, although unlikely, that an emergency situation may arise demanding delivery room care. The procedure begins with real-time B scanning to document presentation. It also permits observation of the fetus for movement and evaluation of relative amniotic fluid volume and location of the placenta. Next, a nonstress test (NST) is performed. We avoid ECV if the NST is nonreactive. An i.v. is started, and a tocolytic agent, generally a betamimetic drug (magnesium sulfate in diabetics), is given to promote uterine relaxation. The operator places one hand over the breech for elevation and the other over the head, and begins to rotate through the shortest arc. Rotation is accomplished slowly, carefully, and avoiding undue force.

This procedure is successful in 70–80% of breech presentations at 37–39 weeks gestation. We are currently evaluating the efficacy of external version for both breech and transverse presentations in early labor when the membranes are intact.

Selective Trial of Labor. Patients with known breech presentation prior to labor represent a high-risk group. Even on obstetric services that permit a trial of labor (TOL), the majority of women with breech presentations will require cesarean section.[20] The overall incidence of cesarean section for all breech presentations averages about 70% at Women's Hospital, LAC/USC. In the term breech, cesarean section rates of 33% for frank breech fetuses have been reported; in another study that allowed a TOL regardless of type of breech, a cesarean section range of 50–60% was noted. We have noted no significant difference between primiparous and multiparous patients in this regard, although our cesarean section rate for primiparous patients is slightly higher than for multiparas.

Our protocol for the management of term breech presentation in labor is the same for both frank and nonfrank breech presentations. As previously noted the protocol outlined has a historic basis (The Sloane Hospital for Women at Columbia University[24,56]) and a current prospective basis (Women's Hospital, LAC/USC Medical Center). The risk of cord prolapse and body prolapse in the first stage of labor is higher in nonfrank than in frank breech presentations, but this complication does not present an unmanageable problem on a service with full emergency services.[20,24,25] Continuous electronic fetal monitoring, frequent clinical evaluation, and the availability of emergency cesarean delivery are essential.

We begin our approach to these patients with a detailed discussion as to the fetal and maternal risks and benefits of a trial of labor or an elective cesarean delivery. Our recent experience with several hundred patients in this category provides the background data that are described to each patient. We believe that the risk to the breech-presenting fetus of a TOL and vaginal delivery is not unreasonable in highly selected circumstances. Neonatal morbidity, comparing groups undergoing carefully monitored labor and assisted breech delivery and cesarean section, is similar.[8,20,24,25,43,60] Maternal morbidity is substantially greater with abdominal delivery.[8,25,43] The risk of fetal/neonatal death secondary to breech delivery exists even with adherence to the protocol and attention to detail; however, this risk is small (approximately 1/500). In our preliminary study, one asphyxiated infant was lost as a result of inadequate resuscitation.[25] Subsequently, we have not lost an infant due to vaginal delivery. The risk of occurrence of fetal injuries at vaginal delivery and cesarean section is similar (1/100:1/500). Thus, the fetal/neonatal risk associated with vaginal delivery must be weighed against the increased maternal morbidity (50%) and maternal mortality (1/10,000) seen with cesarean delivery. The final choice becomes an individual decision that each patient, the family, and the physician must consider.

After informed consent is obtained, the patient is prepared for abdominal delivery. Cesarean section, if elected, is performed, utilizing regional anesthesia if appropriate. If a TOL is elected, ultrasound is performed to exclude obvious neural tube defects. Anencephaly, hydrocephaly, and meningomyelocele are more common in breech presentation.[5,40] Their presence may countermand cesarean section because of limited survival. The management of hydrocephaly is controversial since long-term outlook remains limited. With cesarean section the outlook for these neonates may actually improve. With parental consent, decompression may be performed to allow vaginal delivery in selected cases.

Next, the patient is sent for x-ray evaluation. Significant factors in the x-ray evaluation of the fetus and maternal pelvis include the bony pelvis, evaluation for hyperextension of the head, and the bones of the fetal skull.

We have already noted the importance of excluding patients with borderline pelvis from vaginal delivery of a breech-presenting fetus (i.e., lack of time for the moulding process).[48,56] Entrapment of the aftercoming head by the cervix is less likely than is difficulty in effecting delivery of the aftercoming head due to bony obstruction by a borderline pelvis.[20] The exception is the premature infant in which entrapment by the cervix is the greater risk.[20,21] (See section below entitled Preterm Breech.) The trauma that may be sustained, both to the skull and to the cervical spine, has lethal potential. Thus x-ray pelvimetry is essential to exclude a contracted pelvis.

X-ray pelvimetry appeared in Europe in the late 1800s following Roentgen's discovery of the x-ray. Its long history is punctuated by waxing and waning popularity, along with questions regarding its necessity, usefulness, and risk to the fetus and infant. Many methods of x-ray pelvimetry exist.[17,58] The older methods are relatively cumbersome. Pelvimetry by digital radiography provides less exposure to radiation and is currently being compared with traditional x-ray pelvimetry for accuracy. Decreased x-ray exposure is desirable because of the oncogenic potential of fetal irradiation. The maximum radiation required to perform pelvimetry by computerized tomography (CT) scan is about 20–30% that of traditional methods.[16] Fetal gonadal exposure from traditional x-ray pelvimetry is on the order of 800 millirads.[44] By comparison, a single digital radiograph exposes the fetus to 20–30 millirads. As important as the absolute accuracy or radiation dosage delivered, however, is the correlation of the results of computerized tomographic studies with those of x-ray pelvimetry. The relative cost effectiveness and availability of CT scanning must also be evaluated. Evaluation of the fetus and bony pelvis by CT scanning has the potential to further enhance safe delivery in breech presentation. It seems likely that this technique will gain in popularity in the future if proved accurate and cost effective.

Todd and Steer[56] reported on the delivery of over 1000 term breeches at Columbia Presbyterian Medical Center during the 1950s and 1960s. The ultimate safety of vaginal delivery was directly related to the adequacy of pelvic measurements as obtained by x-ray pelvimetry. When the inlet of the bony pelvis measured 11 cm in the AP and 12 cm in the transverse diameters, the majority (85%) of infants were delivered vaginally and safely. The perinatal mortality was 1 in 200. When either of these critical measurements was not achieved, the majority of infants required cesarean delivery (60%) and the perinatal mortality rate among those infants allowed to deliver vaginally was 12 times greater than in the group with adequate measurements. Twenty years later on the same obstetric service, Gimovsky et al.[24] added an interspinous diameter of greater than 10 cm to Todd and Steer's original recommendations. This simple 10,11,12 rule (Table 24-2) provides the basis for excluding the "borderline" pelvis. Clinical pelvimetry is not sufficient to accomplish this.[48,54] Perinatal morbidity is increased fivefold when x-ray pelvimetry is omitted or when the critical measurements are not equaled or exceeded.

The x-ray must also evaluate the relation between the head and thorax to exclude hyperextension, which occurs in approximately 5% of term breech presentations.[20] The anterior angle between the mandible and the cervical spine is used to judge the degree of flexion or extension of the fetal head. Extension is diagnosed when this angle exceeds 105°– (Fig. 24-8). Extension of the head in breech presentation is often associated with spinal cord trauma and traumatic injury at vaginal delivery.[6] Indeed, these fetuses may be difficult to deliver even at cesarean section. The causes of hyperextension include multiple loops of nuchal cord,[45] fetal neck masses, torticollis,[6] neurological abnormalities of the neck musculature,[2] trisomy 21, anencephaly, and uterine abnormalities such as myomas or septae.[20]

TABLE 24-2. RESULTS OF X-RAY PELVIMETRY FROM A GROUP OF WOMEN UNDERGOING A SUCCESSFUL TRIAL OF LABOR UNDER PROTOCOL

	Minimum Acceptable	Actual (Mean ± 2 SD)
Inlet		
Anteroposterior	≧ 11 cm	11.9 ± 0.8 cm
Transverse	≧ 12 cm	12.8 ± 0.6 cm
Midpelvis		
Interspinous	≧ 10 cm	10.5 ± 0.5 cm

Source: Gimovsky, M. L., Wallace, R. L., Schifrin, B. S., and Paul, R. H.: Randomized management of the nonfrank breech presentation at term: A preliminary report. *Am. J. Obstet. Gynecol.* **146:**34–40, 1983.

If the radiologic criteria are met, the patient returns to the fetal intensive care area for fetal monitoring during labor. Fetal distress is managed similarly to the vertex presentation. However, the breech fetus may become acidotic during labor more rapidly than the cephalic fetus.[15,30,61,62] Pelvic exam should be performed on spontaneous rupture of membranes or with any evidence of abnormal fetal heart rate patterns to exclude prolapse of the umbilical cord. Fetal blood samples may be obtained from the fetal buttocks. Changes in fetal pH or base excess similar to those in cephalic presentation are predictive of fetal distress and may signal the need for imminent delivery. In general, serious abnormalities of FHR in the breech mandate cesarean delivery.[30]

The use of oxytocin in breech labor and delivery is controversial. Induction of labor for toxemia, postdate pregnancy, or abnormal antepartum testing may be considered if the breech is engaged in the pelvis and if the radiologic criteria are met. There is no increased risk to breech presentations induced for these indications.[8,20,24,25] Macrosomia, as well as potential uteroplacental insufficiency such as seen in severe pregnancy-induced hypertension or postmature pregnancy, should be considered as relative contraindications to induction in breech presentation.

Augmentation of labor may present significant risk, but the data are inadequate to yield firm conclusions. Rupture of the membranes to augment breech labor increases risk over that of the breech infant in spontaneous labor.[5] Augmentation with oxytocin in the presence of intact membranes is probably safer. Arrest of active labor in breech presentation may signal the presence of a large fetus.[18] Thus, the arrest of labor may be a signal that cesarean section should be employed. In our experience, the majority of infants with arrest of dilatation or of descent are indeed large. Thus, cesarean section may be preferable to augmentation of labor.[25]

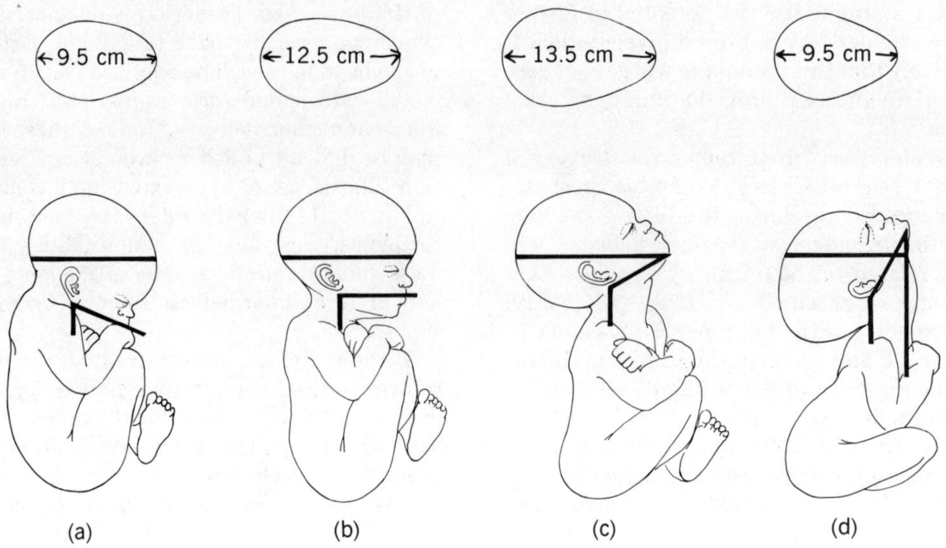

Figure 24-8. Progressive deflexion (hyperextension) of the aftercoming head causes change in the largest effective diameter of the fetal head. (a) Full flexion presents the suboccipitobregmatic diameter. (b) The occipitofrontal diameter results from partial deflexion. (c) Further extension presents the occipitomental diameter. (d) Complete extension presents the trachelobregmatic diameter. See text for details.

We continue to augment labor selectively and collect data.

The second stage of labor ideally should be managed in the delivery room. With an anesthesiologist and a pediatrician present, the patient is prepped and draped in the usual fashion for vaginal delivery. We prefer anesthesia standby with prompt induction of general anesthesia, should circumstance mandate.

After bladder catheterization, pudendal nerve block is utilized. A generous episiotomy (or episioproctotomy) is performed when the buttocks crown. By utilizing continuous electronic fetal monitoring within the delivery room, fetal evaluation is possible virtually to completion of delivery. The membranes are left intact as long as possible. At this point, the inexperienced attendant must consciously suppress any feelings of anxiety. We have preselected an average-sized fetus in an average-sized pelvis who has not had significant fetal distress or serious labor abnormality and, therefore, we may expect safe delivery. The infant is allowed to deliver spontaneously as far as possible. The majority deliver at least to the umbilicus without assistance. At this point, the membranes are ruptured, if intact, and a loop of umbilical cord may be freed. The infant's body should be supported with the left hand by the right-handed obstetrician. The Mauriceau-Smellie-Viet or Wigand-Martin-Winkle maneuver may then be employed. The Piper forceps are especially designed to deal with the aftercoming head and can be used for maintaining flexion, but not for traction. A common error in utilizing Piper forceps is to attempt to apply them before the head has fully descended into the pelvis.

The differences in outcome between breech infants delivered by elective cesarean section or vaginally under the protocol described above are minimal for infants between 1500 and 4000 grams, whether frank or nonfrank presentations, and whether the mother is nulliparous or multiparous. Although we are still studying the 1500–2000 gram group, we consider a patient a definite candidate for a trial of labor if she has attained at least 36 weeks gestation, or if the fetal weight is more than 2000 grams. At LAC/USC Women's Hospital in 1980, the only deaths in term breech infants were associated with lethal congenital anomalies. A head:abdomen ratio of less than 1:1 is desirable.

At LAC/USC, approximately 50% of women

with term breech fetuses are allowed a trial of labor.[8,24,25,43] Approximately one-half of the women who enter the protocol ultimately require cesarean section. The vast majority of these (60%) fail to meet minimal x-ray pelvimetry criteria (Table 24-3).[25] In the absence of strict selection criteria and the use of x-ray pelvimetry, fetal monitoring, and assisted breech delivery, the risk of morbidity for term breech infants undergoing vaginal delivery is approximately five times greater than for a similar group of breech fetuses delivered with adherence to protocol.[23] The risk of perinatal mortality was only marginally greater in this group.

Elective Cesarean Section. Many practitioners elect to deliver the breech-presenting fetus by cesarean section regardless of other considerations.[42,63] This decision involves obstetrical, social, and medicolegal factors. The overwhelming concern is to avoid potentially preventable birth injury and the infrequent, but potentially disastrous, entrapment of the aftercoming head.

Routine cesarean section in breech presentation is most beneficial for (1) patients delivering in facilities not equipped with full-time support services, (2) women delivering breech fetuses of 34 or less weeks of gestation and/or estimated fetal weights less than 2000 grams, (3) any viable breech where hyperextension of the head is demonstrated by x-ray, (4) any patient who desires cesarean section, and (5) double footling breech (highest risk fetus among breech presentation for major labor and delivery problems).

Adequate incisions of the uterus and the abdominal wall are critical to avoid fetal trauma at cesarean section for breech presentation. Entrapment of the aftercoming head in the rectus fascia has led to quadraplegia secondary to traumatic transection of the cervical spinal cord, as well as to stillbirth. Although the data do not prove the necessity for a vertical anterior abdominal wall incision, it is recommended that when employing a Pfannenstiel incision care be taken to guarantee an adequate opening in the anterior fascia. The uterine incision, when transverse, must also be generous. At cesarean section, total breech extraction is performed. This is inherently a more dangerous procedure than assisted breech delivery.[36] When delivering the frank breech at cesarean section, rotation of the hips into the incision usually results in spontaneous flexion. Great care must be exercised

TABLE 24-3. "FAILED" TRIAL OF LABOR*

Reason	Number of Patients	Trial of Labor Failures (%)	Trial of Labor Patients (%)
X-ray evaluation			
Fetal head hyperextended	2	5	3
Pelvimetry			
1 Diameter contracted	18	46	26
2 Diameters contracted	5	13	7
Labor			
Latent-phase arrest (with oxytocin)	2	5	3
Active-phase arrest (with oxytocin)	2	5	3
Active-phase arrest (no oxytocin)	1	3	1
Arrest of descent	1	3	1
Prolapse (first stage)			
Umbilical cord	3	8	4
Body	2	5	3
Excluded after randomization			
Progressed too rapidly	2	5	3
Elective	1	3	1
Total number of patients	39		

*Failed TOL ($n = 39$); total patients in study ($n = 105$).

Source: Gimovsky, M. L., Wallace, R. L., Schifrin, B. S., and Paul, R. H.: Randomized management of the nonfrank breech presentation at term: A preliminary report. *Am. J. Obstet. Gynecol.* **146**:34–40, 1983.

not to use excessive force.[46] In incomplete and footling breeches, delivery is usually straightforward. The assistant should maintain pressure on the fundus and follow the fetal head down to maintain flexion. Extraction should be performed slowly to prevent deflexion of the head and to lessen the incidence of nuchal arms. When a nuchal arm occurs, rotation of the trunk and shoulders is necessary as it is at vaginal delivery. The arm should be flexed onto the chest and swept in cephalad to caudad direction to minimize trauma. The aftercoming head should be delivered with continued pressure on the fundus to maintain flexion. The fingers that maintain flexion on the aftercoming head should be placed on the malar eminences and, where possible, the operator should avoid maintaining flexion by placing a finger in the fetal mouth. Diverticula of the oral pharynx have been described from digital pressure applied in this manner. Lateral pressure to the head should be avoided, since this may result in brachial plexus injury. The aftercoming head should be brought into the operative field by pressure directly on the uterus. Additional uterine relaxation with halothane is only rarely necessary to effect delivery. The uterus should be explored for anomalies after delivery of any breech presentation. The septate uterus as well as myomas and minor uterine anomalies are more frequent with breech-presenting fetuses.[5,20]

One-minute Apgar scores of 3 or less occur more frequently in breech than in vertex delivery. This is true whether delivery is by cesarean section or vaginally.[24,25]

The Oucome for the Breech Infant. Bony injury and peripheral nerve damage are increased in breech delivery.[5,12,20,48] Not generally appreciated is that injury occurs to some breech fetuses at cesarean section. The spectrum of injuries sustained by breech-presenting infants is similar at cesarean section and in patients selected for vaginal delivery (Table 24-4).[20] Erb's palsy, bony fractures, and low five-minute Apgar scores are equal in both groups. Five-minute Apgar scores after the vaginal delivery of carefully selected breech presentations are the same as those seen in vertex deliveries.

Intracranial hemorrhage, neurologic sequelae, bony fractures, and visceral injury all are problems that occur in the breech infant independent of gestational age. The prospective study by Collea et al.[8] on frank breeches suggested that the use of a selective protocol could limit injury and "breech" death. Gimovsky et al.,[25] utilizing a selective protocol for nonfrank breech term infants, demonstrated similar neonatal morbidity in infants selected for trial of labor and those delivered by elective cesarean section. Others have noted similar outcomes, both immediate[28] and long term.[31]

Preterm Breech

Twenty-five percent of all breech fetuses are premature at the onset of labor. The vast majority of these will be born by cesarean section. Comparison of the significant fetal diameters (biparietal, bisacromial, and intratrochanteric) of preterm infants with those of term infants demonstrates that the earlier gestational age fetus is at an even greater disadvantage in negotiating the pelvic outlet than is the term breech (Fig. 24-9) due to the disproportionately greater head circumference relative to abdominal circumference. Other significant negative factors

TABLE 24-4. PERINATAL AND MATERNAL MORBIDITY ASSOCIATED WITH BREECH LABOR AND DELIVERY

Perinatal Morbidity (281 infants >2000 g)	Maternal morbidity (330 deliveries)
Five minute Apgar score <7	245 Cesarean sections
Vaginal delivery 5/78 (6.4%)	1 Cesarean hysterectomy
Cesarean section 6/203 (3.0%)	1 Pseudocholinesterase deficiency
Brachial plexus injury	2 Aspiration pneumonias
Vaginal delivery 2/78 (2.6%)	9 Wound infections
Cesarean section 2/203 (1.0%)	85 Vaginal deliveries
p = NS	No significant morbidity

Data from the Obstetrical Service, LAC/USC Medical Center, Los Angeles, CA.
Source: Gimovsky, M. L. and Paul, R. H.: Singleton breech presentation in labor: Experience in 1980. *Am. J. Obstet. Gynecol.* **143**:733–739, 1982.

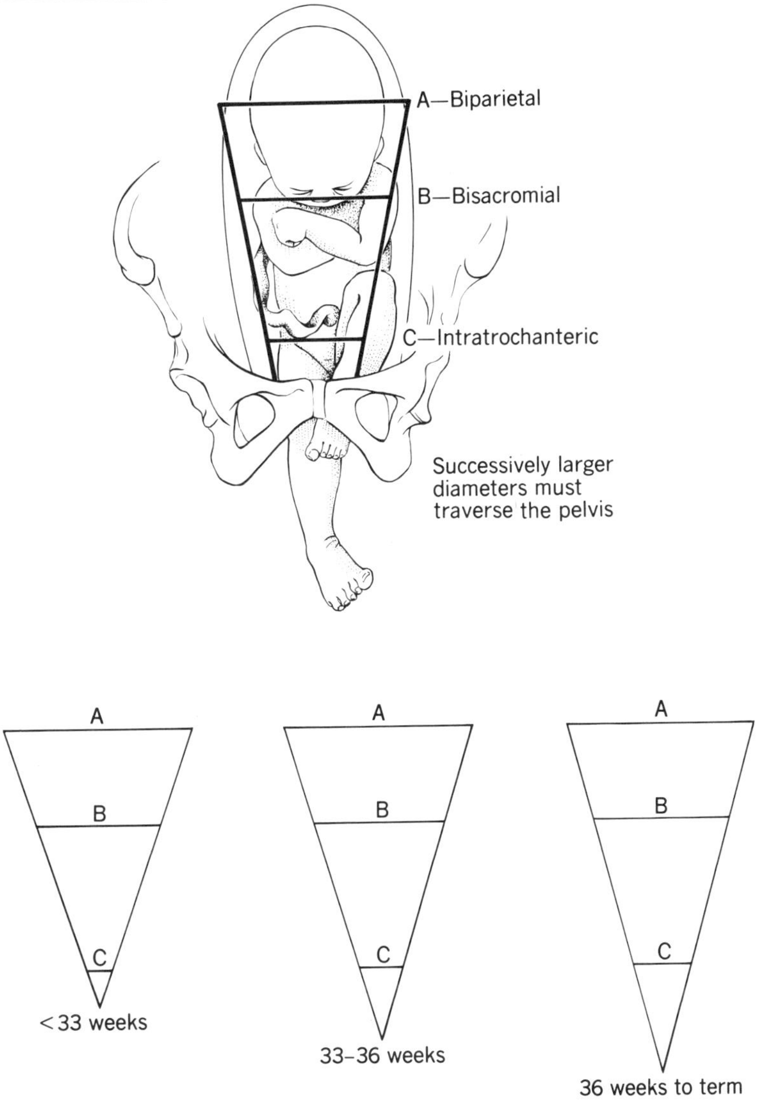

Figure 24-9. The infant in breech presentation may be envisioned as a triangle with the base formed by the biparietal diameter and with the bisacromial and intratrochanteric diameters progressively smaller. The ratios of these diameters decrease with increasing maturity. Thus the relatively smaller body of the premature infant increases the risk of entrapment of the upper body and particularly of the head.

seen in the preterm breech include (1) increased incidence of nonfrank presentations with attendant increased risk of umbilical cord prolapse;[26] (2) increased incidence of premature rupture of membranes, which results in a further loss of effective dilating wedge;[20] (3) decreased ability of the premature infant to tolerate stress in labor;[21,49,59] and (4) the problem of differentiation of the growth-retarded fetus from the premature infant.

The partially dilated cervix, which allows delivery of the smaller fetal diameters, may entrap the head of the premature infant. Only those breech infants weighing less than 1500 grams suffer death or significant depression at birth on the basis of umbilical cord prolapse or head entrapment at delivery.[20] Even when the fetal heart is followed with continuous electronic monitoring, umbilical cord prolapse and resulting fetal distress take a higher toll among preterm infants than among term infants. When the aftercoming head is entrapped, even Dührssen's (cervical) incisions may not allow intact salvage of a preterm breech infant delivered vaginally. The safeguards that have proved efficacious in term breech management (x-ray pelvimetry, fetal monitoring, assisted breech delivery, full anesthesia, and pediatric support) do not protect infants weighing less than 2000 grams. In these small infants, the birth injuries sustained and the neonatal death rates are the same for infants managed with or without benefit of protocol.[21] This outcome is understandable because obstruction offered by the bony pelvis should not play a significant role in delivery trauma for the low-birth-weight fetus. Cervical entrapment of the aftercoming head and soft tissue entrapment are more significant as potential adverse factors. Cesarean section is utilized to a greater extent in the delivery of the preterm infant. Existing data do not prove the benefit of cesarean section to low-birth-weight breech infants.[10,14,21,26,32,33,35] Further review of retrospective data may determine the impact cesarean section has in this group.

External Cephalic Version. External cephalic version performed when labor and delivery seem imminent is a time-honored management for this group of infants. Improved tocolytic drugs may allow ECV in some cases of preterm labor. This would not apply to infants with premature rupture of membranes, placenta previa, placental abruption, or abnormal fetal heart rate testing. Chervenak et al.,[7] using external cephalic version in twin gestations, gained some experience with external cephalic version under tocolysis of low-birth-weight breech infants. They reported one neonatal death among the group of low-birth-weight breech fetuses in an 1100 gram fetus, suggesting increased potential risk of ECV in this group. Perhaps reconstitution of amniotic fluid volume will permit version to become a tenable alternative.

Vaginal Delivery. As noted above, when conducting a trial of labor in breech infants weighing 1500–2000 grams, conduction anesthesia may help to protect the fetus by reducing maternal expulsive efforts during the end of the first stage of labor and delivery and may thus decrease the risk of cord prolapse and the potential for delivering the fetus before complete cervical dilatation.

Fetal monitoring may help to avoid serious asphyxia prior to delivery.[61] Compression of the umbilical cord is associated with an increased tendency to fetal acidosis during labor.[15,30,62] The application of forceps to the aftercoming head decreases mortality among breech infants weighing 1000–2500 grams.[41] A generous episiotomy is desirable.

Among the subgroups of breech infants in which cord prolapse is least likely, that is, frank and complete breeches, a prospective study of trial of labor in infants between 32 and 36 weeks gestational age should be undertaken. Footling and incomplete low-birth-weight breeches are probably best managed by cesarean section.[22]

Cesarean Section. The impact of anesthesia and operative technique must be considered in performing abdominal delivery. General anesthesia may provide better abdominal wall relaxation and allows the addition of halothane, should more uterine relaxation be urgently required. The midline vertical, infraumbilical abdominal wall incision is chosen by most operators for ease in delivery. If there has been no or little labor, the uterine incision should be low vertical. Since the indication for cesarean section is avoidance of trauma, both uterine and abdominal wall incisions must be large enough to permit atraumatic delivery. The preterm breech infant must be handled gently. Delivery by total breech extraction is to be performed with deliberate speed. After delivering the legs and pelvis, the pelvis and abdomen should be covered by a warm, wet towel. The infant should be delivered slowly with steady pressure by the assistant on the fundus to maintain flexion of the aftercoming head. The uterus should always be thoroughly explored after delivery of the placenta. Uterine abnormalities are often associated with preterm uterine activity and with breech presentation. The GU tract should be evaluated and the mother appropriately counseled should a significant uterine anomaly be found.

The Outcome for the Preterm Breech Infant. Among breech infants born at less than 37 weeks of gestation and followed for 1–5 years after birth, the incidence of developmental or neurologic abnormalities was 10-fold greater in premature breech infants (age 33–34 weeks) delivered vaginally as compared to cesarean section. The incidence of CSF bleeding was four times greater among vaginally delivered infants. One-third of the breech infants in whom significant neurologic sequelae occurred were small for gestational age, two infants being 800 grams or less.[32] The frequency of neonatal death among vaginally delivered preterm breeches is greatly increased, even when mean gestational age is 34–35 weeks and mean birth weight is 1950 grams.[14] Deaths occur secondary to asphyxia, hyaline membrane disease, and intracranial hemorrhage.

The incidence of low Apgar scores (less than 7 at 5 min), difficulty with the aftercoming head, peripheral nerve injury, and corrected perinatal mortality is even greater when breech infants weighing less than 1500 grams are delivered vaginally. This is true even when selection and management are meticulous.[12,21,26,35,39] Thus, although 1500 grams is the point at which the change in outcome is most dramatic, lower Apgar scores and increased incidence of neurologic sequelae may be seen in all breeches weighing less than 2000 grams or less than 34 weeks gestational age.[27]

The many causes of compromised outcome among premature infants, vertex or breech, confuse the issue of the benefit to be derived from cesarean section. It is reasonable to assume that the nonasphyxiated infant born with a minimum of birth trauma will be the highest quality survivor. Cesarean section is utilized by most practitioners for delivery of low-birth-weight breech infants.[8,23,38] Until a prospective randomized study is performed, this approach is reasonable. The limited information available concerning the relationship of delivery route to morbidity supports this approach. Those born from breech presentation, regardless of delivery mode, have increased perinatal morbidity and mortality due to increased congenital anomalies,[1,4,5,40,51] obstetrical hemorrhage, premature rupture of membranes, premature labor, and intrauterine growth retardation. Some of these factors may be ameliorated by cesarean section. Perhaps avoidance of labor itself may have the greatest benefit in decreasing morbidity. Follow-up studies of long-term neurologic development are difficult to evaluate because of lack of randomization in obstetric management and lack of sophisticated evaluation. Many reported studies antedated availability of ultrasonic scans, continuous electronic fetal monitoring, and the enhanced survival seen in modern neonatal intensive care units. In favor of cesarean section for the breech infant who weighs less than 2000 grams, is less than 34 weeks gestation, or who is at term and suffers from growth retardation are the following factors: (1) Since the majority of breech presentations weighing less than 2000 grams will be nonfrank, the risk of umbilical cord prolapse is greater than for the term counterpart. (2) Among premature breech infants, the head:abdomen circumference will be proportionately greater than at term, leading to an increased potential for head entrapment. (3) The ability of the premature infant to tolerate asphyxia during labor is severely limited.[49,59]

On balance, until more data are available, the premature breech, particularly the double footling variety, should be delivered by cesarean section. Premature frank and complete breeches between 32 and 34 weeks gestational age represent a group in which trial of labor may be considered. Studies are underway to evaluate the efficacy of an intensively monitored and carefully conducted vaginal delivery in this gestational age/weight group.

THE IMPACT OF SOCIETY AND SOCIAL MORES ON BREECH DELIVERY

Once breech presentation has been diagnosed, the patient and her family usually understand the potential problems that may be encountered. Most women understand that breech presentation presents a significant risk to their baby. The conclusions drawn by the media profoundly influence the millions of women who will deliver infants in any year. This influence is far greater than that of obstetricians and individual patients. We must continue to explain to our patients that the data available suggest that, under some circumstances, vaginal delivery is a reasonable approach to breech presentation.

In an era in which decreasing family size and increasing expectations of a perfect baby and atraumatic birth exist, we must decide whether or not the pressure exerted by the media as well as the threat of litigation will dictate obstetric practice. We stress the importance of encouraging our patients to participate actively in the choice for attempted vaginal delivery or for cesarean section, which carries the risks of major surgery, including hysterectomy, pulmonary embolus, repeat cesarean section, blood transfusion, and postsurgical recuperation. The most significant fetal risks, cervical spine injury and severe birth trauma, are primarily sustained at vaginal delivery. The potential for breech death at vaginal delivery is of the same order of magnitude as the risk of a hysterectomy being required by the mother. How can we equate maternal morbidity (and even perhaps maternal mortality) with risk to the fetus? We clearly can do no more than to explain the risks and to use the available data to help the patient understand why, in any given situation, external cephalic version, a trial of labor, or elective cesarean section may be the optimal choice.

What role does cost:benefit analysis play? Although we endeavor to allow a trial of labor after previous cesarean section at our institution, in most places more than 90% of women with a previous cesarean section are subsequently delivered by repeat cesarean section. Thus the cost is not of a single cesarean section hospitalization and associated fees, but of multiple ones. In a country in which 3,700,000 deliveries occur annually, 120,000 are complicated by breech presentation in labor. If the cesarean section rate remains at the 85–90% level, the ultimate cost is measured in hundreds of millions of health care dollars. The cost in terms of adverse psychological effects of cesarean delivery in comparison to vaginal delivery is an issue that has recently been raised. These costs must be weighed against those incurred as a result of fetal injury.

CONCLUSION

We anticipate decreased utilization of cesarean section for term breech infants as more and more obstetrical units provide comprehensive services, including continuous electronic fetal monitoring, 24-hour availability of anesthesia, and neonatal intensive care.

A potential problem is that lack of experience may produce a generation of obstetricians trained to rely exclusively on cesarean section for breech delivery. The ability of many obstetricians to conduct breech labor and to effect assisted breech delivery is suspect. Reports of birth injuries suffered at cesarean delivery of breech-presenting infants confirm this suspicion. Breech presentation during labor is a high-risk situation and will always require liberal use of cesarean section. However, certain subgroups of breech presentation are at low risk if trial of labor and vaginal delivery are chosen. By utilizing a selective approach, maternal surgical risk and fetal delivery risk should be balanced.

SUMMARY

Term breech infants in frank, complete, incomplete, or single footling presentation are reasonable candidates for trial of labor if strict criteria are satisfied. The double footling breech is likely to be at greater risk for cord prolapse and prolapse of the fetal body through an incompletely dilated cervix and is the most difficult term breech to manage safely through labor and delivery. These diagnoses require that an x-ray be obtained when breech presentation is recognized to document the specific type of breech present. Breech infants at a transitional age, that is, 32–34 weeks in frank or complete presentation, are borderline by size and by shape (head:abdomen ratio) and may in the future be allowed a trial of labor.

CT scanning of the pelvis for mensuration of the significant pelvic diameters may eventually replace traditional x-ray pelvimetry. The measurements obtained by this technique are likely more accurate and deliver less radiation to the patient(s).

Increased utilization of cesarean section has dramatically decreased injury and death during the intrapartum period for breech-presenting infants. We should endeavor to optimize the utilization of cesarean section. Physicians in training should be permitted to develop the skill necessary to effect a safe breech delivery via both vaginal and abdominal routes in order to prepare them to offer reasonable alternatives to their patients.

REFERENCES

1. Axelrod, F., Leistner, H., and Porges, R.: Breech presentation among infants with familial dysautonomia. *J. Pediatr.* **84**:107–108, 1974.
2. Ballas, S. and Toaff, R.: Deflexion of fetal head in breech presentation. *Br. J. Obstet. Gynaecol.* **83**:201–204, 1976.
3. Bird, C. and McElin T.: A six-year prospective study of term breech deliveries utilizing the Zatuchni–Andros prognostic scoring index. *Am. J. Obstet. Gynecol.* **121**:551–555, 1975.
4. Braun, F., Jones, K., and Smith, D. W.: Breech presentation as an indicator of fetal abnormality. *J. Pediatr.* **86**:419–421, 1975.
5. Brenner, W. E., Bruce, R. S., and Hendricks, C. H.: The characteristics and perils of breech presentation. *Am. J. Obstet. Gynecol.* **118**:700–712, 1974.
6. Caterini, H., Langer, A., Sama, J. C., Devanesan, M., and Pelosi, M. A.: Fetal risk in hyperextension

of the fetal head in breech presentation. *Am. J. Obstet. Gynecol.* **123**:632–636, 1975.

7. Chervenak, F., Johnson, R., Berkowitz, R. C., Grannum, P., and Hobbins, J. C.: Is routine cesarean section necessary for vertex-breech and vertex-transverse twin gestations? *Am. J. Obstet. Gynecol.* **148**:1–5, 1984.
8. Collea, J. V., Chein, C., and Quilligan, E. J.: The randomized management of term frank breech presentation. *Am. J. Obstet. Gynecol.* **137**:235–244, 1980.
9. Crawford, B.: An appraisal of lumbar epidural blockade in patients with singleton fetus presenting by the breech. *J. Obstet. Gynaecol. Br. Commonw.* **81**:867–872, 1974.
10. Cruikshank, D. P. and Pitkin, R. M.: Delivery of the premature breech. *Obstet. Gynecol.* **50**:367–369, 1977.
11. Daw, E.: Hyperextension of the head in breech presentation. *Am. J. Obstet. Gynecol.* **119**:564–565, 1974.
12. DeCrespinsny, L. J. C., and Pepperell, R. J.: Perinatal mortality and morbidity in breech presentation. *Obstet. Gynecol.* **53**:141–145, 1979.
13. Douglas, R. G. and Stromme, W. B. (Eds.): *Operative Obstetrics*, 3rd Edition. New York, Appleton-Century-Crofts, 1976, p. 600.
14. Duenhoelter, J., Wells, C., and Reisch, R.: A paired controlled study of vaginal and abdominal delivery of the low birth weight breech fetus. *Obstet. Gynecol.* **54**:310–313, 1979.
15. Eilen, B., Fleischer, A., and Schulman, H.: Fetal acidosis and the abnormal FHR tracing: The term breech fetus. *Obstet. Gynecol.* **63**:233–236, 1984.
16. Federle, M., Cohen, J., and Rosenwein, M.: Pelvimetry by digital radiography: A low dose examination. *Radiology* **143**:733–735, 1982.
17. Fine, E., Brackers, N. M., and Berkowitz, R. C.: An evaluation ofthe usefulness of x-ray pelvimetry. *Am. J. Obstet. Gynecol.* **137**:15–20, 1980.
18. Friedman, E. A.: *Clinical Management of Labor*, 2nd Edition. New York, Appleton-Century-Crofts, 1978.
19. Gimovsky, M. L.: Unpublished data.
20. Gimovsky, M. L. and Paul, R. H.: Singleton breech presentation in labor: Experience in 1980. *Am. J. Obstet. Gynecol.* **143**:733–739, 1982.
21. Gimovsky, M. L. and Petrie, R..: The intrapartum and neonatal performance of the low birth weight vaginal breech delivery. *J. Reprod. Med.* **27**:451–454, 1982.
22. Gimovsky, M. L. and Petrie, R. H.: Optimal method of delivery of the low birth weight breech fetus: An unresolved issue. *J. Calif. Perinat. Assoc.* **4**:34–37, 1983.
23. Gimovsky, M. L. and Petrie, R. H.: Strategy for choosing the best delivery route for the breech baby. *Contemp. OB/GYN* **21** (April):201–215, 1983.
24. Gimovsky, M. L., Petrie, R. H., and Todd, W. D.: Neonatal performance of the selected term vaginal breech delivery. *Obstet. Gynecol.* **56**:687–691, 1980.
25. Gimovsky, M. L., Wallace, R. L., Schifrin, B. S., and Paul, R. H.: Randomized management of the nonfrank breech presentation at term. *Am. J. Obstet. Gynecol.* **146**:34–40, 1983.
26. Goldenberg, R. and Nelson, G.: The premature breech. *Am. J. Obstet. Gynecol.* **127**:240–244, 1977.
27. Granati, B., Rondinelli, M., and Capoti, C.: The premature breech presentation. *Am. J. Perinatol.* **1**:145–147, 1984.
28. Green, J., McLean, F., and Smith, L.: Has an increased cesarean section rate for term breech delivery reduced the incidence of birth asphyxia, trauma and death? *Am. J. Obstet. Gynecol.* **142**:643–648, 1982.
29. Hall, J. and Kohl, S.: Breech presentation: A study of 1456 cases. *Am. J. Obstet. Gynecol.* **72**:977–990, 1956.
30. Hill, J. and Eliot, B.: Intensive care of the fetus in breech labor. *Br. J. Obstet. Gynaecol.* **83**:271–276, 1976.
31. Huchcroft, S., Wearing, M., and Buek, C.: Late results of cesarean and vaginal delivery in cases of breech presentation. *Can. Med. Assoc. J.* **125**:726–731, 1981.
32. Ingemarson, I., Westgren, M., and Svenningsen, N.: Long term follow up of preterm infants in breech presentation delivered by caesarean section. *Lancet* **2**:172–175, 1978.
33. Karp, L. E., Doney, J. R., McCarthy, T., Meis, P. H., and Hall, M.: The premature breech: TOL or C/S? *Obstet. Gynecol.* **53**:88–92, 1979.
34. Kauppila, D.: The perinatal mortality in breech deliveries and observation of affecting factors. *Acta Obstet. Gynecol. Scand.* [*Suppl.*] **39**:1–124, 1975.
35. Kauppilla, O., Gionross, M., Aro, P., Aittoniemi, P., and Kuoppala, M.: Management of low birth weight breech delivery: Should cesarean section be routine? *Obstet. Gynecol.* **57**:289–294, 1981.
36. Kerr, M.: Breech presentation. In: *Munro Kerr's Operative Obstetrics,* 8th Edition. P. Myciscoyh and J. Mori (Eds.). Baltimore, Williams & Wilkins, 1971, pp. 139–187.
37. Kiwisch, F. A.: Zur Lehre von der Extraction des Kindes an den Füssen. *Beitr. Geburtsk. Würzb.* **i**:62–71, 1846.
38. Lyons, E. R. and Papsin, F. R.: Cesarean section in the management of breech presentation. *Am. J. Obstet. Gynecol.* **130**:558–561, 1978.
39. Mann, L. I. and Gallant, J. M.: Modern management of the breech delivery. *Am. J. Obstet. Gynecol.* **134**:611–614, 1979.
40. Mazor, M., Hagay, Z., Leiberman, J. R., Biale, Y., and Insler, V.: Fetal malformations associated with breech delivery: Implications for management. *J. Reprod. Med.*, in press.
41. Milner, R. D. G.: Neonatal mortality of breech deliveries with and without forceps to the after-

coming head. *Br. J. Obstet. Gynaecol.* **72**:783–788, 1975.

42. NIH consensus development task force statement on cesarean childbirth. *Am. J. Obstet. Gynecol.* **139**:902–909, 1981.
43. O'Leary, J.: Vaginal delivery of the term breech. *Obstet. Gynecol.* **53**:341–343, 1979.
44. Osborne, B.: The implications of the reports of the Committee on Radiological Hazards to patients. Symposium, British Institute of Radiology, 1962. *Br. J. Radiol.* **36**:230–237, 1963.
45. Phelan, J., Bethel, M., Devore, G., Gimovsky, M. L., and Platt, L.: Use of ultrasound in breech presentation with hyperextension of the fetal head. A case report. *J. Ultrasound Med.* **2**:373–374, 1983.
46. Pinard, A.: On version by external maneuvers. Traité du palper abdominal an point de vue obstétrical et de la version par manoeuvres externes, précédé d'une préface de M. Pajot, 2nd Edition. Paris, 1889.
47. Piper, E. B. and Bachman, C.: The prevention of fetal injuries in breech delivery. *JAMA* **92**:217–221, 1929.
48. Potter, M. G., Heaton, C. E., and Douglas, G. W.: Intrinsic risk in breech delivery. *Obstet. Gynecol.* **15**:158–162, 1960.
49. Quirk, J., Raker, R., and Petrie, R.: The role of glucocorticoids, unstressful labor and atraumatic delivery in the prevention of RDS. *Am. J. Obstet. Gynecol.* **134**:768–771, 1979.
50. Ranney, B.: The gentle art of external cephalic version. *Am. J. Obstet. Gynecol.* **116**:239–251, 1973.
51. Robinson, G.: Birth characteristics of children with congenital dislocation of the hip. *Am. J. Epidemiol.* **87**:275–284, 1968.
52. Rovinsky, J. J., Miller, J. A., and Solomon, S.: Management of breech presentation. *Am. J. Obstet. Gynecol.* **115**:497–513, 1973.
53. Saling, E. and Muller-Holve, W.: External cephalic version under tocolysis. *J. Perinat. Med.* **3**:115–122, 1975.
54. Steer, C. M.: Unpublished data.
55. Taylor, E. S. (Ed.): *Beck's Obstetrical Practice*, 9th Edition. Baltimore, Williams & Wilkins, 1971, p. 252.
56. Todd, W. D. and Steer, C. M.: Term breech: Review of 1006 term breech deliveries. *Obstet. Gynecol.* **22**:583–595, 1963.
57. VanDorsten, P., Schifrin, B. S., and Wallace, R. L.: Randomized control trial of external cephalic version with tocolysis in late pregnancy. *Am. J. Obstet. Gynecol.* **141**:417–424, 1981.
58. Varner, M., Cruickshank, D., and Laube, D.: X-ray pelvimetry in clinical obstetrics. *Obstet. Gynecol.* **56**:296–300, 1980.
59. Watashsky, D., Hockner-Celnikier, D., and Beller, U.: Neonatal outcome in cesarean section under general anesthesia related to gestational age, induction-delivery, and uterus-delivery intervals. *Isr. J. Med. Sci.* **19**:1059–1063, 1983.
60. Watson, W. J. and Benson, W. L.: Vaginal delivery for the selected frank breech infant at term. *Obstet. Gynecol.* **64**:638–640, 1984.
61. Wheeler, T. and Greene, K.: FHR monitoring during breech labor. *Br. J. Obstet. Gynaecol.* **82**:208–211, 1975.
62. White, P. C. and Cibils, L. A.: Clinical significance of FHR patterns during labor. VII. Breech presentation. *J. Reprod. Med.* **29**:45–51, 1984.
63. Wright, R. C.: Reduction of perinatal mortality and morbidity in breech delivery through routine use of cesarean section. *Obstet. Gynecol.* **14**:758–763, 1959.
64. Zatuchni, A.: Prognostic index for vaginal delivery in breech delivery at term. *Am. J. Obstet. Gynecol.* **93**:237–242, 1965.

25

ABNORMAL PRESENTATIONS—BROW, FACE, TRANSVERSE LIE

Accurate diagnosis of fetal presentation is among the most important elements of the safe conduct of labor and delivery. Ignorance of an abnormal presentation or a casual attitude toward malpresentation can lead to damage or death for either fetus or parturient. This chapter reviews deflection attitudes, abnormal fetal axial presentations, and compound presentation. It considers contributory etiologies, behavior in labor, and principles of clinical management.

Late in gestation or during labor, in 95% of cases, the fetus assumes a longitudinal axis; the fetal head is found at the maternal pelvis, and the fetal head is flexed forward on the neck (Fig. 25-1). When deviation occurs from this normal lie, presentation, or flexion attitude, fetal malpresentation is diagnosed. Malpresentation is associated with increased perinatal risk to mother and fetus. Malpresentation has in the past often resulted in the application of dangerous operative maneuvers intended to effect vaginal delivery. These maneuvers have included destructive fetal procedures and manual and instrumental attempts to convert the malpresentation to a more favorable one. Furthermore, internal podalic version and complete breech extraction have together been proposed as a clinical solution to many positional abnormalities. However, attempts to achieve vaginal delivery of the malpresenting fetus in situations associated with poor progress during labor have carried unacceptably high fetal or maternal morbidity or mortality. These interventions are now strongly discouraged. Cesarean delivery is the safest method of operative delivery in fetal malpresentation when necessary.

Etiologies associated with malpresentations include factors that alter the normal polar shape of the uterine cavity, factors that increase or decrease fetal mobility, and factors that prevent the fetal presenting part from entering the maternal pelvis normally (Table 25-1). Great parity may lead to abdominal wall laxity and some loss of the normal vertical uterine alignment. Polar placentation high in the fundus or in the lower segment also diminishes the probability of a fetus easily assuming a longitudinal lie. Both prematurity and hydramnios allow increased fetal mobility and result in increased probability of noncephalic and/or nonlongitudinal presentation in labor. The decreased fetal muscle tone and strength seen with the autosomal trisomies and with myotonic dystrophy result in decreased fetal mobility and are associated with increased incidence of malpresentations. Amniotic fluid volume relative to the small fetal mass of the premature infant produces a "relative" hydramnios allowing increased fetal mobility and an increased incidence of noncephalic presentation. The small size of the premature infant often permits pelvic engagement, descent, and successful delivery of infants with extreme deflection attitudes. Such success is much less likely with a larger fetus, since deflection attitudes require the passage of a longer diameter of the fetal head than would be the case with a fully flexed head. Finally, the

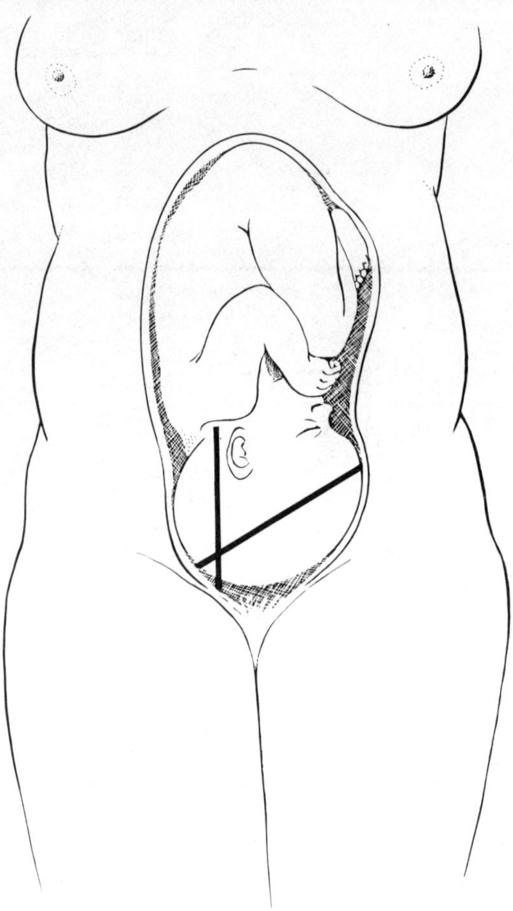

Figure 25-1. In this longitudinal view of the normal fetus, one can see that the long axis of the fetus is aligned with that of the mother and that the occipitofrontal axis of the fetal vertex describes an acute angle as it is flexed on the neck with the axis of the fetal cervical spine.

TABLE 25-1. CLINICAL FACTORS CONTRIBUTING TO MALPRESENTATION

Fetal	Maternal
Hydramnios	Pelvic contracture
Prematurity	Great parity
• Anencephaly	Pelvic tumors
• Hydrocephaly	
Placenta previa	
Multiple gestation	
Cytogenetic abnormality	
• Trisomy 13, 18, 21	
Macrosomia	
Myotonic dystrophy	

cephalopelvic disproportion seen with severe fetal hydrocephalus or with a severely contracted pelvis is often implicated as a factor in malpresentation because engagement of the fetal head is impaired.

It is impossible to identify with confidence the precise mechanism that results in the flexed longitudinal cephalic presentation of the fetus in 95% of cases. The following conclusions can be drawn from our review of the clinical factors associated with deviations from the normal. Early in pregnancy, with a relative abundance of amniotic fluid and free mobility, the fetus is in a state of random unrestricted motion. Sudden rupture of the membranes or labor would result in descent and fixation of whichever fetal pole or part was by chance closest to the maternal pelvis. Therefore, a variety of malpresentations, including breech and abnormal axis, are more often associated with the very premature infant. As pregnancy progresses, the fetus becomes more restricted both by the relative decrease in amniotic fluid and increasingly by the maternal uterus, abdominal wall, spine, and diaphragm. These spatial restrictions tend to align the fetus longitudinally, matching the long axis of the fetus to the vertical long axis of the mother. The fetal vertex stabilizes most often over the pelvis, perhaps because a fundal location would require accommodation to the prominent maternal spine, liver, and diaphragm, whereas the open pelvic girdle is relatively more accepting of the fetal cranium. Clinical factors associated with deviation from the normal, therefore, often include circumstances leading to the loss of these normal spatial restrictions. Great parity with lax abdominal muscles allows ventral uterine deviation away from the maternal spine. Hydramnios allows greater fetal mobility. A low-lying placenta might fill the pelvic inlet and, thereby, decrease the probability of a vertex presentation.

DEFLECTION ATTITUDES

During labor, the fetal head is normally fully flexed at the neck, with the fetal chin against the upper chest. Abnormal attitudes involve deflection or even extension of the fetal head on the spine (Fig. 25-2). These malpresentations are often relatively unstable. Spontaneous conversion to a more flexed position or, alterna-

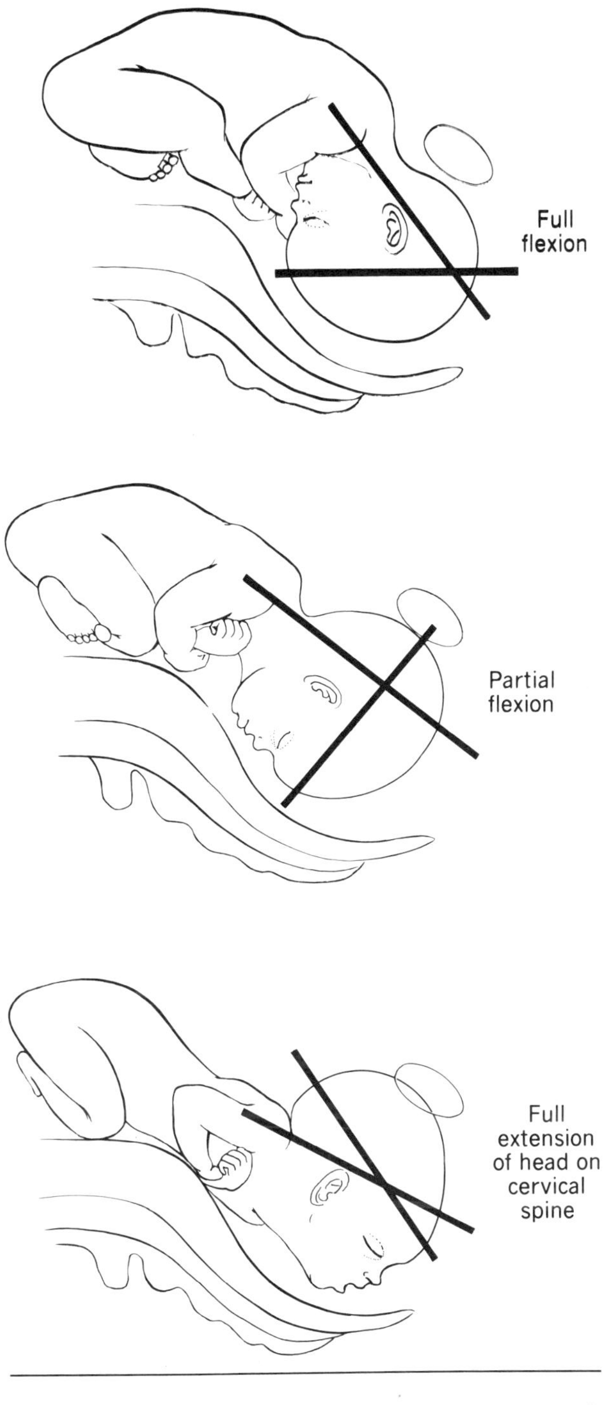

Figure 25-2. These three views illustrate, in the top view, full flexion of the fetal vertex on the cervical spine; in the middle view, partial deflection with the occipitofrontal plane of the fetal head approximately at right angles to the axis of the cervical spine; and, in the lower view, extension of the fetal head on the cervical spine.

tively, further extension of a partially deflexed head to the fully extended position occurs commonly during labor. Etiologies of the two types of deflection attitude are similar. Safe vaginal delivery is possible in the majority of cases, but cautious attention to labor management is mandatory. Experience indicates that the only safe alternative to spontaneous vaginal delivery when a deflection attitude is associated with dysfunctional labor is cesarean birth.

FACE PRESENTATION

A face presentation is diagnosed when a fetus is found in a longitudinal lie, cephalic presentation, with the head fully deflexed or extended on the cervical spine (Fig. 25-3). The fetal occiput will usually be against the fetal upper back.[9] At the time of vaginal examination, the fetal chin is used as the point of designation of the face relative to the maternal pelvis. For example, a fetus presenting by the face whose chin is in the right posterior quadrant of the maternal pelvis would be called a right mentum posterior (RMP) (Fig. 25-4). The average reported incidence of face presentation is about 0.2% or 1:500 livebirths.[6,-14,21,27,31,37,42] Perinatal mortality, corrected for lethal malformations and extreme prematurity, varies from 0.6%[11] to 5%.[18] Cruikshank and White found that the uncorrected perinatal mortality of 28% seen in their series with face presentation dropped to only 1.6% after exclusion of lethal anomalies or birth weights under 1000 g.[16]

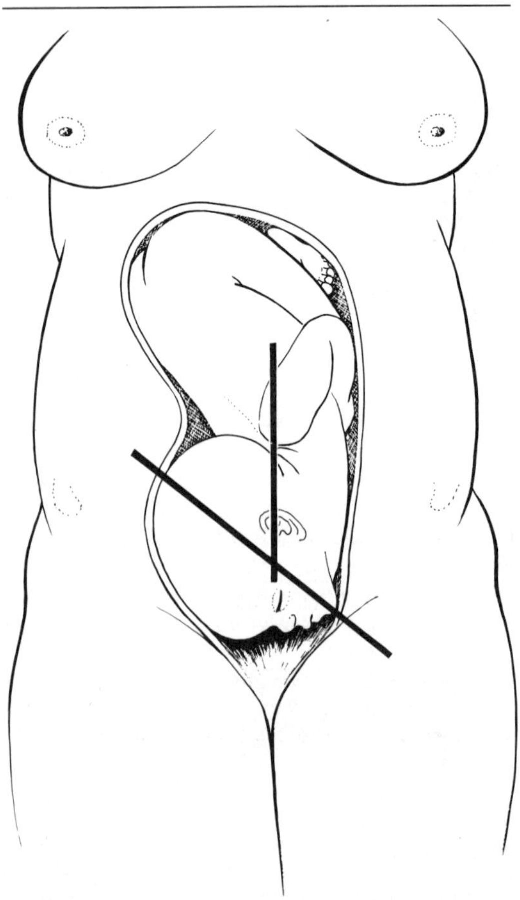

Figure 25-3. This anterior frontal view of a face presentation demonstrates the full deflection of the fetal head on the cervical spine and the entry of the fetal face into the plane of the pelvic inlet.

All clinical factors known to increase the rate of malpresentation in general (Table 25-1) have also been implicated in face presentation specifically, but fetal malformations have appeared more prominently. In fact, a high percentage of infants with a persistent face presentation may be malformed.[9] Anencephaly, for instance, has been reported in 12–60% of cases of face presentation.[9,16,25,44] Frequently observed factors include contracted pelvis or cephalopelvic disproportion.[9,14,37,43] High parity, polyhydramnios, prematurity, and uterine anomalies are also associated with face presentation.[6,14,16,27,31,40] One or another of these etiologic factors is found in up to 90% of cases, especially prematurity, anencephaly, great parity, and cephalopelvic disproportion.[21] However, often no clear etiology is ever found.[15]

Early diagnosis is important to optimal management. Diagnosis can be accomplished by abdominal palpation of the cephalic prominence on the same side of the maternal abdomen as the fetal back (Fig. 25-5), but the diagnosis is more often made at vaginal examination and confirmed by radiography or ultrasound. In practice, fewer than 1:20 infants with face presentation are diagnosed by abdominal examination.[11] Only 10–50% of cases are identified by any means prior to the second stage of labor, and half of all cases remain undiagnosed until delivery.[11,17,18,21,37,44] Early diagnosis, nevertheless, can be important because perinatal mortality is significantly higher with delay in diagnosis. In a series of 41 cases of face or brow presentation, perinatal mortality more than doubled from 10 to 26% with late diagnosis.[14]

MECHANISM OF LABOR

The early mechanism of labor in face presentations is not completely understood. Infants with a face presentation may begin labor in the partially deflexed brow position and extend further as descent into the maternal pelvis occurs. The labor of an infant with a face presentation classically includes engagement, descent, internal rotation usually to a mentum anterior position, and delivery by flexion under the symphysis

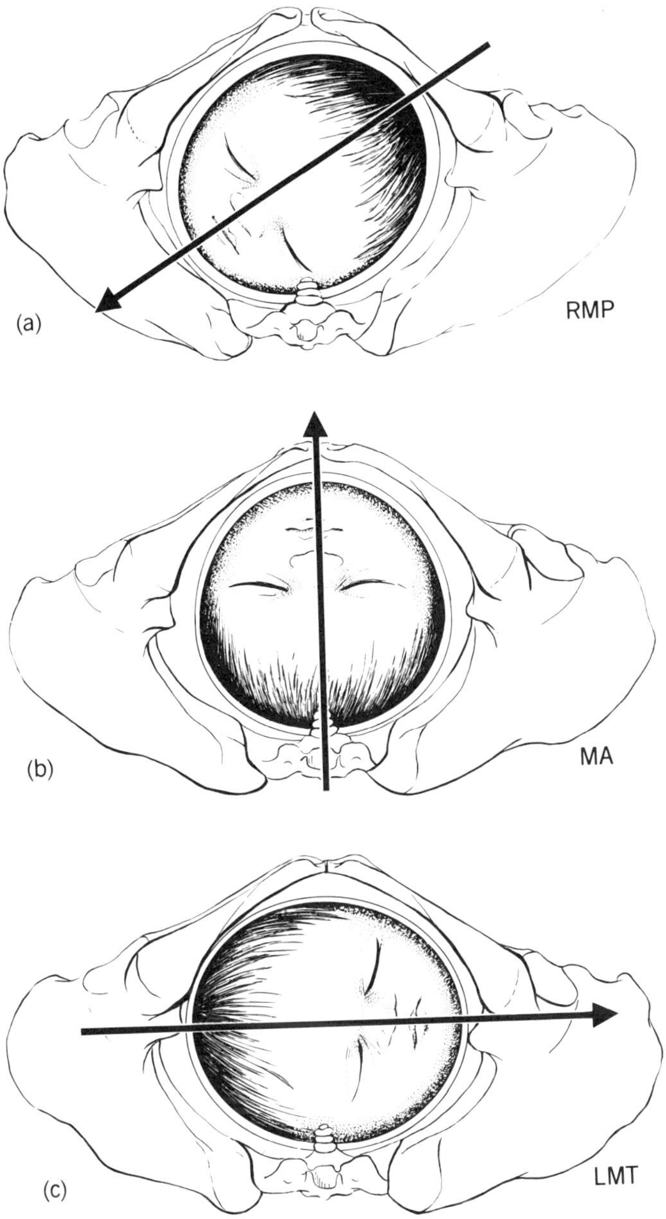

Figure 25-4. These pelvic views of a fetus presenting by the face presentation demonstrate that the fetal chin (mentum) is used as a point of designation. Part (a) demonstrates a right mentum posterior, (b) demonstrates a mentum anterior, and (c) demonstrates a left mentum transverse.

(Fig. 25-6).[14] However, some reports suggest that delivery by flexion under the symphysis may not be so routine and that many infants, in fact, deliver in the extended position.[13] With a very-low-birth-weight infant, internal rotation to mentum anterior (MA) is not strictly necessary for vaginal delivery. The larger the infant, though, the less likely is vaginal delivery to occur from any position except MA.

The size of the infant and the precise position at the time of diagnosis may predict labor performance to a limited extent. At the time of diagnosis 60–80% of infants with face presentation are MA, 10–12% are mentum transverse (MT), and 20–25% are mentum posterior (MP).[11,16,37] In 90–100% of infants with MA, in the absence of cephalopelvic disproportion (CPD), spontaneous or easily assisted vaginal

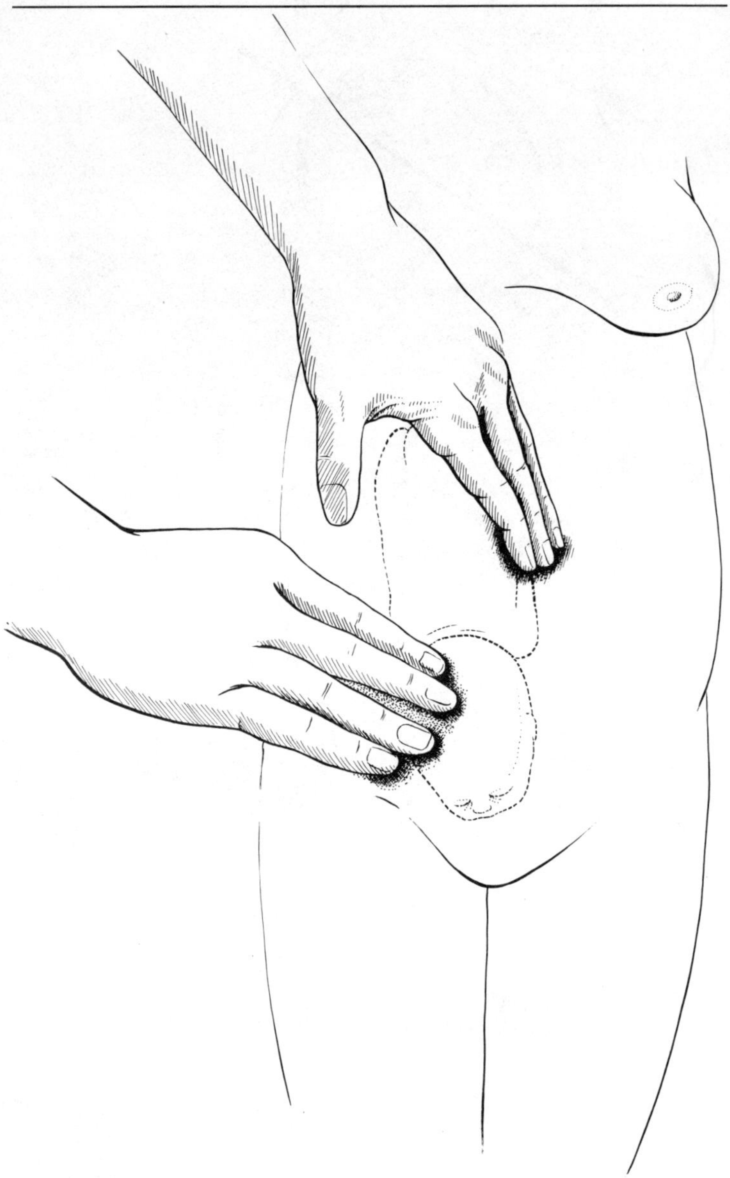

Figure 25-5. A three-dimensional external view of an operator examining the maternal abdomen and finding the cephalic prominence of the fetal head on the same side of the maternal abdomen as the fetal back.

delivery occurs.[2,3,6,11,16] The more deliverable position thus predominates. Furthermore, the majority of infants with MT will rotate to the MA position and deliver vaginally.[6,16] Twenty-five to 33% of infants in the MP position will rotate and deliver in the MA position.[6,16,37] In a series of 40 cases of face presentation in infants over 2500 g and over 36 weeks' gestation, 25% of cases found MP at diagnosis delivered vaginally.[6] Rates of vaginal delivery of infants in the MP position higher than 25% have also been reported.[16]

Persistence of mentum posterior, though, with an infant of normal term size suggests at least relative disproportion, and safe vaginal delivery in these cases is improbable.[43] Overall, 70–80% of infants presenting by the face can deliver spontaneously vaginally or via low forceps, whereas 12–30% will require cesarean delivery.[11,16,18,37] In the case of the term-size infant with persistence of a face presentation, vaginal delivery may occur in only half of cases.[6] Attempts at manual conversion of the face to a flexed attitude or attempts to rotate a posterior

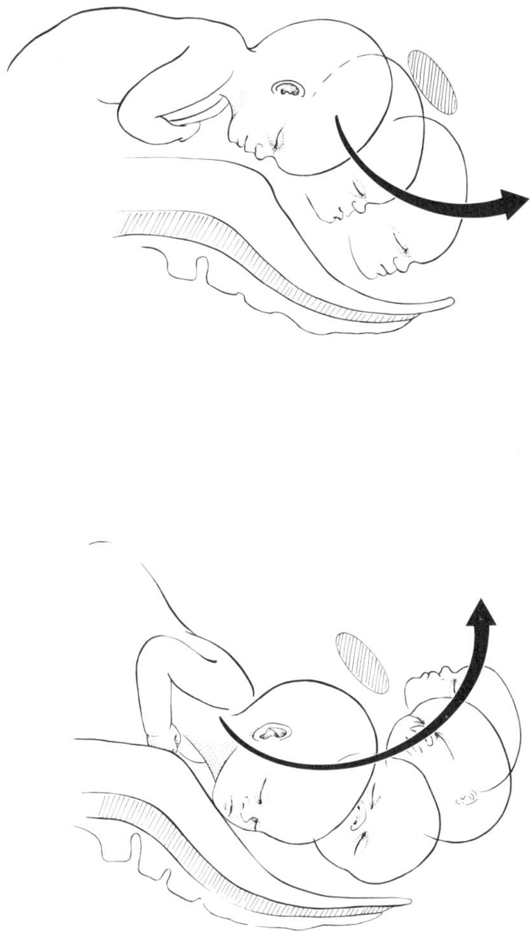

Figure 25-6. These views demonstrate that, as the fetal face engages in the pelvis and descends at first with the chin posterior, rotation occurs and delivery is accomplished as the fetal face exits the pelvic outlet.

position to a more favorable anterior position are rarely successful and both fetal and maternal risks are increased.[6,11,24,43,44] Internal podalic version and breech extraction have been suggested as a remedy for face presentation, but are contraindicated. Fetal losses of up to 60% are associated with such maneuvers. In contrast, when spontaneous delivery or cesarean delivery are the only management options, fetal losses are negligible.[11] Maternal death is rare when spontaneous vaginal delivery or cesarean birth are the only methods used but has been reported in association with version and extraction.[6,11,43,44]

Prolonged labor is a common and ominous feature of face presentation[16,31,40] and is itself associated with a disproportionate number of intrapartum deaths.[14] Therefore, prompt attention to an arrested labor pattern is necessary. The choice between augmentation of a dysfunctional labor or primary cesarean delivery rests on an assessment of the adequacy of prior labor, pelvic size, and fetal condition. In the case of a large pelvis, a small baby, and a hypotonic pattern, augmentation may be considered. Augmentation of an arrested labor with a face presentation should be undertaken only with extreme caution. Fetal distress increases as much as 10-fold with face presentation as compared with the general population.[44] Abnormal fetal heart rate patterns occur more often with face presentation.[6,21] Benedetti et al. observed severe variable decelerations in 29% of cases, and late decelerations in 24%.[6]

Continuous intrapartum electronic fetal monitoring of the fetus with this malposition is necessary for fetal safety. Care must be exercised in placing an internal electrode, however, as occular and other cosmetic damage might result from such a device. If external Doppler heart rate monitoring is inadequate and an internal electrode is considered necessary, the fetal chin is a better location than any part of the upper face.

Neonatal problems associated with face presentation make pediatric consultation and attendance at delivery an important element of optimal care. Laryngeal/tracheal edema occurs with face presentation as a result of the pressures of the birth process. Immediate nasotracheal intubation may be required.[34] Fetal anomalies such as nuchal teratomas or simple goiter sometimes cause these malpresentations and require expert neonatal care.

Successful management, therefore, of a labor complicated by face presentation includes early diagnosis, the use of electronic fetal heart rate monitoring, and cesarean delivery in cases of maternal or fetal distress or arrest of descent or cervical dilatation.[6,21,31,37,43] Cesarean delivery of all term-size infants or infants over 2500 g with MP has been advocated by some authors, but if the fetal heart rate remains normal and steady progress is made, rotation to the MA can occur spontaneously and safe vaginal delivery is possible.[6,16,31]

Pelvimetry might be useful in the management of face presentation in labor, since both CPD and fetal anomalies are common, but if labor is progressive, its utility is uncertain. Adequate pelvimetry does not rule out the need for cesarean delivery and spontaneous vaginal delivery can occur in spite of inadequate dimensions.[16] There is no absolute contraindication to oxytocin augmentation of hypotonic secondary arrest of labor if CPD can be excluded, and the fetus can be reliably monitored.[18,21] CPD, though, is difficult to exclude.

Although reported cesarean delivery rates vary from 7.6–60%,[17,21] safe vaginal delivery may be expected in most cases of face presentation. Cesarean delivery is more often required in the case of the primigravida with a term-size infant in MP position, but in any case of face presentation making steady progress toward delivery, surgical intervention should be reserved.[31] The 50% cesarean rates sometimes reported reflect specifically the fact that the infants were over 36 weeks gestational age and weighed more than 2500 g.[6] When progress is arrested despite adequate labor, or fetal distress is identified, cesarean delivery is the safest management alternative.

BROW PRESENTATION

Brow presentation describes an infant in a longitudinal axis, with a partially deflexed head midway between full flexion and full extension (Fig. 25-7).[9,43] At vaginal examination, the frontal bones and the anterior fontanelle are the point of designation. If the anterior fontanelle is to the maternal right side, for example, with the sagittal suture in the transverse pelvic axis, the fetus is said to present a right frontum transverse (RFT) position (Fig. 25-8). The reported incidence of brow presentation varies between 1:670[38] and 1:3433,[33] averaging approximately 1:1500 deliveries.[1] This wide range of incidence is probably related to timing of diagnosis. Brow may be diagnosed more frequently in early labor, but, since flexion often occurs to more normal attitudes, later diagnosis results in a lower apparent incidence. Less frequently, greater extension occurs during labor and a face presentation results. The lower incidences reported for brow probably indicate persistent brow presentations diagnosed later in labor.

Perinatal mortality rates corrected for lethal anomalies and very low birth weight vary from 1.28% to 8%.[35] Corrected perinatal mortality rates for fetuses presenting by the brow depend on mode of delivery. The highest rate of loss (16%) is associated with manipulative vaginal birth.[29]

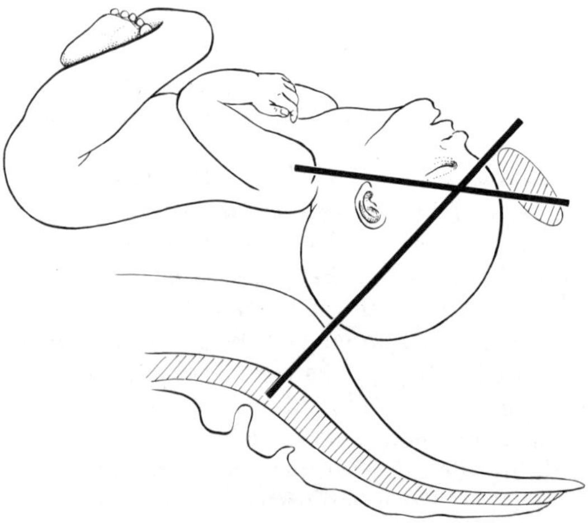

Figure 25-7. This view of a brow presentation demonstrates the partial deflection of the fetal head short of full extension and that the fetal brow is engaging in the pelvic inlet from profile vantage point.

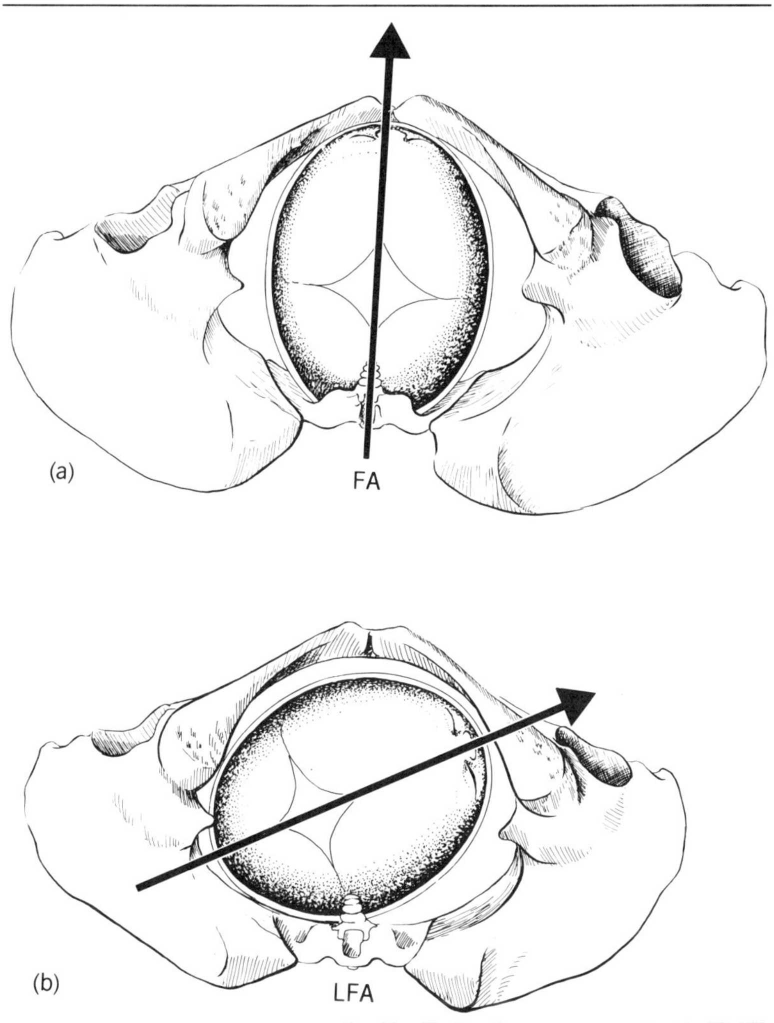

Figure 25-8. In a brow presentation, the anterior fontanelle or frontal bones are used as a point of designation and, therefore, in part (a) one can see that the frontal bones demonstrate a frontum anterior position, whereas in part (b) they are found in a left frontum anterior position.

Causative factors include most of those listed in Table 25-1 and are similar to the clinical circumstances associated with face presentation. Cephalopelvic disproportion, prematurity, and great parity have been implicated in more than 60% of cases of persistent brow.[5,15,16,33,43,46] In general, factors that delay or prevent engagement are more often associated with the persistent brow.

Abdominal diagnosis prenatally or in labor may be possible but is uncommonly accomplished in practice. More often, a brow is detected on vaginal examination.[43] As in the case of face presentation, late diagnosis is the rule. Fifty-two percent of brow presentations may not be detected before the second stage of labor and 47% escape diagnosis until delivery.[5,29,38,46] Frontum anterior is the most common position at the time of diagnosis, occurring about twice as often as either transverse or posterior positions. Whereas the prognostic significance of initial position at diagnosis is limited, the cesarean birth rate is higher with frontum transverse and frontum posterior.[46]

Persistent brow presentation means that the largest (mento-occipital) diameter of the fetal head must engage in the pelvic inlet and negotiate the midplane and outlet.[39] Successful passage of this profile of the fetal head is likely only with a very large pelvis or a small infant or both. However, 30–90% of brow presentations convert spontaneously by flexion or further extension to either a vertex or face presentation and are then managed accordingly.[33,38,43] The earlier the diagnosis is made, the more likely is conversion to occur spontaneously. Less than half of the infants with persistent brow deliver vaginally spontaneously.[16,35]

Prolonged labors occur in 33–50% of cases of brow presentation, and secondary arrest is common.[5,15,16,33,37,38,40,46] Manipulative conversion of the brow to a more favorable position with forceps is contraindicated as are attempts at manual conversion.[1,5,33,38] One unexpected cause of persistent brow presentation may be an open fetal mouth pressed against the vaginal wall, bracing the head and preventing both flexion and extension (Fig. 25-9).[7,33] Borell and Fernstrom report this to be a major cause of persistent brow and report successful manual elevation of the fetal head and closure of the mouth.[7] Such a maneuver risks cord prolapse as well as fetal trauma and may not be preferable to cesarean delivery.

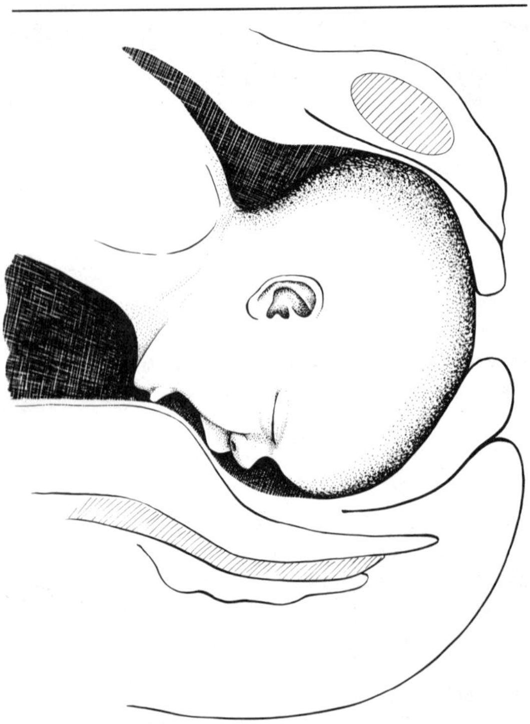

Figure 25-9. This view illustrates how an open fetal mouth can brace a fetal head against the vaginal wall, preventing either flexion or further extension and, therefore, resulting in a persistent brow presentation.

In most cases, as with face presentation, if labor progresses with no observed fetal distress, minimal manipulation is best.[30,33,43] Expectancy is justified only in the presence of a large pelvis, a small infant, and adequate progress.[29] If brow presentation persists with a large baby, successful delivery is unlikely and cesarean might be most prudent.[37,40] However, since spontaneous flexion or extension can occur unpredictably, cesarean intervention prior to any arrest of labor progress or fetal distress is premature. It is important for the obstetrical team to make all preparations for cesarean delivery in order to allow expeditious delivery should circumstances change suddenly.

Safe delivery of an infant over 2500 g as a brow is very unlikely.[43] Pelvimetry in labor has been reported to be useful. Cruikshank and White, for instance, found that 91% of cases with adequate pelvic dimensions converted spontaneously to vertex or face and delivered vaginally, whereas only 20% showing some pelvic contraction did so.[16] Since cephalopelvic disproportion is common with brow presentation and is often considered etiologic, many cases of diminished pelvic dimensions would be expected. Twenty percent of patients with contracted pelvic dimensions on x-ray do deliver successfully vaginally, however, and there is no firm evidence that a carefully monitored trial of labor in a brow presentation is detrimental to either mother or fetus. Therefore, the utility of x-ray pelvimetry remains unsettled.

In the laboring patient, when brow presentation is diagnosed, continuous electronic fetal monitoring should begin. Although limited vaginal manipulation has occasionally been found to be helpful, such intervention is not recommended. Spontaneous conversion and delivery are common in cases of brow presentation diagnosed early in labor, although conversion is much less likely later and uncommon with a small pelvis or a large baby. In the absence of maternal or fetal distress and in the presence of progressive descent and dilatation, manipulation of any kind is unnecessary. Cesarean delivery is indicated when arrest of progress occurs with brow despite good contractions.

When arrest of progress occurs as a result of poor contractions and in the presence of a small fetus, oxytocin augmentation of labor can be considered if continuous uterine and fetal monitoring is available. Contractions should not be allowed to exceed physiologic levels of tonus, frequency, or amplitude. Resumption of contractions should result in prompt and clear progress toward vaginal delivery. If such progress does not occur, cesarean delivery is preferable to prolonged augmentation.

COMPOUND PRESENTATION

A compound presentation is diagnosed when an extremity is found prolapsing beside the fetal head (Fig. 25-10).[8] Reported incidence ranges from 1:377 to 1:1213 deliveries.[8,16,26,47] The upper extremity and the head are the most common combination.[8,16,19,26,47]

This diagnosis should be suspected with any arrest of labor in the active phase or failure to engage in the pelvis during active labor.[47] Diagnosis is made by vaginal examination when the examiner feels an irregular mobile tissue mass adjacent to the presenting part. Ultrasound may be useful in confirming the presence of a prolapsing extremity and in identifying the extremity involved. Delayed diagnosis is common. Half the cases are not diagnosed until the second stage of labor.[26] This may not be detrimental, however, since it is probable that only these persistent cases require significant attention.

Although maternal age, race, parity, and pelvic size have all been implicated in the etiology of compound presentation, prematurity is the most commonly associated clinical finding.[8,16,26,47] The clear implication is that only the very small fetus is likely to demonstrate a persistent compound presentation. External cephalic version late in pregnancy of a fetus in breech position or version of a second twin at the time of delivery may increase the likelihood of a compound presentation. The combination in such cases is most often that of lower extremity and head.[4]

Perinatal mortality is elevated with compound presentation. An overall perinatal mortality rate of 93:1000 and rates of 170–190:1000 when the foot prolapses, have been reported.[16,26] As with other malpresentations, fetal risk increases with the level of manipulative intervention. A fetal mortality of 4.8% is associated with no intervention, 14.4% fetal losses accompany intervention other than cesarean delivery, and a 30% fetal mortality rate has been recorded with internal podalic version and extraction.[26] There is probably some selection bias, since it is more likely that the more difficult cases become candidates for manipulative intervention. Nevertheless, when intervention is necessary cesarean delivery is the only safe choice.

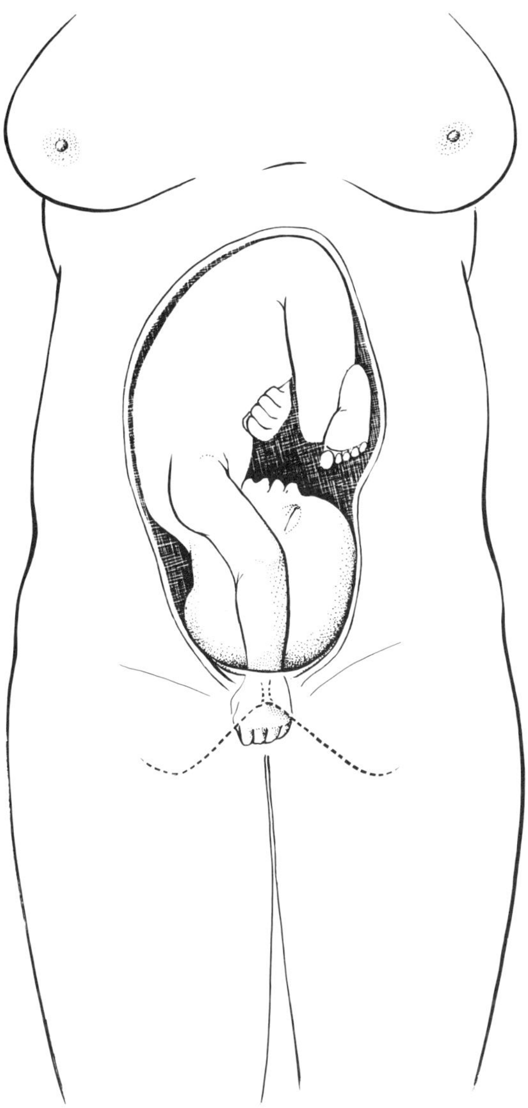

Figure 25-10. Any time an arm or a foot prolapses beside the fetal vertex, this constitutes a compound presentation, as illustrated here.

Fetal risk relates specifically to birth trauma and/or cord prolapse. Cord prolapse occurs in 11–20% of cases and is the most frequent single fetal complication of this malpresentation.[8,16,26,47]

Prolapse of the cord probably occurs more often because the involved extremity splints the vertex and the resulting irregular fetal aggregate incompletely fills the pelvic inlet. Fetal morbidity includes the hypoxic risk of cord prolapse and direct neurological and musculoskeletal damage to the involved extremity.

Nonmanipulation of the prolapsed extremity is the treatment of choice in the case of compound presentation.[8,20,26,47,48] There is no contraindication to labor. The primary indications for surgical intervention are cord prolapse and/or failure to progress.[16] Occult or undetected cord prolapse is possible and, therefore, continuous electronic fetal heart rate monitoring is necessary. Cesarean delivery is the only appropriate clinical intervention other than spontaneous delivery. Both internal version/extraction and attempts to reposition the prolapsed extremity are associated with unacceptably high fetal and maternal morbidity and mortality and are to be avoided.[8,26,47]

Most often, as the fetal head descends during labor, the accompanying extremity retracts. The prognosis, however, is variable. Although as many as 75% of vertex/upper extremity combinations may deliver spontaneously vaginally,[16] spontaneous vaginal delivery of a foot/vertex combination is much less likely. [48] From 2%[8] to 25%[47] of all compound presentations require delivery by cesarean section. Protraction of the second stage of labor occurs frequently with persistent compound presentation and dysfunctional labor patterns are common.[8] As in other malpresentations, spontaneous resolution occurs more often, and surgical intervention is less frequently necessary in cases diagnosed early in labor. Persistent compound presentation is more likely with a small infant, as is the prognosis for successful vaginal delivery. Persistent compound presentation with a term-size infant offers a poorer prognosis for safe vaginal delivery and cesarean delivery is more often required.

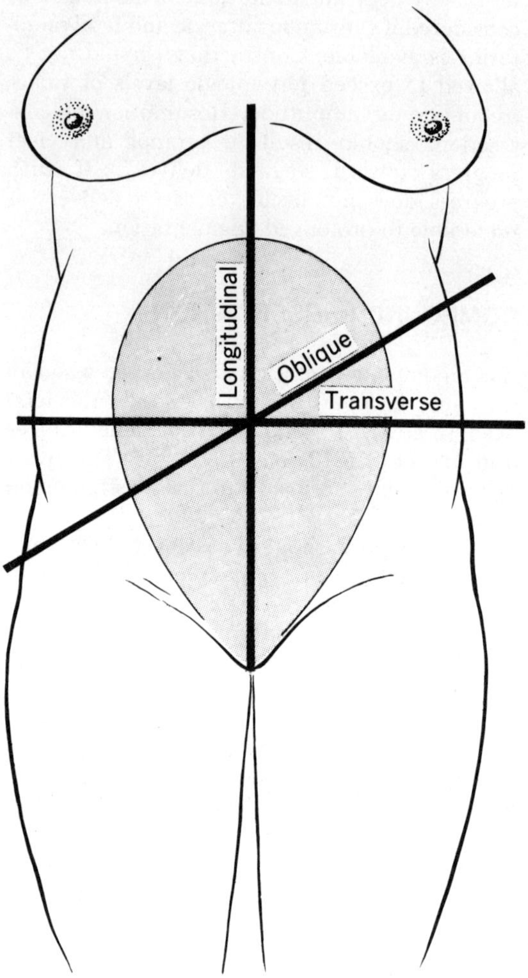

Figure 25-11. The fetal "lie" describes the relationship of the fetal long axis to that of the mother. These axes graphically illustrate the possibilities overlying a pregnant uterus.

ABNORMAL AXIAL LIE

The fetal *lie* describes the relationship of the fetal spine to that of the mother. The normal fetal lie is longitudinal. Lie by itself does not indicate which fetal pole is presenting. Anytime the fetal spine, or long axis, crosses the mother's, the fetus is said to occupy either a transverse or an oblique lie (Fig. 25-11), and either may result in a shoulder or an arm presentation (Fig. 25-12). The presentation is designated *unstable* if the fetal membranes are intact and there is great fetal mobility.[43,49]

Abnormal fetal lie is seen in 1:103[36] to 1:1200[12,45] deliveries with the average approximately 1:300 or 0.33%.[16,22,23,31,43] Abnormal lie occurs in approximately 2% of pregnancies at 32 weeks. This is six times the incidence at term.[32] Abnormal lie must be ruled out in any patient in premature labor if the presenting part cannot be confidently identified by vaginal examination. Ultrasound is an easy technique for confirming fetal position. Persistence of a transverse,

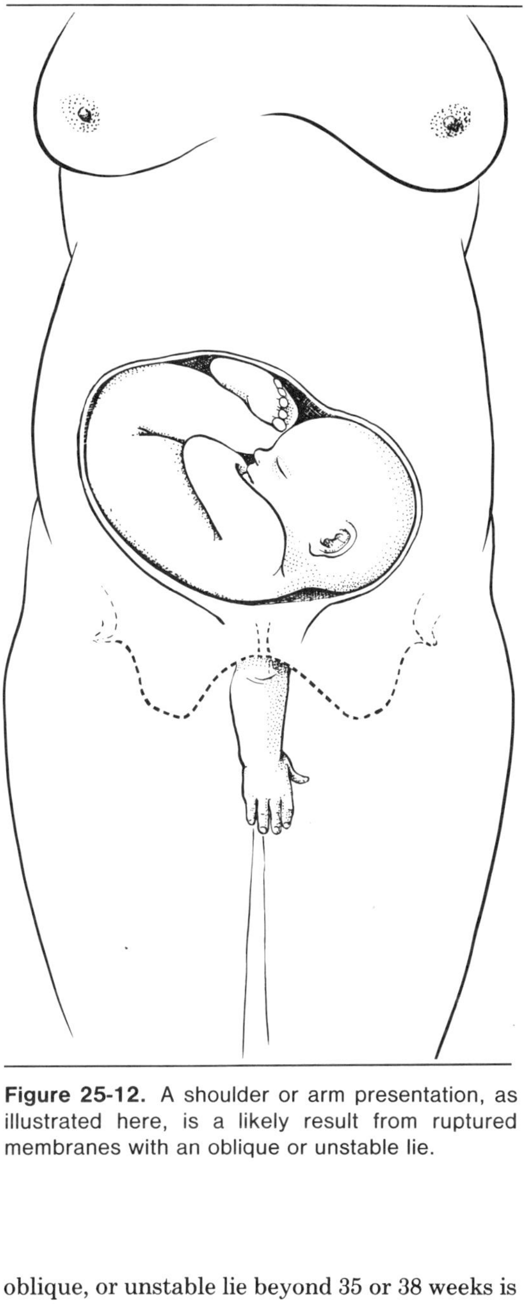

Figure 25-12. A shoulder or arm presentation, as illustrated here, is a likely result from ruptured membranes with an oblique or unstable lie.

oblique, or unstable lie beyond 35 or 38 weeks is potentially of major clinical significance and deserving of attention. Sonography may be used to confirm position, locate the placenta, or search for fetal or uterine malformations that may be associated with the malpresentation.

Unexpected rupture of the membranes without a fetal part filling the pelvic inlet carries a high risk of cord prolapse, fetal distress, and maternal morbidity if neglected. Some clinicians recommend elective hospitalization of patients with these abnormal lies to allow for promptly ruling out or dealing with cord prolapse if the membranes rupture.[22,28,36]

Great parity, prematurity, pelvic contracture, and abnormal placentation are the most commonly reported clinical conditions associated with abnormal lie.[16,22,23,31,32,36] Although Cockburn and Drake reported that in 30–79% of cases no etiology is found,[12] other investigators have observed one of the four factors mentioned above in most cases.[9,31,43] Any factor that destroys the normal vertical polarity of the uterine cavity encourages an abnormal fetal lie.[12,28]

Diagnosis may be accomplished by inspection, palpation, or vaginal examination,[43] but detection is successful in as few as 41% of cases prior to labor.[12] A strong case can be made for sonographic evaluation of all patients in premature labor to establish fetal lie and presentation and to assess morphology and size. A fetal loss rate of 9.2% is associated with early diagnosis, whereas losses of 27.5% can occur when diagnosis is delayed.[12] It is obvious, therefore, that careful attention to the diagnosis of abnormal lie is important to optimal fetal salvage.

Perinatal mortality rates for unstable or transverse lie corrected for lethal malformations or extreme prematurity vary from 3.9%[28] to 24%[49] with maternal mortality as high as 10%. Maternal deaths are most often related to infection following premature rupture of membranes, hemorrhage secondary to abnormal placentation, operative complications, or traumatic vaginal delivery.[23,32] Fetal loss is primarily associated with neglect, prolapsed cord, or traumatic delivery.[32] Cord prolapse occurs 20 times as often with abnormal axis as it does with vertex presentation. The risk of fetal death varies with the type of obstetrical manipulation. Fetal mortality of 0–10% has been reported for cesarean birth, compared to a mortality of 25–90% when internal podalic version and breech extraction are performed.[10,12,23,31,32,45] A 6% fetal mortality is reported for external version and vertex vaginal delivery.[31,32]

If an infant of any size becomes trapped by oligohydramnios in any of these abnormal axes, safe vaginal delivery cannot occur.[23,41,43,45] Although the very premature infant might be physically flexible enough to distort, thereby making vaginal delivery possible, the danger of trauma is so great that any infant considered viable is best delivered by cesarean. A transverse/oblique or unstable lie after 35–38 weeks may benefit from careful evaluation to rule out placenta previa or contracted pelvis.[28] If elective admission for observation near term is not feasible, careful instructions should be given to the patient regarding prompt presentation to the hospital in the event of rupture of membranes or onset of labor.[23] Although external version is often unsuccessful and is not completely free of fetal risk, a careful attempt at external version is a reasonable alternative to expectant observation or primary cesarean section if placenta previa can be excluded and if the fetal heart rate is monitored.[23,45] Tocolysis is recommended to relax the uterus and thus to facilitate the procedure. Intact membranes and the absence of active labor are recommended prerequisites, but external version is possible in early labor or even with ruptured membranes if sufficient fetal mobility remains and cord prolapse can be excluded.[12]

External version followed by artificial rupture of membranes has been suggested, but in the absence of contractions may be dangerous. If the patient does not initiate labor in response to the ruptured membranes, oxytocin augmentation may be necessary.[36] Twenty percent of 254 patients between 38 and 39 weeks had abnormal fetal axial lie, ruptured membranes, or initiated labor before a scheduled elective admission for a stabilizing induction. In those remaining patients in whom cephalopelvic disproportion and placenta previa were excluded, oxytocin induction with fetal monitoring was begun. After contractions were established, external version was attempted and, if successful, amniotomy was performed with a fetal pole over the inlet. Eighty-six of 96 cases managed in this way were delivered vaginally with fetal distress occurring in only four cases. No fetal losses occurred.[22] Prophylactic stabilizing induction is feasible only when the cervix is sufficiently favorable to allow artificial rupture of membranes. Real-time ultrasound can facilitate the procedure by giving the operator continuous information about fetal position. Prior consultation with an anesthesiologist is recommended along with prearrangements for prompt cesarean delivery in the event of fetal distress or cord prolapse, both of which are possible complications. Tocolysis is a useful temporary adjunct in managing cord prolapse.

In cases where external version is impractical, unsuccessful, or unavailable or when rupture of membranes has occurred with an abnormal axial like, cesarean delivery is the treatment of choice.[12,41,49] There is no place for internal podalic version and breech extraction in the management of transverse/oblique lie or unstable presentation, because of the unacceptably high rate of fetal and maternal complications.[36]

Persistent abnormal axial lie, particularly accompanied by ruptured membranes may also alter the technique of cesarean delivery (see Chapter 46). Although the low transverse cervical incision has theoretical and surgical advantages both immediately and for the mother's future potential to delivery vaginally, as many as 25% of transverse uterine incisions require vertical extension in the case of abnormal lie in order to allow access to a head trapped in the muscular fundus.[12,41] Furthermore, in many cases of abnormal lie, there is not a well-developed lower uterine segment. Therefore, in transverse or oblique lie with ruptured membranes and a poorly developed lower segment, a low vertical incision is more appropriate. Another technique utilized is intraoperative, extrauterine version at the time of cesarean. In many cases the fetal lie can be manually corrected after entry into the maternal peritoneal cavity is accomplished, but before the uterine incision is made. Such an approach may result in easier surgical delivery and may allow the use of a low transverse uterine incision more often.[41] However, in the presence of ruptured membranes, oligohydramnios, and a poorly developed lower segment, intraoperative version is not likely to be helpful.

REFERENCES

1. Abell, D. A.: Brow presentation—A review of 70 cases. *S. Afr. Med. J.* **47**:1315–1318, 1973.
2. Abroms, I. F., Bresnan, M. J., Zuckerman, J. E., Fischer, E. G., and Strand, R.: Cervical cord injuries secondary to hypertension of the head in breech presentations. *Obstet. Gynecol.* **41**:369–378, 1973.
3. Adams, C. M.: Review of breech presentation. *S.D. J. Med.* **32**:15–17, 1979.
4. Ang, L. T.: Compound presentation following external version. *Aust. N.Z. J. Obstet. Gynaecol.* **18**:213–214, 1978.
5. Bednoff, S. L. and Thomas, B. E.: Brow presentation. *N.Y. State J. Med.* **67**:803–805, 1967.
6. Benedetti, T. J., Lowensohn, R. I., and Truscott, A. M.: Face presentation at term. *Obstet. Gynecol.* **55**:199–202, 1980.
7. Borell, U. and Fernstrom, I.: The mechanism of labour. *Radiol. Clin. North Am.* **5**:73–85, 1966.
8. Breen, J. L. and Wiesmeier, E.: Compound presentation—A survey of 131 patients. *Obstet. Gynecol.* **1**:419–422, 1968.
9. Browne, A. D. H. and Carney, D.: Management

of malpresentations in obstetrics. *Br. Med. J.* **5393**:295–1298, 1964.
10. Calkins, L. A. and Pearce, E. W. J.: Transverse presentation. *Obstet. Gynecol.* **9**:123–125, 1957.
11. Campbell, J. M.: Face presentation. *Aust. N.Z. J. Obstet. Gynaecol.* **5**:231–234, 1965.
12. Cockburn, K. G. and Drake, R. F.: Transverse and oblique lie of the foetus. *Aust. N.Z. J. Obstet. Gynaecol.* **8**:211–218, 1968.
13. Collea, J. V.: Current management of breech presentation. *Clin. Obstet. Gynecol.* **23**:525–531, 1980.
14. Copeland, G. N., Nicks, F. I., and Christakos, A. C.: Face and brow presentations. *N.C. Med. J.* **29**:507–510, 1968.
15. Cruikshank, D. P. and Cruikshank, J. E.: Face and brow presentation—A review. *Clin. Obstet. Gynecol.* **24**:333–351, 1981.
16. Cruikshank, D. P. and White, C. A.: Obstetric malpresentations—Twenty years' experience. *Am. J. Obstet. Gynecol.* **116**:1097–1104, 1973.
17. Cucco, U. P.: Face presentation. *Am. J. Obstet. Gynecol.* **94**:1085–1091, 1966.
18. Dede, J. A. and Friedman, E. A.: Face presentation. *Am. J. Obstet. Gynecol.* **87**:515–524, 1963.
19. Dignam, W. J.: Difficulties in delivery, including shoulder dystocia and malpresentations of the fetus. *Clin. Obstet. Gynecol.* **19**:577–585, 1976.
20. Douglas, H. G. K. and Savage, P. E.: An unusual case of compound presentation. *J. Obstet. Gynecol. Br. Commonw.* **77**:1036, 1970.
21. Duff, P.: Diagnosis and management of face presentation. *Obstet. Gynecol.* **57**:105–112, 1981.
22. Edwards, R. L. and Nicholson, H. O.: The management of the unstable lie in late pregnancy. *J. Obstet. Gynaecol. Br. Commonw.* **76**:713–718, 1969.
23. Flowers, C. E.: Shoulder presentation. *Am. J. Obstet. Gynecol.* **96**:145–147, 1966.
24. Gold, S.: The conduct and management of face presentations. *J. Int. Coll. Surg.* **43**:253–258, 1965.
25. Gomez, H. E. and Dennen, E. H.: Face presentation—A study of 45 consecutive cases. *Obstet. Gynecol.* **8**:103–106, 1956.
26. Goplerud, J. and Eastman, N. J.: Compound presentation. *Obstet. Gynecol.* **1**:59–66, 1953.
27. Groenig, D. C.: Face presentation—Analysis of 37 cases at Louisville General Hospital. *Obstet. Gynecol.* **2**:495–499, 1953.
28. Hourihane, M. J.: Etiology and management of oblique lie. *Obstet. Gynecol.* **32**:512–519, 1968.
29. Ingolfsson, A.: Brow presentations. *Acta Obstet. Gynecol. Scand.* **48**:486–496, 1969.
30. Jennings, P. N.: Brw presentation with vaginal delivery. *Aust. N.Z. J. Obstet. Gynaecol.* **8**:219–224, 1968.
31. Johnson, C. E.: Abnormal fetal presentations. *Lancet* **84**:317–323, 1964.
32. Johnson, C. E.: Transverse presentation of fetus. *JAMA* **187**:642–646, 1964.
33. Kovacs, S. G.: Brow presentation, Royal Hospital for Women, Paddington (1950-1965), and review of literature. *Med. J. Aust.* **2**:820–824, 1970.
34. Lansford, A., Arias, D., and Smith, B. E.: Respiratory obstruction associated with face presentation. *Am. J. Dis. Child.* **116**:318–319, 1968.
35. Levy, D. L.: Persistent brow presentation—A new approach to management. *South. Med. J.* **69**:191–192, 1976.
36. MacGregor, W. G.: Aetiology and treatment of the oblique, transverse and unstable lie of the foetus with particular reference to antenatal care. *J. Obstet. Gynaecol. Br. Commonw.* **71**:237–244, 1964.
37. Magid, R. and Gillespie, C. F.: Face and brow presentations. *Obstet. Gynecol.* **9**:450–457, 1957.
38. Meltzer, R. M., Sachtleben, M. R., and Friedman, E. A.: Brow presentation. *Am. J. Obstet. Gynecol.* **100**:255–262, 1968.
39. Moore, E. J. T. and Dennen, E. H.: Management of persistent brow presentation. *Obstet. Gynecol.* **6**:186–189, 1955.
40. Mostar, S., Akaltin, E., and Babuna, C.: Deflexion attitudes. *Obstet. Gynecol.* **28**:49–56, 1966.
41. Pelosi, M. A., Apuzzio, J., Fricchione, D., and Gowda, V. V.: The "intra-abdominal version technique" for delivery of transverse lie by low-segment cesarean section. *Am. J. Obstet. Gynecol.* **135**:1009–1011, 1979.
42. Prevedourakis, C. N.: Face presentation—An analysis of 163 cases. *Am. J. Obstet. Gynecol.* **94**:1092–1097, 1966.
43. Pritchard, J. A., and MacDonald, P. C. (Eds.): Dystocia caused by abnormalities in presentation, position or development of the fetus. In: *Williams Obstetrics*, 16th Edition. New York, Appleton-Century-Crofts, 1980, pp. 797–830.
44. Salzmann, B., Soled, M., and Gilmour, T.: Face presentation. *Obstet. Gynecol.* **16**:106–112, 1960.
45. Sandhu, S. K.: Transverse lie. *J. Indian Med. Assoc.* **68**:205–208, 1977.
46. Skalley, T. W. and Kramer, T. F.: Brow presentation. *Obstet. Gynecol.* **15**:616–620, 1960.
47. Weissberg, S. M. and O'Leary, J.A.: Compound presentation of the fetus. *Obstet. Gynecol.* **41**:60–64, 1973.
48. Weissberg, S. M. and Weingold, A. B.: Compound presentation of the fetus. *N.Y. State J. Med.* **47**:936–939, 1967.
49. Yates, M. J.: Transverse foetal lie in labour. *J. Obstet. Gynaecol. Br. Commonw.* **71**:245–248, 1964.

26

MULTIPLE PREGNANCIES

"The rarity of plural births in women and the increased danger to mother and offspring in these circumstances renders such an event in a certain limited sense, a disease or an abnormality."[7] The greater risk to twins has been recognized since ancient times, and indeed such an event was looked on either with veneration or with horror. This is exemplified by the different approaches to twin births by groups living in close proximity in West Africa. In some parts of Nigeria twins were welcomed, in others they were disliked, and in yet others, they were taboo. Possibly this had something to do with the very high twinning rates in Nigeria.

THE INCIDENCE OF TWINNING

The incidence of twinning varies widely throughout the world (Table 26-1), but this variation is only in the dizygotic type arising from two ova (Fig. 26-1). In the monozygotic type, there seems to be a remarkably standard incidence throughout the world.

DIFFERENTIATION OF THE TWO TYPES OF TWINNING

It is sometimes possible to determine whether a given set of twins is monozygotic or dizygotic by examination of the sex and the membranes. If the sexes are different then they must be dizygotic and if there is only one chorionic membrane, then they must be monozygotic, but situations where the sex is the same and the placentation is dichorionic can be associated with either monozygotic or dizygotic twin pregnancies. In such cases, zygosity is determined by examination of genetic markers in the various blood groups and placental and blood enzymes.[5] Finger and palm printing can also be used. Although each member of a pair of monozygotic twins does not have exactly the same prints, the patterns are similar in the two members of the set of twins.

FACTORS INFLUENCING THE INCIDENCE

There does not seem to be any distinguishing feature in the mothers of monozygotic twins, but the mothers of dizygotic twins tend to be older, of higher parity, taller, and heavier than mothers of singletons.[1] There is a well-known, but ill-defined, familial tendency to dizygotic twinning. Several instances of monozygotic twinning occurring in some families have been reported, but this is uncommon and monozygotic twinning is not usually considered to be familial.

Gonadotrophic stimulation of multiple ovulation causes dizygotic twinning. There is some evidence[13] that levels of follicle stimulating hormone are higher in women who have had twin pregnancies than in women who have had singleton pregnancies. Whether taller, heavier women are more likely to produce more follicle stimulating hormone than smaller women is not

TABLE 26-1. INCIDENCE OF DIZYGOTIC TWINNING IN VARIOUS PARTS OF THE WORLD

Place	Population	Monozygous	Dizygous	Total
Nigeria	Yoruba	5.0	49.0	54.0
Nigeria	Ibo	5.0	22.0	27.0
United States	Black	4.7	11.1	15.8
England and Wales	Hospital statistics	3.5	8.8	12.3
United States	White	4.2	7.1	11.3
Bombay	Indian	4.3	6.8	11.1
Singapore	Chinese	6.7	4.2	10.9
Japan	Hospital statistics	3.9	2.9	6.8

Source: Adapted from Nylander.[14]

yet determined, nor is it known whether there is a familial tendency to higher FSH production.

THE MATERNAL RESPONSE TO TWIN PREGNANCY

This is much more marked than in singleton pregnancy and the response to higher multiples is even greater. There is a greater weight gain in twin pregnancies compared to singletons, even in the first trimester of pregnancy.[1] This is in large measure due to water retention.[2] There is also a greater expansion of plasma volume in twin pregnancies compared to singletons (Table 26-2) and the combined birth weights correlate with the amount of plasma volume.[3] The cardiac output is also greater in twin pregnancies than in singletons and the blood pressure is slightly lower in midtrimester in twin pregnancies.[2] Because the increase in the plasma volume is greater than the increase in the red cell volume, the hemoglobin concentration falls. Levels of 10 g/100 ml hemoglobin are quite normal in twin pregnancies by 30 weeks' gestation. The total hemoglobin mass is greater than in singleton pregnancies and the mean corpuscular volume remains about 85. The erythrocyte sedimentation rate and the increase in leucocytes are likewise greater in twin pregnancies than in singletons. Serum concentrations of sodium, potassium, and chloride and the serum osmolality are the same in twin pregnancies as in singletons. Although the total protein concentration falls to about 6.0 g/100 ml in singleton pregnancies and to 5.5 g/100 ml in twin pregnancies, the total intravascular mass of proteins is greater in twin than in singleton pregnancies.[2] There is an increase in glomerular filtration rate[16] and a greater increase in respiratory tidal volume in twin pregnancies[17] compared with singletons.

Many of these changes, if not all, are under the control of placental hormones and it is not surprising, therefore, to find that there is an increased production of about 50% above normal singleton values of estrogens and progesterone and also in placental protein hormones SP_1, PAPP-A, PP_5, HPL, and alpha-fetoprotein.

The maternal response to higher multiple pregnancies is even greater; for example, in quadruplet pregnancy, the plasma volume increases to double that in singleton pregnancies and 50% more than in twin pregnancies.

COMPLICATIONS OF TWIN PREGNANCIES

Many complications of pregnancy are more frequent in twin pregnancies than in singletons. Minor complaints such as alimentary disturbances, including vomiting and constipation, are more frequent and often more marked. Not all complications, however, are either more frequent or more marked in twin pregnancies.

Anemia

The greater expansion of plasma volume produces a lower hemoglobin concentration, but this does not indicate anemia. There is, however, a reduction in both iron and folic acid stores in twin pregnancy,[9] but the incidence of clinically significant anemia is low. We do not recommend routine iron and/or folic acid prophylactically, but rather specific treatment should be given when there is evidence of signif-

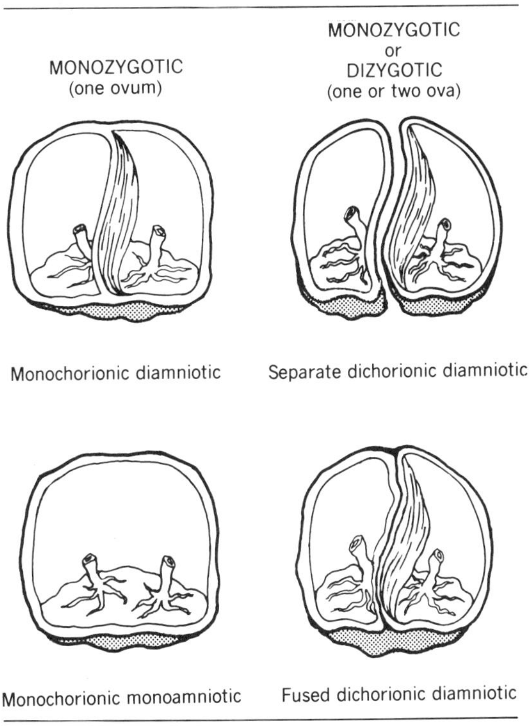

Figure 26-1. Monozygotic twins, derived from a single ovum, share a single placenta to which two umbilical cords are connected. They usually share a single chorion, but each has a separate amnion. Rarely, they share a single amnion. In such instances, fetal mortality is high, due largely to cord accidents. If the embryo splits before the amnion is formed, an amnion arises in response to each embryo. If the embryo splits after the amnion has formed, monoamniotic twins result. However, single-ovum twins may be derived from a zygote that splits so early (8–12 cells) that the relations of the placenta and membranes are exactly those seen in dizygotic twins. Dizygotic twins are always dichorionic and diamniotic. The chorions may be fused or unfused, as may be the placentas.

icant anemia. Any deficiency is likely to be transient and of a self-limiting nature. It is important to emphasize, however, that full blood examination is indicated regularly in twin and other multiple pregnancies.

Antepartum Hemorrhage

Although it is generally considered that antepartum hemorrhage is more frequent with twin pregnancies than with singletons, a careful study of a large number of twin pregnancies showed no greater incidence.[14]

Preeclampsia

There is no doubt that preeclampsia is a common complication of twin pregnancies. In a very large series of 1206 twin births in Aberdeen in which the zygosity was accurately determined by examination of cord blood and placental tissue for blood groups and enzymes, it was found that there was no difference between the incidence of proteinuric preeclampsia in monozygotic compared with dizygotic twin pregnancies. The incidence was found to be high in both types, and particularly in primigravidas (Table 26-3).[5,10] These results indicate that there is a balance between the antigenic differences and circulating immunosuppressive substances in both monozygotic and dizygotic twin pregnancies. This has an important bearing on any immunological theory for the etiology of preeclampsia.

Polyhydramnios

Polyhydramnios is more common in twin pregnancies than in singletons. The incidence of chronic hydramnios is probably the same in monozygotic and dizygotic twin pregnancies, but acute hydramnios is more common in monozygotic twin pregnancies.

Abortion

This is probably more common in twin pregnancies than in singletons but this is difficult to determine because, in many cases, it is not recognized that a twin pregnancy is present. Furthermore, the frequency of occurrence of the "disappearing twin" phenomenon is difficult to determine. It is possible by ultrasound scanning to detect when one twin dies and is absorbed and many such cases are now on record.

Fetal Malformations

As many early abortions are known to be due to abnormalities, it is possible that the greater abortion rate in twin pregnancies could be accounted for by an increased incidence of malformations in twin gestations. The incidence of fetal malformations is higher in twin pregnancies than in singletons, and the incidence of malformations in monozygotic twin pregnancies is twice that in dizygotic. The type of placentation does not influence the incidence of fetal malformation.[6,12]

TABLE 26-2. MEAN (±SD) PLASMA VOLUME (ML) BY COMBINED BIRTH WEIGHT CENTILES IN PRIMIGRAVID TWIN PREGNANCIES (NUMBERS IN PARENTHESES ARE NUMBERS IN EACH GROUP)

	< 25	25–<50	50–<75	≧75
Normotensive and mild preeclampsia (78)	3769* ± 481 (28)	4049 ± 643 (12)	4013 ± 439 (17)	4175* ± 566 (21)
Proteinuric preeclampsia (30)	3952 ± 661 (14)	4092 ± 278 (4)	4240 ± 468 (5)	4112 ± 307 (7)
All (108)	3830* ± 547 (42)	4060 ± 574 (16)	4065 ± 446 (22)	4159* ± 573 (28)

* Statistically significant

TABLE 26-3. INCIDENCE OF PREECLAMPSIA IN MONOZYGOTIC AND DIZYGOTIC TWIN PREGNANCIES BY PARITY

	Proteinuric Preeclampsia		Gestational Hypertension		Normotensive	
	%	No.	%	No.	%	No.
Primigravidas						
Monozygotic (n = 119)	17.65	21	26.89	32	55.46	66
Dizygotic (n = 236)	18.64	44	24.15	57	57.21	135
Multigravidas						
Monozygotic (n = 223)	7.18	16	13.45	30	79.37	177
Dizygotic (n = 628)	8.28	52	17.20	108	74.52	468

Fetal Growth

Fetal growth is less in twins than in singletons and is decreased even more in higher multiples. Discrepancies in birth weight of twins tends to be more marked in monozygotic twins than in dizygotic twins. Fetal growth retardation is, therefore, a common feature of twin pregnancies, but this is not the only reason for them being born small.

Preterm Delivery

Premature delivery is very common in twin pregnancies. Low-birth-weight infants, weighing less than 2500 g, account for over 50% of multiple births compared to less than 10% for singleton births.[15] The cause of preterm delivery is unknown, but some pointers to the cause were found in a recent study[11] which showed that there were differences in the ways in which the preterm labor began and also the frequency of preterm labor, depending on the zygosity and the sex of the babies. In 624 pregnancies with accurately determined zygosity and placentation, there were 176 deliveries before 37 completed weeks of gestation (28.4%). Of these, 72 (11.54%) went into labor with spontaneous uterine contractions, 73 (11.7%) had spontaneous rupture of the membranes before labor, and 31 (4.97%) had induction of labor or cesarean section performed. When the deliveries were divided by zygosity, it was found that preterm deliveries occurred in 33% of monozygotic, but in only 25% of dizygotic pregnancies. The difference was mainly accounted for by the fact that spontaneous rupture of the membranes occurred twice as frequently in monozygotic as in the dizygotic. The incidence of preterm labor was not affected by the type of placentation. The reason for the more frequent occurrence of rupture of the membranes in monozygotic twin pregnancies is not clear, but it seems unlikely that acute hydramnios occurs sufficiently frequently to account for this.

Labor has been shown to occur at an earlier gestational age with male babies than with females.[8] The sex of the babies in twin deliveries, therefore, was studied.[11] Once again, there was a preponderance of males over females in preterm twin deliveries. This sex ratio was associated with both the spontaneous onset of contractions and with spontaneous rupture of the membranes. However, although the preponderance of boys over girls was quite dramatically true of monozygotic twinning, it did not occur with dizygotic twins. Furthermore, no differences in placentation were associated with the sex of the babies. These findings are at present inexplicable, but as the differences are so marked, it would seem that the difference in sex ratio should give useful indications to the causation of preterm labor.

Prevention and Management of Preterm Labor in Twin Pregnancy

Prevention and management of preterm labor in twin pregnancy has given rise to much controversy. There are various claims that preterm onset of labor can be prevented by rest, betasympathomimetic agents, or cervical sutures, but there have been no reports of any properly controlled studies of large series. Alhough unaccustomed activity should be avoided, there does not seem to be any indication for complete rest unless there is marked discomfort or some complication of the twin pregnancy. If preterm labor is suspected or anticipated, possibly by regular examination of the state of the cervix in the last trimester, it is very important that the woman should be in, or very near to, a hospital with good facilities for caring for small babies.

Diagnosis

It is preferable that the diagnosis of twin pregnancy should be made at least by the end of the second trimester, so that arrangements can be made for the proper care of the twins, should they be delivered early. The early diagnosis of multiple pregnancy is more often made nowadays because of ultrasonic scanning, the higher results of screening tests such as alpha-fetoprotein, and by wider utilization of such simple clinical tests as weighing and assessment of uterine size.

Early diagnosis is also important so that the mother can be warned about the possibility of complications arising. It is also important to diagnose twin pregnancy early so that gestational age can be accurately determined.

Perinatal Mortality and Morbidity in Twins

The perinatal mortality in twins is about five or six times higher than in singletons and the perinatal mortality in monozygotic is higher than in dizygotic twins. The main cause of death is low birth weight of the twins due to both growth retardation and preterm labor. Male twins are at greater risk than females and the second twin has a worse prognosis than the first. There is also an increased risk of malpositions and malpresentations in twins compared with singletons. Second twins tend to have a lower Apgar score than do first twins. Assisted breech delivery results in a lower Apgar score than any other type of delivery. Since twins are more liable to asphyxia, it is not surprising that the incidence of cerebral palsy is higher in twins than in singletons.

There are more psychological problems, lower intelligence quotients, and more language and verbal reasoning difficulties in twins than in singletons.

Antenatal Management

Women with twin pregnancies require more antenatal care than those with singletons because of the greater incidence of complications. It seems, however, that rest in the hospital is unlikely to prevent any of the complications, for example, preeclampsia or preterm labor. Nevertheless, these women should be encouraged to take as much rest as possible at home.

The diet taken by women with twin pregnancies need not be any different from that of those with singleton pregnancies. It was found in our Aberdeen studies[4] that good-sized twin babies were produced by mothers taking a diet with an average energy intake of 2000 kcal per day and 65 g of protein. No additional trace element or vitamin supplementations need to be added to the ordinary mixed diet.

When complications arise, it is, of course, necessary to admit these women to a well-equipped maternity hospital. Induction of preterm labor may be necessary if there is severe preeclampsia or severe growth retardation, or some other complication. In some cases, cesarean section may be indicated.

Postmaturity is difficult to deal with in twin pregnancies, because it is not possible to assess the condition of both babies. In view of this, it is commonly believed that twin pregnancies should not go beyond 40 weeks.

Elective cesarean section is not without risk, particularly to the babies (respiratory distress syndrome), but to the mother as well. Routine elective cesarean section is not necessary in twin pregnancies. There should be a clear and definite indication for doing a cesarean section, such as an antenatal complication or the presence of malpresentation.

Cesarean section after the onset of labor may be necessary if complications arise, particularly in malpresentations or cord prolapse. As preterm labor is common in twin pregnancies, the decision as to whether cesarean section is carried out in pregnancies of short gestation will often depend on the adequacy of the neonatology service. If the pregnancy is less than 28 weeks, it is unlikely that cesarean section should be carried out, even though there is malpresentation. Between about 28 and 34 weeks, the risks of vaginal breech delivery, particularly for the second baby, are high and cesarean section may be carried out in these cases. After 34 weeks, vaginal delivery may be carried out, even though one or both babies are presenting by the breech.

Management of Labor

Adequate sedation must be provided and this is commonly carried out with epidural anesthesia. In any case, it is highly desirable that an anesthetist should be available for all twin deliveries. If epidural anesthesia is not available, then pudendal block anesthesia can be administered for delivery of the first baby by forceps or assisted breech, but the patient should, in any case, be prepared for general anesthesia in case this is necessary for the delivery of the second baby.

The condition of the twins should be monitored during labor by cardiotocography if possible.

The first baby is delivered in the usual way employed for delivery of a singleton.

After delivery of the first twin, the lie of the second twin is determined and, if necessary, corrected externally to a longitudinal lie. The fetal heart is checked and a vaginal examination is carried out to rupture the second sac of membranes. Should there be any delay in the onset of uterine contractions, an oxytocin drip should be set up. Indeed, it is preferable that an infusion of suitable fluid should be set up early in labor so that it can be switched to oxytocin as required. The delivery of the second baby is then carried out, either spontaneously or by forceps or ventouse if it is a cephalic presentation, or by assisted breech delivery if the breech is presenting. The oxytocin drip is also useful for the delivery of the placenta or placentas. Occasionally, the first placenta is delivered before the second twin.

Cesarean section should rarely be necessary for the delivery of the second twin, even though it is presenting by the breech or in a transverse or oblique lie. If the lie cannot be corrected by external version, it is usually easy to do so by internal manipulation. It is only in unusual circumstances where the liquor amnii has drained away and the uterus is firmly contracted around the second baby, that cesarean section would be necessary.

An undiagnosed second twin is at considerable risk, particularly if an oxytocic drug has been given after the delivery of the first twin. As soon as the diagnosis is made, the lie is checked and the membranes ruptured. The second twin is then delivered as expeditiously as possible.

Locked twins and conjoined twins are fortunately very rare. When this is suspected, particularly if there is obstructed labor, then wherever possible, delivery by cesarean section should be performed. Otherwise, a difficult destructive operation may be necessary.

Delivery of Triplets and Higher Multiples

As the risks of abnormal presentations and intrauterine growth retardation are increased in higher multiples, recourse to cesarean section is usually made. If conditions seem particularly favorable, vaginal delivery may be attempted for triplets.

As preterm labor is likely to occur, it is possible that the babies may be delivered spontaneously and survive, as happened with the famous Dionne quintuplets. Most higher multiples are nowadays due to inappropriate ovulation stimulation and are likely to be diagnosed early, so that early hospitalization and cesarean section will be carried out when necessary.

REFERENCES

1. Campbell, D. M., Campbell, A., and MacGillivray, I.: Maternal characteristics of women having twin pregnancies. *J. Biosoc. Sci.* **6**:463–470, 1975.
2. Campbell, D. M. and MacGillivray, I.: Maternal physiological responses and birthweight in singleton and twin pregnancy by parity. *Eur. J. Obstet. Gynecol. Reprod. Biol.* **7**:17–24, 1977.
3. Campbell, D. M. and MacGillivray, I.: The importance of plasma volume expansion and nutrition in twin pregnancy. *Acta Genet. Med. Gemellol. (Roma)* **33**:19–24, 1984.
4. Campbell, D. M., MacGillivray, I., and Tuttle, S.: Maternal nutrition in twin pregnancy. *Acta Genet. Med. Gemellol. (Roma)* **31**:221–227, 1982.

5. Corney, G. and Robson, E. B.: Types of twinning and determination of zygosity. In: *Human Multiple Reproduction*. I. MacGillivray, P. P. S. Nylander, and G. Corney, (Eds.). London, W. B. Saunders, 1975, pp. 16–39.
6. Corney, G., MacGillivray, I., Campbell, D. M., Thompson, B., and Little, J.: Congenital anomalies in twins in Aberdeen and Northeast Scotland. *Acta Genet. Med. Gemellol. (Roma)* **32**:31–35, 1983.
7. Duncan, J. M.: On the comparative frequency of twin-bearing in different pregnancies. *Edinburgh Med. J.* **10**:928–929, 1865.
8. Hall, M. and Carr-Hill, R.: The weaker sex? The impact of sex ratio on the onset and management of labour. *Br. Med. J.* **285**:401–403, 1982.
9. Hall, M., Campbell, D. M., and Davidson, R. J.: Anaemia in twin pregnancy. *Acta Genet. Med. Gemellol. (Roma)* **28**:279–282, 1979.
10. MacGillivray, I.: Determinants of birthweight in twins. *Acta Genet. Med. Gemellol. (Roma)* **32**:151–157, 1983.
11. MacGillivray, I., Campbell, D. M., Samphier, M., and Thompson, B.: Preterm deliveries in twin pregnancies in Aberdeen. *Acta Genet. Med. Gemellol. (Roma)* **31**:207–211, 1982.
12. Myrianthopoulos, N. C.: Congenital malformations. The contribution of twin studies. *Birth Defects* **XIV**(6A):151–165, 1978.
13. Nylander, P. P. S.: Serum levels of gonadotrophin in relation to multiple pregnancy in Nigeria. *J. Obstet. Gynaecol. Br. Commonw.* **80**:651–653, 1973.
14. Nylander, P. P. S.: Frequency of multiple births. In: *Human Multiple Reproduction*. I. MacGillivray, P. P. S. Nylander, and G. Corney, (Eds.). London, W. B. Saunders, 1975, pp. 87–97.
15. Potter, E. L.: Twin zygosity and placental form in relation to the outcome of the pregnancy. *Am. J. Obstet. Gynecol.* **87**:566–577, 1963.
16. Swapp, G. H.: Personal communication, 1975.
17. Templeton, A. A., and Kelman, R.: Personal communication, 1975.

SECTION C
MATERNAL PROBLEMS IN PREGNANCY

27

VULVOVAGINITIS IN PREGNANCY

Symptoms referable to the lower genital tract are common in pregnant women. Vulvovaginitis seen during pregnancy is similar to that encountered in nonpregnant women. However, altered response to therapy and concern for fetal effects of treatment regimens mandate a careful approach to diagnosis and therapy.

VULVOVAGINAL PHYSIOLOGY DURING PREGNANCY

Hormonal changes of pregnancy and increased vascularity of the vagina lead to rapid turnover of vaginal epithelial cells rich in glycogen. The cervical mucus becomes opaque and viscid. The average number of species of aerobic bacteria found in the vagina remains relatively constant, but the number of anaerobic species declines slightly. The prevalence of lactobacilli and yeast increases.[6] This trend toward increasing benignity of vaginal flora during pregnancy has led to the teleologic explanation that such flora are less threatening to the fetus traversing the birth canal.[9,10]

The physiologic alterations of pregnancy may cause the patient to complain of unusually heavy discharge when no demonstrable infection is present. Additionally, the increased frequency of yeast colonization may predispose pregnant patients to a slightly increased incidence of monilial vaginitis.

DIAGNOSTIC AIDS

The equipment necessary to successfully evaluate vulvovaginal complaints during pregnancy is simple. The cornerstones of diagnosis of vulvovaginitis are the 0.9% saline and the 10% KOH wet mount. A drop of vaginal discharge mixed with a drop of saline or potassium hydroxide on a microscope slide provides immediate microscopic diagnosis in most cases. In addition to microscopic examination, the "whiff test" in which a 10% KOH slide from a patient with believed *Gardnerella vaginalis* vaginitis emits a "fishy" amine odor is useful.[4]

Litmus pH paper is another useful diagnostic aid. A profuse odorous discharge with pH greater than 5 suggests either *G. vaginalis* or *Trichomonas vaginalis* infection. Diagnosis of pediculosis pubis and various types of vulvar dermatitis is facilitated by the use of a hand-held magnifying glass. A Wood's light may be helpful in the differential diagnosis of erythrasma or tinea fungal infection. A Keyes' punch biopsy tray should be available to allow biopsy to clarify difficult vulvar dermatologic diagnoses.

THERAPEUTIC AIDS

Although the causes of vulvovaginal infection in pregnancy are similar to those in the nonpregnant state, concern for fetal safety dictates special considerations for therapy in some cases. Several therapeutic agents are useful in the treatment of vulvovaginitis.

Acyclovir

Acyclovir is a recently approved inhibitor of herpes virus-specific deoxyribonucleic acid polymerase. The drug reduces the duration of viral shedding and speeds healing of lesions in patients with primary infection. It is effective in treatment of disseminated herpes infection, both in immunocompromised patients and in pregnancy.[7] However, data on the use of this drug in pregnancy are minimal. Its use, therefore, is not recommended for simple primary or recurrent cutaneous infection.

Aluminum Acetate

Burow's solution (5% aluminum acetate) is an effective and safe topical astringent and antiseptic useful in many cases of vulvovaginitis.

Ampicillin

Penicillins have been used extensively during pregnancy with no known teratogenic effects. In the neonate, ampicillin may compete for bilirubin binding sites and may also interfere with neonatal bacterial cultures.

Boric Acid

Boric acid powder utilized in gelatin capsules per vaginam offers an inexpensive and effective alternative to imidazole antifungal agents for the treatment of vulvovaginal candidiasis.[20] Serum boric acid levels after vaginal administration of 600 mg are very low. Animal studies reveal no teratogenic effects.[18]

Clotrimazole

Miconozole and Clotrimazole are imidazole antifungal agents designed for topical application. These drugs have been used extensively in pregnancy with no reported fetal effects.[1]

Corticosteroids

Topical corticosteroids sparingly applied for brief periods of time are without demonstrable ill effects on pregnancy.

Gentian Violet

Gentian violet in 1% aqueous solution is an effective topical antifungal agent that is safe for use during pregnancy.

Laser

Carbon dioxide laser has been safely and effectively used during pregnancy in the treatment of vulvovaginal condylomata acuminata.[2,11]

Lindane

Lindane is the active ingredient in gamma benzene hexochloride. It is highly effective in the treatment of pediculosis pubis. The drug is poorly absorbed through the skin. There is no suggestion of teratogenesis in animals.[1,5]

Metronidazole

Metronidazole is a nitroimidazole agent with a broad spectrum of activity against protozoans and anaerobic bacteria. Its usefulness in the treatment of *Trichomonas vaginalis* and *Gardnerella vaginalis* infections is well documented.[14,15,19] Although there is no evidence of teratogenesis in humans,[17] metronidazole is mutagenic in bacteria and carcinogenic in rodents.[15] This has led some authorities to advise restriction of the use of this drug during pregnancy to cases of amebiasis, giardiasis, or refractory *T. vaginalis* infection after the first trimester.

Podophyllin

Podophyllin is a resinous mixture of plant extracts with colchicine-like effects on rapidly growing tissue.[3] It is commonly used as a topical antiviral agent in the treatment of vulvar condylomata. Systemic absorption may cause maternal and fetal neurotoxicity, and the drug may be teratogenic in early pregnancy.[3,8] This, combined with its relative ineffectiveness in the treatment of condylomata in pregnancy, condemns the use of podophyllin during gestation.

COMMON INFECTIOUS VULVOVAGINITIDES DURING PREGNANCY

As in nonpregnant women, infectious causes of vulvovaginitis in pregnancy fall into four gen-

TABLE 27-1. CHARACTERISTICS OF THE COMMON VULVOVAGINITIDES

	Gardnerella Vaginalis	Trichomonas Vaginalis	Candida Species
Symptoms			
Pruritus	±	++++	++++
Discharge	++++	++++	±
Odor	++++	++++	−
Signs			
Inflammation	−	++++	++
Discharge	++++	++++	++++
Color	Yellow	Green	"Cottage cheese"
pH	>5.0	>5.0	<4.5
Microscopy	Saline; few PMNs; "clue" cells	Saline; many PMNs; motile flagellates	KOH; Budding yeast and hyphae.
Therapy	Boric acid Ampicillin Metronidazole	Clotrimazole Metronidazole	Gentian violet Boric acid Clotrimazole

eral categories: bacterial, viral, fungal, and protozoan/parasitic (See Table 27-1).

Bacterial

Gardnerella Vaginalis. In the annals of microbiology, few organisms have stirred as much interest and taxonomic controversy as *Gardnerella vaginalis* (formerly *Hemophilus vaginalis, Corynebacterium vaginalis*). This small gram-negative bacillus is present in from 10% to 20% of women seen in gynecology clinics and may account for up to 45% of cases of vaginitis.[4]

The organism is transmitted by sexual contact. Kaufman and Gardner have suggested that it is a surface parasite attaching only to desquamated or superficial epithelial cells.[4] Presenting symptoms are usually profuse discharge and foul odor. On physical examination, possibly owing to the noninvasive nature of the infection, there is minimal inflammation with a profuse milky, perhaps frothy, malodorous discharge with a pH above 5. Ten percent KOH wet mount may produce a "fishy" amine odor. Saline wet mount reveals a paucity of white blood cells, numerous squames and bacteria, and squamous cells covered with attached bacteria ("clue cells"). A discharge with these characteristics and no motile trichomonads is diagnostic of *G. vaginalis* vaginitis.

G. vaginalis vaginitis is a benign condition, and therapy in pregnancy should be equally benign. Metronidazole, 500 mg twice daily for seven days, is effective;[14,19] however, the yet unknown risks of metronidazole in pregnancy must be considered. Boric acid powder, 600 mg in a gelatin capsule per vaginam once daily for two weeks, commonly relieves symptoms. If this regimen fails, Ampicillin, 500 mg every six hours for five days, is benign and moderately effective.[14]

Other Bacterial Vulvovaginitides. Bacterial vulvovaginitis is uncommon in reproductive-aged females in the absence of trauma, estrogen deficiency, or an immunocompromised state. One exception is that of erythrasma, a superficial vulvar infection caused by *Corynebacterium minutissimum*. Seen primarily in warm climates, the disease presents as an inflammation of intertriginous areas which is characterized by "coral red fluorescence" visualized under Wood's light. It is treated by local cleansing and erythromycin 250 mg orally four times daily for one week.

Viral

Herpes Genitalis. Herpes genitalis is an epidemic sexually transmitted disease caused by herpes virus hominis type II. Active herpetic vulvovaginitis in the perinatal period can be catastrophic for the neonate. The diagnosis and perinatal management of this disease are discussed in detail in Chapter 38.

Condyloma Acuminatum. Condyloma acuminatum is a sexually transmitted disease caused by human papillomavirus. The condylomata appear on the vulva and perianal regions as small warty growths. There may be associated discharge and irritation if other sexually transmitted diseases are present. The perineal moisture and hormonal milieu of pregnancy may accelerate growth. Diagnosis is usually easy, due to the characteristic appearance of the lesion. Biopsy reveals marked acanthosis with cellular vacuolation and dermal inflammatory infiltrate.[4]

Condylomata can be treated by topical application of podophyllin in benzoin solution. However, the use of this drug is contraindicated in pregnancy. Cryocautery and electrodesiccation are effective and readily available forms of surgical therapy. Recent studies have explored the effectiveness of the carbon dioxide laser during pregnancy.[2,11] Since condylomata acuminata usually regress postpartum, therapy is best delayed until after delivery.

Fungal

Monilial Vulvovaginitis. Approximately 30% of pregnant women harbor *Candida* species in the vagina.[4] As many as 50% of these colonized individuals may intermittently manifest clinical evidence of infection. The high incidence of colonization and infection is believed due to hormonal changes of pregnancy which alter vaginal microbial flora and vaginal epithelial glycogen content.[13]

The commonest presenting complaints of monilial vulvovaginitis are pruritus and vulvar burning. Many patients complain of dysuria and dyspareunia. On physical examination the vulva is intensely erthematous with spread of discontinuous "satellite" lesions onto the mons, inner thighs, and buttocks. Vaginal examination reveals fiery red, friable mucosal tissues with a thick "cottage cheese" pseudomembrane obscuring the cervix and vagina. The vaginal pH is approximately 4.5. A 10% KOH wet mount reveals the characteristic morphology of the offending organism. *Candida* species are characterized by budding yeast and hyphae formation, whereas *Torulopsis glabrata* manifests only budding yeast without filament formation.

Uncomplicated monilial vulvovaginitis can be successfully treated by one of several topical agents. For severe cases, gentian violet applied on two occasions two days apart affords rapid relief. This initial therapy should be followed by 10–14 days of vaginal 2% miconozole, 1% clotrimazole, or boric acid, 600 mg in gelatin capsules.[16,20] Adjunctive symptomatic therapy with topical corticosteroids or aluminum acetate soaks may be helpful during the first 3–4 days of therapy.

Tinea Cruris

Tinea cruris is a fungal infection of the genitocrural folds occurring most often during warm weather. Patients complain of intense pruritis and painful excoriations. The lesion presents as a symmetrical, erythematous, vesicular, advancing margin with central clearing. A heated 10% KOH prep of scrapings from the margin of the lesion reveals hyphae without budding yeast forms. Topical corticosteroid creams and aluminum acetate soaks provide symptomatic relief. One percent clotrimazole eradicates the organism within 10 days to 2 weeks.

Protozoans and Cutaneous Parasites

Trichomonas Vaginalis. *Trichomonas vaginalis* is a unicellular protozoan flagellate that is primarily sexually transmitted. Its prevalence varies from 3% to 5% among middle-class patients to 90% among prostitutes.[4] Like *G. vaginalis* and *Candida* species, the organism may remain latent and produce no obvious infection.

Patients with acute symptomatic trichomoniasis typically complain of vulvar pruritus, profuse foul, frothy discharge, vaginal spotting, and perhaps dysuria and mild lower abdominal pain. Physical examination reveals a fiery red vagina with cervical petechiae (strawberry cervix) and a profuse, foamy sometimes greenish discharge with pH above 5. Saline wet preparation reveals abundant polymorphonuclear cells and motile flagellate organisms.

Due to a fear of the effects of metronidazole during pregnancy, some authorities recommend only symptomatic therapy for pregnant patients with trichomoniasis. However, recent prospective studies have associated trichomoniasis with premature spontaneous rupture of the chorioamnion.[12] Although the study did not demonstrate a causal relationship or effects of therapy, it seems prudent to treat at least those pregnant patients with acute trichomoniasis who have a poor obstetrical history. Clotrimazole alleviates about 50% of cases of trichomoniasis and has been suggested as the initial therapy in pregnancy.[16] For persistent symptomatic trichomoniasis beyond the first trimester, metronidazole 2 g orally is not contraindicated.

Phthirus Pubis

Pediculosis pubis is a sexually transmitted infestation with a crab louse that attaches itself primarily to the hair of the mons and lives on blood. Intense vulvar pruritis without an associated skin lesion is suggestive of the disease. Diagnosis is based on identification of the louse or its nits attached to the base of the pubic hair. Topical application of gamma benzene hexachloride (with 1% lindane) repeated in 24 hours is highly therapeutic.

REFERENCES

1. Berkowitz, R. L., Coustan, D. R., and Mochizuki, T. K.: *Handbook for Prescribing Medications During Pregnancy.* Boston, Little, Brown and Company, 1981.
2. Ferenczy, A.: Treating genital condyloma during pregnancy with the carbon dioxide laser. *Am. J. Obstet. Gynecol.* **148**:9–12, 1984.
3. Friedrich, E. G.: *Vulvar Disease*, Chapters 1, 2, and 3. Philadelphia, W. B. Saunders, 1976.
4. Gardner, H. L. and Kaufman, R. H.: *Benign Diseases of the Vulva and Vagina*, 2nd Edition, Chapters 3,12,13,14,15,17,19, and 23. Boston, G. K. Hall Medical Publishers, 1981.
5. Goodman, L. S. and Gillman, A.: *The Pharmacologic Basis of Therapeutics*, 5th Edition. New York, Macmillan Publishing, 1975.
6. Goplerud, C. P., Ohm, M. J., and Galask, R. P.: Aerobic and anaerobic flora of the cervix during pregnancy and puerperium. *Am. J. Obstet. Gynecol.* **126**:858–868, 1976.
7. Grover, L., Kane, J., Kravitz, J., and Cruz, A.: Systemic acyclovir in pregnancy: A case report. *Obstet. Gynecol.* **65**:284–287, 1985.
8. Karol, M. D., Conner, C. S., Watanabe, A. S., and Murphrey, K. J.: Podophyllum: Suspected teratogenicity from topical application. *Clin. Toxicol.* **16**:283–286, 1980.
9. Larsen, B. and Galask, R. P.: Vaginal microbial flora: Composition and influences of host physiology. *Ann. Intern. Med.* **96**:926–930, 1982.
10. Larsen B. and Galask R. P.: Vaginal microbial flora: Practical and theoretic relevance. *Obstet. Gynecol.* **55**:100S–113S, 1980.
11. Malfetano, J. H., Marin, A. C., and Malfetano, J. H., Jr.: Laser treatment of condylomata acuminata in pregnancy. *J. Reprod. Med.* **26**:574–576, 1981.
12. Minkoff, H., Grunebaum, A. N., Schwarz, R. H., Feldman, J., Cummings, M., Krombleholme, W., Clark, L., Pringle, G., and MacCormack, W. M.: Risk factors for prematurity and premature rupture of membranes: A prospective study of the vaginal flora in pregnancy. *Am. J. Obstet. Gynecol.* **150**:965–972, 1984.
13. Paavonen, J.: Physiology and ecology of the vagina. *Scand. J. Infect. Dis.* **40**:31–35, 1983.
14. Pheifer, T. A., Forsyth, P. S., Durfee, M. A., Pollock, H. M., and Holmes, K. K.: Nonspecific vaginitis: Role of *Haemophilus vaginalis* and treatment with metronidazole. *N. Engl. J. Med.* **298**:1429–1434, 1978.
15. Robbie, J. O. and Sweet, R. L.: Metronidazole use in obstetrics and gynecology: A review. *Am. J. Obstet. Gynecol.* **145**:865–881, 1983.
16. Rein, M. F.: Current therapy of vulvovaginitis: *Sex. Transm. Dis.* **8**:316–320, 1981.
17. Roe, F. J. C.: Toxicologic evaluation on metronidazole with particular reference to carcinogenic, mutagenic, and teratogenic potential. *Surgery* **93**:158–164, 1983.
18. Shepard, T. H.: *Catalog of Teratogenic Agents*, 3rd Edition. Baltimore, Johns Hopkins University Press, 1980.
19. Spiegel, C. A., Amsel, R., Eschenbach, D., Schoenknecht, R., and Holmes, K.: Anaerobic bacteria in nonspecific vaginitis. *N. Engl. J. Med.* **303**:601–607, 1983.
20. Van Slyke, K. K., Michel, V. P., and Rein, M. D.: Treatment of vulvovaginal candidiasis with boric acid powder. *Am. J. Obstet. Gynecol.* **141**:145–148, 1981.

28

SKIN CHANGES AND DISEASES OF PREGNANCY

The dramatic endocrine changes occurring in pregnancy may be associated with both physiologic and pathologic alterations in the skin, hair, and nails. To aid in their recognition and differentiation, pregnancy-related skin changes can conveniently be classified into the following five broad categories: (1) physiologic changes, (2) diseases specifically related to pregnancy, (3) cutaneous tumors influenced by pregnancy, (4) genital infections related to pregnancy, and (5) other skin diseases influenced by pregnancy.[7]

PHYSIOLOGIC CHANGES (TABLE 28-1)

Hyperpigmentation

Increased skin pigmentation is common in pregnancy, occurring in up to 90% of women. The degree is usually mild and generalized, with accentuation on the breast areolae, axillae, perineum, perianal skin, genitalia, and inner thighs. Linea nigra, a darkened streak from the symphysis pubis to the umbilicus that may extend to the xiphoid process, occurs more commonly in women with dark hair and skin. In fact, increased skin pigmentation of pregnancy is much more prone to occur in those women with darker complexions. The darker skin color tends to fade after pregnancy but usually persists on the areolae and may persist in other areas.[2]

Melasma (Chloasma)

The so-called mask of pregnancy is also a very common side effect of the birth control pill. The pigmentation is most common on the upper lip but may occur on the cheeks, forehead, nose, chin, and mandibular area. A malar pattern may be seen.

The cause of melasma is poorly understood, but pregnant women should avoid heavy sunlight exposure to minimize the risk of developing this form of hyperpigmentation.

Jaundice

Physiologic alterations in hepatic function may result in various degrees of jaundice, particularly in the third trimester. Treatment for the jaundice of pregnancy is poor; this condition almost invariably disappears postpartum.

Vascular Changes

Vascular spiders are first noted between the second and fifth months and are present in 67% of white and 11% of black women by the third trimester.[8] They occur most commonly in skin areas drained by the superior vena cava (neck, throat, face, and arms). The spiders show a red central arteriolar puncta that may faintly pulsate. These lesions tend to increase in size throughout pregnancy. Most of the angiomas

TABLE 28-1. PHYSIOLOGIC CHANGES

Hyperpigmentation
Chloasma
Jaundice
Vascular changes
Striae distensae
Sweat gland activity
Edema
Pruritus
Hair and nail changes

disappear after pregnancy, but some faintly persist.

Palmar erythema, presumably due to increased estrogen levels, is a frequent finding, with onset in the first trimester.

Varicosities appear commonly on the legs. Hemorrhoidal varicosities can be very troublesome, causing pain and bleeding.

Vascular tumors, including hemangiomas, hemangioendotheliomas, and glomangiomas, may develop on the skin during gestation.

Cutis marmorata, a transitory bluish-red mottling of the skin over the legs, may occur with exposure to cold. It is due to vasomotor instability, which would also account for the pallor and facial flushing often seen in pregnancy.

Purpura on the legs is fairly common during the final trimester, probably due to increased capillary permeability and fragility.

Striae Distensae

This skin change, also called striae gravidarum, is seen in most pregnant women, particularly in whites, being less common in blacks and Asians. The lesion is characterized by pink to violaceous stripes on the skin of the abdomen, breasts, buttocks, thighs, and inguinal area.

Sweat Gland Activity

Eccrine sweating tends to increase during the latter part of pregnancy and may be associated with an increased incidence of miliaria (heat rash).

Apocrine sweating, which occurs chiefly in the axillae and groin area, tends to decrease during pregnancy.

Sebaceous Gland Activity

There is disagreement on this issue, but complaints of oily skin are common in pregnancy, and this would point to increased activity of the sebaceous glands.

Edema

Nonpitting edema of eyelids, face, ankles, and hands is a frequent association of late pregnancy. The edema tends to improve with daily activity (see Chapter 3).

Pruritus

Itching can cause considerable morbidity during pregnancy and can affect up to 20% of pregnant women. It tends to be particularly bad on the abdomen. Treatment is symptomatic.

Hair

Increased hair growth is seen in most women, particularly in those who are already somewhat hirsute. Luxuriant scalp hair is the norm in pregnancy, with very little fallout noted during the pregnancy. The hair follicles tend to remain in the anagen (growth) phase. Marked thinning of scalp hair with considerable fallout is common after delivery. These women require assurance that the loss of hair will be a temporary problem.

Nails

Changes seen in the nails include transverse grooving, brittleness, and a distal whitening of the nail due to separation from the nail bed (onycholysis).

Mucous Membranes

Gingivitis with gum hypertrophy is commonly seen in pregnancy and tends to clear afer delivery. The cause is not well understood.

SKIN DISEASES OF PREGNANCY

Several skin diseases are increased in incidence during pregnancy and seem to be unique to gestation and the puerperium. Table 28-2 lists these conditions. Most occur with very low frequency; some are even questionable but tend to be perpetuated in the literature. It is my feeling that some of these diseases overlap and that classification may be confusing rather than clarifying.

TABLE 28-2. SKIN DISEASES OF PREGNANCY

Herpes gestationis
Impetigo herpetiformis
Pruritic urticarial papules and plaques of pregnancy (PUPPP)
Papular dermatitis of pregnancy
Prurigo gestationis of Besnier
Toxemic rash of pregnancy
Autoimmune progesterone dermatitis of pregnancy

Herpes Gestationis

Herpes gestationis is a rare autoimmune disease estimated to occur in 1:3000 to 1:10,000 pregnancies.[3] It usually occurs in the second or third trimester and is characterized by severe itching, erythematous papules, plaques, vesicles, and bullae. Initially, the lesions tend to occur on the abdomen, but they rapidly spread to other body areas. When the blisters rupture, the denuded areas become crusted and secondary bacterial infection may occur. The disease may rarely begin or exacerbate in the postpartum period but usually subsides within 3 months of delivery. Herpes gestationis tends to recur in subsequent pregnancies with an earlier onset and a more severe course. It is not well established whether there is an associated increased incidence of fetal morbidity or mortality. Prematurity, stillbirth, and transient blisters in the newborn have been reported.

The blister is subepidermal; direct immunofluorescence shows a band-like deposit of C_3 and IgG at the basement membrane zone.[4] Other laboratory associations include leukocytosis and marked eosinophilia.

Systemic corticosteroids in moderate dosage will usually control the disease. With this therapeutic management there is only minimal fetal risk.

Impetigo Herpetiformis

Considerable controversy exists as to whether or not impetigo herpetiformis is a true dermatosis of pregnancy. The eruption resembles pustular psoriasis. Only about 100 cases have been reported; these women gave no previous history of psoriasis, nor was there a family history of the disease. Fetal mortality was high in reported cases. Most likely this represents pustular psoriasis that happened to develop during pregnancy rather than a true pregnancy-related skin disease.

Pruritic Urticarial Papules and Plaques of Pregnancy (PUPPP)

Holmes and Black propose that this diagnostic term be deleted from classification and, instead, suggest the name, polymorphic eruption of pregnancy.[3] They would also put late-onset prurigo of pregnancy, toxic erythema of pregnancy, and erythema multiforme of pregnancy under this broader classification.

The disease that we think of as PUPPP was first described in 1979 and a number of cases have been reported. Primigravidas constitute a high percentage of cases, the cause is unknown, and the onset is late in pregnancy, with an average time of onset being the 36th week of gestation.[9] The skin lesions start on the abdomen and consist of red papules and urticarial plaques. Prominent striae on the abdomen seem to be affected in this disease. Spread to the thighs, arms, and buttocks is seen in some cases. Itching is a constant finding and may be severe in some women. The disease is self-limited. Maternal and fetal complications do not occur.

There are no consistent abnormal laboratory features. Topical corticosteroids are effective in relieving the pruritus. If the itching is severe, brief tapering courses of systemic corticosteroids are indicated.

Papular Dermatitis of Pregnancy

Spangler et al. first described papular dermatitis of pregnancy in 1962.[6] Since that time, controversy has surrounded this disease because of the reported 27% fetal mortality. The incidence is estimated at 1 in 2400 pregnancies. Clinically, these patients have pruritic red papules on the trunk and extremities. The characteristic biochemical findings are increased urinary human chorionic gonadotropin, reduced plasma cortisol, and reduced urinary estriol. Certain aspects of this disease undoubtedly require reassessment, particularly the high fetal mortality and the overall incidence. Many dermatologists doubt the existence of this disease.

Prurigo Gestationis of Besnier

Prurigo gestationis of Besnier, manifested by pruritic papules occurring quite early in pregnancy, may also simply be called prurigo of pregnancy.[5] The condition is quite common, with an incidence of about 1 in 300 pregnancies. The rash may occur in women who have a tendency toward atopic dermatitis and are more prone to itching. The lesions tend to develop on the extremities but may also be seen on the trunk. Treatment is symptomatic. No maternal or fetal complications are anticipated.

Previously Classified Diseases

In this confusing and overly elaborate classification of skin disease, the following names are reported: toxemic rash of pregnancy, which has nothing to do with toxemia and is probably the same as PUPPP; prurigo annularis, which is probably a variant of prurigo gestationis; and autoimmune progesterone dermatitis of pregnancy, which most likely has no relationship to gestation. Only one case of the latter has been reported in pregnancy.

SKIN TUMORS INFLUENCED BY PREGNANCY

Several skin and mucous membrane tumors are associated with gestation. Some of these may first arise in pregnancy, some may enlarge, and others may increase in number. A red vascular tumor on the gums, granuloma gravidarum or pyogenic granuloma of pregnancy, is seen in 2% of pregnant women. It usually arises about midway through the pregnancy. The tumor recedes and disappears at term or shortly thereafter.

Skin tags on the neck, chest, axillae, and face may develop in some women. They are benign tumors and are often called fibroma gravidarum.

Other vascular tumors, including hemangiomas and gliangiomas, may develop.

Neurofibromas often increase in size and number.

Pigmented nevi usually darken and new nevi often develop. The incidence of malignant change in nevi is not increased; however, pregnancy may adversely affect the course and prognosis of malignant melanoma, particularly in women with Stage II disease. The course of melanoma without metastasis is probably not altered by pregnancy.

GENITAL INFECTIONS RELATING TO PREGNANCY

The usual gamut of sexually transmitted diseases may, of course, also develop during pregnancy. These include chlamydia, gonorrhea, chancroid, syphilis, mycoplasma, warts, molluscum contagiosum, granuloma inguinale, and herpes simplex.

Herpes simplex can cause severe problems in the newborn. The seriousness of neonatal herpes simplex cannot be overemphasized, since infant mortality and the incidence of severe neurologic disease are so high. Positive vaginal cultures or the presence of active genital lesions may mandate abdominal delivery of the infant (see Chapter 38).

Genital warts can attain giant size in pregnancy and may interfere with normal delivery. Treatment with podophyllin is contraindicated.

OTHER SKIN DISEASES INFLUENCED BY PREGNANCY

Lupus Erythematosus

Earlier reports indicate an adverse effect of pregnancy on the course of lupus erythematosus. More recent studies do not substantiate this. Although this issue is somewhat clouded in controversy, there is good evidence to support the fact that pregnancy, in itself, does not adversely affect the mother with lupus erythematosus. However, there is increased risk for the fetus, with a higher-than-normal incidence of stillbirth, spontaneous abortion, prematurity, growth retardation, and the development of lupus in the newborn; this last may be associated with congenital heart block.[1]

Scleroderma

Unless renal disease is present, pregnancy appears to have no adverse effect on patients with scleroderma. Preeclampsia and renal failure are serious complications that may develop in the last trimester. The renal status should be evaluated carefully in all pregnant women having scleroderma.

Dermatomyositis

This disease is rarely aggravated by pregnancy; however, fetal mortality is thought to be increased.

Psoriasis

There is no consistent effect of this disease; most women with psoriasis remain about the same. Some improve dramatically and others experience a flare-up of the psoriasis.

Neurofibromatosis

Pregnancy can be hazardous to women with this autosomal dominant disease. Severe hypertension may develop. There is a 50% chance of the child developing this disease. The new mutation rate in neurofibromatosis tends to be high.

Sarcoidosis

Sarcoidosis tends to improve during pregnancy.

Acne Vulgaris

Acne improves in most women during pregnancy, but this is highly unpredictable. Severe acne flares may occur.

Porphyria

Increased estrogen levels may exacerbate or bring on subsets of this disease, namely, porphyria cutanea tarda, acute intermittent porphyria, and hereditary coproporphyria.

Atopic Dermatitis

The effect of pregnancy on atopic dermatitis is completely unpredictable. Some women definitely improve, some flare, but most remain about the same.

Hidradenitis and Fox–Fordyce Disease

These apocrine gland disorders improve and often temporarily resolve during pregnancy.

REFERENCES

1. Barnett, E. V., Danovitch, G. M., Nissenson, A. R., Conolly, M. E., Lieb, S. M., and Barrett, C. T.: Systemic lupus erythematosus in pregnancy. *Ann. Intern. Med.* **94**:667–677, 1981.
2. Fitzpatrick, T. B., Eisen, A. Z., and Wolff, K.: *Dermatology in General Medicine.* New York, McGraw-Hill, 1979, pp. 1363–1370.
3. Holmes, R. C. and Black, M. M.: The specific dermatoses of pregnancy. *J. Am. Acad. Dermatol.* **8**:405–412, 1983.
4. Katz, S. I., Hertz, K. C., and Yaoita, H.: Herpes gestationis. Immunopathology and characterization of the HG factor. *J. Clin. Invest.* **57**:1434–1441, 1976.
5. Nurse, D. S.: Prurigo of pregnancy. *Australas. J. Dermatol.* **9**:258–267, 1968.
6. Spangler, A. S., Reddy, W., Bardawil, W. A., Roby, C. C., and Emerson, K.: Papular dermatitis of pregnancy. *JAMA* **181**:577–581, 1962.
7. Winton, G. B. and Lewis, C. W.: Dermatoses of pregnancy. *J. Am. Acad. Dermatol.* **6**:977–998, 1982.
8. Wong, R. C. and Ellis, C. N.: Physiologic skin changes in pregnancy. *J. Am. Acad. Dermatol.* **10**:929–940, 1984.
9. Yancey, K. B., Hall, R. P., and Lawley, T. J.: Pruritic urticarial papules and plaques of pregnancy. *J. Am. Acad. Dermatol.* **10**:473–480, 1984.

29

AUTOIMMUNE DISEASES IN PREGNANCY

The normal mammalian immune system aggressively resists invasion by any foreign substance, yet, during pregnancy, it tolerates the fetus, which is antigenically distinct (see Chapter 4). The microenvironment of the placenta is partially responsible for preventing immunologic attack on the fetus, but there is also compelling evidence for generalized down-regulation of the mother's immune system. Evidence for such a diffuse effect includes an increased incidence or severity of opportunistic infections during pregnancy, an alteration in the immunologic effects of pregnancy serum components or blood leukocytes, and an amelioration of disease activity with certain autoimmune processes during pregnancy.

The latter observation would be reason enough to examine more closely the relationship between autoimmune disease and pregnancy, but there is more. Autoimmune disorders affect women more commonly than they do men and tend to do so particularly during the childbearing years. Patients with these disorders may have a slightly decreased reproductive fitness, but the majority can conceive, particularly during times of reduced disease activity. Such pregnancies tend to exhibit a higher-than-normal risk of complications, so an understanding of the disorders is important to optimal prenatal and postpartum care.

The approach of this chapter will be the same for each of the major disorders listed. First there will be a brief introduction to each connective tissue disease followed by four sections of information: clinical presentation, influence of pregnancy on the disease, influence of the disease on pregnancy, and clinical management in pregnancy.

The purpose is not to cover in detail all the autoimmune diseases, but to present important features of those that affect females in the childbearing years. Each of the disorders presented is distinctive in one or more respects. Systemic lupus erythematosus tends to be exacerbated during pregnancy, whereas rheumatoid arthritis usually remits. In some situations, reassurance is all the treatment that is required for the autoimmune disease when it occurs during pregnancy. In others, an alteration in drug therapy may be necessary to protect the developing fetus from teratogenic effects. Rarely, early delivery of the fetus or even therapeutic abortion may be indicated to protect the mother from developing serious complications.

RHEUMATOID ARTHRITIS (RA)

Introduction

This autoimmune disorder is the one most commonly recognized for its tendency to improve during pregnancy. The improvement is so dramatic in some patients that they express the desire for permanent pregnancy. RA may occur at any age but most commonly begins in the third or fourth decades. It affects women three times more frequently than men. Convincing evidence indicates a genetic predisposition to this disease, since it tends to occur sporadically in families and is associated with certain histocompatibility antigens. Autoimmunity in this setting appears to be antibody-mediated, although an attenuation of cell-mediated immunity is also present. Since about 1% of the general population has rheumatoid arthritis, physicians who care for the medical problems of women see this disorder frequently.

Clinical Presentation

Rheumatoid arthritis is a painful, chronic, inflammatory arthritic disorder of synovial joints. It tends to involve the articulating structures on either side of the body in a symmetrical manner. The synovial lining of such joints, which is normally only one or two cells thick, undergoes a rampant, almost malignant proliferation. Such inflammatory panus can be very destructive. The articular cartilage becomes soft and friable. Tendons rupture, ligaments stretch, and the periarticular bone is eroded away. In addition to pain, patients contend with major functional disabilities such as weakness and joint deformity. They may be unable to turn a key in a lock, open a jar, or lift a child in their arms. In most patients, the disorder follows a pattern of remissions and exacerbations of disease activity, but in a small proportion, it develops an aggressive, unrelenting course. Even patients who undergo relatively permanent remissions continue to exhibit some residual disability in the previously affected joints where degenerative articular disease then occurs at an accelerated rate.

The American Rheumatism Association has developed criteria for the diagnosis of RA (Table 29-1). The criteria require typical symptoms to be present for more than six weeks. The joint swelling must be documented by a physician because some patients with nonarthritic disorders may report a sensation of joint swelling that cannot be documented objectively. Increased specificity of these criteria is obtained by a number of exclusions that eliminate other connective tissue diseases and joint space infections. Extensive reviews of the clinical and pathological features of RA are available.[24,46,60]

Patients with RA typically present with persistent fatigue, joint pain, and morning stiffness that tends to improve with the day's activities. Transient joint stiffness, referred to as gelling phenomenon, may occur at any time during the day following a period of rest. Early in the course of the disease, there may be very little apparent abnormality in the affected joints. Eventually characteristic soft tissue swelling is palpable at the proximal interphalangeal joints, the metacarpophalangeal joints, the wrists, elbows, knees, ankles, and metatarsophalangeal joints. Patients may complain of facial pain with chewing due to involvement of the temporomandibular joints and may experience sore throat due to cricoarytenoid involvement. Neck pain is also common because the facet joints of the spine are surrounded by synovial tissue. Even though the severe pain and morning stiffness may recede somewhat, the swelling of the affected joints usually persists throughout the day or even increases with use.

Unfortunately, the disease is not limited to the joints. Most patients with active disease have rheumatoid nodules at their elbows or even in the substance of visceral organs. Other potential systemic manifestations include anemia of chronic disease, inflammatory lung injury, and vasculitis.

About 70% of patients have a circulating IgM autoantibody called rheumatoid factor, which is specific for the Fc portion of self-IgG. Patients who have high titer rheumatoid factor tend to

TABLE 29-1. MODIFIED ARA CRITERIA FOR RHEUMATOID ARTHRITIS

A. Clinical	B. Laboratory
1. Morning stiffness	7. Typical radiographic changes
2. Pain in one joint	8. Positive rheumatoid factor
3. Swelling of one joint	9. Inflammatory synovial fluid
4. Swelling of another joint	10. Typical synovial histology
5. Symmetry of joint involvement	11. Typical nodule histology
6. Subcutaneous nodules	

"Definite RA" = five criteria for six weeks
"Probable RA" = three criteria for six weeks

Source: Adapted from the *Primer on the Rheumatic Diseases*, 8th Edition, pp. 207–208 copyright 1983. Used by permission of the Arthritis Foundation.

have more severe joint disease and a greater frequency of extra-articular manifestations.

In active rheumatoid arthritis, an analysis of joint fluid indicates inflammation if 2000–100,000 white cells/mm^3, including 50–75% neutrophils, are present (Tables 29-2 and 29-3). Not infrequently, patients with active disease develop inflammatory pleural or pericardial effusions that are characterized by a very low glucose concentration relative to that in the serum.

The etiology of rheumatoid arthritis is unknown. It has been speculated that an infectious agent initiates an inflammatory response that is then perpetuated in susceptible individuals. There seems to be a clear familial tendency. Sporadic cases occur throughout a family tree at a frequency greater than expected by chance. In addition, there is a well-documented association of rheumatoid arthritis with the histocompatibility antigens HLAD4 and HLADR4. On the other hand, disease concordance among identical twins is low.

Immunologically, RA appears to be an autoimmune articular disease that, in some patients, spills out into other organ systems for reasons that are unclear. A polyclonal B cell activation results in production of rheumatoid factor and other immunoglobulins so patients tend to be hypergammaglobulinemic. Cell-mediated immune responses by peripheral blood leukocytes are generally lower than normal, perhaps as a result of the massive infiltrative diversion of mononuclear leukocytes into the synovial pannus.

In nonpregnant patients, therapy of rheumatoid arthritis is aimed at controlling pain, inhibiting the inflammatory process, and restoring as much of the lost function as possible. In the early stages of disease, a "basic program" of education, rest, physical therapy, and aspirin is usually initiated. These measures are adequate for some patients, but others need more aggressive therapy. The so-called "remittive agents" used to inhibit the underlying inflammatory process include hydrochloroquine, gold salts, penicillamine, methotrexate, and immunosuppressive drugs such as azathioprine or cyclophosphamide. A typical therapeutic sequence begins with hydroxychloroquine to which an oral or parenteral gold salt may later be added. If that regimen fails to control disease activity

TABLE 29-2. EXAMINATION OF SYNOVIAL FLUID

Test	Normal	Non-inflammatory (Group I)	Inflammatory (Group II)	Septic (Group III)
Color	Colorless	Yellow	Yellow	Gray-green
Clarity	Clear	Clear	Turbid	Opaque
String Sign	>2 cm	>2 cm	<2 cm	<2 cm
WBC (per mm^3)	<200	200–2,000	2,000–100,000	>50,000
PMN (%)	<25%	<25%	>50%	>75%
Glucose (mg/IOO ml)	Nearly equal to blood	Nearly equal to blood	Some lower than blood	Much lower than blood
Gram stain and culture	Negative	Negative	Negative	Often positive

Source: Adapted from the *Primer on the Rheumatic Diseases*, 8th Edition, p. 187 copyright 1983. Used by permission of the Arthritis Foundation.

TABLE 29-3. DISORDERS WITH ABNORMAL SYNOVIAL FLUID FINDINGS

Synovial fluid	Disorders
Noninflammatory	Degenerative joint disease, trauma, neuropathic arthropathy.
Inflammatory	Rheumatoid arthritis, acute gout, acute pseudogout, ankylosing spondylitis, Reiter's syndrome, psoriatic arthritis, arthritis of inflammatory bowel disease, acute rheumatic fever, systemic lupus, scleroderma
Septic	Bacterial infections, mycobacterial infections, some fungal infections
Hemorrhagic	Hemophilia, trauma, neuropathic arthropathy, pigmented villonodular synovitis, intra-articular neoplasm

Source: Adapted from the *Primer on the Rheumatic Diseases*, 8th Edition, p. 187 copyright 1983. Used by permission of the Arthritis Foundation.

after a 6–12 month trial, the gold and hydroxychloroquine might be discontinued and penicillamine or methotrexate substituted. During the administration of "remittive therapy," the basic program would be continued, with the occasional exception that another nonsteroidal anti-inflammatory drug may take the place of aspirin, if aspirin intolerance occurs. The major problem with most of the "remittive" agents is that their degree of effectiveness seems to be directly proportional to the severity of their potential toxicities. A partial summary of the adverse effects associated with each of these drugs is shown in Table 29-4.

Occasionally, local injection of corticosteroids into a joint space is necessary to provide relief from pain and stiffness in that joint for a month or more until "remittive measures" take effect. Local injection of corticosteroids carries a relatively low risk of hazard when careful aseptic technique is used. Rarely, a patient with RA requires low-dose oral corticosteroid therapy to maintain control of extra-articular symptoms.

Influence of Pregnancy on Rheumatoid Disease Activity

In 1938, Hench reported observations of 37 pregnancies in 22 women with active RA.[20] He described a marked improvement of the disease that clearly corresponded with the pregnant state. More recently, Persellin reviewed 296 pregnancies in women with RA. Seventy-four percent of patients experienced some degree of improvement during gestation.[37] Patients who improved reported a gradual reduction in swelling, stiffness, and joint pain accompanied by a generalized feeling of well-being that was a welcome relief from their previous symptoms. The majority of patients improved in the first trimester. A progressively smaller number noted a reduction in symptoms during the second or third trimesters (Fig. 29-1). By the time of delivery, more than 74% of patients were much improved (Fig. 29-2). In contrast, the most aggressive of chemotherapeutic programs can claim only about a 60% response rate.

Unfortunately, all the patients' symptoms returned within one to two months postpartum (Fig. 29-3). Oka[39] studied a smaller number of pregnant rheumatoid patients and obtained similar results. In the postpartum period, disease activity may return to its prepregnant level or may progress even more rapidly than before. Subsequent pregnancies in a single individual tend to follow the same pattern.

Paradoxically, a small number of patients experience worsening of their rheumatoid arthritis symptoms during pregnancy and others experience the initial symptoms of the disease during pregnancy or shortly after parturition (Fig. 29-1). Some authorities therefore view pregnancy as an exacerbating factor [16,39]

One potential explanation for the fact that some patients improve during pregnancy and others do not follows from an improved understanding of the disease and of its distribution in the population. A study of seronegative RA revealed that patients with rheumatoid factor in their serum (seropositive) were clinically and genetically different from the smaller number of patients who were seronegative. The frequency of HLADR4 in the seropositive patients was significantly greater than in a group of control subjects, whereas its frequency in the seronegative rheumatoids was not. In the seronegative rheumatoid population, however, patients who did exhibit HLADR4 had more severe disease than did seronegative patients without DR4. The frequency of seropositive disease (72%) in the study almost exactly parallels the frequency of disease remission during pregnancy, but it is not known whether there is any relationship between the two observations.[2]

Another investigation prospectively studied the course of 10 patients with RA and 13 patients with ankylosing spondylitis throughout pregnancy. Controls included 15 patients with ankylosing spondylitis who did not become pregnant and 31 normal, healthy pregnant individuals. Nine of the 10 rheumatoid arthritis patients improved symptomatically during pregnancy but suffered exacerbations in the postpartum period. In contrast, eight of the ankylosing spondylitis patients were worse during pregnancy and experienced relief postpartum. The nonpregnant spondylitics experienced a gradually progressive increase in their symptoms over the same period of time.[41] This study implies a dissimilarity in outcome of various connective tissue diseases during pregnancy and indicates that the previous retrospective studies were not significantly distorted by their design.

Another study compared a group of RA patients who had become pregnant with a control group of rheumatoid patients who were never pregnant but were matched for age and severity of disease. The study asked whether the brief hiatus in symptoms experienced by most pregnant rheumatoid patients had any effect on the

TABLE 29-4. POTENTIAL PREGNANCY-RELATED RISKS OF DRUGS USED TO TREAT PATIENTS WITH RHEUMATIC DISEASES

Class	Drug	*n**	Relative Risk†	Crosses Placenta	Secreted into Breast Milk	Type of Risk‡	Reference
Analgesics	Acetaminophen	>50,000	Low	+	+	B- Hemolytic anemia	
						F- Fetal liver damage	8,19
						F- Congenital hip dislocation	
	Propoxyphene	>600	Moderate	+	+	F- Clubfoot	
						B- Shortened first-stage labor	
						F- Microcephaly, patent ductus, cataract	8,19
						F- Benign tumors, clubfoot	
						F- Hypospadias	
						F- Withdrawal syndrome	
	Codeine	>50,000	Moderate (High if abused)	+	+	F- Respiratory depression	8
						F- Narcotic addiction	
						F- Genitourinary abnormalities	
						F- Tumors	
						F- Umbilical and inguinal hernias	
						F- Hydrocephalus	
						F- Pyloric stenosis	
NSAID	Aspirin	>54,000	Moderate (High in T-3)	+	+	M- Vaginal hemorrhage	8,19
						F- Intracranial hemorrhage	8,55
						B- Prolonged Labor	
						B- Complicated deliveries	
						F- Growth retardation	
						F- Fetal mortality	
						F- Premature closure DA	
						F- Decreases factor XII	
						B- Salicylism	
						B- Platelet dysfunction	
						F- Hypospadias	
	Fenoprofen	NA	Low (High in T-3)	–	±	B- Prolonged labor	
						F- Premature closure DA	
						F- Pulmonary hypertension	
	Ibuprofen	NA	Low (High in T-3)	NA	±	B- Prolonged labor	
						F- Premature closure DA	
						F- Pulmonary hypertension	
						F- Anencephaly one case	
	Indomethacin	>100	High	+	+	F- Phocomelia	8,38
						F- Agenesis of penis	55
						F- Premature closure DA	
						F- Prolonged labor	
						F- Oligohydramnion	
						F- Meconium staining	
						F- Hemorrhage	
	Meclofenamate	NA	Low (High in T-3)	NA	NA	B- Prolonged labor	8
						F- Premature closure DA	
						F- Pulmonary hypertension	

TABLE 29-4. Continued

Class	Drug	n*	Relative Risk†	Crosses Placenta	Secreted into Breast Milk	Type of Risk‡	Reference
	Naproxen	NA	Low (High in T-3)	+	±	B- Prolonged labor F- Premature closure DA F- Pulmonary hypertension F- Hyperbilirubinemia F- Impaired renal function F- Increased clotting times F- Intracranial hemorrhage	
	Sulindac	NA	Low (High in T-3)	NA	NA	B- Prolonged labor F- Premature closure DA	
	Tolmetin	NA	Low (High in T-3)	NA	NA	B- Prolonged labor F- Premature closure DA F- Pulmonary hypertension	8
	Colchicine	NA	NA	NA	NA	M- Chromosomal abnormalities F- Atypical Down's syndrome F- Azoospermia	8
Xanthene oxidase inhibitor	Allopurinol	NA	NA	NA	NA	None known	55
Immuno-suppressives	Azathioprine	NA	High	+	NA	B- Immunosuppression, lymphopenia F- Pulmonary valvular stenosis F- Preaxial polydactyly F- Transient chromosomal aberrations M- Interference with intra-uterine contraception F- Renal insufficiency F- Decreased IgA levels	8,38
	Chlorambucil	NA	High	±	NA	F- Unilateral renal and urethral agenesis M- Amenorrhea, azoospermia	
	Cyclophosphamide	NA	High	NA	+	B- Pancytopenia F- Low birth weight M- Amenorrhea and azoospermia M- Chromosomal abnormalities	8,55
	Penicillamine	>89	High	NA	N	F- Hypotonia F- Hyperflexion F- Pyloric stenosis F- Impaired wound healing F- Ventricular septal defect, simian crease F- Vein fragility B- Systemic lupus, myositis	

	Methotrexate	>15	High	±	±	M- Gonadal dysfunction F- Oxycephaly F- Low-set ears F- Hypertelorism F- Dextrocardia F- Absence of toes F- Growth retardation F- Anomalous ribs F- Webbed fingers M- Pancytopenia	8
Antimalarials	Chloroquine	NA	High	NA	–	F- Vestibular anomalies F- Neurologic and ophthalmic toxicity	8
Gold salts	Gold thiomalate	NA	High	+	NA	None	8,19
Cortico-steroids	Betamethasone	NA	Moderate	NA	NA	F- Hypoglycemia F- Death in preeclampsia F- Transient leukocytosis	8,55
	Cortisone	>50,000	High	NA	NA	F- Cataracts F- Cyclopia F- Intra-atrial septal defect F- Gastroschisis F- Hydrocephalus F- Cleft lip F- Coarctation aorta F- Clubfoot F- Undescended testicles F- Neonatal adrenal insufficiency	8,19
	Prednisone	NA	Low	NA	+	F- Stillbirths B- Immunosuppression F- Defective spermatogenesis F- Cataracts B- Smaller placentas	8,55
Uricosurics	Probenecid	NA	Low	NA	NA	None	8
Histamine antagonists	Cometidine	NA	Low	+	+	F- Transient liver impairment	8,38
Sedatives	Diazepam	>1800	High	+	+	F- Cleft lip or palate F- Inguinal hernia F- Cardiac defect F- Pyloric stenosis F- Hemangiomas F- Circulatory defects F- Absence of thumbs F- Spina bifida F- Absence of left forearm F- Floppy infant syndrome F- Withdrawal	8,38
Antidepressants	Imipramine	>500,000	High	NA	+	F- Altered thermogenesis F- Bilateral amelia F- Defective abdominal muscles	8

TABLE 29-4. POTENTIAL PREGNANCY-RELATED RISKS OF DRUGS USED TO TREAT PATIENTS WITH RHEUMATIC DISEASES

Class	Drug	*n**	Relative Risk†	Crosses Placenta	Secreted into Breast Milk	Type of Risk‡	Reference
Diuretics	Thiazide	NA	High	NA	NA	F- Diaphragmatic hernia F- Exencephaly F- Cleft palate F- Adrenal hypoplasia F- Renal cystic degeneration F- Withdrawal syndrome F- Urinary retention B- Electrolyte imbalance M- Hyperglycemia F- Hypoglycemia M- Hyperuricemia M- Pancreatitis F- Death 2° electrolyte imbalance in mother F- Decreased birth weight F- Hyponatremia F- Hyperbilirubinemia F- Bone marrow suppression F- Thrombocytopenia	55
	Furosemide	NA	Moderate	NA	NA	F- Hyponatremia F- Hyperuricemia	55
Antihypertensives	Captopril	NA	Moderate	+	+	F- Absent limb F- Absence of skull M- Proteinuria M- Leukopenia	8
	Prazosin	NA	Moderate	NA	NA	NA	8
	Propranolol	NA	Moderate	–	–	F- Growth retardation F- Hypoglycemia F- Bradycardia F- Respiratory distress F- Small placenta	38

* *n* = Estimated number of pregnancies in which drug has been administered.
NA = Data not available.
DA = Ductus arteriosus.
T-3 = Third trimester of pregnancy.
† Relative risk scale:
Very low—Controlled studies demonstrate no apparent risk.
Low—There is a remote but potentially real risk.
Moderate—Animal studies indicate a risk, but no controlled studies to define it better for humans.
High—Known risk that precludes use of drug in pregnancy except in life-threatening maternal disease.
Very High—Known risk of fetal injury that outweighs any possible benefit in the mother.
‡ Individuals at risk of adverse effect coded as F = Fetus, M = Mother, B = Both mother and fetus.

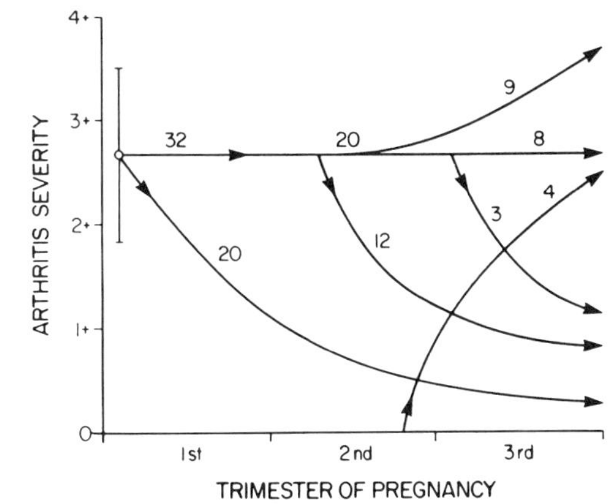

Figure 29-1. The effect of pregnancy on rheumatoid arthritis disease activity. Arrows going away from the baseline identify the numbers of pregnant patients who experienced a change in disease activity. Deviation from above the horizontal indicates worsening; deviation from below the horizontal indicates improvement. See text for details. Reprinted from Neely, N. T., and Persellin, R. H.: Activity of Rheumatoid Arthritis during Pregnancy. Tex. Med. 73:59–63, 1977.

long-term prognosis of rheumatoid arthritis. Despite good clinical remissions during pregnancy and fairly large numbers of subjects in each group, there were no significant differences between groups after 10 years of follow-up.[40]

The mechanism by which pregnancy temporarily ameliorates rheumatoid arthritis is not known. The immunologic changes that accompany normal pregnancy are detailed in Chapter 4. It is not known whether any of those mecha-

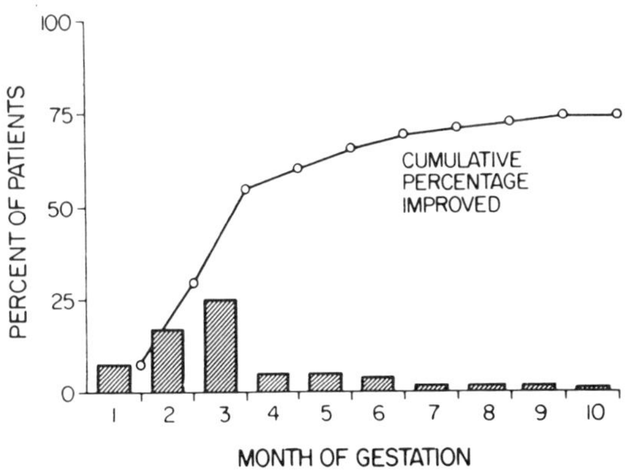

Figure 29-2. Onset of symptomatic improvement in rheumatoid arthritis disease activity during 296 pregnancies. Reprinted from Neely, N. T., and Persellin, R. H.: Activity of Rheumatoid Arthritis during Pregnancy. Tex. Med. 73:59–63, 1977.

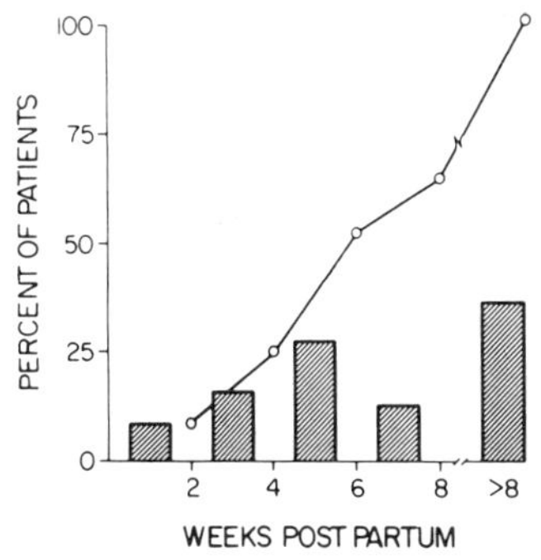

Figure 29-3. Exacerbations of disease activity occurring in the weeks after delivery among rheumatoid arthritis patients who experienced a remission during pregnancy. Reprinted from Neely, N. T., and Persellin, R. H.: Activity of Rheumatoid Arthritis during Pregnancy. Tex. Med. 73:59–63, 1977.

nisms alone or in combination adequately explain the observed improvement. Unger et al.[58] studied 14 RA patients prospectively through a pregnancy in which 10 improved or remained unchanged and 4 worsened. They also measured the serum levels of pregnancy-associated alpha-2-glycoprotein (PAG), which exhibits immunoinhibitory activity in vitro. The average PAG level among the group that improved (1250 ± 730 mg/liter) was significantly higher than that of the group that did not improve (470 ± 304 mg/liter). When the data from all patients were combined, a significant negative correlation between rheumatoid disease activity and serum PAG concentration was noted, suggesting that PAG may be responsible for the observed change. Although that conclusion is a logical one, the concentrations of many other serum factors are increased during pregnancy and would need to be examined in comparable manner.

It has been argued that immunoglobulin G (IgG) with specificity for the paternal alloantigens binds to the placenta and is responsible for the improvement in disease activity during pregnancy. To test that hypothesis, a weakly acidic buffer was used to elute polyclonal immunoglobulin from large numbers of normal placentas. After extensive purification, the IgG preparation was administered parenterally to patients with resultant benefit.[49] It is not known whether parenteral administration of other pregnancy-associated serum components would also result in amelioration of disease activity.

Immune complexes decrease substantially in rheumatoid arthritis patients during pregnancy,[43] but it is not clear whether the decrease results from an increased clearance by the reticuloendothelial system,[47] from a decreased production of antibodies, or from some other mechanism. The rheumatoid factor titer also decreases in an occasional patient, but, in most patients, it does not change, even though the immune complex level falls.

It has been argued pro and con that changes in the steroid hormone levels during pregnancy may be responsible for some of its ameliorating effects. Indeed, clinically apparent improvement in rheumatoid symptoms has been demonstrated during each post-ovulatory phase of the normal menstrual cycle.[30]

Influence of Rheumatoid Arthritis on Pregnancy

One might expect RA patients to have slightly decreased reproductive performance because of their inflammatory disease activity and the disability it imposes on them. There are very little data to support that conclusion, however, except for a preliminary report that indicated lower fertility in rheumatoid women, even antedating the onset of RA symptoms.[29] It is understandable that an RA patient who experiences articular pain with even the slightest movement of affected joints might have difficulty with the physical aspects of sexual intercourse. On the other hand, some patients who achieve orgasm on a regular basis experience temporary relief from their joint symptoms. An even more difficult problem than pain for some rheumatoids is limited motion of the hips. Not infrequently, that has become the last straw in dissolution of marriages already strained by the patient's inability to do her share of the family work. Loving couples who show a willingness to adapt to their circumstances can usually find coital positions suitable to them (Fig. 29-4).

A tendency toward small-for-dates babies has been noted in pregnancies complicated by RA.[9,35] Rarely, the offspring of RA patients exhibit congenital heart block.[34] In general, the disease itself has very little effect on fetal outcome, but that cannot be said for the drugs used in the treatment of nonpregnant rheumatoids.

Aspirin and the other nonsteroidal anti-inflammatory drugs portend significant risk to fetus and mother, particularly during the third trimester when their capacity to inhibit prostaglandin synthesis may interfere with timely labor and delivery (Table 29-4). Prostaglandin synthetase inhibitors can cause premature closure of the fetal ductus arteriosus with resultant chronic pulmonary hypertension. Aspirin has probably been used more than any of the other nonsteroidal drugs during pregnancy and is relatively free of adverse effects, especially when it is not used during the third trimester. Administration of aspirin in the last trimester of pregnancy places the mother at risk of postpartum hemorrhage and the infant at risk for intracranial hemorrhage at delivery because of irreversible inactivation by aspirin of prostaglandin synthetase in platelets.

Among the "remittive" drugs, azathioprine is probably the safest.[51] It has been used in pregnant lupus patients to control disease activity without apparent untoward effects. Normal outcomes have also occurred in a few pregnancies despite continued therapy with gold thiomalate, but its use is not recommended.[6] Gold crosses the placenta and circulates in the fetal blood stream. There is, at present, insufficient experience to confirm its safety, even though no teratogenic effects have been demonstrated in humans.

Penicillamine has been given to approximately 90 pregnant women. Abnormalities noted in the fetuses include hypotonia, hyperreflexia, pyloric stenosis, ventricular septal defect, venous fragility, and congenital connective tissue disease manifestations. It is not recommended in pregnancy. A number of major fetal growth and developmental defects have been seen when methotrexate therapy is continued during pregnancy, so it should not be administered during pregnancy or lactation. Cyclophosphamide has the potential of producing pancytopenia and causes low birth weights. The amenorrhea and azoospermia associated with cyclophosphamide may be permanent or temporary. The determining factor in different individuals is not clear.

Hydroxychloroquine treatment in pregnancy is thought to be responsible for causing vestibular, neurologic, and ophthalmic abnormalities in a number of infants. Corticosteroids cause cleft palate in experimental animals but appear to be safe in human pregnancy, especially when prednisone is used in levels lower than 30 mg/day. Although there is a paucity of data, corticosteroids appear to cross the placenta and to be secreted in breast milk, so evidence of Cushing's syndrome must be searched for in the infant.

Management of Rheumatoid Arthritis During Pregnancy

It is not yet entirely clear what genetic counsel should be given to patients with RA. RA can present in the offspring of rheumatoid patients, but no consistent hereditary pattern has been defined. Therefore, patients have been advised not to modify their family plans for fear of giving the disease to their children. With continued immunogenetic studies, however, it has become clear that HLADR4 is somehow related to the incidence of seropositive disease and to the severity of seronegative disease. The prevalence of RA in first-degree relatives is increased threefold if the index cases have erosive RA. The frequency of active RA is increased in the twins of affected individuals.[52] The pattern of inheritance remains unclear, perhaps because it is polygenic or subject to reduced penetrance.

Female patients who wish to conceive should do so when their disease is sufficiently well controlled that medications with known teratogenic effects can be discontinued in advance without hazard of precipitating an exacerbation of the arthritis. It seems appropriate to utilize aspirin, fenoprofen, ibuprofen, meclofenamate, sulindac, tolmetin, or even low-dose corticosteroids as needed during the first and second trimesters of pregnancy. Gold, penicillamine, plaquenil and the immunosuppressive drugs should be discontinued a month or two in advance of conception to reduce the risk of fetal abnormalities. It is to be anticipated that most patients will experience a remission of their symptoms by the end of the second trimester and will no longer need drug therapy. Nonsteroidal anti-inflammatory drugs should be discontinued some weeks prior to parturition because of their potential effects on hemostasis, duration of labor, and closure of the ductus arteriosus.

The basic program of clinical management for RA patients, which includes rest, physical therapy, and education, should be continued with only minor modifications during pregnancy. Rheumatoid patients may need more rest than normal gravid females, but, on the other hand, if their disease remits during preg-

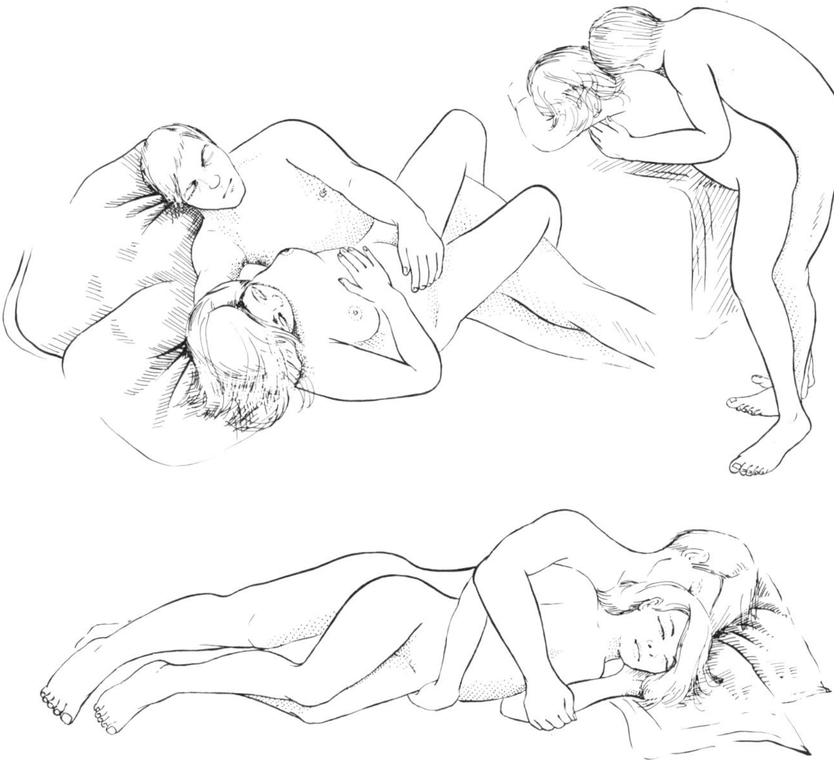

Figure 29-4. Coital positions for rheumatoid arthritis patients with limited hip abduction. Patients are advised to first find a position that is comfortable and then adapt it to sexual activity. (Adapted from *Toward Intimacy: Family Planning and Sexuality Concerns of Physically Disabled Women.* Task Force on Concerns of Physically Disabled Women, New York, Human Sciences Press.)

nancy, they may tolerate considerably more activity than they did before pregnancy. The remission induced by pregnancy may provide an ideal opportunity for patients to use more aggressive physical therapy to regain lost motion in previously affected joints. Patients who have already been disabled by their disease to the extent that they cannot easily tie their shoes or perform other self-help activities may have even greater difficulty during pregnancy as a result of the expanding uterus. Such patients may benefit from consultation with a physiatrist, occupational therapist, or physical therapist to obtain mechanical aids for such tasks.

Women who require analgesia during the last trimester of pregnancy may be given acetaminophen in moderate doses or corticosteroids in low doses without much risk. If corticosteroids are used during pregnancy, a "steroid prep" should probably be given during labor to help manage the stress of delivery. The infant should be observed closely for signs of adrenal insufficiency. If patients with aggressive RA were taking "remittive" drug therapy prior to conception, it seems reasonable to avoid breast-feeding and to reinitiate the previous therapy immediately after delivery to avoid an uncontrolled exacerbation of disease. However, there are no studies to document the effectiveness of such an approach.

Delivery itself need not be altered for most RA patients, but obstetricians should be aware of two potentially complicated situations. Patients who have severe limitation of hip motion may experience great discomfort associated with the procedures and mechanics of vaginal delivery. For such patients, delivery in the lateral position or cesarean section may be the wisest course. Patients who require intubation for general anesthesia may be at risk for cervical cord injury due to C1-2 subluxation. Therefore, all patients with moderately severe RA should have flexion and extension views of the cervical spine performed early in the course of pregnancy and consultation should be sought with an anesthesiologist experienced in protecting the cervical cord.

SYSTEMIC LUPUS ERYTHEMATOSUS (SLE)

Introduction

SLE is a chronic, inflammatory, autoimmune disorder of unknown etiology. Although it may begin at any age, the majority of affected individuals experience their first symptoms during young adulthood. Women are affected nearly nine times more frequently than men. Estimates of its incidence vary with the population studied. In Caucasians, it affects about 5 individuals per 100,000, but, among black females, the annual incidence may be as high as 1 in 500. In general, pregnancy has no long-term effect on the prognosis of the disease, but exacerbations are more common than remissions, particularly in the postpartum period.

Autoimmune injury in lupus is humorally mediated, whereas cell-mediated immunity is decreased. Evidence suggests a variably penetrant familial pattern of inheritance with HLA association. A possible infectious agent is suspected but unproved. Perhaps the most important recent finding is that infants born to lupus patients are at increased risk for congenital heart abnormalities, in addition to transient lupus-like symptoms. Since obstetricians and gynecologists are often the primary care physicians for young women, it is important that they be aware of the manifestations of systemic lupus and the effects of pregnancy on the course of this disorder.

Clinical Presentation

There is such wide variability in the initial symptoms of SLE patients that some specialists believe the term encompasses a whole family of disorders.[44,48,59] The most common symptoms include arthralgias or arthritis, fever, fatigue, weight loss, and rash. Joint pain may be associated with true arthritis, but the number of inflammatory cells in the synovial fluid tends to be lower than seen in association with RA. The joints may develop reducible subluxations due to laxity of the periarticular ligaments, but true erosion of bone is uncommon. Fever is usually low-grade but may be as high as 105 °F. Active lupus must be distinguished from infection because lupus patients are predisposed by their disease and its treatment to recurrent infections. The typical erythematous rash of lupus extends over the nose and cheeks, but may expand to involve wide areas of the body. Lupus patients are very sensitive to sun exposure, which has the potential of exacerbating systemic disease with resultant arthritis and fever.

An American Rheumatism Association committee has developed a set of 11 clinical signs that help to distinguish this disorder from the other connective tissue diseases[56] (Table 29-5).

TABLE 29-5. REVISED ARA CRITERIA FOR SYSTEMIC LUPUS ERYTHEMATOSUS

A. Clinical	B. Laboratory
1. Facial erythema (butterfly rash)	8. Antinuclear antibody
2. Discoid lupus rash	9. LE cells, anti-DNA, anti-Sm or chronic false positive test for syphilis
3. Photosensitivity	10. Hemolytic anemia, leukopenia, lymphopenia, thrombocytopenia
4. Oral or nasopharyngeal ulcers	11. Proteinuria (>3.5 g/24 h) and/or cellular casts in the urine
5. Arthritis without deformity	
6. Pleuritis, pericarditis	
7. Psychosis or convulsions	

SLE is confirmed for research study purposes, if four or more criteria are met.

Source: Adapted from the *Primer on the Rheumatic Diseases*, 8th Edition, 1983, p. 211 copyright 1983. Used by permission of the Arthritis Foundation.

Only four of these criteria must be present to support the diagnosis with reasonable certainty. Lupus characteristically follows a course of remissions and exacerbations. The overall prognosis depends on the type of organ involvement.

The more serious manifestations include glomerulonephritis in about 50%, central nervous system involvement in at least 30%, disseminated infections, and complications of chemotherapy. Patients must be carefully evaluated for hemolytic anemia, leukocytopenia, thrombocytopenia, and blood clotting abnormalities as with the lupus anticoagulant. Pericarditis and pleurisy are benign in most patients, but can cause respiratory insufficiency or circulatory compromise due to large pleural effusions or to constrictive pericarditis. Diffuse vasculitis is sometimes responsible for bowel ischemia or myocardial infarction.

The antinuclear antibody test is positive in almost all lupus patients but is not specific for lupus. The patterns of nuclear fluorescence most frequently seen with lupus are the rim pattern, due to antibody to native DNA, the homogeneous pattern associated with antibody to DNA protein, and occasionally a speckled pattern (Table 29-6). The speckled immunofluorescence pattern of lupus results, in part, from antibody to a nuclear antigen (Sm, after a patient named Smith) that is extractable with aqueous buffers. The Sm antigen, present in about 30% of patients, is not digested by ribonuclease as is RNP, the extractable nuclear antigen associated with mixed connective tissue disease syndrome (MCTD). When lupus is active, increased levels of immune complexes may be found in serum. As a result, complement levels are usually depressed during active disease. The circulating levels of IgG anti-DNA antibody appear to parallel the severity of the renal disease in lupus. Anti-DNA antibody levels thus have prognostic value and can assist in directing appropriate therapy.

The cause of lupus is not known, but very basic immunologic abnormalities have been recognized. Patients usually exhibit polyclonal B cell activation. Among the autoantibodies produced by lupus patients are those directed against red cells, platelets, and suppressor T cells. The resultant decrease in suppressor T cells may be partially responsible for the increased immunoglobulin levels. As noted above,

TABLE 29-6. ANTIBODIES TO NUCLEAR ANTIGENS

Immunofluorescent Pattern	Nuclear Antigen Specificity	Primary Clinical Disorder
Homogeneous nuclear staining	DNA-protein	Systemic lupus Drug-induced lupus
Nuclear rim staining	DNA	Systemic lupus
Speckled nuclear staining	*Buffer extractable	SLE, MCTD, Sjögren's
Nucleolar staining	Unknown	Scleroderma

* Sm antigen—SLE; Mixed connective tissue disease—MCTD; SS_B—SLE and Sjögren's.

cell-mediated immunity is attenuated. It is not yet clear whether the decreased numbers or function of suppressor T cells is the primary defect or the result of circulating antilymphocyte antibody. Genetic studies have indicated an association between lupus and histocompatibility antigens DR2 and DR3.

In nonpregnant patients, most manifestations of lupus such as rash, arthralgias, and fever are usually treated conservatively. Avoidance of sun exposure, use of sun screens, increased rest, avoidance of fatigue, and use of aspirin are usually helpful. The antimalarial hydroxychloroquine has proven useful for controlling the cutaneous manifestations in nonpregnant patients but is considered unsafe in pregnancy. The indications for use of corticosteroids have been clearly defined to include management of proliferative glomerulonephritis, central nervous system involvement, cytopenias, vasculitis, severe serositis, and myopathic disease. When aggressive organ involvement is present, immunosuppressive drugs are usually added to the therapeutic regimen because of their ability to augment the effect of steroids and thus to spare steroid dosage even though risks of substantial toxicity are attendant with use of immunosuppressive drugs. Plasmaphoresis should theoretically be helpful in active disease because of its ability to filter out immune complexes, but opinion regarding its value is mixed.

Drug-induced (Table 29-7) lupus is similar to the spontaneous disease but differs in two respects. It tends more frequently to affect the lung, whereas serious renal disease is less common. In most cases, resolution of clinical symptoms occurs within one to two weeks after discontinuing the offending drug, but the ANA may remain positive for years.

Influence of Pregnancy on Disease Activity

As recently as 10–15 years ago, available data suggested that pregnancy was likely to cause major exacerbations of systemic lupus and to affect adversely the mother's ultimate prognosis, but it now seems that is not the case. Several recent reviews[1,11,15,23,26,53,57,61,66] indicate that long-term maternal outcome is not altered, particularly if pregnancy occurs during a time of clinical disease inactivity. A recent review reported the frequency of adverse effects from pregnancy in women with lupus noted during a 30-year period from 1950 through 1979[11] (Table 29-8). For each of the three decades reported, lupus patients averaged one exacerbation for

TABLE 29-7. DRUGS SUSPECTED OF INDUCING AN LE-LIKE SYNDROME

Antiarrhythmic	Antihypertensive
Practolol	Guanoxan
Procainamide	Hydralazine
	Methyldopa
Antibacterial or antifungal	Reserpine
Griseofulvin	Minoxidil
Isoniazid	
Penicillin	Antithyroid
Sodium aminosalicylate ("PAS")	Methylthiouracil
Streptomycin	Propylthiouracil
Sulfonamides	
Tetracycline	Miscellaneous
	Chlorpromazine
Anticonvulsant	D-penicillamine
Carbamazepine	Methylsergide
Ethosuximide	Oral contraceptives
Mephenytoin	Phenylbutazone
Pheneturide	
Phenytoin	
Primidone	
Troxidone	

Source: Adapted from Hughes, G. R. V., Systemic lupus erythematosus. In:. *Copeman's Textbook of the Rheumatic Diseases*, 5th Edition. J. T. Scott (Ed.). Edinburgh, Churchill Livingston, 1978, p. 910.

TABLE 29-8. EFFECTS OF PREGNANCY ON SLE MORBIDITY AND MORTALITY *

Period	Pregnancies	Exacerbations†	Remissions†	Maternal Deaths†
1950–1959	139	84 (0.6)	48 (0.3)	24 (0.17)
1960–1969	272	142 (0.5)	61 (0.2)	21 (0.08)
1970–1979	277	134 (0.5)	23 (0.08)	3 (0.01)

* Adapted from Cecere, F. A. and Persellin, R. H.: The interaction of pregnancy and the rheumatic diseases. Clin. Rheum. Dis. 7:747–768, 1981.
† Values in parentheses represent mean frequency per pregnancy.

every two pregnancies. The frequency of remissions appeared to decrease slightly by decade. The most dramatic change was seen in the frequency of maternal deaths, which dropped from approximately 17% to only about 1%, apparently as a result of improved medical management of lupus-related complications. Alternatively, there may actually have been a change in the average severity of disease, because milder cases are now being diagnosed through sensitive testing procedures such as the antinuclear antibody test.

Even patients who had previously experienced fairly aggressive renal disease can conceive and maintain a successful pregnancy without undue risk of long-term morbidity if their disease is under control at the time of conception.[15,23,26,61] There is, of course, no guarantee that a clinical remission will persist for a prolonged period of time, so one author[66] has advised patients who desire pregnancy to "seize the moment" and "not insist that a protracted and unnecessary arbitrary period of remission persist before conception."

Exacerbations during pregnancy may involve any organ system but tend to mimic the exacerbations seen in the same patient before pregnancy. The problem has often been to distinguish an exacerbation of lupus renal disease from preeclampsia presenting in a lupus patient (see Chapters 32 and 34). Preeclampsia is a relatively common disorder that can occur at any age but tends to present in young primiparous patients. Both lupus and preeclampsia can cause moderately severe hypertension, proteinuria, and edema, but they can usually be distinguished by clinical and laboratory criteria. For example, preeclampsia is not likely to exhibit the rash or arthritis that commonly accompany exacerbations of lupus. A falling serum complement titer and rising anti-DNA antibody titer also suggest a change in lupus disease activity.

Influence of Disease on Pregnancy

The fertility of lupus patients appears to be substantially decreased during times of increased disease activity, but fairly normal at other times. During lupus exacerbations, patients may fail to ovulate or to exhibit a regular menstrual cycle. There is, therefore, some protection from pregnancy during exacerbations, but it is not sufficiently dependable that contraceptive measures can be ignored when pregnancy is unwanted.

Although pregnancy seems relatively safe for the lupus patient, that is not true for the infant she carries. Fetal wastage is consistently increased among pregnant lupus patients. A number of studies dating back to 1950 compare fetal outcomes with those of the general population identified as non-SLE (Table 29-9). This composite of nearly 1200 lupus pregnancies indicates that fetal wastage is 1.5 to 3-fold higher than in the normal population. It appears from the more recent studies[26,61] that fetal mortality has decreased somewhat with time, but the values presented are averages that obscure the fact that fetal mortality is much higher in patients with active disease. Patients whose lupus manifestations first present during pregnancy exhibit fetal mortality rates as high as 50%. In contrast, fetal mortalities of 14% are noted in patients whose disease is clinically inactive at the time of conception.[26,61]

Infants of lupus mothers more frequently are born prematurely, are small for gestational age and have anomalies such as congenital heart block. Lupus patients who deliver viable infants tend to have more males than females. This contrasts with the sex distribution of the general population and may be due to the disease-remitting effects of androgens produced by the male fetus.

The neonatal lupus syndrome is characterized by the presence of a typical rash, congenital

TABLE 29-9. EFFECTS OF SLE ON FETAL OUTCOME

Population	Pregnancies	Spontaneous Abortions	Stillborns	Neonatal Deaths	Therapeutic Abortions	Fetal Wastage*
SLE†	1045	17	8	1	8	28
Non-SLE		15	9	8.5		10
SLE‡	38	8	5	5		15
SLE§	104	14	0.1	NA	9	17

* $\text{Percent} = 10^2 \times \frac{\text{(spontaneous abortions + stillborns + neonatal deaths)}}{\text{(pregnancies − therapeutic abortions)}}$

† Data from Cecere and Persellin.[11] Includes reported SLE pregnancies from 1950 to 1981.

‡ Data from Varner et al.[61]

§ Data from Jungers et al.[26]

heart disease, and occasionally cytopenia in an infant born to a mother with lupus.[66] The rash presents as annular, erythematous, and scaly plaques, most prominent on the head and neck, which develop from birth up to 12 weeks of age and usually resolve within six months. Histologically, the skin abnormalities are typical of those seen with systemic lupus.

Congenital heart block occurs at a rate of approximately 20% in infants of mothers with connective tissue diseases like systemic lupus, Sjögren's syndrome, and RA, whereas it occurs in only 1% of infants born in the general population.[5,7,21] Occasionally, the mothers of infants born with complete heart block have experienced no clinical symptoms of connective tissue disease before delivery, but 30–60% of them later develop active disease. The mortality rate associated with congenital heart block is relatively low. The 20-year survival is 95%, but some infants require placement of a permanent pacemaker to avoid sudden death. Most infants with congenital heart block have a histologic abnormaliy of the cardiac conduction system in the region of the atrioventricular node, which is either absent or entrapped in excess fibrous tissue. Other abnormalities associated with this disorder include transposition of the great vessels, patent ductus arteriosus, and atrial septal defects.

The circulating antibody to a nuclear antigen called SSA or Ro has been observed[50,63] in association with congenital heart block in infants born to lupus patients. Anti-Ro is composed of IgG antibody capable of crossing the placenta and of circulating in the fetal blood. It is not clear whether anti-Ro is directly involved in producing the congenital heart defects or is simply a maternal serum marker for increased risk. Nevertheless, screening of pregnant lupus patients for the presence of this antibody is warranted because fetal monitoring and early institution of pacemaker therapy may decrease fetal mortality.

The management of systemic lupus in pregnant patients may necessitate the use of aspirin or other nonsteroidal anti-inflammatory drugs, corticosteroids, and immunosuppressive drugs in patients with active disease affecting major organs. In addition, development of systemic hypertension in some patients may require the introduction of antihypertensive medications. It should be noted that all these drugs carry potential risks to both fetus and mother (Table 29-4). Among them, prednisone seems to be one of the more benign. Prednisone may cause a decrease in placental size, induce cataracts, mediate immunosuppression, and raise the risk of transient adrenal insufficiency in the newborn infant, but the cleft palate seen in experimental animals seems not to occur in human fetuses exposed to moderate doses (30 mg/day) of this drug.

Aspirin, which is effective in controlling joint pain experienced by nonpregnant lupus patients, should probably be avoided in pregnant individuals, particularly during the third trimester, because of its tendency to alter prostaglandin synthesis with resultant platelet dysfunction and premature closure of the ductus arteriosus. Chloroquine, which is quite innocuous in the nonpregnant state, has the potential of causing neurologic, ophthalmic, and vestibular anomalies in the developing fetus. Azathioprine has been used with apparent safety through a number of pregnancies, but concern regarding its potential hazards has led most clinicians to use it only when active disease is not adequately controlled by moderate doses of prednisone. Even the antihypertensive drugs must be used with caution. It appears, from available data, that furosemide is a safer diuretic for temperate use in pregnancy than are the thiazides. Captopril, which is often very helpful in the management of severe hypertension in nonpregnant lupus patients, has been blamed for some severe congenital anomalies, in addition to its tendency to cause leukopenia and proteinuria in the mother.

Clinical Management in Pregnancy

The known associations between lupus and HLA DR2/DR3 histocompatibility antigens suggests a theoretical risk of vertical transmission of lupus to an affected patient's offspring. The infant may also be at greater risk of developing lupus later in life because of hyperestrogenic exposure in utero (Ahmed, A., Dauphinee, M. J., and Talal, N.: Unpublished data). Those risks are in addition to the neonatal lupus syndrome that is thought to result from the transplacental infusion of IgG anti-SSA antibodies. Once the patient understands these considerations and still desires pregnancy, she should be advised to wait until a relative lull in disease activity to increase the likelihood of successful outcome.

Conservative measures utilized in the treatment of nonpregnant lupus patients, with the exception of aspirin, should also be observed carefully during pregnancy. Careful monitoring for evidence of active disease will allow patients to be treated with corticosteroids early in their course before serious injury to the mother or infant occurs.

The following recommendations seem to represent a reasonable approach to clinical monitoring, although there are differences of opinion regarding some of the laboratory measures[1,53] (see discussion, reference 15). Most patients should be evaluated regularly by both an obstetrician and a rheumatologist. There should be documentation of organ system involvement at approximately monthly intervals, depending on the patient's status. Laboratory tests should include complete blood count, platelet count, serum creatinine, and urinalysis. A 24-hour urinary protein measurement is useful if proteinuria is present. Serologic tests should measure anti-DNA antibody titers and the level of at least one serum complement component at alternate visits. Serum complement levels tend to rise during normal pregnancy, so even a normal value may accompany increased consumption. A decrease in serum complement or a rising anti-DNA titer might predict an exacerbation of the renal disease. The sedimentation rate, which is a useful measure of disease activity in nonpregnant patients, is less valuable during pregnancy because it rises even in normal pregnant women.

Patients should be monitored for evidence of preeclampsia. Regular fetal surveillance should be initiated once the fetus has reached an age at which it is potentially salvageable by elective delivery. Unfortunately, many lupus patients require administration of corticosteroids during pregnancy. Corticosteroid administration may invalidate interpretation of estriol levels as a marker of fetal well-being.[61] The only controlled study[23] of corticosteroid treatment of pregnant lupus patients indicated that use of steroids decreased the frequency of exacerbations and improved fetal survival. Corticosteroid dosages should be decreased very gradually or not at all throughout the course of pregnancy to prevent exacerbations.

In patients who require more than 30 mg/day of prednisone to maintain control of disease activity, the use of azathioprine in low to moderate doses may be indicated for its steroid-sparing effect. There is still some controversy regarding the potential benefit of larger doses of corticosteroids in the postpartum period. Such prophylaxis seems to us a small price to pay for avoidance of an exacerbation at that stage.

All patients who have taken more than 5 mg of prednisone (or equivalent) per day throughout pregnancy should receive a "steroid prep" during labor and delivery because of the physiologic stress of parturition. Infants should be observed carefully for evidence of congenital lupus syndrome, particularly congenital heart block, and for adrenal insufficiency if their mothers were treated chronically with corticosteroids.

POLYMYOSITIS AND DERMATOMYOSITIS

Introduction

Polymyositis is the term given to a syndrome of autoimmune injury to skeletal muscle.[5,7,21,22] Dermatomyositis is similar except for the presence of a characteristic rash. Both entities exhibit a bimodal age-of-onset pattern with one peak at about eight years of age and another about midway through the fifth decade. In the childhood form, myositis is occasionally associated with vasculitis in which immunoglobulin deposits are found in vessel walls. Dystrophic calcinosis is a fairly common feature. In the adult form, the most troublesome manifestations are related to skeletal muscle injury. These disorders are uncommon in the general population. The annual incidence is 0.5–8 per 100,000 [21] but they may accompany other connective tissue diseases such as scleroderma, lupus, and mixed connective tissue disease.[22] Patients with autoimmune myositis are fourfold more likely to develop a variety of malignancies.[5] As in the other connective tissue diseases, women are affected more frequently than men. The cause of polymyositis is unknown. In contrast to lupus and rheumatoid arthritis, which are primarily humoral immune diseases, its destructive mechanism is cell mediated.

Clinical Presentation

At onset, patients may notice a sudden or an insidious loss of strength in the neck and the proximal muscles of the extremities. If untreated, the weakness can progress to involve the muscles of glutition, the diaphragm, and even distal muscle groups. Prominent weakness of the pharangeal muscles can result in aspiration of food into the lung or its regurgitation through the nose. The symptoms may progress very rapidly until a patient is unable to rise from a chair or lift her head off a bed. Occasionally, these symptoms are associated with muscle soreness resulting from attempts to continue usual activities despite decreased functional muscle mass.

Cutaneous manifestations of dermatomyositis include a reddish-purple discoloration of the eyelids (heliotrope), a scaly, erythematous rash on the knuckles of the hands (goitrins or colloidin patches), and, in some patients, a diffuse sun-sensitive eruption. When myositis is associated with a connective tissue disease, there may be a rough erythematous rash on the palmar surface of the thumb and first two fingers.

Arthritis is an infrequent manifestation but may be due to periarticular deposition of hydroxyapatite. When present, the arthritis tends to accompany a cell-mediated infiltration of lung parenchyma. Joint discomfort may respond to colchicine alone, but, when the lung is involved, corticosteroids should be given in moderate to high doses. If untreated, the lung disease may progress to diffuse fibrosis. Weakness of the diaphragm can lead to alveolar hypoventilation. Infiltration of the myocardium with inflammatory cells can eventually precipitate cardiac arrhythmias or congestive heart failure.

An association of inflammatory myositis with malignancy has long been recognized, but the malignancies tend to occur primarily in the elderly, so malignancy is less likely to be a factor in patients of childbearing age. The types of associated malignancy found in these patients are the same as those found in the general population.

A number of laboratory tests are of value in confirming the diagnosis of inflammatory myopathy. Serum enzymes such as CPK, SGOT, aldolase, and LDH may be elevated in the blood during active myositis. Although any of these enzymes may be normal in the face of active disease, only rarely are they all normal. There is no correlation of ESR with disease activity. An EMG usually shows insertional irritability, low-amplitude polyphasic motor unit potentials, and fibrillations. These findings only indicate the presence of inflammation and loss of muscle fibers, so they can be seen in other myopathic disorders. Further confirmation of autoimmune myositis depends on histologic evaluation of skeletal muscle from involved tissue. Typical histologic features include inflammatory infiltrates, centralization of skeletal muscle nuclei, and muscle fibers that exhibit various stages of degeneration or regeneration.

Most patients with myositis respond dramatically to high-dose corticosteroid therapy, for example, 60 mg/day of prednisone in three divided doses. Within two to four weeks, enzyme levels in the blood begin to fall. Strength gradually improves over a period of weeks to months. As serum enzyme levels decrease, the dose of corticosteroid should be tapered to a single morning dose of 30–40 mg/day and then reduced more slowly over one to two years. lt is not unusual for patients to experience at least one recurrence of symptoms requiring a short-term increase in dosage. Some patients require low doses of prednisone for several years in order to maintain remission. Rarely, another agent such as methotrexate or cyclophosphamide is needed to control steroid-resistant disease.

Influence of Pregnancy on Disease Activity

The published experience regarding pregnancy in patients with polymyositis or dermatomyositis includes 24 women, ranging from 10 to 65 years of age, mean 35.7 years.[18] The onset of polymyositis/dermatomyositis began before the index pregnancy in 17 (71%) of these patients. In 6 women (25%), the onset occurred during pregnancy. One patient (4%) developed her initial symptoms in the postpartum period. (Table 29-10)

Of those patients who had stable polymyositis or dermatomyositis before the pregnancy, half had active disease at the time of conception. Thus, active disease does not prevent conception. All patients who experienced their first symptoms during pregnancy did so within the first trimester. Three of the eight patients who had inactive disease at the time of conception developed exacerbations during their pregnancies, two during the third trimester and one in the postabortion period.

Thus, conception can occur during active myositis. There is little chance that the disease will improve during pregnancy. Patients who become pregnant during inactive disease are fairly likely to experience an exacerbation of myositis. Finally, pregnancy may serve as an inducing factor for the onset of disease in some patients. There are no reports of maternal deaths attributable to pregnancy in patients with myositis nor are there any data to indicate whether the long-term prognosis of myositis is altered by pregnancy.

The primary mechanism responsible for autoimmune myositis is cell-mediated immunity against skeletal muscle antigens. The pathogenesis of this reaction is not clear, but an association with histocompatibility antigens has been reported.[3,17] There is also evidence to suggest that toxoplasma infection may be an inducing factor.[33] It is not clear whether women are more susceptible to toxoplasma infection during pregnancy. It is also not known whether the other complications of toxoplasma infection during pregnancy are related to skeletal muscle injury.

Influence of Disease on Pregnancy

In 18 patients with polymyositis/dermatomyositis, 77 pregnancies antedated the diagnosis of myositis, whereas 10 pregnancies occurred after its onset.[18] Seventeen patients had one or more pregnancies before the onset of PM/DM, giving a fertility rate of 4.5. After the onset of disease, there were only 10 pregnancies in seven sexually active patients, indicating a drop in the fertility rate to 1.7. The average age of onset of myositis in these seven patients was 23 years (range 10–33 years), so it is unlikely that the drop in fertility rate was due to advancing age.

Fetal outcome was markedly affected by coincident myositis.[18] Before onset of the disease, only 7 (9%) of 77 pregnancies ended in spontaneous abortion and two (2.5%) in neonatal deaths, giving a total clinical pregnancy wastage of 11.5%. That rate was normal for the general population at the time of the study. By contrast, the 10 pregnancies that occurred after the onset of myositis exhibited a wastage of 50% due to spontaneous abortions, stillbirths, and neonatal deaths. The level of myositis activity at the time of conception seemed to have little effect on the rate of fetal wastage. Polymyositis and dermatomyositis represent a high risk to the fetus. It is unlikely that the high fetal wastage was due to maternal corticosteroid therapy.

Clinical Management in Pregnancy

There are insufficient data to develop rational genetic counseling for patients with autoimmune myositis. Although there is some evidence for a

TABLE 29-10. EFFECTS OF PREGNANCY ON PM/DM

Onset PM/DM before pregnancy	17	(71%)
Disease active at conception	9	
Improved	2	
Disease inactive at conception	8	
Exacerbation third trimester	2	
Exacerbation postabortion	1	
Onset PM/DM associated with pregnancy	7	(29%)
Onset in first trimester	6	
Onset postpartum	1	
	24	

Source: Adapted from Gutierrez, G., Dagnino, R. and Mintz, G.: Polymyositis/dermatomyositis and pregnancy. Arthritis Rheum. 27:291–294, 1984. Reprinted from Arthritis and Rheumatism Journal, copyright 1984. Used by permission of the American Rheumatism Association.

genetic basis for these diseases, the modes of inheritance and the expected degree of penetrance cannot be predicted with confidence.

Since there was no apparent difference in the rate of fetal wastage, whether the mother's disease was active or inactive at the time of conception, there is no effective approach to planning pregnancy in a myositic patient. Patients should not be taking immunosuppressive drugs and there is theoretic advantage to beginning the pregnancy at a time when low to moderate rather than high doses of corticosteroids are being taken.

The management of polymyositis during pregnancy is similar to management of nonpregnant myositic patients.[7] They should be examined monthly or more frequently for evidence of progressive weakness and elevation of serum muscle enzymes. Early termination of pregnancy should be considered before administering immunosuppressive drugs, if high-dose corticosteroids are ineffective. Documentation of the patient's strength at various times is best accomplished by using objective measures that are not dependent on the relative strength of the examiner, such as: can the patient stand from a squat or from a chair without assistance; can she walk unaided, get in and out of the bathtub without help, or raise her head off the bed without a struggle. As in any pregnancy treated with corticosteroids, a "steroid prep" should be given in the antepartum period and the infant should be observed carefully for evidence of adrenal insufficiency during the first few days of independent life.

PROGRESSIVE SYSTEMIC SCLEROSIS

Introduction

Systemic sclerosis is an uncommon clinical disorder of unknown etiology characterized by thickening of the skin and certain visceral organs due to collagen deposition.[45] It occurs at a rate of 3–12 per 100,000 population and is three times more common in females than males. Available data indicate that pregnancy does not substantially modify the course of the disease, but that fetal demise and/or growth retardation are expected complications.

Clinical Presentation

At onset, patients may notice a puffy swelling of their digits which does not pit. This edematous phase resolves after a variable period of time, leaving the skin tight and shiny. There usually is gradual loss of skin appendages such as hair, sweat glands, and sebaceous glands. As a result, the skin may feel unusually smooth and dry. The diagnosis of scleroderma should not be made on the basis of hand involvement (sclerodactyly) alone. Induration of the skin on the trunk, face, or arms proximal to the wrist should be present before making this diagnosis. Deposits of hydroxyapatite crystals in the skin may be present as subcutaneous nodules that can erode through the skin and periodically drain chalky material. Raynaud's phenomenon is noted in most patients. With repeated ischemic insult and skin tightening, the distal ends of the fingers begin to break down and calcium in the tuft of the distal phalanx is resorbed.

Visceral involvement is often first recognized as dysphagia due to esophageal hypomotility. Dysfunction of the gastroesophageal sphincter allows acid reflux into the esophagus, causing ulceration and stricture formation. Atony of the small bowel may lead to stasis and malabsorption as a result of bacterial overgrowth. Barium studies often reveal dilation of the small bowel and large-mouth diverticulae anywhere along the gastrointestinal tract from the stomach to the colon.

Deposition of collagen in the lung parenchyma makes the lungs stiff and noncompliant. In addition to the increased work necessary for ventilation, the thickened alveolar septae represent a barrier to oxygen perfusion. Respiratory insufficiency and pulmonary hypertension are the ultimate result. Deposits of collagen in the myocardium may cause conduction defects that further compromise a heart already stressed by pulmonary and/or systemic hypertension.

Some patients develop a neuropathy due to compression of axons by thickened connective tissue. The most commonly involved nerve is the fifth cranial nerve, resulting in trigeminal neuralgia. Scleroderma patients may also develop two types of myopathy. One is noninflammatory, whereas the other is indistinguishable from polymyositis. Joint pain is occasionally a problem in scleroderma, but it is usually mild and nondeforming. The periarticular deposits of hydroxyapatite can at times be responsible for local inflammation.

No laboratory test is specific for scleroderma. Patients may exhibit low titers of rheumatoid factor. Nearly 70% have positive ANAs with a speckled or nucleolar pattern. Newer serologic tests for antibodies against nuclear antigens may eventually prove more specific. Excessive collagen deposition can be seen microscopically in the skin and involved visceral organs. Histologic study of the kidneys shows the same form of intimal thickening as seen with systemic hypertension, even in nonhypertensive scleroderma patients.

No treatment is available to prevent deposition of collagen in the tissues of scleroderma patients, although it is reported[45] that penicillamine in high doses can reduce the skin thickness and obviate the pulmonary infiltrative process. In general, therapy depends on management of the reversible complications of the disease. Vasospastic attacks of Raynaud's phenomenon can be minimized by avoidance of cold exposure and judicious use of vasodilator drugs. Moisturizing creams can help keep the skin from cracking. Esophageal stricture due to acid reflux can be prevented by regular administration of antacids and cimetidine and attention to gravity posturing. Malabsorption from bacterial overgrowth in a hypotonic small bowel can often be reversed by administration of a broad spectrum antibiotic, such as tetracycline. The severe hypertensive crises, previously considered universally fatal, have responded to drugs such as captopril, which block activation of the angiotensin system.

Influence of Pregnancy on Disease Activity

Since scleroderma is relatively uncommon, there is little information regarding the influence of pregnancy on its progression. The largest published series[25] includes 337 scleroderma patients, 30 of whom became pregnant after the onset of scleroderma. Pregnancy had no definable effect on the outcome of the disease. Approximately 1/3 of the patients improved during pregnancy, 1/3 stayed the same, and 1/3 got worse. There is some suggestion that some patients have noted softening of their skin during pregnancy,[4,28,31,52,54] but the disease is generally unaffected by pregnancy. A possible exception to that generalization is the experience of some authors who have reported episodes of maternal renal involvement with severe, systemic hypertension and ultimate maternal demise. It is not clear, however, that pregnancy is responsible for these complications, since hypertension is not uncommon in scleroderma in the absence of pregnancy. No data clearly indicate that long-term prognosis of scleroderma is altered by pregnancy.

The mechanism of disease in scleroderma remains controversial. A circulating, low molecular weight factor that is toxic to endothelial cells is thought responsible for the concentric, onion ring-like narrowing of arterial walls such as those in the kidney.[27] If such a factor were present, it might also alter placental weight and thus compromise circulatory support of the fetus.

Influence of Disease on Pregnancy

No clear data indicate whether fertility is modified by progressive systemic sclerosis. Some authors have concluded that the pregnancy rate among affected women is lower than expected.[4,54] One observation offered in explanation of the lower fertility is the occurrence of local scleroderma of the genital areas, including the uterine cervix. It is possible that the disease reduces reproductive fitness through psychosocial mechanisms as much or more than it does via pathophysiologic mechanisms.

The effect of progressive systemic sclerosis on maternal and fetal outcomes was reviewed by Ballou et al. (Table 29-11).[4] In five series involving more than 500 patients, there were 46 individuals who had a pregnancy during the course of their scleroderma. There were two maternal deaths and a number of maternal complications such as preeclampsia, hypertension, uterine rupture, and heart failure. As a result of nonuniform reporting of fetal outcome, the available data are based on the results of 38 pregnancies in which there were 11 term deliveries, 11 premature deliveries, and 16 abortions. Only 16 infants survived, giving an estimated fetal wastage of approximately 50%. However, the majority of the fetal deaths were in the series reported by Slate and Graham,[52] which may inappropriately inflate the summary data.

It is difficult to determine which medications the patients were taking and to what extent those medications were responsible for some of the adverse effects. A number of drugs used in the past to treat scleroderma patients can adversely affect the fetus (see Table 29-4). Even the antihypertensive drugs currently used to control mild elevations of blood pressure and captopril, which has seemed to reverse the severe hypertensive crisis in some patients, are potentially teratogenic. High doses of penicillamine would also be likely to produce adverse effects.

TABLE 29-11. FETAL OUTCOME OF PREGNANCIES IN PATIENTS WITH PROGRESSIVE SYSTEMIC SCLEROSIS

Author	Pregnancies	Term	Premature	Deaths	Abortions	Fetal Wastage*
Leinwand, et al.[31]	2	1	1	0	0	0
Slate and Graham[52]	17	0	4	2	13†	87.5%
Donaldson‡	16	9	4	2	3†	26.7%
Ballou	3	1	2	0	0	0
TOTAL	38	11	11	4	16	50%

$$* \text{ Percent} = 10^2 \times \frac{(\text{spontaneous abortions} + \text{deaths})}{(\text{pregnancies} - \text{therapeutic abortions})}$$

† Includes one therapeutic abortion.

‡ In discussion of reference 52.

Source: Adapted from Ballou, S. P., Morley, J. J. and Kushner, I.: Pregnancy and systematic sclerosis. Arthritis Rheum. 27:295–298, 1984. Reprinted from Arthritis and Rheumatism Journal, copyright 1984. Used with permission of the American Rheumatism Association.

Clinical Management of Pregnancy

There are scattered reports that scleroderma exhibits a familial pattern of occurrence, but the data are insufficient to confirm this. Counseling should perhaps focus more attention on the potential inmediate risks to the woman and her fetus, should she decide to undertake pregnancy. Advanced planning for such a pregnancy might fruitfully involve a careful gynecologic examination to determine whether genital involvement is present and an evaluation of the prospective mother's renal function. There is no obvious way to predict a future hypertensive crisis in scleroderma, so patients must be observed carefully and treated aggressively if hypertension occurs.

In general, management of scleroderma during pregnancy is identical to that in the nonpregnant patient. Since there is no drug that is outstandingly successful in obviating the collagen deposition of scleroderma, it seems prudent to avoid penicillamine and other drugs during gestation. Use of aspirin or acetaminophen to ease the discomfort of joint symptoms seems appropriate as long as aspirin is discontinued early in the third trimester. The patient should be followed closely for evidence of fetal distress so that the mother will not long be subjected to the symptoms occasionally associated with intrauterine demise. Difficult labor due to tight perineal skin has been reported[25] and is probably fairly common among these patients. Despite that, it appears that postpartum healing is normal. There are no predictable perinatal problems with the infants of such mothers, aside from a tendency toward prematurity and low birth weight.

POLYARTERITIS NODOSA

Introduction

This multisystem necrotizing vasculitis that affects primarily the medium-sized arteries throughout the body can be a serious, life-threatening disorder.[14,62] It may occur in persons of either sex and at any age, but it is more common in males between 30 and 60 years of age. The overall annual incidence is approximately 0.2 per 100,000 persons in the general population.

Clinical Presentation

One form of the disease is limited to the skin and remains relatively benign. The systemic form may present with very nonspecific symptoms such as fever, malaise, weakness, anorexia, weight loss, myalgias, arthralgias, and hypertension. The most common neurologic presentation is foot drop resulting from injury to the popliteal nerve. The prognosis for untreated cases of the systemic form ranges from 20% to 80% mortality per year.

The cause of polyarteritis is not known, but several associated conditions are worth mentioning. Up to 30% of patients with this disorder exhibit hepatitis B_s antigenemia, but the course of their disease is not significantly different from that of patients without detectable viral antigen. Patients taking intravenous amphetamines or allergy desensitization prophylaxis are also predisposed to this form of vasculitis. In another group of patients, the typical illness follows an episode of serous otitis media or a Meniere's-like syndrome.

Laboratory abnormalities in polyarthritis include an elevated ESR and normocytic anemia. The patients with hepatitis B antigenemia may also be hypocomplementic. None of these abnormalities is specific for polyarteritis. Other potentially useful studies include EMG and sural nerve biopsy in patients with neuropathy; angiography in patients with renal or abdominal visceral involvement to demonstrate aneurysm formation; and biopsy of muscle, kidney, or liver for histologic evidence of vascular injury.

Treatment for polyarteritis nodosa involves use of high-dose corticosteroids and cyclophosphamide in addition to aggressive antihypertensive therapy to control hypertension.

Influence of Pregnancy on Disease Activity

Current literature includes the descriptions of 10 patients with documented polyarteritis nodosa who became pregnant. Before 1973, there were seven cases reported, all of which resulted in maternal death. Those deaths were due, in part, to preeclampsia which obscured the correct diagnosis until postmortem examination. Another case, reported in 1980, was diagnosed during pregnancy, but attempts to control the process were unsuccessful, so another maternal death occurred. Two cases have now been handled successfully with reasonably good maternal outcome.[10,36] In both cases, the patients had been previously diagnosed and had responded to treatment. They were both asymptomatic or well controlled at the time of conception. As a result, hypertension and proteinuria were not mistaken for preeclampsia. One patient was delivered at 37 weeks when her hypertension and proteinuria became worse. She remained well for about 18 months, but then developed a flare of her disease that proved fatal. The other patient was successfully aborted early in the course of pregnancy with no apparent complications.

Although there is really no dependable information about the long-term effect of pregnancy in these patients, it is likely that antepartum diagnosis and thoughtful medical management represent their only hope. Of the 10 reported cases, only the patient who underwent therapeutic abortion remained alive and well. The mechanism responsible for the high mortality in pregnant women with polyarteritis nodosa is probably not different from that responsible for the high mortality in the absence of pregnancy.

Influence of Polyarteritis Nodosa on Pregnancy

There is no information on the effect of polyarteritis nodosa on fertility. Since most patients with this disorder tend to be quite ill and require regular medical therapy, it is likely that their reproductive fitness is low.

Because maternal outcome during pregnancy in polyarteritis has been so very poor, it is somewhat surprising that six infants from the nine pregnancies survived. Histologic evaluation of the abortus from one patient was normal on gross and light and electron-microscopic examination, disclosing no evidence of vasculitic involvement in the placenta or villous stromal vessels. It would appear, therefore, that the placenta and fetal circulation are protected from the vasculitic disease and that the uterine circulation is not involved, even on the maternal side.

The risks to the fetus from therapy with high-dose corticosteroid and cyclophosphamide are not known, but teratogenicity of the cytotoxic agent is high. In addition, rigorous antihypertensive therapy presents substantial risk (Table 29-4).

Clinical Management of Pregnancy

There is no basis for genetic counseling in patients with polyarteritis nodosa nor has a precedent been established by which a patient and physician can appropriately plan a pregnancy.

Optimal management of pregnancy in patients with polyarteritis nodosa is difficult to outline at this time. Perhaps the safest course is therapeutic abortion[36] while maintaining immunosuppressive and antihypertensive therapy as needed. If pregnancy is to be continued, moderate to high doses of corticosteroids and use of a relatively safe antihypertensive drug, such as furosemide, may provide disease control adequate for both mother and infant to survive. A "steroid prep" should be a part of therapy at labor, delivery, or abortion if corticosteroids have been used on a regular basis prior to or during pregnancy. Infants should be observed closely for evidence of adrenal insufficiency.

TAKAYASU'S ARTERITIS

Introduction

This disorder is sometimes called pulseless disease because, if untreated, it eventually causes obliteration of the aortic arch or its tributaries. It seems to be most common in Orientals and exhibits worldwide distribution. It shows a striking predilection for young women and is, therefore, occasionally encountered during pregnancy.[65]

Clinical Presentation

Constitutional symptoms that manifest themselves before the onset of vascular insufficiency may simulate a number of other connective tissue diseases. Patients report tiredness, headache, arthralgias, dyspnea, fever, and palpitations. With the onset of vascular insufficiency, intermittent claudication, hypertension, syncopy, Raynaud's phenomenon, and abdominal pain are relatively characteristic findings. As the disease progresses, there is a tendency for patients to develop a total absence of pulses in the extremities, usually in an asymmetric pattern relative to the two sides of the body or to upper and lower extremities.

Histologically, the lesions in the vessels may resemble those of giant cell arteritis, but inflammation seems to center about the vasovasorum. Dystrophic calcification in affected vessels may eventually give the appearance of atherosclerosis. The sedimentation rate is moderately elevated, helping to differentiate this disorder from premature atherosclerotic vascular disease. Angiography is most helpful in demonstrating the extent of the disease once the diagnosis is seriously entertained.

The immunological mechanism responsible for Takayasu's arteritis is not known, but HLA antigen associations have been found, including BW52 and CW3 for Type I, which involves the aortic arch, and MB3 and DR4 for Type II, which involves primarily the abdominal aorta and renal vessels.

It is important to document the peripheral pulses and the high blood pressure in all four extremities for use in monitoring therapy. Initially, therapy for active disease should include a corticosteroid, such as prednisone, at a dose of 1 mg/kg/day for up to three months. Thereafter, dosage can be tapered very gradually, using the sedimentation rate and the peripheral pulses to screen for recurrence of active disease. Patients who are less than totally responsive to corticosteroids may benefit from addition of cytotoxic agents such as cyclophosphamide or azathioprine.

Influence of Pregnancy on Disease Activity

The most recent report on the coincidence of Takayasu's arteritis and pregnancy comes from a group in Hong Kong[65] who described the outcome of 30 pregnancies in Takayasu's patients. Eleven pregnancies occurred before the disease was clinically evident and were obstetrically unremarkable. Eleven patients experienced 19 pregnancies after diagnosis of Takayasu's arteritis. Seven women exhibited their first recognized symptoms during routine prenatal examination. There was no evidence to indicate that pregnancy was responsible for the onset of symptoms, but rather it was presumed that the prenatal examination was sufficiently thorough to disclose the additional diagnosis. In most cases, the course of pregnancy was complicated by superimposed symptoms of preeclampsia which were successfully treated with diuretics, methyldopa, and/or beta adrenergic blockers.

Influence of Disease on Pregnancy

There is no evidence that reproductive fitness or fertility is altered in patients with Takayasu's arteritis.

Of the 11 patients experiencing 19 pregnancies after the diagnosis of Takayasu's arteritis, only one patient died during follow-up. That patient had previously undergone surgery to autotransplant both kidneys into the pelvis with a new blood supply from the internal iliac arteries. Her second pregnancy was delivered by cesarean section at 38 weeks because of rising blood pressure and proteinuria. She went home after the delivery but suddenly died 14 days later of acute myocardial infarction. Most of the other patients experienced hypertension during pregnancy but, with careful management, remained otherwise well.

Among the 19 pregnancies, there were three first-trimester spontaneous abortions and one therapeutic abortion. The 15 pregnancies that proceeded beyond the second trimester all resulted in viable infants. Most of them exhibited low birth weight, however, perhaps due to an abnormality in placental blood flow.

It is unclear from the report[65] whether the patients were receiving immunosuppressive therapy or corticosteroids during their pregnancies. Obviously, if cytotoxic drugs are required to maintain pregnancy, there could be resultant teratogenic effects. In addition, the necessary use of regular antihypertensive agents carries risk.

Clinical Management of Pregnancy

Since Takayasu's arteritis exhibits an association with certain histocompatibility antigens, a familial tendency is likely. Genetic transmission has not been sufficiently well documented to serve as a basis for genetic counseling. The high prevalence of this disorder among Orientals also suggests a genetic predisposition, although it is clear from other disorders that cultural habits, nutrition, and other environmental factors can be important to the pathogenesis of a disease process.

Pregnancy is likely to be successful if it occurs early in the course of the disease before vascular involvement has become diffuse. Thereafter, it is more likely to be associated with multiple complications due to ischemic involvement of major organs. Many patients have an unusually short duration of labor, which may be related to the small babies.

The most important factor in managing pregnant patients with Takayasu's arteritis is to control hypertension. That can generally be accomplished with conventional antihypertensive drugs. No specific therapy or precautions are needed for the infants in the perinatal period.

MYASTHENIA GRAVIS

Introduction

This autoimmune disorder usually presents as a gradually progressive weakness of striated muscles.[42] It has a female preponderance of 3:1 and a peak incidence at age 30, but affected individuals range from childhood through octogenarians. It involves about one individual per 100,000 in the general population. As with other autoimmune disorders, there is evidence for a genetic predisposition.

Clinical Presentation

Initial symptoms are related to ptosis in 90% of cases and diplopia resulting from unequal weakness of the ocular muscles. Choking or aspiration of food can result from laryngeal and pharyngeal muscle involvement. The symptoms may progress to other skeletal muscles until gait disturbances and even respiratory compromise become apparent. Respiratory insufficiency can become so profound as to require long periods of care on a respirator.

As with other autoimmune disorders, the course of myasthenia follows an unpredictable pattern of remissions and exacerbations. Patients who develop severe weakness are prone to respiratory infections that can prove fatal. In this way, respiratory insufficiency contributes to the demise of about 10% of patients. Those who survive for 10 or more years will likely continue to experience a benign course.

About 10% of myasthenia patients have a small-cell tumor of the thymus gland which may be pathogenically related, because thymectomy is remittive in some patients. Occasionally, myasthenia is found in association with systemic lupus erythematosus, rheumatoid arthritis, polymyositis, thyrotoxicosis, or malignant neoplasms. It can also be induced by penicillamine.

Myasthenia is believed to result from an IgG antibody binding to the acetylcholine receptor at the myoneural junction and thus competing for binding by acetylcholine.[32] Genetic studies have indicated an association with histocompatibility antigens B8 and DR3.

Treatment of myasthenia involves administration of drugs such as neostigmine that prevent catabolism of acetylcholine by the cholinesterase so that acetylcholine can more effectively compete with the antibody for its receptor on the motor endplate. A difficult differential diagnostic problem is presented by patients on treatment with anticholinesterase drugs, because the major manifestation of both myasthenic crisis (too little acetylcholine) and cholinergic crisis (too much acetylcholine) is progressive weakness. Response to edrophonium chloride, a short and rapidly acting anticholinesterase, can be used to confirm myasthenia as the cause of weakness and to assess the adequacy of stable anticholinesterase therapy.

Immunosuppression with corticosteroids is useful in some patients. The value of thymectomy or thymic irradiation remains controversial, but there is growing optimism that selected patients may benefit dramatically and permanently.[13] The use of other immunosuppressive drugs such as cyclophosphamide or methotrexate or the use of plasmapheresis have been advocated, but these modalities are generally reserved for treatment of the most severe cases.

Influence of Pregnancy on Disease Activity

The effect of pregnancy on the course of myasthenia was evaluated in summarized data from 292 pregnancies involving 202 mothers.[42] The three potential outcomes (1) no change, (2) remission, or (3) exacerbation were equally distributed among the patients. About one-third of the total experienced an exacerbation postpartum. Maternal death due to myasthenia complicated about 4% of the pregnancies. A pregnancy-related exacerbation of myasthenia symptoms was more likely to occur within the first 12–24 months after onset of the disease than later in its course, so delaying pregnancy for two or three years is likely to improve the chances of a benign course.

There are insufficient data to evaluate the risk of administering anticholinesterase drugs during human pregnancy. Most authors advocate their use instead of corticosteroids for reasons that are not clearly stated (see Table 29-4).

Influence of Disease on Pregnancy

Fertility appears to be reduced in myasthenic patients, but the extent of the reduction is not clear. There are documented cases of conception during active phases of the disease.

In the series of 292 pregnancies reviewed by Plauche,[42] 13% of fetuses were aborted (one-third spontaneously) and 2% were stillborn. Eighty-five percent of babies were liveborn but 4% died in the neonatal period. Neonatal myasthenia was noted in 19% of the liveborn infants (presumably due to transplacental transmission of IgG antibody), contributing to some of the neonatal mortality. In most infants, weakness lasted only a few weeks and resolved without serious sequelae. An exacerbation of neonatal myasthenia has been reported to follow breast-feeding and to resolve again when lactation was discontinued.

Clinical Management in Pregnancy

A small proportion of children born to myasthenic mothers later develop the disease, supporting the concept of a genetic predisposition to myasthenia. Despite that and despite the substantial risk of fetal or neonatal demise, it is difficult to argue convincingly against a myasthenic patient bearing children. As noted earlier, postponing conception for two to three years after the onset of disease seems prudent.

Induction of labor during the daytime hours when optimal hospital resources are available may be beneficial. When labor begins, parenteral neostigmine should be used as needed to control muscle weakness. Regional anesthesia is preferable to general anesthesia because myasthenic patients are very sensitive to sedative, narcotic, tranquilizer, and curare-like drugs. Instrumental delivery may be indicated to reduce maternal fatigue.

Careful observation of the mothers during the first few weeks postpartum is important, because about one-third experience a major exacerbation. The neonates are at risk of having myasthenic symptoms for several weeks until the IgG passively acquired from the mother has decayed. They may also develop a cholinergic crisis due to transplacentally acquired neostigmine. If chronic steroid therapy was used for the mother, neonatal adrenal insufficiency must also be considered.

OTHER PERTINENT DISORDERS

Sjögren's Syndrome

This chronic autoimmune disorder is characterized clinically by dry eyes (keratoconjunctivitis sicca), dry mouth (xerostomia), and a connective tissue disease. Any two of the three features is sufficient to establish the diagnosis. The failure of salivary and lacrimal secretions is due to massive infiltration of the respective glands by inflammatory cells. The process is diffuse, as evidenced by a concomitant decrease in secretions from glands in the skin, in the vagina, in the lung and in the gastrointestinal tract.

Sjögren's syndrome occurs as an associated condition in roughly 25% of patients with rheumatoid arthritis, systemic lupus erythematosus, and systemic sclerosis. It also occurs as a primary disease without any other accompanying condition. The fact that nearly one-fourth of all patients who have rheumatoid arthritis also have Sjögren's syndrome makes it a relatively common disorder that affects more than one million people in the United States. Half of all Sjögren's patients have rheumatoid arthritis. Females are affected about nine times more frequently than males.

The most common clinical findings are dry eyes and dry mouth. The patients may lose their teeth early in the course of the disease because of inadequate salivary secretions. The lymphocytic infiltration may progress to a pseudolymphomatosis or even lymphomatosis stage. Articular manifestations in some patients are typical of rheumatoid arthritis, whereas others have joint pain and morning stiffness that does not progress to deformity.

Laboratory findings include elevated sedimentation rate, mild anemia, and polyclonal gammopathy with very high titers of rheumatoid factor and ANA. A hereditary predisposition may exist, since there is a high association between primary Sjögren's syndrome and HLADR3.

Sjögren's syndrome usually remains benign. Treatment is directed at relief of bothersome symptoms. Inadequate lacrimal secretions can be recognized by a positive Schirmer's test and by staining of corneal ulcers with rose bengal. Regular use of ophthalmic drops containing 0.5% methylcellulose will help to prevent corneal ulceration. A glycerine mouthwash containing methylcellulose may be helpful in relieving xerostomia.

There is no published information concerning the effects of pregnancy on Sjögren's disease activity nor on maternal or fetal outcome. Although it may be unwise to generalize, it seems likely that the pattern of involvement with pregnancy would be comparable to that of the associated connective tissue disease.

Ankylosing Spondylitis (AS)

Ankylosing spondylitis is an autoimmune inflammatory disorder of the site at which tendons or ligaments attach to bone (the enthesis). As such, it has the potential of affecting many areas of the body, but it tends most commonly to cause back pain and limitation of back motion. Following a prolonged episode of inflammation in the area of the enthesis, healing takes place with dystrophic calcification. As this process occurs repeatedly, the patients develop spurs or syndesmophytes that can be demonstrated radiologically. Sacroiliitis with erosions or progressive ankylosis of the sacroiliac joint is a common radiographic finding in moderately affected individuals.

Patients typically complain of back pain that awakens them from sleep in the middle of the night. To obtain relief, they must get out of bed and move around for a while before returning to sleep. They are frequently stiff after prolonged stooping or bending at a task and must "work this out" for a few seconds. There may also be aching in the costovertebral or costochondral junction areas. Although the pain is first recognized in the lumbar spine, it may progress rapidly to involve the cervical spine resulting in neck pain and/or limited motion of the neck.

In the past, ankylosing spondylitis was thought to be a male disease, but careful radiographic evaluation of female populations has indicated that the radiographic signs also occur in a substantial proportion of females. Since the preponderance of symptomatic males persists, it is concluded that females are for some reason clinically less bothered by the symptoms even though they have the disease with approximately the same frequency as men. Not infrequently there is a history of a male relative with hunchback or some other chronic back ailment. Approximately 90% of Caucasians with ankylosing spondylitis carry the HLA B27 antigen, but only one-quarter of the 7% of normal Caucasian adults who carry the antigen ever develop symptoms of active disease.

There is very little information regarding pregnancy in patients with ankylosing spondylitis, but since AS does occur in young people of both sexes, pregnancies must occur with significant frequency in affected individuals. One controlled clinical trial[41] compared the effects of pregnancy in rheumatoid arthritis patients with those of pregnancy among ankylosing spondylitis patients. The rheumatoid arthritis patients exhibited definite improvement in disease activity, whereas the ankylosing spondylitis patients tended to become worse. No clear explanation for that finding is apparent except that back pain is a common manifestation of pregnancy in normal females and it would be difficult to distinguish those symptoms from an exacerbation of inflammatory back pain due to ankylosing spondylitis. Another factor for consideration is that ankylosing spondylitis patients may not relax the pubic symphysis or other pelvic structures normally in preparation for vaginal delivery. Medication used in treatment of ankylosing spondylitis consists primarily of nonsteroidal inflammatory drugs (Table 29-4). They should be discontinued early in the third trimester to avoid fetal abnormalities and hemorrhagic complications at delivery.

It appears inappropriate to advise patients with ankylosing spondylitis against having children because the offspring of heterozygotes have only a 50% chance of being HLA B27 positive and positive individuals have only a 25% chance of developing disease. Therefore, there is a predicted one in eight chance of the offspring's developing the disease and an even lower likelihood that a female offspring would be symptomatic.

Reiter's syndrome bears many resemblances to ankylosing spondylitis but is clearly a different disease. It also tends to be symptomatic more frequently in males than in females. Spinal ankylosis is an integral manifestation of the disease, but is not present in all patients. In contrast to ankylosing spondylitis, which causes bony ankylosis of the spine progressing upward from the caudal area, Reiter's syndrome may involve the spine in an asymmetric manner, leaving skip lesions of fairly normal vertebrae between ankylosed areas. Reiter's syndrome is characterized by the tetrad of dermatitis, conjunctivitis, arthritis, and iritis, often exacerbated or induced by a venereal or gastrointestinal infection. No published studies critically examine pregnancy in Reiter's syndrome.

Fibrositis Syndrome

Fibrositis (fibromyalgic) syndrome is perhaps the most common generalized periarticular pain problem presenting to the primary care physician. Estimates have indicated that it may occur in as many as 10% of the general population with a nine to one predilection for females. Patients with this disorder commonly complain of persistent pain all over their bodies. The diagnosis is confirmed by the presence of tenderness at multiple discrete areas such as the insertion of the trapezius muscle to the occiput, the lateral border of the trapezius muscle, the biceps tendon, the lateral epicondyles of the elbows, the costochondral junctions in the chest wall, the presacral fat pad areas, the trochanteric bursi, and the pes anserine bursae medially below the knees.

The term fibrositis is probably a misnomer, because little or no true inflammation is observed histologically. Most patients complain of sleeping poorly and have a variety of sleep abnormalities, including nocturnal bruxism, nocturnal myoclonis, sleep apnea, or a disturbance of stage 4 non-REM sleep. Depression is commonly present in affected individuals and in first-degree relatives. Fibrositis syndrome can exist alone or can be associated with a connective tissue disease, an infection, or thyroid dysfunction. Potentially associated disorders should be sought out.

Fibrositis syndrome is difficult to treat in the nonpregnant patient but generally responds favorably to administration of nonsteroidal agents, reassurance, relaxation therapy, and avoidance of stress-inducing situations. Depressed patients or those having much difficulty with persistent pain may benefit from the use of amitriptyline (25–75 mg), alprazolam (0.5–1.0 mg) or cyclobenzaprine (15–20 mg) at bedtime. Occasionally, local injections of a corticosteroid and an analgesic will relieve severe localized pain. There is no indication for use of systemic corticosteroids in primary fibrositis.

An informal survey of investigators caring for fibrositis patients has indicated no unusual pregnancy-related problems. It is important that the physician not overreact to the patient's symptoms, which may be very dramatically portrayed, and, in some cases, quite physically disabling, because of true somatic pain.

Autoimmune Thyroid Disease

The endocrinology of pregnancy is extensively discussed in other chapters but is only mentioned here because of the interesting way in which autoimmune thyroid injury of the mother and infant can be influenced by pregnancy. The prevalence of thyroid disease in pregnancy is estimated at approximately 0.7%.[12] The incidence is thought to be reduced relative to the general population because thyroid dysfunction can result in reduced fertility for both males and females. Therefore, it is a selective factor reducing the reproductive fitness of affected individuals (see Chapter 36).

Enlargement of the thyroid during pregnancy has been thought of as a normal phenomenon. However, there is little evidence to support that conclusion, so an enlarged gland should prompt an investigation of its cause. The hyperthyroidism of Graves' disease results from excessive thyroid hormone secretion induced by an antibody (long acting thyroid stimulator, LATS) with specificity for the TSH binding site in the thyroid. These antibodies are capable of crossing the placenta and causing neonatal hyperthyroidism.

The antibodies associated with thyroid destruction are not known to cause hypothyroidism in the fetus, so they may not traverse the placental barrier as readily. Antithyroid drugs cross the placenta and prevent LATS from inducing fetal hyperthyroidism. Some patients experience an exacerbation of thyroid dysfunction in the immediate postpartum period due to transient thyroiditis or temporary dysregulation of thyroid hormone output.

Hashimoto's thyroiditis has also been reported with a significant frequency in the postpartum period. It tends to occur three to six months postpartum and can result in hypothyroidism as glandular function is destroyed by cellular infiltration.

Intermittent Hydrarthrosis (Periodic Benign Synovitis)

This uncommon and poorly understood arthritic disorder is characterized by attacks of arthritis followed by symptom-free periods that cycle at regular intervals.[64] Females are affected twice as frequently as males. Ages at onset range from 13 to 45.

At the onset of an attack, patients develop pain, limitation of motion, and swelling of one or more joints (most commonly a knee). Those symptoms persist for a fixed period of time (one to seven days, depending on the patient), before resolving completely. Patients then become symptom free for a fixed time period (one week to two months, depending on the patient) before the cycle begins again. During attacks, palpable synovitis with a mildly inflammatory effusion is found in about 75% of cases. Histologically the synovium exhibits hyperemia, edema, and some inflammatory infiltrate. The ESR is generally normal and unaltered by periodic attacks.

No therapy, including corticosteroids, is successful in controlling the symptoms or their periodicity, but nine out of 10 patients experience complete remissions during pregnancy that last three months or more after delivery.

REFERENCES

1. Abramowsky, C. R.: Lupus erythematosus, the placenta, and pregnancy: A natural experiment in immunologically mediated reproductive failure. In: *Reproductive Immunology*. N. Gleicher (Ed). New York, Alan R. Liss, Inc., 1981, pp. 309-320.
2. Alarcon, G. S., Koopman, W. J., Acton, R. T., and Barger, B. O.: Seronegative rheumatoid arthritis, a distinct immunogenetic disease? *Arthritis Rheum.* **25**:502-507, 1982.
3. Arnett, F. C., Hirsch, T., Bias, W. B., Nishikai, M., and Reichlin, M.: The Jo-1 antibody system in myositis: Relationships to clinical features and to HLA. *J. Rheum.* **8**:925-930, 1981.
4. Ballou, S. P., Morley, J. J., and Kushner, I.: Pregnancy and systemic sclerosis. *Arthritis Rheum.* **27**:295-298, 1984.
5. Barnes, B. E.: Dermatomyositis and malignancy: A review of the literature. *Ann. Int. Med.* **84**:68-76, 1976.
6. Bluhm, G. B.: Treatment of rheumatoid arthritis with gold. *Semin. Arthritis Rheum.* **5**:147-166, 1975.
7. Bohan, A., Peter, J. B., Bowman, R. L., and Pearson, C. M.: A computer-assisted analysis of 153 patients with polymyositis and dermatomyositis. *Medicine (Baltimore)* **56**:255-286, 1977.
8. Briggs, G. G., Bodendorfer, T. W., Freeman, R. K., and Yaffe, S. J.: *Drugs in Pregnancy and Lactation. A Reference Guide to Fetal and Neonatal Risk.* Baltimore, MD, Williams & Wilkins, 1983.
9. Bulmash, J. M.: Rheumatoid arthritis in pregnancy. *Obstet. Gynecol. Annu.* **8**:223-276, 1979.
10. Burkett, G. and Richards, R.: Periarteritis nodosa and pregnancy. *Obstet. Gynecol.* **59**:252-254, 1982.
11. Cecere, F. A. and Persellin, R. H.: The interaction of pregnancy and the rheumatic diseases. *Clin. Rheum. Dis.* **7**:747-768, 1981.
12. Davies, T. F. and Weiss, I.: Autoimmune thyroid disease and pregnancy. *Am. J. Reprod. Immunol.* **1**:187-192, 1981.
13. Eden, R. D. and Gall, S. A.: Myasthenia gravis and pregnancy: A reappraisal of thymectomy. *Obstet. Gynecol.* **62**:328-333, 1983.
14. Fauci, A. S., Doppman, J. L., and Wolff, S. M.: Cyclophosphamide-induced remissions in advanced polyarteritis nodosa. *Am. J. Med.* **64**:890-894, 1978.
15. Fine, L. G., Barnett, E. V., Danovitch, G. M., Nissenson, A. R., Conolly, M. E., Lieb, S. M., and Barrett, C. T.: Systemic lupus erythematosus in pregnancy. *Ann. Int. Med.* **94**:667-677, 1981.
16. Flebo, M. and Snorrason, E.: Pregnancy and the place of therapeutic abortion in rheumatoid arthritis. *Acta Obstet. Gynecol. Scand.* **40**:116-126, 1961.
17. Garlepp, M. J. and Dawkins, R. L.: Immunological aspects of polymyositis/dermatomyositis. *Clin. Rheum. Dis.* **10**:35-51, 1984.
18. Gutierrez, G., Dagnino, R., and Mintz, G.: Polymyositis/dermatomyositis and pregnancy. *Arthritis Rheum.* **27**:291-294, 1984.
19. Heinonen, O. P., Slone, D., and Shapiro, S.: *Birth Defects and Drugs in Pregnancy.* Littleton, MA, Publishing Sciences Group Inc., 1977.
20. Hench, P. S.: The ameliorating effects of pregnancy on chronic atropic (infectious) rheumatoid arthritis, fibrositis and intermittent hydrarthrosis. *Proc. Mayo Clin.* **13**:161-167, 1938.
21. Hodgson, P.: Polymyositis and dermatomyositis in adults. *Clin. Rheum. Dis.* **10**:85-93, 1984.
22. Isenberg, D.: Myositis in other connective tissue disorders. *Clin. Rheum. Dis.* **10**:151-174, 1984.
23. Ivanova, A. V.: Systemic lupus erythematosus and pregnancy. *Akush. Ginekol.* **5**:55-62, 1974.
24. Jacoby, R. K., Jayson, I. V., and Cosh, J. A.: Onset, early stages and prognosis of rheumatoid arthritis: A clinical study of 100 patients with 11-year follow-up. *Br. Med. J.* **2**:96-100, 1973.
25. Johnson, T. R., Banner, E. A., and Winkelmann,

R. K.: Scleroderma in pregnancy. *Obstet. Gynecol.* **23**:467-469, 1964.
26. Jungers, P., Dougados, M., Pelissier, C., Kuttenn, F., Tron, F., Lesavre, P., and Bach, J. F.: Lupus nephropathy and pregnancy. Report of 104 cases in 36 patients. *Arch. int. Med.* **142**:771-776, 1982.
27. Kahaleh, M. B., Shorer, K. H., and LeRoy, E. C.: Endothelial injury in scleroderma. *J. Exp. Med.* **149**:1326-1335, 1979.
28. Karlen, J. R. and Cook, W. A.: Renal scleroderma and pregnancy. *Obstet. Gynecol.* **44**:349-354, 1974.
29. Kay, A. and Bach, F.: Subfertility before and after the development of rheumatoid arthritis in women. *Ann. Rheum. Dis.* **24**:169-173, 1965.
30. Latman, N. S.: Relation of menstrual cycle phase to symptoms of rheumatoid arthritis. *Am. J. Med.* **74**:957-960, 1983.
31. Leinwand, I., Duryee, A. W., and Richter, M. N.: Scleroderma (based on a study of over 150 cases). *Ann. Int. Med.* **41**:1003-1037, 1954.
32. Lisak, R. P.: Myasthenia gravis: Mechanisms and management. *Hosp. Pract.* **18**:101-109, 1983.
33. Magid, F. K. and Kagen, L. J.: Serologic evidence for acute toxic plasmosis in polymyositis/dermatomyositis. Increased frequency of specific anti-toxoplasma IgM antibodies. *Am. J. Med.* **75**:313-320, 1983.
34. McCue, C. M., Mantakas, M. E., Tingelstad, J. B., and Ruddy, S.: Congenital heart block in newborns of mothers with connective tissue disease. *Circulation* **56**:82-90, 1977.
35. Morris, W. I. C.: Pregnancy in rheumatoid arthritis and systemic lupus erythematosus. *Aust. N.Z. J. Obstet. Gynecol.* **9**:136-144, 1969.
36. Nagey, D. A., Fortier, K. J., and Linder, J.: Pregnancy complicated by periarteritis nodosa: Induced abortion as an alternative. *Am. J. Obstet. Gynecol.* **147**:103-106, 1983.
37. Neely, N. T. and Persellin, R. H.: Activity of rheumatoid arthritis during pregnancy. *Tex. Med.* **73**:59-63, 1977.
38. O'Brien, T. E. and Balmer, J. A.: Drugs and the human fetus. *U.S. Pharm.* **6**:44-64, 1981.
39. Oka, M.: Effect of pregnancy on the onset and course of rheumatoid arthritis. *Ann. Rheum. Dis.* **12**:227-229, 1953.
40. Oka, M. and Vainio, U.: Effect of pregnancy on the prognosis and serology of rheumatoid arthritis. *Acta Rheum. Scand.* **12**:47-52, 1966.
41. Ostensen, M. and Husby, G.: A prospective clinical study of the effect of pregnancy on rheumatoid arthritis and ankylosing spondylitis. *Arthritis Rheum.* **26**:1155-1159, 1983.
42. Plauche, W. C.: Myasthenia gravis in pregnancy: An update. *Am. J. Obstet. Gynecol.* **135**:691-697, 1979.
43. Pope, R. M., Yoshinoya, S., Rutstein, J., and Persellin, R. H.: Effect of pregnancy on immune complexes and rheumatoid factors in patients with rheumatoid arthritis. *Am. J. Med.* **74**:973-979, 1983.
44. Reichin, M. and Mattioli, M.: Antigens and antibodies characteristic of systemic lupus erythematosus. *Bull. Rheum. Dis.* **24**:756-760, 1974.
45. Rodnan, G. P., Gablonska, S., and Medsger, T. A.: Classification and nomenclature of progressive systemic sclerosis (scleroderma). *Clin. Rheum. Dis.* **5**:5-13, 1979.
46. Ropes, M. W., Bennett, G. A., Kalec, S., Jacox, R., and Jessar, R. A.: 1958 Revision of diagnosis criteria of rheumatoid arthritis. *Bull. Rheum. Dis.* **9**:175-176, 1958.
47. Rosenthal, M.: Enhanced phagocytosis of the immune complexes in pregnancy. *Clin. Exp. Immunol.* **28**:189-191, 1977.
48. Rothfield, N. F.: *Systemic Lupus Erythematosus: Clinical and Laboratory Aspects, Arthritis and Allied Conditions.* D. J. McCarty (Ed.). Philadelphia, Lea & Febiger, 1979.
49. Sany, J., Clot, J., Bonneau, M., and Andary, M.: Immunomodulating effect of human placenta eluted gammaglobulins in rheumatoid arthritis. *Arthritis Rheum.* **25**:17-24, 1982.
50. Scott, J. S., Maddison, P. J., Taylor, P. V., Esscher, E., Scott, O., and Skinner, R. P.: Connective tissue disease, antibodies to ribonucleoprotein, and congenital heart block. *N. Engl. J. Med.* **309**:209-212, 1983.
51. Sharon, E., Jones, J., Diamond, H., and Kaplan, D.: Pregnancy and azathioprine in systemic lupus erythematosus. *Am. J. Obstet. Gynecol.* **118**:25-28, 1974.
52. Slate, W. G. and Graham, A. R.: Scleroderma and pregnancy. *Am. J. Obstet. Gynecol.* **101**:335-340, 1968.
53. Smolen, J. S. and Steinberg, A. D.: Systemic lupus erythematosus and pregnancy: Clinical, immunological and theoretical aspects. In: *Reproductive Immunology.* N. Gleicher (Ed.) New York, Alan R. Liss, Inc., 1981, pp. 283-302.
54. Stenchever, M. A. and Ng, A. B. P.: Scleroderma of the uterine cervix. *Am. J. Obstet. Gynecol.* **107**:965-966, 1970.
55. Stern, L. (Ed.): Drugs and the management of chronic diseases. In: *Drug Use in Pregnancy.* Boston, MA, Adis Health Science Press, 1984, pp. 193-211.
56. Tan, E. M., Cohen, A. S, Fries, J. F., Masi, A. T., McChange, D. J., Rothfield, N. F., Shaller, J. G., Talal, N., and Winchester, R. J.: Revised criteria for the classification of systemic lupus erythematosus. *Arthritis Rheum.* **25**:1271-1277, 1982.
57. Tozman, E. C. S., Urowitz, M. B., and Gladman B. D.: Systemic lupus erythematosus and pregnancy. *J. Rheum.* **7**:624-632, 1980.
58. Unger, A., Kay, A., Griffin, A. J., and Panayi, G. S.: Disease activity in pregnancy—associated α2-glycoprotein in rheumatoid arthritis during pregnancy. *Br. Med. J.* **286**:750-752, 1983.
59. Urman, J. D. and Rothfield, N. F.: Corticosteroid treatment in systemic lupus erythematosus: Survival studies. *JAMA* **238**:2272-2276, 1977.

60. Utsinger, P. D. Zvaifler, N. J., and Ehrlich, G. E. (Eds.): *Rheumatoid Arthritis: Etiology, Diagnosis, Management.* Philadelphia, J. B. Lippincott Co., 1985.
61. Varner, M. W., Meehan, R. T., Syrop, C. H., Strottmann, M. P., and Goplerud, C. P.: Pregnancy in patients with systemic lupus erythematosus. *Am. J. Obstet. Gynecol.* **145**:1025–1040, 1983.
62. Verztman, L.: Polyarteritis nodosa. *Clin. Rheum. Dis.* **6**:279–317, 1980.
63. Vetter, V. L. and Rashkind, W. J.: Congenital complete heart block and connective tissue disease. *N. Engl. J. Med.* **309**:237–238, 1983.
64. Weiner, A. D. and Ghormley R. K.: Periodic benign synovitis. *J. Bone Joint Surg.* [*Am.*] **38**:1039–1055, 1956.
65. Wong, V. C. W., Wang, R. Y. C., and Tse, T. F.: Pregnancy in Takayasu's arteritis. *Am. J. Med.* **75**:597–601, 1983.
66. Zurier, R. B.: *SLE and Pregnancy in the Clinical Management of Systemic Lupus Erythematosus.* P. H. Schur (Ed.). New York, Grune & Stratton, 1983, pp. 211–220.

30

HEMATOLOGICAL COMPLICATIONS IN PREGNANCY

ANEMIAS IN PREGNANCY

Hemoglobin is the principal protein used in the transport of oxygen. Reductions of hemoglobin/hematocrit values below a designated normal range identify the anemic patient. Screening tests during pregnancy allow diagnosis of many cases of anemia that might otherwise remain undiscovered. In addition, the nutritional and metabolic demands of pregnancy often result in a preexisting subclinical pathophysiological process becoming evident. Anemia is therefore among the more common medical complications encountered by the obstetrician.

Classification of Anemias

Anemias are categorized either by using the underlying pathophysiology (impaired production, shortened red blood cell survival, blood loss) as described in Table 30-1, or by using morphological findings and/or quantitative red blood cell indices. The latter classification employs the data available to the obstetrician at the time anemia is initially diagnosed (Table 30-2). This scheme provides information as to possible etiologies and suggests directions for further diagnostic tests and is more practical for use by obstetricians.

Laboratory Evaluation—Routine Prenatal Screening and Evaluation of Results

The WHO scientific group defines anemia in pregnancy as a hemoglobin concentration of less than 11.0 g/dl.[90] Other studies demonstrate that hemoglobin concentrations below 10.5 g/dl are abnormal (±2 SD).[16] A hematocrit below 31% in pregnancy is indicative of anemia. Defining anemia solely on the basis of a decreased hematocrit and/or hemoglobin can result in diagnostic errors. Both hemoglobin and hematocrit values are dependent on the plasma volume of the patient and the method by which the sample is obtained and evaluated. Should anemia present during antepartum laboratory screening, examination of the peripheral smear should be performed. The peripheral smear may provide significant information as to the etiology of the anemia. Evidence of leukemias, iron deficiency, folate deficiency, microangiopathic hemolytic anemias, and so on may be quite obvious on examination of the peripheral smear.

Morphological evaluation of the peripheral smear, or preferably by quantitative red blood cell indices obtained with automated methods (Coulter, SMA, etc.), should be obtained during antepartum screening. Except at extremes of cell size, automated quantitative indices are su-

TABLE 30-1. PATHOPHYSIOLOGIC MECHANISMS OF ANEMIA

- I. Decreased red blood cell production
  - A. Metabolic/nutritional
    - Iron deficiency
    - Folate deficiency
    - B_{12} deficiency
  - B. Marrow failure
    - Aplastic anemia
    - Myelophthistic anemia
    - Chronic inflammation/disease
    - Endocrinopathies
    - Drugs
- II. Increased red blood cell destruction (see table 30-4)
  - A. Red blood cell abnormalities
    - Spherocytosis and other membrane abnormalities
    - G6PD and other enzyme deficiencies
    - Hemoglobinopathies
  - B. Extrinsic abnormalities
    - Immune
    - Microangiopathic
    - Splenomegaly
    - Bacterial (clostridia)
- III. Blood loss
  - A. Acute
    - Abruptio
    - Previa
    - Trauma
  - B. Chronic
    - Gastrointestinal tumors
    - Ulcers

TABLE 30-2. MORPHOLOGICAL CLASSIFICATION OF ANEMIA

- I. Microcytic/hypochromic indices
  - Iron deficiency
  - Thalassemias
  - Hemoglobinopathies
- II. Normocytic indices
  - A. Red blood cell loss (increased reticulocyte count)
    - 1. Acute blood loss
    - 2. Hemolytic anemias (see Table 30-4)
      - Intravascular
      - Extravascular
  - B. Decreased production (decreased reticulocyte count)
    - 1. Chronic disease/inflammation
    - 2. Marrow depression/infiltration
    - 3. Sideroblastic anemias
    - 4. Red blood cell aplasia/hypoplasia
- III. Macrocytic indices
  - A. Nutritional deficiency
    - Folate
    - B_{12}
  - B. Malabsorption
    - Crohn's disease
    - Sprue
    - Fish tapeworm
    - Pernicious anemia

perior to the peripheral smear, especially in reproducibility. Red blood cell size and chromicity provide important clues to the mechanism underlying an anemia. Further evaluation should include determination of the platelet count (qualitative or quantitative) and white blood cell count.

Antepartum screening should also include determination of blood type, Rh, and an indirect Coombs' test. Although such screening is primarily for hemolytic disease of the fetus, a rare case of maternal hemolytic anemia may be discovered.

Sickle cell screening should be utilized in all patients at risk for either sickle cell trait or sickle cell disease.

The reticulocyte count provides an assessment of the bone marrow response to anemia. The reticulocyte count must be corrected for both the degree of anemia and for the effect of erythropoietin in the premature delivery of marrow reticulocytes (shift cells) to circulation. The values for the second correction factor (CF_2) are given in Table 30-3. The formula for determination of the reticulocyte production index is

$$\text{Corrected Reticulocyte Count} = \text{Observed Reticulocyte Count} \times \frac{\text{Patient Hgb}}{\text{Ideal Hgb}} \div CF_2$$

Anemias with Low MCV/Low Reticulocyte Count

Iron Deficiency. The most common cause of microcytic/hypochromic anemia during pregnancy is iron deficiency (Table 30-2). Microcytes appear early in iron deficiency anemia. The MCV provides both a sensitive sign and a means of differentiating a falling or borderline hematocrit from the "hemodilution" of pregnancy. Serum ferritin levels are indicative of reticuloendothelial iron stores. These values are insensitive to recent iron ingestion. Ferritin levels below 10–12 ng/liter are indicative of iron deficiency.[25] A serum iron concentration less than 60 ng/100 ml and an iron binding capacity greater than 300 ng/100 ml are considered diagnostic of iron deficiency, although each can be misleading. Such studies are unnecessary for patients presenting with a microcytic/hypochromic anemia, low serum ferritin, and low corrected reticulocyte counts.

TABLE 30-3. RETICULOCYTE COUNT—SECOND CORRECTION FACTOR

Hematocrit	Second Correction Factor (CF_2)
45	1.0
35	1.5
25	2.0
15	2.5

Oral iron is the mainstay of therapy in iron deficiency anemia. Therapy should be instituted as a three-times-daily (t.i.d.) regimen of one of the compounds described in Table 30-4. Although iron is best absorbed when taken on an empty stomach, gastrointestinal side effects may necessitate taking iron supplements with meals.

Response to oral iron therapy is evidenced by a reticulocytosis beginning between the fifth and seventh day of therapy and peaking between days 10 and 14 of therapy.[7] Hemoglobin levels begin to rise on the seventh to tenth day. The maximum rate of increase is approximately 0.3 g/dl per day.[7] Hemoglobin levels usually rise at a rate of 1 g/dl per week.

Failure to respond appropriately to oral iron therapy necessitates that the obstetrician first determine patient compliance. Serum iron levels may be obtained after the first week of therapy. If a compliant patient fails to respond appropriately, other etiologies of anemia must be sought. Iron deficiency combined with other etiologies (folate deficiency, thalassemia, hemoglobinopathy, chronic disease, etc.) may present as anemia refractory to iron therapy.

Parenteral iron therapy in the form of iron dextran should be reserved for the rare patient who either cannot tolerate or cannot absorb oral iron. Iron dextran should be injected as a 0.25 ml test dose the first day, followed by 2.0–5.0 ml/day until the desired dosage is administered. An approximation of iron requirements can be calculated from various formulas.[7,26]

Iron dextran has been given intravenously (i.v.) in several hundred milliliters of normal saline over 60 minutes. This route of administration causes less pain than does intramuscular (i.m.) injection. The dosing schedule remains controversial as does the use of i.v. versus i.m. therapy. Response to parenteral iron therapy is no more rapid than to oral therapy. In addition to being more expensive and painful, parenteral therapy carries the risks of anaphylaxis, local side effects (inflammation discoloration), or sys-

TABLE 30-4. IRON MEDICATIONS

Generic name	Common Strength (mg)	Elemental Iron (mg)
Tablets/Capsules		
Ferrous sulfate	325	65
Ferrous gluconate	320	37
Ferrous fumarate	330	110
Liquids		
Ferrous sulfate	220 mg/5 ml	44 mg/5 ml
Ferrous gluconate	300 mg/5 ml	34 mg/5 ml
Parenteral		
Iron dextran	50 mg/ml	50 mg/ml

temic toxicity (headache, hemolysis, etc.). Parenteral iron therapy offers little except in the rare obstetrical patient who cannot tolerate or absorb oral therapy.

Thalassemias often present with microcytic hypochromic indices. The decrease in indices may be far in excess of the decreased hemoglobin/hematocrit. Hemoglobin E, a hemoglobinopathy present in Orientals, is a rare cause of a microcytic hypochromic anemia with indices appearing far worse than the evidenced anemia. These disorders are differentiated from iron deficiency by demonstrating normal iron studies and abnormal hemoglobin electrophoresis.

Normocytic Normochromic Anemia

Normocytic normochromic anemias may result from underproduction of erythrocytes or from increased erythrocytic destruction (hemolytic anemia) occurring either within or outside the reticuloendothelial (RE) system. The corrected reticulocyte count differentiates the two basic processes.

Underproduction of Erythrocytes—Inappropriate Reticulocyte Response. The differential diagnosis for a suppressed or absent erythrocytic marrow response is shown in Tables 30-1 and 30-2. The anemias of liver disease, renal disease, and hypothyroidism are diagnosed by the appropriate clinical and laboratory findings. The perinatal and maternal outcomes and management for such anemias are determined by the underlying pathophysiology. The anemias of other chronic disease (infection, autoimmune, malignancy) demonstrate low serum iron, low total iron binding capacity (TIBC), normal or increased ferritin, and normal or increased iron stores. The outcome and management are determined by the underlying process.

Sideroblastic anemias are a diverse group resulting from numerous etiologies, both inherited and acquired (malignancies, collagen-vascular, etc.). Abnormal heme production results in iron loading of perinuclear mitochondria. Special iron stains demonstrate these ringed sideroblasts. Serum ferritin is elevated whereas serum iron is low. Management and outcome are dependent on the underlying process.

Pure red blood cell hypoplasia/aplasia has been reported during pregnancy with rapid resolution during the puerperium.[44,66] Serum from affected patients inhibits erythropoiesis in normal erythropoietic cell cultures. Infants born to affected mothers are hematologically normal. Steroids and transfusions have been used in the antepartum management of these patients. Worsening anemia despite therapy may mandate early delivery with a resultant increase in perinatal morbidity and mortality. The disorder may or may not recur in subsequent pregnancies.[44]

Marrow infiltration resulting from metastatic cancer, leukemias, and hematologic malignancies results in teardrop erythrocytes, nucleated red blood cells, and a left shift with myelocytes. Marrow infiltration is rare in pregnancy and can be diagnosed by marrow aspiration. Management and outcome depend on the underlying disorder.

Increased Rate of Red Cell Destruction—Hemolysis. Premature destruction of erythrocytes may occur within the reticuloendothelial system (extravascular destruction) or within the vascular system (intravascular lysis). Clues to location and etiology may be gained from laboratory studies. Intravascular hemolysis results in hemoglobinemia, decreased free haptoglobin, and hemoglobinuria.

Extravascular Hemolysis. Extravascular hemolysis is the most common site of destruction. Extravascular hemolysis is evidenced by decreased erythrocyte survival, normal or slightly decreased serum-free haptoglobin and lack of hemoglobinemia and hemoglobinuria. Extravascular hemolysis may present with an elevated indirect serum bilirubin and serum LDH. The pathophysiology of extravascular hemolysis may be divided into intrinsic erythrocyte disorders and extrinsic disorders. The differential diagnoses are shown in Table 30-5. The hemoglobinopathies are discussed below.

Glucose-6-phosphate dehydrogenase (G6PD) deficiency is transmitted as a sex-linked trait occurring in 12% of North American blacks and 2–9% of Greeks.[7,82] Most female carriers are asymptomatic and carry two populations of red blood cells—those deficient for G6PD and those normal in G6PD.

A few heterozygous females are symptomatic, presumably as the result of inactivation of the X chromosome with the normal G6PD gene in the majority of marrow erythrocyte precursors (Lyon hypothesis). Individuals with the Mediterranean variety have a lower level of enzyme activity than blacks and thus have more severe clinical manifestations. Lowered erythrocytic levels of G6PD result in decreased intracellular NADPH and reduced glutathione which protect cellular membrane thiol (SH) groups from oxidant stress. A severe acute oxidant stress may therefore disrupt the erythrocyte cellular membrane resulting in intravascular hemolysis. The deficiency in G6PD also results in an inability of erythrocytes to protect the heme of sulfhydryl groups from oxidation. Oxidized heme precipitates forming Heinz bodies visible on the peripheral smear. Precipitation of hemoglobin reduces red blood cell deformability resulting in damage within the microcirculation and subsequent destruction within the reticuloendothelial system. The management of G6PD is directed at the avoidance of oxidative agents, including sulfonamides, phenacetin, vitamin K, nalidixic acid, probenecid, nitrofurans, PASA, and antimalarials. Patients presenting with a hemolytic episode should be managed with fluids to maintain urine output. Transfusions are seldom indicated because the episodes are self-limited. Screening of a patient for G6PD deficiency immediately after a hemolytic episode may result in a false negative result, as only older erythrocytes may present with the deficiency.

TABLE 30-5. HEMOLYTIC ANEMIAS

Intravascular
- Microangiopathic hemolytic anemia
- Paroxysmal nocturnal hemoglobinuria
- Acute G6PD
- Clostridial sepsis
- Physical trauma and burns

Extravascular
- Intrinsic abnormalities
  - Hemoglobinopathies
  - G6PD
  - Spherocytosis
  - Elliptocytosis
- Extrinsic abnormalities
  - Autoimmune hemolytic anemias
  - Secondary immune hemolytic anemia
    - Drugs/medications
    - Lymphoproliferative disorders
    - Collagen-vascular disease
  - Hypersplenism

Other intrinsic abnormalities resulting in extravascular hemolytic anemias include membrane abnormalities, for example, hereditary spherocytosis and elliptocytosis. Spherocytosis occurs in approximately 1:4500 patients. Although usually evident in infancy, it may not manifest until adulthood. Family history may be important; however, 20% of patients present without such a history.[7] Autoimmune spherocytosis must be excluded by appropriate laboratory studies. Treatment may necessitate splenectomy in the nonpregnant state; however, splenectomy should be avoided if possible during pregnancy. The outcome of pregnancy is dependent on the severity of the intrinsic membrane abnormalities.

Antibodies or complement directed at red blood cell surface antigens result in sequestration and destruction of affected erythrocytes by the RE system. The diagnosis of autoimmune hemolytic anemia is established by the demonstration of antibodies attached to the erythrocyte surface (direct Coombs') or the presence of such antibodies within the serum (indirect Coombs'). Such antibodies can be subcategorized as warm (IgG class) or cold (IgM). IgG antibodies cross the placenta whereas IgM antibodies do not.

Immune hemolytic anemia may be either autoimmune (idiopathic) or secondary, as described in Table 30-5. The management and outcome of patients with secondary immune hemolytic anemia depend on the underlying pathophysiology, with one important additional consideration. If the antibody is of the IgG class, there is the possibility of the development of fetal hemolytic disease. Management should include fetal evaluation (testing/sonograms) and amniotic fluid evaluation.

Pregnancy-associated autoimmune hemolytic anemia resolves in the puerperium.[72] The antibody class must be identified. Should the antibody prove to be IgG, appropriate fetal evaluation, including testing, sonography, and amniotic fluid studies should be obtained. Studies should also be obtained to exclude possible causative etiologies, for example, mononucleosis, mycoplasma pneumonia, collagen-vascular disease, and neoplastic diseases. There is no correlation between the degree of maternal anemia/hemolysis and the extent of fetal involvement. Difficulty in obtaining compatible blood must be anticipated and early orders for crossmatching given.

In some cases of pregnancy-associated hemolytic anemia, no identifiable immune or intracorpuscular or extracorpuscular defects can be dscovered.[80] These cases resolve in the puerperium and the hemolytic anemia tends to recur in subsequent pregnancies. All patients respond to steroids. The maternal and neonatal outcome is good, although transient mild neonatal hemolysis is evident in some of the offspring.

Intravascular Hemolysis. Hemoglobinemia, hemoglobinuria, and saturation of serum haptoglobin indicate intravascular hemolysis. The differential diagnosis of intravascular hemolysis is shown in Table 30-5. During later gestation, microangiopathic hemolytic anemia must be considered as it is known to result from severe preeclampsia.

Paroxysmal nocturnal hemoglobinuria (PNH) is a chronic disease resulting from increased sensitivity to complement-mediated hemolysis. It often presents as iron deficiency anemia accompanied by abdominal pain or as an acute hemolytic event. Pregnancy in such patients carries a significant incidence of thromboembolic events in the immediate puerperium.[27,31,91] Such patients should be advised against pregnancy. Oral contraceptives should be avoided. Therapeutic dosages of heparin with full anticoagulation should be utilized in the intrapartum–postpartum interval.[27,31] Transfusions of cross-matched, washed, packed red blood cells may be necessary for treatment of severe anemia.

Hemoglobinopathies and Thalassemias. Hemoglobin is a tetrameric protein consisting of heme and polypeptide chain subunits. Each heme unit is an iron molecule surrounded by four pyrrole rings. The four polypeptide chains surround the heme unit. These polypeptide chains together make up the globin portion of hemoglobin. Globin is usually composed of two pairs of genetically determined polypeptide chains. Normal adult hemoglobin is composed of:

1. Hemoglobin A (95%) $\alpha_2\ \beta_2$.
2. Hemoglobin A (2–3.5%) $\alpha_2\ \delta_2$.
3. Fetal hemoglobin (1.5–3%) $\alpha_2\ \gamma_2$.

The stereochemistry of the globin molecule, which is determined by the sequence of amino acids in the polypeptide chains, affects oxygen affinity, buffering capability, and cytoplasmic solubility. Alterations in amino acid sequencing are genetically directed and are described as hemoglobinopathies. A single gene locus on each chromosome 11 directs for the production of beta chains. Beta chain variants are thus inherited in classic mendelian fashion. To date, over 200 variations in beta chain sequencing have been determined.

Alpha chain genetics are less well defined. It appears most populations have two alpha chain loci on each chromosome 16, but many black populations exhibit only one locus on each chromosome 16.[18,82] Variations in alpha chain sequencing are not as clinically important and/or as common as beta chain substitutions.

Thalassemias (Fig. 30-1) result from decreased or absent synthesis of specific polypeptide chains. Reduced synthesis of one of the component chains results in the production of abnormal tetramers and decreased hemoglobin production. The gene for beta thalassemia is closely linked to the locus for the beta chain sequence on chromosome 11. The gene for beta chain production affects only the CIS gene, resulting in either no beta chain production (B^o gene) or reduction in beta chain production (B^+ gene).[18] Because of their close proximity, the beta chain production genes and sequencing genes are considered as alleles and their inheritance follows classical mendelian genetics.

The genetic locus for alpha thalassemia is closely linked to the genetic loci for alpha chain amino acid sequencing. In patients with alpha-thal-1, both CIS loci for alpha chain production are inactivated. A fetus homozygous for alpha-thal-1 produces no alpha chains resulting in production of Hgb Barts (γ_4) and hydrops fetalis.

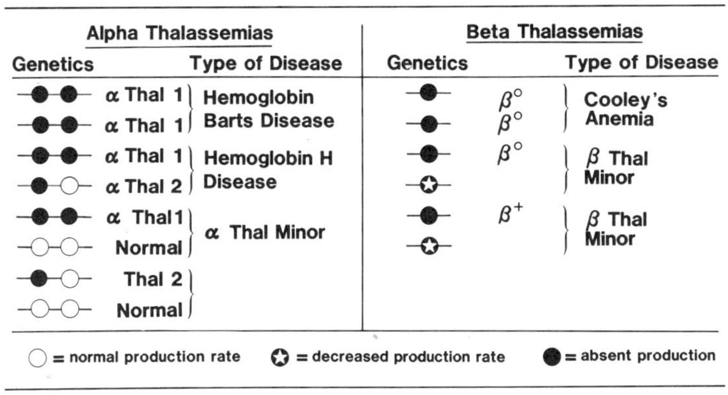

Figure 30-1. The genetics of alpha and beta thalassemias.

Infants heterozygous for alpha-thal-1 are born with 5–20% Hgb Barts and are considered to have a form of thalassemia minor. Only one of the two CIS alpha chain genes is inactivated by the alpha-thal-2 gene. Patients homozygous for alpha-thal-2 will still have two functioning genes (one in each chromosome) and are only mildly affected (form of thalassemia minor). Blacks seldom carry the alpha-thal-1 gene and therefore seldom demonstrate hemoglobin H disease or hydrops fetalis due to nonproduction of alpha chains (hemoglobin Barts).[18] The alpha-thal-1 disease however, is frequently carried by Southeast Asians resulting in a significant incidence of hemoglobin H disease and hydrops fetalis in this population.

Hemoglobin H (B_4) disease occurs in patients heterozygous for the alpha-thal-1 and alpha-thal-2 genes. Such patients are affected with splenomegaly, microcytic anemia, and hemolytic episodes precipitated by sulfonamides. Patients with hemoglobin H disease present with severe anemia and are transfusion dependent.

Pregnancy and Sickle Cell Disease. Sickle cell "disease" includes patients with SS disease (sickle cell anemia), Hgb SC disease, and HgbS-Bthal disease. The incidence of sickle cell trait (heterozygous for Hgb S) is about 1 in 12 (8–9%) in American blacks.[82] The incidences of the various hemoglobinopathies and thalassemias in American blacks are given in Table 30-6. Sickle cell disorders also exist in patients from Mediterranean or Middle Eastern regions, but to a lesser extent than in blacks.

The clinical manifestations of sickle cell anemia result from the substitution of valine for glutamic acid at position six of the beta chain, which contains a total of 146 amino acids. In the oxygenated state, hemoglobin S functions as hemoglobin A. Deoxygenation results in alteration in the globin stereochemistry and formation of hydrophobic bands between the alpha chains of adjacent hemoglobin molecules. Continued hydrophobic bounding results in the formation of microfilaments that coalesce to form microcables (see Fig. 30-2). Microcables aggregate to form cables at which time a sickled erythrocyte

TABLE 30-6. FREQUENCIES OF HEMOGLOBINOPATHIES AND THALASSEMIAS IN AMERICAN BLACKS

Phenotype Frequencies		Gene Frequencies	
Hb AS	8%	Hb^{s}_{β}	0.04
HbAC	3%	Hb^{c}_{β}	0 015
β Thal heterozygote	1.5%	Hb β Thal	0.0075
HPFH	0.1%	HPFH	0.005
Hb S-S	1:525		
Hb S-C	1:833		
Hb S/HPFH	1:25,000		
Hb S-β Thal	1:1,667		
Hb C-C	1:4,444		
β Thal homozygote	1:17,778		

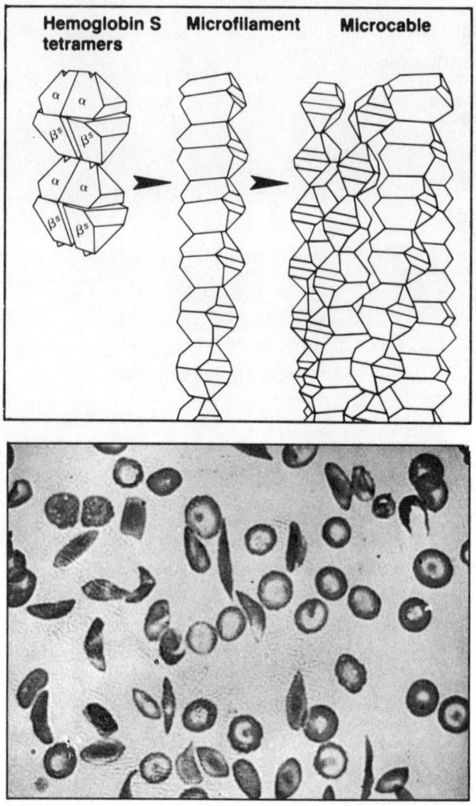

Figure 30-2. Sickling process. (Reprinted from Morrison, J.C., Ruvinsky, E. D., and Nicholls, E. T.: Sickling and pregnancy: A worrisome combination. Contemp. OB/GYN 18:125–132, 1981, with permission of *Contemporary OB/GYN* and the Medical Economics Company.)

is formed. Should the process continue, irreversible damage is inflicted on the erythrocyte resulting in its destruction by the reticuloendothelial system. Such sickled cells lack normal plasticity with resultant obstruction of the microcirculation and production of many of the classic signs and symptoms of a sickle crisis.

Sickle cell disease resulting from Hgb SS presents early in childhood. Until recent years, the majority of afflicted patients either died from complications prior to reaching reproductive age or were infertile and/or incapacitated during the reproductive portion of their shortened life span. Recent advances in the management of such patients has resulted in increased numbers presenting for obstetrical care. Patients with sickle cell disease due to Hgb SC characteristically have fewer crises than their Hgb SS counterparts and often are relatively asymptomatic prior to the onset of significant stress. Stresses such as infection, trauma, or pregnancy can lead to catastrophic events in patients with Hgb SC disease, however. Patients with Hgb S-thalassemia usually present with mild asymptomatic iron refractory anemia unless stressed (trauma, infection, or pregnancy), at which time they behave in a manner similar to Hgb SS disease.

Sickle cell disease at one time increased maternal and perinatal morbidity and mortality so much that the patients were advised against pregnancy and for sterilization.

Table 30-7 details the maternal mortality and morbidity associated with various types of sickle disease as reported in recent studies within the United States. The perinatal morbidity and mortality from these same studies are shown in Table 30-8. The risk of significant maternal morbidity remains elevated. Perinatal mortality is elevated (7.9%), as are the incidences of prematurity (~20%) and IUGR (14.3%).

Patients with sickle cell disease (Hgb SS, SC, S-Thal) should be advised of the associated maternal and perinatal risks. This counseling should ideally occur prior to conception, but many patients first have their sickle cell disease (especially SC, S-Thal) diagnosed by routine antepartum screening. Genetic counseling should be proffered such patients (including patients with sickle cell trait) and paternal screening obtained when appropriate.

Antepartum visits should be at least bimonthly until 24 weeks and then weekly until delivery, unless clinical circumstances dictate more frequent evaluation. A hemoglobin/hematocrit (and hemoglobin electrophoresis for patients receiving prophylactic partial exchange transfusions [PPET]) should be obtained at each interval visit. Careful evaluation of fetal growth and well-being is essential. Fetal testing should be instituted with either nonstress test (NST) or contraction stress test (CST) at a gestational age at which abnormal results would be acted on.[58] Folic acid 1 mg b.i.d. should be given pregnant patients with sickle cell disease. Iron therapy should be reserved for patients demonstrating iron deficiency (serum ferritin, total serum iron, or iron binding capacity). Timing of delivery should be based on obstetrical considerations.

Conventional management uses transfusions only for severe or recurrent crisis and for significant anemia (hemoglobin less than 7.0–7.5 mg/dl). Such transfusions can be either partial exchange or packed red blood cells (PRBC), depending on the clinical setting.

The efficacy of prophylactic transfusions in

TABLE 30-7. MATERNAL COMPLICATIONS IN SICKLE CELL DISEASE

Study (Year)	Patients	Number of Pregnancies	Maternal Deaths	Pulmonary (Pneumonia, Emboli)	Urinary Tract Infection/Hematuria	Toxemia	Crisis
Charache et al.[11] (1980)							
SS	28	43	1	7	6	6	NA
SC	10	24	0	3	2	4	NA
ST	4	7	0	0	4	1	NA
TOTAL	42	74	1	10	12	11	NA
Cunningham et al.[15] (1983)							
SS		48	0	10	9	NA	33
SC		52	0	7	8	NA	15
ST		8	0	0	1	NA	3
TOTAL		108	0	17	18	NA	51
Miller et al.[53] (1981)							
SS		39	0	7	0	2	6
SC		16	0	2	1	3	0
ST		9	0	0	0	0	1
TOTAL		64	0	9	1	5	7
Morrison et al.[55] (1980)							
SS	41	41	0	3	1	NA	2
SC	25	25	0	1	1	NA	1
ST	9	9	0	0	1	NA	0
TOTAL	75	75	0	4	3	NA	3
Total Studies							
SS		171	1 (0.6%)	27 (15.8%)	16 (9.4%)	8/82 (9.8%)	41/128 (32.0%)
SC		117	0	13 (11.1%)	12 (10.3%)	7/40 (17.5%)	16/93 (17.2%)
ST		33	0	0	6 (18.2%)	1/16 (6.3%)	4/26 (15.4%)
TOTAL		321	1 (0.3%)	40 (12.5%)	34 (10.6%)	16/138 (11.6%)	61/247 (24.7%)

TABLE 30-8. PERINATAL COMPLICATIONS WITH SICKLE CELL DISEASE

Study (Year)	Total Pregnancies	Infants to Viability	Spontaneous Abortion	Neonatal Death	Stillborn	IUGR	Weight <2500 g	PNM
Charache et al.[11] (1980)								
SS	43	33	10	2	2	5	9	4
SC	24	21	3	0	0	2	7	0
ST	7	7	0	0	0	0	1	0
TOTAL	74	61	13	2	2	7	17	4
Cunningham et al.[15] (1983)								
SS	48	48	NA	2	6	13	5	8
SC	52	52	NA	1	4	9	5	5
ST	8	8	NA	0	0	2	1	0
TOTAL	108	108	NA	3	10	4	11	13
Miller et al.[53] (1981)								
SS	39	33	5	3	1	6	16	4
SC	16	16	1	0	1	1	6	1
ST	9	9	0	0	0	1	1	0
TOTAL	64	58	6	3	2	8	23	5
Morrison et al.[55] (1980)								
SS	44	41	3	1	0	1	3	1
SC	26	25	1	0	1	1	1	1
ST	9	9	0	0	0	0	1	0
TOTAL	79	75	4	1	1	2	5	2
Total Studies								
SS	174	155	18/107 (16.8%)	8 (5.5%)	9 (5.8%)	25 (17.1%)	33 (22.6%)	17 (11%)
SC	118	114	5/66 (7.6%)	1 (0.9%)	6 (5.3%)	13 (12.0%)	19 (17.5%)	7 (6.1%)
ST	33	33	0/27 (0%)	0 (0%)	0 (0%)	3 (9.0%)	4 (12.1%)	0 (0%)
TOTAL	325	302	23/200 (11.5%)	9 (3.1%)	15 (5.0%)	41 (14.3%)	56 (19.5%)	24 (7.9%)

reducing maternal and perinatal complications in pregnancies compromised by maternal sickle cell disease has not been completely defined. Proponents theorize that maintaining the hematocrit and hemoglobin A percentage above defined limits will decrease the incidence of crisis and infection in the mother and also decrease perinatal compromise (specifically perinatal mortality [PNM], intrauterine growth retardation [IUGR], prematurity). The theoretical risks and benefits of prophylactic transfusions are shown in Table 30-9.

Prophylactic partial exchange transfusions reduce the risk of volume overload associated with red blood cell transfusions. Such procedures may employ the manual exchange methods,[54] isovolumetric calculations and procedures,[60] or automated erythrocytopheresis systems.[39] Whichever method is used, prophylaxis is begun before maternal and fetal compromise becomes evident. There is no consensus as to when to begin prophylaxis.[57] Some units begin transfusions with the first prenatal visits and others in the third trimester. The majority of complications occur after 28 weeks.[54] Prophylaxis is therefore usually begun at 28 weeks gestation,[14,54] provided maternal complications (crisis, severe anemia, infection, etc.) have not necessitated transfusions earlier. Once begun, prophylactic transfusions are timed to maintain a preselected hematocrit and/or percentage of hemoglobin S. Patients are rechecked weekly and retransfused if they become symptomatic (crisis or anemia) or if the hematocrit falls below a preselected level (25–30%) or the percentage of hemoglobin S rises above a preselected level (50–60%).

Most, but not all, initial studies appear to demonstrate a reduction in maternal morbidity and in perinatal morbidity/ mortality with PPET management (Table 30-10).[11,15,53,55] However, these studies are not randomized but rather are comparisons to data obtained retrospectively from different eras. Much of the improvement noted may actually be due to improved obstetrical and neonatal care. PPET therapy has several significant complications. Isoimmunization secondary to antigens not normally tested in blood banking may result in a patient for whom it is virtually impossible to obtain compatible blood. Formation of isoantibodies could also potentially result in fetal hemolytic disease. Hepatitis is a very real possibility, especially when banked blood must be utilized. Iron overload and hemochromatosis are theoretical risks but unlikely in such short-

TABLE 30-9. PROPHYLACTIC TRANSFUSIONS

Proposed Benefits
- Decreased erythropoiesis
- Decreased incidence sickling crisis
- Decreased incidence of anemia
- Decreased maternal morbidity
- Decreased perinatal morbidity/mortality
- Increased sense of well-being

Proposed Risks
- Hepatitis
- Transfusion reaction
- Isoimmunization
  - Difficulty in obtaining blood in future
  - Hemolytic disease of the newborn
- Volume overload
- Iron overload

term management. Table 30-10 details some results of prophylactic transfusions along with the outcomes and complications.

No definitive recommendation for or against prophylactic exchange transfusion can be given. Although there is a reduction in immediate maternal morbidity and an apparent reduction in perinatal complications, consideration must be given to the risks of potentially serious complications (Table 30-10). The rate of hepatitis appears to be quite low. However, there is a significant incidence of isoimmunization (10%) in patients managed with prophylactic transfusions. How this rate of isoimmunization compares with that in conventionally managed patients is unknown.

The rates of perinatal mortality, intrauterine growth retardation, and prematurity all appear to be decreased with prophylactic transfusions (Table 30-10). Again, these improvements are in comparison to historical controls. Improvements in obstetrical and neonatal management account for an unknown percentage of the reported decreases in perinatal mortality, growth retardation, and prematurity.

Patients with sickle cell disease should be informed of the short-term and long-term risks and benefits associated with conventional and prophylactic transfusion therapy. Patients to be treated with prophylactic transfusions should receive only buffy-coat-poor washed single volunteer donor red blood cells for which extensive cross-matching has been performed.

Should a sickle cell crisis present, precipitating causes (infection, trauma, etc.) must be identified and treated. Patients should receive immediate hydration with volume expanders and adequate analgesia (narcotics, acetamino-

TABLE 30-10. PROPHYLACTIC TRANSFUSIONS VERSUS CONVENTIONAL MANAGEMENT

Study (Year)	Pregnancies Treated	Maternal Morbidity	Perinatal Mortality	Perinatal IUGR	Perinatal LBW or Premature	Transfusion Hepatitis	Complications Isoimmunization
Cunningham et al.[15] (1983)							
Conventional	54	35/54	12/54	14/54	8/54	—	—
P. transfusion	54	10/54	1/54	10/54	3/54	2/54	6/54
Miller et al.[53] (1981)							
Conventional	39	22*	4/35	5/35	14/35	—	—
P. transfusion	25	15*	4/26	3/26	9/26	0/24	9/24
Morrison et al.[55] (1980)							
Conventional	—	—	—	—	—	—	—
P. transfusion	75	11/75	2/75	2/75	5/75	2/75	1/75
Total							
Conventional		35/54† (64.8%)	16/89 (18%)	19/89 (21.3%)	22/89 (24.7%)	—	—
P. transfusion		21/129‡ (16.3%)	7/155 (4.5%)§	15/155 (9.7%)§	17/155 (11.0%)§	4/153 (2.6%)	16/153 (10.5%)

* Contains patients with multiple etiologies.
† Cunningham et al.
‡ Cunningham et al. and Morrison et al.
§ Difference between conventional and PPET significant ($p<0.05$).

phen). Antisickling agents (urea, thiocyanate) have not been approved for use in pregnancy and should be avoided because of their potential side effects. Oxygen therapy is utilized (4 L by nasal catheter), although its efficacy has never been proved.

In patients for whom PPET is used, crisis is an indication for initiating such therapy or for retransfusion. Exchange transfusion should be considered for patients managed with conventional therapy should the crisis be severe, recurrent crisis develop, or if significant anemia is discovered.

Laboring patients with sickle cell disease should be placed in the semi-Fowler lateral recumbent position with continuous electronic monitoring of the fetal status. Adequate hydration must be maintained throughout labor. Some clinicians advocate the addition of alkali to the intravenous fluids (10% NaCitrate 20 ml or Nabicarb 50 ml in each liter), although the efficacy of alkali therapy remains in question and most clinicians do not use it. Oxytocin induces no ill effects in patients with sickle cell disease. Adequate pain relief should be provided. Epidural anesthesia is excellent provided hypotensive episodes are avoided. Hypoxia should be avoided in the sickle cell patient. The method of delivery should be based on obstetrical considerations. Partial exchange transfusion should be considered in patients with severe disease prior to undergoing general anesthesia, although this may not be possible for the patient undergoing emergent cesarean delivery.

Sickle cell patients are at increased risk for thromboembolic disorders and consideration should be given to intrapartum heparin or dextran prophylaxis, especially in patients with other risk factors (parity, age, operative delivery, obstetrical complications, or blood transfusions). In the puerperium, sickle cell patients are at increased risk for endomyometritis and urinary tract infections and must be carefully observed.

Sickle Cell Trait. Sickle cell trait (Hgb AS) has a benign clinical course, both in the nonpregnant and pregnant patient. The increased incidence of hematuria and bacteriuria and pyelonephritis in patients with the trait warrant careful antepartum screening. Should the maternal antepartum sickle cell screen prove positive, hemoglobin electrophoresis of both the mother and father should be obtained and appropriate genetic counseling provided.

Pregnancy and Beta Thalassemias. Cooley's anemia or beta thalassemia major is a homozygous state in which few, if any, beta chains are produced. In utero, the fetal production of hemoglobin ($\alpha_2\gamma_2$ = HgbF) protects it from clinical disease. At approximately three months of age, the infant becomes anemic, develops hepatomegaly, and may require blood transfusions every 3–4 weeks.[3] Pregnancy is infrequent because the vast majority of patients with Cooley's anemia die by age 20 and those who do survive have impaired fertility. A few patients with Cooley's anemia with high hemoglobin F levels can be expected to achieve pregnancy. Due to the high erythropoietic state, these patients must be carefully managed with folic acid supplements.

The clinical appearance of beta thalassemia minor (heterozygous thalassemias) depends on the production rate of the affected beta chain. Perinatal and maternal outcomes are strongly related to the degree of anemia and/or associated hemoglobinopathies. Appropriate paternal evaluation should be obtained. Iron supplements should be reserved for patients with demonstrated iron deficiency. Folate supplementation should be provided to all patients.[3]

Alpha Thalassemias. In hemoglobin Barts (γ_4) disease, the absence of all four alpha genetic loci results in the nonproduction of alpha chains. Such fetuses die of hydrops fetalis.[3] There is a 50% incidence of severe toxemia in the mothers of such infants. This disease is uncommon in the black population but is the most common cause of hydrops in patients from Southeast Asia.

Hemoglobin H (β_4) disease is the result of deletion of three of four alpha chain genetic loci and is the most severe form of alpha thalassemia compatible with extrauterine life. As with hemoglobin Barts, this disease is rarely seen in the black population but is more common in patients from Southeast Asia. Pregnancy can be complicated by severe anemia requiring numerous transfusions. Hgb H (β_4) is considered unstable and oxidative agents (salicylates, nitrofurans, sulfas) must be avoided.

Alpha thalassemia minor (deletion of two genes) results in a mild hypochromic, microcytic anemia with little apparent effect on maternal or perinatal outcome. These thalassemias are usually discovered after iron deficiency and beta thalassemias have been ruled out as a cause of a microcytic hypochromic anemia.

Macrocytic Anemias

The etiology of megaloblastic anemia in pregnancy is nearly always folate deficiency. Vitamin B_{12} deficiency is rare. During pregnancy, dietary intake of folate should be 800 ng each day. Total body stores (mainly in the liver) may be adequate for 2–3 months if no folate is taken orally. Folate deficiency manifests itself by the events detailed in Fig. 30-3. Pregnancy may accelerate the sequence of events and complicating factors such as hemoglobinopathies and multiple gestations may put a further load on folate requirements. Patients with malabsorptive states or epileptic patients on dilantin, primidone, or phenobarbital may have difficulties absorbing ingested folate, necessitating careful monitoring of folate levels.

Folate deficiency is determined by the presence of macrocytosis and lowered folate levels. Serum folate is known to decrease during the course of normal gestation.[10,18] Hypersegmentation (five lobes) of the nuclei of polymorphonuclear leukocytes (PMN) is suggestive of folate deficiency, but 25% of normal pregnancies also demonstrate some hypersegmentation. Hypersegmentation indices have also been utilized to describe the degree of hypersegmentation.[7] Therapy for folate deficiency should be at least 1 mg folate per day (orally or parenterally). A response as evidenced by reticulocytosis should be evident within one week. Iron deficiency may coexist with folate deficiency.

Vitamin B_{12} stores are usually on the order of 3000 ng with total fetal demands of only 50 ng.[18] Decreased body stores in pregnant patients may exist in vegetarians, patients with malabsorption, and in rare patients with pernicious anemia. Should macrocytic indices be discovered in a pregnant patient, B_{12} levels should be obtained and interpreted in light of known decreases in serum and red blood cell B_{12} concentrations during pregnancy.[10,18] Urinary excretion of methylmalonic acid is increased in vitamin B_{12} deficiency. A thorough history may reveal the classic triad of weakness, sore tongue and tingling in the extremities. Anorexia and diarrhea may be other presenting symptoms. Physical exam may demonstrate loss of vibratory sense in the lower extremities, loss of a fine coordination of the fingers, incoordination of the lower extremities, and a glazed tongue. Associated autoimmune disease should be sought out. If malabsorption and sprue are excluded, the diagnosis is probably pernicious anemia. In this situation, the Schilling test is diagnostic but must be postponed until the puerperium. Treatment should consist of daily intramuscular injections of 100 μg hydroxycobalamin for one week, followed by every-other-day injections of 100 μg B_{12} for two weeks. Once remission is obtained, 1 mg B_{12} is given intramuscularly monthly throughout the course of pregnancy.

The expected outcome of pregnancies complicated by macrocytic anemia is dependent on the underlying etiology, the time of diagnosis, and the degree of hematologic correction. Dietary deficiencies are easily corrected with good outcomes. The outcome of B_{12} deficiencies with associated autoimmune diseases are dependent on the course of the autoimmune disorder.

3 weeks → **fall in serum folate**

5 weeks → **hypersegmentation of PMNs**

17 weeks → **rbc folate decreases**

18 weeks → **megaloblastic anemia**

Figure 30-3. Calendar of events in folate deficiency.

PLATELETS

Physiological Changes in Pregnancy

Platelet concentration decreases during the course of normal gestation.[67,78] This decrease is likely due to dilutional effects. A minimal decrease in platelet survival time may contribute slightly to the decreased platelet concentration.[69,86] Platelet lifespan throughout normal gestation is about nine days (± one day). This is not true in pregnancies complicated by preeclampsia, however, as decreased survival time has been demonstrated.[69] The range of the decrease (between the first trimester and term) varies from the 20% decline found by Pitkin and Witte (longitudinal study)[67] to a 12.5% decrease determined by Sejeny and colleagues in a cross-sectional study.[78] While the platelet concentrations appear to decline, it should be noted that the number of total circulating platelets actually increases due to the increase in circulating blood volume.

Platelet function may be somewhat altered

during the course of normal gestation. A prostaglandin balance system mediated by platelet thromboxane (proaggretory) and vascular endothelial production of prostacyclin (antiaggretory) is theorized to be important in normal platelet homeostasis. There appears to be a disturbance or resetting of this balance late in gestation. Platelet aggregability increases and prostacyclin metabolite levels increase as pregnancy progresses.[45]

THROMBOCYTOPENIA

A maternal platelet count below 100,000 should be considered abnormal and an etiology sought.

It is convenient to categorize the etiologies of thrombocytopenia under the major headings of decreased production, decreased survival, or increased utilization (see Table 30-11).

Thrombocytopenia most often presents clinically with a history of easy bruising, bleeding gums and/or previous menorrhagia. Patients with decreased platelet counts who are clinically asymptomatic are often discovered on routine screening during pregnancy. With normal platelet function, excessive bleeding at surgery is not expected for counts exceeding 50,000/cu mm and spontaneous bleeding rarely occurs with counts above 20,000/cu mm.

Evaluation of Thrombocytopenia

The history should include the time of onset of clinical symptoms, previous episodes, previous bleeding with surgery or trauma, previous bruising or bleeding gums, and so on. A medication/drug history for agents resulting in marrow suppression and for those capable of producing immunologically mediated thrombocytopenia should be sought. Family history should be scrutinized for similar presentations and for relatives with collagen-vascular diseases. On physical examination, the liver, spleen, and lymph nodes should be carefully evaluated for evidence of hypersplenism, lymphoproliferative disorders, and so on. Stigmata of collagen-vascular disease should be noted. Evidence of recent viral illness should be sought and acute and convalescent titers obtained if deemed appropriate from the history of exposure. This is especially true for infectious mononucleosis and rubella (which could significantly affect further management).

A platelet count should be obtained for any patient with a report of decreased platelets on a complete blood count. For counts <100,000/cu mm, a peripheral smear provides significant information as to the possible etiology. Increased concentration of megathrombocytes is indicative of increased marrow activity in response to either decreased platelet survival time or increased platelet utilization. It must be remembered, however, that if the insult (decreased platelet survival or increased utilization) is acute, the marrow may not have had time to respond. A predominance of old, small platelets with few megathrombocytes is indicative of a production or marrow defect. Thrombocytopenia with a normal incidence of megathrombocytes on peripheral smear can exist in any of the three major categories noted in Table 30-11.

The morphology of the other blood components may add information as to the underlying mechanism of the thrombocytopenia. Erythrocytic indices may evidence a megaloblastic process, as would hypersegmentation of polymorphonuclear cells.

Schistocytes and helmet cells are suggestive of a microangiopathic process with associated platelet consumption. Finally, evidence of acute or chronic myelogenous disease may be present.

Acute thrombocytopenia should be evaluated with clotting studies (thrombin time, activated partial thromboplastin time, prothrombin time, fibrinogen, fibrin split products) to rule out disseminated intravascular coagulation.

Template bleeding times are a function of both platelet numbers and platelet function. Young large platelets are hemostatically the most effective, and older smaller platelets are

TABLE 30-11. THROMBOCYTOPENIA

I.	Decreased production
	Nutritional (folate, etc.)
	Metabolic/drugs (EtOH, etc.)
II.	Decreased survival
	Autoimmune (ITP)
	Secondary immune (drugs, SLE, etc.)
III.	Consumption
	Acute blood loss
	Microangiopathic hemolytic anemias
	Severe preeclampsia
	TTP/hemolytic uremic syndrome
	DIC
	Sepsis
	Hypersplenism

much less active. Patients with an increased population of megathrombocytes will have decreased bleeding times in proportion to their platelet counts. Platelet function can be significantly altered by ingestion of antiplatelet medications such as aspirin.

Bone marrow examination can demonstrate a megakaryocyte response or myeloproliferative disorders, production defects, or marrow infiltration. An adequate number of megakaryocytes with thrombocytopenia can occur in production defects resulting from megaloblastic anemia, paroxysmal nocturnal hemoglobinuria, and hereditary thrombocytopenias (e.g., Wiskott–Aldrich syndrome). Megakaryocyte suppression may be evidence of ingestion of medications such as synthetic estrogens, thiazides, or alcohol.

Collagen-vascular disease (especially systemic lupus erythematosus [SLE]) must be ruled out in every case of thrombocytopenia with megathrombocytes and megakaryocytes. About 10% of patients with SLE develop an immune-mediated thrombocytopenia.[7]

Antiplatelet antibody levels (both platelet-associated and circulating) should be obtained in patients presenting with thrombocytopenia with megathrombocytes on peripheral smears. The importance of these levels in the management of immune mediated thrombocytopenia is discussed below.

Preeclampsia is at the forefront of the differential diagnosis for thrombocytopenic pregnant patients presenting after the 20th week of gestation (see Chapter 32).

Immune Thrombocytopenic Purpura (ITP). ITP is an immunologically mediated destructive thrombocytopenia in which antibodies are directed against platelet antigens. These antibodies are most often of the IgG class. As the only class of immunoglobulin with significant transplacental passage, IgG antibodies have important implications for the offspring of an affected pregnancy.

The disease process focuses within the reticuloendothelial system, specifically the spleen, bone marrow, and liver. The spleen is the primary site of both antibody production and (in most patients) of sequestration and destruction of antibody-coated platelets. The bone marrow serves as a source of intramedullary platelet destruction and antibody production. The bone marrow becomes the primary site of both processes in splenectomized patients. The large reticuloendothelial system within the liver can result in significant platelet sequestration and destruction, especially in those patients with high levels of circulating antiplatelet antibodies.

ITP can be classified in terms of underlying immunological disorder (see Table 30-12) as either primary or secondary. Secondary immune thrombocytopenia is associated with numerous disease processes. SLE (or other collagen-vascular diseases) and acute viral infections are most common in women of reproductive age. Pregnancy with concomitant leukemia or lymphoma is somewhat rare (see Chapter 41). Numerous medications produce immune-mediated thrombocytopenia, most often by serving as haptens. The more commonly implicated medications (quinidine, quinine) are seldom used in patients of reproductive age. However, almost any medication may cause an immune-mediated thrombocytopenia. The management and prognosis of gestation complicated by secondary ITP is most closely related to the underlying mechanism or disease, not to the existence of immune thrombocytopenia. Intrapartum screening of potentially thrombocytopenic infants should be conducted, regardless of the underlying disease process.

Clinically, ITP presents in three time modes (see Table 30-13). Acute ITP, as seen by the obstetrician, is most often secondary to acute viral illness. Although the majority of acute episodes resolve, between 7% and 28% become chronic.[34] Chronic and intermittent ITP can be of either primary or secondary immunologic origin.

Primary immune thrombocytopenic purpura is an autoimmune disorder with autoantibodies (usually IgG class) directed against any one of a diverse set of platelet antigens. Included are ABO blood group antigens (RH is not expressed on platelets), histocompatibility antigens (class I), HLA antigen, platelet specific antigens, and glycoproteins. The complexity of the antigen systems and potential cross reactivities of antibodies complicate the management of affected

TABLE 30-12. IMMUNE THROMBOCYTOPENIC PURPURA

Primary
Autoimmune
Secondary
Acute viral infection
Medications
Collagen-vascular disorders
Lymph or proliferative disease

TABLE 30-13. CLINICAL PRESENTATION OF ITP

Acute
- Most commonly sequela to viral illness
- 7–28% become chronic

Intermittent
- Episodes of thrombocytopenia with intervals of clinical *and* immunological remission

Chronic
- Episodes of clinical exacerbation and remission of purpura.
- *No* remission of underlying immunological disorder

pregnancies. The presence of maternal antibody within the fetal circulation gives no indication as to its affinity for fetal platelet antigens.

Primary immune thrombocytopenia, although relatively uncommon in general, is one of the more common hematological disorders encountered by the obstetrician because of its tendency to affect women in their reproductive years. The incidence and clinical course of the disease are not altered by pregnancy. A significant proportion of patients are first diagnosed during pregnancy as a result of screening tests. Many patients have a subclinical immune process with decreased platelet counts and platelet survival times.[35] Routine semiquantitative platelet counts (as occur in pregnancy screening) identify patients with subclinical immunological disease.

The diagnosis of primary ITP is largely a diagnosis of exclusion. The patient presenting with purpura must meet the criteria presented in Table 30-14. Before a definitive diagnosis of ITP can be made, all medication that could result in secondary ITP must be discontinued. Measurement of antiplatelet antibody levels (both platelet-bound and free-circulating) help to establish the diagnosis.

Maternal Considerations. Maternal mortality as high as 10% was reported in the 1950s, the decade in which steroids were incorporated into the management of ITP. There has been only one maternal death related to ITP subsequent to 1951.[63] The incidence of maternal antepartum bleeding is not statistically different from that in the nonaffected population. Postpartum hemorrhage occurs in 5–26% of afflicted pregnancies.[33,38] A strong correlation exists between maternal platelet counts and the incidence of postpartum hemorrhage. Because of the normal myometrial mechanical hemostatic mechanism, postpartum bleeding from the placental site usually causes little concern. Most postpartum hemorrhage in ITP patients occurs at operative sites or from lacerations. Appropriate predelivery evaluation and therapy, minimal trauma at delivery, and hemostatic surgical techniques are important.

TABLE 30-14. DIAGNOSIS OF MATERNAL AUTOIMMUNE (PRIMARY) ITP

- Thrombocytopenia (100,000 per cu mm)
- CBC normal (except platelets)
- Megakaryocytes in bone marrow
- No other disease processes found (SLE, leukemia, viral infection, etc.)
- No medications capable of serving as haptens
- Platelet associated or serum antiplatelet antibodies detected

Management of Maternal ITP. The management of maternal primary ITP during pregnancy is the same as in nonpregnant patients. Corticosteroids, splenectomy, and immunosuppression form the basis of therapy. Recently, high-dose immunoglobulin has been incorporated for patients with refractory or life-threatening disease. Remission of purpura, *not immunologic cure*, is the therapeutic goal.

Corticosteroids are usually effective in raising the platelet count, with the effects being dose dependent.[34] Steroids are the medical equivalent of splenectomy, because they prevent sequestration of damaged or antibody-coated platelets in the spleen. Steroids also enhance capillary resistance. Effects are usually noted within the first 24–48 hours although delays of 3–4 days before significant inhibition of splenic sequestration are not unusual. Effective response is seen in 36–44% of patients treated with 0.5–1 mg/kg/d of prednisone. Increasing the dose to 1.5–2 mg/kg/d of prednisone induces some response in 70–80% of initially treated patients.[34] Long-term steroid therapy does not affect the natural history of ITP; in fact, protracted high-dose steroid ingestion may produce significant thrombocytopenia.

No association has been demonstrated between prednisone treatment and human anomalies. Intrauterine growth retardation has been linked to prednisone use in case studies. Small placentas with decreased glycogen stores have been seen in renal transplant patients on prednisone. The difficulty is separating those complications resulting from medications from complications resulting from the underlying disease process. Theoretically, adrenal insufficiency may be present in the neonate but the risk appears minimal, most likely due to the low fetal levels of active drug.

For patients who either do not respond to steroids or cannot be tapered to sufficiently low doses, splenectomy is the next therapeutic measure. A favorable response to steroids is an indication that the spleen is the primary site of platelet destruction and that the patient will probably benefit from splenectomy. A number of patients who do not respond to steroids will benefit from splenectomy, however. The platelet life span returns to normal (9 days) within 65 hours after splenectomy.[6] The response is clinical not immunological. The antiplatelet antibodies remain!

Overall response to splenectomy varies between 50% and 85%.[34] Splenectomy results in only a 30% response rate in patients with high levels of antiplatelet antibodies and resultant hepatic sequestration and destruction of platelets.[19,34] Approximately 10–12% of patients initially responsive to splenectomy will relapse, the majority within the first year.[19]

Splenectomy is to be considered in all chronic forms (>6 months' duration) regardless of the site of platelet destruction. The spleen is normally the site of sequestration of 40% of the platelets. Splenectomy is therefore expected to increase circulating platelets, regardless of the principal site of destruction. The major risks associated with splenectomy include infection and bleeding.

During pregnancy, splenectomy should be reserved for patients with purpura in whom steroids fail to improve clinically significant thrombocytopenia. Splenectomy performed during pregnancy has the additional risks of abortion, premature labor, and significant maternal hemorrhage.[33] Splenectomy during pregnancy carries increased maternal morbidity and perinatal mortality rates.[33,38] Elective splenectomy should be avoided in pregnant patients. Therapeutic splenectomy should be performed when indicated, regardless of gestational age.

Immunosuppressive agents (azathioprine, cyclophosphamide, and vinca alkaloids) are reserved for patients refractory to combined steroids and splenectomy. These agents are effective in only about one-third of refractory patients treated and may require two months before their effect is fully realized.[33] Data on immunosuppressive agents in treatment of ITP during pregnancy are minimal. The greatest experience with immunosuppression during pregnancy has been with organ transplant patients. A recent review of renal transplant patients demonstrated no adverse effect on fetal development in patients treated with cyclophosphamide or azathioprine in doses to 1.5 mg/kg/day.[18] The experience with vinca alkaloids is even more limited, although four women receiving vinblastine during the first trimester had normal offspring.[4] Patients requiring immunosuppressive agents prior to gestation should probably be continued on them. There is little indication for initiation of such therapy in the first trimester, however.

Recent advances in the managements of ITP have incorporated high-dose parenteral immunoglobulins (0.4 g/kg/d x 4 days).[32] The mechanism of remission with this therapy is still undetermined but is most likely secondary to overwhelming the reticuloendothelial system's ability to catabolize IgG. Pregnant patients undergoing immunoglobulin therapy have demonstrated rapid responses in maternal platelet counts.[49,62,83,88] Data currently available do not appear to support significant intrapartum benefit from such therapy. High-dose immunoglobulin therapy should be reserved for cases of unremitting, life-threatening maternal thrombocytopenia or in the emergent preoperative management of such patients.

Prophylactic platelet transfusions only increase the likelihood of additional antiplatelet antibodies and should be reserved for acute perioperative management or management of severe maternal hemorrhage.

Perinatal Considerations. The placenta facilitates transport of maternal IgG into the fetal circulation. The transport of maternal autoantibodies sets the stage for destruction of fetal platelets, with the potential for significant perinatal morbidity and mortality.

Perinatal mortality is between 10% and 15% in those pregnancies complicated by ITP.[18,33,46,64,77] The most common complication is intracranial hemorrhage (ICH).[33,64,77] The incidence of intrauterine demise in pregnancies complicated by ITP is significant. About 50% of the perinatal mortality occurs prior to the onset of labor.[76] Significant neonatal bleeding does not occur if the fetal platelet count is above 50,000/cu mm. Serious bleeds occur in 28% and mild bleeds in 21% of fetuses with platelet counts below 50,000/cu mm. Mild bleeds also occur in 21% of neonates with counts between 50,000 and 100,000/cu mm.[76] Thus a perinatal platelet count of 50,000/cu mm is the critical value for obstetrical decisions.

Perinatal Thrombocytopenia. The overall incidence of neonatal thrombocytopenia is 33–70% in pregnancies complicated by ITP. The nadir of neonatal platelet counts occurs 2–6 days postpartum in affected pregnancies. Although this is relevant for the neonatologist, it is the intrapartum fetal status that counts in obstetrical management decisions. The overall incidence of intrapartum fetal thrombocytopenia of less than 50,000 platelets/cu mm is about 24%. There is poor correlation between maternal and infant platelet counts.[77] Management protocols based solely on maternal platelet count overdiagnose fetal thrombocytopenia in 72% of cases and underdiagnose it in 26% (Table 30-15). The percentage of thrombocytopenic infants is roughly the same whether the maternal platelet count is above or below 100,000/cu mm (Table 30-15).

The incidence of neonatal thrombocytopenia correlates with the severity of maternal disease. Mothers requiring no therapy deliver infants with neonatal thrombocytopenia about 10% of the time, whereas infants born to splenectomized mothers have a 50% incidence of thrombocytopenia at birth.[77] However, perinatal management cannot be based on these observations.

Both platelet-bound antibody (PA-IgG) and circulating unbound antiplatelet antibody (C-IgG) levels are positively correlated with neonatal platelet counts of less than 50,000 (Tables 30-16 and 30-17). Although elevated antibody levels are imperfectly predictive of a thrombocytopenic infant (predictive value of an abnormal test is 33% and 41% for bound and unbound levels, respectively), low levels of PA-IgG are predictive of a fetus with a platelet count greater than 50,000 (96% predictive value negative). This screening test may prove to be very important, especially in splenectomized patients. The predictive value of PA-IgG, however, may be altered by maternal steroid ingestion. Corticosteroids decrease PA-IgG with a concomitant increase in circulating unbound antiplatelet antibody.[12] Maternal therapy thus must be considered in utilizing this screening test.

Amniotic fluid IgG levels provide no clinically useful information.[77]

Intrapartum Management. The avoidance of intracranial trauma during vaginal delivery was proposed to decrease the incidence of intracranial hemorrhage in infants with thrombocytopenia. However, basing such therapy on maternal platelet counts would result in unnecessary elective operative deliveries in about 80% and one-quarter of infants allowed vaginal delivery would be thrombocytopenic (Table 30-15).

Intrapartum scalp platelet counts accurately predict fetal/neonatal thrombocytopenia. Absolute numbers are not as important as is establishing that the count is greater or less than 50,000/cu mm. Scalp samples yielding borderline values (40,000–60,000/cu mm) present a

TABLE 30-15. MATERNAL PLATELET COUNTS AND FETAL THROMBOCYTOPENIA

Maternal Platelet Count (per cu mm)	Incidence of Fetal Platelet Count (per cu mm)	
	<50,000	>50,000
<100,000	28%	72%
$n = 39$	$n = 11$	$n = 28$
>100,000	26%	74%
$n = 53$	$n = 14$	$n = 39$
Sensitivity 44%	Predictive value positive 28%	
Specificity 58%	Predictive value negative 74%	

Source: References 35, 43, 46, and 77.

TABLE 30-16. PLATELET ASSOCIATED ANTIPLATELET ANTIBODY LEVELS AND PERINATAL THROMBOCYTOPENIA

	Neonatal Platelet Count	
PA-IgG	**>50,000**	**>50,000**
Increased	33%	67%
$n = 12$	$n = 4$	$n = 8$
Normal	4%	96%
$n = 27$	$n = 1$ *	$n = 26$
TOTAL	13%	87%
$n = 39$	$n = 5$	$n = 34$

Sensitivity 80% Predictive value positive = 33%
Specificity 76% Predictive value negative = 96%
Chi-square = 6.81 ($p < 0.05$)

* Not on steroids
Source: Reference 37.

clinical dilemma. The greatest technical difficulty encountered in fetal scalp sampling is clotting prior to transfer. To date, no complications (including fetal hemorrhage) have been reported in sampled pregnancies.[5,77] Although the most definitive screening mechanism available, fetal scalp platelet sampling requires a sufficiently dilated cervix, ruptured membranes, and a vertex presentation at a station low enough to allow sampling. This technique, while offering significant information for intrapartum management, does not address antepartum or early intrapartum fetal demise, which account for 50% of the perinatal mortality in this population.

All pregnancies complicated by ITP, *whether in remission or active*, should have intrapartum fetal scalp platelet concentrations determined. Having once identified the fetus with significant thrombocytopenia, the question of management by cesarean section arises. The benefits of abdominal delivery have not been established by rigorously controlled studies.[33,43] However, there appears to be adequate justification for the abdominal delivery of a thrombocytopenic (<50,000/cu mm) infant. For example, the incidence of retinal hemorrhage is between 17% and 33% for vaginal deliveries, as compared to between 0 and 2% for cesarean sections.[74] Subarachnoid hemorrhage (venous origin) of limited extent is believed to occur in a significant percentage of term vaginal deliveries. What are the consequences of subjecting a thrombocytopenic infant to central nervous system small vessel damage?[42,92]

Patients recently treated with steroids should receive an initial intrapartum intravenous bolus of 100 mg hydrocortisone followed by 100 mg hydrocortisone every six hours into the puerperium. Patients undergoing operative delivery should receive the same regimen.

Although some authors[9,48] state that, if fetal scalp platelet counts cannot be obtained, abdominal delivery should be proffered if the maternal platelet count is less than 100,000/cu mm or the mother has previously undergone splenectomy for management of ITP, we do not agree with this concept. As discussed above, this management may undertreat a significant portion of thrombocytopenic infants (25–30%). Another approach would be to perform a cesarean on all patients with ITP if fetal platelet counts cannot be obtained. This approach may add significantly to maternal morbidity and mortality. The development of antiplatelet antibody level testing may prove useful in the future management of ITP in pregnancy. At the present time,

TABLE 30-17. CIRCULATING ANTIPLATELET ANTIBODY AND PERINATAL THROMBOCYTOPENIA

	Neonatal platelet count	
Circulating IgG	**<50,000**	**>50,000**
Increased	41%	59%
$n = 17$	$n = 7$	$n = 10$
Normal	11%	89%
$n = 27$	$n = 3$	$n = 24$
TOTAL	23%	77%
	$n = 10$	$n = 34$

Sensitivity 70% Predictive value positive = 41%
Specificity 70% Predictive value negative = 89%
Chi-square = 5.38 ($p < 0.05$)

Source: References 12 and 77.

patients with pregnancies complicated by ITP should continue to be managed in facilities with capabilities for fetal scalp platelet sampling.

Meticulous hemostasis, whether at repair of episiotomies or lacerations or at cesarean delivery, is critical. Platelet infusions should be given to any preoperative antepartum patients with platelet counts less than 50,000/cu mm. The need for platelet infusions in the puerperium should be determined clinically.

Antepartum Fetal Therapy. Even if abdominal delivery proves efficacious in reduction of neonatal mortality, 50% of the perinatal mortality associated with autoimmune thrombocytopenia occurs prior to labor.

Although some clinicians advocate the antepartum use of steroids that readily cross the placenta (betamethasone, dexamethasone) to treat the fetus, no adequately controlled clinical trials exist to support such therapy. For pregnancies complicated by autoimmune thrombocytopenic purpura that is steroid dependent, a switch to betamethasone or dexamethasone during the latter weeks appears theoretically justified, especially in pregnancies with initially high PA-IgG levels and subsequent elevation of unbound antibody levels after initiation of steroid therapy. The benefits and risks associated with a short course of steroids at term in pregnancies with non-steroid-dependent maternal ITP are unknown at the present time.

Review of the literature does reveal a decrease in the incidence of perinatal thrombocytopenia, although this decrease is not statistically significant (Table 30-18). The majority of the patients in these reviewed pregnancies were treated with prednisone, which is known for low fetal to maternal plasma levels. Future considerations and studies should be directed toward fetal antepartum therapy with betamethasone or dexamethasone.

High-dose immunoglobulin therapy has proved useful for the acute management of severely thrombocytopenic patients, both pregnant and nonpregnant. However, mothers who respond rapidly may still deliver thrombocytopenic infants.[2,49,62] Therefore, the initial data are not suggestive of fetal benefit. We recommend that high-dose immunoglobulin therapy be based on maternal indications alone until further data are available.

Conclusion. Primary autoimmune ITP presents a significant risk to mother and fetus. Maternal management should be based on established treatments used in the nonpregnant state.

Pregnancies complicated by maternal ITP should be managed in facilities with capabilities to obtain fetal scalp platelet counts. Intrapartum management should include measurements of fetal platelet counts. Fetuses with platelet counts below 50,000/cu mm have a 25–30% incidence of significant hemorrhage. Vaginal delivery may be afforded to those infants with counts above 50,000/cu mm.

A significant proportion of the perinatal mortality occurs prior to the onset of labor. Maternal platelet-associated antiplatelet antibody levels appear to be the best antepartum screening parameter.

Secondary ITP is managed according to the underlying disease process.

Thrombotic Thrombocytopenic Purpura. Thrombotic thrombocytopenic purpura (TTP) is a rare disorder. Fewer than 400 cases are reported. The incidence is higher in females than in males, with a predominance in patients 10–40 years of age. Approximately 30 cases have been reported with concomitant pregnancy.

The etiology of TTP is unknown, and the disorder probably results from numerous un-

TABLE 30-18. MATERNAL STEROIDS AND NEONATAL THROMBOCYTOPENIA

	Neonatal Platelet Count	
	<50,000	>50,000
Maternal steroids	19%	81%
$n = 52$	$n = 10$	$n = 42$
No maternal steroids	38%	62%
$n = 45$	$n = 15$	$n = 25$

Chi square = 3.76 ($0.05 < p < 0.10$)

Source: References 35, 43, 46, and 77.

derlying mechanisms. TTP presents with a pentad of findings. Of these, purpura, microangiopathic hemolytic anemia, and transient neurological abnormalities are always present and renal disease and fever are often encountered.

The underlying pathophysiology of TTP is either primary endothelial damage with resultant platelet thrombus formation, microangiopathic hemolytic anemia and end-organ damage, or platelet thrombus formation resulting from either a stimulus or disruption of normal antiaggregation factors that leads to the formation of platelet aggregates.[61] Such aggregates may collect in the microcirculation with resultant endothelial and end-organ damage.

Histological evaluation (usually by gingival biopsy) in patients with TTP demonstates hyaline microthrombi occlusion of the arterioles and capillaries. Such lesions are not pathognomonic, but merely consistent with the diagnosis of TTP.

The outlook for a pregnancy complicated by TTP is guarded for both mother and fetus.[50] The perinatal salvage rate is not much higher than 30%, although recent case reports have demonstrated a more favorable prognosis.

The clinical presentation of TTP in pregnancy significantly overlaps that of eclampsia/preeclampsia. The presentation of microaggregates of platelets, hemolytic anemia, and end-organ disease in severe preeclamptics has been documented by many authors (see Chapter 32). When acute preeclampsia/eclampsia is managed as TTP, the maternal mortality rate is over 80%, far in excess of that seen in preeclampsia/eclampsia.[75] Because of the increased mortality associated with treating preeclampsia/eclampsia as TTP, we continue to treat patients with such clinical presentations as severe pre-eclamptics, with delivery effected by appropriate means.

If the occasional patient presents with no stigmata of preeclampsia/eclampsia, the diagnosis of TTP syndrome may be made by exclusion. Management is empirical. Early institution of plasma infusion and/or exchange transfusion may result in marked improvement.

Antiplatelet drugs (ASA, dipramidole, and sulfinpyrazone) are also used. These drugs preferentially inhibit thromboxane A_2 (TXA_2) synthesis. Although this inhibition has a beneficial effect, theoretically they may also inhibit an already deficient mechanism for prostaglandin I_2 (PGI_2). The potential availability of synthetic PGI_2 for infusion may dramatically alter the course of this often fatal disorder.

COAGULATION ABNORMALITIES IN PREGNANCY

The plasma protein factors involved in the coagulation cascade (Fig. 30-4) are all altered during pregnancy. Fibrinogen levels increase by 50%, to levels averaging 450 mg/dl. Factors XI and XIII decrease during pregnancy, to levels approximately 50–70% of nonpregnant levels. All other protein coagulation factors increase during gestation. Antithrombin III levels have been previously described as being decreased in pregnancy.[36] Recent data using a sensitive plasma-based assay revealed no significant changes in plasma antithrombin III levels throughout the course of normal pregnancy or in the early puerperium.[87]

Coagulation defects complicating pregnancy may result from either acquired or inherited disorders.

Inherited Coagulation Defects

Von Willebrand's disease, which accounts for 10% of all inheritable coagulation disorders, is the most common clinically significant disorder encountered in the pregnant patient. This disease is transmitted as an autosomal dominant. The severity of symptoms varies among affected family members. The disorder may present with epistaxis, menorrhagia, ecchymosis, and significant post-traumatic or postoperative hemorrhage. The prolonged bleeding time associated with von Willebrand's disease sets it apart from other hemophilia-like diseases. Other laboratory findings are decreased platelet agglutination and decreased Factor VIII levels (both procoagulant and antigenic activities).

With the exception of increased postpartum hemorrhage, perinatal and maternal outcomes are not altered. Measurement of Factor VIII levels during early parturition identifies patients requiring intrapartum prophylaxis. Factor VIII levels exceeding 30% of nonpregnant normals do not require therapy, provided a significant bleeding/consumptive complication does not occur (abruptio placentae, placenta previa, operative mishap, lacerations, etc.).

Management of intrapartum or postpartum hemorrhage requires either cryoprecipitate or plasma transfusion. Both correct Factor VIII deficiency and the prolonged bleeding time. Factor VIII concentrates (antihemophiliac factor [AHF]) have no effect on the prolonged bleeding time. The correction of the bleeding time by plasma lasts less than 12 hours after

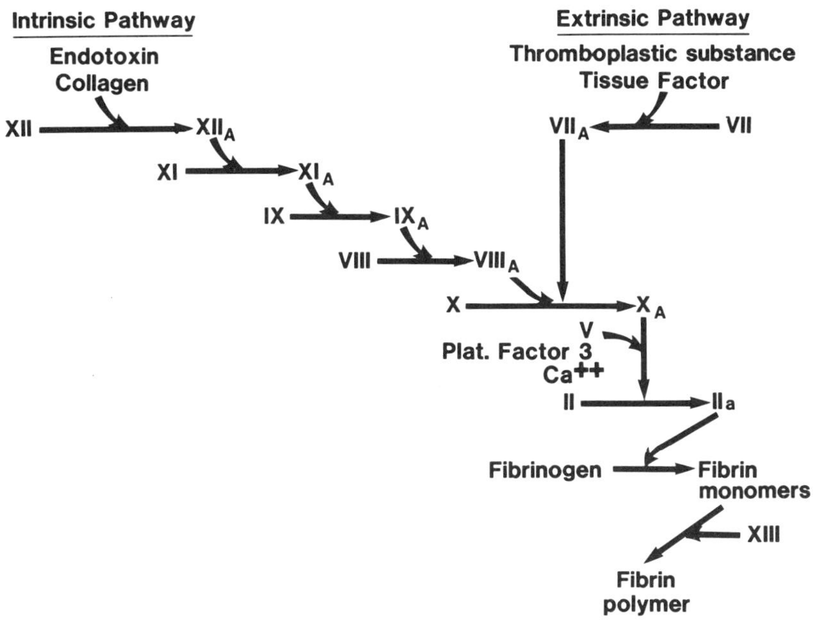

Figure 30-4. Coagulation cascade.

transfusion. Factor VIII correction, however, is evident for a much longer interval.

Transfusion of plasma into a patient with von Willebrand's disease results in production of new Factor VIII. For maintenance of Factor VIII levels, daily transfusion is used (once for intrapartum prophylaxis and continued for 3–5 days for management of intrapartum/postpartum hemorrhage). The quantity of plasma (cryoprecipitate) is determined from the response to the initial transfusion. If correction of bleeding time is also required, a twice-daily infusion schedule should be used.[36]

Hemophilia A (classic hemophilia, Factor VIII) and *Hemophilia B* (Christmas Factor, Factor IX) are inherited as sex-linked recessives. In the nonpregnant state, post-traumatic or postoperative hemorrhage may be expected in 10–30% of carrier females. The significant rises in Factors VIII and IX during gestation protect the majority of these patients. Management of bleeding episodes associated with either type of hemophilia utilizes cryoprecipitate or the appropriate factor concentrate.

Although the majority of female carriers are unaffected, identification is important in anticipation of possible hemorrhagic complications and for genetic counseling. Abnormalities of the antigen to procoagulant activities for Factor VIII are diagnostic for carriers of Hemophilia A.[18,36] Hemophilia B carriers may be more difficult to identify.[36]

Although hereditary deficiencies of Factor XI and XIII are extremely rare, the physiological decrease of these factors during normal gestation may potentiate clinical manifestations. Therapy should be based on proper replacement.

Acquired Disorders—Circulating Anticoagulants

Any patient presenting with an acute bleeding diathesis, abnormal coagulation studies, and no previous history of a bleeding disorder should be evaluated for a circulating anticoagulant. An abnormal mixed plasma coagulation test (1:1 normal to patient) is diagnostic of such anticoagulants.

The most common circulating inhibitors involve inhibitors to Factor VIII. Such inhibitors have been described in collagen-vascular diseases, ulcerative colitis, Hemophilia A, and in the puerperium.[71] Clinical presentation is similar to severe Hemophilia A, but hemorrhage into tissues and ecchymosis is common with the inhibitor. Patients with pregnancy-associated Factor VIII anticoagulant usually present between 2 and 4 months postpartum but can present up to one year postpartum.[70]

Patients with systemic lupus erythematosus (SLE) have a 5–10% incidence of circulating anticoagulants, evidenced by a prolonged activated partial thromboplastin time (aPTT). The majority of these patients do not have significant bleeding tendencies. Patients with lupus anticoagulant have a significantly increased incidence of perinatal mortality. Interestingly, thrombotic rather than hemorrhagic events are the major complicating factors in such pregnancies, with placental thromboses the predominant cause of fetal death.[47] Patients with SLE should be screened for the circulating anticoagulant. Therapy with long-term glucocorticoids and aspirin has been demonstrated to improve perinatal outcome.[47] Intrapartum and postpartum prophylaxis against thromboembolic events should be considered for these patients.

The management of the pregnant or puerperal patient with a circulating anticoagulant should involve a hematologist knowledgeable in the coagulation changes associated with pregnancy. The basic principles of therapy include the following: (1) administration of inhibited factor, (2) removal of inhibitor (plasmaphoresis), (3) bypass site of inhibited factor (prothrombin complexes), and (4) suppression of inhibitor synthesis (immunosuppressive agents, steroids).[70]

THROMBOEMBOLIC DISORDERS IN PREGNANCY

Pathogenesis

The three predisposing factors associated with thromboembolic disorders were initially described by Virchow in 1856 and were subsequently designated "Virchow's Triad." The triad is blood hypercoagulability, venous stasis of blood, and damage or interruption of vein wall integrity. The first two components of Virchow's Triad are known physiological alterations during normal pregnancy. Damage to venous intimal cells can be expected from the trauma of either spontaneous or operative delivery.

The coagulation cascade is demonstrated in Fig. 30-4. The final common pathway of both the extrinsic and intrinsic systems is activation of factor X. Fibrin monomers, formed by the action of activated factor X_A on fibrinogen, subsequently polymerize and precipitate. During pregnancy, all trace protein coagulation factors except factors XI and XIII increase. The naturally occurring circulating coagulation inhibitor antithrombin III (heparin cofactor) has been reported to decrease[36] and remain unchanged[87] during normal pregnancy. Changes in the fibrinolytic activity during gestation are also debatable.[24,36]

Venous stasis of the lower extremities increases gradually throughout gestation with a rapid increase in stasis noted at parturition.[13] Factors implicated include mechanical obstruction resulting from the gravid uterus and decreased venous tone[52] resulting from hormonal effects on vascular smooth muscles. Decreased venous tone may also be responsible for the increased incidence of venous varicosities during pregnancy.

Parturition carries the additional risks of (1) increased coagulability due to release of tissue thromboplastin at the time of placental separation; (2) increased stasis due to engagement of the fetal head, patient positioning, and/or immobilization; and (3) damage to veins secondary to spontaneous delivery or operative delivery.

Pulmonary embolism most often results from dislodgement of thrombi from the lower extremities. Fully 95% of pulmonary emboli in nonpregnant patients result from thrombi in the deep veins of the lower extremities, with the majority originating in the proximal veins.[81] About 25% of antepartum patients with deep venous thrombosis in the lower extremities who are not anticoagulated develop pulmonary emboli.[85] The majority of patients presenting with antepartum and puerperal pulmonary emboli probably have previously undiagnosed deep venous thrombophlebitis.

Incidence

The incidence of thromboembolic disorders associated with pregnancy is 0.1–12 per 1000 pregnancies.[1,8,18,40,59] Not all studies separate superficial from deep venous thrombosis. The majority of the studies use only clinical criteria for the diagnosis of thrombosis. The poor reliability of clinical parameters is well known.

In studies using objective diagnostic criteria, the incidence of antepartum deep venous thrombosis is 0.13[40] to 0.78[8] per 1000. Although predisposing factors are described for the antepartum patient, her risk of developing thrombosis is not significantly increased over nonpregnant women on oral contraceptives. Whether the recurrence risk is greater in the antepartum patient with a remote history of a thromboembolic disorder cannot be determined from the literature. As in the nonpregnant patient, there appears to be a predisposition for thrombosis in patients with blood type A.[8]

Thrombosis is significantly increased in the postpartum patient with the ratio of postpartum to antepartum thrombosis being 3:1 to 6:1.[1,59,84] The increased risk evidenced in the puerperal patient is dependent on method of delivery, the existence of major obstetrical complications, and the use of blood transfusions. About one-quarter of patients presenting with puerperal deep venous thrombosis have an obstetrical complication.[1]

Pulmonary embolism associated with pregnancy is a potentially catastrophic but very rare event. However, with improvement in the management of other life-threatening events such as hemorrhage, sepsis, and preeclampsia, it has become a major cause of maternal morbidity and mortality. In Britain, pulmonary embolism is the leading cause of maternal death.[18] A maternal death resulting from pulmonary embolism occurs once in 1500–2500 cesarean deliveries.[18] Arro and Juergens found the overall incidence of pulmonary embolism to be 1:2488 pregnancies with an antepartum incidence of 1:10,779 (3 patients) and a postdelivery incidence of 1:3233 (10 patients).[1]

Diagnosis—Clinical Presentation and Diagnostic Procedures

Superficial Thrombophlebitis. Superficial thrombophlebitis is relatively easy to diagnose clinically. The thrombosed vein is palpable as a tender cord beneath the skin. Often there is a surrounding area of inflammation and/or erythema.

Deep Venous Thrombophlebitis. Clinical suspicion of deep venous thrombophlebitis (DVT) is usually aroused by the symptoms and physical findings described in Table 30-19. The error in diagnosis is as high as 50%.[8,40,41,70] The commonly reported presenting signs and symptoms have poor predictive value (see Table 30-19). If objective studies are performed on all clinically suspicious patients, only 2 of 17 (12%) patients presenting antepartum and 9 of 12 (75%) patients presenting postpartum have objective evidence of DVT.[40] Thus, although the often cited clinical signs and symptoms of DVT are sensitive for deep thrombosis, they are overpredictive. The left lower extremity is most often involved in patients presenting with antepartum DVT.[1,8] This phenomenon is believed to be secondary to crossing of the left common iliac vein by the common iliac artery. Puerperal DVT has no predilection for either lower extremity.

TABLE 30-19. DIAGNOSTIC ACCURACY OF PHYSICAL SIGNS OF DVT

Sign	False Positive* (%)	True Positive* (%)
Ankle edema	48	40
Difference in calf circumference	11	35
Leg tenderness	29	62
Homans' sign	16	42
Local hyperthermia	13	33
Palpable thrombi	2	10

* False- and true-positive values are in comparison with results of contrast venography.

Source: Modified from Richards, K., Armstrong, J., Tikoff, G., Hershgold, E., Booth, J., and Rampton, J.: Noninvasive diagnosis of deep venous thrombosis. *Arch. Int. Med.* **136:**1091–1096, 1976.

Objective studies include radionucleotide studies (^{125}I fibrinogen), impedance plethysmography (IPG), Doppler flow studies, thermography, and the venogram.

^{125}I fibrinogen scanning is accurate in detecting calf and lower thigh thrombosis but is inaccurate in documenting proximal or pelvic vein thrombosis. It is contraindicted in pregnancy or during breast-feeding. It can be a valuable diagnostic test in the non-breast-feeding puerperal patient.

Impedance plethysmography (IPG) is accurate in the diagnosis of proximal and pelvic thrombosis, provided that the thrombosis is large enough to impede venous return. This procedure is based on the relationship of blood volume to electrical impedance within the calf. With the patient in a left pelvic tilt position, a pneumatic cuff is applied to the involved thigh and inflated to a pressure of 45 cm H_20. This allows venous blood to collect within the calf. Electrodes with a fixed current are then applied. Sudden release of the cuff allows drainage of the venous system, provided that no venous occlusion exists. The sudden change in blood volume produces a corresponding change in calf impedance and thus in measured voltage in accordance with Ohm's law ($V = IR$). Proximal thrombosis retards the venous drainage. Abnormal results are determined by plotting the initial increase in voltage against the rate of return. IPG is not useful in suspected thrombosis of calf veins. False positive tests may be obtained in tense patients, in pregnant patients lying supine with resultant venous occlusion, and in conditions resulting in decreased venous return (e.g., pericarditis, cardiac failure).

Doppler flow studies are sensitive indicators of proximal thrombosis but require subjective evaluation by a skilled interpreter. In an appropriately staffed vascular laboratory, they can be extremely useful.

Venography, although potentially the most definitive procedure, has inherent disadvantages. It is invasive, uncomfortable and costly, and carries the risk of dye reactions and postinjection thrombophlebitis. It can be difficult to obtain adequate studies, especially of the external iliac and common iliac veins, sometimes necessitating femoral venography for definitive studies. The internal iliac system, which may be the site of major thrombosis in the postcesarean patient, is not visualized by routine venography.

In summary, impedance plethysmography or Doppler flow studies should be used in all patients suspected of having proximal venous thrombosis. Radionucleotide studies should not be used in the antepartum or breast-feeding postpartum patient. Venography should be reserved for patients in whom a definitive diagnosis cannot be obtained by IPG or Doppler studies and in whom the risk of anticoagulation therapy outweighs the cost and risk of the procedure. The importance of obtaining objective evidence prior to initiation of long-term therapy is demonstrated by the poor predictive value of the clinical criteria (especially in the antepartum patient) and the potential adverse side effects of therapy.

Pulmonary Embolism

As with deep venous thrombosis, there are no specific or pathognomonic symptoms or physical findings. Chest pain is a common initial presenting symptom. In nonpregnant patients with pulmonary embolism, the vast majority present with dyspnea or tachypnea (20 respirations per minute). Dyspnea, hemoptysis, or pleuritic pain are present in nearly all patients. Tachycardia occurs in about 50% of patients.[81]

Arterial blood gases may be useful if the PaO_2 is low; however, a small pulmonary embolism may present with a PaO_2 greater than 80 mmHg. The chest x-ray may be important for its negative findings in an acutely dyspneic patient. However, consolidation, pleural effusion, or elevated diaphragm occur in a majority of patients with acute pulmonary embolism [81]

The ECG is highly sensitive but has low specificity. The most common changes are nonspecific ST and/or T wave changes and axis changes. Most nonpregnant patients with acute pulmonary embolism present with abnormal ECGs.[81]

The ventilation/perfusion lung scan (V/Q scan) is highly suggestive of pulmonary embolism if the perfusion component demonstrates defects in regions of normal ventilation. Such scans should be employed in any patient in whom pulmonary embolism is suspected. In the antepartum patient, the potential radiation effects to the fetus are minimal and are far outweighed by decisions for maternal/fetal management and therapy.

Pulmonary arteriography should be reserved for patients in whom satisfactory ventilation/perfusion scans cannot be obtained or properly interpreted (chronic pulmonary disease or cardiac disease). Serious morbidity occurs in 2–4% of patients undergoing arteriography.

Therapy of Acute Thromboembolic Events

General Concepts. Prevention of pulmonary emboli (either initial episodes or recurrence) and reduction of long- and short-term morbidity associated with venous obstruction are the goals of treatment of thromboembolic disorders. Although these goals could readily be realized by removal of the formed thrombus, thrombolytic therapy is not used in the majority of patients presenting with thromboembolic disorders. Anticoagulant therapy is aimed at preventing the progression of the thrombus formation. To provide prophylaxis against embolic complications, anticoagulated patients should be placed at bedrest to allow for fixation of the previously formed thrombus. The patient's own fibrinolytic activity and the recanalization of obstructed veins and formation of collaterals reduce the incidence of postphlebitic syndrome. Postphlebitic syndrome is more common in heparinized patients suffering proximal as compared to calf thrombi.

Anticoagulation may be approached by (1) interference with fibrin formation (heparin, coumadin), (2) interference with platelet function (ASA, etc.), and (3) acceleration of lysis of formed thrombus. Heparin and coumadin are the fundamental therapeutic modalities. Heparin is the drug of choice in the acute setting and for long-term management of antepartum patients.

Heparin. Heparin is a negatively charged mucopolysaccharide with a molecular weight of approximately 20,000. Heparin obtains its anticoagulation properties from its ability to combine with antithrombin III and thus to increase the binding of this alpha$_2$ globulin to thrombin with inhibition of the formation of fibrin monomers. Heparin also inhibits the activation of factor IX (Christmas factor).

Heparin infusion adequate to prevent formation of a thrombus results in a Lee White clotting time of 2.5 times normal. Adequate anticoagulation is obtained with circulating heparin levels of 0.3 units/ml, which usually correspond with aPTT and thrombin clotting time (TCT) values 1.5–2.5 times control values.

The half-life of infused heparin is approximately 60 minutes.[23] Approximately 20% of an infused heparin dose is recovered from the urine, with the hepatic enzymes most likely degrading the remainder. Heparin has other pharmacological effects, including release of lipoprotein lipase from the endothelium and interference with aldosterone release.

Heparin must be given either intravenously or subcutaneously. Intramuscular injections should never be used because of the risk of hematoma formation.

The greatest risk associated with heparin is hemorrage, with incidences cited between 4% and 33%.[73] The risk of hemorrhage is increased if antiplatelet medications are being given, if coagulation defects exist, and if intermittent rather than continuous intravenous heparin is given.[73] Heparin levels greater than 0.6 units/ml are associated with significant hemorrhage. Such levels are most likely to occur in patients treated with intermittent intravenous heparin. Although intermittent and continuous infusions have been found to be equally efficacious in achieving therapeutic results, the risk of major hemorrhage is increased seven times in patients treated with intermittent boluses.[73]

Mild bleeding while on heparin therapy usually necessitates interruption or decreasing heparin dosages. For patients demonstrating life-threatening hemorrhage or patients undergoing emergency surgery, heparin may be reversed by protamine sulfate. The full neutralizing dose of protaimine sulfate is 1 mg per 100 units of heparin. Care must be taken to consider the half-life of heparin when attempting to reverse its effects with protamine, because protamine sulfate excess can produce anticoagulation. Protamine must be slowly infused over 20–30 minutes to avoid hypotensive responses.

Monitoring of aPTT or similar clotting studies is not efficacious in preventing hemorrhagic complications. Such monitoring should be used to demonstrate that adequate anticoagulation has been achieved.[68]

Subcutaneous heparin is variably absorbed and should not be used in the acute management of thromboembolic disorders. It can play a significant role, however, in the long-term and prophylactic management of patients, especially the antepartum patient.

In addition to hemorrhage, heparin can result in alopecia, allergic reactions, thrombocytopenia, and osteoporosis. Thrombocytopenia presents with decreasing platelet counts three to eight days after initiation of therapy with a nadir two to three days later. Recovery of platelet counts begins within five days.[81] The etiology of the thrombocytopenia is undetermined. Significant thrombocytopenia may necessitate discontinuation of heparin therapy. Mild episodes may be observed while heparin therapy is continued.

Bone demineralization resulting from prolonged heparin therapy is dose related and occurs in all patients treated for prolonged intervals (>10 weeks).[17,29,89] It is unknown if the demineralization reverses after discontinuation of therapy.[17] The precise mechanism of this side effect is unknown. Heparin is known to complex with calcium ions and also may potentiate parathyroid hormone activity.

Coumadin. Although heparin is a direct anticoagulant with in vivo and in vitro activity, coumadin indirectly affects the coagulation cascade by decreasing hepatic production of the coagulation factors. It is utilized in long-term management of thromboembolic disorders, after initial therapy of the acute episode with heparin. Coumadin is a vitamin K antagonist that inhibits the synthesis of vitamin K-dependent clotting factors (II, VII, IX, X). Due to the relatively long half-lives of factors II, IX, and X, coumadin must be given over a period of days before an adequate state of anticoagulation is obtained.

Coumadin is metabolized in the liver and has a half-life of approximately four hours.[84] Unlike heparin which can be rapidly reversed with protamine, coumadin requires infusion of clotting factors II, VII, IX, and X for rapid reversal.

Initial dosages of coumadin are 5–10 mg/day without a loading dose. Coumadin is routinely begun after the acute thrombus has organized (4 days).

Coumadin crosses the placenta, whereas heparin does not. Hall and coworkers,[28] in a review of 418 pregnancies in which coumadin derivatives were used, found that one-sixth of the liveborn infants were abnormal, one-sixth of the pregnancies resulted in stillbirth or abortion, and two-thirds were apparently normal. Warfarin embryopathy results from administration of coumadin derivatives during the first trimester (specifically between the sixth and ninth weeks), with the most persistent anomalies being nasal hypoplasia and epiphyseal stippling.[23,28] Exposure to coumadin derivatives in the second and third trimesters results in a 3% incidence of central nervous system anomalies.[28] Warfarin has not been detected in breast milk or the plasma of breast-feeding infants.[18] Biscoumacetate has been demonstrated in the breast milk and should be avoided in the breast-feeding patient.[18]

Aspirin. Antiplatelet medications such as aspirin derive their therapeutic activity from inhibition of prostaglandin synthesis. Considering the importance of prostaglandins in the regulation of uterine blood flow, myometrial activity, patency of the fetal ductus arteriosus, and fetal/neonatal pulmonary vascular resistance, it is currently recognized that use of aspirin in pregnancy should be reserved for the rare patient in which traditional therapy is contraindicated.

Fibrinolysis. Fibrinolytic therapy has been described in antepartum patients presenting with pulmonary emboli and/or DVT. In pulmonary emboli, such therapy is known to return pulmonary function to normal, whereas anticoagulation does not.[79] Streptokinase is superior to heparin in the management of the nonpregnant patient with a proximal venous thrombosis of less than one week's duration.[22] Streptokinase minimally crosses the placenta with no fibrinolytic effects evidenced in the fetus.[51,65]

Streptokinase cannot be utilized within 10 days of surgery or delivery. Impending delivery (within 10 days of therapy) is a major contraindication to its use.[18]

Management—Deep Venous Thrombophlebitis. Diagnosis of deep venous thrombophlebitis mandates immediate initiation of bedrest and anticoagulation. The affected limb should be elevated, preferably with the patient in the Trendelenburg position. This avoids venous obstruction due to acute angulation that often occurs when only the involved extremity is elevated by a pillow. Bedrest should continue until symptoms have begun to resolve, adequate anticoagulation has been obtained for at least two days, and there is no evidence of recurrence or progression of the thrombus.

Anticoagulation should be begun with intravenous (preferably continuous) heparin. Since it is known that higher heparin levels are required to stop the propagation of thrombus than are required to inhibit thrombus initiation, a loading dose of 5000 units (or 70 units/kg) intravenously is appropriate in patients presenting with proximal thromboembolism.

Continuous intravenous heparin should be based on laboratory values, preferably heparin levels (0.3 units/ml) or, if these are unavailable, activated PTT (1.5–2 times control) Fifteen to 20 μ/kg/hr should be given as an initial dose and adjusted in accordance with the laboratory values. Laboratory studies should be obtained every 4–6 hours until stabilization of dose has occurred. Once the active process and propagation of the thrombotic event have arrested, the circulating levels of thrombin should be expected to be decreased with resultant increased half-life and activity of heparin, possibly resulting in lowered requirements for heparin. The monitoring of the aPTT is to assure adequate anticoagulation. Such monitoring does not decrease the incidence of hemorrhagic complications associated with heparin therapy.[68] Heparin therapy and full anticoagulation, as evidenced by a therapeutically prolonged aPTT, should be continued for 7–10 days.

In the puerperal patient, coumadin therapy may begin on the second or third day of anticoagulation. The required antithrombotic effects may not be seen until six days after therapy has begun. Heparinization and full anticoagulation should continue during early coumadin treatment. Initial dosages of coumadin should be in the range of 5–10 mg daily (preferably in the evening), with alterations to maintain the PT 1.5–2 times the control value. Loading doses are not recommended, because the rates of decline in the activities of factors II, IX, and X are not increased with a loading dose.[81] Avoidance of a loading dose bypasses the complication of excessive anticoagulation due to the dose-dependent decline in factor VII activity. At the conclusion of the "dual anticoagulation" interval, heparin may be discontinued, provided adequate coumadin anticoagulation is evidenced by a prolonged PT. The literature reveals no consensus as to the duration of anticoagulation after an acute postpartum thrombophlebitis. Individualization is necessary. The patient with a deep venous thrombosis occurring after an operative delivery, hemorrhage, and numerous transfusions presents a different long-term risk than does the patient with a history of previous thromboembolic event with a proximal thrombosis after uncomplicated vaginal delivery. A conservative recommendation is that patients developing acute puerperal thrombophlebitis be anticoagulated for a total of three months. After daily PT evaluations have established a steady-state condition, the PT should be measured at least weekly for a month, then at least monthly. All such patients should be warned and informed of the possible serious drug interactions with the medications listed in Table 30-20.

The *acute* management of antepartum DVT differs little from that of the nonpregnant patient. The importance of establishing a definitive diagnosis with objective studies due to the poor predictive value of clinical evaluation has

TABLE 30-20. WARFARIN-DRUG INTERACTIONS

Drugs that Increase Warfarin Effect	Drugs that Decrease Warfarin Effect
Allopurinol	Barbiturates
Anabolic steroids	Carbamazepine
Chloral hydrate	Cholestyramine
Chloramphenicol	Contraceptives, oral
Cimetidine	Glutethimide
Clofibrate	Griseofulvin
Disulfiram	Rifampin
Metronidazole	
Miconazole	
Nalidixic acid	
Phenylbutazone	
Quinidine, quinine	
Salicylates (>2 g/day)	
Sulfinpyrazone	
Sulfonamides	
Thyroid hormones	
Triclofos sodium	
Vitamin E	

Source: Reference 41.

been stressed above. The obstetrician's ability to obtain a definitive diagnosis is compromised by the contraindication to radionucleotide studies and the desire to avoid irradiation of the fetus. When one considers the long term risk of anticoagulation both in the present and in possible subsequent pregnancies, a strong argument for definitive diagnosis can be made. The vast majority of deep venous thrombi can now be identified by impedance or Doppler studies. There will remain a rare patient with a calf or thigh thrombosis that necessitates venography (with fetal shielding). The risks of inappropriate long-term anticoagulation outweigh the risk of even venography.

Anticoagulation should begin as described above with an initial loading dose followed preferably by a continuous intravenous infusion. Difficulties can arise in monitoring the effects of heparin in the antepartum patient. The effect of heparin on the most commonly used laboratory test (aPTT) can be modified by the high levels of factor VIII that occur in the pregnant patient, thus giving the appearance of a heparin-resistant state.[36] It has been suggested that this complication may be overcome by using the patient's own pretreatment aPTT as the control, or by use of the thrombin clotting time. If available, the heparin assay provides the most accurate assessment of adequate anticoagulation (heparin level 0.2–0.4 units/ml).

Long-term anticoagulation with warfarin-like medications in the antepartum patient is debatable at best. These medications are contraindicated in the first trimester due to the possibility of warfarin embryopathy. The inability to monitor fetal effects and the apparent risk of intrauterine fetal hemorrhage make their use in the second trimester questionable. Third trimester usage is contraindicated by the inability to reverse fetal effects rapidly during labor, with the potential for significant intra/postpartum hemorrhage. Heparin is the antepartum anticoagulant of choice.

Previous long-term antepartum prophylactic heparin regimens employed either fixed-dose subcutaneous or intermittent intravenous heparin via indwelling catheters. Fixed low-dose heparin is ineffective in preventing recurrent deep venous thrombosis in nonpregnant patients.[30] Intermittent intravenous infusion on an outpatient basis is inconvenient (indwelling catheter placement and maintenance) and has significant potential complications (hemorrhage, infection/sepsis).

In a high-risk, nonpregnant population, a dose-adjusted subcutaneous regimen is as effective as coumadin in preventing recurrence while decreasing the incidence of hemorrhagic complications associated with warfarin.[30] Subcutaneous heparin is administered every 12 hours. The total dose is calculated from the total intravenous heparin dose required to maintain the aPTT at 1.5–2 times the control value. The mid-interval aPTT is again checked after initiation of subcutaneous therapy. The changing of coagulation factor concentrations during the progression of gestation requires close monitoring. Again it must be noted that increasing levels of factor VIII associated with pregnancy influence certain aPTT systems presenting a seemingly heparin-resistant state. Thrombin clotting times or heparin assays should be used in such situations.

Patients presenting with antepartum thromboembolic events should receive secondary prophylaxis for at least three months after the acute event, or until at least one week postdelivery (if fully ambulatory), whichever is the longer interval.

Patients on long-term prophylactic heparin should be continued on heparin prophylaxis during the intrapartum and the immediate postpartum interval.

Management—Pulmonary Embolism. In consideration of the life-threatening nature of pulmonary embolism, therapy should be initiated when sufficient clinical suspension is aroused, without waiting for the results of definitive objective evaluations. Heparin therapy should be initiated with a 10,000 unit bolus followed by continuous intravenous therapy. The bolus achieves rapid anticoagulation and decreases the pulmonary vasoconstriction resulting from the release of amines. The half-life of heparin is decreased in patients with pulmonary emboli as compared to those with deep venous thrombosis.[81] Moderate dosages of heparin have proved adequate in approximately 95% of nonpregnant patients with thrombophlebitis. High-dose therapy which consists of administration of between 2000 and 4000 units/hr (50,000–100,000 units/24 hours) may be preferred.[81,84] Whichever regimen is used, coagulation tests should document adequate anticoagulation (every two to six hours until desired effect, then daily). Heparin levels (0.3–0.4 units/ml), aPTT (1.5–2 times control), or thrombin time (1.5–2 times control) should be obtained. The pregnancy-associated increased levels of factor VIII and the effects such increases have on certain aPTT systems may be especially confusing in the antepartum patient with a pulmonary embolus. Use of thrombin time or heparin levels may be required to determine if a "heparin-resistant" state associated with the pulmonary embolism exists. Subsequent management of the pregnancy-associated pulmonary embolus should continue as described for deep venous thrombophlebitis.

Recurrent emboli despite evidence of adequate anticoagulation may necessitate surgical intervention with interruption of the inferior vena cava. Such emergent procedures in nonpregnant patients are associated with a 30% operative mortality, with ligation apparently having a much higher mortality rate than plication.[81] In addition, postoperative complications are more common in those patients undergoing ligation compared to those undergoing plication.[81] Plication is thus preferred, except in those patients with recurrent septic emboli. Vena caval filters, while eliminating the risk associated with a major operative procedure, carry the risk of migration. Filters should be considered in the acutely ill patient with evidence of recurrent emboli.

In the United States thrombolytic therapy continues to be reserved for patients with massive pulmonary embolism with resultant cardiorespiratory compromise.

Embolectomy is reserved for patients with cardiopulmonary collapse due to massive pulmonary embolism.

Management—Antepartum Patients with a Remote History of Thromboembolic Disorders

Most clinicians agree that patients presenting with a history of pregnancy-associated thromboembolic events should receive prophylaxis in the present pregnancy. The management of those with a history of a thromboembolic disorder not associated with pregnancy is debated. Some clinicians advocate prophylaxis throughout pregnancy and the puerperium. Others use only intrapartum and postpartum prophylaxis. No study delineates the risk of recurrences. In addition, the clinician is often confronted with the previous diagnosis made solely on a clinical basis.

We recommend that patients with a well-documented history of pregnancy-associated thromboembolic events receive prophylaxis with low-dose subcutaneous heparin (5000–

10,000 units every 12 hours) throughout the course of pregnancy and continued one to two weeks postpartum.

Patients with a history of thromboembolic disorders unassociated with pregnancy should receive low-dose heparin prophylaxis intrapartum and during the first postpartum week. Whether to administer prophylaxis during the antepartum period must be based on the clinician's assessment of how firm the previous diagnosis was, how remote was the event, does the patient appear to be at increased risk (e.g., primigravida with history of numerous DVT and/or PE), and consideration of the potential adverse side effects of long-term low-dose heparin.

Use of intrapartum intravenous dextran has both theoretical and clinical support. Dextran does have the potential to produce anaphylactic reactions and should not be used in an unconscious patient or in a patient with a significant potential for an allergic reaction. A physician should be immediately available at the beginning of a dextran infusion. Infusion should begin with a dose of 600 mg/kg during the first three to four hours, then 300 mg/kg/24 hours. Dextran and heparin should not be given simultaneously, because dextran increases the effects of heparin. Dextran prophylaxis should be considered in patients with a remote history of thromboembolic disorders undergoing abdominal delivery.

Puerperal Pelvic Vein Thrombophlebitis (Ovarian Vein Thrombophlebitis and Enigmatic Fever)

The puerperal patient (especially after an operative delivery) is at increased risk for thrombophlebitis originating in the pelvic veins. Such patients present with either acute ovarian vein thrombophlebitis or enigmatic fever.[20]

The diagnosis of pelvic vein thrombophlebitis may be exceptionally difficult. Routine noninvasive studies (Doppler, IPG) and ascending venography offer little, if any, information. Specialized phlebography studies have been used. Extrinsic compression of a ureter on intravenous pyelogram (IVP) is indirect evidence of ovarian vein thrombosis. Computerized tomography may provide additional information.[20] Enigmatic fever will likely continue to be a diagnosis of exclusion.

Therapy should consist of antibiotics and heparinization for a course of 7–10 days. Long-term prophylaxis with anticoagulants is not required in the majority of patients.

Many puerperal patients with pelvic vein thrombophlebitis are diagnosed at exploratory laporotomy (80–85%).[20] Should either of the two described entities be discovered intraoperatively, the question arises as to what, if any, surgical therapy should be undertaken. Most patients respond to anticoagulation. Should operative intervention be selected at the time of intraoperative diagnosis or for patients not responding to conservative medical management, ligation of the involved vessels (without excision) should be undertaken, followed by postoperative anticoagulation and antibiotics. Reproductive abilities may be impaired in patients undergoing ovarian vein or vena cava interruption.[20]

REFERENCES

1. Aaro, L. A. and Juergens J. L.: Thrombophlebitis associated with pregnancy. *Am. J. Obstet. Gynecol.* **109**:1128–1133, 1970.
2. Adderley, R. J., Rogers, P. C., Shaw, D., and Wadsworth, L. D.: High-dose intravenous therapy with immune globulin before delivery for idiopathic thrombocytopenic purpura. *Can. Med. Assoc. J.* **130**:894–896, 1983.
3. Alger, L. S., Golbus, M. S., and Laros, R. K.: Thalassemia and pregnancy: Results of an antenatal screening program. *Am. J. Obstet. Gynecol.* **134**:662–673, 1979.
4. Armstrong, J. G., Dyke, R. W., and Fouts, R. J.: Delivery of a normal infant during the course of oral vinblatine sulfate for Hodgkins disease. *Ann. Intern. Med.* **61**:106–107, 1964.
5. Ayromlooi, J.: A new approach to the management of immunologic thrombocytopenic purpura i pregnancy. *Am. J. Obstet. Gynecol.* **130**:235–236, 1978.
6. Baldini, M.: Idiopathic thrombocytopenic purpura. *N. Engl. J. Med.* **274**:1245–1251, 1966.
7. Beeson, P. and McDermott, W. (Eds.): *Textbook of Medicine*. Philadelphia, W. B. Saunders, 1975.
8. Bergquist, A., Bergquist, D., and Hallbook, T.: Deep vein thrombosis during pregnancy: A prospective study. *Acta Obstet. Gynecol. Scand.* **62**:443–448, 1983.
9. Carloss, H. W., McMillan, R., and Crosby, W. H.: Management of women with immune thrombocytopenic purpura. *JAMA* **244**:2756–2758, 1980.
10. Chararin, I., Rothman, D., Ward, A., and Perry, J.: Folate status and requirement in pregnancy *Br. Med. J.* **2**:390–394, 1968.
11. Charache, S., Scott, J., Niebyl, J., and Bonds, D.: Management of Sickle Cell Disease in Pregnant Patients. *Obstet. Gynecol.* **55**:407–410, 1979.

12. Cines, D. B., Busak, B., Tomaski, A., Mennuti, M., and Schreiber, A. D.: Immune thrombocytopenic purpura and pregnancy. *N. Engl. J. Med.* **306**:826–831, 1982.
13. Clarke-Pearson, D. L. and Jelovsek, F. R.: Alterations of occlusive cuff impedance plethysmography in the ostetrical patient. *Surgery* **89**:594–598, 1981.
14. Cunningham, F. G., Pritchard, J. A., Mason, R., and Chase, G.: Prophylactic transfusions of normal red blood cells during pregnancies complicated by sickle cell hemoglobinopathies. *Am. J. Obstet. Gynecol.* **135**:994–1001, 1979.
15. Cunningham, F. G., Pritchard, J. A., and Mason, R.: Pregnancy and sickle cell hemoglobinopathies: Results with and without prophylactic transfusions. *Obstet. Gynecol.* **62**:419–424, 1983.
16. DeLeevw, N. K. M., Lowestein, L., and Hsieh, Y. S.: Iron deficiency and hydremia in normal pregnancy. *Medicine* **45**:291–315, 1966.
17. deSwiet, M., Dorrington Ward, P., Fidler, J., Horsman, A., Katz, D., Letsky, E., Peacock, M., and Wise, P. H.: Prolonged heparin therapy in pregnancy causes bone demineralization. *Br. J. Obstet. Gynaecol.* **90**:1129–1134. 1983.
18. deSwiet, M. (Ed.): *Medical Disorders in Obstetrical Practice.* Oxford, Blackwell Scientific Publications, 1984.
19. Difino, S. M., Lachant, N. A., Kirshner, J. J., and Gottlieb, A. J.: Adult idiopathic thrombocytopenic purpura: Clinical findings and response to therapy. *Am. J. Med.* **69**:430–442, 1980.
20. Duff, P. and Gibbs, R. S.: Pelvic vein thrombophlebitis: Diagnostic dilemma and therapeutic challenge. *Obstet. Gynecol. Surv.* **38**:365–373, 1983.
21. Doan, C. A., Bouroncle, B. A., and Wiseman, B. K.: Idiopathic and secondary thrombocytopenic purpura: Clinical study and evaluation of 38 cases over a period of 28 years. *Ann. Intern. Med.* **53**:861–876, 1960.
22. Elliot, M. D., Immelman, E. J., Jeffery, P., Benata, S. R., Funstein, M. R., Smith, J. A., Shepstone, B. J., Ferguson, A. D., Jacobs, P., Walker, W., and Louw, J. H.: A comparative randomized trial of heparin versus streptokinase in the treatment of acute proximal venous thrombosis: An interim report of a prospective trial. *Br. J. Surg.* **66**:838–843, 1979.
23. Fillmore, S. J. and McDevitt, E.: Effects of coumadin compound on the fetus. *Ann. Intern. Med.* **73**:731–735, 1970.
24. Fletcher, A. P., Alkjaersig, N. K., and Burstein, R.: The influence of pregnancy upon blood coagulation and plasma fibrinolytic enzyme function. *Am. J. Obstet. Gynecol.* **134**:743–751, 1979.
25. Goodlin, R. C.: Why treat "Physiologic" anemias of pregnancy? *J. Reprod. Med.* **27**:639–646, 1982.
26. Goodman, L. S. and Gilman, A. (Eds.): *The Pharmacological Basis of Therapeutics*, 5th Edition. New York, Macmillan, 1975.
27. Greene, M. F., Frigoletto, F. D., Claster, S., and Rosenthal, D.: Pregnancy and paroxysmal nocturnal hemoglobinuria: Report of a case and review of the literture. *Obstet. Gynecol. Surv.* **38**:591–596, 1983.
28. Hall, J. G., Paul, R. M., and Wilson, K. M.: Maternal and fetal sequelae of anticoagulation during pregnancy. *Am. J. Med.* **68**:122–140, 1980.
29. Howel, R., Fidler, J., Letsky, E., and deSwiet, M.: The risks of antenatal subcutaneous heparin prophylaxis: A controlled study. *Br. J. Obstet. Gynaecol.* **90**:1124–1128, 1983.
30. Hull, R., Delmore, T., and Carter, C., Adjusted subcutaneous heparin versus warfarin sodium in the long-term treatment of venous thrombosis. *N. Engl. J. Med.* **306**:189–194, 1982.
31. Hurd, W. W., Miodovnik, M., and Stys, S. J.: Pregnancy associated with paroxysmal nocturnal hemoglobinuria. *Obstet. Gynecol.* **60**:742–746, 1982.
32. Imbach, P., Barandun, S., d'Apuzzo, V., Baumgartner, C., Hirt, A., Morell, A., Rossi, E. Schöni, Vest, M., and Wagner, H. P.: High-dose intravenous gamma globulin for idiopathic thrombocytopenic purpura in childhood. *Lancet* **1**:1228–1231, 1981.
33. Kagan, R. and Laros, R.: Immune thrombocytopenia. *Clin. Obstet. Gynecol.* **26**:537–546, 1984.
34. Karpatkin, S.: Autoimmune thrombocytopenic purpura. *Blood* **56**:329–343, 1980.
35. Karpatkin, M., Porges, R. F., and Karpatkin, S.: Platelet counts in infants of women with autoimmune thrombocytopenia: Effect of steroid administration to the mother. *N. Engl. J. Med.* **305**:936–938, 1981.
36. Kelton, J. G. and Hirsh, J.: *Medical Complications in Pregnancy*, 2nd Edition. G. N. Burrow and T. F. Ferris (Eds.). Philadelphia, W. B. Saunders, 1982, pp. 169–186.
37. Kelton, J. G., Inwood, M. J., Barr, R. M., Effer, S. B., Hunter, D., Wilson, W. E., Ginsburg, D. A., and Powers, P. J.: The prenatal prediction of thrombocytopenia in infants of mothers with clinically diagnosed immune thrombocytopenia. *Am. J. Obstet. Gynecol.* **144**:449–454, 1982.
38. Kessler, I., Lancet, M., Borenstein, R., Berrebi, A., and Mogilner, B. M.: The obstetrical management of patients with immunologic thrombocytopenic purpura. *Int. J. Gynaecol. Obstet.* **20**:23–28, 1982.
39. Key, T. C., Horger, E. O., Walker, E. M., and Mitchum, E. N.: Automated erythrocytopheresis for sickle cell anemia during pregnancy. *Am. J. Obstet. Gynecol.* **138**:731–737, 1980.
40. Kierkegaard, A.: Incidence and diagnosis of deep vein thrombosis associated with pregnancy. *Acta Obstet. Gynecol. Scand.* **62**:239–243, 1983.
41. Klotz, T. A.: DVT: Diagnostic advances, therapeutic guidelines. *Contemp. OB/GYN* **19**:18–34, 1982.
42. Kryc, J. J. and Corrigan, J. J.: Idiopathic thrombocytopenic purpura during pregnancy: A pediat-

ric viewpoint. *Am. J. Pediatr. Hematol. Oncol.* **5**:21–25, 1983.

43. Laros, R. K. and Kagan, R.: Route of delivery for patients with immune thrombocytopenic purpura. *Am. J. Obstet. Gynecol.* **148**:901–905, 1984.
44. Lehman, G. and Alcoff, J.: Reversible pure red cell hypoplasia in pregnancy. *JAMA* **247**:1170–1171, 1982.
45. Lewis, P. J., Boylan, P., Friedman, L. A., Hensby, C. N., and Downing, I.: Prostacyclin in pregnancy. *Br. Med. J.* **11**:1581–1582, 1980.
46. Logaridis, T. E., Doran, T. A., Scott, J. G., Gare, D. G., and Comtesse, C.: The effect of maternal steroid administration of fetal platelet count in immunologic thrombocytopenic purpura: Management of pregnancy and mode of delivery. *Am. J. Obstet. Gynecol.* **145**:147–151, 1983.
47. Lubbe, W. F., Palmer, S. J., Butler, W. S., and Liggins, G. C.: Fetal survival after prednisone suppression of maternal lupus-anticoagulant. *Lancet* **1**:1361–1368, 1983.
48. Martin, J. N., Morrison, J. C., and Files, J. C.: Autoimmune thrombocytopenic purpura: Current concepts and recommended practices. *Am. J. Obstet. Gynecol.* **150**:86–96, 1984.
49. Mizunuma, H., Takahashi, Y., Taquchi, H., Arai, A., Igarashi, M., Morita, K., Omine, M., and Maekawa, T.: A new approach to idiopathic thrombocytopenic purpura during pregnancy by high dose immunoglobulin G infusion. *Am. J. Obstet. Gynecol.* **148**:218–219, 1984.
50. May, H. V., Harbert, G. M., and Thorton, W. N. J.: Thrombotic thrombocytopenic purpura associated with pregnancy. *Am. J. Obstet. Gynecol.* **126**:452–458, 1976.
51. McTaggart, D. R. and Ingram, T. G.: Massive pulmonary embolism during pregnancy treated with streptokinase. *Med. J. Aust.* **1**:18–20, 1977.
52. McCausland, A. M., Hyman, C., Winsor, T., and Trolter, A. D.: Venous distensibility during pregnancy. *Am. J. Obstet. Gynecol.* **81**:472–479, 1961.
53. Miller, J. M., Horger, E. O., Key, T. C., and Walker, E. M.: Management of sickle hemoglobinopathies in pregnant patients. *Am. J. Obstet. Gynecol.* **141**:237–241, 1981.
54. Morrison, J. and Wiser, W. L.: The use of prophylactic partial exchange transfusion in pregnancies associated with sickle cell hemoglobinopathies. *Obstet. Gynecol.* **48**:516–520, 1976.
55. Morrison, J. C., Schneider, J. M., Whybrew, W. D., Bucovaz, E. T., and Menzel, D. M.: Prophylactic transfusions in pregnant patients with sickle hemoglobinopathies: Benefit versus risk. *Obstet. Gynecol.* **56**:274–280, 1980.
56. Morrison, J. C., Ruvinsky, E. D., and Nicholls, E. T.: Sickling and pregnancy: A worrisome combination. *Contemp. OB/GYN* **18**:125–132, 1981.
57. Morrison, J. C., Blake, P. G., and Reed, C. D.: Therapy for the pregnant patient with sickle hemoglobinopathies: A national focus. *Am. J. Obstet. Gynecol.* **144**:268–269, 1982.
58. Morrison, J. C., Blake, P. G., McCoy, C., Martin, J. N., and Wiser, W. L.: Fetal health assessment in pregnancies complicated by sickle hemoglobinopathies. *Obstet. Gynecol.* **61**:22–24, 1983.
59. Moseley, P. and Kerstein, M. D.: Pregnancy and thrombophlebitis. *Surg. Gynecol. Obstet.* **150**:593–599, 1980.
60. Nagey, D. A., Alawode, N. A., Pupkin, M. J., and Crenshaw, C.: Isovolumetric partial exchange transfusion in the management of sickle cell disease in pregnancy II. Simplified ambulatory technique. *Am. J. Obstet. Gynecol.* **147**:693–696, 1983.
61. Najean, Y., Ardaillou, N., Dresch, C., and Bernard, J.: The platelet destruction site in thrombocytopenic purpuras. *Br. J. Haematol.* **13**:409–426, 1967.
62. Newland, A. C., Boots, M. A., and Patterson, K. G.: Intravenous IgG for autoimmune thrombocytopenia in pregnancy. *N. Engl. J. Med.* **310**:261–262, 1984.
63. Noriega-Guerra, L., Aviles-Miranda, A., de la Cadena, 0. A., Espinosa L. M., Chavez J. P., and Pizzuto J.: Pregnancy in patients with autoimmune thrombocytopenic purpura. *Am. J. Obstet. Gynecol.* **133**:439–448, 1979.
64. O'Reilly, R. A. and Taber, B.: Immunologic thrombocytopenic purpura and pregnancy. *Obstet. Gynecol.* **51**:590–597, 1978.
65. Pfeifer, G. W.: Distribution and placental transfer of ^{131}I-streptokinase. *Aust. Ann. Med. Suppl.* **19**:17–18, 1970.
66. Picot, C., Triadou, P., Lacombe, C., Casa de val, N., and Girot, R.: Relapsing pure red-cell aplasia during pregnancy. *N. Engl. J. Med.* **311**:196, 1984.
67. Pitkin, R. M. and Witte, D. L.: Platelet and leukocyte counts in pregnancy. *JAMA* **242**:2696–2698, 1979.
68. Pitney, W. R., Pettit, J. E., and Armstrong, L.: Control of heparin therapy. *Br. Med. J.* **4**:139–141, 1970.
69. Rakozi, I., Tallian, F., Bagdany, S., and Gati, I.: Platelet lifespan in normal pregnancy and preeclampsia as determined by a non radioisotape technique. *Thromb. Res.* **15**:553–556, 1979.
70. Ramsay, L. E.: Impact of venography in the diagnosis and management of deep vein thrombosis. *Br. Med. J.* **286**:698–699, 1983.
71. Reece, E. A., Romero, R., and Hobbins, J.: Coagulopathy associated with Factor VIII inhibitor. *J. Reprod. Med.* **29**:53–58, 1984.
72. Sacks, D. A., Platt, L. D., and Johnson, C. S.: Autoimmune hemolytic disease during pregnancy. *Am. J. Obstet. Gynecol.* **140**:942–946, 1981.
73. Salzman, E. W., Deykin, D., Shapiro, R. M., and Rosenberg, R.: Management of heparin therapy—controlled prospective trial. *N. Engl. J. Med.* **292**:1046–1050, 1975.
74. Schenker, J. G. and Gombos, G. M.: Retinal hem-

orrhage in the newborn. *Obstet. Gynecol.* **27**:521–524, 1966.

75. Schwartz, M. L. and Brenner, W. E.: The obfuscation of pre-eclampsia by thrombotic thrombocytopenic purpura. *Am. J. Obstet. Gynecol.* **131**:18–24, 1978.
76. Scott, J. R., Cruikshank, D. P., Kochenour, N. K., Pitkin, R. M., and Warenski, J. C.: Fetal platelet counts in the obstetrical management of immunologic thrombocytopenic purpura. *Am. J. Obstet. Gynecol.* **136**:495–499, 1980.
77. Scott, J. R., Rote, N. S., and Cruikshank, D. P.: Antiplatelet antibodies and platelet counts in pregnancies complicated by autoimmune thrombocytopenic purpura. *Am. J. Obstet. Gynecol.* **145**:932–936, 1983.
78. Sejeny, S., Easthan, R., and Baker, S.: Platelet counts during normal pregnancy. *J. Clin. Pathol.* **28**:812–813, 1975.
79. Sharma, G. V. and Burlesco, V. A.: Effect of thrombolytic therapy on pulmonary-capillary blood volume in patients with pulmonary embolism. *N. Engl. J. Med.* **303**:842–845, 1980.
80. Starksen, N. F., Bell, W. R., and Kickler, T. S.: Unexplained hemolytic anemia associated with pregnancy. *Am. J. Obstet. Gynecol.* **146**:617–622, 1983.
81. Stein, P. D. and Willis, P. W.: Diagnosis prophylaxis and treatment of acute pulmonary embolism. *Arch. lntern. Med.* **143**:991–994. 1983.
82. Sutton, H. E.: *An Introduction to Human Genetics*, 3rd Edition. Philadelphia, Saunders College, 1980.
83. Tchernia, G., Dreyfus, M., Laurian, Y., Derychke, M., Miaca, C., and Kerbrat, G.: Management of immune thrombocytopenia in pregnancy: Response to infusions of immunoglobins. *Am. J. Obstet. Gynecol.* **148**:225–226, 1984.
84. Tawes, R. L., Kennedy, P. A., Harris, E. J., Brown, W. H., Scribner, R. G., Sydorak, G. R., and Beare, J. P.: Management of deep venous thrombosis and pulmonary embolism during pregnancy. *Am. J. Surg.* **144**:141–145, 1982.
85. Villasanta, U.: Thromboembolic disease in pregnancy. *Am. J. Obstet. Gynecol.* **93**:142–160, 1965.
86. Wallenburg, H. C. S. and Kessel, P. H.: Platelet lifespan in normal pregnancy as determined by a non radioisotope technique. *Br. J. Obstet. Gynaecol.* **85**:33–36, 1978.
87. Weiner, C. P. and Brandt, J.: Plasma antithrombin III activity in normal pregnancy. *Obstet. Gynecol.* **56**:601–603, 1980.
88. Wenske, C., Gaedicke, G., Kuenzlen, E., Heyes, H., Mueller-Eckhardt, C., Kleihauer, E., and Lauritzen, C.: Treatment of idiopathic thrombocytic purpura in pregnancy by high-dose intravenous immunoglobin. *Blut* **46**:347–353, 1983.
89. Wise, P. H. and Hall, A. J.: Heparin-induced osteopenia in pregnancy. *Br. Med. J.* **1**:110–111, 1980.
90. World Health Organization: Nutritional Anemias. Technical report series, No. 503, 1972.
91. Wozniak, A. J. and Kitchens, C. S.: Prospective hemostatic studies in a patient having paroxysmal nocturnal hemoglobinuria, pregnancy and cerebral venous thrombosis. *Am. J. Obstet. Gynecol.* **142**:591–593, 1982.
92. Zalneraitis, E. L., Young, R. S. K., and Krishnamoorthy, S.: lntracranial hemorrhage in utero as a complication of isoimmune thrombocytopenia. *J. Pediatr.* **95**:612–614, 1979.

31

CARDIAC DISEASE

Fewer than 2% of pregnant women have heart disease, a decline from previous eras, due to a decrease in rheumatic fever. The ratio of rheumatic heart disease to congenital heart disease has changed from 20:1 to about 3:1.[113]

Major advances in cardiology and in cardiothoracic surgery have led to the development and refinement of new and precise diagnostic techniques and therapeutic modalities. Medical management of cardiac disease in pregnancy is often effective. However, it may require a delicate manipulation of drugs that have complex interactions with mother and fetus. If medical management is unsuccessful, an excellent outcome can still be obtained by utilizing closed or open cardiac surgery during pregnancy. The administration of anticoagulants also requires special consideration regarding the risk/benefit ratio for the mother and the fetus (see Chapter 30).

As a consequence, the obstetrician is faced with a bewildering array of medical and surgical approaches to patients with heart disease. This chapter reviews these clinical situations and presents basic concepts of the diagnosis and management of heart disease in pregnancy.

HEMATOLOGIC AND CARDIOVASCULAR ALTERATIONS IN PREGNANCY

The changes in blood volume, plasma volume and red blood cell mass during pregnancy are reflective of the volume expansion that is imposed by the pregnancy (Fig. 31-1) (see Chapter 3). Plasma volume increases an average of 40–50% by the 32nd week, after which the volume plateaus until term. The plasma volume increment is related to the total mass of the conceptus and to birth weight in primigravidas.[60,117] A larger increase in volume is associated with twins (67% above normal) and an even greater expansion is associated with triplets (96.3% above normal).[101]

Total red blood cell mass increases by 20–40%, primarily during the late second and third trimester (Fig. 31-1). The change in red blood cell mass lags behind plasma volume expansion to produce the "physiological anemia of pregnancy." This is not a true anemia, but rather a dilutional effect. After 32 weeks, the dilutional effect decreases as red blood cell mass continues to increase slowly and plasma volume expansion reaches a plateau.

Cardiac output has been studied extensively. Most studies were done prior to 1975.[102,118-125] The resting cardiac output of the pregnant woman increases early in pregnancy to a peak value of 30–50% above normal by the 28th to 32nd week. Almost maximal levels are achieved by the 20th to 24th week of gestation (Fig. 31-2).[60,125] The cardiac workload in multiple pregnancy is about equal to that in singleton pregnancy. It occurs earlier and remains higher at term, thus adding to the overall cardiac stress.[102]

There is a gradual decline in the cardiac output as term is approached, which is probably

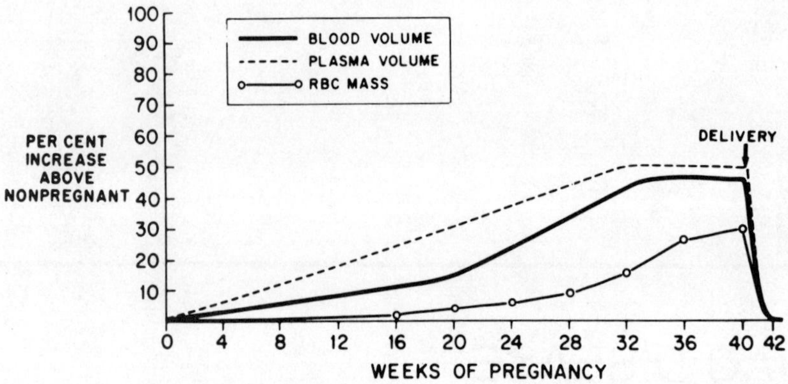

Figure 31-1. Changes in blood volume, plasma volume, and red cell mass during pregnancy. (Reprinted from Scott, D. E.: Anemia in pregnancy. Obstet. Gynecol. Annual. R. M. Wynn (Ed.), 1972, pp. 219–244, by permission of Appleton-Century-Crofts, New York.)

due in part to the obstructive effects of the increasing uterine mass on the vena cava.[55] Decreased stroke volume in the last trimester also contributes to the decreasing cardiac output (Fig. 31-2). Since vena cava obstruction must occur in all women who assume the supine position during the third trimester, the fact that only a few patients manifest the "supine hypotensive syndrome" must be due to the development of an adequate collateral circulation in most patients, probably via the ascending lumbar and azygous venous systems or via the ovarian veins.[11]

Cardiac output increases with exercise throughout pregnancy.[7,47] Whereas exhaustive exercise may have a deleterious effect on the fetus, exercise in moderation is probably safe for the fetus of a healthy mother.[72] Suboptimal increased demand on cardiac output with exercise, such as might occur in patients with mitral stenosis, could result in the development of pulmonary edema.[113,124]

Significant changes may occur in cardiac output with the onset of labor. These changes are variable and depend on the position of the patient and the anesthesia employed at the time that the measurements are performed.[119,120] Cardiac output may increase up to 25% during the first stage of labor and up to 50% during the second stage of labor.[120] These increases are dampened when regional anesthesia is employed.[120,122] When the patient is on her left side, under regional anesthesia, cardiac output will usually remain relatively constant during and immediately after a contraction.[119] Following vaginal delivery, cardiac output may increase by 60–80%, unless regional anesthesia is used for delivery.[122]

Delivery by cesarean section may circumvent some of the widely fluctuating hemodynamic changes associated with labor and vaginal delivery. The surgery itself adds the risks and hazards of a major operative procedure. Epidural anesthesia is the anesthetic method of choice for cesarean section, because it blunts the hemodynamic changes during the operative procedure and during the immediate postpartum period.[118]

DIAGNOSIS OF CARDIAC DISEASE IN PREGNANCY

Cardiac disease associated with pregnancy is of major concern because pregnancy itself constitutes a "cardiac stress test." If the patient is not physiologically competent to handle this stress, her life will be endangered and the fetus will also suffer, because maternal defense mechanisms ultimately favor the survival of the mother at the expense of the fetus.

Normal pregnant patients commonly display a variety of symptoms suggetive of heart disease, such as dyspnea, orthopnea, chest discomfort or heaviness, fatigability, dizzy spells or syncope. When severe dyspnea, paroxysmal nocturnal dyspnea, or progressive orthopnea occur, especially if they limit the patient's activ-

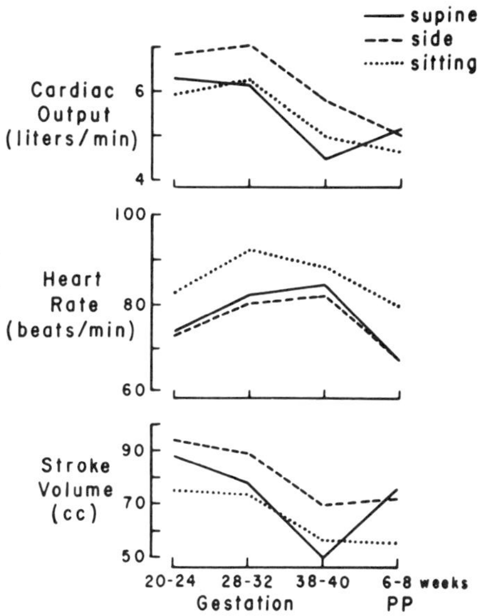

Figure 31-2. Effects of time in gestation and of maternal position on maternal cardiovascular system. Data were obtained at three periods during gestation and once postpartum. (Reprinted from Ueland, K., Novy, M. J., Peterson, E. N. and Metcalfe, J.: Maternal cardiovascular dynamics. IV. The influence of gestational age on the maternal cardiovascular response to posture and exercise. Am. J. Obstet. Gynecol. 104:856–864, 1969, by permission of the C. V. Mosby Company.)

ity, consideration should be given to the possibility of heart disease. If palpitations and syncope occur together, cardiac arrhythmia should be suspected. Chest pain that follows the referral pattern of angina pectoris should alert the physician to the possibility of true myocardial ischemia or infarction.

The findings on physical examination of the pregnant patient may be confusing, in that peripheral edema, distended neck veins, an S3 gallop, cardiomegaly, and basal rales in the lung fields may be present in patients without heart disease.[77] During normal pregnancy, the heart is pushed upward and rotated forward by the elevation of the diaphragm. This moves the apex beat upward and lateral from its normal position.[60] This displacement may give the impression of cardiac enlargement on physical examination and on the chest x-ray. The left cardiac border may appear straightened and the pulmonary artery may be more prominent. On the lateral x-ray view, increased prominence of the left atrium and resultant indentation of the esophagus may incorrectly suggest mitral stenosis.

The first heart sound often is split and increased in intensity. Rapid filling of the ventricles during early diastole accentuates the normal third sound, which can usually be heard after the 20th week of gestation. Occasionally, a diastolic murmur is heard transiently along the left sternal border. A systolic murmur of variable intensity, probably due to increased blood flow, may be heard along the left sternal border beginning early in the second trimester and persisting until about one week postpartum. Late in pregnancy, a presystolic murmur that originates in the internal mammary artery may be heard, along with a continuous murmur derived from the venous engorgement of the breasts. These sounds generally disappear one week after delivery. The presence of a systolic murmur, grade III/VI intensity or greater, should be considered indicative of possible heart disease. Any diastolic murmur in pregnancy is considered significant.

Electrocardiographic (ECG) changes in pregnancy are generally attributable to the upward displacement of the heart. The electrical axis shifts 15 degrees to the left. The T-wave may be flattened or negative in lead III, with nonspecific ST-wave depression in other leads. Low voltage QRS complexes and deep Q-waves occasionally may appear in lead III.

The ECG and the chest x-ray are of limited diagnostic utility. Invasive techniques may be indicated if the patient is seriously ill. Certainly, consideration of cardiac surgery requires a more definitive identification of the type and extent of the cardiac lesions. Cardiac catheterization usually is required for accurate preoperative evaluation. The balloon flotation pulmonary artery catheter (Swan–Ganz) provides an accurate cardiac hemodynamic assessment and is useful for monitoring cardiac patients in labor.

Recent advances in medical ultrasound have made a variety of noninvasive tests available. M-mode and two-dimensional echocardiography are of value in evaluating anatomy and function of the cardiac chambers and valves.[37] Doppler echocardiography is also useful for noninvasive assessment of valvular abnormalities and intracardiac shunts.[37] Radionuclide cardiac imaging gives an assessment of left ventricular function and morphology and provides information about intracardiac shunts (e.g., atrial or ventricular septal defects). The calculated dose of irradiation to the fetus with this technique is 0.8 rads or less.[37] Contrast echocardiography is also useful in evaluation of valvular disease and minimizes the need for radiation during cardiac catheterization.[38] Measurement of maximal oxygen consumption during exercise may prove useful in detecting potentially serious heart disease.[37] The measurement of the vital capacity (VC) or the forced expiratory volume (FEVl) in patients at each office visit may detect impending cardiac failure.

CLASSIFICATION OF PATIENTS WITH HEART DISEASE

The functional classification proposed by the New York Heart Association offers a simple clinical method for assessing the status of a cardiac patient (Table 31-1).[32] Generally, most maternal morbidity and mortality occurs in Class III and IV patients. In such patients, pregnancy should be discouraged or, if they are pregnant, therapeutic abortion should be considered. In selected patients, surgical correction of a cardiac defect may allow a subsequent pregnancy with minimal risk.

The majority of cardiac patients can enjoy a successful pregnancy outcome. Exceptions to this statement include individuals with pulmonary hypertension, Marfan's syndrome, Eisenmenger's syndrome, complicated coarctation of the aorta, some individuals with cardiomyopathy, patients with a poor functional result after corrective surgery, and patients with advanced coronary artery disease.

TABLE 31-1. FUNCTIONAL CLASSIFICATION

Class I.	Patients with cardiac disease but without resulting limitations of physical activity. Ordinary physical activity does not cause undue fatigue, palpitation, dyspnea, or anginal pain.
Class II.	Patients with cardiac disease resulting in slight limitation of physical activity. They are comfortable at rest. Ordinary physical activity results in fatigue, palpitation, dyspnea, or anginal pain.
Class III.	Patients with cardiac disease resulting in marked limitations of physical activity. They are comfortable at rest. Ordinary physical activity results in fatigue, palpitation, dyspnea, or anginal pain.
Class IV.	Patients with cardiac disease resulting in inability to carry on any physical activity without discomfort. Symptoms of cardiac insufficiency or of the anginal syndrome may be present even at rest. If any physical activity is undertaken, discomfort is increased.

GENERAL PRINCIPLES OF MANAGEMENT

Once the diagnosis of cardiac disease has been firmly established, complete assessment of the patient's functional and therapeutic status should be carried out. A thorough evaluation of maternal and fetal risks should be outlined and a plan of management developed. The basic principles in the treatment of the pregnant cardiac patient are reduction of the maternal cardiac work load and maintenance of blood flow to the fetal-placental unit.

The obstetrician should develop a team that includes a cardiologist, a cardiothoracic surgeon, an anesthesiologist, and a pediatrician. A plan of management that includes all aspects of the patient's care should be developed with the direct involvement of the patient to insure complete compliance.

The functional classification of the patient's cardiac status will define the level of physical activity that is permissible. Physical activity in Classes I and II should remain below the level at which symptoms have appeared.

Infections place an additional burden on cardiac patients and may precipitate congestive heart failure. In the presence of valvular lesions or prostheses, antibiotics should be administered at delivery and in the puerperium to protect against the development of subacute bacterial endocarditis (SBE).[77]

Emotional and psychologic stress may alter cardiovascular parameters sufficiently to endanger the cardiac. Chronic fatigue, anemia, and personal habits, such as alcoholism, smoking, or the use of addictive drugs, add an unnecessary burden to the pregnant cardiac.

MANAGEMENT OF HEART DISEASE BY ETIOLOGY

Acquired Heart Disease

Mitral Valve Disease

Mitral Stenosis. Mitral stenosis is rheumatic in origin. lt is probably the most common and most significant acquired heart lesion seen in the pregnant patient. The hemodynamic defect in mitral stenosis is obstruction to blood flow from the left atrium into the left ventricle during diastole. When the pressure gradient in the left atrium required to overcome the stenotic opening exceeds 25 mmHg, there is transudation of fluid into the pulmonary alveolar walls, resulting in pulmonary edema and hemoptysis.[116] This sequence of events is even more likely in pregnant patients with mitral stenosis, because of the increased heart rate and cardiac output of pregnancy. Elevation of left atrial pressure also increases the risk of development of atrial fibrillation, with subsequent formation of an atrial thrombus and embolization.[116] Since the elevated atrial pressure is required to maintain the cardiac output in mitral stenosis, any sudden shift in blood volume distribution can cause a dangerous fall in cardiac output. These factors explain the increased maternal and fetal morbidity and mortality seen with this lesion. Indeed, unrecognized mitral stenosis may cause sudden death in a patient who has no prior history of heart disease.

Management of mitral stenosis begins with a thorough knowledge of the disease process and its pathophysiologic ramifications during pregnancy. When severe stenosis of the mitral valve is identified, mitral commissurotomy should be performed, ideally prior to conception. Restriction of physical activity, prevention of pulmonary congestion and avoidance of fatigue are the goals of therapy. Should pulmonary congestion occur, physical activity should be restricted severely. Digitalization may be indicated to decrease the heart rate and to protect against a rapid ventricular response should atrial fibrillation develop. In severe cases, a sodium restricted diet (i.e., 2 grams per day) and judicious use of diuretics are necessary. Hospitalization and complete bedrest may greatly improve the maternal and fetal outcome in severe mitral stenosis. Should such measures be unsuccessful, closed commissurotomy of the mitral valve, or rarely valve replacement, may be necessary.[82] Anticoagulation with heparin is usually indicated in patients with atrial fibrillation, or in those who have experienced embolic phenomena. Rheumatic fever prophylaxis is indicated, since this is the only valvular lesion that is exclusively rheumatic in origin.

Mitral Insufficiency. Mitral insufficiency is generally well tolerated by most patients. Although it may have a variety of causes, rheumatic fever prophylaxis during pregnancy and prophylaxis for subacute bacterial endocarditis (SBE) is indicated at labor and delivery. Endocarditis itself may cause mitral regurgitation. If congestive heart failure occurs, especially if unresponsive to medical therapy, mitral valve replacement should strongly be considered. Most patients in whom corrective mitral valve surgery is performed during pregnancy enjoy a good outcome.[46,82,92]

Aortic Valve Disease

Aortic Stenosis. This lesion is more common in men than in women and is rare in pregnancy.[6] Patients with aortic stenosis are usually asymptomatic and almost never develop congestive heart failure. The major pathophysiology stems from inability to maintain adequate cardiac output due to obstruction of the outflow tract of the left ventricle. As a consequence, any significant decrease in venous return or any additional demand for increased cardiac output causes an absolute or relative decrease in cardiac output and leads to symptoms of cerebral ischemia. When this occurs, the fetus may also be placed in jeopardy due to associated decrease in uterine blood flow. Major reductions in cardiac output may result in sudden dyspnea, chest pain, syncope, or sudden death. This is not uncommon during the intrapartum period in association with hypotension secondary to regional anesthesia. Regional anesthesia must be used cautiously, if at all, in these patients. In patients with severe aortic stenosis, the maternal mortality rate may be as high as 40% if pregnancy is interrupted as opposed to 17% if pregnancy is allowed to continue. The perinatal mortality associated with aortic stenosis is 31%.[6]

Aortic Insufficiency. This lesion is also uncommon and is rarely associated with congestive heart failure. Medical treatment is usually successful. Aortic valve replacement prior to pregnancy is the therapy of choice. However, the valve can be replaced during pregnancy if necessary. Antibiotic prophylaxis is indicated at labor and delivery. Endocarditis itself may result in aortic insufficiency and may necessitate valve replacement during pregnancy and in the early puerperium when medical therapy is ineffective.[19,35,92,93]

Pulmonary Valve and Tricuspid Valve Disease. Disease involving these valves is rare and seldom causes significant hemodynamic changes. The tricuspid valve may occasionally require replacement. Tricuspid disease is almost always associated with concomitant severe disease of the aortic and mitral valves, unless it is related to right-sided endocarditis, which is a drug addiction-related problem.[106]

Cardiomyopathies. Although reports of congestive heart failure following pregnancy appeared as early as 1849, it was in 1937 that Hull and Hafkesbring first called attention to a new "toxic" postpartal heart disease.[57] The existence of this condition as a distinct entity has been doubted by some authorities due to lack of an etiologic factor. However, the modern consensus holds that the syndrome of peripartum cardiomyopathy does indeed exist.[126] This syndrome is defined as occurring in the peripartum period in a patient with no previous history of heart disease and in whom no specific etiology can be identified.[14,27,80] Possible etiologies that have been advanced are (1) hypertensive disease, (2) beri-beri heart disease, (3) idiopathic myocardial degeneration, (4) viral myocarditis, (5) autoimmune myocarditis, and (6) familial causes.[81,94]

Peripartum cardiomyopathy occurs in 1:1300 to 1:4000 pregnancies.[80,94,110,126] It is more common in older multiparous women and is more frequent in black patients in the United States,[14,27,57] although it has been reported in Orientals and whites. The maternal mortality rate is 30–60%, and the fetal mortality rate is about 10%.[78]

The role of nutrition in peripartum cardiomyopathy is uncertain, as is the significance of the hypertension present in a number of patients.[27] It is possible that toxemia is a predisposing factor to development of cardiomyopathy. Associated multiple gestation (twins) has been noted in 7–10% of cases.[27,94,110] Both an autoimmune and a viral etiology have been implicated in cases that appear to be indistinguishable from peripartum cardiomyopathy.[126] In such instances, transvenous endomyocardial biopsy may be utilized.[81] This procedure appears to be a safe and valuable aid in the clinical management of acute and chronic cases.

The onset of dyspnea, edema, tachyarrhythmias, cough, and orthopnea, secondary to an enlarged heart and congestive heart failure, usually occurs during the second postpartum month but has been noted from the seventh month of pregnancy up to six months postpartum. Renal failure may be a component of the clinical picture.[98]

Cardiac findings at autopsy consist of a grossly enlarged heart with dilatation of all heart chambers and a pale, flabby myocardium. Endocardial thickening and mural thrombi may be present. Histologic examination reveals edema, tissue necrosis, and lymphocytic infiltration.[27]

The prognosis for future childbearing in patients who survive a peripartum myocardiopathy is poor. Fifty to 80% of these patients experience cardiac failure in subsequent pregnancies with a mortality as high as 60%.[18,127] The outlook is better for patients whose heart size has returned to normal within six months and who do not have cardiomegaly at the onset of pregnancy.[27] If congestive heart failure is present antepartum, the prognosis is poor for both mother and fetus.[18,27,78]

Treatment consists of bedrest, a salt-restricted diet, diuretics for those with congestive heart failure, and usually digitalization. Digitalis levels should be measured frequently, because digitalis toxicity is frequent in patients with postpartum cardiomyopathy.[18] Anticoagulation is indicated, because of the increased risk of embolic phenomena as a result of intracardiac mural thrombi.[126] Immunosuppressive therapy using corticosteroids and azathioprine has been utilized.[81] A long-term benefit of this treatment has not been verified.

Congenital Heart Disease

Pregnancy associated with congenital heart disease is more common today due to advances in corrective heart surgery. Complete understanding of the cardiac defect and of the corrective surgical procedure is essential to management. In general, 2–4% of the offspring of these patients are at risk for a similar heart lesion.[86] In some forms of congenital heart disease, the risk may be over 14%.[130]

Coarctation of the Aorta. Simple coarctation of the aorta is rare. Pregnancy may be undertaken without undue risk to the mother after surgical correction. The fetal risks may be increased. A complicated coarctation of the aorta is associated with an increased maternal mortality rate. The most frequent associated cardiac defect is a bicuspid aorta valve,[44,113] which can be the seat of bacterial infection. There is an occasional association with congenital cerebral aneurysm.[113] A weakening of the aorta or an atrial septal defect[13] may also be present.

The pregnancy increase in cardiac output

may be poorly tolerated in patients with coarctation of the aorta. Strict limitations of physical activity are indicated throughout pregnancy. The postpartum period is especially dangerous. Deaths in the early postpartum period are secondary to aortic rupture, congestive failure, cerebral vasculature accidents, and endocarditis.[116] M-mode and cross-sectional echocardiography are helpful in identifying patients at high risk.[13] SBE prophylaxis is recommended for labor and delivery. Cesarean section is indicated only for obstetrical reasons.[113]

Septal Defects. Left-to-right shunting is associated with septal defects. If the defect is large and shunting severe, pulmonary hypertension and right ventricular failure may occur. In most instances, the defect is small or has been corrected surgically prior to pregnancy. In these cases, pregnancy is well tolerated and antibiotic prophylaxis is not indicated.

Atrial septal defects are especially well tolerated in pregnancy. Ventricular septal defects are associated with loud murmurs and usually are detected early in life. Spontaneous closure occurs in approximately 50% of patients with small defects.[78] Large defects may require surgical correction.

Tetralogy of Fallot. The component defects of this disorder are (1) pulmonary stenosis, (2) intraventricular septal defect, and (3) aortic displacement. These defects result in right ventricular hypertrophy, varying degrees of right-to-left shunting, and an admixture of venous and arterial blood. The degree of pulmonary stenosis present is the major determinant of right-to-left shunting, the magnitude of cyanosis, and the pulmonary blood flow.[116]

Pregnancy is dangerous to patients with tetralogy of Fallot. As peripheral vascular resistance falls during pregnancy, right-to-left shunting and cyanosis increase.[116] Poor prognostic signs include elevation of the maternal hematocrit above 60% and/or an arterial oxygen saturaton less than 80%. Any sudden decrease in venous return to the heart is hazardous, thus supine hypotension syndrome or other sudden positional changes should be avoided. Conduction anesthesia must be used cautiously in these patients to avoid episodes of hypotension, but regional anesthesia allays anxiety, reduces pain, and dampens the fluctuations in the cardiac output that accompany normal labor.

In contrast to those with a cyanotic heart disease problem, patients with noncyanotic congenital heart defects have a reasonably good outcome with a live birth rate of 77% and little or no maternal mortality.[130] If no cyanosis is present after corrective surgery, infant birth weights are higher than are those in patients who manifest cyanosis. The rate of stillbirths is lower in patients who return to good cardiac function after corrective surgery.

The management of the patient with tetralogy of Fallot in labor includes (1) oxygen administration, if cyanosis is present; (2) SBE prophylaxis; (3) avoidance of a sudden decrease in the venous return to the heart secondary to maternal position (e.g., supine hypotension syndrome); (4) appropriate use of analgesia or anesthesia (e.g., regional anesthesia); (5) electrocardiographic monitoring of the mother (and when indicated, monitoring by Swan–Ganz catheter); and (6) electronic monitoring of the fetus to detect fetal distress. Patients with cyanotic heart disease, past or present, are more apt to have cephalopelvic disproportion. Should cesarean section be necessary, the surgery is usually well tolerated.[130]

Patent Ductus Arteriosus. Patent ductus arteriosus that persists into adult life is usually small and is well tolerated. SBE prophylaxis is indicated in labor.

Eisenmenger's Syndrome. This complex of findings has a grave prognosis in pregnancy. Maternal mortality is 30–60%.[43,95] Eisenmenger's syndrome consists of pulmonary hypertension, with a reversed or bidirectional shunt occurring at the aorticopulmonary, atrial, or ventricular septal areas. The pathophysiology is initiated by an increase in pulmonary vascular resistance in a patient with a septal defect and a left-to-right shunt. As pulmonary vascular resistance continues to rise, the shunt reverses to right-to-left and cyanosis appears. A ventricular septal defect is the most common shunt abnormality and is associated with a maternal mortality of 60%.[43] When the shunt is atrial, mortality decreases to 44%, and if the shunt is due to a patent ductus arteriosus, maternal mortality is 41%.[43] Cesarean section or other operative procedures are especially hazardous. One study reported that three of four pregnant women who were delivered by cesarean section died. A death also occurred in a patient who underwent hysterotomy for pregnancy termination.[43]

With all congenital heart defects involving right-to-left shunts or bidirectional shunts, any change in hemodynamics that adversely affects venous return (and thus cardiac output) or increases shunting must be avoided. Hypoventilation and bronchospasm must be avoided because they may cause impaired oxygenation of capillary blood. This results in increased pulmonary vascular resistance because of vasoconstriction, increased right-to-left shunting, and decreased pulmonary blood flow. For these reasons, sedatives and narcotics in labor and the postpartum period may have adverse effects. Rapid deterioration of a patient following intra-amniotic injection of prostaglandin $F_{2\alpha}$ has been reported.[95]

The patient should assume the left lateral decubitus position when lying down and should avoid the supine position throughout the latter part of pregnancy. Wrapping the legs may aid in preventing sequestration of fluid in the extremities. Regional anesthesia, if utilized, must be administered very cautiously to avoid hypotension. Because intravascular pulmonary thrombosis may occur in patients with Eisenmenger's syndrome, anticoagulation for 10 days postpartum has been suggested.[116] Others disagree with this approach, because of bleeding complications.[95] Although the maternal mortality rate is very high in some reports, a large series has not yet been published. In one report that reviewed the outcome with and without corrective surgery, eight patients with Eisenmenger's syndrome did well.[130]

Pulmonary Hypertension. Pregnancy is contraindicated in patients with pulmonary hypertension. The risk of death for mother and fetus is extremely high, whether the hypertension is primary or secondary.[79] Maternal mortality is as high as 50% if the process is primary and 60% if it is secondary to Eisenmenger's syndrome.[43,79] The pathophysiology involved is essentially the same as in Eisenmenger's syndrome. Exercise is poorly tolerated. Strict limitation of exercise is mandatory. Anticoagulation should be considered in the immediate puerperium.[116] The functional capacity prior to pregnancy may be misleading, since asymptomatic patients with pulmonary hypertension may still be at high risk during pregnancy.[116] After delivery, augmentation of the venous return from the lower extremities and the uterus may lead to acute right ventricular failure and circulatory collapse.[79]

All forms of anesthesia are hazardous to patients with pulmonary hypertension. Spinal and epidural block have been avoided in these patients. The investigational use of morphine and other opiates in the spinal and epidural spaces is promising because these drugs may provide pain relief without motor or sympathetic blockade.[1,56] Intrathecal administration of 1 mg or less of morphine is effective for prolonged pain relief, but additional anesthesia is required for a surgical incision.[1] Side effects of maternal respiratory depression, urinary retention, nausea and vomiting, severe pruritus, and somnolence have been troublesome.[56] The pain relief after epidural injection of opiates has been unpredictable. The dose required is often more than 7.5 mg of morphine. Vascular absorption of the drug from the epidural space is the same as that after intramuscular injection. Epidural injection of 5 mg of morphine in 10 ml of diluent provides long-lasting analgesia after cesarean section. This technique is useful in all cardiac patients, and most of all in patients with pulmonary hypertension, whether primary or secondary.

Isolated Pulmonary Stenosis. Isolated pulmonary stenosis is rarely associated with pregnancy because most patients with significant stenosis have undergone elective valvotomy in childhood. Pregnancy outcome is generally good, but the patient with severe stenosis may develop right heart failure. If this occurs, pulmonary valvotomy in pregnancy has been successful. Severe pulmonary stenosis should be corrected surgically prior to pregnancy.[113]

Developmental Abnormalities

Mitral Valve Prolapse. The incidence of mitral valve prolapse in young adults is about 5–10%, although a 17% incidence of mid-to-late systolic clicks or murmurs has been reported.[75,78] The diagnosis usually is based on the finding of a late systolic click associated with a late systolic murmur. The severity of mitral valve prolapse can be determined by cross-sectional echocardiography.[13] Associated cardiac arrhythmia or mitral insufficiency should be managed appropriately. Prophylactic antibiotics should be utilized during labor and delivery, especially if mitral insufficiency is present.[78]

Idiopathic Hypertropic Subaortic Stenosis (IHSS). This autosomal dominant inherited cardiac lesion produces aortic outflow obstruction. The patient may present with a history of chest pain or pressure, syncope, and shortness of breath. A loud systolic murmur may be present along the left sternal border, which may increase in intensity during a Valsalva maneuver. The murmur may decrease in intensity or may disappear during pregnancy. M-mode echocardiography may detect asymmetric septal hypertrophy (i.e., thickening of the septum as compared to the posterior ventricular wall) and an abnormal anterior motion of the mitral valve leaflet during systole. The outcome of pregnancy is generally good. However, some patients have a significant increase in symptoms, especially syncope, dyspnea, and chest pain.[66,91,-115] Beta-adrenergic blocking agents are useful in treating these symptoms and in treating tachyarrhythmias.[116] Prophylactic antibiotics are indicated during labor and delivery.

Marfan's Syndrome. Marfan's syndrome is an autosomal dominant disorder. However, it may arise de novo. It is a congenital form of mesodystrophy, a systemic anomaly that is limited to the mesodermal structures. Marfan's syndrome is characterized by cardiovascular abnormalities (cystic medial degeneration with diffuse or dissecting aneurysms of the thoracic aorta), ocular problems (ectopia lentis), abnormalities of the skeletal system (arachnodactyly, excessive length of long bones, and "spider" feet), and pulmonary disease (cystic disease of the lungs).

The classic form of the disease is recognized readily, but the diagnosis may be difficult to establish on occasion. Presence of an aortic aneurysm and subluxation of the ocular lens generally suggest the diagnosis. Because this syndrome is the major cause of dissecting aneurysm in people under 40 years of age, the association with pregnancy is especially lethal.[78,116] Pregnancy interruption should be considered for patients with Marfan's syndrome.[77,84]

In patients who desire to continue pregnancy, efforts are directed toward avoidance of increased intravascular pressure by strict bedrest throughout pregnancy, continuous epidural anesthesia during labor and delivery, and use of low forceps to shorten the second stage of labor and to minimize Valsalva maneuvers at delivery. Beta-adrenergic blocking agents can be used to decrease heart rate and to diminish pressure on the weakened aortic walls during labor and delivery.[77,84,116] Antibiotic prophylaxis is indicated at labor and delivery because mitral valve prolapse and aortic regurgitation frequently are associated with this syndrome.

Other Cardiac Conditions

Deaths have occasionally been reported in association with rare conditions involving cardiac function. One such example was death due to a cardiac rhythm disturbance in a patient who had pseudoxanthoma elasticum.[10]

HEART VALVE SURGERY AND PREGNANCY

Valvotomy

Selection of patients for mitral valve surgery should take into account the additional cardiovascular load that pregnancy imposes on the mother. Generally, patients who have symptoms with activity are ideal candidates, whereas patients who have symptoms at rest are poor surgical risks. Because pregnancy places a burden on patients with mitral stenosis, which often may lead to cardiac failure by the fourth or fifth month, cardiac surgery ideally should be performed prior to pregnancy.

Closed-heart valvotomy carries no greater mortality rate during pregnancy than in the nonpregnant state. The operative mortality for closed mitral valvotomy is 3%; the 6-year survival is 90%, and the 12-year survival is 78%.[23] Class IV patients do quite well with closed mitral surgery. The success rate is high and the maternal mortality is low in pregnancy even when congestive heart failure and persistent pulmonary edema are present at the time of valvotomy.[40]

Following closed mitral valvotomy, a number of hemodynamic parameters of cardiac function should improve. Usually, left atrial pressure as well as pulmonary artery pressure decrease. Pulmonary vascular resistance falls toward normal and cardiac output increases.[39] Symptomatic improvement from the corrective surgery should be recognized during the first three months to one year and should remain at the improved level for many years. Re-stenosis of the valve may occur in some patients and may require reoperation at a later date.

Heart Valve Prostheses

Replacement of the mitral, aortic, or tricuspid valve may be the procedure of choice in patients with stenosis or insufficiency. In each instance, cardiopulmonary bypass is utilized to allow direct visualization of the cardiac valve during replacement. A mechanical valve, such as the Starr–Edwards ball-valve, or a heterograft (i.e., xenograft) consisting of a glutaraldehyde-preserved tissue valve of porcine origin, such as the Hancock valve, or a fresh antibiotic-treated homograft may be used.[12,20,28,50,68,88,103]

Mechanical Valves. Women with prosthetic heart valves pose many problems during pregnancy, depending on the type of valve and its location. A large clinical experience with mechanical prostheses exists.[20,50,68,103] A number of types of mechanical valves of different sizes are available. The three most common rigid cardiac valve prostheses are (1) caged-ball (Starr–Edwards), (2) caged-disk (Beall–Surgitool), and (3) tilting-disk (Bjork–Shiley).[50] Mechanical valves are durable and reliable but carry a risk of thromboembolism of 3–6%.[90] Thrombosis and subsequent valvular malfunction may occur at any time after insertion and occur with both the caged-ball and the tilting-disk prostheses.[46,68,71,103] Valve thrombosis is seen most often in patients with a Bjork–Shiley mitral prosthesis. Heparin may not be as effective as coumarin in preventing this potentially disastrous complication of mechanical valve prosthesis.[71,89,103]

Aortic valve replacement is associated with an operative mortality of 5%.[90] Operative mortality for mitral or multiple valve replacement is 10%. Repeat valve replacement has a higher morbidity and mortality than does the initial operation.[90]

Aortic valve replacement is associated with excellent functional results. Pregnancy outcome is good. Mitral valve and multiple valve replacement are also associated with a good functional result, but exercise response is impaired and medical complications are more common.[58,68,103] Pregnancy outcome in patients with mitral or multiple valve replacement is poor and is related to the requirement for long-term anticoagulation. Successful pregnancy has been reported in patients with triple-valve replacement.[5,30,33,85]

Bioprosthetic Valves. The major advantage of tissue valves is the low risk of thromboembolism (i.e., less than 2%) which eliminates the need for anticoagulation in most instances.[12,28,87,88] Aspirin administered as an antiplatelet factor is effective.[88] Aspirin is as effective as warfarin in preventing emboli in patients with atrial fibrillation after porcine valve placement.[87] Neither aspirin nor dipyridamole should be substituted for coumarin drugs or heparin in patients with mechanical prostheses.[89,103] Bioprosthetic grafts are not as durable and high failure rates are reported in children and in patients under 35 years of age.[64] Although the porcine valve is easily produced and thus readily available, the failure rate in young patients increases when the valve is in place more than five years.[64,90] Valve calcification and subsequent malfunction have been reported. The reason for valve calcification is unknown.[12] Homografts are available for aortic and mitral placement. These valves also display a high incidence of late-graft deterioration. Homografts are not as readily available as porcine heterografts. Lack of availability of an assortment of sizes is a major problem.[28] In general, pregnancy outcome in patients with bioprostheses has been good.[12,28,88] Lack of durability and valve calcification must be overcome before bioprostheses can be accepted unequivocably as the valves of choice in women during the reproductive years.

Open Heart Surgery in Pregnancy

Pregnancy may have a successful outcome following open heart surgery.[46,51,132] Fetal bradycardia has been noted during cardiopulmonary bypass for mitral valve correction, but the infants were delivered with good Apgar scores.[65] In addition to bradycardia, late decelerations and loss of beat-to-beat baseline variability during cardiopulmonary bypass have been reported.[8,69,114,129] The abnormal fetal heart rate pattern may disappear when the bypass flow rate is increased.[129] One of the most unusual reports described a cesarean section on a patient on cardiopulmonary bypass with a good outcome for mother and fetus.[76] Although the number of reported cases of open heart surgery during pregnancy is not large, it appears that this complex surgery can be performed with some degree of safety in all three trimesters of pregnancy.

ANTICOAGULATION IN PREGNANCY

Many patients with valvular cardiac defects and most, if not all, patients with mechanical valve prostheses require chronic anticoagulation to reduce or eliminate the possibility of thromboembolism and its sequellae. Pregnancy adds significantly to the complexity of anticoagulation, because of the pregnancy-related alterations in the blood-coagulation mechanism and because of the maternal and fetal complications that may result from the administration of anticoagulants during pregnancy. (See Chapter 30 for detailed discussion.)

Coumarin Derivatives

Coumarin derivatives are contraindicated or rarely indicated in pregnancy. Preconceptional counseling may reduce the number of fetuses exposed to coumarin compounds. If pregnancy is contemplated, the patient should be changed to heparin prior to conception. In the event that unplanned pregnancy occurs, oral anticoagulation should be discontinued immediately and heparin substituted. If oral anticoagulant administration is discontinued prior to the onset of pregnancy or with the first missed menses, warfarin embryopathy could probably be reduced significantly or eliminated.

Heparin

Heparin cannot be absorbed by the oral route and therefore must be given parenterally, which adds to the inconvenience of utilizing this agent. Its half-life is 60 minutes and its anticoagulant effect occurs immediately. Heparin therapy should be monitored using the activated partial thromboplastin time, the thrombin clotting time, or a heparin assay.

The therapeutic dose of heparin may need to be increased in pregnancy, since a low-dose regimen in one study failed to provide adequate anticoagulation in a group of patients with mechanical valve prostheses.[128] The ideal "safe and effective" dose of heparin has not been determined. An appropriate dose probably lies somewhere between the mini-dose and full heparinization.

MANAGEMENT OF ARRHYTHMIAS

As pregnancy progresses, plasma volume increases and plasma protein concentration decreases, resulting in a reduction of the protein binding of many drugs. Since glomerular filtration rate is also increased, large quantities of some medications may be lost in the urine. In addition to specific pregnancy changes, large amounts of medication may be transferred to the fetal compartment.[70] The rate of placental transfer may be increased if the drug has a high lipid solubility, a low degree of ionization, and low molecular weight (i.e., less than 600 daltons).[100,108] The size of the placental membrane surface area that is exposed to the drug as well as the rate of blood flow also affect the amount of drug absorbed into the fetal compartment. As a result of these factors, the therapeutic dose of a drug may be alerted markedly throughout pregnancy.[100] Medications used in the treatment of maternal heart disease are also transferred to the fetus, with the potential of adverse side effects.

The basic concept that a pregnant woman should not take any more medications than absolutely necessary is also valid in treatment of cardiac arrhythmias. Careful consideration of the effects of the drug, as well as the need for the drug, should be made in each case. For example, in the case of asymptomatic premature beats, drug therapy is not indicated.

Tachyarrhythmias are the most common arrhythmias in pregnant women. In many cases, adequate control of the patients' environment may eliminate the need for medications. For example, avoidance of caffeine-containing substances (e.g., cola, tea, coffee) and of antiasthmatic preparations or decongestants and minimization of anxiety-producing situations and undue fatigue, often eliminate the need for drug therapy. If medications are required, the drugs usually used to control tachyarrhythmias (paroxysmal supraventricular tachycardia, atrial flutter, or atrial fibrillation) may be used. Electrical cardioversion also may be used without danger to mother or fetus.[109]

Bradyarrhythmias are secondary to an atrioventricular (A-V) block or may occur as a result of disease of the sinoauricular (S-A) node, which paces an atrial rate that is too slow to produce adequate ventricular response. The most common cause of permanent bradycardia is complete A-V block, either congenital or acquired. The acquired form is often a result of open heart surgery. Occasionally, a pacemaker may be required because of Adams–Stokes attacks.[2] Pregnancy outcome is generally excellent in patients with permanent bradycardias if the heart is otherwise normal.[2,62]

Antiarrhythmic Medications

Cardiac Glycosides. Cardiac glycosides are both inotropic and antiarrhythmia agents. Digoxin is the best studied and has an excellent safety record for mother and fetus.[100] Because digoxin crosses the placenta, it has been used to treat fetal tachycardia and congestive heart failure.[63] Maternal serum levels are similar to those in the newborn.[63,99] Digoxin is not teratogenic. As with many medications used in treatment of heart disease, serum levels are lower in the pregnant than in the nonpregnant state. As a consequence, many patients require a significantly increased dosage during pregnancy. Serum digoxin determinations are essential if a therapeutic level is to be maintained.

Quinidine. Quinidine has been used in obstetrics for decades. Quinidine is one of the safest and most widely used antiarrhythmic drugs.[100] It is not teratogenic. Quinidine is used most commonly to maintain sinus rhythm after conversion of atrial fibrillation or atrial flutter. It is also effective in treating ventricular arrhythmias associated with Wolff–Parkinson–White syndrome.

Lidocaine. Lidocaine, by intravenous infusion, is the therapy of choice for ventricular arrhythmias. It has proved to be safe in early pregnancy. The incidence of adverse effects when used during labor and delivery[52] is very low except in the presence of fetal acidosis, in which instance fetal cardiac and CNS toxicity has been reported.[15]

Procainamide. Procainamide may be the drug of choice for patients who cannot tolerate quinidine. Patients on chronic therapy may develop a lupus-like syndrome replete with antinuclear antibodies. A unique use of procainamide has been conversion of a supraventricular arrhythmia in a fetus in whom digoxin and propranolol had been used unsuccessfully.[34]

Disopyramide. Disopyramide is a newer antiarrhythmia agent that has indications for use similar to those of quinidine but has fewer gastrointestinal side effects. It is useful in ventricular tachyarrhythmias resistant to other agents. Since it has a negative inotropic effect, it should not be used in patients with congestive heart failure.[100] At the present time, use in pregnancy is limited.

Beta-Adrenergic Blocking Agents. Beta-adrenergic blocking agents have been used extensively in pregnancy in the management of hypertension,[36,105] thyrotoxicosis,[17] idiopathic hypertrophic subaortic stenosis,[115] and fetal cardiac rhythm disturbances.[34] They are effective in management of atrial and ventricular premature beats and supraventricular and ventricular tachycardias. They are administered chronically in patients with a long QT syndrome.[16] Propranolol has been incriminated as a cause of intrauterine fetal growth retardation. The evidence for this is not firm. Other adverse effects in the newborn are apnea, bradycardia, and hypoglycemia.[48] The experience with metaprolol and atenolol, both selective beta-1-blockers, is limited but encouraging. A selective beta-1-blocker theoretically should be more specific and safer, since the potential for increase in uterine tone associated with nonselective blockade should be eliminated. No fetal developmental anomalies have been reported with this class of medication.

Calcium Channel Blocking Agents. Verapamil is the best known drug of this group. It is effective in converting paroxysmal supraventricular tachycardias to sinus rhythm. The drug is less effective in atrial flutter or atrial fibrillation. Verapamil is used for hypertension and angina. High dosages may precipitate cardiac failure. Verapamil has been utilized in treating fetal supraventricular tachycardia in utero.[131] Calcium entry blockers theoretically should inhibit uterine contractions. Little clinical information is available regarding the use of these drugs in pregnancy.

Cardioversion

Recurrent arrhythmias resistant to pharmacologic therapy may occur during pregnancy. Electric cardioversion may be performed safely at all stages of pregnancy.[29,109] Cardioversion does not precipitate premature labor. The fetal heart rate is maintained during cardioversion, since the electrical energy reaching the fetal heart is small.

DIURETICS AND PREGNANCY

Diuretics in general, and specifically thiazide diuretics, should be used very selectively in pregnancy. Even short-term administration has been associated with a reduced metabolic clearance rate of dehydroisoandrosterone sulfate[41] and a mean decline of 450 cc in blood volume,[121] implying a potential to decrease uterine blood flow and placental perfusion. Other maternal side effects include hyperglycemia,[67] hemorrhagic pancreatitis,[83] hypokalemia,[96] and thrombocytopenia. Numerous neonatal problems may occur secondary to maternal thiazide administration. Hyponatremia has been found in neonates of hyponatremic mothers, and fetal bradycardia responsive to parenteral potassium therapy was noted in a patient with diuretic-induced hypokalemia.[3,4] Maternal hyperglycemia secondary to thiazide therapy may result in neonatal hypoglycemia.[67] Since undesirable side effects are associated with diuretics, these drugs should be used only for specific maternal indications such as congestive heart failure and pulmonary edema. Furosemide is an excellent medication for impending cardiac failure, frank failure, or pulmonary edema. The drug reduces preload and stimulates diuresis.

MYOCARDIAL INFARCTION AND ATHEROSCLEROTIC HEART DISEASE

Myocardial infarction is rare in pregnancy. The incidence is 1:10,000 live births.[42,59] The maternal mortality is 28–32%. [24,42,59] It is lowest during the first trimester but rises to 67% in the last month of pregnancy and remains as high as 50% in the puerperium.[42,59] The majority of deaths occur at the time of initial infarction or in patients delivered within two weeks of an infarction. [49] Mortality rate is age related. It is about 50% in patients under 35 years of age, but only about 10.5% in older patients.[42]

Angiocardiography should be performed postinfarction[24] and before another pregnancy is undertaken. If occlusive atherosclerotic disease is present, the likelihood of recurrent infarction may be increased.[24,59] In addition to coronary disease, ventricular aneurysm, with or without cardiac valve incompetence, may be detected with angiography.[31,97] The ten-year survival of symptomatic patients with ventricular aneurysm is only 46%. If the patient is asymptomatic, survival is 90% at the end of one year.[45] Surgical correction is therefore indicated in patients who have symptomatic ventricular aneurysms.

There are numerous reports of normal coronary arteries found on angiography after myocardial infarction in pregnancy or the puerperium.[9,21,22,54,104,107] It has been proposed that the etiology of the infarction in such cases was spasm of the coronary arteries, and that this spasm may be drug induced. Another explanation for the presence of normal coronary arteries after a myocardial infarction in the puerperium is embolization with subsequent recanalization.[9]

A dissecting aneurysm of the coronary artery may occur, usually during the postpartum period.[61,111] The event is nearly always fatal, but a survival has been reported.[111]

The management of myocardial infarction in the peripartum period is primarily medical. Angina pectoris, embolic phenomena and congestive heart failure are usually amenable to conventional therapy. A recent report describes myocardial infarction and cardiac arrest in the second trimester in a patient who subsequently was delivered uneventfully at 38 weeks.[112]

The management of myocardial infarction during pregnancy or parturition mandates that myocardial oxygen demand/consumption be limited throughout pregnancy and particularly at parturition. Invasive monitoring techniques should be utilized at labor and delivery. The hemodynamic status is kept stable by utilizing regional anesthesia. Parenteral nitrate may be administered to patients with angina at rest. Cesarean section should be reserved for obstetric indications, because maternal mortality is higher with cesarean section than with vaginal delivery.[49]

Surgical intervention (i.e., coronary bypass and/or ventricular aneurysm resection) should be carried out in selected cases, especially if medical management fails, regardless of the trimester of pregnancy. Coronary artery bypass in the second trimester can result in an uneventful pregnancy and delivery.[74]

Although vaginal delivery is preferred, prolonged induction or difficult labor should not be permitted. Although cesarean section may eliminate some of the hemodynamic disadvantages of labor and delivery, it adds the additional stress of an operative procedure and the potential for serious complications, during surgery and postoperatively (infection, embolism, aspiration, wound dehiscence, and excessive blood loss). The ideal anesthetic for patients with atherosclerotic heart disease is controlled continuous epidural regional block that provides relief from pain and anxiety and maintains hemodynamic stability. A single epidural injection of morphine provides excellent pain relief in the early puerperium if operative delivery has been performed.[56]

The prognosis for patients who have undergone coronary bypass surgery is unknown. It is probably dependent on the extent of the disease that necessitated the bypass and the postoperative patency of the coronary vessels. Nonpregnant patients who have undergone coronary bypass have usually tolerated general anesthesia and another operative procedure well.[26,73] Patients with a prior coronary bypass have a lesser risk of myocardial infarction during subsequent anesthesia and surgery than do patients who have coronary disease and have not had coronary bypass.[26]

INVASIVE CARDIAC MONITORING (See Chapter 49)

Invasive cardiac monitoring is important in management of the high-risk cardiac patient.[25] The basic monitoring device is the balloon flotation pulmonary artery catheter (Swan–Ganz) with appropriate expanding computer attachments. This catheter provides continuous venous and pulmonary artery pressure and intermittent pulmonary capillary wedge pressure (PCWP). In addition, cardiac output can be determined by thermodilution. With the addition of such data to the usual clinical and laboratory data (blood pressure, urine output, heart rate and rhythm, arteriovenous oxygen differences, and acid–base status), a precise and comprehensive evaluation of cardiopulmonary function is available.

Pulmonary edema of cardiac origin can be differentiated quickly from that of lung injury by finding an elevated PCWP.[25] Other areas of cardiac function that can be assessed with the Swan–Ganz catheter are preload, afterload, and the contractile state of the myocardium.[25] Knowledge of ventricular filling pressure information and cardiac output allows calculation of the optimal preload. Preload can be increased by administration of crystalloid, colloid, or blood or decreased by administration of a diuretic (e.g., furosemide) or by phlebotomy (rarely). Afterload, defined as ventricular wall tension during systole, is dependent on systemic and pulmonary vascular resistances. Vasodilators reduce afterload. Reduction of vascular resistance with hydralazine increases cardiac output in patients with severe pregnancy-induced hypertension.[53] Alpha-adrenergic medications increase afterload. The contractile, or inotropic, state of the myocardium is defined by the force and velocity of ventricular function, when preload and afterload are held constant. If contractile force is inadequate and is not corrected by adjustments of the preload and afterload, a beta-sympathomimetic agent may improve the situation. Dopamine or isoproterenol may be chosen for short-term correction, and digoxin may be used for either acute or chronic therapy.

The information obtained from invasive monitoring is most valuable and useful during labor and delivery and in the early puerperium. If operative delivery is necessary, the information provided by the Swan–Ganz catheter becomes critical. It not only allows exact administration of intravenous fluids and medications but aids in controlling the anesthetic. For example, the level of an epidural block may be altered to attain the least fluctuation (increase) in cardiac output. Such "fine tuning" of regional anesthesia can prevent a cardiovascular crisis, such as acute cardiac failure or pulmonary edema.

REFERENCES

1. Abboud, T. K., Raya, J., Noueihed, R., and Daniel, J.: Intrathecal morphine for relief of labor pain in a parturient with severe pulmonary hypertension. *Anesthesiology* **59**:477–479, 1983.
2. Abramovici, H., Faktor, J. H., Gonen, Y., Brandes, J. M. and, Amikam, S.: Maternal permanent bradycardia: Pregnancy and delivery. *Obstet. Gynecol.* **63**:381–383, 1984.
3. Alstatt, L. B.: Transplacental hyponatremia in the newborn infant. *J. Pediatr.* **66**:985–988, 1965.
4. Anderson, G. G. and Hanson, T. M.: Chronic fetal bradycardia: Possible association with hypokalemia. *Obstet. Gynecol.* **44**:896–898, 1974.
5. Andrinopoulos, G. C. and Arias, F.: Triple heart valve prosthesis and pregnancy. *Obstet. Gynecol.* **55**:762–764, 1980.
6. Arias, F. and Pineda, J.: Aortic stenosis and pregnancy. *J. Reprod. Med.* **20**:229–232, 1978.
7. Bader, R. A., Bader, M. E., Rose, D. J., and Braunwald, E.: Hemodynamics at rest and during exercise in normal pregnancy as studied by cardiac catheterization. *J. Clin. Invest.* **34**:1524–1536, 1955.
8. Bahary, C. M., Ninio, A., Gorodesky, I. G., and Neri, A.:. Tococardiography in pregnancy during extracorporal bypass for mitral valve replacement. *Isr. J. Med. Sci.* **16**:395–397, 1980.
9. Beary, J. F., Summer, W. R., and Buckley, B. H.: Postpartum acute myocardial infarction: A rare occurrence of uncertain etiology. *Am. J. Cardiol.* **43**:158–161, 1979.
10. Berde, C., Willis, D. C., and Sandberg, E. C.: Pregnancy in women with pseudoxanthoma elasticum. *Obstet. Gynecol. Surv.* **38**:339–344, 1983.
11. Bieniarz, J., Yoshida, T., Romero-Salinas, G., Curuchet, E., Caldeyro-Barcia, R., and Crottogini, J. J.: Aortocaval compression by the uterus in late human pregnancy. IV. Circulatory homeostasis by preferential perfusion of the placenta. *Am. J. Obstet. Gynecol.* **103**:19–31, 1969.
12. Bortolotti, U., Milano, A., Mazzucco, A., Valfre, C., Russo, R., Valente, M., Schivazappa, L., Thiene, G., and Gallucci, V.: Pregnancy in pa-

tients with a porcine valve bioprosthesis. *Am. J. Cardiol.* **50**:1051–1054, 1982.

13. Bresnahan, D. R., Askenazi, J., and Lesch, M.: Noninvasive assessment of cardiovascular function. *Clin. Obstet. Gynecol.* **24**:711–742, 1981.
14. Brockington, I. F.: Postpartum hypertensive heart failure. *Am. J. Cardiol.* **27**:650–658, 1971.
15. Brown, W. U., Bell, G. C., and Alper, M. H.: Acidosis, local anesthetics, and the newborn. *Obstet. Gynecol.* **48**:27–30, 1976.
16. Bruner, J. P., Barry, M. J., and Elliott, J. P.: Pregnancy in a patient with idiopathic long QT syndrome. *Am. J. Obstet. Gynecol.* **149**:690–691, 1984.
17. Bullock, J. L., Harris, R. E., and Young, R.: Treatment of thyrotoxicosis during pregnancy with propranolol. *Am. J. Obstet. Gynecol.* **121**:242–245, 1975.
18. Burch, G. E., McDonald, C. D., and Walsh, J. J.: The effect of prolonged bed rest on postpartal cardiomyopathy. *Am. Heart J.* **81**:186–201, 1971.
19. Cavalieri, R. L., Watkins, L., Abraham, R. A., Berkay, H. S., and Niebyl, J. R.: Acute bacterial endocarditis with postpartum aortic valve replacement. *Obstet. Gynecol.* **59**:124–125, 1982.
20. Chen, W. W., Chan, C. S., Lee, P. K., Wang, R. Y., and Wong, V. C.: Pregnancy in patients with prosthetic heart valves: An experience with 45 pregnancies. *Q. J. Med.* **51**:358–365, 1982.
21. Ciraulo, D. A. and Markovitz, A.: Myocardial infarction in pregnancy associated with a coronary artery thrombus. *Arch. Intern. Med.* **139**:1046–1047, 1979.
22. Cohen, W. R., Steinman, T., Patsner, B., Snyder, D., Satwicz, P., and Monroy, P.: Acute myocardial infarction in a pregnant woman at term. *JAMA* **250**:2179–2181, 1983.
23. Commerford, P. J., Hastie, T., and Beck, W.: Closed mitral valvotomy: Actuarial analysis of results in 654 patients over 12 years and analysis of preoperative predictors of long-term survival. *Ann. Thorac. Surg.* **33**:473–479, 1982.
24. Cortis, B. S. and Gensini, G. G.: Can the risks of myocardial infarction in pregnancy be reduced? *Bull. Texas Heart Inst.* **4**:49–60, 1977.
25. Cotton, D. B. and Benedetti, T. J.: Use of the Swan-Ganz catheter in obstetrics and gynecology. *Obstet. Gynecol.* **56**:641–645, 1980.
26. Crawford, E. S., Morris, G. C., Howell, J. F., Flynn, W.F., and Moorhead, D. T.: Operative risk in patients with previous coronary artery bypass. *Ann. Thorac. Surg.* **26**:215–221, 1978.
27. Demakis, J. G., Rahimtoola, S. H., Sutton, G. C., Meadows, W. R., Szanto, P. B., Tobin, J. R., and Gunnar, R. M.: Natural course of peripartum cardiomyopathy. *Circulation* **44**:1053–1061, 1971.
28. Denbow, C. E., Matadial, L., Sivapragasam, S., and Spencer, H.: Pregnancy in patients after homograft cardiac valve replacement. *Chest* **83**:540–542, 1983.
29. DeSilva, R. A., Graboys, T. B., Podrid, P. J., and Lown, B.: Cardioversion and defibrillation. *Am. Heart J.* **100**:881–895, 1980.
30. Diab, F., Strasburg, E. R., and Barnard, M. S.: Pregnancy after the insertion of three cardiac valve prostheses. *S. Afr. Med. J.* **49**:1182–1184, 1975.
31. Diro, M., Beydoun, S. N., Jaramillo, B., O'Sullivan, M. J., and Kieval, J.: Successful pregnancy in a woman with a left ventricular cardiac aneurysm. A case report. *J. Reprod. Med.* **28**:559–563, 1983.
32. *Diseases of the Heart and Blood Vessels—Nomenclature Criteria for Diagnosis*, 6th Edition. New York Heart Association, Inc. Boston, Little, Brown & Co., 1964, pp. 112–113.
33. Duffy, B. L.: Pregnancy and triple heart valve prosthesis. *Anaesth. Intensive Care* **10**:59–61, 1982.
34. Dumesic, D. A., Silverman, N. H., Tobias, S., and Golbus, M. S.: Transplacental cardioversion of fetal supraventricular tachycardia with procainamide. *N. Engl. J. Med.* **307**:1128–1131, 1982.
35. Eilen, B., Kaiser, I. H., Becker, R. M., and Cohen, M. N.: Aortic valve replacement in the third trimester of pregnancy: Case report and review of the literature. *Obstet. Gynecol.* **57**:119–121, 1981.
36. Eliahou, H. E., Silverberg, D. S., Reisin, E., Romem, I., Mashiach, S., and Serr, D. M.: Propranolol for the treatment of hypertension in pregnancy. *Br. J. Obstet. Gynaecol.* **85**:431–436, 1978.
37. Elkayam, U. and Gleicher, N.: Cardiac problems in pregnancy. I. Maternal aspects: The approach to the pregnant patient with heart disease. *JAMA* **251**:2838–2839, 1984.
38. Elkayam, U., Kawanishi, D., Reid, C. L., Chandraratna, P. A., Gleicher, N., and Rahimtoola, S. H.: Contrast echocardiography to reduce ionizing radiation associated with cardiac catheterization during pregnancy. *Am. J. Cardiol.* **52**:213–214, 1983.
39. Ellis, F. H., Kirklin, J. W.,Parker, R. L., Burchell, H. B., and Wood, E. H.: Mitral commissurotomy: An overall appraisal of clinical and hemodynamic results. *Arch. Intern. Med.* **94**:774–784, 1954.
40. El-Maraghy, M., Abou Senna, I., El-Tehewy, F., Bassiouni, M., Ayoub, A., and El-Sayed, H.: Mitral valvotomy in pregnancy. *Am. J. Obstet. Gynecol.* **145**:708–710, 1983.
41. Gant, N. F., Madden, J. D., Siitteri, P. K., and MacDonald, P. C.: The metabolic clearance rate of dehydroisoandrosterone sulfate. III. The effect of thiazide diuretics in normal and future preeclamptic pregnancies. *Am. J. Obstet. Gynecol.* **123**:159–163, 1975.
42. Ginz, B.: Myocardial infarction in pregnancy. *J. Obstet. Gynaecol. Br. Commonw.* **77**:610–615, 1970.
43. Gleicher, N., Midwall, J., Hoffberger, D., and Jaffin, H.: Eisenmenger's syndrome and pregnancy. *Obstet. Gynecol. Surv.* **34**:721–741, 1979.

44. Goodwin, J. F.: Pregnancy and coarctation of the aorta. *Clin. Obstet. Gynecol.* 4:645–664, 1961.
45. Grondin, P., Kretz, J. G., Bical, O., Donzeau-Gouge, P., Petitclerc, R., and Campeau, L.: Natural history of saccular aneurysms of the left ventricle. *J. Thorac. Cardiovasc. Surg.* **77**:57–64, 1979.
46. Guidozzi, F.: Pregnancy in patients with prosthetic cardiac valves. *S. Afr. Med. J.* **65**:961–963, 1984.
47. Guzman, C. A. and Caplan, R.: Cardiorespiratory response to exercise during pregnancy. *Am. J. Obstet. Gynecol.* **108**:600–605, 1970.
48. Habib, A. and McCarthy, J. S.: Effects on the neonate of propranolol administered during pregnancy. *J. Pediatr.* **91**:808–811, 1977.
49. Hankins, G. D., Wendel, G. D., Leveno, K. J., and Stoneham, J.: Myocardial infarction during pregnancy: A review. *Obstet. Gynecol.* **65**:139–146, 1985.
50. Harrison, E. C. and Roschke, E. J.: Pregnancy in patients with cardiac valve prostheses. *Clin. Obstet. Gynecol.* **18**:107–123, 1975.
51. Harthorne, J. W., Buckley, M. J., Grover, J. W., and Austen, W. G.: Valve replacement during pregnancy. *Ann. Intern. Med.* **67**:1032–1034, 1967.
52. Heinonen, O. P., Slone, D., and Shapiro, S.: *Birth Defects and Drugs in Pregnancy.* Littleton, Publishing Sciences Group, Inc., 1977, p. 361.
53. Henderson, D. W., Vilos, G. A., Milne, K. J., and Nicol, P. M.: The role of Swan-Ganz catheterization in severe pregnancy-induced hypertension. Am. J. *Obstet. Gynecol.* **148**:570–574, 1984.
54. Henion, W. A., Hilal, A., Matthew, P. K., Lazarus, A. R., and Cohen, J.: Postpartum myocardial infarction associated with normal coronary arteries. *N.Y. State J. Med.* **82**:57–62, 1982.
55. Howard, B. K., Goodson, J. H., and Mengert, W. F.: Supine hypotensive syndrome in late pregnancy. *Obstet. Gynecol.* **1**:371–377, 1953.
56. Hughes, S. C.: Intraspinal narcotics in obstetrics. *Clin. Perinatol.* **9**:167–175, 1982.
57. Hull, E. and Hafkesbring, E.: "Toxic" postpartal heart disease. *New Orleans Med. Surg. J.* **89**:550–557, 1937.
58. Hultgren, H., Hubis, H., and Shumway, N.: Cardiac function following mitral valve replacement. *Am. Heart J.* **75**:302–312, 1968.
59. Husaini, M. H.: Myocardial infarction during pregnancy: Report of two cases with a review of the literature. *Postgrad. Med. J.* **47**:660–665, 1971.
60. Hytten, F. and Chamberlain, G.: *Clinical physiology in obstetrics.* Boston, Blackwell Scientific Publications, 1980, pp. 4, 8, 45, 295.
61. Jewett, J. F.: Committee on maternal welfare. Two dissecting coronary-artery aneurysms post partum. *N. Engl. J. Med.* **298**:1255–1256, 1978.
62. Kenmure, A. C. and Cameron, A. J.: Congenital complete heart block in pregnancy. *Br. Heart J.* **29**:910–912, 1967.
63. Kerenyi, T. D., Meller, J., Steinfeld, L., Gleicher, N., Brown, E., Chitkara, U., and Raucher, H.: Transplacental cardioversion of intrauterine supraventricular tachycardia with digitalis. *Lancet* **2**:393–394, 1980.
64. Kirklin J. W.: The replacement of cardiac valves. *N. Engl. J. Med.* **304**:291–292, 1981.
65. Koh, K. S., Friesen, R. M., Livingstone, R. A., and Peddle, L. J.: Fetal monitoring during maternal cardiac surgery with cardiopulmonary bypass. *Can. Med. Assoc. J.* **112**:1102–1104, 1975.
66. Kolibash, A. J., Ruiz, D. E., and Lewis, R. P.: Idiopathic hypertrophic subaortic stenosis in pregnancy. *Ann. lntern. Med.* **82**:791–794, 1975.
67. Ladner, C. N., Pearson, J. W., Herrick, C. N., and Harrison, H. E.: The effect of chlorothiazide on blood glucose in the third trimester of pregnancy. A preliminary report. *Obstet. Gynecol.* **23**:555–560, 1964.
68. Larrea, J. L., Nunez, L., Reque, J. A., Aguado, M. G., Matorras, R., and Minguez, J. A.: Pregnancy and mechanical valve prostheses: A high-risk situation for the mother and the fetus. *Ann. Thorac. Surg.* **36**:459–463, 1983.
69. Levy, D. L., Warriner, R. A., and Burgess, G. E.: Fetal response to cardiopulmonary bypass. *Obstet. Gynecol.* **56**:112–115, 1980.
70. Levy, G.: Pharmacokinetics of fetal and neonatal exposure to drugs. *Obstet. Gynecol.* **58**:9S–16S, 1981.
71. Lewis, B. S., Agathangelou, N. E., Dos Santos, L. A., and Antunes, M. J.: Real time 2-dimensional echocardiographic visualization of a thrombus on a Bjork–Shiley mitral valve prosthesis. Emergency cesarean section and mitral valve replacement in late pregnancy. *Am J. Cardiol.* **51**:908–909, 1983.
72. Lotgering, F. K., Gilbert, R. D., and Longo, L. D.: The interactions of exercise and pregnancy: A review. *Am. J. Obstet. Gynecol.* **149**:560–568, 1984.
73. Mahar, L. J., Steen, P. A., Tinker, J. H., Vlietstra, R. E., Smith, H. C., and Pluth, J. R.: Perioperative myocardial infarction in patients with coronary artery disease with and without aorta-coronary artery bypass grafts. *J. Thorac. Cardiovasc. Surg.* **76**:533–537, 1978.
74. Majdan, J. F., Walinsky, P., Cowchock, S. F., Wapner, R. J., and Plzak, L.: Coronary artery bypass surgery during pregnancy. *Am. J. Cardiol.* **52**:1145–1146, 1983.
75. Markiewicz, W., Stoner, J., London, E., Hunt, S. A., and Popp, R. L.: Mitral valve prolapse in one hundred presumably healthy young females. *Circulation* **53**:464–473, 1976.
76. Martin, C., Pernoll, M. L., Boruszak, A. N., Jones, J. W., and LoCicero, J.: Cesarean section while on cardiac bypass: Report of a case. *Obstet. Gynecol.* **5**:41S–45S, 1981.

77. McAnulty, J. H., Metcalfe, J., and Ueland, K.: General guidelines in the management of cardiac disease. *Clin. Obstet. Gynecol.* **24**:773–788, 1981.
78. McAnulty, J. H., Metcalfe, J., and Ueland, K.: Heart disease and pregnancy. In: *The Heart*, 5th Edition. J. W. Hurst (Ed.). New York, McGraw-Hill, 1983, pp. 1527, 1530–1532.
79. McCaffrey, R. M. and Dunn, L. J.: Primary pulmonary hypertension in pregnancy. *Obstet. Gynecol. Surv.* **19**:567–591, 1964.
80. Meadows, W. R.: Postpartum heart disease. *Am. J. Cardiol.* **6**:788–797, 1960.
81. Melvin, K. R., Richardson, P. J., Olsen, E. G., Daly, K., and Jackson, G.: Peripartum cardiomyopathy due to myocarditis. *N. Engl. J. Med.* **307**:731–734, 1982.
82. Miller, M., Buchanan, N., Cane, R. D., and Kinsley, R.: Two mitral valve replacements during the course of a single pregnancy. *Intensive Care Med.* **4**:41–42, 1978.
83. Minkowitz, S., Soloway, H. B., Hall, J. E., and Yermakov, V.: Fatal hemorrhagic pancreatitis following chlorothiazide administration in pregnancy. *Obstet. Gynecol.* **24**:337–342, 1964.
84. Murdoch, J. L., Walker, B. A., Halpern, B. L., Juzma, J. W., and McKusick, V. A.: Life expectancy and causes of death in the Marfan syndrome. *N. Engl. J. Med.* **286**:804–808, 1972.
85. Nagorney, D. M. and Field, C. S.: Successful pregnancy 10 years after triple cardiac valve replacement. *Obstet. Gynecol.* **57**:386–388, 1981.
86. Nora, J. J. and Nora, A. H.: Th evolution of specific genetic and environmental counseling in congenital heart diseases. *Circulation* **57**:205–213, 1978.
87. Nunez, L., Aquado, M. G., Celemin, D., Iglesias, A., and Larrea, J. L.: Aspirin or coumadin as the drug of choice for valve replacement with porcine bioprosthesis. *Ann. Thorac. Surg.* **33**:354–358, 1982.
88. Nunez, L., Larrea, J. L., Aguado, M. G., Reque, J. A., Matorras, R., and Minguez, J. A.: Pregnancy in 20 patients with bioprosthetic valve replacement. *Chest* **84**:26–28, 1983.
89. Oakley, C.: Pregnancy in patients with prosthetic heart valves. *Br. Med. J.* **286**:1680–1682, 1983.
90. Oakley, C. M.: Long-term complications of valve replacement. *Br. Med. J.* **284**:995–997, 1982.
91. Oakley, G. D., McGarry, K., Limb, D. G., and Oakley, C. M.: Management of pregnancy in patients with hypertrophic cardiomyopathy. *Br. Med. J.* **1**:1749–1750, 1979.
92. O'Donnel, D., Gillmer, D. J., and Mitha, A. S.: Aortic and mitral valve replacement for bacterial endocarditis in pregnancy. A case report. *S. Afr. Med. J.* **64**:1074, 1983.
93. Payne, D. G., Fishburne, J. I., Rufty, A. J., and Johnston, F. R.: Bacterial endocarditis in pregnancy. *Obstet. Gynecol.* **60**:247–250, 1982.
94. Pierce, J. A., Price, B. O., and Joyce, J. W.: Familial occurrence of postpartal heart failue. *Arch. Intern. Med.* **111**:651–655, 1963.
95. Pitts, J. A., Crosby, W. M., and Basta, L. L.: Eisenmenger's syndrome in pregnancy. Does heparin prophylaxis improve the maternal mortality rate? *Am. Heart J.* **93**:321–325, 1977.
96. Pritchard, J. A. and Whalley, P. J.: Severe hypokalemia due to prolonged administration of chlorothiazide during pregnancy. *Obstet. Gynecol.* **81**:1241–1244, 1961.
97. Roberts, A. D., Low, R. A., Rae, A. P., and Hillis, W. S.: Left ventricular aneurysm complicating acute myocardial infarction occurring during pregnancy. Case report. *Br. J. Obstet. Gynaecol.* **90**:969–970, 1983.
98. Robson, J. S., Martin, A. M., Ruckley, V. A., and MacDonald, M. K.: Irreversible post-partum renal failure. A new syndrome. *Q. J. Med.* **37**:423–435, 1968.
99. Rogers, M. C., Willerson, J. T., Goldblatt, A., and Smith, T. W.: Serum digoxin concentrations in the human fetus, neonate and infant. *N. Engl. J. Med.* **287**:1010–1013, 1972.
100. Rotmensch, H. H., Elkayam, U., and Frishman, W.: Anti-arrhythmic drug therapy during pregnancy. *Ann. Intern Med.* **98**:487–497, 1983.
101. Rovinsky, J. J. and Jaffin, H.: Cardiovascular hemodynamics in pregnancy. I. Blood and plasma volumes in multiple pregnancy. *Am. J. Obstet. Gynecol.* **93**:1–15, 1965.
102. Rovinsky, J. J. and Jaffin, H.: Cardiovascular hemodynamics in pregnancy. II. Cardiac output and left ventricular work in multiple pregnancy. *Am. J. Obstet. Gynecol.* **95**:781–786, 1966.
103. Salazar, E., Zajarias, A., Gutierrez, N., and Iturbe, I.: The problem of cardiac valve prostheses, anticoagulants, and pregnancy. *Circulation* **70** (Suppl. 1):169–177, 1984.
104. Salem, D. N., Isner, J. M., Hopkins, P., and Konstam, M. A.: Ergonovine provocation in post partum myocardial infarction. *Angiology* **35**:110–114, 1984.
105. Sandstrom, B.: Antihypertensive treatment with adrenergic beta-receptor blocker metoprolol during pregnancy. *Gynecol. Obstet. Invest.* **9**:195–204, 1978.
106. Saravolatz, L. D., Burch, K. H., Quinn, E. L., Cox, F., Madhavan, T., and Fisher, E.: Polymicrobial infective endocarditis: An increasing clinical entity. *Am. Heart J.* **95**:163–168, 1978.
107. Sasse, L., Wagner, R., and Murray, F. E.: Transmural myocardial infarction during pregnancy. *Am. J. Cardiol.* **35**:448–452, 1975.
108. Schanker, L. S.: Passage of drugs across body membranes. *Pharmacol. Rev.* **14**:501–530, 1962.
109. Schroeder, J. S., and Harrison, D. C.: Repeated cardioversion during pregnancy. Treatment of refractory paroxysmal atrial tachycardia during 3 successive pregnancies. *Am. J. Cardiol.* **27**:445–446, 1971.
110. Seftel, H. and Susser, M.: Maternity and myo-

cardial failure in African woman. *Br. Heart J.* **23**:43–52, 1961.

111. Shaver, P. J., Carrig, T. F., and Baker, W. P.: Postpartum coronary artery dissection. *Br. Heart J.* **40**:83–86, 1978.

112. Stokes, I. M., Evans, J., and Stone, M.: Myocardial infarction and cardiac arrest in the second trimester followed by assisted vaginal delivery under epidural analgesia at 38 weeks gestation. Case report. *Br. J. Obstet. Gynaecol.* **91**:197–198, 1984.

113. Szekely, P. and Snaith, L.: *Heart Disease and Pregnancy.* London, Churchill Livingston, 1974, pp. 54, 149–150, 164, 167–168.

114. Trimakas, A. P., Maxwell, K. D., Berkay, S., Gardner, T. J., and Achuff, S. C.: Fetal monitoring during cardio pulmonary bypass for removal of a left atrial myxoma during pregnancy. *Johns Hopkins Med. J.* **144**:156–160, 1979.

115. Turner, G. M., Oakley, C. M., and Dixon, H. G.: Management of pregnancy complicated by hypertrophic obstructive cardiomyopathy. *Br. Med. J.* **4**:281–284, 1968.

116. Ueland, K.: Cardiovascular diseases complicating pregnancy. *Clin. Obstet. Gynecol.* **21**:429–442, 1978.

117. Ueland, K.: Maternal cardiovascular dynamics. VII. Intrapartum blood volume changes. *Am. J. Obstet. Gynecol.* **126**:671–677, 1976.

118. Ueland, K., Akamatsu, T. J., Eng, M., Bonica, J. J., and Hansen, J. M.: Maternal cardiovascular dynamics. VI. Cesarean section under epidural anesthesia without epinephrine. *Am. J. Obstet. Gynecol.* **114**:775–780, 1972.

119. Ueland, K. and Hansen, J. M.: Maternal cardiovascular dynamics. II. Posture and uterine contractions. *Am. J. Obstet. Gynecol.* *103*:1–7, 1969.

120. Ueland, K. and Hansen, J. M.: Maternal cardiovascular dynamics. III. Labor and delivery under local and caudal analgesia. *Am. J. Obstet. Gynecol.* **103**:8–18, 1969.

121. Ueland, K., McAnulty, J. H., Ueland, F. R., and Metcalfe, J.: Special considerations in the use of cardiovascular drugs. *Clin. Obstet. Gynecol.* **24**:809–823, 1981.

122. Ueland, K. and Metcalfe, J.: Circulatory changes in pregnancy. *Clin. Obstet. Gynecol.* **18**:41–50, 1975.

123. Ueland, K., Novy, M. J., and Metcalfe J.: Cardiorespiratory responses to pregnancy and exercise in normal women and patients with heart disease. *Am. J. Obstet. Gynecol.* **115**:4–10, 1973.

124. Ueland, K., Novy, M. J., and Metcalfe, J.: Hemodynamic responses of patients with heart disease to pregnancy and exercise. *Am. J. Obstet. Gynecol.* **113**:47–59, 1972.

125. Ueland, K., Novy, M. J., Peterson, E. N., and Metcalfe, J.: Maternal cardiovascular dynamics. IV. The influence of gestational age on the maternal cardiovascular response to posture and exercise. *Am. J. Obstet. Gynecol.* **104**:856–864, 1969.

126. Veille, J.: Peripartum cardiomyopathies: A review. *Am. J. Obstet. Gynecol.* **148**:805–818, 1984.

127. Walsh, J. J., Burch, G. E., Black, W. C., Ferrans, V. J., and Hibbs, R. G.: Idiopathic myocardiopathy of puerperium (postpartal heart disease). *Circulation* **32**:19–31, 1965.

128. Wang, R. Y., Lee, P. K., Chow, J. S., and Chen, W. W.: Efficacy of low dose, subcutaneously administered heparin in treatment of pregnant women with artificial heart valves. *Med. J. Aust.* **2**:126–128, 1983.

129. Werch, A., Lambert, H. M., Cooley, D., and Reed, C. C.: Fetal monitoring and maternal open heart surgery. Letter to the Editor. *South. Med. J.* **70**:1024, 1977.

130. Whittemore, R., Hobbins, J. C., and Engle, M. A.: Pregnancy and its outcome in women with and without surgical treatment of congenital heart disease. *Am. J. Cardiol.* **50**:641–651, 1982.

131. Wolff, F., Breuker, K. H., Sclensker, K. H., and Bolte, A.: Prenatal diagnosis and therapy of fetal heart rate anomalies: With a contribution on the placental transfer of Verapamil. *J. Perinat. Med.* **8**:203–208, 1980.

132. Zitnik, R. S., Bradenburg, R. O., Sheldon, R., and Wallace, R. B.: Pregnancy and open heart surgery. *Circulation* **39** (Suppl. 1):257–262, 1969.

32

HYPERTENSIVE DISORDERS OF PREGNANCY

The hypertensive disorders of pregnancy, both acute and chronic, regardless of cause, are among the most serious medical complications that the pregnant patient encounters. The incidence of these problems is remarkably constant among developed countries but varies in different population groups. Hypertensive diseases complicate 8–10% of all pregnancies. Preeclampsia/eclampsia constitute some 6–8%. The remainder of the hypertensive diseases in pregnancy are caused by chronic hypertension. The majority of pregnancies complicated by hypertensive diseases do reasonably well; however, there is a potential for death to both the mother and the fetus.

CLASSIFICATION OF HYPERTENSIVE DISORDERS

Vascular derangements may antedate or accompany pregnancy and are manifested by elevated blood pressure readings along with both normal and abnormal findings in other organ systems. Classification of hypertensive disorders has never proved to be completely satisfactory; however, the one that is used most commonly is that proposed by the Committee on Terminology of the American College of Obstetricians and Gynecologists.

1. True preeclampsia (glomeruloendotheliosis)
2. Chronic hypertension
   a. Essential
   b. Due to other causes
   c. With superimposed preeclampsia
3. Transient hypertension (occurs in labor and early postpartum)

This classification is simplified from a more complicated classification:

I. Preeclampsia (toxemia, pregnancy-induced hypertension, acute hypertension in pregnancy, gestational hypertension)
II. Chronic hypertensive diseases
   A. Primary (essential, idiopathic)—the most common form of hypertension
   B. Secondary (related to a known cause)
      1. Renal/parenchymal disease, such as glomerulonephritis, chronic pyelonephritis, interstitial nephritis, polycystic kidney; renal vascular; lupus erythematosus, and so on.
      2. Adrenal gland:
         Cortical—Cushing's disease, hyperaldosteronism;
         Medullary—pheochroocytoma
      3. Other:
         Thyrotoxicosis, coarctation of aorta, and so on.
III. Chronic hypertensive disease with superimposed preeclampsia
IV. Transient hypertension—occurs during labor or in the immediate postpartum period (most likely an aberrant form of preeclampsia)

The classification of hypertension appears to be more straightforward than it actually is. It is made on clinical grounds with some laboratory backup. The problem of the inaccuracy of clinical diagnosis was underscored by renal biopsy studies done at Chicago Lying-In Hospital which showed poor correlation between the renal biopsy diagnosis and the clinical diagnosis. The International Society for the Study of Hypertension in Pregnancy has spent much time during the past two years in trying to achieve worldwide agreement on the classification of hypertensive diseases in pregnancy. For practical purposes, only the clinical diagnosis is of value because renal biopsies are no longer routinely performed. Certain criteria must be met before renal biopsies are done. Unless an electron microscope is available, renal biopsy is of little value, because light microscopy is inadequate for accurate comparison. Electron microscopy and immunologic staining are necessary to make a precise diagnosis of renal pathology. We still do renal biopsies but reserve them for the patient in whom we suspect a specific renal disease or in whom the diagnosis seems unusually obscure. There are few, if any, indications to perform renal biopsy during pregnancy. The usual time that renal biopsy is done is postpartum. Most commonly, we have done this at the time of cesarean section, utilizing a vertical skin incision and general anesthesia. Upon completion of the delivery of the baby and repair of the uterus, and prior to closure of the peritoneum, large packs and retractors are used for visualization of the right abdominal gutter over the region of the right kidney. A disposable breast biopsy needle is used for at least two biopsies. One biopsy specimen is studied by conventional means. The other is deposited in glutaraldehyde for electron microscopic and immunofluorescent studies. The value of the renal biopsy is for future pregnancies and follow-up. In the University of Chicago study of renal biopsies, less than 1% of patients had a clinical diagnosis of chronic renal disease, whereas more than 15% of patients had chronic renal disease as diagnosed by electron microscopy by biopsy. The findings of this study were later extended. No correlation was found between levels of hypertension, proteinuria, plasma, creatinine, or blood urea nitrogen and lesions seen by electron microscopy. Eighty-two percent of preeclamptic patients were primigravidas with the renal lesion of preeclampsia. No primigravida with hypertension had a normal renal biopsy. Fifty percent of patients who had heavy proteinuria, that is, more than 3.5 grams/24 hours, had preeclampsia. The greatest error in classification of disease involves patients with chronic hypertension and those with renal disease (Table 32-1).[11,29]

PREECLAMPSIA AND ECLAMPSIA

Various terms have been used to describe preeclampsia. They all mean the same entity. They are acute hypertension in pregnancy, toxemia, preeclampsia, and pregnancy-induced hypertension. We prefer the term preeclampsia because it is more understood worldwide. The Europeans prefer the term gestational hypertension. Once the patient has preeclampsia plus a seizure, she is then said to have eclampsia. Preeclampsia has been with us since the beginning of time. Thousands of pages and many

TABLE 32-1. RENAL PATHOLOGY (ELECTRON MICROSCOPY); 176 PREGNANT HYPERTENSIVE PATIENTS

Diagnosis	Number	Primigravidas	Multiparas
Preeclampsia*	96	79	17
With nephrosclerosis	13	6	7
With renal disease	3	1	2
With both	2	1	1
Nephrosclerosis	19	3	16
With renal disease	4	2	2
Renal disease	31	12	19
Normal histology	8	0	8
TOTAL	176	104	72

*Only glomerular endotheliosis on biopsy.

Source: Fisher, K., Luger, A., Spargo, B. H., and Lindheimer, M. D.: Hypertension in pregnancy; clinical pathological correlations and late prognosis. *Medicine* **60**:267–276, © by Williams & Williams 1981.

books have been devoted to this enigma of unknown etiology, which is seen in the last trimester of pregnancy and is usually associated with progressive development of edema, hypertension, and proteinuria. In general, eclampsia is the most severe form of the disease and is associated with loss of maternal life between 0 and 17% and of the life of the baby or fetus in from 8% to 38% of cases in the world today. Eclampsia means to strike forth or to come with a lightning impulse. However, this seldom is the case. Eclampsia usually is preceded by preeclampsia of various degrees. The real problem rests with our inability to make a diagnosis of impending disease. It has always been our contention that the severe forms of the disease are usually preventable. The onset of the disease is often subtle and the casual observer will fail to make an early diagnosis.

Hypertensive diseases in pregnancy continue to be the leading cause of maternal death in the world today. In the United States it is second, exceeded only by death due to hemorrhage. In most underdeveloped countries, hypertension is the major cause of death. The challenge for the clinician is to recognize individuals at high risk for the disease, to institute appropriate preventive measures, and then to eliminate the severe forms. Theoretically, severe forms should occur only under unusual circumstances and perhaps in individuals who have a genetic predisposition for the disease.

DEFINITION OF TERMS

Preeclampsia is principally a disease of the first viable pregnancy. Its onset in the late second trimester or third trimester of pregnancy is associated with progressive development of edema or abnormal weight gain, hypertension, and, lastly, proteinuria. Preeclampsia also can develop in the patient who has chronic hypertension. It often occurs earlier and may be more severe in this setting. The major goal in taking care of the woman who has chronic hypertension is prevention of preeclampsia because fetal and maternal morbidity and mortality may be increased four to five times above normal. This group of patients may indeed display the highest maternal mortality. As this disease of unknown etiology progresses from mild to significant preeclampsia, a reversible renal lesion designated glomeruloendotheliosis is identified. Once glomeruloendotheliosis is present, the renal lesion cannot be reversed by medical care. Only delivery will cure the situation. Once significant glomeruloendotheliosis is present, proteinuria of greater than 2+ usually is found.

Patient Profile

Certain maternal conditions are associated with an increased incidence of preeclampsia. These groups include:

1. Pregnancies that have a larger volume of placental tissue (hyperplacentosis), such as those associated with diabetes mellitus, Rh disease, or multiple gestation, have a higher propensity for preeclampsia.
2. Recently, when we reviewed our data at Ohio State University, we found that patients with congenital anomalies, that is, double uterus, septate uterus, and so on, also have a higher incidence of preeclampsia (as high as 30%). The hyperplacentosis and congenital anomaly patients have a propensity to develop preeclampsia that is two to four times greater than the expected incidence of 6%.
3. Patients with chronic renal and chronic cardiovascular diseases and those with a genetic history of hypertension in pregnancy in their siblings or mother also have a higher propensity for preeclampsia.
4. It is to be underscored that the first viable pregnancy in an individual should be considered as high risk and potential for preeclampsia.
5. It is unwise to make a diagnosis of preeclampsia unless the patient is nulliparous, less than 25 years of age, has progressive onset of edema, hypertension, and proteinuria, and is completely normal 4–6 weeks postpartum.

It is unusual for preeclampsia to be present without abnormal weight gain or overt edema. When the blood pressure reaches 140/90 mmHg, or when there has been a 30 mmHg increase in systolic or a 15 mmHg increase in diastolic over midtrimester values, a diagnosis of mild preeclampsia can be entertained. This type of preeclampsia is usually insignificant as far as maternal and fetal outcome is concerned, but when proteinuria develops, then the disease warrants major concern. Severe preeclampsia is diagnosed when the blood pressure reaches 160/110 mmHg, when proteinuria exceeds 5 grams/day, or when there is evidence of symptomatic end organ damage with such symptoms as headache, visual disturbances, epigastric pain, oliguria, or renal failure. These findings should alert the physician for major concern. Eclamptic seizures are the worst maternal complications. They can occur with blood pressures in the high normal range but usually occur when the blood pressure exceeds 140/90. A common cause of maternal death in these patients is cerebral edema, but aspiration of gastric contents and congestive heart failure, along with other end organ derangement, also are key factors in death.

PATHOPHYSIOLOGY

Preeclampsia disrupts normal homeostatic mechanisms. The disruption eventually results in disturbed pathophysiology, which may then manifest itself in different ways. The major disturbed pathophysiology includes: (1) a disease of the arterioles with vasospasm resulting in hypertension; (2) alterations in cardio-vascular reactivity resulting in increased response to pressor agents (endogenous and exogenous); (3) a renal lesion, known as glomeruloendotheliosis, clinically resulting in proteinuria, oliguria, and disturbed renal function; this lesion is reversible and does not cause permanent renal damage; (4) central nervous system irritability, clinically seen as clonus, cerebral edema, or convulsions; if convulsions occur, the term eclampsia is used; (5) uteroplacental bed constriction of distal spiral arteries and increased tissue norepinephrine that clinically may result in intrauterine growth retardation, stillbirth, or relative tissue hypoxia; (6) a decrease in cardiovascular volume that is manifested clinically by an increase in hematocrit; and (7) a catabolic disease clinically recognized as negative nitrogen balance when such patients are studied on a metabolic ward.

Target Organs

The major target organs involved in preeclampsia are: (1) the cardiovascular system, with vasospasm resulting in hypertension and altered cardiovascular reactivity; (2) the kidney with proteinuria and/or oliguria as a result of glomeruloendotheliosis; (3) the uteroplacental bed where there is a decrease in uterine blood flow resulting in a propensity for intrauterine growth retardation and relative fetal hypoxia. The secondary organs involved may well be significant in the severity of the disease. These are the liver, where hepatocellular damage can be seen and may be identified by aberrations in liver function tests; the reticuloendothelial system, where there may be a decrease in platelets, an increase in fibrin split products, and relative disseminated intravascular coagulopathy; and, lastly, the brain, where edema and hemorrhage may take place. A given patient may have a propensity for one factor and others may not be too involved or there may be involvement in various combinations of all organ systems.

Laboratory Studies

The garden variety preeclamptic patient usually will have normal laboratory studies except perhaps for an elevated hematocrit identifying hemoconcentration due to a filled, constricted but diminished blood volume. As the disease progresses, more positive findings may be seen. In an individual patient, a specific target organ system may be involved that will result in abnormal laboratory findings, and these must be searched for. Tables 32-2 and 32-3 identify some useful parameters that should be evaluated in patients who have hypertensive diseases.

Table 32-3 identifies the area that we think gives the highest yield for a diagnosis of preeclampsia. When uric acid is elevated, if the clinical picture is compatible and confirmatory, in the absence of benzothiadiazine diuretics, preeclampsia is likely. Serum free iron normally decreases in pregnancy. However, in patients with preeclampsia there is slight hemolysis and this creates increased free iron. The antithrombin III determination, which we have studied extensively, is one of the most sensitive laboratory tests and oftentimes will tell when a patient has impending or mild preeclampsia, in which case antithrombin III is decreased below 70%. We rank antithrombin III as the most sensitive test, but it is to be emphasized that no single test will identify a patient with preeclampsia. It is important to understand the deranged homeostatic mechanisms and then to look for the organ system involved.[9,10,23,31-33]

ETIOLOGY

The exact etiology of preeclampsia/eclampsia is unknown. Since humans have walked erect, we have had the development of preeclampsia/eclampsia. The basic requirement for the development of preeclampsia and eclampsia is chorionic villi. When all else fails in therapy, the products of conception should be removed and

TABLE 32-2. LABORATORY CLUES TO PREECLAMPSIA

	Hematocrit	Electrolytes	Serum Proteinuria
Normal pregnancy	Normal to decreased	Normal	0.4–0.6
Mild preeclampsia	Normal to decreased	Normal	0.4–0.6
Severe preeclampsia	Increased	Normal	0.6–0.8
Eclampsia	Increased	Normal	0.8 or greater

	Liver Enzymes	Fibrinogen and Split Products	Proteinuria
Normal pregnancy	Normal	Normal	0
Mild preeclampsia	Normal	Normal	Trace
Severe preeclampsia	Normal	Normal to increased	2–3+
Eclampsia	Increased	Occasional decrease in fibrinogen and increase in split products	4+

TABLE 32-3. MOST USEFUL LABORATORY INDICATORS OF PREECLAMPSIA

	Uric Acid	Serum Free Iron	Antithrombin III	Platelet Catecholamines (NE)
Normal pregnancy	Normal	Normal to decreased	More than 80%	Normal
Mild preeclampsia	Normal	Normal to decreased	Less than 80%	Slightly elevated
Severe preeclampsia	Increased	Increased	Less than 70%	Elevated
Eclampsia	Increased	Increased	Less than 70%	Elevated

the disease then abates. Many hypotheses proposed by investigators who felt that they had discovered the specific etiology of eclampsia have been tested and failed. The many theories of etiology have included placental toxins, catecholamines, endocrine abnormalities, nutrition, immunology bad breeders, and most recently parasites. None of these reveals the etiology of the disease. The precise cause remains unknown. Recently, two geneticists have reviewed Chesley's third generation follow-up studies[5] of his original eclamptic study patients from Margaret Hague Maternity Hospital and have proposed a recessive gene theory for these eclamptic patients.[6]

The Chesley data deal with the offspring of mothers who had eclampsia. A significantly increased incidence of preeclampsia or eclampsia during the first pregnancy of daughters of eclamptic mothers is demonstrated. This tends to support the maternal recessive gene theory and offers a rational explanation for repeated preeclampsia.

Incidence of Preeclampsia and Mortality

The accuracy of classification and reporting is obviously the hallmark of true incidence and, if done incorrectly, negates comparisons of one country or one population group to another. It may well be better to use the broad term "hypertensive diseases in pregnancy," since a diagnosis of true preeclampsia may be difficult, and then to use a subcategory under that diagnosis if laboratory or renal biopsy data seem accurate. The general incidence figures in the United States for preeclampsia are 6% ± 1.5% and vary, depending on the number of first pregnancies and the accuracy of reporting. Originally, it was thought that the incidence figures in the black population were greater in the United States, but, in actuality, this may have nothing to do with the black race, but rather with the availability of health care. The higher incidence of preeclampsia in adolescents is most likely due to their inability to seek early health care and to take pregnancy seriously. It has been demonstrated amply by maternal and infant care projects in the United States that poor pregnant women, when given adequate planned prenatal health care, have incidence figures similar to those of middle class individuals. The best example of this was the maternal and infant care project established for 12 adjacent rural counties around Augusta, Georgia, in the mid-1960s. The incidence of eclampsia fell from 1 of 100 deliveries to no more than 1 eclamptic per year in the same health care system. Early hospitalization, coupled with identification of patients prone to develop the disease, lowered the incidence of eclampsia. Hence, prenatal care alters the incidence of severe disease, but may be unrelated to development of mild disease. There is probably no way to determine the true incidence figures of hypertensive diseases in the population. If edema is eliminated because it is a "soft" end point and only hypertension above 140/90 and/or proteinuria in a primigravid woman are considered criteria, the diagnosis of preeclampsia would be more certain.

Fetal mortality in the most severe form of the disease (eclampsia) varies between 10% and 35%, but, in a developed country with good health care, at least 90% of the offspring should be born alive, regardless of gestational age. Since the entry of the neonatal intensive care unit into the health care system during the past 15 years, the survival of the small baby should increase further and expectancy of salvage should be greater. Currently, at the Ohio State University, if a baby weighs 1250 grams or more and comes from a toxemic mother who has been transported to Ohio State University while pregnant, the chance of survival is greater than 93%. It is our recommendation that all mothers who are 34 weeks of gestation or less be transported to a tertiary care center. Interestingly, 50% of the fetuses of multiparous patients who have eclampsia die, as contrasted to less than 38% in all other pregnancies with eclampsia, indicating that the multiparous patient most likely has underlying cardiovascular or renal disease and should have intensive aggressive management.[19]

It has been our contention for many years that the type of treatment also determines survival of the fetus and morbidity and mortality in the mother. The treatment for severe preeclampsia and eclampsia is parenteral magnesium sulfate to prevent seizures and liberal use of hydralazine to control blood pressure. Our first report of treatment of the eclamptic patient in 1965 and the Pritchard and Stone report in 1967 of a larger series of eclamptic patients utilized similar therapy. To this day these reports continue to have identified the best maternal mortality (0) and the best fetal salvage (90%) in the treatment of eclampsia.[25,38]

MANAGEMENT—GENERAL AND PREVENTION

The main theme of all pregnancies is to promote good maternal-fetal health, prevent complications, and deliver a surviving child. The theme in the 1980s should be prevention of disease and diagnosis of insidious and impending problems.The following information should be imparted to the pregnant woman in an effort to diminish the incidence of preeclampsia and to promote general fetal welfare:

1. The patient should accept the responsibility for her pregnancy in a serious fashion and should subjugate her own personal pleasures to the welfare of her fetus. Ths means the elimination of caffeine, nicotine, and alcohol during pregnancy. Having faith in her physician and the health care team should achieve a degree of tranquility, lack of anxiety, and expectation of a planned and wanted child.
2. The patient should understand that nutrition is the cornerstone of an exemplary pregnancy and that it is necessary to achieve at least a 0, or preferably a positive nitrogen balance, by ingesting a minimum of 1 gram of protein/kg of body

weight/day. An adequate intake of protein should be surrounded with a well balanced diet in which the pregnant woman eats the desired amount of food on four or five occasions each day. Additional iron supplementation is needed in pregnancy, since sufficient iron cannot be obtained in the diet.

3. Instruct her to rest in bed at least 1½ hours a day, preferably at noontime, on her side to increase uterine blood flow and provide additional nutrition and oxygenat on for her fetus. If she works, she should obtain a minimum of 30 minutes of rest during her lunch hour, then, in addition, at least one hour of bed rest when she returns home from work. It is essential that this be done daily and that she understand that the position of health for her fetus is when she is in the lateral recumbent position. The lateral recumbent position helps to achieve homeostasis by increasing renal blood flow and glomerular filtration rate, which, in turn, presents additional sodium to the kidney for mild diuresis; this feedback then works to decrease vascular reactivity. Additionally, bed rest in the lateral recumbent position increases uterine blood flow, which, in turn, provides additional fetal nutrition and oxygenation, part of which is due to the diminution in endogenous catecholamines that allows less vascular constriction. It may well be that bed rest is the single most important feature in the quality of health care for the pregnant woman. Bed rest is not easy to achieve, since more than 40% of the work force are females, and it is difficult, especially for the multiparous patient, to accomplish this goal. Nonetheless, bed rest should still be promoted as a major theme in prenatal care.

TYPES OF THERAPY

Various empirical forms of therapy for preeclampsia/eclampsia have been used since the beginning of the description of this disease and will continue to be empiric until the specific etiology of the condition is known. Some forms of therapy may be harmless and others drastic. Studies have compared therapy in different countries, most recently between the United Kingdom and the United States by utilizing a detailed questionnaire on management of pregnancy hypertension complicated by preeclampsia. The questionnaire was sent to three groups of physicians in the United States: obstetricians in private practice, obstetricians in academic departments, and nephrologists in academic departments. The response from the questionnaire was compared to a previous questionnaire utilized for consultant obstetricians in the United Kingdom.[18] The results of the questionnaire revealed major differences and some similarities in the method of management of hypertensive diseases of pregnancy between obstetricians in the United States and obstetricians in the United Kingdom. The United States nephrologists closely resembled and modeled the British obstetricians in treating severe preeclampsia and in the amount of drugs used. The one common denominator of all American obstetricians, whether academic or practicing, was the use of magnesium sulfate as the primary agent to treat severe preeclampsia/eclampsia (98–100). The drug most frequently used to control hypertension was hydralazine. The consultant obstetricians from the United Kingdom do not use magnesium sulfate as their anticonvulsant medication. Only 2% of them indicated this use.

Diet and Diuretics

Advocates for a high protein diet to prevent preeclampsia are many, but few data confirm such statements. Well women can develop preeclampsia on low, moderate, or high protein intake diets.[21] Our balance studies on normal pregnant patients, as well as those with eclampsia, indicate that a normal pregnant woman needs at least 1 gram of protein/kg of body weight/day to replace the protein needed for her developing products of conception. This is the diet that we recommend.[36] Our metabolic studies indicate that the eclamptic patients did not have a sufficient nitrogen intake to create a positive or zero nitrogen balance. They were actually all in negative nitrogen balance. A number of years ago, salt restriction was thought important in prevention of preeclampsia, but no data support this contention. Actually, our salt-loading studies in normal patients, mild preeclamptic patients, and moderate to severe preeclamptic patients confirm that normal patients and mild preeclamptic patients can excrete all their ingested salt. When renal involvement is present in severe preeclampsia, the clinical condition worsens when excessive amounts of salt are ingested.[35]

There is no longer any conflict about the use of diuretics in pregnancy. The double-blind studies that have been done demonstrate that the use of diuretics will not prevent eclampsia. The reasons are too numerous to enumerate. Chesley has devised 11 reasons why diuretics should not be used; suffice it to say they are not useful.[4]

Invasive Human Hemodynamic Monitoring

The central venous pressure catheter and the Swan–Gaz catheter may be useful to a limited extent in women who have severe disease. They are reserved for the person who has an unstable hemodynamic system, who is severely ill, and who does not respond to the usual and customary therapy. Some studies have concluded that pregnant women with preeclampsia are unable to cope with the circulating volume necessary to maintain a cardiac index and ventricular filling pressure, and that patients with preeclampsia do not have the capacity for complete vasodilation.[13]

Primary Therapy for Preeclampsia/Eclampsia

Once a clinical diagnosis of preeclampsia is made, the patient deserves hospitalization to extricate herself from the environment in which she became ill. As noted earlier, there is a general sequence of events in the development of preeclampsia, the first being edema, next an incremental increase in blood pressure, and, lastly, proteinuria. If the symptoms do not occur in this sequence, the diagnosis may be questionable or another disease may also be present. The only symptom of mild preeclampsia is edema. Symptoms such as headache, blurred vision, scotomata, and epigastric pains are not symptoms of mild preeclampsia, but of moderate to severe disease. The following therapeutic regimens are useful.

Mild Preeclampsia

1. Treatment should not take place in the home or in the environment in which the disease developed, but should be in an optimal hospital or domiciliary setting.
2. The patient should be on complete bed rest on her side with bathroom privileges.
3. A diet adequate to provide more than 1 gram of protein/kg of body weight/day with no limitation of sodium intake.
4. Phenobarbital, 30 mg q.i.d., as a sedative, to enable the patient to rest better in bed, but this is not essential.
5. Daily weights, noting that the patient should lose at least 2 kg of weight in the first three days of therapy.
6. Fluid intake and output should be measured to assure an adequate diuresis that should occur within the first 48 hours of hospitalization, demonstrated by a diminution in weight and a decrease in the patient's blood pressure.
7. The blood pressure should be determined at least 4 times a day. Laboratory work should consist of baseline studies including a CBC, daily hematocrit for the first 4 days, daily urine protein; initially, blood urea nitrogen and serum creatinine, along with an antithrombin III, serum free iron and uric acid, as well as platelet count, fibrinogen level, liver profile studies, and electrolytes. It is assumed that these will be normal, but they are used for a baseline in case the disease worsens. As a generalization, the patient should be improved in 3–5 days and may be allowed up more during this time before she is permitted to return home. If she does return home, she should be seen at least twice a week for evaluation of any condition that may worsen. The status of the pregnancy, including gestational age, should be evaluated. If the patient is beyond 36 weeks of gestation and fetal maturity is present, serious consideration should be given to termination of pregnancy.

If the patient is 38 or more weeks gestation, induction of labor should take place. If there is uncertainty as to gestational age, further evaluation utilizing ultrasound and amniocentesis may be in order, as well as antepartum biophysical testing (NST, OCT). If the patient is less than 38 weeks gestation, individualization is necessary. The patient should remain in the hospital for a minimum of 5 days. If she is then sent home, it is necessary that she be seen twice a week. She should be encouraged to continue bed rest at home. If these criteria cannot be met, the patient should remain in the hospital until delivered. She may not respond to therapy and, if so, may proceed to severe preeclampsia, at which time therapy must be more aggressive.

Severe Preeclampsia

It is necessary to meet one or more of the following criteria in order to make the diagnosis of severe preeclampsia:

1. Systolic blood pressure of 160 or diastolic blood pressure of 110, taken two times, recorded 6 hours apart, with the patient at bed rest.
2. Proteinuria of greater than 5 grams in 24 hours, or 3 to 4+ protein on dipstick.
3. Oliguria, defined as urinary output of less than 400 cc in 24 hours.
4. Cerebral or visual disturbances, including eye changes.
5. Pulmonary edema or cyanosis.

Headaches, epigastric pain, or visual disturbances, especially scotomata, all imply worsening disease. Therapy should be aggressive and pregnancy termination considered. The five most common complications that should be avoided in the patient who has severe preeclampsia are:

1. A seizure. (The diagnosis of eclampsia must then be made.)
2. A cerebrovascular accident.
3. Placental abruption.
4. A diminution in platelets with disseminated intravascular coagulopathy.
5. Intrapartum or neonatal distress or death.

It is often said that severe preeclampsia and eclampsia are different diseases, but this concept may not be correct. Some patients who have severe preeclampsia are more ill than some patients who have eclampsia. Whether the patient has severe preeclampsia or eclampsia, the treatment is identical. These entities constitute a serious medical emergency, requiring the utmost priority by the health care team. As a generalization, the patient with severe preeclampsia/eclampsia needs to be delivered within a reasonable period of time. The tendency to or the occurrence of convulsions must be controlled. Once convulsions occur, the delivery schedule should be accelerated. It is probably inappropriate to carry a patient who has severe disease for any protracted period of time, even though the infant is severely premature. The severe vasospasm allows minimal to no additional intrauterine growth of the baby and only maturity may be achieved. The one thing known to cure the mother is removal of the products of conception. The patient who has severe preeclampsia will have hemoconcentration. Serial hematocrits are diagnostic. The hematocrit should decrease with improvement. The blood urea nitrogen and serum creatinine usually are normal but may be slightly elevated.

Treatment of Severe Preeclampsia Without Hyperreflexia

1. Hospitalization.
2. Bed rest in the lateral recumbent position with bathroom privileges.
3. Diet supplying more than 1 gram of protein/kg of body weight/day and restriction of salt intake since the patient has a renal lesion and will retain ingested sodium.
4. Phenobarbital, 30 mg q.i.d. for sedation.
5. Daily weight.
6. Record fluid intake and output.
7. Blood pressure at least four times a day.
8. Baseline laboratory data to include serial hematocrits every 8 hours until stable. Additional laboratory data to include platelet count, fibrinogen level, and liver profile studies, as well as blood urea nitrogen and serum creatinine, antithrombin III, serum free iron, and uric acid and electrolytes.
9. Nonstress test every other day with fetal kick counts during two 1-hour periods a day. Fetal kick counts of greater than 6/hour indicate fetal health.
10. Ultrasound for placental evaluation.

The outcome is dictated by the weeks of gestation and the absence of hypoxia in the fetus. If the patient is more than 34 weeks' gestation, in all probability she should be induced, but if less than 34 weeks, selective evaluation should be utilized. It usually is not necessary to give antihypertensive medications to these patients unless the diastolic pressure is persistently greater than 100 mmHg. Magnesium sulfate is given only if the patient is hyperreflexic, but if in doubt it should be given. Diuresis should be expected within 48 hours, and if not, serious consideration should be given to termination of pregnancy. Prior to termination of pregnancy, amniocentesis should be done to determine pulmonary maturity. If there is an urgency for delivery, but delivery can wait a minimum of 24–36 hours, consideration can be given to treatment with corticosteroids (betamethasone, 12 mg i.m. on two occasions 12 hours apart), followed by a minimum wait of 24 hours after the last dose prior to termination of prgnancy. We have not seen enhancement of hypertension by corticosteroids and we have now treated more than 100 patients in this fashion.[15]

Severe Preeclampsia with Hyperreflexia

The regimen outlined above is instituted, and the following additional measures are taken:

1. Intravenous magnesium sulfate is given by pump, loading dose to saturate body tissues of 4–6 grams given over a period of at least 10 minutes and, following this, 1–2 grams are given every hour. A simplified method of giving the medication is to add 20 grams of magnesium sulfate to 1000 ml of D5W with half normal saline and to allow the infusion to run in at a controlled rate.
2. Reflexes are checked every hour and should be present but hypoactive.
3. Urinary output is checked every hour. Usually this is done by utilizing a Foley catheter. Output should exceed 30 ml/hour. Aggregate totals of urine should exceed 100 ml every 4 hours.
4. Diuretics are not given.
5. Antihypertensive medications should be utilized if the diastolic pressure is consistently greater than 100 mmHg or if cerebral symptoms are present. Hydralazine is given parenterally in an intravenous bolus utilizing 5 mg in the initial injection. Following the bolus injection, a decision can be made in 20 minutes as to whether or not the patient needs additional hydralazine. If so, 100 mg of hydralazine are added to a 200 ml plastic bag of normal saline. Infusion with a control device is utilized to control blood pressure. We use an automatic blood pressure monitor to record the blood pressure and to assist in nursing care. If antihypertensive medication is given, it is important not to diminish the diastolic pressure to less than 80 or fetal distress may ensue.
6. Fetal monitoring is essential.

If the patient is ill, in all probability she should be delivered as soon as possible by induction with oxytocin, especially if the cervix is favorable. If the cervix is unfavorable, we utilize prostaglandin gel (2 mg) every 12 hours to soften the cervix prior to institution of an oxytocin infusion beginning at 0.5–1 milliunit/min. Preeclamptic patients often have additional uterine activity that can be augmented by the prostaglandin gel. If the patient does not deliver within 12 hours, cesarean section should be considered seriously. Electronic fetal monitoring is necessary. As soon as possible, rupture the membranes and insert an internal scalp clip monitor. Pay careful attention to the ominous signs of decreased variability of the fetal heart rate and the presence of meconium in amniotic fluid. Our basis for using intravenous medications is that intramuscular medications are not absorbed as rapidly in a patient who has generalized edema and diminished blood volume. If nursing care is not adequate, utilization of the intramuscular route is quite satisfactory for the use of both magnesium sulfate and hydralazine.[38]

There is no contraindication to the administration of an epidural anesthesia if this is controlled carefully and the level is raised gradually. Spinal anesthesia should *not* be used for delivery, especially in patients who have had antihypertensive medications. Oftentimes, local injection or a pudendal block is all that is needed for vaginal delivery. Paracervical block is probably contraindicated in patients with hypertensive diseases due to the diminished blood flow. If this is the only analgesia available, then use half the usual dose and concentration.

Eclampsia

The patient who develops eclampsia must be considered as one of the most severely ill patients for whom an obstetrician cares. Management requires acute intensive care for mother and fetus by a skilled health care team. If this is not possible, the patient should be referred to a tertiary care center for care. During convulsions, use a padded tongue blade to avoid oral trauma. The convulsion should be controlled with magnesium sulfate, 4–6 grams, given intravenously over 5–10 minutes. Diazepam, sodium amytal, phenytoin sodium, or other anticonvulsant medications are not used because they depress the fetus and mother. After the convulsion, do the following:

1. Insert a plastic airway and give oxygen.
2. Place the patient in Trendelenberg position to prevent aspiration.
3. Suction the nasal and oral passages to remove any secretions.
4. If the stomach is full, rid the stomach contents through a nasogastric tube. Be-

fore removal of the tube, instill an adequate amount of an antaci such as sodium citrate to increase gastric pH. Do not do this until the patient has been controlled with magnesium sulfate, because the manipulation may precipitate another seizure.

5. Start an intravenous line of D5W in order to replace urinary output and insensible loss. Alternate i.v. fluids with D5W and saline or Ringer's lactate. Replace fluids by output and insensible loss.
6. Insert a Foley catheter and record hourly intake and output.
7. Laboratory tests should include a 24-hour urine for protein. Urinary specific gravity should be tested periodically at the bedside and protein checked every 6–8 hours. The hematocrit should be followed closely every 6–8 hours. Additional laboratory data include blood urea nitrogen, serum creatinine and electrolytes, as well as liver enzymes, platelets, and other baseline studies as needed. A portable chest x-ray may be appropriate if there is a suspicion that the patient may have aspirated.
8. Periodic clotting studies for platelets, fibrinogen and fibrin-split products with identification of insipient disseminated or intravascular coagulopathy are in order and, if positive, should be of serious concern.
9. Following the convulsion, continue magnesium sulfate, 1–2 grams per hour intravenously in D5W. If hyperactive reflexes are present (and these should be checked every hour), the dose of magnesium sulfate should be increased. If reflexes are absent or if oliguria is present, the dose of magnesium sulfate should be diminished and may even need to be stopped temporarily.
10. It is necessary to keep calcium gluconate or calcium chloride at the bedside in case of a magnesium overdose. The dose, if necessary, is 1 gram intravenously.
11. Reflexes, urinary output, and respirations should be checked hourly. Urinary output should be at least 30 ml/hour and respirations greater than 12/min to avoid overadministration of magnesium, and the reflexes should be present but hypoactive.
12. Continue the magnesium sulfate for at least 12–24 hours after delivery as seizure activity may recur at that time, and then gradually decrease.
13. Blood levels for magnesium are obtained if an overdose occurs or if a seizure occurs in spite of therapy. A cord blood magnesium may assist the neonatal team. Usually, it is not necessary to use blood magnesium levels to monitor routine therapy. This can be done in selected cases.

Decision for Delivery

The indications for delivery of the eclamptic patient are principally fetal but are also maternal if the mother is ill. The decision becomes difficult, especially if the pregnancy is quite premature, that is, less than 30 weeks of gestation, but delivery should be anticipated. Once the patient has been treated and stabilized, it is essential to sample the amniotic fluid for the presence of both meconium and surfactant. Usually, this is done in the severely preeclamptic patient and not necessarily in the eclamptic patient unless there is no NICU available. The easiest screening test we've found that quickly gives data on pulmonary maturity is optical density at 650 ηm. If the value is greater than 0.12, the baby will have a mature L/S ratio or will not have RDS. Many years ago, we observed that the intrauterine stress that takes place in these patients in some way activates and promotes the development of pulmonary surfactant so that fewer of these babies have RDS than do their counterparts of comparable gestational age. Once the patient has received magnesium sulfate, had adequate hydration, the maternal and fetal situations are well evaluated, and the blood pressure is controlled, the decision can then be made, usually within 4 hours, as to what ultimately should be done for the patient. Most patients can be induced cautiously with intravenous oxytocin and amniotomy. They respond to oxytocin more readily than does the usual patient because the uterus is more sensitive. Hence, caution should be the watchword in starting oxytocin at a rate of no more than 1 milliunit/min.[37] If the fetus is less than 1200 grams and the cervix is unfavorable, serious consideration should be given to cesarean section.

Prognosis

The woman who has preeclampsia need not be concerned that this will cause any permanent cardiovascular damage with resultant hypertension later in life. Our follow-up studies have shown that only those who have a genetic history of hypertension have hypertension after age 50, otherwise there is no propensity for hypertension later in life.[2] The lesion of glomeruloendotheliosis in the kidney is also reversible and goes away soon after delivery has been accomplished. There is one category of patients who may be predisposed to recurrent severe preeclampsia/eclampsia:. those who have a maternal genetic component for the disease as characterized by previous obstetric history, positive maternal history, or siblings who have had similar problems. This is an unusual situation, but it is impossible to reassure all patients who have eclampsia in their first pregnancy that they will never have it again, even though that was the contention a number of years ago.

The major complications of the disease should be avoided, such as (1) abruptio placentae, (2) decompensation of the hematopoietic system with disseminated intravascular coagulopathy with or without hypofibrinogenemia, and (3) maternal cerebrovascular accident. If these are avoided, the prognosis is excellent for the mother and she should have a good recovery.

The prognosis for the fetus is dependent principally on the presence or absence of prematurity. The more premature the baby, the more difficult recovery will be, but probably unrelated to the fact that the mother had preeclampsia/eclampsia unless an unusual number of respiratory depressing agents are used. In the absence of hypoxia during the labor–delivery process, the fetal and newborn prognosis should be excellent.

CHRONIC HYPERTENSION IN PREGNANCY

Chronic hypertension implies a disease state antedating pregnancy. A difference of opinion exists between the nonobstetrician and the obstetrician in understanding the complex interrelationships of hypertension in pregnancy. The nonobstetrician tends to be concerned about blood pressures that are much higher than the obstetrician encounters, and, accordingly, concern for the fetus may not exist. Hypertension is diagnosed if the sustained elevation of arterial blood pressure is greater than 140/90 mmHg in both the pregnant and nonpregnant state. During pregnancy, peripheral resistance is decreased and a lowering of the blood pressure may be seen during the second trimester of pregnancy. If the diastolic blood pressure is greater than 80 mmHg in the second trimester of pregnancy, chronic hypertension should be suspected. A more appropriate way of measuring blood pressure is to utilize the mean arterial blood pressure, which basically accounts for the pressure in vessels, organs, and in the placenta for perfusion. Perinatal mortality increases with increased mean arterial pressure and is increased significantly when mean arterial pressure is greater than 90 mmHg in the second trimester of pregnancy.[24] The commonly used formula[3] for mean arterial pressure is

$$\text{MAP} = \frac{S(\textit{systolic}) + 2(\textit{diastolic})}{3}$$

Examples of rather modest blood pressures that achieve a reading of 90 mmHg mean arterial blood pressure would be 110/80, 120/74, and 130/70, which to the untrained observer are all within normal limits, but for the pregnant patient may be significant.

Classification

Our classification of severity of hypertension in gravidas uses, in the first and second trimesters, the diastolic as well as the mean arterial blood pressure in mild, moderate, and severe hypertension (Table 32-4). Other criteria include cardiac size, EKG evaluation, funduscopic examination, and renal function. This classification may be too complicated for the average clinician but is helpful in identifying more than one parameter in chronic hypertension.

The more severe the disease, the worse the perinatal outcome. The sicker the mother, the more chance she has of mortality, especially if superimposed preeclampsia intervenes.

Fetal Effects

The effects on the fetus of women who have chronic hypertension run the gamut from no effects to one in which the fetus ends as a stillborn. Fetal well-being relates to unobstructed blood flow through the uteroplacental bed and the ability of the spiral arteries to dilate in an appropriate fashion and to remain dilated throughout pregnancy. It is most likely that there is never a truly normal uteroplacental bed in a woman who has chronic hypertension; hence, dysmaturity of fetal growth and development are common[14] and relate principally to undetected small degrees of antepartum fetal

TABLE 32-4. CLASSIFICATION OF SEVERITY OF HYPERTENSION IN GRAVIDAS BY DIASTOLIC AND MEAN ARTERIAL PRESSURE AS WELL AS PRESSURE END-ORGAN EFFECTS

	First and Second Trimesters		Third Trimester	
I. By blood pressure	*D*	*MAP*	*D*	*MAP*
Mild	80	90	90	95
Moderate	90	100	100	105
Severe	110	120	110	120

II. By other clinical criteria

	Cardiac	Fundoscopy	Renal
Mild	Normal cardiac size Normal EKG	Normal or minimal (KWI*)	Normal renal function (30–50% ↑ GFR† with pregnancy)
Moderate	± Cardiac enlargement; EKG evidence of left ventricular hypertrophy; few symptoms	Spastic or sclerotic changes (KW I, II)	Renal function decreased (GFR that of normal nonpregnant woman)
Severe	Cardiac enlargement usually evident; EKG evidence of left ventricular hypertrophy and ischemia; some symptoms (i.e., headache and palpitations)	Above, and occasionally hemorrhages and exudates (KW III)	Decreased renal function
Malignant	Above symptoms + those of cardiac failure; ischemic pain and/or encephalopathy	Frank hemorrhages and exudates; papilledema (KW IV malignant phase)	Rapidly decreasing renal function; hematuria proteinuria

* Keith Wagener classification.
† Glomerular filtration rate.
D, diastolic; MAP, mean arterial pressure.
Source: Zuspan, F. P.: Chronic hypertension in pregnancy. Cl. Obstet. Gynecol. 27:854–873, 1984.

hypoxia. A common synergistic cause of intrauterine growth retardation in chronic maternal hypertension is smoking and this of course, should be stopped.[1,20] Other factors correlated with the degree of fetal growth are (1) maternal hypertension, (2) contraction of blood volume (hence, no diuretics), (3) plaque formation in the radial or low spiral arteries of the uteroplacental bed, and (4) the amount of norepinephrine in the uteroplacental bed associated with vasoconstriction. It is my contention that a large portion of a "normal placenta" can be nonfunctional before changes affect the fetus. The first change that is seen is in the small-for-gestational-age newborn. Changes in fetal growth and development are difficult to diagnose prior to the 30th week of gestation but should still be suspected if a patient has hypertension. If the fetus develops intrauterine growth retardation, the risk of perinatal mortality increases eightfold.[30] It has been our observation, as well as others', that these small fetuses that have had chronic intrauterine stress have enhanced pulmonary maturity and often do better than expected.[12] One of the most significant factors in adverse fetal outcome in women who have chronic hypertension is the presence of preeclampsia. If preeclampsia is superimposed on chronic hypertension, the fetal morbidity and mortality are at least five times greater than expected from the chronic hypertensive who does not have preeclampsia.[19]

A remaining problem for the fetus is the presence of abruptio placentae, which further compromises fetal circulation. This may be small in magnitude or it may be acute, sudden, and large in amount. It is more significant in women who have mild or severe chronic hypertension and this further impedes the already compromised function placenta. Table 32-5

TABLE 32-5. INCIDENCE OF ABRUPTIO PLACENTAE AT CHICAGO LYING-IN HOSPITAL

Non-toxemic patients	0.8%
Preeclampsia	
Mild	1.5%
Severe	1.0%
Hypertensive disease	
Mild	3.0%
Severe	6.3%

summarizes the experience at Chicago Lying-In Hospital

It is imperative that a woman who has chronic hypertension and complains of abdominal pain is carefully investigated to rule out abruptio placentae. Ultrasound and clinical observations are the appropriate ways to determine the presence or absence of an abruptio placentae. We have been able to make a diagnosis of abruptio placentae by ultrasound on as little as a 75 cc bleed. The most important thing is to have a high degree of suspicion and then to try to prove the diagnosis.

Diagnosis and Management

The diagnosis of hypertension should be determined in the nonpregnant patient by a persistent elevation of blood pressure on serial examinations, preferably days apart. The examiner should report three numbers for the blood pressure determination, representing I, IV, and V, respectively, of the sounds of Korotkoff, for example, 140/80/50. The true diastolic blood pressure probably lies somewhere between the fourth and fifth sound. Recording of the three numbers then means something specific for comparison and the patient can easily understand this. A thigh blood pressure cuff should be used on women with large arms greater than 35 cm in circumference. If the blood pressure cuff is too small, it will yield a false elevation of the blood pressure. The blood pressure changes throughout the day. The lowest blood pressure reading will be during sleep, the next lowest when the patient awakens, and the highest in the afternoon after activity. We are most concerned about the highest blood pressure and blood pressure when she first arises, then again in the early afternoon before rest. It is not unusual for patients to have labile blood pressures varying from normotensive to hypertensive, depending on their environments and their lifestyles. The importance of identifying labile blood pressure is to appreciate the highest reading and to suggest the necessity for investigation to rule out pheochromocytoma as a cause of labile blood pressures. All blood pressures should be determined with the patient lying in the lateral recumbent position so that the effect of the uterus will not interfere with the blood pressure determination. We stress this when patients do self blood pressure determinations. In this way, we can compare a 12-week self-determined blood pressure to a 40-week self-determined blood pressure.

For the past nine years, we have utilized self blood pressure instructions in all pregnant patients who have chronic hypertension. Our studies have shown that only one-third of the blood pressures in the office will be similar to the home blood pressures. Hence, erroneous conclusions can be drawn from utilizing only office blood pressures at least two-thirds of the time.[27] Serial blood pressures done at home are important. Instructions are for blood pressures to be taken three days per week. One of those days should be a nonworking day such as Saturday or Sunday. Alterations in blood pressures can be evaluated and correlated with environmental situations and work habits. It is important for the patient to understand what makes her blood pressure increase so that she can avoid triggering and exasperating influences. We ask the patient to record any unusual events associated with an abnormal elevation of her blood pressure. The patient is taught self blood pressure determination by our nurse, utilizing a dual stethoscope. It takes a minimum of an hour for the patient to understand how to take her pressure and to feel reassured that she is doing it correctly.

The history should search for acute episodes of vasomotor symptoms that might suggest pheochromocytoma associated with labile hypertensive episodes. A history of urinary tract infection or childhood kidney trouble is important in assessing underlying renal parenchymal disease. As stated above, less than 1% of patients have the clinical diagnosis of chronic renal parenchymal disease made, whereas by renal biopsy and electron microscopy studies, at least 15% have chronic renal disease. History apparently is not helpful in making this definitive diagnosis unless it is positive. A family history strongly positive for hypertension usually supports the genetic component of this disease in the patient. Other associated diseases that may be significant are collagen diseases and diabetes.

Physical examination should be complete,

including funduscopic examination and a careful evaluation of heart size to assess any end organ damage. Auscultation over the renal arteries may reveal the continuous bruit of renal vascular hypertension. Palpation of femoral and radial artery pulses should be done simultaneously to rule out coarctation of the aorta. The initial examination may include evaluation of the blood pressure in all extremities. This should be done on at least one occasion. If the patient is suspected of having hypertension and it is present in the initial office reading, self blood pressure determinations are taught to the patient.

Initial laboratory evaluation need not be extensive, but should include a careful urinalysis, looking for proteinuria as well as bacteria by means of culture. We recently have been utilizing test tapes that are positive for nitrites as well as leukocytes, but we still think that the urine of these individuals should be sent to the laboratory for culture and determination of protein. The laboratory tests basically are to rule out chronic renal disease, pheochromocytoma, and end organ involvement from hypertension. The blood urea nitrogen, serum creatinine, creatinine clearance, serum electrolytes, and an ultrasound examination of the kidneys are sufficient to rule out renal disease, short of renal biopsy. If hypertension is significant, an EKG and chest x-ray are in order. The one screening tool that we always utilize is urinary catechols and VMA to rule out pheochromocytoma.

The history and physical examination and laboratory data (Table 32-6) can all be done on an outpatient basis. Answers should be obtained on all these determinations within a week of the time that the patient is first seen so that appropriate counseling can be done. Counseling includes evaluation of blood pressure determinations that the patient has done and helping her to understand her own stress. Ideally, the patient should be seen prior to the initiation of pregnancy, but this is oftentimes not the case and the first evaluation will be when she is pregnant. The changing peripheral vascular resistance, the enlarging uterus, and the activity pattern of the patient will dictate the response of the blood pressure. It is important to realize in the pregnant patient that what is said today may well not be correct a month from now because changes in physiology take place rapidly as pregnancy progresses.

Early ultrasound determination for fetal growth and development is essential (Table 32-7). We prefer to have the first ultrasound done between 10 and 14 weeks of gestation so that the crown–rump measurement will confirm the estimated date of confinement. Chronic hypertensive patients should be delivered before term or at term. It is inappropriate to let these patients go beyond term. If the timely diagnosis of intrauterine growth retardation is to be made, a second ultrasound determination is done between 20 and 26 weeks' gestation and a third at 32–34 weeks' gestation when the first suspicion of intrauterine growth retardation usually is aroused. The amount of fluid present around the fetus is a good index of fetal health if it is adequate. We utilize biophysical measurements

TABLE 32-6. GUIDELINES FOR DIAGNOSIS AND FETAL EVALUATION

History
Hypertension
Renal disease in childhood
Repeated urinary tract infections
Sibling and mother having hypertension during pregnancy

Physical Examination
General examination
Funduscopic examination
Self-determination of blood pressure

Laboratory Diagnosis
Urine—24-hour protein or protein:creatinine ratio spot urine
Urine culture
Urine sediment
BUN, serum creatinine
Creatinine clearance
Serum electrolytes
Ultrasound renal evaluation
EKG
Chest x-ray
Urine catechols, VMA

TABLE 32-7. ANTENATAL FETAL ASSESSMENT

Ultrasound—first determination, 10–14 weeks
second determination, 20–26 weeks
third determination, 32 weeks

Amniocentesis—for fetal maturity studies

Biophysical testing

Non stress testing (NST)
Nipple stimulation test
Contraction stress test (CST)
Fetal kick counts

Estrogen:creatinine ratio—urine

as the major way of evaluating fetal health in these patients, beginning at the 32nd week of gestation and done on a weekly basis. The patient is taught to count fetal movements. Fetal kick count is done for two 1-hour periods each day with the patient lying on her side. If the fetal kick count exceeds six or more per hour, we reassure the patient that this means good fetal health. If the fetal kick count is done much before the 34th week of gestation, oftentimes the patient will not perceive movement because of the generous amount of amniotic fluid. The fetal kick count assures two things: first, that the patient will lie on her side for two 1-hour periods a day, and second, that she will develop further bonding with her baby by identifying movement. Additionally, a nonstress test is done on a weekly or biweekly basis, noting fetal accelerations. If there is a suspicion of a compromised fetal–placental unit, nipple stimulation testing is done following the nonstress test. A washcloth is warmed and applied to one nipple for 60 seconds. Then the patient is instructed to massage her nipple with the washcloth to create uterine contractions from release of oxytocin, which should occur 3/10 minutes. If no decelerations are noted and if the contractions have been achieved, this is considered a satisfactory test. If nipple stimulation is done and decelerations are noted, it is necessary that a contraction stress test then be done in a hospital environment. We prefer not to do a contraction stress test initially in hospital because it is expensive and we think that the nonstress test and nipple stimulation test suffice for at least 90% of patients. Additionally, we have obtained a spot urine examination on each visit for the estrogen:creatinine ratio. As long as it remains above 10, we feel reasonably comfortable that a satisfactory fetal–placental unit is present. The absolute value and numbers of the estrogen:creatinine ratio are unimportant. The important part is the trend. The ratio should continue to increase as gestation progresses. The biochemical measurements are probably the least reliable basis for management decisions and the biophysical measurements the most important.

Management of the Nonpregnant Patient

The nonpregnant patient should be counseled for her next pregnancy. Work-up is similar to that previously outlined. An important issue in counseling is that the patient should come away from the consultation with some degree of guarded optimism. The idea of going through another prenancy generates great anxiety in a woman who has lost a baby and almost died herself. The interval between the last pregnancy and conception should be at least six months. Appropriate time should be allowed to work the patient up and to help her to achieve an understanding of her problem prior to conception. It is essential that the patient have a specific understanding of what she must do during pregnancy. The physician's obligation is to guide her through this regimen. If consultation is needed from a nephrologist for a renal biopsy, the best time to do this is in the nonpregnant state. The patient should be instructed in self blood pressure determination when she is not pregnant. It will then be easy for her to continue when she becomes pregnant and will diminish her anxiety about her blood pressure. Any other problems should be corrected. For example, if she is overweight, the achievement of a close-to-normal height:weight ratio is desirable prior to conception. If she has chronic hypertension, it is highly desirable for her to get used to a low sodium intake. If she has chronic urinary tract infections, the cause should be sought with a careful work-up. Consideration should be given to chronic urinary antiseptic treatment. She should be instructed in a good diet containing at least 1 gram of protein/kg of body weight/day which should include adequate minerals and vitamins, as well as supplemental iron to replenish any iron stores that she may have lost. It is useful to instruct the patient that an hour of bed rest in the afternoon is highly desirable if she does not work. She must ultimately get in the habit of doing this during pregnancy because this is the only known phenomenon that increases blood flow to her uterus and kidneys. Patients should be seen on two or three occasions for complete evaluation before a decision is made to initiate pregnancy. All this should be handled in a very serious manner because the subject is of deepest emotional concern to the patient and her spouse. During the evaluation, contraception should be prescribed. The most logical method is a barrier contraceptive.

Management of the Pregnant Patient

The hypertensive patient should begin prenatal care as early after a missed period as possible. The physician should establish good rapport with the patient early because she will need to be followed at least every two weeks and perhaps weekly throughout her pregnancy. A strong relationship develops between the patient and her obstetrician. This can be utilized for support and guidance during pregnancy. Her first visit should include the usual prenatal tests (see Chapter 6), as well as baseline blood urea nitrogen, serum creatinine, urine culture, urine protein, and serum electrolytes. Creatinine clearance should be measured early in pregnancy and repeated every two months if renal disease is suspected. If significant hypertension (greater than 140/90) is present, a baseline electrocardiogram and chest x-ray are important. An ultrasound examination at 10–12 weeks of gestation is essential to date the pregnancy as accurately as possible and to confirm that it concurs with the menstrual history. The patient is sent to a dietitian for evaluation of the adequacy of her diet and estimation of her sodium intake. If the patient has significant proteinuria, protein intake should be increased to 1.5 grams of protein/kg of body weight/day. lf the patient is taking a diuretic medication this is eliminated gradually over a period of two weeks. Usually, she is instructed to salt her food to taste. If inappropriate retention of fluid is noted, this is modified. The kidney regulates sodium metabolism over a wide range of daily salt intakes. Unless there is superimposed severe preeclampsia or some other significant renal lesion, the kidney usually can excrete ingested sodium without difficulty. Approximately 20% of women have an enhancement or an exaggeration of their hypertension with sodium loading. A low-salt diet is advisable in this group.

Bed Rest

The single most important part of management of chronic hypertension during pregnancy is two hours of bed rest per day with one of these hours at noon. This poses a problem for the 40% of working women who have chronic hypertension. We instruct the patient to carry her lunch to work. A note is given to the patient, advising her employer that one hour of bed rest during her lunch hour is essential. She lies on her side during this period of time. She is advised to have one hour of additional rest when she returns home. It is essential to have the husband come in early in pregnancy so that this can be discussed with him, and he understands that she must rest one hour before she prepares dinner. Compliance is necessary for both partners. We have found during nine years of instructing patients to follow this rest regimen, coupled with self blood pressure determination, that they have much more energy later in the day and are better able to cope with problems that may arise. It is difficult to measure the direct benefits of bed rest, but presumably bed rest improves uteroplacental perfusion and nutrient supply to the fetus. Bed rest increases renal blood flow and glomerular filtration rate, resulting in the presentation of more sodium to the kidney with consequent mild diuresis and sodium loss. This, in turn, decreases or stabilizes cardiovascular reactivity and helps to maintain a stable or lowered blood pressure. Bed rest also diminishes endogenous excretion of amines (epinephrine from the adrenal gland and norepinephrine from the sympathetic nervous system), which further decreases cardiovascular reactivity. The net end result of all these mechanisms appears to be increased uterine blood flow which enhaces fetal well-being.[7,22]

Antihypertensive Drugs

Diuretic medications have already been discontinued in the chronic hypertensive patient who is pregnant. The next decision is whether or not antihypertensive drugs will benefit the patient and her fetus. The drug that has been tested in the largest number of randomized studies is methyldopa and this is our drug of choice. Many anecdotal and retrospective studies have reported use of a variety of antihypertensive drugs in women who have chronic hypertension during pregnancy. Two of the randomized studies that have been done have used methyldopa. One by Leather et al.[17] reported on a small group of patients in which 23 patients were assigned randomly to an antihypertensive treatment and 24 to a control group. A larger study by Redman et al.[28] of 243 patients randomly assigned indicates a significant improvement in fetal salvage in the group treated with the antihypertensive agent. However, when the data are analyzed critically, the significant difference derives from the fact that nine babies in the control group died in the midtrimester; none died in the last trimester. It is our contention that this may not be significant. It remains to be proved that antihypertensive drugs are effective in improving fetal salvage. We are still undecided on this issue. The primary reason for antihypertensive drugs is to prevent maternal complications and to stabilize fluctuations in maternal blood pressure. The one drug that has been proved effective is methyldopa. No others have been evaluated in randomized double-blind prospective studies. There is urgent need to investigate other drugs, especially beta blockers, in large, randomized, prospective studies. The studies done in Europe and Australia thus far appear to show no significant differences among the agents studied. Importantly, none of the studies to date have used self blood pressure determinations to diminish the anxiety the patients manifest during prenatal visits and to separate the variations between the office recordings and the home recordings; hence, we still do not know. The interpretation of therapy based on an office blood pressure reading is difficult because many patients started on antihypertensive drugs may not need them. Efficacy is inferred by a response from the spuriously high office blood pressure and not by the true response from a home-monitored blood pressure.[27]

Beta Blockers

Propranolol was the first significant beta blocker used in treating hypertension in nonpregnant women. There has been a great debate about the use of propranolol in pregnancy because some say it causes intrauterine growth retardation. These individuals fail to recognize that hypertension also causes intrauterine growth retardation. Many women have been treated with beta blockers. They appear to be safe. Propranolol tends to augment the action of other antihypertensive agents and is often used in conjunction with agents such as methyldopa or oral hydralazine. Unfortunately, oral hydralazine does not work well over a sustained period of time in pregnant individuals because of tachyphylaxis. Hydralazine usually increases renin secretion. Propranolol may be used in conjunction with hydralazine to offset the marked increase in cardiac output elicited by hydralazine alone and also to suppress the release of renin evoked by hydralazine. the combination of propranolol and hydralazine in pregnancy has not been studied in randomized trials.[8,26]

Alpha- and Beta-Adrenergic Blockade

Labetalol has both alpha- and beta-adrenergic blocking properties. It is said to owe its antihypertensive property chiefly to blockade of alpha-adrenergic receptors of the arteriolar smooth muscle and concurrent blockade of beta-adrenergic receptors. A hypertension symposium held in Nottingham, England, in 1983 summarized treatment with labetalol in pregnancy, All the studies were small, but it is encouraging that no major adverse effects were found. In one study, labetalol reduced blood pressure more efficiently than methyldopa and also significantly decreased the urinary sodium:potassium ratios.[16] Currently, labetalol has been introduced into the United States. It would be best to wait until the current, ongoing, randomized double-blind trials of labetalol versus methyldopa are reported. The current state of drug therapy for pregnant women with chronic hypertension is summarized in Table 32-8.

TABLE 32-8. ANTIHYPERTENSIVE DRUGS USED IN CHRONIC HYPERTENSION IN PREGNANCY

Drug	Action	Average Dose
Methyldopa	Inhibition of vasoconstricting impulses from vaso-regulating center in medulla oblongata, inhibition of impulses from hypothalamus	500 mg t.i.d.
Propranolol	Beta-adrenergic blockade usually associated with decreased cardiac output	20–40 mg q.i.d.
Labetalol	Alpha- and beta-adrenergic blockade	100 mg t.i.d.
Hydralazine	Direct relaxation of arterioles, action on vascular smooth muscle	20–40 mg q.i.d.

(Diuretics are not indicated and have no beneficial effect.)

Suggested Protocol for Drug Use in the Chronic Hypertensive Patient

1. Work up and rule out renal disease and pheochromocytoma. Start self blood pressure determinations.
2. Advise two hours of bed rest daily with blood pressure taken before and after rest to reinforce its efficacy.
3. If blood pressure shows no effect after 5–7 days and blood pressure is consistently greater than 140/90, start methyldopa, 500 mg t.i.d. Continue bed rest program.
4. See patient weekly or biweekly.
5. If organ systems deteriorate in spite of adequate therapy, hospitalize and re-evaluate.
6. Start biophysical testing at 32 weeks and do weekly or biweekly.
7. Identified incipient preeclampsia by watching for increased blood pressure, proteinuria, increased uric acid, or a decrease in antithrombin III below 70%.
8. Evaluate fetal growth by ultrasound and clinical measurements.
9. Do not let the pregnancy go beyond term. Induce if fetal growth ceases or if organ failure intercedes.

A roll test is done on each visit from the 24th week of gestation on. The patient lies on her left side. Her blood pressure is taken in the upper arm and then she rolls on her back. As long as the increase in diastolic blood pressure is less than 20, in all probability preeclampsia will not intercede. If the roll test becomes positive, it is unpredictable what will happen. The suspicion of incipient preeclampsia comes from clinical and laboratory tests. The most solid indications are the clinical tests:

1. An increase in baseline blood pressure. This is identified easily if the patient is doing self blood pressure determinations. She may well be the first to alert the physician to a gradual increase in her basal blood pressures.
2. Edema. It is normal for pregnant women to have dependent edema, but if the edema is more than that or there is sudden weight gain over a period of a week, incipient preeclampsia should be suspected.
3. Symptoms such as blurred vision, headache, or epigastric pain should alert the clinician that preeclampsia may be present.

Laboratory Studies to Help Determine Preeclampsia

1. *Uric Acid.* Uric acid normally is decreased during pregnancy because of increased glomerular filtration rate. Once involvement of the kidney occurs in preeclampsia with glomeruloendotheliosis, uric acid increases. Serial determinations are helpful.
2. *Proteinuria.* If the patient does not have proteinuria during pregnancy, the onset of proteinuria is significant. If a constant amount of protein is present in the urine initially, an increase in protein heralds the onset of preeclampsia. We often ask our patients to use a dip-stick for albumin at home in conjunction with self blood pressure monitoring.
3. *Antithrombin III.* Two reports, one in the United States and the other in Europe, confirmed that antithrombin III decreases in preeclampsia. The studies demonstrate a high likelihood of preeclampsia if antithrombin III is less than 70% of normal. The converse is not true, because some patients with preeclampsia have normal antithrombin III levels. The basis for this determination is the change in fibrin-split products.
4. *Ultrasound.* Ultrasound is utilized to identify intrauterine growth retardation and degrees of oligohydramnios. Serial determinations are essential. Intrauterine growth retardation signals rather severe diminution in uterine blood flow. If preeclampsia intercedes, the vasoconstriction becomes even worse.

All these tests warn the physician that careful observation of the patient and added concern are warranted. If the patient has chronic hypertension and has any hint of preeclampsia, she should be hospitalized immediately and treated with complete bed rest and observation. What is done next depends on h individual situation.

Some patients suffer an exacerbation of hypertension earlier than is desirable (less than 32 weeks of gestation). In these patients the decision to terminate pregnancy may be forced. We have now treated more than 100 patients with glucocorticoids in an effort to enhance pulmonary maturity after demonstrating immature surfactant in the amniotic fluid in patients who needed to be delivered within 2–3 days.[15,34] We did not find any increase in hypertension in any of the patients treated with hydrocortisone (1 gram q. 8 h x 4). Whether or not glucocorticoids help diminish the severity of respiratory distress syndrome is not known. It can only become known by observing thousands of patients, which is impossible for one investigator to achieve.

Therapy for the Patient Who Has Chronic Hypertension with Superimposed Preeclampsia

Preeclampsia superimposed on chronic hypertension poses a major problem for mother and fetus. An increased incidence of neonatal deaths, stillbirths and intrapartum deaths, as well as maternal mortality, is seen in this group of patients. The patient requires excellent acute care and must be hospitalized. The degree of preeclampsia dictates the urgency for delivery. As a general rule, once a chronic hypertensive patient develops preeclampsia, this cannot be reversed. Delivery should take place within a reasonable period of time.

The primary therapy is to treat the patient as though she has preeclampsia alone, with administration of magnesium sulfate to prevent eclampsia and parenteral hydralazine to control blood pressure. The methods of administration of hydralazine in severe preeclampsia have been outlined previously. It is essential to assume that this patient is very fragile and needs the utmost care. The mother should be monitored with an ultrasound blood pressure monitor and the fetus should be monitored electronically. These patients should deliver vaginally if oxytocin induction is possible. However, if induction is not feasible or is unsuccessful, delivery should be achieved by cesarean section utilizing general anesthesia.

REFERENCES

1. Arias, F.: Expansion of an inravascular volume and fetal outcome in patients with chronic hypertension and pregnancy. *Am. J. Obstet. Gynecol.* **123**:610–616, 1975.
2. Bryans, C. I., Jr., Southerland, W. L., and Zuspan, F. P.: Eclampsia: A long-term follow-up study. *Obstet. Gynecol.* **21**:701–707, 1963.
3. Burton, A. C.: *Physiology and Biophysics of the Circulation.* Chicago, Year Book Medical Publishers, 1965.
4. Chesley, L. C.: The control of hypertension in pregnancy. *Obstet. Gynecol. Annu.* **10**:69–106, 1981.
5. Chesley, L. C., Annitto, J. D., and Cosgrove, R. A.: The familial factor in toxemia of pregnancy. *Obstet. Gynecol.* **32**:303–311, 1968.
6. Cooper, D. W. and Liston, W. A.: Genetic control of severe pre-eclampsia. *J. Med. Genet.* **16**:409–416, 1979.
7. Curet, L. B. and Olson, R. W.: Evaluation of a program of bed rest in the treatment of chronic hypertension in pregnancy. *Obstet. Gynecol.* **53**:336–340, 1979.
8. Eliathou, H. E., Silverberg, D. S., Reisin, E., Romem, I., Masiach, S., and Serr, D. M.: Propranolol for the treatment of hypertension in pregnancy. *Br. J. Obstet. Gynaecol.* **85**:431–436, 1978.
9. Entman, S. S., Moore, R. M., Richardson, L. D., and Killam, A. P.: Elevated serum iron in toxemia of pregnancy. *Am. J. Obstet. Gynecol.* **143**:398–404, 1982.
10. Fadel, H. E., Northrop, G., and Misenhimer, H. R.: Hyperuricemia in pre-eclampsia. A reappraisal. *Am. J. Obstet. Gynecol.* **125**:640–647, 1976.
11. Fisher, K. A., Luger, A., Spargo, B. H., and Lindheimer, M. D.: Hypertension in pregnancy; clinical pathological correlations and late prognosis. *Medicine* **60**:267–276, 1981.
12. Gluck, L. and Kulovich, M. V.: Lecithin-sphingomyelin ratios in amniotic fluid in normal and abnormal pregnancy. *Am. J. Obstet. Gynecol.* **115**:539–546, 1973.
13. Grooenendijk, R., Trimbos, J. B. M. J., and Wallenburg, H. C. S.: Hemodynamic measurements in preeclampsia. Preliminary observation. *Am. J. Obstet. Gynecol.* **150**:232–236, 1984.
14. Gruenwald, P.: Growth of the human fetus. II. Abnormal growth in twins and infants of mothers with dibetes, hypertension or isoimmunization. *Am. J. Obstet. Gynecol.* **94**:1120–1132, 1966.
15. Iams, J. D., Semchyshyn, S., O'Shaughnessy, R., Moynihan, V., and Zuspan, F. P.: Blood pressure response in hypertensive pregnancies treated with cortisol. *Clin. Exp. Hypertens.* **2**:923–932, 1980.
16. Laming, G. C. and Symonds, E. M.: Comparison of alpha beta blocking drugs, Labetalol and Aldomet, in the treatment of pregnancy induced hypertension. In: *Pregnancy Hypertension.* B. B. Sammour, E. M. Symonds, F. P. Zuspan, and N. El-Tomi (Eds.). Cairo, Ain Shams University Press, 1982, pp. 359–372.
17. Leather, H. M., Humphreys, D. M., Baker, P., and Chadd, M. A.: A controlled trial of hypotensive agents in hypertension in pregnancy. *Lancet* **2**:488–490, 1968.
18. Lewis, P. J., Bulpitt, C. J. and Zuspan, F. P.: A comparison of current British and American practice in the management of hypertension in pregnancy. *Br. J. Obstet. Gynecol.* **1**:78–81, 1980.

19. Lopez-Llera, M. and Linares, G. R.: Factors that influence maternal mortality in eclampsia. In: *Hypertension in Pregnancy.* M. D. Lindheimer, A. I. Katz, and F. P. Zuspan (Eds.). New York, John Wiley & Sons, 1976, pp. 41–49.
20. MacGillivray, I. and Campbell, D. M.: A prospective study of factors affecting intrauterine growth. In: *Hypertension in Pregnancy.* M. C. Lindheimer, A. I. Katz, and F. P. Zuspan (Eds.). New York, John Wiley & Sons, 1976, pp. 23–29.
21. MacGillivray, I. and Johnstone, F. D.: Dietary protein and preeclampsia. In: *Hypertensive Disorders of Pregnancy.* F. K. Beller and I. MacGillivray (Eds.). Stuttgart, Georg Thieme, 1978, pp. 81–82.
22. Mathews, D. D., Agarwal, V., and Shuttleworth, T. P.: A randomized controlled trial of complete bed rest versus ambulation in the management of proteinuric hypertension during pregnancy. *Br. J. Obstet. Gynaecol.* **89**:128–131, 1982.
23. O'Shaughnessy, R., Adams, K., Lehman, E., Scott-Tibbs, G., and Zuspan, F. P.: Plasma and platelet catecholamines in normal and preeclamptic pregnancy. Proceedings of the 3lst Annual Meeting of the Society for Gynecologic Investigation, San Francisco, CA, 1984, p. 200 (Abstract 331P).
24. Page, E. W. and Christianson, R.: The impact of mean arterial pressure in the middle trimester upon the outcome of pregnancy. *Am. J. Obstet. Gynecol.* **125**:740–746, 1976.
25. Pritchard, J. A. and Stone, S. R.: Clinical and laboratory observations on eclampsia. *Am. J. Obstet. Gynecol.* **99**:754–765, 1967.
26. Pruyn, S. C., Phelan, J. P., and Buchanan, G. C.: Long-term propranolol therapy in pregnancy: Maternal and fetal outcome. *Am. J. Obstet. Gynecol.* **135**:485–489, 1979.
27. Rayburn, W. F., Zuspan, F. P., and Piehl, E. J.: Self-monitoring of blood pressure during pregnancy. *Am. J. Obstet. Gynecol.* **148**:159–162, 1984.
28. Redman, C. W. G., Bellin, L. J., Bonner, J., and Gunsted, M. K.: Fetal outcome in trial of antihypertensive treatment in pregnancy. *Lancet* **2**:753–756, 1976.
29. Spargo, B., McCartney, C. P., and Winemiller, G.: Glomerular capillary endotheliosis in toxemia of pregnancy. *A.M.A. Arch. Pathol.* **68**:593–599, 1959.
30. Usher, R. H.: Clinical and therapeutic aspects of fetal malnutrition. *Pediatr. Clin. North Am.* **17**:169–183, 1970.
31. Weiner, C. P. and Brandt, J.: Plasma antithrombin III activity in normal pregnancy. *Obstet. Gynecol.* **56**:601–609, 1980.
32. Weenink, G. H., Treffers, P. E., Vijn, P., Smorenberg-Schoorl, M. E., and ten Cate, J. W.: Plasma antithrombin III levels in preeclampsia. *Clin. Exp. Hypertens. [B]* **2**:145–162, 1983.
33. Weiner, C. P. and Brandt, J.: Plasma antithrombin III activity: An aid in the diagnosis of preeclampsia–eclampsia. *Am. J. Obstet. Gynecol.* **142**:275–281, 1982.
34. Zuspan, F. P.: Problems encountered in the treatment of pregnancy induced hypertension. A point of view. *Am. J. Obstet. Gynecol.* **131**:591–597, 1978.
35. Zuspan, F. P. and Bell, J. D.: Variable salt-loading during pregnancy with preeclampsia. *Obstet. Gynecol.* **18**:530–534, 1961.
36. Zuspan, F. P. and Goodrich, S.: Metabolic studies in normal pregnancy. I. Nitrogen metabolism. *Am. J. Obstet. Gynecol.* **100**:7–14, 1968.
37. Zuspan, F. P., Talledo, E., and Rhodes, K.: Factors affecting delivery in eclampsia. The condition of the cervix and uterine activity. *Am. J. Obstet. Gynecol.* **100**:672–685, 1968.
38. Zuspan, F. P. and Ward, M. C.: Improved fetal salvage in eclampsia. *Obstet. Gynecol.* **26**:893–897, 1965.

33

DIABETES MELLITUS

Over the past 50 years, great advances have been made in the care of pregnancies complicated by diabetes mellitus. The understanding of maternal metabolism and the pathophysiology of diabetes in pregnancy as well as the development of new therapeutic techniques have helped reduce fetal and neonatal mortality from approximately 65% before the discovery of insulin to 2–5% at present. If one excludes deaths due to major congenital malformations, the perinatal mortality rate in pregnancies of diabetic women receiving optimal care is equivalent to that observed in normal pregnancies. The incidence of insulin-dependent diabetes in pregnancy is 0.1–0.5%. Gestational diabetes occurs in 3–12% of obstetrical patients, depending on the patients screened and the diagnostic criteria utilized.

Pathophysiology of Diabetes in Pregnancy

During pregnancy, maternal metabolism adjusts to provide adequate nutrition for both the mother and her growing fetus. (See Chapter 3.) In early pregnancy, increasing placental production of estrogen and progesterone lead to β cell hyperplasia and increased insulin secretion in response to a glucose load.[28] Glycogen deposition in peripheral tissues is increased and accompanies a fall in hepatic glucose production. Insulin-dependent diabetic women commonly experience periods of hypoglycemia in the first trimester. This phenomenon can be explained by increased peripheral utilization of glucose as well as decreased caloric intake due to nausea and vomiting early in gestation. The heightened hypoglycemia associated with maternal fasting during pregnancy has been described as "accelerated starvation."[13] Compensatory mechanisms that offset these changes include increased protein catabolism and accelerated renal gluconeogenesis from amino acid precursors.

Human placental lactogen (hPL), a polypeptide hormone produced by the syncytiotrophoblast, stimulates lipolysis in maternal adipose tissue.[29] The resultant release of glycerol and fatty acids reduces maternal glucose utilization and spares this fuel for the fetus.

The actions of hPL are responsible, in part, for the "diabetogenic state" of pregnancy, which is characterized by an exaggerated rate and amount of insulin release associated with decreased sensitivity to insulin at the cellular level.[60] Hormones that partially antagonize this response include free cortisol, estrogen, progesterone, and prolactin. With placental growth, larger amounts of these contrainsulin factors are synthesized. These hormones contribute to the observed impaired glucose tolerance by promoting insulin resistance in peripheral tissues and also profoundly affect hepatic glucose metabolism. As pregnancy advances, hepatic glycogen storage decreases and glucose production by the liver increases. In normal pregnancies, maternal β cell hyperplasia and associated increased production of insulin maintain glucose levels between 60 and 120 mg/dl. A woman with overt diabetes cannot respond to the "diabetogenic stress" of pregnancy and needs additional insulin therapy throughout gestation. The heightened requirement for exogenous insulin is roughly equivalent to the increase in endogenous insulin seen in normal gestations.

If a pregnant patient has borderline pancreatic reserve, her endogenous insulin production may be inadequate. Diabetes may then be revealed for the first time during gestation. Unlike known pregestational insulin-dependent patients, obese gestational diabetics with presumed peripheral insulin resistance may experience large increases in their insulin requirement during pregnancy. These patients also often have increased levels of fasting triglycerides and elevated serum LDL and HDL levels.[24]

Glucagon, which has both glycogenolytic and gluconeogenic actions, does not appear to contribute greatly to the "diabetogenic stress" of pregnancy. Levels of this hormone change little throughout gestation.[51] The glucagon response to glucose administration appears to be suppressed in normal pregnant women, resulting in more prolonged hyperglycemia and hyperinsulinemia after feeding. In this way, periods of "facilitated anabolism" offset the "accelerated starvation" of the fasting state.[13]

The placenta is essentially impermeable to protein hormones such as insulin, glucagon, growth hormone, and hPL. Maternal glucose reaches the fetus by carrier-mediated facilitated diffusion. There is a close correlation between fetal glucose uptake and maternal blood levels as well as the maternal–fetal concentration gradient.[2] Fetal blood glucose levels usually remain 20–30 mg/dl lower than those of the mother. Amino acids are actively transposed to the fetal compartment. Ketoacids appear to diffuse across the placenta freely and may serve as fetal fuel during periods of maternal starvation.[9]

As a direct result of maternal glucose homeostasis, fetal glucose levels are normally maintained within narrow limits. In pregnancy complicated by diabetes mellitus, periods of maternal hyperglycemia produce fetal hyperglycemia.[41] Even with optimal therapy, daily glucose excursions are greater in patients with diabetes mellitus than in normal patients. The fetal pancreas responds to this hyperglycemia with β cell hyperplasia and resultant fetal hyperinsulinemia.[54]

Improved understanding of the importance of maternal control in relation to fetal outcome has played a major role in reducing perinatal mortality due to intrauterine death. Fetal hypoxemia occurs in association with hyperinsulinemia and hyperglycemia.[4] Hyperglycemia, in the presence of minimal degrees of hypoxemia, may result in lactic acidosis and fetal death.[43]

Fetal macrosomia is a direct consequence of fetal hyperinsulinemia. Increased deposition of fat, protein, and glycogen may lead to excessive neonatal birth weights in up to one-fourth of pregnancies complicated by diabetes.[15] It has been hypothesized that glucose serves as a primary precursor for α-glycerophosphate used in fetal triglyceride synthesis.[53]

Like the fetus, the placenta and umbilical cord may be increased in size in pregnancy complicated by diabetes mellitus. Histologic examination of the placenta reveals large and edematous villi with thickened basement membranes.[11] In patients with vascular disease, the placenta may be small with decidual vessels narrowed by hyaline change and fibrinoid necrosis.[7] This finding is more often observed in pregnancies associated with intrauterine growth retardation.

Classification and Risk Assessment

In 1949, Priscilla White pointed out that age at onset of diabetes, duration of diabetes, and the severity of vascular disease influence perinatal outcome.[58] This classification scheme has assumed tremendous importance and wide application (Table 33-1). The use of White's classification allows obstetricians to focus on those patients who are at greater risk during pregnancy and to compare perinatal outcomes from different institutions.

Class A diabetes mellitus includes patients who have demonstrated carbohydrate intolerance during a 100 g three-hour oral glucose tolerance test (GTT). Because these patients demonstrate primarily postprandial hyperglycemia, they may be managed by dietary regulation alone. If the fasting blood sugar is elevated, insulin therapy will most often be required. Patients with Class A diabetes usually have normal fasting glucose values.

Gestational diabetes is a form of latent diabetes in which the stress of pregnancy reveals glucose intolerance. Following pregnancy, carbohydrate metabolism usually returns to normal. The term gestational diabetes fails to specify whether the diabetes can be controlled by diet alone or the patient requires insulin. This distinction is important. Patients who are

TABLE 33-1. WHITE CLASSIFICATION OF PREGNANT DIABETIC WOMEN

Class	Diabetes Onset Age (years)		Duration (years)	Vascular Disease	Insulin Needs
A	Any		Any	0	0
B	>20		<10	0	+
C	10–19	or	10–19	0	+
D	<10	or	>20	+	+
F	Any		Any	+	+
H	Any		Any	+	+
R	Any		Any	+	+
T	Any		Any	+	+

normoglycemic while fasting have a significantly lower perinatal mortality rate and do not display an increased incidence of intrauterine fetal death.[15] Gestational diabetics who require insulin therapy for fasting or postprandial hyperglycemia may have poorer outcomes than those who can be controlled by diet alone.

Patients requiring insulin are designated by the letters B, C, D, R, and F (Table 33-1). Class B patients are those whose onset of disease is after age 20. They have had diabetes less than ten years and have no vascular complications. Gestational diabetics who require insulin are often referred to as Class B, despite the fact that they generally do not require insulin after delivery.

Class C diabetes includes patients who have the onset of their disease between the ages of 10 and 19 or have had the disease for 10–19 years. Vascular disease is not present.

Class D includes women with disease of 20 years duration or greater, or whose onset occurred before age 10. Class D also designates women who have benign retinopathy, which includes microaneurysms, exudates, and venous dilatation.

Class F describes patients with renal disease. This includes those with impaired creatinine clearance and proteinuria of at least 400 mg/24 hours measured during the first trimester. The presence of hypertension is a poor prognostic sign.[30] Several studies have failed to demonstrate a permanent worsening of diabetic nephropathy as a result of pregnancy. Recently, a new group of patients has been described, Class T, women with nephropathy who have undergone renal transplantation.

Class R diabetes designates patients with proliferative retinopathy. There is no difference in the prevalence of retinopathy in women who have or have not been pregnant. Proliferative retinopathy that has been treated with laser therapy usually remains quiescent during pregnancy. If progressive neovascularization occurs, laser photocoagulation with careful follow-up has helped to maintain many pregnancies until fetal pulmonary maturation has been achieved.[25]

Class H describes patients with diabetes mellitus and coronary atherosclerosis. During pregnancy, these women are at increased risk for fatal myocardial infarction.[48]

The perinatal risk and, therefore, the plan of care for the obese patient with gestational diabetes differs from that for the young primigravida with a long history of diabetes and vasculopathy. Class A patients are at lowest risk for poor fetal outcome. Classes B and C require intensive education and supervision to optimize their chances for a good outcome. If they are not well controlled, high perinatal morbidity and mortality may be encountered. Classes D, F, and R require careful antepartum surveillance of both fetal and maternal well-being.

The Danish internist, Jorgen Pedersen, described important prognostically bad signs in pregnancies complicated by diabetes mellitus.[42] The perinatal mortality rate is increased substantially if patients develop pyelonephritis, ketoacidosis, or preeclampsia. Noncompliance and neglect also increase risk.

Detection of Diabetes in Pregnancy.

Diabetes mellitus complicates 2–3% of all pregnancies. Gestational diabetes constitutes 90% of these cases. Patients with gestational diabetes are at significant risk for developing glucose intolerance later in life. More than 50% of these women develop diabetes in the 15 years following pregnancy.[39] Gestational diabetes is a designation restricted to pregnant women whose impaired glucose tolerance is detected during pregnancy.[12] The diabetogenic stress of pregnancy is most often encountered late in gestation. In most cases, these patients have a normal fasting glucose concentration, and their carbohydrate intolerance must be unmasked with a glucose challenge. In the past, glucose tolerance was determined in a subgroup of patients thought to be at increased risk for developing gestational diabetes. This group included patients with a family history of diabetes, unexplained stillborn, malformed infant, or macrosomia. Obesity, hypertension, glycosuria, and maternal age over 25 were other indications for screening.[40] Glycosuria is common in pregnancy as a result of the increased glomerular filtration rate.

Approximately 50% of all patients with gestational diabetes fail to demonstrate the risk factors cited above.[31] Therefore, it has been recommended by the American Diabetes Association that *all* pregnant women be screened for gestational diabetes. The preferred method is that every patient at 24–28 weeks' gestation receives a 50 g oral glucose load followed by a glucose determination one hour later.[40] Women with a previous history of gestational diabetes may be screened earlier in pregnancy. Plasma values 140 mg/dl on the screening test require a full 100 g oral GTT. Approximately 15% of patients with an abnormal screening value demonstrate an abnormal three-hour GTT. The critical plasma glucose values for the GTT are fasting 105 mg/dl, one hour 190 mg/dl, two hour 165 mg/dl, and three hour 145 mg/dl. Two of these values must be met or exceeded to establish the diagnosis of gestational diabetes. The patient must have a normal fasting value and two abnormal postprandial glucose determinations to be designated Class A.[58] In patients with an initially normal GTT, but significant risk factors, including a previous history of gestational diabetes, a repeat test may be performed at 32–34 weeks' gestation. Glycosylated hemoglobin, an index of glucose control over previous weeks and months, has not proved to be of value in screening for gestational diabetes.[47]

Treatment of the Insulin-Dependent Patient.

Home glucose monitoring combined with aggressive insulin therapy has made it possible to maintain physiologic maternal glucose levels between 60 and 120 mg/dl. Patients should monitor their glucose control using glucose oxidase impregnated reagent strips and a glucose reflectance meter. Several studies of pregnant patients have shown excellent results using multiple injection therapy complemented by different methods of home glucose monitoring.[27,55] Glucose determinations are made in the fasting state and before lunch, dinner, and bedtime. Fasting levels should be 60–90 mg/dl with levels before meals no greater than 105 mg/dl. Postprandial values may also be helpful and should not exceed 120 mg/dl two hours after eating. During pregnancy, most insulin-dependent patients require multiple insulin injections. A combination of intermediate acting and regular insulin before breakfast and at dinner time is the most common regimen.[32] As a general rule, the amount of intermediate-acting insulin taken in the morning will exceed that of regular by a two to one ratio. Patients usually receive two-thirds of their total insulin dose at breakfast and the remaining one-third at suppertime. An alternative regimen is to administer separate injections of regular insulin at dinner time and intermediate-acting insulin at bedtime to reduce nocturnal hypoglycemia.[32] The latter may occur when the mother is in a relative fasting state while placental and fetal glucose consumption continue.

Caloric intake must be tailored to match the patient's activity level and insulin regimen. Most patients consume three meals and several snacks.[19] Dietary composition should be 50–60% carbohydrate, 20% protein, and 25–30% fat with less than 10% saturated fats, up to 10% polyunsaturated fatty acids, and the remainder derived from monounsaturated sources.[38] Caloric intake is based on ideal prepregnancy weight and desired weight gain during gestation. Patients should consume approximately 35 kcal/kg body weight. Obese women may be managed with an intake as low as 1600 calories per day. Weight reduction generally is not advised. If ketonuria develops, the caloric prescription may be increased. This often requires additional insulin therapy.

For some patients, hospitalization may be necessary early in gestation to achieve the desired glucose control. The need for careful attention to taking the prescribed insulin and proper dietary intake is reinforced. Patients are taught how they should manage hypo- or hyperglycemia. These teaching efforts should gradually enable the patient to feel that she has taken charge of her diabetic control. Vasculopathy may be detected during an early ophthalmologic examination. At the same time, baseline renal function is established by assaying a 24-hour urine collection for creatinine clearance and protein. An electrocardiogram and a urine culture are also obtained.

Despite multiple insulin injections and dietary adjustments, a small group of patients may require continuous subcutaneous infusion (CSII) pump therapy to maintain adequate control.[46] The initiation of this treatment usually requires hospitalization. Basal infusion is established at approximately one unit per hour with bolus infusions given with meals and snacks. Adjustments are based on frequent glucose determinations by the patient. This therapy requires both intensive supervision and a highly motivated, compliant patient. The risk of nocturnal hypoglycemia may be further increased in pregnant women employing CSII. Therefore, patients who fail to demonstrate normal counter-regulatory responses to hypoglycemia should probably be discouraged from using an insulin pump. Ketoacidosis has been observed in association with pump failure or maternal infection.[33]

After the initial hospitalization, most patients are followed with outpatient visits at one to two week intervals. At each visit, control is assessed and adjustments in insulin dosage are made. However, the patient should be instructed to call at any time if periods of hypoglycemia (<50 mg/dl) or hyperglycemia (>200 mg/dl) occur. A glycosylated hemoglobin level may be determined in each trimester to assess overall control. Fetal growth is evaluated by serial ultrasound examinations at four to six week intervals. In the third trimester, pregnancy-induced hypertension may become evident, necessitating hospitalization. This complication has been observed in up to 25% of pregnancies complicated by diabetes mellitus.[41] Ophthalmologic examinations are performed during each trimester but are done more often if retinopathy is detected.

During the third trimester, when the risk of sudden intrauterine death is increased, a program of fetal surveillance is initiated. Antepartum fetal monitoring tests have been used primarily to reassure the obstetrician and to avoid unnecessary premature intervention.[26] In the patient who is well controlled and exhibits no vasculopathy or significant hypertension, such testing allows for further fetal maturation in utero.

Estriol assays were the first tests widely employed for fetal monitoring in pregnancies complicated by diabetes mellitus.[20] Rising estriol values were rarely associated with sudden intrauterine deaths. Although estriol assays yield few false negative results, false positive results are more common. The frequency of abnormal estriol values is 15–20%. Therefore, management employing estriol testing alone would lead to a high rate of unnecessary intervention for presumed fetal distress. In well-controlled patients without vascular disease, estriol assays may not be necessary for antepartum fetal assessment.[6,10]

The contraction stress test (CST) is an important tool in the assessment of fetal well-being in pregnancies complicated by diabetes.[18] In a well-controlled patient, a negative CST predicts fetal survival for at least one week. Positive contraction stress tests, observed in approximately 10% of insulin-dependent diabetic patients, are associated with increased perinatal mortality, late decelerations during labor, low Apgar scores, respiratory distress syndrome, and fetal growth retardation. The CST has a significant false positive rate of up to 60%.

The nonstress test (NST) has become the preferred antepartum heart rate screening test in patients with diabetes mellitus. If the NST is nonreactive, a CST must be performed. Antepartum heart rate monitoring is begun at approximately 28–30 weeks' gestation and should be performed twice weekly. Two studies have demonstrated an increased fetal death rate with NST monitoring performed only once each week.[1,35] In patients with vascular disease or poor control, in whom the incidence of abnormal tests and intrauterine deaths is greatest, testing often is performed daily.

Maternal monitoring of fetal activity is a practical method and a useful means of assessing fetal condition.[44] Although this technique has not been studied solely in pregnancies complicated by diabetes, it appears that maternal assessment of fetal activity is comparable to heart rate testing and may be more sensitive than estriol assays. Patients record fetal activity over a 12-hour period, usually from 9 A.M. until 9 P.M. At least 10 movements should be noted during this interval. If fewer than 10 movements are recorded during this interval, heart rate testing is performed. Patients may also count fetal movement for 30–60 minute periods each day.

Ultrasound has become the most important tool available for evaluating fetal growth, estimating fetal weight, and detecting hydramnios and malformations.[45] Determinations of maternal serum alpha-fetoprotein at 16 and 18 weeks gestation should be employed in association with ultrasonography in an attempt to detect neural tube defects.[37] Macrosomia is the leading risk factor for shoulder dystocia and traumatic delivery. Antenatal detection of macrosomia could significantly reduce the incidence of traumatic delivery and birth asphyxia. Therefore, evaluation of fetal size at term is important to select those patients best delivered by elective cesarean section. In most infants weighing more than 4000 g, the chest diameter will be at least 1.4 cm greater than the biparietal diameter.[8] The disproportionate increase in the size of the chest reflects an enlarged liver with a higher glycogen content.[22]

Management protocols developed during the past decade utilized both biochemical and biophysical techniques for fetal evaluation. Hospitalization frequently was undertaken at 32–34 weeks in patients with insulin-dependent diabetes.[18] Estriol collections were obtained daily and a CST was performed weekly. Despite the high incidence of false positive results, preterm intervention based on suspected fetal jeopardy was uncommon. Delivery was accomplished only if all parameters of antepartum assessment suggested impending fetal demise. Perinatal mortality rates using such protocols were generally below 5% and fetal death rates were no higher than those in the general population.

With home monitoring techniques now available to maintain maternal normoglycemia, protocols that are less rigorous and far less costly have been developed.[21] A select group of pregnant women with diabetes can be treated as outpatients throughout pregnancy. The assessment of maternal glycemia using home testing and the availability of outpatient heart rate testing have made this possible. Perinatal outcome does not appear to be compromised by this management. Patients with poor glycemic control and vascular complications are hospitalized and may require daily fetal surveillance.

The Timing of Delivery

Delivery should be delayed until fetal maturation has taken place, providing that the diabetes is well controlled and that antepartum surveillance remains normal. Studies have suggested that hyperinsulinemia may be associated with delayed pulmonary maturation and an increased incidence of respiratory distress syndrome (RDS).[49] Therefore, before any elective delivery, amniocentesis should be performed to document fetal pulmonary maturity. Although the value of the lecithin/sphingomyelin ratio (L/S) has been questioned in pregnancies complicated by diabetes mellitus, many series report a low incidence of RDS in patients with mature L/S ratios. In one large study, an L/S ratio of 2.0 or greater was associated with a 3% risk of hyaline membrane disease, a result identical to that observed in the nondiabetic population.[17]

The presence of the acidic phospholipid phosphatidylglycerol (PG) serves as a final marker of fetal pulmonary maturation. Several reports describe RDS in a significant percentage of infants of diabetic patients with mature L/S ratios but without PG present.[23] Therefore, caution is warranted in planning elective delivery of patients with an L/S between 2.0 and 3.0 but absent PG. If antepartum assessment remains reassuring, delivery may be delayed for another week. Most important, the clinician must be familiar with the laboratory analysis of amniotic fluid in his or her institution and the subsequent neonatal outcome at various L/S ratios in the presence or absence of PG.

When antepartum testing suggests fetal compromise, delivery must be considered. If amniotic fluid analysis yields an L/S of 2.0 or greater, delivery should be accomplished. When the L/S ratio is immature, the decision to proceed with delivery is individualized. When heart rate testing suggests fetal compromise, assessment of a fetal biophysical profile may prove helpful and may reduce unnecessary interventions. It is important not only to use the results of antepartum testing when considering intervention but also to assess the clinical features of that pregnancy. These include the patient's glucose control, blood pressure, renal function, and ophthalmologic status.

The route of delivery of the patient with diabetes must be individualized. When fetal distress is strongly suggested by heart rate testing, delivery by cesarean section often is performed. If a patient reaches 38 weeks' gestation with a mature lung profile and is at significant risk for intrauterine demise because of poor control or a history of a prior stillbirth, delivery is accomplished.[18] In these cases elective cesarean section is performed if the cervix is not favorable for induction. In most institutions, the cesarean section rate, including repeat cesarean sections for patients with insulin-dependent diabetes mellitus, is approximately 50%.

During labor, continuous fetal heart rate

monitoring is mandatory. Labor is allowed to progress as long as normal rates of cervical dilatation and descent are documented. An arrest pattern in labor should alert the physician to the possibility of cephalopelvic disproportion and fetal macrosomia. About 25% of macrosomic infants delivered after a prolonged second stage have shoulder dystocia.[3] Operative vaginal delivery significantly increases the risk of this dreaded complication. (See Chapter 45.) In general, a patient who fails to demonstrate significant cervical change after 6–8 hours of oxytocin stimulation may be best delivered by cesarean section.

Several approaches have been utilized to maintain normal maternal glucose levels during labor and delivery.[5] Neonatal hypoglycemia is related directly to maternal glucose levels during labor as well as to the degree of antepartum control. The frequency of neonatal hypoglycemia increases significantly if the mean maternal blood glucose level exceeds 90 mg/dl.[50] Regardless of the method used, it is important to utilize a flow sheet that summarizes glucose values, insulin dosage, and other metabolic parameters. Originally, White recommended that one-third to one-half of the *prepregnancy* dose of insulin be administered subcutaneously on the morning of induction in the form of intermediate-acting insulin.[57] Glucose levels were then monitored and supplemental regular insulin was given as needed.

Clinicians now prefer to use a continuous infusion of insulin and glucose during labor and delivery.[56,59] Five units of regular insulin are added to 500 ml of 5% dextrose that is mixed with 5 ml of 25% albumin. Albumin decreases insulin adherence to glass or plastic surfaces. This mixture is then administered at a rate of 100 ml/h. Alternatively, 10 units of regular insulin may be added to 1000 ml of solution containing 5% dextrose without albumin. An infusion rate of 100–125 ml/h will result in good glucose control in most cases. Maternal glucose levels are determined every one to two hours at the bedside, using home glucose monitoring techniques.

When cesarean section is to be performed, the procedure should be scheduled for the early morning. The patient is given nothing by mouth after midnight and the usual morning insulin dose is withheld. Epidural anesthesia is preferred because it allows the anesthesiologist to evaluate the mental status of the patient and to detect early signs of hypoglycemia. Following surgery, glucose levels are monitored every two hours and an intravenous solution of 5% dextrose is administered.

After delivery, insulin requirements usually are significantly lower than pregnancy or even prepregnancy needs. The objective of "tight control" used in the antepartum period is relaxed. Glucose values of 150–200 mg/dl are considered satisfactory. Patients delivered vaginally, who are able to eat a regular diet, are given one-half of their prepregnancy dose of NPH insulin on the morning of the first postpartum day. Frequent glucose determinations are made throughout the day, and supplemental regular insulin is given as needed. The amount of NPH insulin prescribed on the following morning is increased by an amount equal to two-thirds of the additional regular insulin. Most patients are stabilized on this regimen within a few days after delivery.

The patient who has been delivered by cesarean section often requires no additional insulin on the day of delivery. On the first and second postoperative days, regular insulin may be administered to maintain glucose values below 200 mg/dl. As the diet is advanced, the amount of NPH insulin required is calculated based on the regular insulin requirement of the preceding day.

Women with diabetes should be encouraged to breast-feed. Dietary adjustments for breastfeeding are made as in nondiabetic patients. However, the insulin dose may be somewhat lower in lactating women.

Management of the Patient with Gestational Diabetes

Women with gestational diabetes usually do not require hospitalization. Patients are begun on a diet program of 2000–2500 calories daily with the exclusion of simple sugars.[17] Fasting and two hour postprandial glucose levels are monitored weekly. If the fasting plasma glucose level exceeds 105 mg/dl and/or postprandial values are greater than 120 mg/dl, insulin therapy is begun. These patients may benefit from receiving highly purified porcine insulin or human insulin which reduces antibody formation.

Patients with well-controlled gestational diabetes are at low risk for intrauterine death. They may be followed safely until 40 weks' gestation as long as fasting and postprandial glucose values remain normal.[15] At 40 weeks, fetal surveillance is begun with weekly NSTs. Patients with a history of prior stillbirth as well as those who develop pregnancy-induced hyper tension should undergo fetal surveillance with twice-weekly NSTs commencing no later than 34 weeks' gestation. As in patients with insulin-dependent diabetes, ultrasound may be helpful in selecting the macrosomic fetus that is best delivered by cesarean section. Antepartum fetal surveillance in patients with gestational diabetes requiring insulin is accomplished in a manner similar to other insulin-dependent patients.

Congenital Malformations in the Pregnancy Complicated by Diabetes Mellitus.

Improved understanding of maternal metabolism, advances in techniques to regulate maternal glycemia, and improved methods for antepartum fetal surveillance have markedly reduced perinatal morbidity and mortality arising from intrauterine deaths, trauma, and RDS. The most frequent cause of perinatal loss in pregnancies complicated by insulin-dependent diabetes is fatal congenital malformation.[14] Infants of diabetic mothers have an increased incidence of severe malformations involving major organ systems.[36] The frequency of major congenital malformations observed in the offspring of insulin-dependent diabetics is 6–8%, as compared to 2–3% in the general population. The incidence of major anomalies is not increased in women with gestational diabetes. Reports of higher malformation rates in infants of patients with gestational diabetes may reflect that the patients under study actually had pregestational overt diabetes.

Anomalies observed in infants of diabetic mothers, including the caudal regression syndrome, renal agenesis, transposition of the great vessels, and anencephaly, must arise during the first seven weeks of gestation. Elevated hemoglobin A_{1c} concentrations early in pregnancy, reflecting poor control at conception and during embryogenesis, correlate with an increased incidence of malformations.[34] With the increasing evidence that poor control of the blood sugar levels is responsible for the congenital malformations seen in pregnancies complicated by diabetes, it is apparent that preconception counseling should be instituted. The obstetrician can explain to the nonpregnant patient techniques for home glucose monitoring and the need for proper dietary management. Physicians who care for young women with diabetes must also be made aware of the importance of such counseling.

Family Planning

Contraception remains an important consideration in the care of the young woman with diabetes.[52] Thromboembolic and vascular occlusive diseases are increased greatly in insulin-dependent diabetic women using combined oral contraceptives. Therefore, combined oral contraceptives are contraindicated. Women with a history of gestational diabetes should not use combined oral contraceptives, as they may develop carbohydrate intolerance while on "the pill." The progestin-only pill has been employed safely as a contraceptive in diabetic women.

The intrauterine device (IUD) may have an increased failure rate in patients with diabetes mellitus, but this observation remains controversial. The diaphragm and other barrier methods pose the least risk to the diabetic patient, although they are not as effective as either oral contraceptives or the IUD. Surgical sterilization should be discussed after the couple has completed their family.

Conclusion

The risk of mortality for the offspring of pregnant women with diabetes mellitus has been reduced substantially during the past decade. A reduction in the increased incidence of congenital malformations remains an important goal for the future. Physiologic glucose levels at the time of conception and early embryonic development appear to reduce the risk of malformations. Improved diabetic control during gestation also will reduce the risk of neonatal morbidity.

REFERENCES

1. Barret, J. M., Salyer, S. L., and Boehm, F. H.: The non-stress test: An evaluation of 1000 patients. *Am. J. Obstet. Gynecol.* **141**:153–157, 1981.
2. Beard, R. W., Turner, R. C., and Oakley N. W.: Fetal response to glucose loading. *Postgrad. Med. J.* **47**:68–78, 1971.
3. Benedetti, T. J. and Gabbe, S. G.: Shoulder dystocia: A complication of fetal macrosomia and prolonged second stage of labor with midpelvic delivery. *Obstet. Gynecol.* **52**:526–529, 1978.
4. Carson, B. S., Philipps, A. F., Simmons, M. A., Battaglia, F. C., and Meschia, G: Effects of a sustained insulin infusion upon glucose uptake and oxygenation of the ovine fetus. *Pediatr. Res.* **14**:147–152, 1980.
5. Cohen, A. W. and Gabbe, S. G.: Intrapartum management of the diabetic patient. *Clin. Perinatol.* **8**:165–172, 1981.

6. Dooley, S. L., Depp, R., Socol, M. L., Tamura, R. K., and Vaisrub, N.: Urinary estriols in diabetic pregnancy: A reappraisal. *Obstet. Gynecol.* **64**:469–475, 1984.
7. Driscoll, S. G.: The pathology of pregnancy complicated by diabetes mellitus. *Med. Clin. North Am.* **49**:1053–1068, 1965.
8. Elliot, J. P., Garite, T. J., Freeman, R. K., McQuown, D. S., and Patel, J. M.: Ultrasonic prediction of fetal macrosomia in diabetic patients. *Obstet. Gynecol.* **60**:159–162, 1982.
9. Felig, P.: Maternal and fetal fuel homeostasis in human pregnancy *Am. J. Clin. Nutr.* **26**:998–1005, 1973.
10. Fern, P. E., Grunert, G. M., and Lewis, S. B.: Urinary estriols: Are they of value in normoglycemic diabetic pregnancy? *Diabetes Care* **5**:316–318, 1982.
11. Fox, H.: Pathology of the placenta in maternal diabetes mellitus. *Obstet. Gynecol.* **34**:792–798, 1969.
12. Freinkel, N.: Gestational diabetes 1979: Philosophical and practical aspects of a major health problem. *Diabetes Care* **3**:399–401, 1980.
13. Freinkel, N., Metzger, B. E., Nitzan, M., Hare, J. W., Shambaugh, G. E., III, Marshall, R. T., Surmaczynska, B. Z., and Nagel, T. C.: Accelerated starvation and mechanisms for the conservation of maternal nitrogen during pregnancy. *Isr. J. Med. Sci.* **8**:426–439, 1972.
14. Gabbe, S. G.: Congenital malformations in infants of diabetic mothers. *Obstet. Gynecol. Surv.* **32**:125–132, 1977.
15. Gabbe, S. G., Demers, L. M., Greep, R. O., and Villee, C. A.: Placental glycogen metabolism in diabetes mellitus. *Diabetes* **21**:1185–1191, 1972.
16. Gabbe, S. G., Lowensohn, R. I., Mestman, J. H., Freeman, R., and Goebelsman, U.: The lecithin/sphingomyelin ratio in pregnancies complicated by diabetes mellitus. *Am. J. Obstet. Gynecol.* **128**:757–760, 1977.
17. Gabbe, S. G., Mestman, J. H., Freeman, R. K., Anderson, G. V., and Lowensohn, R. I. : Management and outcome of class A diabetes mellitus. *Am. J. Obstet. Gynecol.* **127**:465–469, 1977.
18. Gabbe, S. G., Mestman, J. H., Freeman, R. K,, Goebelsmann, U. T., Lowensohn, R. I., Nochimson, D., Cetrulo, C., and Quilligan, E. J.: Management and outcome of diabetes mellitus classes B-R. *Am. J. Obstet. Gynecol.* **129**:723–732, 1977.
19. Gabbe, S. G. and Quilligan, E. J.: General obstetric management of the diabetic pregnancy. *Clin. Obstet. Gynecol.* **24**:91–105, 1981.
20. Goebelsmann, U., Freeman, R. K., Mestman, J. H., Nakamura, R. M., and Woodling, B. A.: Estriol in pregnancy. II. Daily urinary estriol assays in the management of the pregnant diabetic woman. *Am. J. Obstet. Gynecol.* **115**:795–802, 1973.
21. Golde, S. H., Montoro, M., Good-Anderson, B., Brousard, P., Jacobs, N., Loesser, C., Trujillo, M., Walla, C., Phelan, J., and Platt, L. D.: The role of non-stress tests, fetal biophysical profile, and CSTs in the outpatient management of insulin-requiring diabetic pregnancies. *Am. J. Obstet. Gynecol.* **148**:269–273, 1984.
22. Grandjean, H., Sarramon, M. F., DeMouzon, J., Reme, J. M., and Pontonnier, G.: Detection of gestational diabetes by means of ultrasonic diagnosis of excessive fetal growth. *Am. J. Obstet. Gynecol.* **138**:790–792, 1980.
23. Hallman, M. and Teramo, K.: Amniotic fluid phospholipid profile as a prediction of fetal maturity in diabetic pregnancies. *Obstet. Gynecol.* **54**:703–707, 1979.
24. Hollingsworth, D. R. and Grundy, S. M.: Pregnancy-associated hypertriglyceridemia in normal and diabetic women:. Differences in insulin-dependent, non-insulin-dependent and gestational diabetes. *Diabetes* **31**:1092–1097, 1982.
25. Horvat, M., Maclean, H., Goldberg, L., and Crock, G. W.: Diabetic retinopathy in pregnancy: A 12-year prospective study. *Br. J. Ophthalmol.* **64**:398–403, 1980.
26. Jorge, C. S., Artal, R., Paul, R. H., Goebelsmann, U., Gratacos, J., Yeh, S. Y., Golde, S. H., and Mestman, J. H.: Antepartum fetal surveillance in diabetic patients. *Am. J. Obstet. Gynecol.* **141**:641–645, 1981.
27. Jovanovic, L. and Peterson, C. M.: Management of the pregnant, insulin-dependent diabetic woman. *Diabetes Care* **3**:63–68, 1980.
28. Kalkhoff, R. K., Kissebah, A. H., and Kim, H.-J.: Carbohydrate and lipid metabolism during normal pregnancy: Relationship to gestational hormone action. In: *The Diabetic Pregnancy. A Perinatal Perspective.* I. R. Merkatz and P. A. J. Adam (Eds.). New York, Grune & Stratton, 1979, pp. 3–21.
29. Kaplan, S. L.: Human chorionic somatomammotropin secretion, biologic effects and physiologic significance. In: *The Endocrine Milieu of Pregnancy, Puerperium and Childhood.* R. B. Jaffe (Ed.). Columbus, OH, Ross Laboratories, 1974, pp. 75–80.
30. Kitzmiller, J. L., Brown, E. R., Phillippe, M., Stark, A. R., Acker, D., Kaldany, A., Singh, S., and Hare, J. W.: Diabetic nephropathy and perinatal outcome. *Am. J. Obstet. Gynecol.* **141**:741–751, 1981.
31. Lavin, J. P., Barden, T. P., and Miodovnik, M.: Clinical experience with a screening program for gestational diabetes. *Am. J. Obstet. Gynecol.* **141**:491–494, 1981.
32. Lewis, S. B., Murray, W. K., Wallin, J. D., Coustan, D. R., Daane, T. A., Tredway, D. R., and Navins, J. P.: Improved glucose control in nonhospitalized pregnant diabetic patients. *Obstet. Gynecol.* **48**:260–267, 1976.
33. Lock, D. R. and Rigg, L. A.: Hypoglycemic coma associated with subcutaneous insulin infusion

by portable pump. *Diabetes Care* **4**:389–391, 1981.
34. Miller, E., Hare, J. W., Cloherty, J. P., Dunn, P. J., Gleason, R. E., Soeldner, J. S., and Kitzmiller, J. L.: Elevated maternal HbA_{1c} in early pregnancy and major congenital anomalies in infants of diabetic mothers. *N. Engl. J. Med.* **304**:1331–1334, 1981.
35. Miller, J. M., Jr.: Antepartum fetal heart rate testing in diabetic pregnancy (class B-F). Third Annual Meeting of the Society of Perinatal Obstetricians, San Antonio, Texas, January, 1983, p. 18.
36. Mills, J. L.: Malformations in infants of diabetic mothers. *Teratology* **25**:385–394, 1982.
37. Milunsky, A., Alpert, E., Kitzmiller, J. L., Younger, M. D., and Neff, R. K.: Prenatal diagnosis of neural tube defects. VIII. The importance of serum alpha-fetoprotein screening in diabetic pregnant women. *Am. J. Obstet. Gynecol.* **142**:1030–1032, 1982.
38. Nuttall, F. Q. and Brunzell, J. D.: Principles of nutrition and dietary recommendations for individuals with diabetes mellitus: 1979. American Diabetes Association. *Diabetes* **28**:1027–1030, 1979.
39. O'Sullivan, J. B.: Body weight and subsequent diabetes mellitus. *JAMA* **248**:949–952, 1982.
40. O'Sullivan, J. B., Mahan, C. M., Charles, D., and Dandrow, R. V.: Screening criteria for high risk gestational diabetic patients. *Am. J. Obstet. Gynecol.* **116**:895–900, 1973.
41. Pedersen, J.: *The Pregnant Diabetic and Her Newborn*, 2nd Edition. Baltimore, Williams & Wilkins, 1977.
42. Pedersen, J., Pedersen, L. M., and Andersen, B.: Assessors of fetal perinatal mortality in diabetic pregnancy. *Diabetes* **23**:302–305, 1974.
43. Philipps, A. F., Dubin, J. W., Matty, P. J., and Raye, J. R.: Arterial hypoxemia and hyperinsulinemia in the chronically hyperglycemic fetal lamb. *Pediatr. Res.* **16**:653–658, 1982.
44. Rayburn, W., Zuspan, F., Motley, M. E., and Donaldson, M.: An alternative to fetal heart rate testing. *Am. J. Obstet. Gynecol.* **138**:223–226, 1980.
45. Reece, E. A. and Hobbins, J. C.: Ultrasound's role in diabetic pregnancies. *Contemp. OB/GYN* **23**:87–108, 1984.
46. Rudolf, M. C., Coustan, D. R., Sherwin, R. S., Bates, S. E., Felig, P., Genel, M., and Tamborlane, W. V.: Efficacy of insulin pump in the home treatment of pregnant diabetics. *Diabetes* **30**:891–895, 1981.
47. Shah, B. D., Cohen, A. W., May, C., and Gabbe, S. G.: Comparison of glycohemoglobin determination and the one-hour oral glucose screen in the identification of gestational diabetes. *Am. J. Obstet. Gynecol.* **144**:774–777, 1982.
48. Silfen, S. L., Wapner, R. J., and Gabbe, S. G.: Maternal outcome in Class H diabetes mellitus. *Obstet. Gynecol.* **55**:749–751, 1980.
49. Smith, B. T., Giroud, C. J. P., Robert, M., and Avery, M. E.: Insulin antagonism of cortisol action on lecithin synthesis by cultured fetal lung cells. *J. Pediatr.* **87**:953–955, 1975.
50. Soler, N. G., Soler, S. M., and Malins, J. M.: Neonatal morbidity among infants of diabetic mothers. *Diabetes Care* **1**:340–350, 1978.
51. Spellacy, W. N.: *Maternal and Fetal Metabolic Interrelationships in Carbohydrate Metabolism in Pregnancy and the Newborn.* H. W. Sutherland and J. M. Stowers (Eds.). Edinburgh, Churchill Livingston, 1975, pp. 42–57.
52. Steel, J. M. and Duncan, L. J. P.: Contraception for the insulin-dependnt diabetic woman: The view from one clinic. *Diabetes Care* **3**:557–560, 1980.
53. Szabo, A. J., Opperman, W., Hanover, B., Gugliucci, D., and Szabo, O.: Fetal adipose tissue development: Relationship to maternal free fatty acid levels. In: *Early Diabetes in Early Life.* R. A. Camarini-Davalos and H. S. Cole (Eds.). New York, Academic Press, 1975, pp. 167–176.
54. Van Assche, F. A., Hoet, J. J., and Jack, P. M. B.: The endocrine pancreas of the pregnant mother, fetus, and newborn. In: *Fetal Physiology and Medicine.* R. W. Beard and P. W. Nathanielsz (Eds.). London, W. B. Saunders, 1976, pp. 121–157.
55. Varner, M. W.: Efficacy of home glucose monitoring in diabetic pregnancy. *Am. J. Med.* **75**:592–596, 1983.
56. West, T. E. T. and Lowy, C.: Control of blood glucose during labour in diabetic women with combined glucose and low dose insulin infusion. *Br. Med. J.* **1**:1252–1254, 1977.
57. White, P.: Pregnancy and diabetes: Medical aspects. *Med. Clin. North Am.* **49**:1015–1024, 1965.
58. White, P.: Pregnancy complicating diabetes. *Am. J. Med.* **7**:609–616, 1949.
59. Yeast, J. D., Porreco, R. P., and Ginsberg, H. A.: The use of continuous insulin infusion for the peripartum management of the diabetic pregnancy. *Am. J. Obstet. Gynecol.* **131**:861–864, 1978.
60. Yen, S. S. C.: Endocrine regulation of metabolic homeostasis during pregnancy. *Clin. Obstet. Gynecol.* **16**:130–147, 1973.

34

RENAL DISEASE

Pregnancy is associated with major anatomical and physiological changes. The renal tract figures particularly prominently in these alterations, some of which have already been discussed in Chapter 3. Many of these changes are of such an unusual nature and magnitude that the unwary obstetrician may fail to realize their importance when interpreting data from gravidas with renal disease or may incorrectly diagnose renal disorders where only the extremes of adaptation (such as excess proteinuria) are displayed. Bearing in mind background physiology and various diagnostic pitfalls, this chapter focuses on urinary tract infection, chronic renal disease, dialysis and renal transplantation in relation to pregnancy.

INFECTION OF THE URINARY TRACT

The increased nutrient content of urine and the stasis associated with ureteropelvic dilatation (and/or partial ureteral obstruction) predispose pregnant women to symptomatic urinary infection. Two clinical syndromes are recognized: lower urinary tract infection, or cystitis, and upper tract infection, or acute pyelonephritis.

Covert Bacteriuria

Covert or asymptomatic bacteriuria designates true bacteriuria in the absence of symptoms or signs of acute urinary tract infection.[14]

Diagnostic Criteria. The growth of bacteria from culture of urine may represent either contamination of the urine with urethral or perineal organisms or true bacteriuria resulting from multiplication of bacteria within the urinary tract. The entities are distinguished on the basis of colony counts from a freshly obtained, cleanly voided midstream urine specimen (MSU). The threshold for a positive urine culture is 100,000 colonies per ml of urine. Exceptionally lower counts ($<10^5$/ml), especially when coliform bacteria are cultured consistently, may be significant. Still, two consecutive MSUs containing the same organism in numbers greater than 100,000 colonies per ml of urine define true bacteriuria, as does a single suprapubic aspiration with any bacterial growth. The bacteriology is similar in pregnant and nonpregnant populations. Seventy-five percent of the infecting organisms are *Escherichia coli*. Other significant organisms include enterococci, streptococci, coagulase-negative staphylococci, and other gram-negative enteric bacilli. A number of presumptive tests based on changes in chemical indicators exist, but these are not reliable enough for clinical practice.

Covert bacteriuria is a heterogeneous entity. Several methods have been used to try to differentiate between upper and lower urinary tract bacteriuria; for example, renal biopsy, ureteral catheterization, bladder washout tests, urinary concentration tests, and serum antibody tests. The first two methods are too invasive for clinical practice and the remainder are insufficiently precise to confidently localize infections. The utility of another predictor of the presence and site of a urinary tract infection, the determination of antibody-coated bacteria in the urine, also remains equivocal.[44]

Significance and Implications. The reservoir of young women with covert bacteriuria acquired during childhood is about 5%, but only 1.2% are infected at any one time. The incidence increases after puberty and is approximately equal in both the pregnant and nonpregnant populations (2–10%). During pregnancy, 30–40% of the infected group, if left untreated, develop acute symptomatic urinary tract infection. Thus, treating gravidas with covert bacteriuria should prevent approximately 60–70% of all potential cases of symptomatic urinary tract infection in pregnancies. About 2% of those with initial negative cultures, however, develop acute infections, and this accounts for the remaining 30–40% of all cases of acute urinary tract infection in pregnancy.

Why do some women with covert bacteriuria develop upper urinary tract infection during gestation? Perhaps they represent a special population at greater risk, not only for acute urinary tract infection but also for other pregnancy problems. However, because there is no difference in pregnancy outcome among women with treated covert bacteriuria of presumed renal origin (diagnosed by the antibody-coated bacteria technique, with a 20% false-positive rate), those with treated bladder infection, and noninfected control subjects, this hypothesis has been questioned.[45] The available data suggest that the putative association of asymptomatic bacteriuria with increased fetal loss, prematurity, preeclampsia and anemia is not proved.[14,30]

Although most authorities encourage routine screening for asymptomatic bacteriuria, others[20] argue that this is not justified because bacteriuric patients do not necessarily develop urinary tract infection and the majority of patients with infection do not have bacteriuria on routine screening. There is also evidence that a combination of bacteriuria in pregnancy with a history of urinary tract infection selects women at greatest risk for infection. In such women, the likelihood of developing symptomatic urinary infection is ten times greater than in those with neither feature and four times greater than in those with asymptomatic bacteriuria alone.[20] Thus, even those who oppose routine culturing would screen women with historical evidence of infection.

Management in Pregnancy. Until more data are available, we agree with the majority who believe that covert bacteriuria in pregnancy *must* be eradicated. The choice of drug should be based on the sensitivity of the cultured organism(s), taking into account acceptability of the antibiotic use in pregnant women. At least 60% of patients with bacteriuria have bladder involvement alone. Although nonpregnant women might be treated with single doses, a 10–14 day course is still recommended during gestation. *Reinfection* is recurrent bacteriuria that involves a different strain of bacteria after successful eradication of the initial infection, invariably limited to the bladder and occurring at least six weeks after therapy. *Relapse* is the recurrence of bacteriuria due to the same organism, usually within six weeks of the initial infection. About 25% of gravidas will have a recurrence and need a second course of treatment, but only about 40% of these will have the covert bacteriuria cleared (Fig. 34-1). Persistent infections may merit continuous treatment to the time of delivery.

Management in the Long Term. As the interval between treatment of bacteriuria in pregnancy and postdelivery follow-up increases, the influence of the initial course of treatment on the incidence of bacteriuria becomes less noticeable. Ten or more years after an initial episode of bacteriuria of pregnancy, the prevalence of bacteriuria in women not treated during pregnancy (25%) is virtually the same as in those women who were treated (29%). Women never bacteriuric during pregnancy have remote bacteriuria rates of about 5%.

The use of postpartum intravenous urography (IVU) is controversial.[43] About 20% of patients with covert bacteriuria have urological abnormalities demonstrated on IVU. This percentage is increased among patients who develop acute infections during pregnancy (40%) or whose infections are refractory to treatment (60%). The significance of an x-ray abnormality is uncertain, however, as it may be unrelated to or a result of the infection, rather than a predisposing factor. In fact, many of the detected abnormalities are inconsequential or not amenable to surgical treatment. We recommend, therefore, that before an IVU is undertaken, the patient should meet the following additional criteria: (1) history of acute infections before

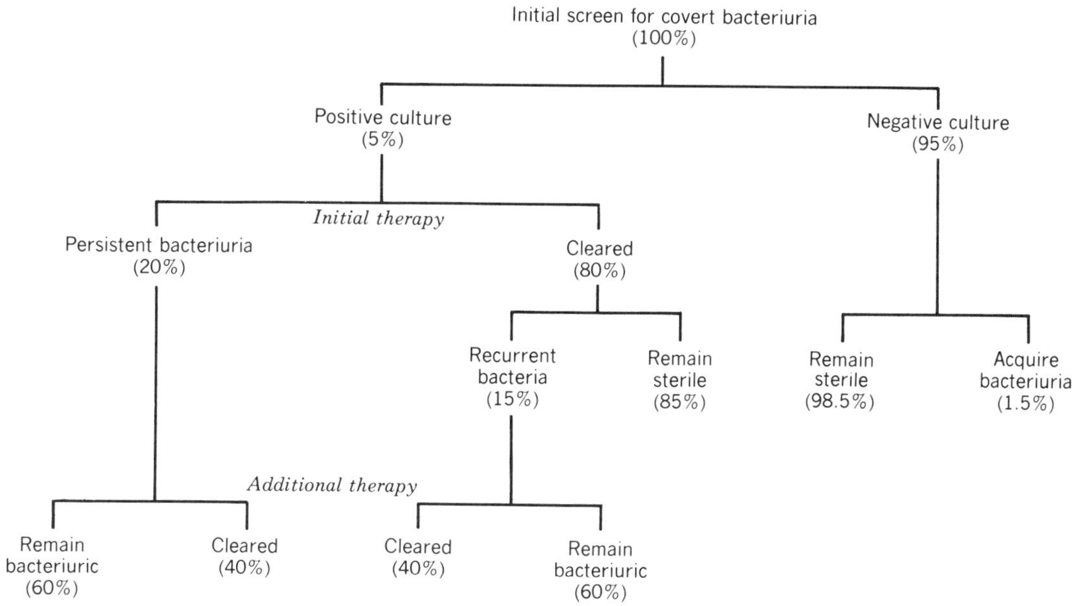

Figure 34-1. Natural history of covert bacteriuria and the effect of treatment during pregnancy, based on initial screening at first antenatal attendance. Approximate percentages are given in parentheses.

the index pregnancy, (2) difficulty in eradicating the bacteriuria during the pregnancy, (3) episode(s) of acute symptomatic urinary tract infection during pregnancy, and (4) persistence or recurrence of covert bacteriuria or acute infection after delivery.

Acute Urinary Tract Infection

Gravidas often complain of or will admit to frequency of micturition, urgency, dysuria, or nocturia, singly or in combination. These symptoms are not necessarily diagnostic of urinary tract infection and can be elicited from women with sterile urine.[100]

Acute Cystitis. This occurs in about 1% of gravidas of whom 60% have a negative initial screening.[14] The symptoms are often difficult to distinguish from those due to pregnancy itself. Features indicating a true infection include hematuria, dysuria, and suprapubic discomfort, as well as a positive urine culture. The bacteriology is the same as in women with covert bacteriuria. Similar treatment is recommended with the aims of abolishing symptoms and preventing occurrence of acute pyelonephritis.

Acute Pyelonephritis. This is the most common urinary tract complication of pregnancy, occurring in 1–2% of all pregnancies. Its presentation in the gravida is similar to that in the nonpregnant woman with fever, flank pain, nausea, and vomiting with or without frequency, urgency, and dysuria. Physical examination usually confirms the presence of pyrexia and loin tenderness on the affected side. Causative organisms are similar to those in the general population. *Escherichia coli* represents approximately 70%. Other gram-negative enteric organisms are less frequent sources of infection. Approximately 25% of patients experience a transient decrease in glomerular filtration rate and a rise in blood creatinine.[30]

Acute pyelonephritis may or may not play a role in the etiology of anemia, hypertension, and intrauterine deaths, but upper tract infections certainly may mimic and/or precipitate premature labor.[45] Maternal sepsis occurs in approximately 10% of all cases. Some even develop septic shock, usually in association with instrumentation of the infected urinary tract. In fact, gravidas are more vulnerable to endotoxins than nonpregnant women, which is one reason they tolerate acute pyelonephritis poorly.

Treatment of acute pyelonephritis requires early hospitalization and adequate intravenous hydration. After appropriate cultures are obtained, treatment with broad spectrum intravenous antibiotics should be started. Antibiotic therapy should be adjusted to organism sensitivities when known. Most patients treated appropriately respond clinically within 48 hours. Lack of clinical improvement by 72 hours suggests inadequate or improper antibiotic use or underlying anatomical urinary tract condition. The overall recurrence rate is estimated at approximately 20%. After resolution of an episode of acute pyelonephritis, the patient should be treated for at least three weeks and then should be followed with frequent urine cultures.[76] Continuous antimicrobial suppression with close follow-up until term may be used in the noncompliant patient or where an underlying urinary tract abnormality is present or suspected, if assessment of this can safely be postponed until the puerperium.[14]

Acute pyelonephritis may occasionally be confused with acute hydronephrosis and hydroureter, which should be suspected when recurrent episodes of loin pain or low abdominal pain radiating to the groin are associated with repeat sterile MSUs. Obstruction may occur at varying levels at or above the pelvic brim. On occasion, and due to the physiological changes of pregnancy, compensated pelviureteric junction obstruction becomes decompensated and symptomatic. Diagnosis can be confirmed using limited excretory urography (1–3 films) or sonar scanning. Positioning of the patient in lateral recumbency may relieve the obstruction, but if this fails, ureteral catheterization or nephrostomy may be necessary. In a typical case, the pain is relieved rapidly by ureteric catheterizaton whether or not the urine is sterile or infected. Antibiotics should be given if appropriate. Corrective surgery is best delayed until the postpartum period.

Rarely, there is spontaneous rupture of the renal pelvis, usually due to an obstructed kidney. This condition, which is difficult to diagnose, requires prompt surgical intervention.

CHRONIC RENAL DISEASE

There are conflicting views regarding pregnancy in women with renal disease.[3,7,17,39,56,58,62,64,65,67–71,96,101,102] The majority view is that, with the exception of certain specific disease entities such as renal polyarteritis nodosa and scleroderma, obstetric outcome is usually successful, provided renal function is at most moderately compromised and hypertension is absent or minimal. Furthermore, there is a consensus that, in such instances, pregnancy does not have an adverse effect on the natural history of the renal disease.

Renal Function in Normal Pregnancy

Glomerular filtration rate (GFR), measured as 24 hour creatinine clearance, increases shortly after conception. Serum levels of creatinine and urea nitrogen (SUN), which average 0.82 mg/100 ml and 13 mg/100 ml, respectively, in nonpregnant women, decrease to mean values of 0.58 mg/100 ml and 9 mg/100 ml in gravidas.[27] Near term, a 15–20% decrement in GFR occurs which affects blood creatinine minimally.

Values of creatinine of 0.85 mg/100 ml and BUN of 15 mg/100 ml, which are acceptable in nonpregnant subjects, are suspect in pregnancy. However, caution is necessary when assessing renal function by serum creatinine levels alone, as an individual may lose up to 50% of renal function, still be symptom free, and have a serum creatinine level of less than 1.5 mg/100 ml. When renal function is compromised severely, a small decrement in GFR causes a marked rise in serum creatinine.

Although serum creatinine, its reciprocal or its logarithm, often is used to estimate or even calculate GFR (in relation to age, height, and weight), this approach should not be used in pregnancy. This is because body weight or size does not reflect kidney size. Ideally, evaluation of renal function in pregnancy should be based on the clearance rather than the blood concentration of creatinine. Creatinine levels may increase by up to 0.18 mg/100 ml shortly after ingesting cooked meat (because cooking converts preformed creatine into creatinine); the timing of the blood sample during a clearance period must take meals and their content into account.[60]

Urinary protein excretion increases during pregnancy. It should not be considered abnormal until it exceeds twice the nonpregnant norms at one's institution.

Implication of Renal Dysfunction

Conceiving and sustaining a viable pregnancy are related to the degree of functional impairment rather than to the underlying renal lesion. Fertility is diminished as renal function falls.

When preconception serum creatinine and urea nitrogen levels exceed 3 mg/100 ml and 30 mg/100 ml, respectively, normal pregnancy is rare. There are exceptions. Successes have been documented in women with moderate to severe disease, including some treated with chronic ambulatory peritoneal dialysis as well as hemodialysis.[23,25,54,92]

Preconception Counseling

Ideally, pregnancy is probably best restricted to women whose preconception blood creatinine levels are 2 mg/100 ml or less and who have a diastolic blood pressure of 90 mmHg or less. Some clinicians recommend that pregnancy not be undertaken when blood creatinine exceeds 1.5 mg/100 ml. Whatever level is utilized, one should recognize that degrees of impairment that do not cause symptoms or appear to disrupt homeostasis in nonpregnant individuals certainly can jeopardize pregnancy. The question has to be asked, "Is a pregnancy advisable?" If a woman with chronic renal disease wishes to have a family, the sooner she starts, the better, because, in some of these women, renal function will continue to decline with time.

Balance Between Effect of Disease on Pregnancy and Effect of Pregnancy on Disease

Clinicians do not always have the occasion to counsel women with chronic renal disease prior to conception. A patient with suspected or known renal disease often presents with pregnancy as a "fait accompli" and then the question has to be asked, "Does the pregnancy continue?" In view of the radically different obstetric and long-term outlooks in women with different degrees of renal insufficiency, it is important to consider the impact of pregnancy by categories of renal functional status prior to conception.[65]

Preserved/Mildly Decreased Renal Function and Minimal Hypertension

Perspective. Women with chronic renal disease, but normal or only mildly decreased renal function at conception, usually have a successful obstetric outcome and pregnancy does not adversely affect the course of their disease. Although true for most patients, some authors suggest that this statement be tempered somewhat in lupus nephropathy, membranoproliferative glomerulonephritis, and perhaps IgA and reflux nephropathies, which appear more sensitive to intercurrent pregnancy.[64,86,102] Where renal disease is detected for the first time during pregnancy (often because of discovering proteinuria or hypertension during the prenatal exam, followed by a definitive biopsy diagnosis in the puerperium), it usually is surmised that renal function was relatively preserved before gestation brought an underlying mild lesion to clinical expression.[102]

Most women with nephropathy show increments in GFR, but the increases are usually less than those of normal pregnant women. Increased proteinuria is the most common renal effect of pregnancy, occurring in almost 50% of pregnancies (although rarely in women with chronic pyelonephritis), and it can be massive (often exceeding 3 g in 24 hours), frequently leading to nephrotic edema. The prevalence of hypertension, renal functional abnormalities, and proteinuria, as well as their severity, are considerably lower between pregnancies and during long-term follow-up. When renal failure does supervene, it rarely bears any temporal relationship to pregnancy but rather reflects the inexorable course of a particular renal disease.

Lessons from the Literature. The above generalizations are supported by data from a number of recent studies in which the nature of each disease was established by renal biopsy and sufficient data were available to evaluate long-term renal prognosis.[3,56,58,62,102] In the study of Katz and colleagues,[64] all women had normal or at most slightly impaired renal function (serum creatinine, $\leqq$ 1.4 mg/dl) before conception. Proteinuria was present in one-third and hypertension in 20%, but both were mild in most cases. Five of 89 patients eventually progressed to renal failure, but each had a disease that carried an ominous prognosis (e.g., amyloidosis, polycystic kidney disease, focal glomerulosclerosis, crescentic glomerulonephritis, and chronic diffuse glomerulonephritis) and would likely have progressed similarly, regardless of the intervening pregnancy, which in most cases preceded the functional deterioration by years (Tables 34-1 and 34-2; Figs. 34-2 and 34-3).

Similar conclusions were reached by another group of workers[102] who surveyed 86 women during 123 pregnancies. In their survey, the most common diagnoses were IgA nephropathy and Alport's syndrome (Table 34-5). More than

TABLE 34-1. PREGNANCY OUTCOME RELATED TO TYPE OF DISEASE

Biopsy Diagnosis	Patients	Pregnancies	Fetal Deaths*	Neonatal Deaths	Preterm Deliveries	Small-for-Dates-Infants	Birth Weight of Live Infants†			
							<1500g	<2000g	<2500g	<2500g
Diffuse glomerulonephritis	26	33	3	3	13	9	6	3	6	13
Focal glomerulonephritis	12	26	2	2	1	6	0	1	7	18
Membranoproliferative glomerulonephritis	4	4	9	9	9	1	9	9	1	3
Membranous nephropathy	7	10	0	0	1	1	0	0	2	5
Lipoid nephrosis	3	6	0	0	1	4	0	0	4	2
Focal glomerulosclerosis	1	1	0	0	0	0	0	0	0	1
Interstitial nephritis (pyelonephritis)	21	26	1	1	4	2	0	1	4	20
Arteriolar nephrosclerosis	8	8	0	0	3	3	2	2	0	4
Others‡	7	7	1	0	1	1	1	0	1	4
Totals	89	121§	7	6	24	27	9	7	25	70
Percent			6	5	20	24	8	6	23	63

* Stillbirths and second trimester spontaneous abortions.
† Birth weights available for only 111 of the 116 live infants.
‡ Includes sickle cell nephropathy (2 cases) and polycystic disease, IgA nephropathy, diabetic glomerulosclerosis, renal amyloidosis, and bilateral renal artery stenosis (1 case of each).
§ Two sets of twins.
Source: Modified from Katz, A. I., Davison, J. M., Hayslett, J. P., Singson, E., and Lindheimer, M. D.: Pregnancy in women with kidney disease. Kidney International **18**:192–206, 1980, with permission.

TABLE 34-2. IMMEDIATE AND REMOTE EFFECTS OF PREGNANCY IN WOMEN WITH KIDNEY DISEASE

	Course During Pregnancy or Postpartum					Status at the End of Follow-up				
	Patients	Pregnancies	H/T*	Decreased RF†	Increased Proteinuria‡	Patients	H/T	Decreased RF†	ESRD§	Increased Proteinuria‡
Diffuse glomerulonephritis	26	33	11	11	24	23	1	3	2	7
Focal glomerulonephritis	12	26	6	2	9	11	0	2	0	0
Membranoproliferative glomerulonephritis	4	4	0	1	3	4	0	0	0	4
Membranous nephropathy	7	10	0	0	8	7	0	0	0	6
Minimal change lesion	3	6	0	0	2	3	0	0	0	0
Focal glomerulosclerosis	1	1	0	0	1	1	—	—	1	—
Interstitial nephritis	21	26	3	1	2	19	0	0	0	2
Arteriolar nephrosclerosis	8	8	5	2	3	6	0	0	0	2
Others#	7	7	3	2	5	6	—	—	2	2
Totals	89	121	28	19	57	80	1	5	5	23
Percent			23	16	47		1	6	6	29

* Blood pressure ≧160/110 mmHg; or increased ≧30/20 mmHg above prepregnancy levels (H/T = Hypertension).

† BUN, 25 mg/dl or serum creatinine, ≧1.5 mg/dl, or increase ≧50% above prepregnancy in either of these two measurements (RF = Renal function).

‡ 24 hour protein excretion, >3 g or 100% above prepregnancy levels, or ≧1 g/d or ≧2+ (≧0.3 g/d or ≧1+ at the end of follow-up) if prepregnancy measurements not available or negative.

§ ESRD (patient on maintenance hemodialysis or after transplantation). Patients are not counted in the other categories (e.g., H/T, proteinuria, etc.).

Includes sickle cell nephropathy (2 cases) and polycystic disease, IgA nephropathy, diabetic glomerulosclerosis, renal amyloidosis, and bilateral renal artery stenosis (1 case of each).

Source: Modified from Katz, A. I., Davison, J. M., Hayslett, J. P., Singson, E., and Lindheimer, M. D.: Pregnancy in women with kidney disease. Kidney International **18**:192–206, 1980, with permission.

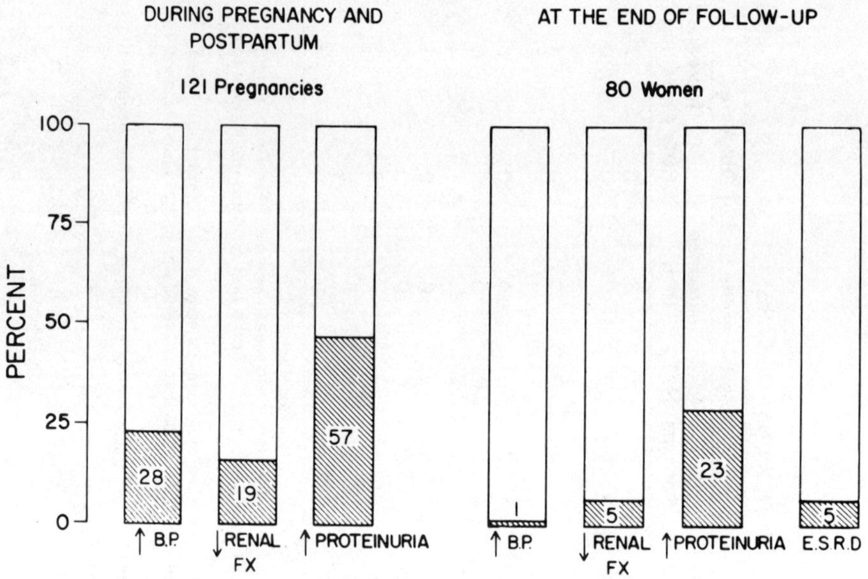

Figure 34-2. Course of pregnancy in 89 women during pregnancy and immediately postpartum (3 bars on left side) and 80 of these women who were followed up after the pregnancy (4 bars on right side). Numbers contained within bars are individual pregnancies (on left) and individual women (on right). FX = Renal function. E.S.R.D. = End-stage renal failure. (Data calculated from Katz et al.[64] and previously published by Katz, A. I. and Lindheimer, M. D.: Effect of pregnancy on the natural course of kidney disease. Semin. Nephrol. 4: 252–259, 1984.)

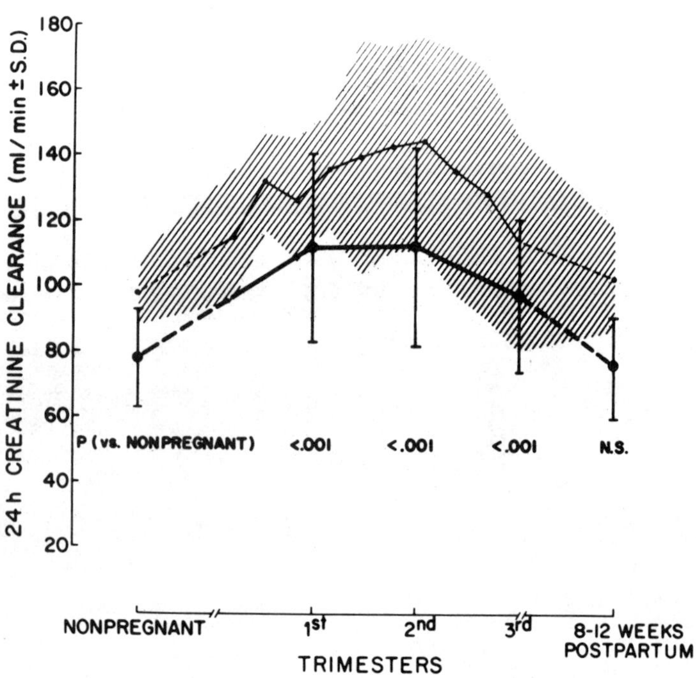

Figure 34-3. Serial 24 hour creatinine clearances (mean ± SD) during 33 pregnancies in 26 women with chronic renal disease. Studies undertaken before pregnancy, in each trimester of pregnancy and 8–12 weeks after delivery (solid line). Measurements from 10 healthy women similarly studied (mean ± SD) are shown by hatched area. (From Katz, A. I., Davidson, J. M., Hayslett, J. P., Simpson, E., and Lindheimer, M. D.: Pregnancy in women with kidney disease. Kidney Int. 18: 192–206, 1980.)

half the pregnancies were uneventful, while 24 were complicated by hypertension (reversible in 13 cases in which it was attributed to superimposed preeclampsia). Deterioration of renal function (defined as an increase of 50% or more in blood creatinine) was observed in 10 women, but six recovered their lost function. Of four pregnancies complicated by permanent functional impairment, two were in women with membranoproliferative glomerulonephritis and one each with amyloidosis and Alport's syndrome. No data on renal function before conception were available, but the unusually high number (41%) of renal abnormalities detected for the first time during pregnancy suggests that kidney function was relatively preserved before the putative gestation which apparently brought an underlying mild lesion to clinical expression. In most patients, pregnancy did not modify the natural history of glomerular disease, but women with membranoproliferative glomerulonephritis had a higher propensity to renal functional deterioration, and women with IgA nephropathy tended to develop hypertension that persisted after pregnancy. More recently, however, reports have appeared that even women with these underlying diseases tend to have successful pregnancy outcomes.[17,62,96,102]

Moderate Renal Insufficiency. Prognosis is more guarded where renal function is moderately impaired before pregnancy (blood creatinine 1.4 mg/100 ml). It is difficult to draw firm conclusions about pregnancy in these women, chiefly because the number of cases reported is still small.[65] In one series, a high incidence of renal morbidity occurred early in gestation; nearly half (5 of 11) developed serious deterioration of renal function culminating in terminal renal failure several months postpartum.[67] Due to this experience and the fact that apparent deterioration also was seen in an occasional patient with stable renal function, this group of investigators has adopted a rather pessimistic approach to pregnancy in women with both mild and moderate renal disease.

Another study of the influence of pregnancy on chronic renal disease specifically examined the influence of the level of kidney function before pregnancy or when first seen in gestation.[8] No immediate loss of renal function could be detected in 29 patients whose blood creatinine levels were less than 1.5 mg/dl. In contrast, four of eight patients with initial blood creatinine levels above 1.6 mg/dl experienced a significant further increase in blood creatinine during pregnancy, which was complicated in virtually every case. Four patients in this group progressed to end-stage renal failure within 18 months of delivery. These authors, and others since,[56,58,62] emphasized that uncontrolled hypertension is a very important factor in the overall deterioriation (Table 34-4). Our final recommendation was that pregnancy is best avoided in women who have lost 50% of their kidney function.

Recent studies have reopened the question. Hou et al. recorded a successful obstetrical outcome in 92% of the gestations in 22 women with creatinine levels of 1.7–2.7 mg% whose pregnancies were allowed to go beyond the second trimester. However, many of these patients had hectic blood pressure and in 25% there was an accelerated decline in renal function (Table 34-3). Thus although fetal survival is now improved in such women, maternal risks, especially complications of poorly controlled hypertension, preclude encouraging such women to conceive or to continue gestations already in progress.

Severe Renal Insufficiency. Most women with severe renal insufficiency are amenorrheic or anovulatory. Therefore, the likelihood of conceiving, let alone having a normal pregnancy and delivery, is low but not, as some have been misled to believe, impossible.[37] Data on such patients are very limited, so it is difficult to evaluate whether pregnancy has an adverse effect on their disease. However, it is our opinion that the risk of maternal complications (severe preeclampsia, bleeding, etc.) is greater than the probability of a successful obstetric outcome.

Management in Pregnancy

Renal Function. If renal function deteriorates at any stage of pregnancy, reversible causes, such as urinary tract infection, subtle dehydration, or electrolyte imbalance, occasionally precipitated by inadvertent diuretic therapy, should be sought. Near term, a 15–20% decrement in function, which affects blood creatinine minimally, is permissible (Fig. 34-3). Failure to detect a reversible cause of a significant decrement is grounds to end the pregnancy by elective delivery. When proteinuria occurs and persists, but blood pressure is normal and renal function is preserved, the pregnancy can be allowed to continue.

TABLE 34-3. CHRONIC RENAL DISEASE AND PREGNANCY: IMMEDIATE AND REMOTE EFFECTS

	Number of Women	Number of Pregnancies	Course During Pregnancy or Postpartum			Preterm Deliveries	Small-for-Dates Infants	Fetal Deaths	Neonatal Deaths	Status at End of Follow-up			
			H/T*	Increased Proteinuria	Decreased RF*					Time (years)	H/T	Increased Proteinuria	Decreased RF
Barcelo and Lopez[3]	48	63	17 (27%)	14 (22%)	6 (10%)	7 (11%)	5 (7%)	2 (3%)	1 (2%)	2	4 (6%)	4 (6%)	—
Hou et al.[56†]	22	24	14 (58%)	16 (65%)	5 (21%)	14 (58%)	—	2 (8%)	2 (8%)	—	4 (18%)	—	6 (25%)
Imbasciati et al.[58†]	15	15	10 (66%)	—	4 (26%)	6 (40%)	4 (26%)	2 (13%)	0	3	6 (40%)	—	4 (26%)
Jungers et al.[62‡]	122	240	160 (66%)	48 (20%)	—	41 (17%)	—	49 (20%)	12 (5%)	1	28 (23%)	— (6%)	7
Katz et al.[64]	89	121	28 (23%)	57 (47%)	19 (16%)	24 (20%)	27 (24%)	7 (6%)	6 (5%)	5.3	1 (29%)	23 (6%)	5
Surian et al.[102]	86	123	24 (20%)	—	10 (8%)	17 (14%)	7 (6%)	12 (10%)	5 (4%)	1	11 (9%)	—	4 (3%)

* Abbreviations as in Table 34-2.
† Women in these series had nonpregnant plasma creatinine levels >1.4 mg% (125 μmol/liter)
‡ Some women in this series had nonpregnant plasma creatinine levels >1.4 mg% (125 μmol/liter).
Source: figures calculated from data in Refs. 3, 56, 58, 62, 64, and 102.

TABLE 34-4. CHRONIC RENAL DISEASE AND PREGNANCY: EFFECT OF BLOOD PRESSURE AND/OR NEPHROTIC SYNDROME ON FETAL MORTALITY IN 240 PREGNANCIES IN 122 WOMEN*

	Fetal Mortality		
	Hypertension†	Nephrotic Syndrome	Both
Absent throughout pregnancy	18	12	10
Present at some time during pregnancy	34	20	40
Present from first trimester and controlled	20	20	—
Present from first trimester and uncontrolled	100	20	—
Present only during third trimester	12	12	—

*Calculated from data of Jungers et al.,[62] whose series contained several women who had moderate renal insufficiency.
†Hypertension not specifically defined.

Blood Pressure. Most of the specific risks of hypertension appear to be mediated through superimposed preeclampsia. There is still controversy about the incidence of preeclampsia in those women with preexisting renal disease. The diagnosis cannot be made with certainty on clinical grounds alone, because hypertension and proteinuria may be manifestations of the underlying renal disease. Treatment of mild hypertension (diastolic blood pressure less than 95 mmHg in the second trimester or less than 100 mmHg in the third) is not necessary during normal gestation, but many would treat gravidas with underlying renal disease more aggressively, believing this preserves function.[91]

Assessment of Fetal Well-Being and Timing of Delivery. Fetal surveillance is needed because renal disease can be associated with intrauterine growth retardation and, when complications do arise, the judicious moment for intervention is influenced by fetal status. Current technology should minimize intrauterine fetal death and neonatal morbidity and mortality from prematurity. Regardless of gestational age, most babies weighing 1500 g or more survive better in a special care nursery than in a hostile intrauterine environment. Delivery before 38 weeks may be necessary if there are signs of impending intrauterine fetal death, if renal function deteriorates substantially, if uncontrollable hypertension supervenes, or if eclampsia occurs.

Problems with Particular Renal Diseases

Various problems are associated with particular kidney diseases (Table 34-5). The crux of the clinical situation with any disease is the balance between fetal prognosis and maternal prognosis—the effect of a particular disease on pregnancy and the effect of pregnancy on that disease.

Chronic Pyelonephritis. This also is called tubulointerstitial disease. Gestational prognosis is similar to that for patients with glomerular disease, in that outcome is best in patients with adequate renal function and normal blood pressure. Compared to the nonpregnant state, there is an increased frequency of symptomatic infections in gravidas, but, overall, they have a more benign antenatal course than do women with glomerular disease.[64]

Urolithiasis (Stone Disease). The prevalence in pregnancy is 0.03–0.05%, which is about the same as in the nonpregnant population.[21,31,48,73] The composition of recovered calculi from gravidas is similar to that of the general population and, therefore, likely secondary to the same etiologies.

Diagnostic Pitfalls. Renal and ureteric calculi are among the most common causes of nonuterine related abdominal pain severe enough to warrant in-patient assessment in pregnancy. Despite the classical right-sided ureteropelvic dilatation, stones and, hence, symptoms occur equally frequently on right and left sides.

There is a valid reluctance on the part of obstetricians to consider x-ray examination. It has been proposed[85] that in the first instance clinical criteria including microscopic hematuria, recurrent urinary tract symptoms, and sterile urine

TABLE 34-5. EFFECTS OF PREGNANCY ON PREEXISTING RENAL DISEASE

Renal Disease	Effects
Chronic pyelonephritis (infectious tubulointerstitial disease)	Bacteriuria in pregnancy can lead to exacerbation.
Urolithiasis	Infections can be more frequent, but ureteral dilatation and stasis do not seem to affect natural history.
Permanent urinary diversion	Might be associated with other malformations of the urogenital tract. Urinary tract infection common during pregnancy. Renal function may undergo reversible decrease. No significant obstructive problem but cesarean section often needed for abnormal presentation.
Chronic glomerulonephritis and noninfectious tubulointerstitial disease	Usually no adverse effect in the absence of hypertension. One view is that glomerulonephritis is adversely affected by the coagulation changes of pregnancy. Urinary tract infections may occur more frequently.
Systemic lupus erythematosus (SLE)	Controversial; prognosis most favorable if disease in remission >6 months prior to conception. Steroid dosage should be increased postpartum.
Periarteritis nodosa	Fetal prognosis is dismal and maternal death often occurs.
Scleroderma	If onset during pregnancy then can be rapid overall deterioration. Reactivation of quiescent scleroderma may occur postpartum.
Diabetic nephropathy	No adverse effect on the renal lesion, but there is increased frequency of infection, edema, and/or preeclampsia.
Polycystic disease	Functional impairment and hypertension usually minimal in childbearing years.
After nephrectomy, solitary and pelvic well tolerated	Might be associated with other malformations of urogenital tract. Pregnancy dystocia rarely occurs with a pelvic kidney.

cultures when pyelonephritis is suspected, should be sought. The presence of two of these criteria suggests a diagnosis of calculi in at least 50% of gravidas. Ultrasonic examination, followed by an intravenous urogram, limited to 1–3 exposures, is advisable in such instances. It is essential that the ureteropelvic dilatation occurring normally with pregnancy not be misinterpreted as evidence of an obstructing calculus. Particular attention should be paid to the caliber of the ureter below the pelvic brim, as dilatation of the pelvic ureter is evidence in favor of obstruction (or reflux in the absence of stone). Associated chronic pyelonephritis should also be sought.

Obstetric Outcome. Few significant adverse effects on pregnancy or the fetus occur as the result of renal stones. There is no significant difference in the number of infections, rate of spontaneous abortions, premature delivery, maternal hypertension, or cesarean section. Furthermore, there is no difference in these complications in patients developing stone disease before or after onset of pregnancy, except for a slight increase in the incidence of urinary infections in patients with nephrolithiasis. However, these generalizations refer to women with the more common calcium calculi. Little is known of the natural history of the more ominous struvite (infectious) stones. Patients with the latter form of stone disease may do more poorly.

Management and Long-Term Evaluation. In pregnancy, approximately 50% of ureteral calculi pass spontaneously (compared with 80% in the general population) and a conservative approach should be adopted initially. This consists primarily of adequate hydration, appropriate antibiotic therapy, and pain relief. While the latter usually is provided by systemic analgesics, continuous segmental epidural block (T11 to L2) has been used successfully, especially in nonpregnant patients with ureteric colic, and may even favorably influence spontaneous passage of stones.[90] Spinal block can be confined to the segments relevant to pain relief, which will allow the patient to micturate without difficulty and move without assistance. This will decrease the risk of thromboembolic complications.

One-half of pregnant patients with stones require surgical intervention (although, in one series, many patients were managed entirely conservatively[21]). Surgery is best performed in the second trimester, and, if possible, one should temporize until then or until after delivery.

The long-term evaluation and treatment of these patients are similar to those of the general population. Recurrent stone formers should undergo evaluation for a metabolic etiology of their disease after delivery.[21,88] There appears to be little risk to subsequent pregnancies, with the exception of a slight increase in the risk of infections.

Permanent Urinary Diversion. This procedure still has widespread applicability in the management of congenital defects of the lower urinary tract, even though its use for the treatment of neurogenic bladders has declined since the introduction of self-catheterization. During pregnancy, the most common complication for these patients is urinary infection ranging from covert bacteriuria to severe acute pyelonephritis.[5] Decrements in renal function during pregnancy are commonplace but usually are transient and related to underlying infection and/or intermittent obstruction. The site of obstruction is variable. With an ileal conduit, the expanding uterus can cause elevation and compression with outflow obstruction, whereas with a ureterosigmoid anastomosis (rarely used nowadays), ureteric obstruction can occur. Changes usually reverse after delivery.

Premature labor occurs in 20%. Antibiotics given prophylactically throughout pregnancy may reduce this incidence.[5] The mode of delivery is related to obstetric factors and not to the presence of the urinary diversion. Vaginal delivery is safe with both ileal conduit and ureterosigmoid anastomosis, bearing in mind that, in the latter group of patients, continence is dependent on an intact anal sphincter which should be protected during vaginal delivery with an adequate mediolateral episiotomy. Abnormal presentation probably accounts for a cesarean section rate of 25%, with minor genital tract abnormalities contributing to the obstetric problems.

Acute and Chronic Glomerulonephritis. Only rarely does acute poststreptococcal glomerulonephritis complicate pregnancy and, on occasion, it has been mistaken for preeclampsia. Outcome in both mother and fetus is usually favorable.

The natural history of chronic glomerulonephritis in pregnancy is difficult to assess because of inadequate data in the literature pertaining to this disease. In many instances, the degree of functional impairment, the blood pressure prior to conception, and the exact histology of the renal lesion are not given or are obscure. The minority view is that most glomerular diseases are aggravated due to the hypercoagulable state that accompanies pregnancy, and that patients are more prone to superimposed preeclampsia or hypertensive crises earlier in pregnancy.[39,67] Most pregnancies are successful.[17,64,96,102] The predominant view is that renal function is more apt to decrease in women with diffuse glomerulonephritis and possibly membranoproliferative glomerulonephritis than in patients with focal lesions. Increases in blood pressure also occur more readily. Fortunately, these complications are usually transient and do not persist postpartum.

Hereditary nephritis is an uncommon disorder that may exacerbate or first manifest during pregnancy. In an even rarer variant of this disease, the patients have disordered platelet morphology and function. Pregnancy has been successful from a renal viewpoint, but in women with the platelet variant, the deliveries can be complicated by bleeding diatheses.

Systemic Lupus Erythematosus (SLE). The predilection of SLE to affect women in the childbearing age makes the coincidence of this disease and pregnancy a very important clinical combination. Widespread disturbance of the immunological system and multiple organ involvement in SLE, the complex clinical picture, and the immunology of pregnancy form the basis of a vast literature and many controversies.[35,86] With regard to the effects of pregnancy on SLE, transient improvements, no change, and relapses all have been reported.[40,52,53,59,61,65,86,89,104]

Lessons from the Literature. A consensus of opinion is emerging due to several recent studies. Hayslett and Lynn performed a mail survey and analyzed 65 pregnancies in 47 patients with lupus nephropathy.[53] They observed that the course during pregnancy and postpartum correlated better with the activity of the disease in the six months preceding conception than with the type of renal lesion.[53] The likelihood of a successful pregnancy was higher if SLE was in remission during this period; nevertheless, one-third of such gravidas (10 women) experienced a clinical exacerbation, including relapse of the nephropathy in the form of nephrotic syndrome or renal insufficiency. Importantly, in eight of these patients observed for more than three months after delivery, there was complete or partial remission of the exacerbation. The course of pregnancy was more problematic in gravidas with active disease at conception or those in whom SLE first appeared during pregnancy, but even in these groups, most patients improved after delivery.

Fine and colleagues have been involved with 39 patients with SLE.[40] These women did not conceive where there was even a moderate degree of renal functional impairment. During 52 pregnancies, two-thirds had minimal or no functional abnormality and one-third experienced mild dysfunction only. No measurable deterioration of renal function could be detected in 40 of the 52 pregnancies, and in seven others there was a transient decline that was totally reversible. In the remaining five patients, kidney function worsened, remaining depressed during the first year of follow-up, with one patient dying two months after delivery.

The experience of Jungers and colleagues was with 36 patients (104 pregnancies) where, in most, the pregnancy preceded the onset of SLE.[61] In the group with prepregnancy SLE (26 pregnancies), clinical exacerbation was considerably more frequent if the disease was active at the time of conception than if it was not (66% vs. 9%), but renal functional deterioration was uncommon and similar in the two subgroups (1/15 and 1/11, respectively). In contrast, three of nine gestations in which SLE appeared first during pregnancy or postpartum were complicated by the nephrotic syndrome and a substantial increase in serum creatinine. Altogether, in the 36 pregnancies during which SLE antedated the pregnancy or occurred during gestation (all had normal kidney function at conception), renal function deteriorated in five. In three patients, it was reversed by high-dose steroid therapy, but in two women, the nephropathy progressed to renal failure requiring dialysis.

Imbasciati and colleagues have analyzed data from 26 pregnancies in 19 patients with SLE and biopsy-diagnosed renal involvement.[59] The variable course of the nephropathy was clearly evident and, moreover, it could not always be predicted either from the renal biopsy or from the activity of SLE before conception. Although most of the gravidas did well, with either no change in renal function or only modest proteinuria and/or microhematuria, three patients experienced moderate worsening of renal function (persistent in one and reversed in two others by steroids administered postpartum). More alarming, however, was the occurrence of acute renal failure after delivery in four gravidas, three of whom apparently experienced the onset of lupus nephropathy during gestation. Two of these women recovered, but the other two died in renal failure of disseminated intravascular coagulation and sepsis.

Serum Factors and Their Significance. Placental transmission of lupus serum factors (perhaps the so-called LE-anticoagulant) has been documented.[35] Although the LE-anticoagulant was first described in patients with SLE, it has since been observed in patients with other conditions and even in patients without any identifiable disorder.[12,57,81] Intrauterine fetal death is common in gravidas with circulating LE-anticoagulant. The placentas in such cases show extensive thrombotic and arteriosclerotic changes. [1,81] Because treatment with steroids and aspirin may lead to successful pregnancies, it is important to screen all women with SLE and perhaps also women with a history of recurrent intrauterine fetal deaths or thrombotic episodes[1,12,57,81] for LE-anticoagulant in order to identify this cohort.

Congenital cardiac anomalies are increased in the babies of women with SLE and other maternal connective-tissue disease, even if maternal pathology is dormant. This appears related to placental transmission of a maternal antibody to soluble tissue ribonucleoprotein, anti-Ro(SS-A), which is detectable in almost all cases of isolated congenital complete heart block.[98] The prevalence of anti-Ro(SS-A) in patients with SLE is 25–30%. It may also have other associations, particularly recurrent abortion. Paradoxically, the mother's heart is usually unaffected, even though the antibody is present in her system at a higher concentration than in the fetus. Immunofluorescence techniques reveal that maternal autoantibody deposition initiates an immunologically based inflammatory response that subsequently causes congenital heart block as well as endocardial fibroelastosis and certain kinds of congenital heart disease.[80] There are several possible explanations for the variable susceptibility of the fetal heart and the relative escape from damage of the maternal heart. The fetal heart may be more vulnerable to antibody-mediated damage than the maternal heart, it may possess phase-specific antigens, or it may lack access to maternal blocking antibodies of the IgA or IgM class (not transferred to the fetus) which stop an IgG antibody from causing maternal damage. Maternal lupus may not become apparent clinically or serologically for many years after the birth of a baby with heart block.[63]

Preconception Counseling. Renal failure is one of the more ominous complications of SLE.[22] Other serious manifestations include cerebral and cardiac involvement. There are also complications associated with treatment. Thus, decisions regarding pregnancy should take into account the nature of previous manifestations, the date of most recent disease activity and assessment of just how important it is to the patient and her partner to have a baby.

The majority of pregnancies succeed, especially if the maternal disease is in sustained, complete clinical remission for at least six months prior to conception. This applies even if the patient had severe pathological changes in her original renal biopsy and heavy proteinuria in the early stages of her disease. Continued signs of disease activity and/or increasing renal dysfunction reduce the likelihood of an uncomplicated pregnancy.

Polyarteritis Nodosa. In contrast to SLE, the outcome of pregnancy in patients with renal involvement due to polyarteritis nodosa is unpredictable but mainly very poor, largely because of associated hypertension that is frequently malignant.[86] Not only is fetal prognosis dismal, but many cases end with maternal deaths.[4] Whether this reflects selective reporting or the nature of the disease is questionable. These dismal observations must be borne in mind when counseling potential mothers or when making decisions to go on with pregnancy. Therapeutic termination as an alternative management appears to have less risk for the mother.[87]

Scleroderma. The combination of scleroderma and pregnancy is unusual. This infrequent disease occurs most often during the fourth and fifth decades and patients with scleroderma are relatively infertile.[86] Whenever scleroderma has its onset in pregnancy, there is a greater tendency for deterioration. Patients with scleroderma and no evidence of renal involvement prior to conception have developed severe kidney disease in gestation. There are also instances when pregnancy has been uneventful and successful but marked reactivation occurred unexpectedly in the puerperium.[99] Most maternal deaths involve rapidly progressive scleroderma with severe pulmonary complications and infection.

Diabetic Nephropathy. Because of the frequency of diabetes among obstetric patients, it is important to examine the effects of pregnancy on renal lesions in such women. Many patients seen by the obstetrician have had diabetes since childhood and, therefore, probably already harbor microscopic changes in their kidneys. Nevertheless, renal complications are uncommon during pregnancy apart from the increased pevalence of bacteriuria and increased susceptibility to symptomatic urinary tract infection. The frequency of peripheral edema and preeclampsia is also increased.

There has been controversy about the effect of pregnancy on the kidney lesion. Earlier studies indicated that pregnancy adversely affected renal function, but these gravidas had been subjected to severe salt restriction and/or prophylactic diuretics and had moderately severe functional impairment before pregnancy. In contrast, more recent studies found no evidence that pregnancy precipitated deterioration of renal function. Nephrotic-range proteinuria and hypertension are present by the third trimester in more than 50% of women known to have diabetic nephropathy before conception (Class F), but both abnormalities abate in most patients after delivery. Creatinine clearance generally remains stable during pregnancy. Importantly, the rate of any medium-term decrease in creatinine clearance after delivery is similar to that expected spontaneously in this disease.

The approach toward treatment of severe diabetic nephropathy has become considerably more active in recent years.[68,108] Incorporation into dialysis programs, with transplantation the ultimate goal, is now the treatment of choice. This adds a new dimension to the management of diabetes mellitus generally, without even considering the prospects for pregnancy.

Polycystic Renal Disease. This condition may remain undetected during pregnancy, but careful questioning of pregnant women for a history of familial problems coupled with the use of ultrasonography may lead to earlier detection. These patients do well when functional impairment is minimal and hypertension absent, which is often the case during childbearing years. However women with or destined to develop polycystic kidney disease have a higher incidence of hypertension in pregnancy, compared to relatives who have not inherited the dominant gene.[84]

Single Kidney Situation. Some patients have either congenital absence of one kidney or marked unilateral hypoplasia, but most have had a nephrectomy because of pyelonephritis (with or without abscess), hydronephrosis, unilateral tuberculosis, congenital abnormalities, or tumor.[70,106]

When counseling a woman who has had a nephrectomy, it is important to know the indication for and the time since the surgery. There is no difference if the right or left kidney remains, as long as it is located in the normal anatomical position. If function is normal and stable, all such women seem to tolerate pregnancy well.

In patients who had a nephrectomy for an infectious and/or renal structural problem, sequential prepregnancy investigation may be needed to detect persistent infection. If serious infection occurs in a solitary kidney during pregnancy and does not respond quickly to antibiotics, termination may have to be considered to preserve renal function. Ectopic kidneys (usually pelvic) are much more vulnerable to infection and are associated with decreased fetal salvage, probably because of other associated malformations of the urogenital tract.

Nephrotic Syndrome in Pregnancy

Nephrotic syndrome more commonly occurs in the third trimester of pregnancy rather than in the first two trimesters. The usual cause is preeclampsia.[41] This form carries a poorer fetal prognosis than preeclampsia with less heavy proteinuria, but maternal prognosis is similar. Virtually all causes of nephrotic syndrome seen in nongravid individuals have also been described during gestation, including nephropathy, proliferative or membranoproliferative glomerulonephritis, lipoid nephrosis, lupus nephropathy, hereditary nephritis, diabetic nephropathy, renal vein thrombosis, amyloidosis, and secondary syphilis. Steroids should not be withheld in pregnancy, but prior to initiation of such therapy, histological confirmation that one is dealing with a corticoid-responsive lesion should be sought.

If renal function is adequate and hypertension is absent, there should be few complications during pregnancy. Physiological changes occurring during pregnancy however, may, simulate exacerbation of the clinical condition. For example, levels of serum albumin usually decrease by 1 g/100 ml in normal pregnancy. Further decreases that can occur in nephrotic syndrome may enhance fluid retention. In addition, the physiological increments in renal blood flow and/or increments in renal vein pressure due to the enlarging uterus may enhance protein excretion. Despite edema, diuretics should not be given, because these gravidas have a decreased intravascular volume. Diuretic therapy could further compromise uteroplacental perfusion or aggravate the tendency to thrombotic episodes.

Overview and Conclusions.

In patients with chronic renal disease, a balance must be struck between pregnancy outcome and the impact pregnancy has in the long term. Crucial determinants are the functional status of the kidneys at conception, the presence or absence of hypertension, and the nature of the renal lesion. If a patient wants to know if pregnancy will have a successful outcome, the answer is a qualified yes, provided her renal dysfunction is minimal. If dysfunction is moderate, there is still a fair chance that pregnancy will succeed, but the risks are much greater than in normal pregnancy. These statements have to be tempered somewhat in certain nephropathies that appear to have more problematical outcome during pregnancy. This is most true of collagen disorders affecting the kidney. Pregnancy outcome in the presence of focal glomerular sclerosis, reflux nephropathy, IgA nephropathy, and mesangioproliferative glomerulonephritis is disputed.

Pregnancy does not adversely affect the natural history of the underlying renal lesion if kidney dysfunction is minimal and hypertension is absent at conception, again with the exception of certain collagen disorders. Another factor to be considered in long-term prognosis is the sclerotic effects that hyperfiltration might have in the residual (intact) glomeruli in kidneys of patients with moderate renal insufficiency, which could cause further progressive loss of renal function.[13] Similarly, compensatory renal hypertrophy in the single kidneys of uninephrectomized subjects is another form of hyperfiltration which might, over many years, lessen the lifespan of the remaining kidney. This hypothesis is provocative and certainly cannot be ignored, since a gravida with renal disease, like a healthy pregnant woman, often experiences months of physiological hyperfiltration as part of the overall maternal adaptation to pregnancy.

PREGNANCY AND DIALYSIS PATIENTS

Perspectives

Despite reduced libido and relative infertility, women on hemodialysis can conceive and must therefore use contraception if they wish to avoid pregnancy.[37] Although conception is not common (an incidence of 1 in 200 patients has been quoted), its true frequency is unknown, because most pregnancies in dialysed patients probably end in early abortion. Furthermore, there is a high therapeutic abortion rate in this group of patients, suggesting that those who become pregnant do so inadvertently, probably because they are unaware that pregnancy is possible.[72,92]

Despite occasional delivery of a viable infant, most authorities do not advise attempts at pregnancy or its continuation once present if the patient has severe renal insufficiency.[24,54,72,92,95] Clinicians are reluctant to publish unsuccessful cases as well as those that end in disaster, so that the true incidence of successful gestations is probably less than suggested in the few selective reports. These women are prone to volume overload and severe exacerbations of their hypertension and/or superimposed preeclampsia. They also have high fetal wastage at all stages of pregnancy. Gestation poses excessive risks for the mother, with an uncertain (but very low) chance of producing a healthy infant, and therefore should be discouraged.

Management During Pregnancy

Women with severe renal insufficiency frequently present for care in advanced pregnancy because conception was not suspected. Irregular menstruation is common in dialysis patients and missed periods usually are ignored. Urine pregnancy tests are unreliable (even if there is any urine available). One must rely on sonar to confirm and to date these gestations. During pregnancy, scrupulous attention must be paid to fluid balance, blood pressure control, nutritional status, hemoglobin levels, ongoing reviews of drug therapy, increased duration and frequency of dialysis sessions, and meticulous fetal surveillance.[72,74] Because progressive anemia is usually evident in these patients, elective predelivery blood transfusion may be advisable as a safeguard against obstetrical complications.

Cesarean section should only be necessary for obstetrical reasons, but it may be argued that elective section in all cases would eliminate the potential problems of labor. Preterm labor is generally the rule. The use of cesarean section under these circumstances might be considered beneficial as well.

Management in the Long Term

Little is known about the long-term aftermath of pregnancy. In most cases reported in the literature the women remained reasonably well afterwards with little or no change in their hemodialysis regimens.

Chronic Ambulatory Peritoneal Dialysis (CAPD)

Maintenance or resumption of reproductive function may occur in many women with chronic renal dysfunction having CAPD.[68] There are now isolated case reports of women on CAPD carrying pregnancy to the stage of potential viability or to successful delivery. CAPD does not necessarily interfere with the natural progress of pregnancy or with recovery from cesarean section. Nevertheless, pregnancy in these patients is not wise, bearing in mind all the circumstances. It should be remembered that peritonitis is the worst complication of CAPD and accounts for the majority of therapy failures.[47]

PREGNANCY AND RENAL TRANSPLANTATION

After transplantation, renal and endocrine functions rapidly return and normal sexual activity usually ensues.[10,37,51] Approximately 1 in 50 women of childbearing age with a functioning renal transplant becomes pregnant. Forty percent of all conceptions do not succeed beyond the initial trimester due to spontaneous or therapeutic abortions, and a small increase in the incidence of ectopic pregnancy. Ninety percent of pregnancies that continue past the first trimester end successfully. Almost 1500 pregnancies are on record in women with a renal allograft, but, of course, many pregnancies, successful and unsuccessful, go unreported.[29,83] There is a report of a transplant performed with the surgeons unaware that the recipient was in the second trimester of pregnancy. The fact that mother, baby, and kidney came to no harm does not negate the importance of contraception counseling for all renal failure patients and of ruling out pregnancy prior to transplantation.[16]

Preconception Counseling

The return of fertility and the possibility of conception in women of childbearing age who have transplants dictates appropriate counseling to all such patients. Contraceptive advice should be routine. Couples who want a child should be encouraged to discuss all the implications, including the harsh realities of maternal prospects for survival. All involved must appreciate the possibility that the patient may not live to participate in the long-term care of her child.

Individual centers formulate their own specific guidelines. Nevertheless, certain intractable facts must not be ignored. Most advise that it is best to wait 18 months to two years post-transplant. This has turned out to be good advice because, by then, the patient certainly will have recovered from the major surgery and any sequelae, graft function will have stabilized, and immunosuppression will be at maintenance levels. Thus potential teratogenic and suppressive effects and the risks of low birth weight or small-for-dates babies will be minimal. A suitable set of comprehensive guidelines is given here,[28] bearing in mind that the criteria listed below are only relative indications: (1) good general health for two years before transplantation, (2) stature compatible wth good obstetric outcome, (3) no proteinuria, (4) no significant hypertension, (5) no evidence of graft rejection, (6) no evidence of pelvicalyceal distention on a recent intravenous urogram, (7) stable renal function—plasma creatinine of 2 mg/ 100 ml or less (preferably less than 1.5 mg%), and (8) drug therapy reduced to maintenance levels: prednisone, 15 mg/day or less and azathioprine, 2 mg/kg body weight/day or less. Safe doses of cyclosporin A have not yet been established because of limited clinical experience.[42]

Management in Pregnancy

Pregnant renal transplant patients must be considered at high risk (Table 34-6). Antenatal care should be hospital-based and should be supplemented with attention to renal function surveillance, blood pressure control, bone disease, anemia, detection of any infection (however trivial), and assessment of fetal well-being. Serial immunological surveillance, as yet in its infancy and of unknown value, also has been used to assess progress in pregnancy.[11]

Graft Rejection During Pregnancy

Immunosuppressive therapy usually is maintained at prepregnancy levels, but adjustments may be needed if maternal leukocyte or platelet counts decrease. When white blood cell counts are maintained within physiologic limits for pregnancy, the neonate usually is born with a normal blood count.[26] Azathioprine liver toxicity has been noted occasionally during pregnancy and responds to dose reduction.[18] The most sensitive method of monitoring azathioprine dosage is measurement of red blood cell 6-thioguanine nucleotide (6-TG nucleotide). This metabolite of both azathioprine and 6-mercaptopurine is the best index of bioavailability.[77]

Serious rejection episodes occur in 9% of pregnant renal allograft recipients, where gestation is beyond the second trimester.[29,83] This incidence of rejection is no greater than that expected for nonpregnant allograft recipients, but it might be considered high because it is generally assumed that the privileged immunological state of pregnancy benefits the transplant. Furthermore, there are reports of reduction or cessation of immunosuppressive

TABLE 34-6. POINTS TO REMEMBER IN PRENATAL CARE OF PREGNANT RENAL TRANSPLANT RECIPIENTS

Hospital-based management in conjunction with nephrologists
Surveillance of renal function
Allograft rejection and its differential diagnosis
Hypertension/preeclampsia
Surveillance of fetal well-being/intrauterine growth retardation
Maternal infection
Premature rupture of membranes
Preterm labor
Decision on timing and route of delivery
Effects of drug therapy on fetus and neonate

therapy during pregnancy without rejection episodes.[26,66,94]

Whether pregnancy influences the course of subclinical chronic rejection, a problem present in most recipients, is unknown.[50] No factors consistently predict which patients will develop rejection during pregnancy. There is no relationship to prior rejection episodes, HLA types, transplant-pregnancy time interval, or problems in previous pregnancies.

Difficulties can arise in distinguishing rejection from acute pyelonephritis, recurrent glomerulopathy, and possibly severe preeclampsia. Renal biopsy, which can be undertaken safely during pregnancy, is often necessary for definitive diagnosis. Ultrasonography alone may be very helpful (alterations in the echogenicity of the renal parenchyma and the presence of an indistinct corticomedullary boundary are indicative of rejection).[78] It can be very difficult to differentiate between allograft rejection and cyclosporin nephrotoxicity.

At least twenty "successful" pregnancies have been reported to the pharmaceutical company that supplies cyclosporin A. However, through 1985, there were only two or three published reports of (noncomplicated) pregnancies in patients taking cyclosporin A.[42,79] Cyclosporin A is supposedly more effective than conventional immunosuppression, but evaluations are urgently needed in gravidas, because numerous adverse effects are attributed to this drug in nonpregnant transplant recipients, including renal and hepatic toxicity, tremor, convulsions, and neoplasia.[6,33,34,105]

Renal Function

The better the renal function before pregnancy, the more satisfactory the obstetrical outcome.[25] In patients with satisfactory renal function before pregnancy, there may be a decline in GRF as well as appearance of significant proteinuria during the third trimester. These are usually transient and normal function returns postpartum (Fig. 34-4). Permanent impairment of renal function is seen occasionally, especially where compromised prior to conception.

Hypertension

There is a 30% chance of developing preeclampsia but, since the diagnosis usually is made by clinical criteria, it may be incorrect. In the absence of a renal biopsy, it may be difficult to distinguish preeclampsia from rejection, acute

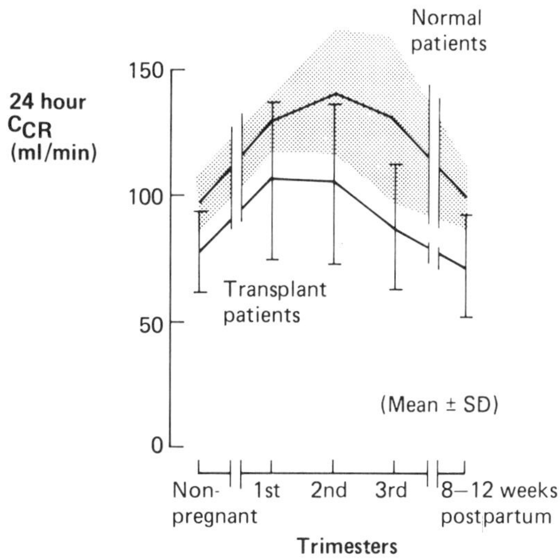

Figure 34-4. Serial 24 hour creatinine clearances (mean ± SD) during 10 pregnancies in 8 women with renal allograft studies undertaken before pregnancy, in each trimester of pregnancy and 8-12 weeks after delivery (solid line). Measurements from 10 healthy women similarly studied (mean ± SD) are shown by hatched area. (Data calculated from Davison, J. M.: The effect of pregnancy on renal function in renal allograft recipients. Kidney Int. 27: 74–79, 1985.)

pyelonephritis, and even recurrent glomerulopathy. Blood uric acid levels and 24 hour urinary protein excretion are often well above the norms for pregnancy in normotensive pregnant allograft recipients. Elevated values do not necessarily signify preeclampsia or herald its onset (Fig. 34-5). Moreover, although many of the hypertensive syndromes occurring in pregnancy transplant recipients are quite severe, there is only one report of a patient in whom the condition progressed rapidly to eclampsia.[109] Incidentally, a subsequent pregnancy was normotensive and uneventful.[110]

Timing and Route of Delivery

The factors already discussed in relation to chronic renal disease also apply here. Timing depends on balancing fetal intrauterine jeopardy against neonatal morbidity and mortality, bearing in mind at all times the mother's well-being.

The transplanted kidney very rarely produces mechanical dystocia during labor and does not sustain apparent mechanical injury during vaginal delivery. Cesarean section is

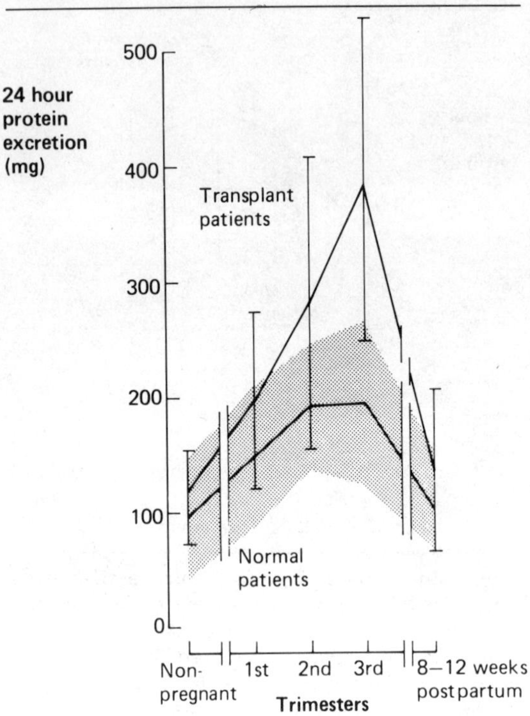

Figure 34-5. Serial 24 hour total protein excretion during 10 pregnancies in 8 women with renal allografts (mean ± SD). Studies undertaken before pregnancy, in each trimester of pregnancy and 8–12 weeks after delivery (solid line). Measurements from 10 healthy women similarly studied (mean ± SD) are shown by hatched area. (From Davison, J. M.: The effect of pregnancy on renal function in renal allograft recipients. Kidney Int. 27: 74–79, 1985.)

usually necessary only for purely obstetrical reasons. Regardless of the route of delivery, steroids must be augmented. Prophylactic antibiotics should be used for any surgical procedure, however trivial, for example, episiotomy.

Neonatal Problems

There are hazards for the neonate.[29] Preterm delivery occurs in 50% and intrauterine growth retardation in at least 20%. Although there are no frequent or predominant congenital abnormalities, one or more complications occur in about 35% of offspring, including respiratory distress syndrome, leukopenia, thrombocytopenia, adrenocortical insufficiency, cytomegalovirus, and other infections, as well as development of HB Ag carrier state (Table 34-7).

TABLE 34-7. POINTS TO REMEMBER IN NEONATES OF RENAL TRANSPLANT RECIPIENTS

Preterm delivery
Respiratory distress syndrome
Adrenocortical insufficiency
Septicemia
CMV infection
HB Ag carrier state
Immunological/hematological problems
Thymic hypoplasia
Depressed hemopoiesis
Reduced lymphocyte PHA-reactivity
Chromosome aberrations in lymphocytes
Reduced T-lymphocytes
Reduced immunoglobulin levels

Infectious Hepatitis

Renal transplant recipients may have been exposed to multiple transfusions at hemodialysis, and some may carry hepatitis B virus. Whereas women developing acute hepatitis in late pregnancy or within two months after delivery often transmit HB Ag to their offspring, the risk to children of asymptomatic carriers is much lower, and antigenicity is most likely to occur in infants whose mothers were also HB Ag positive.[9]

When HB Ag is transmitted to the baby, it invariably disappears within a few weeks after birth, only to be found later in life if active infection develops. This suggests that many HB Ag-positive neonates have been infected (i.e., with their mother's blood or vaginal secretions) at delivery and that this maternally acquired antigen is cleared before a fresh infection is contracted (alternatively, it may "incubate" outside the blood system). Further evidence of perinatal infection is that most cord blood specimens are HB Ag negative or have very low HB Ag titers, even among infants who become HB Ag carriers.[9,46]

Without prophylaxis, a high percentage of infants of HB Ag-positive mothers become carriers within two to three months of birth, an interval that again suggests that infection first occurred during labor or delivery. Furthermore, if infection occurs during pregnancy, immunoprophylaxis initiated at birth would be unlikely to prevent acquisition of the carrier state by the infant. However, hepatitis B immune globulin (HBIG) or hepatitis B virus vaccine (HBVV) given within a few hours of birth is highly effective in reducing the HB Ag carrier state in 50–70% of infants, but not if administration is delayed beyond 48 hours.[2,9,36,46] HBIG and HBVV combined are highly effective in preventing perinatal transmission of HB Ag infection. Over 90% of infants born to HB Ag-positive carrier mothers are protected, a much better rate than achieved with either HBIG or HBVV alone.[9] Most of the remaining 10% who become carriers, despite combined therapy, are presumed to have had in utero infections that were already established at birth.

Breast-Feeding. There are substantial benefits to breast-feeding. It has been argued that the baby has been exposed to azathioprine and its metabolites throughout pregnancy and that their concentrations in mothers' milk are minimal, and, therefore, breast-feeding should be allowed.[38,49] Little is known about the quantities of azathioprine and its metabolites in breast milk and about which levels are biologically trivial or substantial. Until these problems are resolved, breast-feeding should not be encouraged.

Long-Term Pediatric Assessment

Azathioprine can cause transient gaps and breaks in the chromosomes of lymphocytes.[29] These defects disappear spontaneously in 5–32 months, but such anomalies may not be as temporary in tissues not yet studied (Fig. 34-6). The sequelae could be eventual development of malignancies in affected offspring or abnormalities in the next generation. There are some disturbing animal observations. For instance, fertility problems affect the female offspring of mice that have received low doses of 6-mercaptopurine, the major metabolite of azathioprine (equivalent to 3 mg/kg).[93] These offspring subsequently prove sterile, or, if they conceive, have smaller litters and more dead fetuses than do unexposed dams. Thus, exposure in utero may not affect otherwise normal females until they embark on their reproductive careers.

Follow-up After Pregnancy

Renal Outlook. Long-term impact, in terms of renal prognosis and patient well-being, is difficult to quantify. The majority experience suggests that it is safest to wait two years after transplantation before becoming pregnant. Pregnancy does not seem to cause any irreversible decline in renal function.[29,83] A recent study, based on a comparison of very small groups of renal cadaver transplant recipients who did and did not become pregnant, concluded that pregnancy had no effect on graft function or survival.[107]

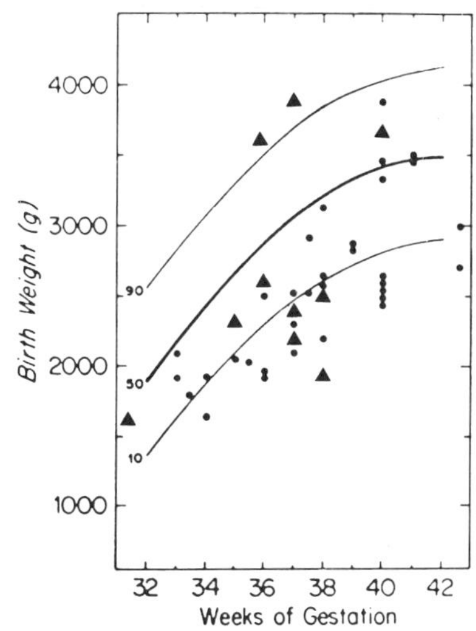

Figure 34-6. Birth weights and gestational ages of babies born to mothers receiving azathioprine throughout pregnancy. Only adequately documented cases are included and those with chronic medical disorders known to be associated with short gestation and/or intrauterine fetal growth retardation are excluded. (Modified from Scott.[97]) Tenth, 50th and 90th centiles are shown (Thomson et al.[103]). Ten infants born to renal transplant mothers in Newcastle upon Tyne (1976–1981) are shown.

Gynecological Considerations. Long-term immunosuppression (usually with azathioprine and steroids) increases the risk of developing malignancy 35-fold.[55] This is probably due to loss of immune resistance, chronic immunosuppression allowing tumor proliferation and prolonged antigenic stimulation of the reticuloendothelial system.[32] The genital tract is an important site for cancer. Reports of cervical change range from cellular atypia to invasive squamous cell carcinoma. Carcinoma of the vulva has also been noted in young patients.[19] Regular pelvic examinations and cervical cytology are essential in these women. Lastly, unusual malignancies have been reported and include reactivation of latent choriocarcinoma[75] and metastases from occult choriocarcinoma in a cadaver kidney [82]

Contraception Counseling. Oral contraceptives can produce subtle changes in the inmune system, but this does not necessarily contraindicate their use. Low-dose estrogen-progestogen preparations can be prescribed, although some authorities avoid them because of the possibility of causing or aggravating hypertension or further increasing the incidence of thromboembolism. If oral contraceptives are prescribed, careful and frequent surveillance is needed.

An intrauterine contraceptive device (lUD) may aggravate menstrual problems, which, in turn, may obfuscate signs and symptoms of abnormalities of early pregnancy, such as threatened abortion or ectopic pregnancy. The increased risk of pelvic infection associated with the IUD makes this method worrisome in an immunosuppressed patient. In any case, the efficacy of these devices may be reduced by immunosuppressive and anti-inflammatory agents, possibly due to modification of the leukocyte response.[15] Nevertheless, many patients request this method. Careful counseling and follow-up are essential.

REFERENCES

1. Abramowski, C. R., Vegas, M. E., Swinehart, B. A., and Gyves, M. T.: Decidual vasculopathy of the placenta in lupus erythematosus. *N. Engl. J. Med.* **303**:66–72, 1980.
2. Baker, D. A. and Polk, B. F.: Hepatitis B: A controllable disease. *Obstet. Gynecol.* **62**:105–108, 1983.
3. Barcelo, P. and Lopez, J.: Glomerulonefritis y embarazo. Proceedings of 15 Curso d Nefrologia para post graduados sobre Rinon y Embarazo. Reuniones y Congresos, S.A., Fundacion Puigvert, Madrid, 1984, pp. 89–91.
4. Barkett, G. and Richards, R.: Periarteritis nodosa and pregnancy. *Obstet. Gynecol.* **59**:252–254, 1982.
5. Barret, R. J. and Peters, W. A.: Pregnancy following urinary diversion. *Obstet. Gynecol.* **62**:582–586, 1983.
6. Beaman, M., Parvin, S., Veitch, P. S., and Walls, J.: Convulsions associated with cyclosporin A in renal transplant recipients. *Br. Med. J.* **290**:139–140, 1985.
7. Bear, R. A.: Pregnancy in patients with chronic renal disease. *Can. Med. Assoc. J.* **18**:663–665, 1978.
8. Bear, R. A.: Pregnancy in patients with renal disease: A study of 44 cases. *Obstet. Gynecol.* **48**:13–18, 1976.
9. Beasly, R. P., Hwang, L-U., and Lee, G-Y.: Prevention of perinatally transmitted hepatitis B virus infections with hepatitis B immune globulin and hepatitis B vaccine. *Lancet* **2**:1099–1102, 1983.
10. Billet, A., Davis, A., Linhardt, G. E., Queral, L. A., Dagher, F. J., and Williams G. M.: The effects of bilateral renal transplantation on pelvic hemodynamics and sexual function. *Surgery* **95**:415–419, 1984.
11. Birkeland, S. A. and Kristoffersen, K.: Immune monitoring of pregnancy in renal transplanted patients. *Am. J. Reprod. lmmunol.* **5**:72–77, 1984.
12. Boey, M. L., Colaco, C. B., Gharavi, A. E., Elkou, K. B., Loizou, S., and Hughes, G. R. V.: Thrombosis in systemic lupus erythematosus: Striking association with presence of circulating lupus anticoagulant. *Br. Med. J.* **287**:1021–1023, 1983.
13. Brenner, B. M., Meyer, T. W., and Hostetter, T. H.: Dietary protein intake and the progressive nature of kidney disease: The role of hemodynamically medicated glomerular injury in the pathogenesis of progressive glomerular sclerosis in aging, renal ablation and intrinsic renal disease. *N. Engl. J. Med.* **307**:652–659, 1982.
14. Brumfitt, W.: The significance of symptomatic and asymptomatic infection in pregnancy. *Contrib. Nephrol.* **25**:23–29, 1981.
15. Buhler, M. and Papiernik, E.: Successive pregnancies in women fitted with intrauterine devices who take anti- inflammatory drugs. *Lancet* **1**:483, 1983.
16. Burleson, R. L., Sunderji, S. G., Aubry, R. H., Clark, D. A., Marbarger, P., Cohen, R. S., Scruggs, B. F., and La Graff, S.: Renal allotransplantation during pregnancy. *Transplantation* **36**:334–335, 1983.
17. Cameron, J. S. and Hicks, J.: Pregnancy in patients with pre-existing glomerular disease. *Contrib. Nephrol.* **37**:149–156, 1984.
18. Campos, H., Kreiss, H. A., Rioux, P., and Crosnier, R.: Azathioprine withdrawal in renal transplant recipients. *Transplantation* **38**:29–31, 1984.
19. Caterson, R. J., Furber, J., Murray, J., McCarthy, W., Mahony, J. F., and Sheil, A. G. R.: Carcinoma of the vulva in two young renal llograft recipients. *Transplant. Proc.* **16**:559–561, 1984.
20. Chng, P. K. and Hall, M. H.: Antenatal prediction of urinary tract infection in pregnancy. *Br. J. Obstet. Gynaecol.* **89**:8–11, 1982.
21. Coe, F. L., Darks, J. H., and Lindheimer, M. D.: Nephrolithiasis during pregnancy. *N. Engl. J. Med.* **298**:324–326, 1978.
22. Correia, P., Cameron, J. S., Lian, J. D., Hicks, J., Ogg, C. S., Williams, D. G., Chantler, C., and

Haycock, D. G.: Why do patients with lupus nephritis die? *Br. Med. J.* **290**:126–131, 1985.

23. Coward, R. A., Allick, N. P., Warrel, D. W., Grimes, D., and Kirkpatrick, H.: Successful pregnancy in severe chronic renal failure not requiring dialysis. *Br. Med. J.* **281**:839, 1980.
24. David, A. S. and Newling, D. W.: Successful pregnancy following hemodialysis and pyelopathy. *Nephron* **34**:64–67, 1983.
25. Davison, J. M.: The effect of pregnancy on renal function in renal allograft recipients. *Kidney Int.* **27**:74–79, 1985.
26. Davison, J. M., Dellagrammatikas, H., and Parkin, J. M.: Maternal azathioprine therapy and depressed haemopoiesis in the babies of renal allograft recipients. *Br. J. Obstet. Gynaecol.,* in press.
27. Davison, J. M. and Dunlop, W.: Changes in renal hemodynamics and tubular function induced by normal human pregnancy. *Semin. Nephrol.* **4**:197–206, 1984.
28. Davison, J. M., Lind, T., and Uldall, P. R.: Planned pregnancy in a renal transplant recipient. *Br. J. Obstet. Gynaecol.* **83**:518–527, 1976.
29. Davison, J. M. and Lindheimer, M. D.: Pregnancy in women with renal allografts. *Semin. Nephrol.* **4**:240–251, 1984.
30. Davison, J. M., Sprott, M. B., and Selkon, J. B.: The effect of covert bacteriuria in schoolgirls on renal function at 18 years and during pregnancy. *Lancet* **2**:651–655, 1984.
31. Drago, J., Rohner, T., and Chez, R.: Management of urinary calculi in pregnancy. *Urology* **20**:578–583, 1982.
32. Editorial: Cancer in organ transplant recipients. Part of an induced immune deficiency syndrome. *Br. Med. J.* **288**:659–660, 1984.
33. Editorial: Cyclosporin nephrotoxicity. *Ann. Intern. Med.* **99**:851–854, 1983.
34. Editorial: Cyclosporin and neoplasia. *Lancet* **1**:1083, 1983.
35. Editorial: Lupus anticoagulant. *Lancet* **1**:1157–1158, 1984.
36. Editorial: Prevention of perinatally transmitted hepatitis B infection. *Lancet* **1**:939–941, 1984.
37. Emmanouel, D. S., Lindheimer, M. D., and Katz, A. I.: Endocrine function in uraemia. In: *The Systemic Consequences of Renal Failure.* G. Eknoyan and G. Knochel (Eds.). New York, Grune & Stratton, 1984, pp. 177–196.
38. Fagerholm, M. I., Coulan, C. B., and Moyer, T. P.: Breast feeding after renal transplantation. 6-Mercaptopurine content of human breast milk. *Surg. Forum* **31**:447–449, 1980.
39. Fairley, K. F., Whitworth, J. A., and Kincaid-Smith, P.: Glomerulonephritis: II. In: *Glomerulonephritis and Pregnancy.* P. Kincaid-Smith, T. H. Mathew, and E. L. Becker (Eds.). New York, John Wiley & Sons, 1973, pp. 997–1011.
40. Fine, L. G., Barnett, E. V., Danovitch, G. M., Nissenson, A. R., Conolly, M. E., Lieb, S. M., and Barrett, C. T.: Systemic lupus erythematosus in pregnancy. *Ann. Intern. Med.* **94**:667–677, 1981.
41. Fisher, K., Luger, A., Spargo, B. H., and Lindheimer, M. D.: Hypertension in pregnancy: Clinical-pathological correlations and remote prognosis. *Medicine* **60**:267–274, 1981.
42. Flechner, S. M., Katz, A. R., Rogers, A. J., Van Buren, C., and Kahan, B. D.: The presence of cyclosporine in body tissues and fluids during pregnancy. *Am. J. Kidney Dis.* **5**:60–63, 1985.
43. Fowler, J. E. and Pulaski, E. T.: Excretion urography, cystography and cystoscopy in the evaluation of women with urinary tract infection. *N. Engl. J. Med.* **304**:462–464, 1982.
44. Gargan, R. A., Brumfitt, W., and Hamilton-Miller, J. M. T.: Antibody-coated bacteria in urine: Criterion for a positive test and its value in defining a higher risk of treatment failure. *Lancet* **2**:704–706, 1983.
45. Gilstrap, L. C., Leveno, K. J., Cunningham, F. G., Whalley, P. J., and Roark, M. L.: Renal infection and pregnancy outcome. *Am. J. Obstet. Gynecol.* **141**:709–716, 1981.
46. Goudeau, A., Lesage, G., Denis, F., Chiron, J. P., Yvonnet, B., Barin, F., Coursaget, P., and Diop Mar, I.: Lack of anti-HBc Igm in neonates with HBsAg carrier mothers argues against transplacental transmission of hepatitis B virus infections. *Lancet* **2**:1103–1104, 1983.
47. Grefberg, N., Danielson, B. G., and Nilsson, P.: Peritonitis in patients on continuous ambulatory peritoneal dialysis. *Scand. J. Inf. Dis.* **16**:187–193, 1984.
48. Gregory, M. C. and Mansell, M. A.: Pregnancy and cystinuria. *Lancet* **2**:1158–1160, 1983.
49. Grekas, D. M., Vasiliou, S. S., and Lazarides, A. N.: Immunosuppressive therapy and breast feeding after renal transplantation. *Nephron* **37**:68, 1984.
50. Guttman, R. D.: Renal transplantation. *N. Engl.J. Med.* **301**:975–981, 1038–1048, 1979.
51. Handelsman, D. J., McDowell, I. F. W., Caterson, I. D., Tiller, D. J., Hall, B. M., and Turtle, J. R.: Ovarian function after renal transplantation: Comparison of cyclosporin A with azathioprine and prednisone combination regimens. *Br. J. Obstet. Gynaecol.* **91**:802–807, 1984.
52. Hayslett, J. P.: Effect of pregnancy in patients with SLe. *Am. J. Kidney Dis.* **2** (Suppl):223–228, 1982.
53. Hayslett, J. P. and Lynn, R. I.: Effect of pregnancy in patients with lupus nephropathy. *Kidney Int.* **18**:207–220, 1980.
54. Hensel, A., Pauls, A., von Herrath, D., and Schaefer, K.: Successful hemodialysis for acute renal failure in late pregnancy. *Am. J. Nephrol.* **2**:98–101, 1982.
55. Hoover, R. and Fraumeni, J. R.: Risk of cancer in renal transplant recipients. *Lancet* **2**:55–57, 1973.
56. Hou, S. H., Grossman, S. D., and Madias, N. E.: Pregnancy in women with renal disease and mod-

erate renal insufficiency. *Am. J. Med.* **78**:185–194, 1985.

57. Hughes, G. R. V.: Thrombosis, abortion, cerebral disease and the lupus anticoagulant. *Br. Med. J.* **287**:1088–1089, 1983.
58. Imbasciati, E., Pardi, G., Bozetti, P., Massa, E., Capetta, P., Airoldi, M. L., Pagliari, B., and Ambroso, G. C.: Pregnancy in women with chronic renal failure. Proceedings of the 4th World Congress of the International Society for the Study of Hypertension in Pregnancy, 1984, p. 78.
59. Imbasciati, E., Surian, M., Battino, S., Cosci, P., Colussi, G., Ambroso, G. C., Massa, E., Minetti, L., Pardi, G., and Ponticelli, C.: Lupus nephropathy and pregnancy. A study of 26 pregnancies in patients with systemic lupus erythematosus and nephritis. *Nephron* **36**:46–51, 1984.
60. Jacobsen, F. K., Christensen, C. K., Mogensen, C. E., and Heilskow, H. C. S.: Evaluation of kidney function after meals. *Lancet* **1**:319, 1980.
61. Jungers, P., Dougados, M., Pelissies, C., Kuttenn, F., Tron, F., Lesavre, P., and Bach, J. F.: Lupus nephropathy and pregnancy. *Arch. Intern. Med.* **142**:771–776, 1982.
62. Jungers, P., Forget, D., Henry-Amor, M., Droz, D., and Giufeld, J. P.: Chronic primary glomerulonephritis and pregnancy. Proceedings of the 4th World Congress of the International Society for the Study of Hypertension in Pregnancy, 1984, p. 7.
63. Kasinath, B. S. and Katz, A. I.: Delayed maternal lupus after delivery of offspring with congenital heart block. *Arch. Intern. Med.* **142**:2317, 1982.
64. Katz, A. I., Davison, J. M., Hayslett, J. P., Singson, E., and Lindheimer, M. D.: Pregnancy in women with kidney disease. *Kidney Int.* **18**:192–206, 1980.
65. Katz, A. I. and Lindheimer, M. D.: Effect of pregnancy on the natural course of kidney disease. *Semin. Nephrol.* **4**:252–259, 1984.
66. Kauffman, J. J., Digman, W., Goodwin, W. E., Martin, D. C., Goldman, R., and Maxwell, H. M.: Successful normal childbirth after kidney transplantation. *JAMA* **200**:162–165, 1967.
67. Kincaid-Smith, P., Whitworth, J. A., and Fairley, K. F.: Mesangial IgA nephropathy in pregnancy. *Clin. Exp. Hypertes.* **2**:821–838, 1980.
68. Kioko, E. M., Shaw, K. M., Clark, A. D., and Warren, D. J.: Successful pregnancy in a diabetic patient treated with continuous ambulatory peritoneal dialysis. *Diabetes Care* **6**:298–300, 1983.
69. Kitzmiller, J. L., Brown, E. R., Phillipe, M., Stark, A. R., Acker, D., Kaldany, A., Singh, S., and Hare, J.: Diabetic nephropathy and perinatal outcome. *Am. J. Obstet. Gynecol.* **141**:741–751, 1981.
70. Klein, E. A.: Urologic problems of pregnancy. *Obstet. Gynecol. Surv.* **39**:605–615, 1984.
71. Klockars, M., Saarikosi, S., Ikonen, E., and Kuhlback, B.: Pregnancy in patients with renal disease. *Acta Med. Scand.* **207**:207–214, 1980.
72. Kobayashi, H., Matsumoto, Y., Otsubo, O., and Nait, F.: Successful pregnancy in a patient undergoing chronic hemodialysis. *Obstet. Gynecol.* **57**:382–386, 1981.
73. Lattanzi, D. R. and Cook, W. A.: Urinary calculi in pregnancy. *Obstet. Gynecol.* **56**:462–470, 1980.
74. Lee, C. C. and Marbury, T. C.: Drug therapy in patients undergoing hemodialysis. Clinical pharmacokinetic considerations. *Clin. Pharmacokinet.* **9**:42–66, 1984.
75. Lelievre, G., Ribet, M., Gosselin, B., Sequiedt, P., Lepoutre, E., and Tacquet, A.: Chorio-carcinoma apres transplantation. *J. Urol. Nephrol. (Paris)* **84**:345–346, 1978.
76. Lenke, R. R., Vandorsten, J. P., and Schifrin, S.: Pyelonephritis in pregnancy: Prospective randomized trial to prevent recurrent disease evaluating suppressive therapy with nitrofurantoin and close surveillance. *Am. J. Obstet. Gynecol.* **146**:953–957, 1983.
77. Lennard, L., Brown, C. B., Fox, M., and Maddocks, J. L.: Azathioprine metabolism in kidney transplant recipients. *Br. J. Clin. Pharmacol.* **18**:693–700, 1984.
78. Levzow, B. L.: The appearance of renal transplant rejection with ultrasound. *Med. Ultrasound* **6**:43–52, 1982.
79. Lewis, G. J., Lamont, C. A. R., Lee, H. A., and Slapak, M.: Successful pregnancy in a renal transplant recipient taking cyclosporin A. *Br. Med. J.* **286**:603, 1983.
80. Litsey, S. E., Noonan, J. A., O'Connor, W. N., Cottrill, C. M., and Mitchell, B.: Maternal connective tissue disease and congenital heart block. *N. Engl. J. Med.* **312**:98–100, 1985.
81. Lubbe, W. F., Butler, W. S., Palmer, S. J., and Liggins, G. C.: Lupus anticoagulant in pregnancy. *Br. J. Obstet. Gynaecol.* **91**:357–363, 1984.
82. Manifold, I. H., Champion, A. E., Goepel, J. R., Rainsewak, S., and Mayor, P. E.: Pregnancy complicated by gestational trophoblastic disease in a renal transplant recipient. *Br. Med. J.* **287**:1025–1026, 1983.
83. Meir, P. R. and Makowski, E. L.: Pregnancy in the patient with a renal transplat. *Clin. Obstet. Gynecol.* **27**:902–913, 1984.
84. Milatinovic, J., Agoda, L. Y., Phillips, L. A., and Bryant, J. I.: Fertility and pregnancy complications in women with autosomal dominant polycystic kidney disease. *Obstet. Gynecol.* **61**:566–570, 1983.
85. Miller, D. R. and Kakkis, J.: Prognosis, management and outcome of obstructive renal disease in pregnancy. *J. Reprod. Med.* **27**:199–201, 1982.
86. Mor-Yosef, S., Navot, D., Rabinowitz, R., and Schenker, J. G.: Collagen disease in pregnancy. *Obstet. Gynecol. Surv.* **39**:67–83, 1984.
87. Nagey, D. A., Fortier, K. J., and Linder, J.: Pregnancy complicated by periarteritis nodosa: Induced abortion as an alternative. *Am. J. Obstet. Gynecol.* **147**:103–105, 1983.

88. Pak, C.: Medical management of nephrolithiasis. *J. Urol.* **128**:1157–1160, 1982.
89. Paul, R. H.: Pregnancy outcome in women with systemic lupus erythematosus. *Obstet. Gynecol.* **63**:686–692, 1984.
90. Ready, B. L. and Johnson, E. S.: Epidural block for the tratment of renal colic during pregnancy. *Can. Anaesth. Soc. J.* **28**:77–79, 1981.
91. Redman, C. W. G.: The management of hypertension in pregnancy. *Contrib. Nephrol.* **4**:270–282, 1984.
92. Registration Committee of the European Dialysis and Transplant Association: Successful pregnancies in women treated by dialysis and kidney transplantation. *Br. J. Obstet. Gynaecol.* **87**:839–845, 1980.
93. Reimers, T. J. and Sluss, P. M.: 6-Mercaptopurine treatment of pregnant mice: Effects on second and third generations. *Science* **201**:65–67, 1978.
94. Rifle, G. and Traeger, J.: Pregnancy after renal transplantation. An international survey. *Transplant. Proc.* **7**:723–728, 1975.
95. Rotellar, C., Ferragut, A., and Borrull, J.: Pregnancy in a patient on regular hemodialysis. *Nephron* **35**:66–67, 1983.
96. Rovati, C., Perrino, M. L., Barbiano de Belgiojoso, G., Surian, M., Radaelli, L., and Minetti, L.: Pregnancy and course of primary glomerulonephritis. *Contrib. Nephrol.* **37**:182–189, 1984.
97. Scott, J. R.: Fetal growth retardation associated with maternal administation of immunosuppressive drugs. *Am. J. Obstet. Gynecol.* **128**:668–676, 1977.
98. Scott, J. S., Maddison, P. J., Taylor, P. V., Esschere Scott, O., and Skinner, R. P.: Connective-tissue disease, antibodies to ribonucleoprotein and congenital heart block. *N. Engl. J. Med.* **09**:209–212, 1983.
99. Smith, C. A.: Progressive systemic sclerosis and post-partum renal failure complicated by peripheral gangrene. *J. Rheumatol.* **9**:455–460, 1982.
100. Stanton, S. L., Kerr-Wilson, R., and Harris, V. G.: The incidence of urologic symptoms in normal pregnancy. *Br. J. Obstet. Gynaecol.* **78**:897–901, 1980.
101. Strauch, B. S. and Hayslett, J. P.: Kidney disease and pregnancy. *Br. Med. J.* **4**:578-582, 1974.
102. Surian, M., Imbasciati, E., Cosci, P., Banfi, G., Barbiano di Belgiojoso, G., Brancaccio, D., Minetti, L., and Ponticelli, C.: Glomerular disease and pregnancy: A study of 123 pregnancies in patients with primary and secondary glomerular diseases. *Nephron* **36**:101–105, 1984.
103. Thomson, A. M., Billewicz, W. Z., and Hytten, F. E.: The weight of the placenta in relation to birthweight. *J. Obstet. Gynaecol. Br. Commonw.* **76**:865–872, 1969.
104. Varner, M. W., Meehan, R. T., Syrop, C. H., Strottman, M. P., and Goplerud, C. P.: Pregnancy in patients with systemic lupus erythematosus. *Am. J. Obstet. Gynecol.* **145**:1025–1040, 1983.
105. Verani, R. R., Flechner, S. M., Van Buren, C. T., and Kahan, B. D.: Acute cellular rejection or cyclosporin A nephrotoxicity? A review of transplant renal biopsies. *Am. J. Kidney Dis.* **4**:185–191, 1984.
106. Waltzer, W. C.: The urinary tract in pregnancy. *J. Urol.* **125**:271–276, 1981.
107. Whetam, J. C. G., Cardelle, C., and Harding, M.: Effect of pregnancy on graft function and graft survival in renal cadaver transplant patients. *Am. J. Obstet. Gynecol.* **145**:193–197, 1983.
108. Wilczek, H., Gunnarsson, R., Lundgren, G., and Ost, L.: Improved results of renal transplantation in diabetic nephropathy. *Transplant. Proc.* **16**:623–627, 1984.
109. Williams, P. F. and Jelen, J.: Eclampsia in a patient who had had a renal transplant. *Br. Med. J.* **2**:972, 1979.
110. Williams, P. F. and Johnstone, M.: Normal pregnancy in renal transplant recipient with a history of eclampsia and intrauterine death. *Br. Med. J.* **285**:1535, 1982.

35

GASTROINTESTINAL PROBLEMS AND JAUNDICE

Pregnancy results in a myriad of physiologic changes in the gastrointestinal tract. These changes often mimic disease, alter anatomical relationships, and influence results of laboratory tests. The diagnosis of gastrointestinal disease in pregnancy is therefore difficult. Furthermore, complications of pregnancy may present with gastrointestinal complaints so that an entire new set of diagnostic possibilities must be considered. Because intra-abdominal disease can mimic or initiate labor, the presence of intra-abdominal disease can be obscured during pregnancy.

To evaluate a pregnant patient with a gastrointestinal disturbance, the physician must understand gestational physiologic changes and the alterations in the clinical presentation of intra-abdominal disease in pregnancy. Otherwise, errors and delays in diagnosis and management will occur with concomitant perinatal and maternal complications.

GASTROINTESTINAL PROBLEMS

Nausea and Vomiting of Pregnancy

Nausea and vomiting may occur in up to 60% of pregnant women and are often considered to be presumptive evidence of pregnancy. Commonly, the symptoms begin early in the first trimester and disappear by the second trimester.

Although the physiology of nausea and vomiting in the nonpregnant patient is well understood, the etiology of nausea and vomiting in pregnancy is unclear. Most clinicians accept a psychogenic component to pathologic nausea and vomiting. Psychologic disturbances or personality alterations are common in patients with hyperemesis. Patients with hyperemesis may display hysterical personalities, below-normal intelligence, and/or strong maternal dependence.[13] Beside psychologic factors, physiologic alterations have been associated with pathologic nausea and vomiting in pregnancy.

Because the onset of nausea and vomiting parallels the rise in serum chorionic gonadotropin (hCG), this hormone has been implicated in hyperemesis.[8] The higher rate of nausea and vomiting in pregnancies with elevated hCG (i.e., twins, gestational trophoblastic disease) further suggests a relationship between this hormone and hyperemesis gravidarum. Some authors have linked variations in estrogen and progesterone levels to the nausea and vomiting of pregnancy, but no clear evidence supports this theory. Adrenal insufficiency may result in nausea, and some patients with pregnancy-associated emesis have responded to steroid administration. ACTH treatment sometimes results in improvement of hyperemesis.[15] Indirect evidence thus suggests a pituitary aberration with a glucocorticoid abnormality as a cause of hyperemesis; however, recent studies of pituitary and adrenocortical function revealed no abnormalities in patients with hyperemesis.[8]

Treatment of uncomplicated nausea and vomiting of pregnancy is controversial. Administration of drugs during embryogenesis carries a risk for teratogenicity. A combination of doxylamine and pyridoxine was a commonly prescribed antiemetic in pregnancy. Because of the high percentage of pregnant women with nausea and vomiting, this drug was probably the most common prescription drug administered in early pregnancy. Concern arose about its possible teratogenic effect. Although a recent study demonstrated no increase in the rate of congenital anomalies in women receiving this agent,[18] the drug has been removed from the market. Experience with other antiemetic preparations in pregnancy is sporadic, and possible side effects are not defined. Therefore, these preparations should be avoided if possible. At present, there is no accepted treatment for nausea and vomiting of pregnancy.

About 0.35% of pregnant women develop hyperemesis gravidarum manifested as severe, persistent vomiting that results in fluid and electrolyte abnormalities and nutritional deficiences.[15] Hyperemesis gravidarum occurs more frequently in first pregnancies. Significant weight loss, ketosis, and ketonuria may occur in severe cases. These derangements can result in hepatic, renal, and neurological damage.

Initial assessment of the patient suspected of hyperemesis gravidarum should include a history of the frequency and severity of vomiting (although this may be exaggerated by patients) and an evaluation of skin turgor and moisture of the mucous membranes to assess fluid loss. Other serious causes of nausea and vomiting such as appendicitis, intestinal obstruction, and cholecystitis should be excluded. Laboratory evaluation should include urinalysis, serum electrolyte evaluation, and, in ill patients, measurement of arterial blood gas and serum ketones to evaluate for ketoacidosis. Abnormalities in these parameters should instigate further evaluation of renal, hepatic, and hematologic status. A combined acid–base disorder may be present. Starvation may result in ketoacidosis whereas vomiting may result in alkalosis (as hydrogen ions move intracellular to compensate for the efflux of potassium from cells caused by the potassium lost in vomiting).

Patients without metabolic abnormalities may be helped by reassurance and dietary changes, but patients with electrolyte abnormalities or ketosis should be hospitalized. Fluid and electrolyte replacement are the mainstays of treatment. In severe cases, antiemetics may be utilized. At first, oral intake is limited, but slowly, it may be increased. Slow recovery with relapses is common. Counseling to resolve family conflicts may be helpful. Recording of weight daily is an excellent method of evaluating progress. Complications are rare with appropriate treatment, but renal and hepatic abnormalities may occur. Hematemesis, Mallory–Weiss syndrome, and acid aspiration also have been reported. In severe cases with persistent weight loss and/or ketosis, parenteral hyperalimentation may be required. When this disease is appropriately treated and the metabolic abnormalities corrected, hyperemesis gravidarum does not seem to predispose to subsequent maternal or fetal complications.

Reflux Esophagitis

Reflux esophagitis results in the common complaint of heartburn in pregnant patients. Up to 70% of pregnant women may report heartburn with the highest rates occurring in late pregnancy. For reasons that are unclear, the rate is higher in Caucasians (78.8%) than in Blacks (9.8%).[3] Both an increase in intra-abdominal pressure from the enlarging uterus and a decrease in lower esophageal sphincter (LES) pressure have been proposed as the cause of reflux. During pregnancy, LES pressure progressively diminishes. The maximal reduction occurs near term.[33] Progestational agents can mimic this effect of pregnancy.[34] Although causality is not proved, progesterone is probably important in decreasing LES pressure since it is a smooth-muscle relaxant.

Extensive laboratory tests are usually unnecessary for the diagnosis of reflux esophagitis. The symptomatology of reflux esophagitis and improvement with empiric therapy are sufficient to arrive at the diagnosis. Patients with reflux esophagitis classically complain of substernal burning, discomfort, or pain—more severe after meals or when recumbent. Radiation of the pain to the neck or back may occur. Activities that increase intra-abdominal pressure often aggravate the problem. "Water brash," a sudden reflux of clear, acidy fluid into the mouth, is a common complaint.

Simple changes in lifestyle often ameliorate the symptomatology of reflux esophagitis. Elevation of the bed, dividing food into multiple, smaller meals, and avoiding late meals help to prevent symptoms. Significant improvement of symptoms and prevention of recurrences can be achieved with antacid administration. Initial therapy usually requires frequent doses that can be tapered as symptoms disappear. In pregnant women who require sodium restriction, care should be exercised in the selection of the antacid preparation since some have a high sodium content.

There is little experience in pregnancy with the new pharmacologic agents (such as cimetidine) that decrease acid secretion. In the nonpregnant patient, cimetidine results in symptomatic improvement of reflux esophagitis.[4] This drug does not affect LES pressure but prevents stomach acid production. Reported complications include arrhythmia and cardiac arrest. An important concern is that cimetidine appears to cross the placenta and reaches significant levels in the fetus.[23] Fetal effects, if any, are not clearly known. Because of the excellent response to antacids, the high cost and possible complications of drugs such as cimetidine, there appears to be little indication to use the acid-reducing drugs in pregnant patients with reflux esophagitis.

Peptic Ulcer Disease

Gastric and duodenal ulcers are grouped under the title peptic ulcer disease although they differ in many respects. All ulcers are more common in males than in females. Gastric ulcers, which are associated with gastric carcinoma, are extremely rare in the childbearing years. Duodenal ulcers are four times more common than stomach ulcers. The rate of duodenal ulcers in American women is 0.08%. In pregnant women, the rate may be lower since gestation appears to ameliorate peptic ulcer disease. Eighty-eight percent of women with peptic ulcer disease report symptomatic improvement during pregnancy.[5] The rate of complications from peptic ulcer disease diminishes with gestation, and bleeding, perforation, or obstruction are rarely seen.

The pathophysiology of peptic ulcer disease is complex but can be attribued to breakdown of mucosal protective mechanisms, acid hypersecretion, and alterations in gastric emptying. Little data exist to explain the improvement that many patients experience in pregnancy, but two factors are thought to be influential. During pregnancy, plasma histaminase levels are elevated, and histamine destruction in the stomach may result in decreased acid production.[6] The few studies of gastric acid secretion in pregnancy, however, show either no alteration or a slight decrease in gastric acid. Another factor is the slowing of gastrointestinal function which results in delayed stomach emptying. The slower passage of stomach contents into the intestine may contribute to a decreased rate of duodenal ulcers.

Because the symptomatology and response to treatment are similar, peptic ulcer disease in pregnancy often is confused with reflux esophagitis. Classically, patients with peptic ulcer disease complain of epigastric pain, especially on an empty stomach. Being awakened at night by the pain is common, and food or antacids offer symptomatic relief. In nonpregnant patients, an upper GI series confirms the diagnosis, but radiation is unnecessary in pregnant women. Treatment with antacids usually resolves the symptoms. If further evaluation is required, endoscopy to visualize the gastric and duodenal mucosa is useful. Patients with severe disease, with gastrointestinal bleeding, or who fail to respond to antacids are candidates for endoscopy.

Outside gestation, therapy for peptic ulcer disease utilizes H_2-histamine receptor antagonists (such as cimetidine) to diminish acid production markedly. Because of the limited experience and possible complications of these drugs in pregnancy, plus the good response to antacids, the use of these blockers in gestation, except under unusual circumstances, is questionable. (See Reflux Esophagitis.)

Pregnant women with peptic ulcer disease respond well to diet modification and antacid administration. Major dietary changes are unnecessary, but avoidance of foods that worsen the symptoms, as well as of caffeine, alcohol, and tobacco is appropriate. Antacids should be administered 1 and 3 hours after each meal and at bedtime. Dosage varies according to the acid-neutralization capacity of the antacid, but the quantity should be sufficient to relieve and prevent symptoms. Neutralization of 150 mEq of acid is ideal, but these large amounts of antacid may result in diarrhea. With antacid therapy, 78% of ulcers heal within four weeks.[29] Lack of response, worsening of the disease, or development of a complication mandates reevaluation and modification of the treatment regimen.

Inflammatory Bowel Disease

Chronic inflammatory bowel disease includes two disorders: regional enteritis (Crohn's disease) and ulcerative colitis. The cause of these diseases is unknown. Familial, infectious, autoimmune, and psychogenic etiologies have been proposed. Although some clinicians consider these two diseases as a continuum affecting different areas of the bowel, the pathophysiology, symptomatology, and complications are sufficiently dissimilar to warrant that each be considered separately.

Regional Enteritis—Crohn's Disease. The chronic inflammatory process of regional enteritis is composed of a lymphocytic and plasma cell infiltrate usually involving all layers of the bowel and occasionally extending into the mesentery. Granuloma formation and fibrosis may be seen. The involved bowel thickens, stenoses, and often becomes adherent to other loops of bowel with possible fistula formation. The most commonly involved area is the distal ileum, but 50% of patients have both ileal and colonic involvement. Isolated colonic involvement also is reported.

Clinical presentation may vary depending on the involved area of bowel. A typical history reveals right lower quadrant pain, diarrhea, fatigue, weight loss, and low-grade fever. Blood in the stool is not uncommon. Symptoms usually have been present for several years, and because of the adherent bowel loops, a mass may be palpable. The clinical picture may be confused with appendicitis, and some patients are initially diagnosed at laparotomy. Intestinal obstruction may occur in 20–30% of patients, but it is usually incomplete and does not necessarily require surgery. Malabsorption, fistulas, and abscesses may complicate the clinical course.

Outside gestation, diagnosis involves sigmoidoscopy, possibly with biopsy, and radiologic studies of the small and large intestine. Pregnancy hampers the ability to obtain a diagnosis, since x-ray exposure should be avoided, and sigmoidoscopy may be difficult with an enlarged uterus.

The treatment of regional enteritis varies according to the severity of disease. Nutritional balance and vitamin supplementation are important. For patients with diarrhea, an antidiarrheal preparation such as dephenoxylate may be indicated. Patients with diarrhea and cramps may benefit from codeine. Both these drugs should be avoided in patients with evidence of ileus or intestinal obstruction.

Patients with more severe disease or those who do not respond to these initial measures may require corticosteroids. Steroids should be administered for the acute episode until remission, and then the dose should be tapered slowly. Continuous prolonged therapy does not alter the rate of recurrences. Steroid dosage in pregnant patients should be similar to those in nonpregnant patients. If the patient is receiving steroids, the dosage should be increased at the time of labor and delivery.

Sulfasalazine, a compound broken to 5-aminosalicylate and sulfapyridine in the gut, has been effective in some patients with regional enteritis.[32] Few data exist to evaluate the safety of this compound in pregnancy, and, theoretically, there may be some risk to the fetus. Animal studies with sulfasalazine did not demonstrate teratogenicity, but other sulfonamides have been implicated in congenital anomalies. Hyperbilirubinemia or kernicterus has been noted in preterm neonates born to women given sulfonamides in pregnancy. However, this has not been reported with sulfasalazine.[22] Sulfasalazine alters folate absorption and metabolism, which may have deleterious effects on the mother or fetus.[12] Use of this drug in pregnancy should therefore be reserved for patients who fail other therapeutic modalities. These theoretical complications have not been seen in studies. Women with inflammatory bowel disease who receive steroids with or without sulfasalazine display the same rate of maternal and perinatal complications as do women who receive no medication for their inflammatory bowel disease.[26]

The clinical course of regional enteritis is not affected by pregnancy. The recurrence rate and severity of disease are not changed by gestation. Patients may experience either an exacerbation or an improvement in the puerperium. There are no clear prognostic criteria for any individual patient.[8]

Crohn's disease that begins during gestation may increase perinatal mortality.[25] However, preexisting regional enteritis does not change perinatal morbidity or mortality.[27] In some patients with perirectal fistula, vaginal delivery may be difficult and/or result in further fistula formation. Proper evaluation of the perirectal extent of disease will help the physician to decide when abdominal delivery is indicated.

Ulcerative Colitis. The inflammatory process of ulcerative colitis is more superficial than that of regional enteritis. Superficial ulcers with only mucosal involvement are common. The rectum, sigmoid, and descending colon are the usual areas of involvement. Fibrosis, perforation, and toxic megacolon may develop. Patients with severe, long-standing disease have a higher risk of colonic carcinoma, which may be due to chronic colonic inflammation.

Prominent features in patients with ulcerative colitis include abdominal pain and cramps, diarrhea (usually bloody), tenesmus, fever, and weight loss. Physical exam may reveal left lower quadrant tenderness, but this finding often is not present. Sigmoidoscopy is very helpful in establishing a diagnosis. Superficial ulcerations, increased friability, and an inflammatory exudate are classic findings. Colonic biopsy confirms the diagnosis, but care must be exercised because perforation may occur. The biopsy should be taken low in the rectum to minimize the risk of perforation. In nonpregnant patients, a barium enema is useful to evaluate the extent of disease. Because of radiation risk to the fetus, fiberoptic colonoscopy is the diagnostic procedure of choice in pregnant women.

The treatment of ulcerative colitis is basically the same as that for regional enteritis. Antidiarrheal agents, steroids, and sulfasalazine in selected cases are the mainstays of therapy. Dehydration (from diarrhea), perforation, and toxic megacolon may occur in these patients and may be life threatening. Proctocolectomy may be necessary in severe disease, toxic megacolon, perforation, or stricture.

Patients with ulcerative colitis do not have higher rates of perinatal morbidity or mortality than does the overall population, so the effect of ulcerative colitis on pregnancy is limited.[36] The effect of pregnancy on ulcerative colitis, however, may not be as benign. Pregnancy may result in a recurrence in patients with inactive disease, especially in the first trimester or the immediate puerperium. However, the overall recurrence rate is probably no higher than in nonpregnant controls. The consensus holds that the course of ulcerative colitis is not altered by pregnancy.[8]

Gastrointestinal Bypass Surgery

The number of women who have undergone major abdominal surgery to correct massive obesity is small. Many of these women, however, are in the reproductive-age group and may become pregnant after the surgery.

In one procedure, the jejunoileal bypass, the jejunum is connected to the lower ileum so that the ingested food is exposed to only a fraction of the absorptive portion of the small intestine. The procedure results in decreased absorption of fats and carbohydrates, which leads to rapid weight loss. Unfortunately, this "relative malabsorption" also applies to needed nutrients and minerals, such as calcium, magnesium, and some vitamins. Complications of the procedure include electrolyte imbalance, diarrhea, and hepatic insufficiency. Jejunoileal bypass does not worsen maternal or perinatal outcome.[37] However, isolated patients demonstrate severe malabsorption and severe electrolyte imbalances. Therefore, patients who have had bypass surgery should be observed and managed as high risk in pregnancy.

The Acute Abdomen in Pregnancy

Besides the usual diseases that result in acute abdominal pain in the nonpregnant patient, certain complications of pregnancy present with acute abdominal pain. Both sets of diagnostic possibilities must be considered in a pregnant patient with acute abdominal pain. Some causes of the acute abdomen are summarized in Table 35-1. This chapter considers only problems arising from the gastrointestinal tract.

Appendicitis

Appendicitis, a common cause of an acute abdomen in gestation, occurs in 0.4–1.4 per 1000 pregnancies.[1] Unruptured appendicitis is associated with a maternal mortality of 0.1%. Maternal mortality rises to 4% with rupture.[10] Increased awareness and prompt treatment

TABLE 35-1. GASTROINTESTINAL CAUSES OF ACUTE ABDOMINAL PAIN IN PREGNANCY WITH TREATMENT OPTIONS

Immediate surgery
Appendicitis
Intestinal obstruction
Perforated viscus
Strangulated hernia
Volvulus
Possible surgery after evaluation or with complications
Cholecystitis
Diverticulitis
Gastrointestinal hemorrhage
Pancreatitis
Peptic ulcer disease
Medical therapy
Gastroenteritis
Regional enteritis
Ulcerative colitis

have reduced maternal mortality and morbidity. The fetus is not affected directly by appendicitis, but contiguous spread of inflammation or the development of peritonitis may result in uterine irritability, premature labor, and delivery. Such events, in preterm gestation, might result in fetal complications or perinatal death. Perinatal mortality in uncomplicated appendicitis is 8.5% but may be as high as 35–70% with peritonitis, gangrene, or perforation.[10]

The natural history of appendicitis varies, but, classically, the patient complains of periumbilical pain with radiation into the right lower quadrant, anorexia, nausea, vomiting, and constipation. On physical exam, the examiner notes low-grade fever, point tenderness in the right lower quadrant, and tenderness on rectal exam. Laboratory tests often reveal a moderate leukocytosis. During gestation, the clinical presentation is obscured because the physiologic changes of pregnancy alter the usual diagnostic criteria.

The abdominal pain of appendicitis has two components. The initial component, periumbilical pain, results from stretching and inflammation of the capsule of the appendix (visceral peritoneum). As the inflammation extends onto the parietal peritoneum, the pain radiates to the involved peritoneum—usually in the right lower quadrant. Therefore, the location of the radiated pain component, varies depending on the position of the appendix. In the pregnant patient, the position of the appendix varies throughout gestation. As the pregnant uterus enlarges, the intra-abdominal contents are displaced cephalad. The appendix rotates in an arc cephalad, laterally, and posteriorly so that by term the appendix is out of the right lower quadrant and in the area of the flank—above the level of the iliac crest in 93% of patients (Fig. 35-1) [2]

The location of the radiated pain may vary with the position of the appendix from the right lower quadrant to the flank. Near term, the radiation of pain and the point of maximum tenderness may be in the flank. Because of its posterior rotation, in some pregnant patients the appendix may not be near the parietal peritoneum. These patients may demonstrate neither radiation of pain nor a point of maximum tenderness.

Pregnancy alters other diagnostic criteria. Although anorexia is very common in nonpregnant patients with appendicitis, anorexia is infrequent in pregnant patients with appendicitis. Nausea, vomiting, and constipation—important symptoms in appendicitis—are normal complaints of pregnancy. A careful, detailed history must be obtained to separate the normal gastrointestinal symptomatology of pregnancy from that of appendicitis.

The normal elevation of the peripheral leukocyte count in pregnancy obscures the interpretation of this diagnostic test. In term pregnancy, normal peripheral leukocyte levels may rise to 16,000/mm^3. Labor is associated with higher values.[17] Therefore, care must be exercised to interpret this laboratory test correctly in the pregnant woman.

The differential diagnosis of appendicitis in pregnancy includes pyelonephritis, urolithiasis, and cholecystitis. In pyelonephritis, pain and tenderness occur in the flank and costovertebral angle. The bacteriuria and pyuria seen with pyelonephritis support the diagnosis, but an occasional patient may have pyuria secondary to an inflamed appendix close to the ureter. The level of fever may help differentiate appendicitis and pyelonephritis. Unless rupture and/or peritonitis have occurred, it is rare to see temperatures of 102°F or more in patients with appendicitis. Such temperatures are common with pyelonephritis.

Overt or microscopic hematuria in patients with urolithiasis differentiates this disease from appendicitis. The character and radiation of pain from renal stones is different from that of appendicitis. Patients with ureteral stones usually complain of pain in the flank with radiation into the groin. Paroxysms of pain often occur. When urolithiasis is suspected, a single film IVP may be indicated to document the diagnosis.

The treatment of appendicitis is surgical. The complications of appendicitis in the pregnant patient directly correlate with delays in diagnosis and therapy. Physicians should maintain a high index of suspicion and should resort to prompt surgical intervention to obtain optimal results. Fetal loss and maternal complications relate more to the severity of disease than to surgical intervention. Occasional negative findings at laparotomy should be expected. Because of the difficulty in diagnosis and the possibility that another condition is the source of the pain, laparotomies on pregnant women usually are done through vertical midline or right paramedian incisions. Uncomplicated appendicitis per se does not require antibiotics. A ruptured appendix or an appendiceal abscess mandates use of antibiotics effective against bowel flora. Cesarean section at laparotomy should be re-

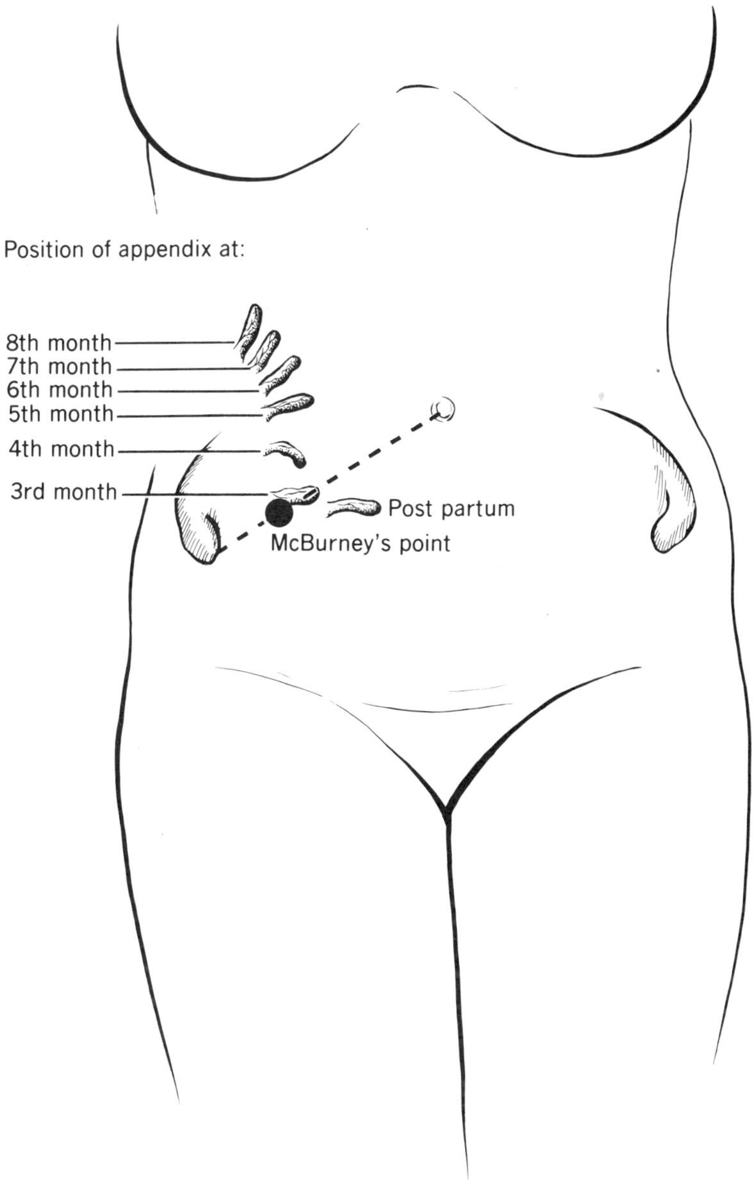

Figure 35-1. Changes in the position of the appendix in the pelvis and abdomen as pregnancy progresses.

served only for patients with a concurrent fetal or maternal indication.

Acute Cholecystitis

Cholecystitis, an inflammation of the gallbladder, usually is caused by a relative or complete obstruction of the cystic duct by gallstones. Ninety percent of patients with cholecystitis have demonstrable gallstones. Cholesterol is the common component of the stones in the Western hemisphere.[10] Women are at higher risk for development of cholesterol stones, and pregnancy appears to accelerate cholesterol stone growth. Three factors predispose to increased stone growth in pregnancy. Pregnancy progesterone levels appear to relax smooth muscle with a decrease in gallbladder tone and emptying. Resultant bile stasis predisposes to stone growth. Increased esterified and free blood cholesterol in pregnancy results in higher cholesterol saturation in the bile. Bile salts, substances important to the maintenance of cholesterol in solution, decrease in pregnancy. The combination of higher cholesterol levels coupled with diminished bile salts and increased bile stasis form an ideal environment for stone growth.

Signs and symptoms of acute cholecystitis are similar in the pregnant and nonpregnant state. The most common complaints are right upper quadrant or midepigastric pain. Pain may be colicky or constant. Radiation to the back or scapula is usual. The patient frequently reports a history of gallstones or prior episodes of cholecystitis. Nausea, vomiting, and anorexia are common, but these symptoms may be confused with the normal changes of pregnancy. Right upper quadrant tenderness is classic, but rebound tenderness usually is not seen unless perforation or abscess formation occurs. An enlarged, tender gallbladder rarely is found in pregnant patients. Leukocytosis may be present. Although the diagnosis can be confirmed with an oral cholecystogram or intravenous cholangiogram, these tests usually are not done in pregnancy to avoid radiation to the fetus. In the pregnant patient with suspected cholecystitis, diagnostic ultrasound of the gallbladder should be performed to document gallstones. Ultrasound is accurate in diagnosis of stones as much as 96% of the time.[16]

The differential diagnosis of cholecystitis includes: acute hepatitis, appendicitis, perforated duodenal ulcer, acute pancreatitis, and acute pyelonephritis.

Treatment of the pregnant patient with cholecystitis differs little from management of the nonpregnant patient. Initial therapy attempts to decrease gastrointestinal contents by utilizing nasogastric suction and ceasing oral intake. Fluid balance is maintained with intravenous crystalloids and colloids, as necessary. Narcotics are often necessary for pain relief. If the patient does not respond or develops sepsis, antibiotics should be added. In occasional patients who do not respond to conservative measures, cholecystectomy is indicated. Less than 3% of pregnant women with cholecystitis require surgery during an acute episode. After delivery, elective surgery may be indicated.

Pancreatitis

Pancreatitis occurs in 0.01–0.1% of pregnant women. Early studies of pancreatitis in pregnancy reported high maternal mortality; however, a recent review notes a good prognosis for mother and fetus with prompt diagnosis and treatment.[9]

An insult to the pancreas initiates a cycle of events that results in pancreatitis. The insult results in the release of proteolytic enzymes, normally contained in granules, into the pancreatic parenchyma. These enzymes digest the pancreatic cells with further enzyme release. To ameliorate the disease, this cycle of progressive tissue destruction must be stopped.

In nonpregnant patients, common initiating insults are chronic alcoholism, gallstones, or trauma. Most pregnant patients do not identify a clear predisposing insult. Other causes of pancreatitis in pregnancy include gallstones, infection, and toxemia.

Pregnancy does not alter the clinical presentation of pancreatitis. The most common complaints are epigastric pain that radiates to the back, nausea, and vomiting. Physical examination reveals epigastric tenderness and occasionally fever. Rebound tenderness may be present in advanced disease. Because the presenting signs and symptoms are nonspecific, laboratory tests are utilized to confirm the diagnosis.

The serum amylase test is commonly utilized for diagnosis of pancreatitis. This test may be difficult to interpret. Other conditions such as intestinal obstruction, liver trauma, common duct stones, and peptic ulcer disease, can elevate the serum amylase. Furthermore, normal pregnancy may increase, decrease, or not alter the concentrations of amylase.[10] Use of serum amylase alone may result in false negative interpretations. Peak levels of serum amylase occur 6–12 hours after the onset of pancreatitis, and often return to normal by 24–72 hours. If the patient is late in seeking medical care or if blood collection is delayed, the test may yield a false-negative result.

The ratio of amylase clearance to creatinine clearance percent (Cam/Ccr %) is a more useful test for pancreatitis. The Cam/Ccr is elevated in pancreatitis and remains elevated for up to 7 days after the onset of symptoms. Ninety-four percent of nonpregnant patients with pancreatitis display elevated Cam/Ccr, whereas only 58% demonstrate elevated serum amylases.[28] In nonpregnant patients without pancreatitis, the Cam/Ccr is normally below 4%, whereas nonpregnant patients with pancreatitis have ratios from 6–15%. Care must be exercised in interpreting this test in pregnancy because of the normal increase in creatinine clearance. The increased creatinine clearance results in lower normal values for the ratio in pregnant women. Normal pregnant women between 12 and 28 weeks have Cam/Ccr ratios between 2 and 3. After 28 weeks, the ratio normally rises to 3–4.[11] The ratio that indicates pancreatitis may therefore be lower in pregnant than nonpregnant patients. If positive, the Cam/Ccr is useful in pregnancy; negative results may not exclude pancreatitis.

Management of pancreatitis consists of elimination of oral intake, nasogastric suction, pain relief, and crystalloids and colloids to maintain intravascular volume. The disease is self-limiting. Ninety percent of patients respond to conservative management within 3–5 days. In severe cases, a peritoneal, toxic, pancreatic exudate that requires surgical removal may develop. Drainage improves the prognosis in severely ill patients.

Serum calcium levels are a useful prognostic tool, but levels normally may be decreased in pregnancy. A poor prognosis may be expected if severe hypocalcemia (less than 7 mg%) is present.[9]

JAUNDICE IN PREGNANCY

Jaundice is seen in 1 of every 1500 gestations. This rate varies with the patient population, and there are rates reported as high as 2%. The most common causes of jaundice in pregnancy are viral hepatitis (40% of cases), cholestasis of pregnancy (20%), and other pregnancy complications (10%).[19]

The Liver in Pregnancy

The liver is a major metabolic organ of the body. Pregnancy alters this organ's activity. In pregnancy, the synthesis, catabolism, and therefore concentrations of circulating proteins produced by the liver are altered. Exogenous estrogen administration mimics some of these changes. The elevated estrogens of pregnancy are thought responsible for many of the alterations. Specific changes include a lowered serum albumin that results mainly from dilution by the increased blood volume. Albumin breakdown is more rapid in pregnancy, but there is a compensatory increase in synthesis. Several other carrier proteins such as ceruloplasmin and transferrin are elevated in a late pregnancy.

Important changes occur in the coagulation proteins (see Chapter 30).

Some of the tests of liver function are elevated in pregnancy. Because the placenta produces an alkaline phosphatase, the levels of this enzyme commonly are elevated in gestation. Near term, 42% of patients have an elevated alkaline phosphatase.[24] Differential tests may be performed to separate placental (heat stable) from liver (heat labile) alkaline phosphatase, but with the availability of other liver tests that remain unchanged in pregnancy, separation of alkaline phosphatase activity is hardly ever necessary. The serum glutamic oxaloacetic transaminase (SGOT) and serum glutamic pyruric transaminase (SGPT) do not vary over gestation and are useful tests of liver function in pregnancy. Gamma-glutamyl transpeptidase (GGT) and lactic dehydrogenase usually rise in late pregnancy and may not be useful.[14]

Bilirubin levels are not altered in normal pregnancy. Bilirubin deposition in the skin and/or sclera results in a yellow pigmentation called jaundice. Individual variations exist, but when serum bilirubin exceeds 2.0–2.5 mg per 100 ml, jaundice is apparent. Catabolism of hemoglobin in senescent red blood cells accounts for 80–85% of bilirubin.

After it is released from red blood cells, bilirubin becomes tightly bound to albumin and is transported to the liver. Hepatic uptake occurs and the unconjugated bilirubin (water insoluble) is rendered water soluble by conjugation with a glucuronide. The conjugated bilirubin then is excreted into bile. Once in the intestine, some of the conjugated bilirubin is metabolized to urobilinogen, which may be reabsorbed by the gut. The remainder of the urobilinogen and the conjugated bilirubin are expelled in the feces. Normally, the urine does not contain bilirubin, but with an elevated serum bilirubin, conjugated bilirubin may be filtered by the renal glomeruli and excreted in the urine. Unconjugated bilirubin is not excreted in urine.

In the pregnant woman, unconjugated bilirubin may cross the placenta. Elevated levels of unconjugated bilirubin have been reported in the newborn of a mother with end-stage hepatic cirrhosis, but large studies have not been reported.[35]

Causes of Jaundice in Pregnancy

Viral hepatitis is the most frequent cause of jaundice in pregnancy. There are three distinct types of viral hepatitis—hepatitis A, B, and non-A, non-B.

Viral hepatitis A commonly occurs in lower socioeconomic populations and in underdeveloped countries. Poor hygiene may predispose to this disease which usually is transmitted by the fecal–oral route. During the prodromal phase and early in the course of the disease, patients with hepatitis A are infectious. The duration of infectivity and the viremia is short. The clinical presentation includes fatigue, nausea, and anorexia. Myalgias, pruritus, and fever are uncommon. Jaundice is usually mild and may not be recognized easily. Symptoms usually last for 10–15 days. During this time, the SGOT and SGPT are elevated. Levels of 1000–2000 are usual. Viral hepatitis A is confirmed with the finding of hepatitis A antibody (HAB). Treatment is symptomatic and includes proper diet and oral–fecal isolation. During the viremia, the blood is also infectious. Patients with severe anorexia or vomiting may require hospitalization for fluid and electrolyte therapy. Immune serum globulin administration to close household contacts may be useful to prevent spread. The disease is self-limiting, and the chronic or carrier state is rare. Pregnancy does not alter the course of the disease nor does the disease alter pregnancy. Transmission of the virus to the fetus is rare and may occur only when the mother has the disease near delivery.

Clinically, hepatitis B is similar to hepatitis A. Hepatitis B, however, is more serious because chronic disease, carrier state, and transmission to the neonate may occur. Transmission is by contact with infected blood although other body fluids such as semen, vaginal secretions, and saliva have been implicated in transmission. The highest rates of infection are reported in drug abusers, homosexuals, health care personnel, and patients treated with blood products (hemophiliacs). The clinical presentation consists of nausea, vomiting, anorexia, and jaundice. In some patients, right upper quadrant pain, arthralgias, and skin rashes may occur. The SGOT and SGPT usually are elevated. Various antibody and antigen markers are useful in this disease. The hepatitis B surface antigen (HBsAg), thought to be viral coat material, commonly is found in the serum of patients 10–14 days prior to onset and during the clinical disease. The "e" antigen (HBeAg), which is related closely to the intact viral particle, usually is seen early in the disease and is a good indirect measure of the infectious state of the patient. Except in chronic carriers of hepatitis B, the "e" antigen disappears as clinical symptomatology improves (6–8 weeks). Antibodies to core (HBcAb) antigen appear during clinical disease and persist for years. Antibodies to surface antigens (HBsAb) also persist for years but do not become elevated until after recovery from the acute illness.

Treatment of hepatitis B consists of nutrition, antiemetics, and maintenance of fluid and electrolyte balance. Isolation precautions must be exercised with body fluids, especially blood.

Maternal complications from hepatitis B are infrequent. The mortality rate in developed countries is not increased compared to nonpregnant women. In undeveloped countries with malnourished populations, the rate of fulminant hepatitis in gestation with resultant mortality is increased and may reach 40%.[20]

Neonatal transmission of hepatitis B is a significant problem. In hyperendemic areas, like the Far East, perinatal transmission is a major cause of persistent hepatitis B infection. In the United States, certain ethnic groups are at high risk for perinatal transmission, and other women are at high risk for transmission because of occupation; therefore, the Committee on Infectious Diseases of the American Academy of Pediatrics has recommended screening for hepatitis in certain population groups. Table 35-2

TABLE 35-2. WOMEN WHO SHOULD BE SCREENED FOR HEPATITIS B IN PREGNANCY[7]

I. *Ethnic groups at risk*
   - Asian
   - Pacific Islander
   - Alaskan Eskimo

II. *Birthplace exposure*
   - Haiti
   - Sub-Saharan Africa

III. *Occupational risk*
   - Hemodialysis worker
   - Worker in institutions for the mentally retarded
   - Worker with frequent exposure to blood products

IV. *Socio-medical risk*
   - Hemodialysis patient
   - Household or sexual contact with a hemodialysis patient
   - Persons rejected as blood donors
   - Persons who have received multiple transfusions
   - Household contact with a hepatitis B carrier
   - History of multiple episodes of venereal disease
   - History of intravenous use of illicit drugs

lists these high-risk groups. Screening should utilize the tests for HBsAg and HBeAg.[7] If a pregnant patient has an acute episode of hepatitis B in the first or second trimester, the risk of transmission to the newborn is 10%. If the acute disease occurs in the third trimester, the risk of transmission is about 65%.[14] In women who are chronic carriers, the HBeAg test predicts the risk of neonatal transmission. HBeAg positive mothers have a 75–95% transmission rate to the newborn as compared to less than 5% for HbeAg negative women.[31] Neonatal disease usually occurs 40–100 days after birth. The most common method of transmission appears to be from blood or vaginal secretions at birth. Transplacental transmission rarely occurs. Hyperimmune serum (HBIG) may prevent or modify neonatal disease and should be administered to neonates at high risk.

Little is known about non-A, non-B hepatitis in the nonpregnant or pregnant patient. The clinical presentation is similar to hepatitis B, but there are no antigenic or antibody markers to identify this disease. The incubation period is long. The mode of transmission is by the parenteral and sexual routes. The majority of patients with post-transfusion hepatitis have non-A, non-B disease.

Cholestasis of Pregnancy

The second most frequent cause of jaundice in pregnancy is cholestasis of pregnancy. Cholestasis of pregnancy occurs in 0.01–0.05% of gestations. The frequency varies by population. In Chile and Scandinavia, rates as high as 2.4% are reported.[30] Because of the higher rates in certain populations and the common finding of affected relatives in women with this disease, a hereditary predisposition has been suggested. The disease often recurs with subsequent pregnancies. Estrogen may play a role in the disease, since many of the patients who have cholestasis of pregnancy develop similar symptoms when taking oral contraceptives containing estrogens.

Pruritus is the predominant symptom of cholestasis of pregnancy. The majority, but not all women, with the disease have mild jaundice. Pruritus and jaundice may start at any time in gestation and quickly disappear after delivery. Characteristically, the patient does not have other symptoms. Liver function tests are mildly elevated with SGOT and SGPT levels below 250. Some patients have a prolonged prothrombin time due to a decrease in vitamin K-dependent coagulation factors. Serum bile acids usually are elevated. Serum bilirubin is elevated, usually to less than 5 mg/100 ml. A rare case has a bilirubin above 10 mg/100 ml. Like the clinical symptoms, laboratory tests return to normal shortly after delivery.

Cholestasis of pregnancy has little permanent effect on the mother. Maternal outcome is not altered by the disease. Perinatal outcome is worsened significantly by cholestasis of pregnancy, due to premature deliveries which occur in 30–60% of patients.[20]

Treatment attempts to relieve pruritus by decreasing skin and serum bile acid levels.[21] Cholestyramine, 12–18 grams/day, is administered. With relief, the dose is lowered to 6–9 grams/day. Patients who receive cholestyramine should also be given parenteral vitamin K supplementation, because this exchange resin interferes with vitamin K absorption.

No permanent liver damage occurs. Histologic liver changes are minimal at the height of the illness. Reported changes include dilated centrilobular canaliculi with bile plugs and occasional macrophages with granules. The portal areas are normal and no hepatocellular damage is present.

Acute Fatty Liver of Pregnancy

Acute fatty liver of pregnancy, an extremely rare but commonly fatal disease, is characterized by a marked fatty infiltration and vacuolization of hepatocytes. The patient usually presents in the third trimester with vomiting, abdominal pain, and jaundice. Tachycardia commonly is seen, as are signs and symptoms of preeclampsia. Laboratory tests reveal severe hypoglycemia, elevated bilirubin (usually 10 mg/100 ml), and slightly elevated SGOT and SGPT. A prolonged prothrombin time and an elevated white count are usual. Shock, acidosis, and renal failure may follow. Multiorgan disease occurs because of vacuolization of cells in the kidney, pancreas, and central nervous system.

Ten percent to 35% of patients survive with vigorous management, but optimal therapy is not established.[14] Therapy is aimed at symptomatic treatment of hepatic and renal failure. Treatment of hypoglycemia, hypertension, electrolyte imbalances, and clotting abnormalities plus airway maintenance are important. Delivery immediately after stabilization may be helpful.

Excessive doses of tetracycline administered to pregnant women may result in a clinical and histologic picture similar to acute fatty liver of pregnancy. Tetracycline-induced disease rarely should be seen since tetracycline is contraindicated in pregnancy because of its fetal effects.

Jaundice may occur in pregnant women for other reasons, such as common duct stones, drug ingestion, hemolytic disorders, and sepsis. These are rare and require treatment of the instigating event.

REFERENCES

1. Babaknia, A., Parsa, H., and Woodruff, J. D.: Appendicitis during pregnancy. *Obstet. Gynecol.* **50**:40–44, 1977.
2. Baer, J. L., Reis, R. A., and Arens, R. A.: Appendicitis in pregnancy with changes in position and axis of the normal appendix in pregnancy. *JAMA* **98**:1359–1364, 1932.
3. Bassey, O. O.: Pregnancy heartburn in Nigerians and Caucasians with theories about aetiology based on manometric recordings from the aesophagus and stomach. *Br. J. Obstet. Gynaecol.* **84**:439–443, 1977.
4. Behar, J., Brand, D. L., Brown, F. C., Castell, D. O., Cohen S., Crossley R. J., Pope C. E., II, and Winans, C. S.: Cimetidine in the treatment of symptomatic gastroesophageal reflux. A double blind controlled trial. *Gastroenterology* **74**: 441–448, 1978.
5. Clark, D. H.: Peptic ulcer in women. *Br. Med. J.* **1**:1254–1257, 1953.
6. Clark, D. H. and Tankel, H. I.: Gastric acid and plasma histaminase during pregnancy. *Lancet* **2**:886–887, 1954.
7. Committee on Infectious Diseases, American Academy of Pediatrics: Prevention of hepatitis B virus infections. *Pediatrics* **75**:362–364, 1985.
8. Conover, W. B. and Key, T. C.: Maternal gastrointestinal diseases in pregnancy. In: *Maternal-Fetal Medicine: Principles and Practice*, R. K. Creasy and R. Resnik (Eds.). Philadelphia, W. B. Saunders, 1984, pp. 951–992.
9. Corlett, R. C., Jr. and Mishell, D. R., Jr.: Pancreatitis in pregnancy. *Am. J. Obstet. Gynecol.* **113**:281–290, 1972.
10. DeVore, G. R.: Acute abdominal pain in the pregnant patient due to pancreatitis, acute appendicitis, cholecystitis, or peptic ulcer disease. *Clin. Perinatol.* **7**:349–369, 1980.
11. DeVore, G. R., Bracken, M., and Berkowitz, R. L.: The amylase/creatinine clearance ratio in normal pregnancy and pregnancies complicated by pancreatitis, hyperemesis gravidarum, and toxemia. *Am. J. Obstet. Gynecol.* **136**:747–754, 1980.
12. Dobbins, J. W. and Spiro, H. M.: Gastrointestinal complications. In: *Medical Complications During Pregnancy*. G. N. Burrow and T. F. Ferris (Eds.). Philadelphia, W. B. Saunders, 1982, pp. 259–277.
13. Fairweather, D. V. I.: Nausea and vomiting in pregnancy. *Am. J. Obstet. Gynecol.* **102**:135–175, 1968.
14. Fallon H. J.: Liver diseases. In: *Medical Complications During Pregnancy*. G. N. Burrow and T. F. Ferris (Eds.). Philadelphia, W. B. Saunders, 1982, pp. 278–301.
15. Feldman, M.: Nausea and vomiting. In: *Gastrointestinal Disease: Pathophysiology, Diagnosis, Management*. M. H. Sleisenger and J. S. Fordtran (Eds.). Philadelphia, W. B. Saunders, 1983, pp. 160–176.
16. Ferrucci, J. T., Jr.: Body ultrasonography. Part II. *N. Engl. J. Med.* **300**:590–602, 1979.
17. Hytten, F. E. and Lind, T.: *Diagnostic Indices in Pregnancy*. Basel, CIBA-GEIGY, 1973.
18. Jick, H., Holmes, L. B., Hunter, J. R., Madsen, S., and Stergachis, A.: Drug use and congenital disorders. *JAMA* **246**:343–346, 1981.
19. Krejs, G. J.: Jaundice during pregnancy. *Semin. Liver Dis.* **3**:73–82, 1983.
20. Krejs, G. J. and Haemmerli, U. P.: Jaundice during pregnancy. In: *Diseases of the Liver*, 5th Edition. L. Schiff and E. R. Schiff (Eds.). Philadelphia, J. B. Lippincott, 1982, pp. 1561–1580.
21. Laatikainen, T.: Effect of cholestyramine and phenobarbital on pruritus and serum bile acid levels in cholestasis of pregnancy. *Am. J. Obstet. Gynecol.* **132**:501–506, 1978.
22. Lennard-Jones, J. E. and Powell-Tuck, J.: Drug treatment of inflammatory bowel disease. *Clin. Gastroenterol.* **8**:187–271, 1979.
23. McGowan, W. A.: Safety of cimetidine in obstetric patients. *J. R. Soc. Med.* **72**:902–907, 1979.
24. McNair, R. D. and Jaynes, R. V.: Alterations in liver function during normal pregnancy. *Am. J. Obstet. Gynecol.* **80**:500–505, 1960.
25. Martinbeau, P. W., Welch, J. S., and Weiland, L. H.: Crohn's disease and pregnancy. *Am. J. Obstet. Gynecol.* **122**:746–749, 1975.
26. Mogadam, M. Dobbins, W. O., III, Korelitz, B. I., and Ahmed, S. W.: Pregnancy in inflammatory bowel disease: Effect of sulfasalazine and corticosteroids on fetal outcome. *Gastroenterology* **80**:72–76, 1981.
27. Mogadam, M., Dobbins, W. O., III, and Korelitz, B.I.: The safety of corticosteroids and sulfasalazine in pregnancy associated with inflammatory bowel disease. (Abstract) *Gastroenterology* **78**:1224, 1980.
28. Murray, W. R. and Mackay, C.: The amylase creatinine clearance ratio in acute pancreatitis. *Br. J. Surg.* **64**:189–191, 1977.
29. Peterson, W. L., Sturdevant, R. A. L., Frankl, H., Richardson, C. T., Isenberg, J. I., Elashoff, J. D., Sones, J. Q., Gross, R. A., McCallum, R. W., and Fordtran, J. S.: Healing of duodenal ulcer with antacid regimen. *N. Engl. J. Med.* **297**:341–345, 1977.
30. Reyes, H.: The enigma of intrahepatic cholestasis

of pregnancy: Lessons from Chile. *Hepatology* **2**:87–96, 1982.

31. Stevens, C. E., Neurath, R. A., Beasley, R. P., and Szmuness, W.: HBeAg and anti-HBe detection by radioimmunoassay: Correlation with vertical transmission of hepatitis B virus in Taiwan. *J. Med. Virol.* **3**:237–241, 1979.
32. Summers, R. W., Sessions, J. T., Switz, D. M., and Singleton, J. W.: National Cooperative Crohn's disease study (NCCDS): Response of subgroups to drug treatment. (Abstract) *Gastroenterology* **74**:1100, 1978.
33. VanThiel, D. H., Gavaler, J. S. Joshi, S., Sara, R. K., and Stremple, J.: Heartburn of pregnancy. *Gastroenterology* **72**:666–668, 1977.
34. VanThiel, D. H., Gavaler, J. S., and Stremple, J.: Lower esophageal sphincter pressure in women using sequential oral contraceptives. *Gastroenterology* **71**:232–234, 1976.
35. Waffarn, F., Carlisle S., Pena, I., Hodgman, J. E., and Bonham, D.: Fetal exposure to maternal hyperbilirubinemia. *Am. J. Dis. Child.* **136**:416–417, 1982.
36. Willoughby, C. P. and Truelove, S. C.: Ulcerative colitis and pregnancy. *Gut* **21**:469–474, 1980.
37. Woods, J. R., Jr. and Brinkman, C. R.: The jejunoileal bypass and pregnancy. *Obstet. Gynecol. Surv.* **33**:697–705, 1978.

36

THYROID DISEASE IN PREGNANCY

Pregnancy mimics many aspects of clinical thyroid disease. Changes in thyroid function during pregnancy include goiter, increased total serum concentrations of thyroxine, increased thyronine binding globulins (TBG), decreased T_3 resin uptake, increased basal metabolic rate, but with normal serum concentrations of free thyroxine as indicated by either a normal free thyroxine index or free thyroxine by equilibrium dialysis. These changes are part of the normal physiology of pregnancy and reflect increased cardiac work, fetal oxygen consumption, and the effects of estrogen on hepatic protein synthesis.[23]

THYROID FUNCTION TESTS

Maternal Compartment

Circulating thyroxine is 99.97% bound to plasma proteins. The bound fraction is inactive. The free thyroxine fraction (0.03%) is biologically active. In pregnancy, circulating total thyroxine concentration is increased by thyronine binding globulins which are found in concentrations approximately twice those of the nonpregnant state. Other thyroid binding proteins, thyronine binding prealbumin and albumin, may be decreased slightly in concentration. Serum triiodothyronine (T_3) is 99.95% bound to plasma proteins. The total serum T_3 level also is increased in pregnancy. Free levels of both thyroxine and triiodothyronine are within the normal range. In the nonpregnant state, all aspects of thyroidal activity are regulated by thyroid stimulating hormone (TSH), a glycoprotein hormone with a molecular weight of about 28,000 daltons. TSH, like other anterior pituitary hormones, is composed of separate alpha and beta subunits. LH, FSH, hCG, and TSH all share identical alpha subunits. The beta subunits confer biologic and immunologic characteristics specific to each hormone. In pregnancy, hCG has a thyrotrophic effect that may partially replace that of TSH during the first trimester,[21] the period in which hCG is at its greatest concentration. However, an overall reciprocal relationship of TSH and hCG is not seen throughout pregnancy.[6]

The pituitary gland increases in size during pregnancy. This has been attributed to an increase in the number of lactotroph cells during the second and third trimesters. Serum prolactin concentrations increase throughout pregnancy in response to increasing serum concentrations of estrogen. Pituitary responsiveness to thyrotropin releasing hormones (TRH) has been studied serially throughout pregnancy and in the puerperium.[47] Serum prolactin levels increase consistently throughout pregnancy. The prolactin and the TSH response to TRH stimulation are similar in each trimester of pregnancy, but the response during pregnancy is relatively smaller than is the nonpregnant response. There does not appear to be an increase in secretory reserve of the pituitary with increasing gestational age.

In vitro studies indicate that the placenta and chorion possess monodeiodinase activity. The T_4 to T_3 pathway is more active than is the T_4 to reverse T_3 pathway. These observations are consistent with the low T_4:T_3 ratio noted in the last trimester as compared with the first few postpartum days.[4]

Total and free T_3 increase in maternal sera during active labor. TRH administered to the mother during active labor results in a brisk TSH release by the fetus, but a blunted fetal prolactin release. Overall response of the maternal pituitary to TRH as measured by release of TSH and prolactin is significantly lower during labor than in the first three trimesters of pregnancy or in nonpregnant women, suggesting that the changes in free T_3 concentrations present at term may inhibit pituitary responsiveness significantly.[34]

Fetal Compartment

In the fetus, the hypothalamic–pituitary–thyroidal axis develops independently, beginning at about the fourth week and continuing in phases throughout pregnancy.[18,19] Thyroid hormones, T_4, T_3, reverse T_3, and TSH, do not cross the placental barrier in significant concentrations. Significant amounts of TRH may cross the placenta; however, there is no evidence that maternal TRH has a significant regulatory influence on the fetal pituitary–thyroidal axis. Embryogenesis of the thyroid occurs during the first trimester with hypothalamic maturation extending from the first to the third trimester.

Maturation of the fetal thyroid system function occurs from about midgestation to term, with full maturation of the thyroid system completed at about four weeks postpartum (Table 36-1). Concentrations of thyroxine and free thyroxine increase in fetal blood throughout the third trimester. Serum T_3 is unmeasurable until approximately 30 weeks' gestation, increasing to a concentration of 50 ng/dl at term. A sharp rise (three to six times the antepartum concentration) in serum T_3 occurs in the immediate neonatal period and has been called the physiologic thyrotoxicosis of the newborn. Conversely, re-

TABLE 36-1. RELATION OF THYROID-SYSTEM ONTOGENESIS AND THYROID DYSFUNCTION IN THE NEONATE

Phases and Events of Thyroid Ontogenesis	*Clinical Disorders of Thyroid Function*
Phase 1: Embryogenesis	
Anatomic and biochemical development of the thyroid gland	Thyroid dysgenesis Agenesis, hypoplasia, or ectopy Dyshormonogenesis Defective TSH responsiveness
Anatomic and biochemical development of the pituitary gland	Pituitary aplasia or hypoplasia TSH deficiency
Phase II: Hypothalamic Maturation	
Biochemical and anatomic development of the hypothalamus	Hypothalamic dysplasia TRH deficiency
Phase III: Maturation of Thyroid-system Function	
Hypothalamic-pituitary function	
Iodothyronine feedback control of TRH and pituitary TSH secretion	Transient hypothyroxinemia
Thyroid-gland function	
TSH control of thyroid function	Transient hyperthyrotropinemia
Thyroid autonomy	Transient hypothyroidism Iodine deficiency Iodine excess Antithyroid compounds
Peripheral T_4 metabolism	Hypotriiodothyroxinemia TBG abnormalities
Iodothyronine receptors and tissue responsiveness	Peripheral thyroid-hormone unresponsiveness

verse T_3 concentrations are elevated slightly during the last trimester, declining sharply as term is approached.

Measurable thyroid hormone concentrations in amniotic fluid have been reported since 1963, with continued debate regarding the significance and interpretability of amniotic fluid thyroid hormone concentrations. There is no significant correlation between amniotic fluid thyroid hormone concentrations and either maternal or cord serum hormones, neonatal serum hormone concentrations, or the clinical status of the neonate.[22] Amniotic fluid TSH and T_4 levels can be elevated significantly in pregnancies complicated by anencephaly in which no pituitary tissue is identifiable in the fetus.

Cord serum TSH and thyroglobin levels in newborns decline with increasing birth weight. Term newborn infants have cord serum thyroglobulin concentrations significantly lower than those in infants born prematurely, but greater than the levels seen in adults or pregnant women at delivery.[37]

Dexamethasone produces a reduction in plasma TSH levels and a reduced response of the pituitary to TRH. Dexamethasone also decreases serum concentrations of T_4 and T_3 with a concomitant increase in serum reverse T_3 in the nonpregnant state. The effects of dexamethasone on fetal and maternal T_4, T_3, reverse T_3, and TSH levels were studied in pregnant women receiving dexamethasone to enhance fetal lung maturation.[36] Thyroid hormone concentrations in maternal and umbilical plasma were compared at term. T_4 and TSH did not vary significantly between groups, but T_3 and reverse T_3 were both markedly higher in cord blood, suggesting that dexamethasone induced increased fetal thyroid T_3 secretion. The increase in T_3 in umbilical blood following dexamethasone is the opposite of that recorded in nonpregnant adults in whom dexamethasone induces a fall in serum T_3 concentrations.

GOITER

Goiter, an enlargement of the thyroid gland, has the same etiology in pregnancy as in the nonpregnant state, with the exception that pregnancy itself is associated with a slight increase in thyroid size. The etiology of the physiologic goiter of pregnancy is unknown but may reflect the thyrotropic effects of hCG, the fall in free T_4 that accompanies the estrogen-mediated increase in thyronine-binding globulin, or increased renal clearance of iodide that occurs in the first trimester.[23] The thyroid gland is normally 20–30 grams in size, with a soft texture and a smooth surface. The goiter that accompanies Graves' disease has similar characteristics but may be two to three times normal size. The size of the goiter is greater in younger women with Graves' disease. The prevalence of simple goiter, multinodular goiter, and Hashimoto's thyroiditis in pregnancy is not different from that in the nonpregnant state. The goiter associated with suppurative thyroiditis rarely is seen in the modern antibiotic era.

Riedel's struma is a rare condition that is associated with a hard, diffusely irregular goiter. Painless thyroiditis and painful thyroiditis may be seen in pregnancy. Thyroid malignancy is an uncommon cause of goiter in pregnancy because of the age and sex distribution of thyroid malignancy. However, with the advent of fine-needle aspiration biopsy of thyroid nodules, the diagnosis of thyroid malignancy will be made more commonly during pregnancy than it has been in the past. The overwhelming majority of goiters that occur in pregnancy are of benign origin, either from autoimmune thyroid disease such as Hashimoto's thyroiditis or from single or multiple benign nodules.

Iodine deficiency goiter has been much studied in this century, but cases are now present only in isolated areas in the world.[32,41] Iodine excess is now a problem in the United States and may be responsible for the increasing prevalence of thyroid cancer. Iodine may precipitate hypo- or hyperthyroidism in patients with subclinical autoimmune thyroid disease.

HYPOTHYROIDISM

Maternal Compartment

Hypothyroidism is defined as an absence of or a decrease in functioning thyroid tissue. Hashimoto's thyroiditis is the most common cause of hypothyroidism in the pregnancy-age group. This diagnosis may be suspected by the appearance of a firm goiter of about twice normal size with an irregular, bosselated surface. A pyramidal lobe may be present. The diagnosis of Hashimoto's thyroiditis is established by a positive antithyroid antibody titer greater than 1:5,000 for antithyroglobin or antimicrosomal antibodies. Other common causes of hypothyroidism in pregnancy include end-stage Graves' disease following ablative therapy with ^{131}I or surgery, or end stage disease following medical therapy in the Graves' patient. Less commonly, a nontoxic multinodular goiter may produce hypothyroidism. Hypothyroidism is rarely secondary to metastatic cancer, tuberculosis, amyloid, sarcoid, or other infiltrative processes. A decrease in thyroid function may occur in women receiving antithyroid drugs, such as methimazole or propylthiouracil, or in patients who have partial defects in thyroid hormone synthesis, such as Pendred's syndrome or other defects in the thyroid hormone synthetic pathway.[38]

Hypothyroidism due to pituitary insufficiency, "secondary hypothyroidism," or hypothalamic dysfunction, "tertiary hypothyroidism," may occur. These disorders usually are associated with tumors of the hypothalamic pituitary axis or other infiltrative central nervous system disorders. Rarely, patients with monotrophic TSH deficiency are described. Finally, a syndrome of peripheral resistance to thyroid hormones has been described, the Refetoff–DeGroot syndrome, in which thyroid hormone concentrations in the plasma are normal or elevated, but clinical features of hypothyroidism are present.

The usual clinical features of hypothyroidism may be masked by the increased metabolic rate attendant to pregnancy. The abnormalities of the central nervous system, including hearing loss, increased sensitivity to cold, increased somnolence, and decreased mentation, may be less well expressed in the pregnant woman than in the nonpregnant woman. Other features of hypothyroidism, including constipation, decreased appetite, and hypoglycemia, are also features of normal pregnancy. Muscle manifestations of hypothyroidism, such as weakness, muscle cramps, and hypotonia, may be construed to be part of normal pregnancy. The periorbital puffiness and other skin changes also may be confused with the physiologic state of pregnancy.

The anticipated clinical findings of hypothyroidism may be either diminished or exacerbated by the pregnancy state. The cutaneous manifestations of hypothyroidism, such as cold intolerance, thickening of the skin, edema of the extremities and face, malar flush, pallor, alopecia, and yellowish discoloration of the skin, may be more marked in the pregnant than in the nonpregnant state. Cardiovascular findings associated with hypothyroidism in pregnancy include bradycardia, low voltage electrocardiogram, cardiomegaly, and slight pericardial effusion. ENT findings such as hoarseness, chronic nasal discharge, and hearing loss may be anticipated. The gastrointestinal manifestations of hypothyroidism such as enlargement of the tongue, mucosal atrophy, slight ascites, and constipation may be enhanced in the pregnant state.

Neuromuscular abnormalities such as carpal tunnel syndrome, which occurs spontaneously in the euthyroid pregnant woman, may be anticipated. There may be slowness of speech and the recovery phase of the deep tendon reflex may be delayed. The normochromic normocytic anemia of hypothyroidism may be expressed more commonly in the pregnant woman. Patients with one form of autoimmune disease, such as Hashimoto's thyroiditis, should be suspected of having other components such as diabetes mellitus and Addison's disease or Schmidt's syndrome.[15] When thyroid replacement is begun, the need for steroid replacement should be anticipated. None of the aforementioned findings is noted invariably in the pregnant woman with hypothyroidism, although the presence of any one abnormality should suggest hypothyroidism and the diagnosis should be pursued.

The question of fertility in the hypothyroid woman has been examined. The data are inconclusive, although there has been speculation that both libido and fertility are diminished. Pregnancy in the hypothyroid woman has been carried successfully to term. Maternal hypothyroidism may improve during the last trimester due to placental transfer of fetal thyroid hormone.[25] It is unclear whether there is an increased risk of fetal hypothyroidism in children born to hypothyroxinemic mothers, but the available data suggest that babies born to hypothyroid mothers are normal at one year postpartum.

Laboratory test abnormalities in hypothyroid pregnancy should include, in all patients, a low T_4 level, with the exception of the rare patient with Refetoff–DeGroot syndrome. The T_3 level may be normal or low and the TSH determination may be low, normal, or high, depending on whether the hypothyroidism is of primary thyroidal origin or of hypothalamic or pituitary origin, T_3 resin uptake generally will be diminished. Other laboratory abnormalities may include elevated serum cholesterol. The erythrocyte sedimentation rate will be elevated, reflecting both pregnancy and hypothyroidism. Most patients will have a relative anemia; antithyroid antibodies may or may not be present. The electrocardiogram may show low voltage.

The treatment of hypothyroidism in pregnancy requires thyroid hormone replacement in all patients (Table 36-2). This is given as levothyroxine in a dose calculated to raise the total T_4 level to the high normal range consistent with the normal pregnant state. The increase in thyroid-binding proteins attendant to pregnancy creates a large population of unoccupied binding sites for thyroid hormones. Therefore, levothyroxine replacement dosage should be greater in pregnancy, for example, than in the elderly nonpregnant patient with hypothyroidism. A dose of 100–150 μg of levothyroxine per day should be given initially, with the usual maintenance dose between 150 and 175 μg of levothyroxine per day. Thyroid preparations containing T_3, such as dessicated thyroid extract, and artificial ratios of T_4 and T_3 are not indicated in pregnancy.

The serum concentration of thyroxine will correct rapidly, usually within one to two weeks. If the TSH level is elevated, it should be anticipated that it will return to the normal range more slowly, probably requiring 6–8 weeks of levothyroxine replacement. If secondary or tertiary hypothyroidism is present, steroids must be administered prior to beginning levothyroxine replacement until the pituitary adrenal axis can be evaluated.

Fetal Compartment

The phases of thyroid ontogenesis have been well summarized.[19,20] Thyroid organogenesis begins at an approximate fetal age of 24 days, with follicle formation at approximately 70 days and initiation of iodine concentration and hormonogenesis at 74 days. The fetal thyroid is not susceptible to radioactive iodine or to excessive iodine or antithyroid drugs until the 10–12 week of gestation. Maternal thyroid hormones such as T_4, T_3, and TSH do not cross the placental barrier to any significant degree during pregnancy. However, a slight gradient may exist from fetal to maternal compartment. Fetal demands for thyroid hormone are satisfied by fetal thyroid function.[7] Fetal serum thyroxine levels steadily increase during the last trimester of pregnancy. At term, fetal concentrations of T_4 and TBG are not significantly different from those of the mother, although the fetal serum T_3 concentration is much less than is the maternal concentration and the reverse T_3 concentration in fetal serum is much greater than that in maternal serum. Amniotic fluid T_4 concentrations are lower than fetal serum T_4. The amniotic fluid reverse T_3 level is significantly higher than the serum reverse T_3 concentration in the fetus, especially during the first two trimesters. Measurements of amniotic fluid thyroid hormones may or may not prove useful in establishing the level of thyroid function in the fetus.[28] Kourides and coworkers have reported a 26 week fetus in which ultrasonography demonstrated a goiter.[26] Serial sampling of amniotic fluid between the 26th and 38th weeks of gestation demonstrated an elevated TSH level, but amniotic fluid concentrations of T_4, T_3, and reverse T_3 were not different from those of euthyroid fetuses. Goitrous hypothyroidism was present at birth, and therapy was instituted on the first day of life with normal growth and development established during the first year of life with thyroid supplementation. Therefore, amniotic fluid TSH may be useful in establishing a diagnosis of intrauterine primary hypothyroidism, whereas earlier positive reports of the usefulness of measuring amniotic fluid reverse T_3 for diagnosis of fetal hypothyroidism have not been confirmed. Fetal hypothyroidism diagnosed in utero has been treated successfully in several instances with intra-amniotic injection of thyroxine.[29]

Fetal hypothyroidism occurs most commonly (82%) from thyroid dysgenesis; 7% of the fetuses are goitrous and 10% of cases of fetal hypothyroidism are secondary to hypopituitarism. Other causes of fetal hypothyroidism include inadvertent administration of an ablative dose of radioactive iodine after 12 weeks' gestation. Familial neonatal transient hypohyroidism may be secondary to maternal TSH inhibitor immunoglobulins.[30] IgG-blocking antibodies for the TSH receptor have been identified in the neonate of a woman with Hashimoto's thyroiditis. Such IgG antibodies may produce hypothyroidism in both mother and fetus.[43]

Neonatal screening for hypothyroidism has been reviewed by The Newborn Thyroid Screening Committee of the American Thyroid Association.[20] Of one million neonates screened

TABLE 36-2. TREATMENT OF HYPOTHYROIDISM IN PREGNANCY

1. Levothyroxine 150–175 μg/day
2. TSH measured to rule out pituitary or hypothalamic disease
3. Other autoimmune diseases, especially pernicious anemia, diabetes mellitus, and Addison's disease must be considered.

for hypothyroidism, 1 in 4000 was hypothyroid. Of these, less than 1% were suspected clinically. Low thyroid-binding globulin levels were found in 1 in 9000 neonates. Measurement of plasma thyroglobulins in the neonate is useful to help clarify the thyroid abnormality once hypothyroidism has been diagnosed.[11] The recommended diagnostic approach is measurement of thyroxine in capillary blood at the second to third day of life. T_4 levels in cord blood also may be measured; however, T_4 measurement alone is inadequate. Capillary blood TSH measurement for confirmation is required in 1.5%–3% of cases. The average time until treatment was instituted varied between two and eight weeks.

Neonatal thyroid function tests are significantly different from those seen prior to birth. A transient rise in serum TSH concentrations occurs immediately after birth and is presumed related to a change in the fetal body temperature. Serum T_4 increases over the first two days of life and then gradually declines to the normal adult range at the end of one week. A physiologic thyrotoxicosis of the newborn has been described in which T_3 concentrations peak at the end of the first day at about two to three times the normal adult maximum and then gradually return to the upper part of the normal range at 48–72 hours following birth. Serum reverse T_3 levels gradually decline to the normal adult range at the end of the first week of life. Preterm infants are at increased risk for primary hypothyroidism. Both healthy and sick preterm infants have low serum concentrations of total and free T_4 and T_3. The TSH response to TRH is attenuated. This state of tertiary hypothyroidism is transient and resolves progressively with age.[13] It is unclear whether thyroxine replacement is beneficial in very-low-birth-weight hypothyroxinemic infants.[9]

HYPERTHYROIDISM

Maternal Compartment

The causes of hyperthyroidism are not different in pregnant women from those identified in nonpregnant women. Graves' disease is the most common cause of hyperthyroidism in pregnancy. Grave's disease is an autoimmune disorder produced by thyroid-stimulating immunoglobulins and characterized by a diffuse toxic goiter, ophthalmopathy (an infiltrative process involving the eye muscles and retroorbital fat pads), and an infiltrative dermopathy. Occasionally, Graves' disease appears as T_3 toxicosis in which the T_3 concentration is increased prior to a rise in serum T_4. Graves' disease is aggravated in early pregnancy. An amelioration of thyrotoxicosis commonly occurs in the second half of pregnancy. Relapse frequently occurs in the postpartum period and can be predicted by a rapid rise of the free T_4 index in early pregnancy.[1]

Other causes of hyperthyroidism in pregnancy include toxic adenoma, toxic multinodular goiter, Hashimoto's thyroiditis resulting in hyperthyroidism and called Hashitoxicosis, thyrotoxicosis factitia which should be suspected in women who are thyrotoxic but who have no palpable goiter, either painful or painless thyroiditis, and trophoblastic tumors such as choriocarcinoma or hydatidiform mole, associated with high titers of hCG and a corresponding thyrotropic effect. Pituitary tumors secreting TSH may cause hyperthyroidism. Struma ovarii is a rare cause of hyperthyroidism. Thyroid cancer in which the tumor burden in the body is great may produce sufficient thyroid hormone to cause hyperthyroidism.

Clinical manifestations of hyperthyroidism are widely variable. Every manifestation of hyperthyroidism should not be anticipated in every patient, although the presence of any manifestation should suggest the possibility of hyperthyroidism. Patients with hyperthyroidism have cutaneous manifestations including hyperhydrosis, alopecia, onycholysis, and thyroid achropachy or clubbing of the fingers and the toes, which is always associated with exophthalmic Graves' ophthalmopathy. Pruritus, a common complaint in hyperthyroidism, may be more marked in pregnancy. Graves' eye disease may vary from no signs or symptoms to severe involvement of the extraocular muscles to loss of vision if the optic nerve is compressed sufficiently. Cardiac manifestations include tachycardia, increased cardiac output, and pulmonic flow murmur. Head and neck manifestations may include unilateral vocal cord paralysis and nasal discharge. Gastrointestinal manifestations such as diarrhea, abdominal pain, hepatic dysfunction with abnormal liver function tests, and dysphagia may be present. Neuromuscular manifestations such as proximal weakness, muscle atrophy, tremor of the extremities and tongue, thyrotoxic myopathic disorders, hyperkalemic periodic paralysis, and myasthenia gravis may appear.

Blood manifestations include anemia and

relative leukopenia. Adrenal function may be suppressed. Other autoimmune diseases commonly are associated with Graves' disease and should be sought in pregnant women with hyperthyroidism, such as vitiligo, diabetes mellitus, myasthenia gravis, rheumatoid arthritis, idiopathic thrombocytopenic purpura, and chronic active hepatitis.

Thyroid function test abnormalities include an increased serum T_3 in all patients with hyperthyroidism. The T_4 concentrations generally are increased. The resin T_3 uptake may return toward the midnormal range. T_4 levels are not elevated in patients with T_3 toxicosis and patients with thyrotoxicosis factitia secondary to thyroxine or T_3 ingestion. The erythrocyte sedimentation rate is increased in patients with subacute thyroiditis. Patients with trophoblastic tumors have hCG levels elevated beyond the normal range for pregnancy.

Thyroid stimulating immunoglobulins are elevated and may be measured to establish a diagnosis of Graves' disease in difficult cases. Detection of elevated maternal thyroid stimulating immunoglobulins in the third trimester predicts neonatal hyperthyroidism (Table 36-3) [48] The measurement should be obtained as late in pregnancy as possible. Patients with TSH-producing pituitary tumors have increased concentrations of TSH and an abnormal sella turcica. Radioisotope studies are contraindicated in pregnancy. However, a thyroid uptake and scan unwittingly performed in pregnancy is not an indication for therapeutic abortion.

The therapy of Graves' disease in pregnancy has been the subject of much debate. In the first half of this century, prior to the availability of antithyroid drugs such as propylthiouracil and methimazole, hyperthyroidism in pregnancy was treated surgically.[5,45] The Mayo clinic has reported an extensive series of subtotal thyroidectomies performed during the second trimester with excellent results.[16] At present, a course of antithyroid drug therapy is considered indicated in virtually all women with pregnancy complicated by hyperthyroidism (Table 36-4). Methimazole has been associated with congenital scalp defects such as aplasia cutis; therefore, propylthiouracil may be preferable for use in pregnancy.[35] The reported experience suggests that, in patients who can be managed with less than 200 mg of propylthiouracil per day, the risk of fetal goiter is minimal. Propylthiouracil crosses the placenta and, if given to the mother in high concentrations, suppresses the fetal thyroid. A starting dose of propylthiouracil, 300 mg daily in three divided doses, provides control of hyperthyroidism in most patients. The dose of propylthiouracil may be decreased rapidly in most patients. Thyroid function is followed with serial thyroid function tests and clinical evaluation. The goal of antithyroid therapy is to reduce the thyroid levels to the range consistent with normal pregnancy, which is the upper portion of the normal range for total thyroxine. In general, the propylthiouracil dose can be tapered after four to eight weeks of therapy to as little as 50–100 mg daily, which will maintain the pregnant woman in the euthyroid state. Antithyroid drugs should be used alone, without levothyroxine as adjunctive therapy. The addition of levothyroxine appears to require an increase in the dose of the antithyroid drug.[33] Such patients should be followed very closely throughout pregnancy. Agranulocytosis should be considered as a potential complication of propylthiouracil therapy, although it is a rare complication given the relatively low dose used.[10] Pregnancy does not significantly alter the pharmacokinetics of propylthiouracil.[42]

Propranolol and other beta blockers are relatively contraindicated in pregnancy. If required to control severe tachyarrhythmia, they may be used but should be discontinued as soon as clinically indicated. The contraindication to beta blockers is greater during the last trimester and during labor because of fetal depression.[31] Phenobarbital is a safe and useful sedative in pregnancy complicated by hyperthyroidism and has the advantage of enhancing hepatic microsomal degradation of thyroid hormone. Surgery may still have a place in the treatment of hyperthyroidism in pregnancy, although in my personal experience, every patient has been managed successfully with conservative medical therapy. Iodine is contraindicated in pregnancy, because it crosses the placenta and will suppress the fetal thyroid, producing hypothyroidism and goiter in the fetus.

Thyroid crisis may occur in the pregnant hyperthyroid patient. The clinical features of thyroid storm include high output failure, hyperpyrexia, nausea, vomiting, and agitation. The management of thyroid storm in pregnancy should not be different from that in the nonpregnant state, including a full blocking dose of propylthiouracil, 1200 mg per day in eight divided doses, iodide, 2 mg over 24 hours by continuous i.v. infusion, propranolol, water-soluble vitamins, digoxin, and diuretics as indicated for management of congestive heart failure. Treatment of any concomitant illnesses should be un-

TABLE 36-3. TSAb VALUES IN PREGNANT WOMEN WITH GRAVES' DISEASE IN RELATION TO THE DEVELOPMENT OF NEONATAL HYPERTHYROIDISM

Family	Mother			Neonate	
Number	Diagnosis	Therapy	TSAb (%)	Diagnosis	TSAb (%)
1	Hashimoto's	T_4	1187 (0.1 mg IgG; 1st pregnancy)	I. Hyperthyroid (diagnosed at 4 months)	3063 (5 mg IgG, 4 months)
			1333 (0.1 mg IgG; 2nd pregnancy)	II. Hyperthyroid (at 45 days)	1180 (cord, 0.2 mg IgG)
2	Graves'	Methimazole	2576	Hyperthyroid	NT
3	Graves'	PTU	2536	Hyperthyroid	941
4	Hashimoto's, Graves' ophthalmopathy	T_4	2429 (1st pregnancy)	I. Hyperthyroid, died	725
			2011 (2nd pregnancy)	II. Hyperthyroid	561 (cord)
5	Graves'	PTU	1267	Hyperthyroid	NT (LATS positive)
6	Graves'	PTU	917	Hyperthyroid	619 (cord)
7	Graves'	PTU	811	Hyperthyroid	315 (cord)
8	Graves', p^{131}I Rx	T_4	503	Hyperthyroid	NT
9	Graves' euthyroid p subtotal thyroidectomy	PTU	293	I. Euthyroid, hyperactive	227
		None	Negative	II. Euthyroid	Negative
10	Graves', p^{131}I Rx euthyroid	None	285	Euthyroid	Negative
11	Graves' p subtotal thyroidectomy	T_4	276	Euthyroid	NT
12	Graves'	PTU	273	Euthyroid	228 (cord)
13	Graves'	PTU	176	Euthyroid	NT
14	Graves'	Methimazole	Negative	Euthyroid	NT
15	Graves'	PTU	Negative	Euthyroid	Negative
16	Graves'	PTU	Negative	Euthyroid	Negative
17	Graves'	PTU	Negative	Euthyroid	Negative

PTU, propylthiouracil.
NT, not tested.
p, after.
TSAb, thyroid stimulating immunoglobulins expressed as percent increase in tissue cAMP levels.

TABLE 36-4. TREATMENT OF HYPERTHYROIDISM IN PREGNANCY

1. Propylthiouracil 300 mg/day initially and reduce dose to <200 mg/day as soon as possible
2. Phenobarbital 15 mg q.i.d. as a sedative and to enhance hepatic clearance of thyroid hormone
3. Rest with frequent naps and decreased work
4. Propranolol only if needed for initial control of symptoms, but not in the last trimester
5. Surgery only if medical therapy has failed in a hospital setting and then in the second trimester

dertaken. The maternal mortality may be as high as 20%.

Fetal Compartment

Clinical characteristics of neonatal thyrotoxicosis include tachycardia, tachypnea, hyperactivity, irritability, and bounding pulse. The eyes may be prominent, with periorbital edema; a goiter may be present. Other features include difficulty gaining weight, hepatosplenomegaly, hyperactive reflexes, prematurity, and congestive heart failure.

The thyroid stimulating immunoglobulins known to cause Graves' disease in the mother cross the placenta and may induce fetal hyperthyroidism. Neonatal thyrotoxicosis is positively correlated with maternal serum concentrations of thyroid stimulating immunoglobulins at term.[14] There are few reports of efforts to treat fetal thyrotoxicosis prenatally. Robinson reported serial measurements of fetal heart rate in a woman with pregnancy complicated by Graves' disease with high titers of thyroid stimulating immunoglobulin.[39] The fetal heart rate was titrated into the normal range with increasing doses of antithyroid drugs administered to the mother. Neonatal thyrotoxicosis was present at delivery.

The human placenta blocks the transfer of T_4 and T_3 between the mother and fetus by inner ring deiodinase activity, which metabolizes T_4 and T_3 to inactive products. Propylthiouracil partially inhibits this mechanism,[17] as well as blocking the fetal thyroid. Therefore, propylthiouracil may protect the fetus from hypothyroidism by enhancing placental transfer of T_4 and T_3.

Neonatal thyroid function has been studied after propylthiouracil therapy in the treatment of maternal Graves' disease.[8] It is unclear whether fetal goiter observed in cases where the mother received more than 200 mg of propylthiouracil per day is the direct result of propylthiouracil or of thyroid stimulating immunoglobulins. The infants of women treated for hyperthyroid Graves' disease with the smallest dose of propylthiouracil that will control their hyperthyroidism exhibit slight decreases in T_4 concentrations and slightly elevated serum TSH levels at birth. The clinical significance of these modest abnormalities is not known. The conclusion to be drawn is that the smallest possible dose of propylthiouracil that controls maternal hyperthyroidism should be used.

Intellectual impairment and craniosynostosis have been reported in neonatal thyrotoxic children.[12] The etiology of craniosynostosis in this syndrome is unclear. A correlation has been established between craniosynostosis and subsequent intellectual impairment. Relatively normal physical growth is noted in children with neonatal thyrotoxicosis with a relatively high incidence of intellectual impairment.

ANTITHYROID TREATMENT DURING LACTATION

Breast-feeding generally has been contraindicated in women who are receiving antithyroid drugs, either methimazole or propylthiouracil. The fear of possible adverse effects of antithyroid drugs in nursing mothers stems from studies which show that only minute quantities of propylthiouracil pass into milk; however, methimazole appears to pass freely into breast milk. Carbimazole is converted to methimazole in vivo. Lamberg and colleagues have reported 11 women treated for hyperthyroidism with carbimazole or propylthiouracil.[27] Breast-feeding was permitted if the dose did not exceed 15 mg of carbimazole or 150 mg of propylthiouracil daily. Neonatal serum T_4 and TSH levels were measured during breast-feeding and did not differ significantly from the normal neonatal range.

HYPEREMESIS GRAVIDARUM AS A MANIFESTATION OF HYPERTHYROIDISM

The first trimester of pregnancy frequently is complicated by nausea and vomiting that may diminish the total food intake and result in weight loss and dehydration. The causes of hyperemesis gravidarum are unclear; however, both multiple pregnancies and trophoblastic tumors predispose to hyperemesis gravidarum. Increased thyroxine concentrations were noted in 73% of 32 pregnancies complicated by hyperemesis gravidarum.[49] The free T_3 index was increased in four of 11 patients with elevated serum T_4 levels. A blunted response of TSH to TRH was noted in five patients with hyperthyroxinemia. None of the patients had goiter, exophthalmos, or a previous history of hyperthyroidism. Hyperthyroxinemia returned to the normal range in one to four weeks without antithyroid therapy. The symptoms of hyperemesis in patients with intractable hyperemesis gravidarum resolve when thyroid function is returned to the normal range with propylthiouracil.[50] There is a relative block in conversion of T_4 to T_3 in patients with hyperthyroxinemia and hyperemesis gravidarum suggestive of similar abnormalities seen in the euthyroid sick syndrome. In the latter, a form of T_4 toxicosis is present. The diagnosis of hyperthyroidism is substantiated by a blunted response of TSH to TRH. It is unclear whether patients with hyperemesis gravidarum and hyperthyroxinemia require antithyroid therapy with propylthiouracil. If a diagnosis of hyperthyroidism is established on the basis of laboratory and clinical findings, a brief course of treatment with antithyroid drugs is not unreasonable; however, the dosage should be tapered as rapidly as possible since many patients' T_4 levels return to normal without any treatment.

POSTPARTUM THYROID DYSFUNCTION

Fluctuations in thyroid hormone concentration during the puerperium have been described frequently. Hypothyroidism is relatively common in the postpartum period. This dysfunction usually represents an exacerbation of subclinical autoimmune thyroid disease, which may be present in 5–10% of the postpartum population.[24] Thyrotoxicosis is also a common complication in the postpartum period, occurring three to eight months after delivery. It is not unusual for a woman to experience transient thyrotoxicosis followed by transient hypothyroidism in the postpartum period. Postpartum thyroid dysfunction is not related to parity, age, or breast-feeding. However, it may be more common in women who give birth to female offspring.[2] Goiter is not present in all patient with postpartum thyrotoxicosis; therefore, postpartum women with symptoms of hypermetabolism should have thyroid function tests performed whether a palpable goiter is present or not.

The clinical characteristics of patients at risk for transient postpartum hypothyroidism include thyroid enlargement in the first four months postpartum, a goiter prior to pregnancy, and positive titers of antithyroid antibodies.[2] A spontaneous return to the euthyroid state may be expected five to ten months postpartum. As the euthyroid state resumes, the goiter decreases in size but may not resolve completely. In patients with clinical characteristics of hypothyroidism, a 6–12 month course of thyroid hormone replacement is warranted. However, it is anticipated that the levothyroxine may be withdrawn at the end of that time with return to normal thyroid function. Painless postpartum thyroiditis may present as severe hypertension.[44]

Circulating thyroid stimulating immunoglobulins may be increased in patients with Graves' disease when they suffer a relapse of hyperthyroidism after delivery.[46] However, thyroid stimulating immunoglobulins may not be detected at the time of postpartum relapse in women who were in clinical remission before and during pregnancy and in whom hyperthyroidism recurred three to five months following delivery. It is not clear that thyroid stimulating immunoglobulins have a role in initiating hyperthyroidism in such patients.

THYROID NODULES

Thyroid nodules occur very commonly in the general population and are found in 5% of autopsy examinations. Of these, approximately 4% are malignant. Because radioisotope scanning is contraindicated in pregnancy, the usual separation of nodules by those that are hyperfunctioning or hot, those that are warm, and those nodules that are cold by scan cannot be established. Therefore patients should be separated into those considered to be at high risk for thyroid cancer and those who are of lesser risk. The principal risk factors for carcinoma include a history of prior head and neck radiation exposure, for example, for an enlarged thymus in infancy or for treatment of acne or enlarged tonsils or adenoids or as part of radiation therapy for other malignancies such as Hodgkin's

TABLE 36-5. REASONS FOR RADIATION THERAPY

Thymic enlargement	Keloids	Tuberculosis adenitis
Cervical adenitis	Eczema	Hemangioma
Sinusitis	Nevi	Laryngeal polyp
Tonsillar enlargement	Ringworm	Enlarged tongue
Toxic goiter	Acne	Peribronchitis
Colloid goiter		Pertussis

disease (Table 36-5).[3] Solitary nodules are more likely to be malignant than are multiple nodules. A family history of medullary thyroid cancer should be sought. Other evidence of malignancy should be identified, such as palpable lymph nodes in the neck or evidence of hematogenous spread to the lung or other tissues.

In addition, the character of the nodule on physical examination is important. Thyroid cancers are firmer and may be fixed to underlying tissues. Patients may complain of symptoms of dysphagia or dysphonia. If a patient has significant risk factors for carcinoma, a more aggressive approach to the nodule should be undertaken (Table 36-6).

A fine-needle aspiration of a thyroid nodule can be performed simply and safely in pregnancy. With the assistance of an expert cytologist, a diagnosis of benign versus malignant cytology from the nodule can be established with approximately 95% predictive accuracy. Ultrasound is not particularly useful. Although ultrasound will distinguish between solid and cystic lesions, papillary thyroid cancer may have a cystic component.

Papillary carcinoma is the most common form of thyroid cancer.[51] The tumor may appear as either a pure papillary lesion or as a mixed papillary follicular lesion, both of which behave as papillary cancer. Metastasis occurs through the lymphatic system. Generally, early metastasis is seen locally in the neck. Papillary cancer occurs most commonly in women under age forty. Follicular carcinoma comprises approximately 18–25% of thyroid cancers.[52] It is most common in women in the childbearing years, age 20–50, and metastasizes through the blood. Anaplastic carcinoma is much less likely to be seen in the pregnant population. It is a disease primarily of the elderly and is only slightly more common in women than in men. It comprises approximately 18% of thyroid cancers and is associated with very poor prognosis and death by rapid local invasion of the neck. Medullary cancer may occur at any age as an autosomal-dominant disorder and may be associated with other components of the multiple endocrine neoplasia syndrome such as pheochromocytoma and parathyroid hyperplasia. A tumor marker, calcitonin, is associated with this disease. Any pregnant woman suspected of having medullary thyroid cancer on the basis of a family history and/or suspicious cytologic findings should be screened with blood calcitonin measurements.

TABLE 36-6. TREATMENT OF THYROID NODULE IN PREGNANCY

1. Assess risk factors for benign vs. malignant lesion
2. Fine-needle aspiration if significant risk factors present
3. Serum calcitonin if medullary thyroid cancer suspected
4. Thyroidectomy and removal of gross nodes in second trimester
5. Decision in third trimester of surgery vs. levothyroxine suppression, 150–175 μg/day, made on individual basis

Many thyroid stimulators are present in pregnancy, including human chorionic gonadotropin, which has been shown to have about 1/1000 the thyroid stimulating activity of TSH. Other thyrotropins isolated from the placenta have been studied. Whether or not thyroid cancer is affected by TSH or other thyrotropins in humans is not known. However, one of the mainstays of therapy in thyroid cancer is suppression of TSH. Therefore, significant concern is present regarding the coexistence of the known thyroid stimulators of pregnancy and thyroid cancer. There is no evidence of activation of metastasis or recurrence of thyroid cancer during pregnancy in women treated for thyroid cancer prior to pregnancy. In patients first diagnosed as having thyroid cancer during pregnancy, the clinical course of disease is not different than the course in the nonpregnant population.[40] Available evidence suggests that pregnancy does not worsen or accelerate the course of thyroid cancer.

If thyroid cancer is identified, thyroidectomy should be considered and is best timed during the second trimester. If a diagnosis of a well-differentiated papillary cancer is established by fine-needle cytology, suppressive levothyroxine therapy should be initiated, utilizing doses of 150–175 mg of levothyroxine daily. In cases in which papillary cancer is found to be metastatic to the neck, such that extensive surgery is required, and if the diagnosis is established in the third trimester, a careful decision regarding the timing of the surgery should be made. Every case must be considered individually.

REFERENCES

1. Amino, N., Tanizawa, O., Mori, H., Iwatani, Y., Kurachi, K Kumahara, Y., and Miyai, K.: Aggravation of thyrotoxicosis in early pregnancy and after delivery in Graves' disease. *J. Clin. Endocrinol. Metab.* **55**:108–112, 1982.
2. Amino, N., Mori, H., Iwatani, Y., Tanizawa, O., Kawashima, M., Tsuge, I., Ibarogi, K., Kumahara, Y. and Miyai, K.: High prevalence of transient postpartum thyrotoxicosis and hypothyroidism. *N. Engl. J. Med.* **306**:849–852, 1982.
3. Asteris, G. T. and DeGroot, L. J.: Thyroid cancer: Relationship to radiation exposure and to pregnancy. *J. Reprod. Med.* **17**:209–216, 1976.
4. Banovac, K., Bzik, L., Tislaric, D., and Sekso, M.: Conversion of thyroxine to triiodothyronine and reverse triiodothyronine in human placenta and fetal membranes. *Horm. Res.* **12**:253–259, 1980.
5. Barnes, H. V. and Gann, D. S.: Choosing thyroidectomy in hyperthyroidism. *Surg. Clin. North Am.* **54**:289–307, 1974.
6. Braunstein, G. D. and Hershman, J. M.: Comparison of serum pituitary thyrotropin and chorionic gonadotropin concentrations throughout pregnancy. *J. Clin. Endocrinol. Metab.* **42**:1123–1126, 1976.
7. Burrow, G. N.: Maternal-fetal considerations in hyperthyroidism. *Clin. Endocrinol. Metab.* **7**:115–125, 1978.
8. Cheron, R. G., Kaplan, M. M., Larsen, P. R., Selenkow, H. A., and Crigler, J. F., Jr.: Neonatal thyroid function after propylthiouracil therapy for maternal Graves' disease. *N. Engl. J. Med.* **304**:525–528, 1981.
9. Chowdhry, P., Scanlon, J. W., Auerbach, R., and Abbassi, V.: Results of controlled double-blind study of thyroid replacement in very low-birth-weight premature infants with hypothyroxinemia. *Pediatrics* **73**:301–305, 1984.
10. Cooper, D. S.: Antithyroid drugs. *N. Engl. J. Med.* **311**:1353–1362, 1984.
11. Czernichow, P., Schlumberger, M., Pomarede, R., and Fragu, P.: Plasma thyroglobulin measurements help determine the type of thyroid defect in congenital hypothyroidism. *J. Clin. Endocrinol. Metab.* **56**:242–245, 1983.
12. Daneman, D. and Howard, N. J.: Neonatal thyrotoxicosis:. Intellectual impairment and craniosynostosis in later years. *J. Pediatr.* **97**:257–259, 1980.
13. Delange, F., Dalhem, A., Bourdoux, P., Lagasse, R., Glinoer, D., Fisher, D. A., Walfish, P. G., and Ermans, A. M.: Increased risk of primary hypothyroidism in preterm infants. *J. Pediatr.* **105**:462–469, 1984.
14. Dirmikis, S. M. and Munro, D. S.: Placental transmission of thyroid-stimulating immunoglobulins. *Br. Med. J.* **2**:665–666, 1975.
15. Drucker, D., Shumak, S., and Angel, A.: Schmidt's syndrome presenting with intrauterine growth retardation and postpartum Addisonian crisis. *Am. J. Obstet. Gynecol.* **149**:229–230, 1984.
16. Emslander, R. F., Weeks, R. E., and Malkasian, G. D., Jr.: Hyperthyroidism and pregnancy. *Med. Clin. North Am.* **58**:835–845, 1974.
17. Fay, M., Roti, E., Fang, S. L., Wright, G., Braverman, L. E., and Emerson, C. H.: The effects of propylthiouracil, iodothyronines, and other agents on thyroid hormone metabolism in human placenta. *J. Clin. Endocrinol. Metab.* **58**:280–286, 1984.
18. Fisher, D. A.: Thyroid physiology in the fetus and newborn.: Current concepts and approaches to perinatal thyroid disease. *Prog Clin. Biol. Res.* **10**:221–233, 1976.
19. Fisher, D. A. and Klein, A. H.: Thyroid development and disorders of thyroid function in the newborn. *N. Engl. J. Med.* **304**:702–712, 1981.
20. Fisher, D. A., Dussault, J. H., Foley, T. P., Jr., Klein, A. H., LaFranchi, S., Larsen, P. R., Mitchell, M. L., Murphey, W. H., and Walfish, P. G.: Screening for congenital hypothyroidism: Results of screening one million North American infants. *J. Pediatr.* **94**:700–705, 1979.
21. Harada, A., Hershman, J. M., Reed, A. W., Braunstein, G. D., Dignam, W. J., Derzko, C., Friedman, S., Jewelewicz, R., and Pekary, A. E.:. Comparison of thyroid stimulators and thyroid hormone concentrations in the sera of pregnant women. *J. Clin. Endocrinol. Metab.* **48**:793–797, 1979.
22. Hollingsworth, D. R. and Alexander, N. M.: Amniotic fluid concentrations of iodothyronines and thyrotropin do not reliably predict fetal thyroid status in pregnancies complicated by maternal thyroid disorders or anencephaly. *J. Clin. Endocrinol. Metab.* **57**:349–355, 1983.
23. Innerfield, R. and Hollander C. S.: Thyroidal complications of pregnancy. *Med. Clin. North Am.* **61**:67–87 1977.
24. Jansson, R., Bernander, S., Karlsson, A., Levin, K., and Nilsson, G.: Autoimmune thyroid dysfunction in the postpartum period. *J. Clin. Endocrinol. Metab.* **58**:681–687, 1984.

25. Kennedy, A. L. and Montgomery, D. A. D.: Hypothyroidism in pregnancy. *Br. J. Obstet. Gynaecol.* **85**:225–230, 1978.
26. Kourides, I. A., Berkowitz, R. L., Pang, S., Van Natta, F. C., Barone, C. M., and Ginsberg-Fellner, F.: Antepartum diagnosis of goitrous hypothyroidism by fetal ultrasonography and amniotic fluid thyrotropin concentration. *J. Clin. Endocrinol. Metab.* **59**:1016–1018, 1984.
27. Lamberg, B. A., Ikonen, E., Osterlund, K., Teramo, K., Pekonen, F., Peltola, J., and Valimaki, M.: Antithyroid treatment of maternal hyperthyroidism during lactation. *Clin. Endocrinol.* **21**:81–87, 1984.
28. Landau, H., Sack, J., Frucht, H., Palti, Z., Hochner-Celnikier, D., and Rosenmann, A.: Amniotic fluid 3,3',5'-triiodothyronine in the detection of congenital hypothyroidism. *J. Clin. Endocrinol. Metab.* **50**:799–801, 1980.
29. Lightner, E. S., Fismer, D. A., Giles, H., and Woolfenden, J.: Intra-amniotic injection of thyroxine to a human fetus. Evidence for conversion of T4 to reverse T3. *Am. J. Obstet. Gynecol.* **127**:487–490, 1977.
30. Matsuura, N., Yamada, Y., Nohara, Y., Konishi, J., Kasagi, K., Endo, K., Kojima, H., and Wataya, K.: Familial neonatal transient hypothyroidism due to maternal TSH-binding inhibitor immunoglobulins. *N. Engl. J. Med.* **303**:738–741, 1980.
31. McDevitt, D. G.: Propranolol in the treatment of thyrotoxicosis: A review. *Postgrad. Med. J.* **52** (Suppl. 4):157–161, 1976.
32. Medeiros-Neto, G. A., Walfish, P. G., Almeida, F., Maia, E., Gomes, E. F., Kiy, Y., Knobel, M., Ginsberg, J., and Chopra, I .J.: 3,3',5'-Triiodothyronine, thyroxine, triiodothyronine, and thyrotropin levels in maternal and cord blood sera from endemic goiter regions of Brazil. *J. Clin. Endocrinol. Metab.* **47**:508–511, 1978.
33. Mestman, J. H., Manning, P. R., and Hodgman, J.: Hyperthyroidism and pregnancy. *Arch. Intern. Med.* **134**:434–439, 1974.
34. Miyamoto, J.: Prolactin and thyrotropin responses to thyrotropin-releasing hormone during the peripartal period. *Obstet. Gynecol.* **63**:639–644, 1984.
35. Mujtaba, Q. and Burrow, G. N.: Treatment of hyperthyroidism in pregnancy with propylthiouracil and methimazole. *Obstet. Gynecol.* **46**:282–286, 1975.
36. Osathanondh, R., Chopra, I. J., and Tulchinsky, D.: Effects of dexamethasone on fetal and maternal thyroxine, triiodothyronine, reverse triiodothyronine, and thyrotropin levels. *J. Clin. Endocrinol. Metab.* **47**:1236–1239, 1978.
37. Penny, R., Spencer, C. A., Frasier, S. D., and Nicoloff, J. T.: Cord serum thyroid-stimulating hormone and thyroglobulin levels decline with increasing birth weight in newborns. *J. Clin. Endocrinol. Metab.* **59**:979–985, 1984.
38. Prout, T. E.: Thyroid disease in pregnancy. *Am. J. Obstet. Gynecol.* **122**:669–676, 1975.
39. Robinson, P. L., O'Mullane, N. M., and Alderman, B.: Prenatal treatment of fetal thyrotoxicosis. *Br. Med. J.* **1**:383–384, 1979.
40. Rosvoll, R. V. and Winship, T.: Thyroid carcinoma and pregnancy. *Surg. Gynecol. Obstet.* **121**:1039–1042, 1965.
41. Silva, J. E. and Silva, S.: Interrelationships among serum thyroxine, triiodothyronine, reverse triiodithyronine, and thyroid-stimulating hormone in iodine-deficient pregnant women and their offspring: Effects of iodine supplementation. *J. Clin. Endocrinol. Metab.* **52**:671–677, 1981.
42. Sitar, D. S., Abu-Bakare, A., and Gardiner, R. J.: Propylthiouracil disposition in pregnant and post-partum women. *Pharmacology* **25**:57–60, 1982.
43. Takasu, N., Mori, T., Koizumi, Y., Takeuchi, S., and Yamada, T.: Transient neonatal hypothyroidism due to maternal immunoglobulins that inhibit thyrotropin-binding and post-receptor processes. *J. Clin. Endocrinol. Metab.* **59**:142–146, 1984.
44. White, W. B. and Andreoli, J. A.: Painless postpartum thyroiditis seen initially as severe hypertension. *Am. J. Obstet. Gynecol.* **148**:346–347, 1984.
45. Worley, R. J. and Crosby, W. M.: Hyperthyroidism during pregnancy. *Am. J. Obstet. Gynecol.* **119**:150–155, 1974.
46. Yabu, Y., Amino, N., Mori, H., Miyai, K., Tanizawa, O., Takai, S. I., Kumahara, Y., Matsuzuka, F., and Kuma, K.: Postpartum recurrence of hyperthyroidism and changes of thyroid-stimulating immunoglobulins in Graves' disease. *J. Clin. Endocrinol. Metab.* **51**:1454–1458, 1980.
47. Ylikorkala, O., Kivinen, S., and Reinla, M.: Serial prolactin and thyrotropin responses to thyrotropin-releasing hormone throughout normal human pregnancy. *J. Clin. Endocrinol. Metab.* **48**:288–292, 1979.
48. Zakarija, M. and McKenzie, J. M.: Pregnancy-associated changes in the thyroid-stimulating antibody of Graves' disease and the relationship to neonatal hyperthyroidism. *J. Clin. Endocrinol. Metab.* **57**:1036–1040, 1983.
49. Bouillon, R., Naesens, M., Van Assche, F. A., DeKeyser, L., DeMoor, P., Renaer, M., DeVos, P., and DeRoo, M.: Thyroid function in patients with hyperemesis gravidarum. *Am. J. Obstet. Gynecol.* **143**:922–925, 1982.
50. Dozeman, R., Kaiser, F. E., Cass, O., and Pries, J.: Hyperthyroidism appearing as hyperemesis gravidarum. *Arch. Intern. Med.* **143**:2202–2203, 1983.
51. Mazzaferri, E. L., Young, R. L., Oertel, J. E., Kemmerer, W. T., and Page, C. P.: Papillary thyroid carcinoma: The impact of therapy in 576 patients. *Medicine* **56**:171–196, 1977.
52. Young, R. L., Mazzaferri, E. L., Rahe, A. J., and Dorfman, S. G.: Pure follicular thyroid carcinoma: Impact of therapy in 214 patients. *J. Nucl. Med.* **21**:733–737, 1980.

37

NEUROLOGICAL DISORDERS IN PREGNANCY

Pregnancy and neurological disease do not coincide very often. When they do, most obstetricians and most neurologists are unfamiliar with the combined problems. The gravida is subject to the same spectrum of neurological disease as the nonpregnant woman, particularly now that older women are embarking on pregnancy. The 35-year-old pregnant for the first time is not uncommon, and the 40-year-old primigravida is no longer quite so unusual. Moreover, improved neurological diagnosis and new modalities of therapy have permitted survival and reproduction in women afflicted with neurological illness. Concomitantly, obstetrical care has made explosive progress, adapting techniques of critical-care medicine to the woman who is both pregnant and sick. Technological advances have fueled this progress in obstetrics and neurology, allowing more women with neurological disease to attempt pregnancy. As a result, obstetricians will encounter more patients with neurological disease and must be able to care for them effectively.

NEUROLOGICAL DIAGNOSIS IN PREGNANCY

The gross neurological examination in the pregnant woman is unchanged from the nonpregnant. The cranial nerves are not affected, although rarely there may be visual field changes due to the physiological hypertrophy of the pituitary gland in normal pregnancy. Motor and sensory functions are unchanged. Reflexes and coordination are not affected directly, although edema, an altered center of gravity, and a different body image may cause some clumsiness during gestation. No cognitive changes occur, except for emotional lability in some patients. Hormonal and psychological factors vary in each individual, producing a variety of emotional responses to pregnancy.

Specific neurodiagnostic tests are unaltered by pregnancy and are not harmful to mother or fetus. Electroencephalography, electromyography, evoked potential tests, and even electroconvulsive therapy are not contraindicated. Computerized axial tomography (CAT) scanning has augmented neurodiagnosis spectacularly. CAT scanning is appropriate in pregnancy with shielding of the fetus and without the use of contrast material containing iodine, if possible. Myelography and angiography may be necessary in certain circumstances. The fetus cannot be shielded completely during myelography or abdominal angiography. Fetal shielding is possible during carotid angiography, which usually is reserved for serious diagnostic problems in gravid women.

CLASSIFICATION OF NEUROLOGICAL DISORDERS IN PREGNANCY

Pregnancy-associated neurological disease may be classified as inflammatory, neoplastic, vascular, nonspecific, specific to pregnancy, neuropathies, and fetal neurological disorders.

This classification includes primary neurological disorders that may be altered by pregnancy or in which management must be altered due to the gestation. Also considered are systemic disorders that may present with neurologic involvement during pregnancy. In addition, neurological symptoms are seen with preeclampsia/eclampsia, which is therefore a pregnancy-specific neurologic illness.

The effects of neurologic disorders on the mother and the clinical management must be considered in relation to mother and fetus. The diagnosis and treatment of fetal nervous system disease, an expanding new field, also must be explored. Advances in medicine in recent years have enlarged the population of women who may expect a successful outcome of pregnancy. Patients of mature age with preexisting neurological disorders and vascular diseases now comprise a growing proportion of obstetrical patients.

INFLAMMATORY DISEASES

Meningitis

Infections of the meninges are the infections most commonly accompanied by neurological symptoms. Viral and bacterial meningitis present in pregnancy as they do in the nonpregnant state. Their influence on pregnancy is secondary to systemic effects. Associated coma with resultant fetal hypoxia may occur but is a rare complication. The most common bacterial organisms include meningococcus, pneumococcus, and H. influenza. Cytomegalovirus and respiratory viruses also are common causes of meningitis. The patient presents with meningeal signs and symptoms of systemic infection. Prompt diagnosis and treatment are essential. Untreated tuberculous meningitis, usually seen in less developed nations, is associated with a high incidence of neonatal tuberculosis.[86] Currently used effective drugs, including isoniazid, ethambutol, and rifampin, do not appear to have adverse effects on the fetus.[80] Their use in pregnancy is recommended.

Syphilis

Secondary and tertiary syphilis may present with a wide variety of neurological symptoms. Diagnosis and treatment early in pregnancy are important. The spirochetes cross the placenta as early as the ninth week in untreated patients.[30] Treatment is directed at both mother and fetus. The earlier the diagnosis is made and therapy given, the better the prognosis for the mother and the lower the risk of fetal abnormality.

Myasthenia Gravis

Myasthenia gravis must be considered in the differential diagnosis whenever a pregnant patient complains of excessive fatigue and weakness. Although fatigue and weakness are common complaints in uncomplicated pregnancy, serious disorders must be ruled out. Myasthenia gravis occurs in all ages and both sexes, but females are affected twice as often as males. The highest incidence is in the third decade of life.[64] The disease is characterized by fluctuating muscle weakness involving the entire skeletal muscle system, but primarily craniofacial muscles. The disease is believed to originate in a defect at the myoneural junction at the level of the acetylcholine receptors. Administration of anticholinesterases such as neostigmine, pyridostigmine, and edrophonium reverse the clinical process but do not cure the disease. Edrophonium usually is administered in small amounts for diagnosis. Antinuclear, anti-endplate, and antimuscle antibodies have been demonstrated in myasthenic patients. Immunoglobulins from myasthenics have been shown to produce weakness.[5] Thymic tumors and hyperplasia are common. Thymectomy often improves the symptoms. Thymectomy often is employed in the nonpregnant state, especially in managing malignant thymoma, but is not indicated in pregnancy. There are many effects of the disease on the young female patient. Fertility rates in myasthenic patients are unchanged.[68] Pregnancy has an unpredictable effect on the disease process. In one study, one-third improved in pregnancy, one-third were unaffected, and one-third suffered exacerbations.[65] The course varies from one pregnancy to the next.[67] Pregnancy does exacerbate the disease process in some patients. Labor and delivery are remarkable only for the patient's increasing fatigability during the second stage with resultant increased incidence of forceps delivery.[67] Respiratory difficulty may occur; however, it is treatable with neostigmine. Magnesium sulfate is contraindicated in myasthenia gravis,[15] as is any drug with a curare-like effect, such as diethyl ether, curare, quinine, and aminoglycoside antibiotics.[32] Myasthenia crisis may be associated with stress such as labor, infection, or any superimposed illness. Crisis presents as severe weakness, including respiratory insufficiency. This must be distinguished from cholinergic crisis secondary to overmedication with anticholinesterases. Cholinergic crisis also may present with severe weakness but often is accompanied by nausea, tearing of the eyes, abdominal cramps, and diarrhea. Edrophonium given intravenously improves myasthenic crisis but not cholinergic crisis.

Recent reports have cited respiratory crisis in association with betamethasone administered to accelerate fetal lung maturation and with hypokalemia from beta-sympathomimetics used as tocolytic agents.[11] The antiacetylcholinesterase agents have a known oxytocic action, which may contribute to premature labor in myasthenic patients. Enemas are not advisable in these patients and anesthesia must be modified to avoid ether and procaine, because the hydrolysis of these agents by plasma cholinesterase is inhibited. Narcotics, tranquilizers, barbiturates, and other potential respiratory depressants should be avoided. Conduction anesthesia is preferred for labor. Neostigmine, 60 mg/d, or pyridostigmine, 240 mg/d, may be needed in labor[78] along with analgesia.

There is transplacental passage of acetylcholine receptor antibodies to the fetus in utero. This transfer is believed responsible for the syndrome of neonatal myasthenia, although the newborn may produce some antibody also.[40] The incidence of neonatal myasthenia is 4–20%.[61] The maternal course is not predictive of which infant is most likely to present with the syndrome. All fetuses of myasthenic patients must be considered at risk. The premature infant born of a myasthenic is especially at risk for severe RDS due to the combined effects of myasthenia and surfactant deficiency. The neonatal disease can appear as late as four days of age but usually presents within the first day of life. There have been reports of postpartum exacerbations of myasthenia gravis related to breast-feeding.[27] These are presumed to be triggered by associated fatigue and malnutrition. Anticholinesterases taken by the mother may be secreted in breast milk, as may be the antibodies. Neither has posed clinical problems in the neonate.

With prompt treatment of the myasthenic symptoms, the prognosis for mother and infant is good.

Multiple Sclerosis

Multiple sclerosis is a disease of uncertain etiology. Epidemiologic data include a specific geographic pattern favoring middle latitudes, with alterations according to migratory patterns, an increase in familial occurrence, and an association with dogs. These observations favor an infectious source, presumably a slow virus, which is contracted early in life. Infection triggers an autoimmune reaction, attacking myelin, with multiple symptoms such as weakness, diplopia, vertigo, and sensory disturbances. Multiple sclerosis has no primary effect on pregnancy.[70] The management of the patient is influenced by secondary complications. Diagnosis is confirmed by identification of gamma globulin elevation above 13–15% of the total protein in the spinal fluid, with mononuclear pleocytosis.[1] Therapy with ACTH and prednisone may be helpful during short-term exacerbations of the disease, but these are not always useful long-term. Treatment of symptoms and supportive measures are the basis of therapy. The disease is characterized by periods of exacerbation and remission, uninfluenced by pregnancy, although postpartum exacerbation may occur.[70] Half of all relapses in a pregnancy year occur in the first three months postpartum. Once the progressive nature of the disease has been taken into consideration and the patient has elected pregnancy, the course of pregnancy, labor, and delivery is affected only by the nonspecific effects of the disease. Recommendations have been made against nursing postpartum as in myasthenics. However, studies comparing nursing and non-nursing mothers for postpartum deterioration of multiple sclerosis do not support this recommendation.[71] Affected children are more frequent than in the population at large, but the data are compatible with common exposure as well as with a hereditary etiology.[12,13,49]

Guillain–Barré Syndrome

Guillain-Barre syndrome or idiopathic polyneuritis is a syndrome that usually follows infection, presumably of viral origin, but may occur without preceding cause. It is rare in pregnancy[79] and is characterized by rapidly progressive weakness of the extremities, more prominent distally than proximally, which may go on to respiratory insufficiency. The course of the disease is short, usually 2–3 weeks, but complete recovery may take months. Respiratory support for the mother may be required if the weakness proceeds to paralysis. Sensory symptoms may be present as well. Autonomic symptoms of hypertension, perspiration, flushes, tachycardia, cardiac arrhythmias, and, rarely, hypotension all may be seen.

Treatment is supportive. The course is not affected by pregnancy. Relapses may occur years after the initial disease in a small number of patients, occasionally associated with pregnancy.[35] Some patients may respond to corticosteroid therapy, but this is controversial.[33] The disease does not appear to affect the fetus except as secondarily related to maternal hypoxia and is not an indication for pregnancy termination. Obstetrical care should be as in the unaffected patient, unless there is severe weakness or respiratory insufficiency.

NEOPLASTIC DISEASES

Tumors

Primary nervous system tumors are rare in women of childbearing age, as are brain metastases secondary to other tumors. Clinical signs and symptoms may be precipitated by pregnancy. The treatment of these tumors is not affected by pregnancy insofar as chemotherapeutic and radiotherapeutic regimens are considered, except for possible teratogens. As in nonpregnant patients, diagnosis is based on signs and symptoms of a space-occupying central nervous system lesion, such as headache, diplopia, and papilledema, as well as sensory or motor deficits.[20] The CAT scan is very useful in diagnosis of such tumors.

Most tumors do not appear to be influenced by pregnancy. However, the course of some benign neoplasms, such as meningiomas, neurofibromas, acoustic neuromas, and angiomas, may be exacerbated by pregnancy.[3,20,53]

Several malignant neoplasms with a propensity toward brain metastases are of clinical importance in women of childbearing age. These include breast and lung cancer and choriocarcinoma. Focal neurological symptoms may be produced by these metastatic lesions. Delay in diagnosis may occur due to misinterpretation of symptoms as due to preeclampsia or eclampsia. Treatment should not be delayed because of pregnancy. Symptoms of progressive deterioration may signal the need for emergency treatment or even abortion in order to provide definitive therapy. When the patient with a brain tumor is to be delivered, vaginal birth using epidural anesthesia is acceptable, although cesarean delivery has been advocated to keep intracranial pressure at a minimum.[74]

Pituitary Adenoma

The pituitary gland normally is enlarged in pregnancy and may enlarge suddenly from rapid growth of an associated pituitary adenoma. This may precipitate neurological symptoms secondary to compression of the optic chiasm with resultant visual field defects and persistent headache. Only 5–10% of women with hyperprolactinemia alone, and therefore pituitary microadenomas, develop signs of tumor growth in pregnancy.[84] There are no adverse effects on the fetus from the adenoma or bromocriptine treatment, despite profound lowering of fetal blood prolactin levels when bromocriptine is administered.[95] Thus, surgical ablation is reserved for macroadenomas in symptomatic women.[45] Treatment of the symptomatic tumor takes precedence and often dictates the need for cesarean delivery. Patients with elevated intracranial pressure should not bear down in second stage labor due to marked increases in intracranial pressure with such expulsive effort. For such patients, conduction anesthesia and forceps or cesarean delivery are indicated.

Pseudotumor Cerebri

This syndrome occurs primarily in young women, especially those who are obese, with symptoms that mimic brain tumors.[19] The patient typically presents with headaches, visual changes, diplopia, or dizziness. Neurological exam reveals papilledema. Large increases in cerebrospinal fluid (CSF) pressure are noted. CSF studies demonstrate increased outflow resistance with slight decrease in formation.[1] The cerebral ventricles are normal or small in size. The syndrome is reported infrequently in pregnant women.[19,72] The disease is not affected adversely by pregnancy and does not appear to influence neonatal outcome.[19] Management includes repeated lumbar puncture to maintain CSF levels. Diuretics and steroids are used in chronic cases.

The diagnosis is made by CAT scan, showing the absence of an intracranial tumor and a normal lumbar puncture except for increased pressure. Pseudotumor cerebri remits spontaneously but slowly. If not treated, there is some risk of optic atrophy, so medical therapy is indicated. Obstetrical management is unaffected, although use of epidural anesthesia and outlet forceps to limit the effects of bearing down are advisable. Rarely, the syndrome recurs in another pregnancy.

VASCULAR DISORDERS

Headache

Headache is a common complaint in pregnancy, as in the nonpregnant patient. Persistent or recurrent headache is an indication for diagnostic assessment. A thorough examination, including ophthalmological and neurological evaluation, should be performed. The history should elicit information concerning the location of the pain, associated symptoms such as visual changes or aura, and past history of migraine headaches and hypertensive disease. Treatment of tension headaches and migraine should be limited to simple analgesics if possible. Ergot alkaloids, used commonly to treat migraine in the nonpregnant patient, should be avoided, because of their associated oxytocic action. This is especially true for ergonovine. Propranolol is the drug most commonly used to treat migraine in pregnancy. Foods such as aged cheeses and cured meats, chocolate, herring, chicken livers, and alcohol, which is a nonspecific vasodilator, should be avoided.

Occasionally patients with migraine will present with severe headache associated with transient neurologic deficit. These patients must undergo further evaluation using CAT scan, and, if necessary, cerebral angiography to rule out a cerebrovascular accident.

Cerebrovascular Accident

Cerebrovascular accidents occur more frequently in pregnant patients with hypertensive disease, diabetes, arteritis, and atherosclerosis. The pathologic process may include abnormalities of vessels, as in aneurysm or arteriovenous malformation with rupture, occlusion by a thrombus or embolus, failure of cerebral blood flow due to blood pressure changes, altered permeability of a vascular wall, as in preeclampsia, or change in blood viscosity, as seen in sickle cell disease. Arterial cerebral vascular occlusions are reported to have a better initial prognosis than those of venous origin. This is probably because significant brain edema arises from the thromboembolic venous obstruction, although the long-term morbidity is less in venous lesions (Table 37-1).

TABLE 37-1. EVALUATION OF THE GRAVIDA WITH CEREBROVASCULAR ACCIDENT

Clinical condition
Headache, seizures, motor and sensory deficits
Papilledema
Consciousness
Preexistent medical conditions
Preeclampsia/eclampsia
Predisposing factors
Laboratory tests
Hemogram, platelet count, sedimentation rate
Blood glucose
Serology, BUN, electrolytes, creatinine
Urinalysis
Procedures
CAT scan of head
Lumbar puncture
EEG
Chest x-ray
ECG
Echocardiogram
Cerebral angiography
Pelvic sonography

Subarachnoid hemorrhage secondary to ruptured aneurysm or arteriovenous (A-V) malformation may account for up to 12% of maternal deaths. Management of an intact aneurysm or A-V malformation that is diagnosed during pregnancy is surgical.[54,77] The treatment of the pregnant patient who has sustained a cerebral hemorrhage or infarct is supportive. Anticonvulsants, such as phenobarbital and diphenylhydantoin, should be administered prophylactically, despite possible fetal risk. Blood pressure should be maintained with hydralazine or aldomet. Cerebral edema can be controlled with dexamethasone. Physical therapy should be started as soon as possible after the patient has been stabilized. The well-known teratogenic risks associated with the use of anticonvulsants such as diphenylhydantoin must be weighed against their need in stabilizing a seriously ill patient. The fetal hydantoin syndrome of limb defects, growth and mental retardation, and facial anomalies is unlikely in these patients, because the drug is employed for a comparatively brief period of pregnancy. Moreover, even with prolonged use, the prevalence of the syndrome is only about 10%.[38] Both diphenylhydantoin and phenobarbital to some degree have an effect on the fetal brain, depressing synthesis of vitamin K-dependent clotting factors. For this reason, neonates of treated mothers should receive vitamin K. Phenobarbital may be an enzyme inducer in the fetal liver, improving bilirubin conjugation. Fetal and neonatal concerns do not prohibit prophylactic use of these drugs in the gravida who has suffered a cerebral vascular accident.

Arterial Occlusion. Cerebral vascular accident from arterial occlusion is more common in pregnancy[18] than in nonpregnant women and is more frequent than venous occlusion. The middle cerebral or carotid arteries often are involved. There may be no evident predisposing factors, or risk factors such as diabetes or hypertension may be superimposed on the hypercoagulability of pregnancy. Arterial occlusion is most common in the latter half of pregnancy and in the puerperium. The patient usually presents with the acute onset of neurological symptoms, frequently without headache. Common symptoms are speech, gait, motor, and sensory deficits and ataxia. Rarely, seizures, obtundation, or loss of consciousness may occur. A CAT scan negative for intracranial hemorrhage, lumbar puncture negative for increased pressure and xanthochromia, and a positive arteriogram confirm the diagnosis. Specific diagnosis of underlying disease is necessary. Full evaluation must be carried out in order to provide appropriate management and to decide on the use of anticoagulants or endarterectomy in a gravid patient (Table 37-2).

Recovery is usually slow, with some degree of persistent residual deficit. When seizures or coma are present, prognosis is guarded. Obstetrical management is not dictated by the arterial thrombus. Vaginal delivery without prolonged second stage or strenuous bearing down is preferred over abdominal delivery. The unstable patient is at increased risk in either case, but abdominal delivery is probably more hazardous to her than is vaginal birth.

TABLE 37-2. CAUSES OF CEREBRAL ARTERY OCCLUSION IN PREGNANCY

Hypercoagulability
Severe anemia
Sickle cell disease
Smoking
Arteriosclerosis
Vasculitis
Hypertension
Preeclampsia
Polycythemia
Thrombotic thrombocytopenic purpura
Hyperviscosity
Syphilis
Septicemia
Cardiomyopathy
Valvular heart disease
Paradoxical embolism via patent foramen ovale

Venous Occlusion. Cerebral venous occlusion is less frequent than arterial occlusion but is more prevalent in pregnancy than in the nonpregnant state. The incidence is estimated at about 1/3000 pregnancies,[10,85] with most of these occurring during the second postpartum week. Predisposing factors are dehydration, hypercoagulability, septicemia, vascular endothelial damage, facial or mastoid infection, venous stasis, anemia, and possibly retrograde embolism from pelvic sepsis or phlebitis.[10,85]

Impaired sensorium, headache, and seizures are the most common presentations. Fluctuating lower extremity or upper extremity motor defects, dysphasia, and severe bilateral headache may be prominent after seizures are controlled.

Four major syndromes are related to specific cerebral vein thrombosis. *Cavernous sinus thrombosis* is rare in pregnancy and is related to infection of the face, orbit, or sinuses. It often involves cranial nerves that pass through the cavernous sinus (III, IV, V, and VI) with visual symptoms present. *Lateral sinus thrombosis* usually follows mastoid or ear infection and rarely is seen in pregnancy. It may produce significant papilledema and substantial increase in intracranial pressure. *Sagittal sinus thrombosis* presents with headache, papilledema, and hypertension. Some of these patients go on to suffer seizures, coma, and paraplegia, with a very poor prognosis. The seizures are usually focal, which helps in discriminating between this syndrome and eclampsia. *Cortical venous thrombosis* is more common but sometimes spreads into the sagittal sinus or cerebellar veins. Presentation is usually severe progressive headache followed by dysphasia, weakness, or focal numbness, sometimes progressing to focal seizures. Rarely, the focal seizures may become generalized and progress to stupor or coma, if the thrombus spreads or there is progressive cerebral infarction.

The diagnosis of cerebral venous thrombosis is made by clinical evaluation for underlying medical disease and CAT scan, lumbar puncture, and careful study of the venous phase of a cerebral angiogram. Mortality is 25–30%. Subarachnoid hemorrhage, progression of symptoms, and coma are poor prognostic signs. Residual neurological deficit is variable but usually is less severe than that seen with arterial occlusion.

Management is similar to that for arterial thrombosis, emphasizing control of seizures, lowering blood pressure and intracranial pressure, supportive care, and physical therapy. Delivery may be vaginal when the lesion is stabilized. Bearing down is to be avoided. Patients with recent thrombosis may be better managed by cesarean birth in order to avoid propagation or hemorrhage. Heparinization has been advocated but remains controversial in patients with cerebral venous thrombosis.[24] There are insufficient data to show significant benefit in the pregnant patient. In an uncontrolled study, 10 of 42 heparin-treated patients died, 10 survivors had recurrent seizures, and another 10 had residual focal neurological findings. One of the deaths was related to heparin-induced hemorrhage.[85] In view of the lack of clear benefit and the potential for obstetrical hemorrhage, heparinization is not recommended for the gravida. It may be considered in specific cases in the puerperium.

Carotid Cavernous Fistula. Carotid cavernous fistula occurs more commonly in pregnancy. It may develop spontaneously or secondary to trauma, usually in the last trimester or postpartum.[94] It is rare and in pregnancy is usually a spontaneous shunt between small branches of the internal carotid artery and the cavernous sinus. Symptoms include unilateral frontal headache with ipsilateral conjunctival hyperemia, exophthalmus, and diplopia due to lateral rectus palsy. The diagnosis usually is made by carotid angiogram. During pregnancy, no treatment is indicated unless progressive symptoms of increased proptosis, loss of vision, sensory, motor, or speech deficits develop. Clipping of the affected carotid branches may be indicated if deterioration occurs, despite the increased risks of this procedure during pregnancy. If there is no progression, the symptoms may regress, and the fistula may close spontaneously over several months postpartum.

Intracranial Hemorrhage

The incidence of cerebral hemorrhage is essentially that of subarachnoid hemorrhage, since only 10–15% of patients have a cause other than arteriovenous malformation or aneurysm.[21] It occurs in 1–5/10,000 pregnancies, with a mortality of up to 30%. A-V malformations are the more common cause of cerebrovascular hemorrhage in pregnancy, especially in women 25 years old or less. A history of unilateral headaches, seizures, or bruit makes the diagnosis of A-V malformation more likely. Diagnosis is made by CAT scan, lumbar puncture, and angiogram. The incidence of bleeding is highest in the first half of pregnancy, with an increased risk of intrapartum recurrent bleeding. Thus, untreated lesions require delivery without bearing down. This may be by vaginal or abdominal route, using regional anesthesia. A short second stage and low forceps with epidural block are the preferred methods.

Women with cerebral aneurysms are usually over 30 years of age. They classically bleed in the second and third trimesters and bleed again in labor or postpartum especially. Both aneurysm and A-V malformation may present with headache, nausea, stiff neck, and Brudzinski or other meningeal signs. Diagnosis is the same for both, as is treatment. Sedation, stabilization of blood pressure and vital functions, and steroids for cerebral edema are indicated. Surgical treatment or embolization of the malformation or aneurysm is the therapy of choice. The modality chosen depends on accessibility of the lesion and stability of the patient. Postoperatively, vaginal delivery may be anticipated. Forceps and regional anesthesia are utilized to prevent second stage expulsive efforts. Untreated aneurysms or A-V malformations may rupture or rebleed during the straining of second stage labor. Thus, forceps and regional anesthesia are preferred to spontaneous birth. In patients with A-V malformation or aneurysm who have bleeding in the third trimester, or in whom rapid labor and delivery are not expected, cesarean birth with regional anesthesia is advisable.

Perinatal mortality associated with maternal cerebral hemorrhage from A-V malformation is about 16% and from aneurysm about 10%, primarily due to precarious maternal condition.[77]

SEIZURE DISORDERS

Epilepsy is the most common seizure disorder and one of the most common neurological diseases. It complicates 0.3–0.6% of pregnancies and has many causes: hypoxia, metabolic derangement, head trauma, and diseases such as diabetes, systemic lupus erythematosus, and meningitis.[7,58] Despite multiple possible causes, it is usually idiopathic.

Management of a seizure disorder requires careful evaluation of the patient. When the onset of seizures first occurs in pregnancy, work-up includes a detailed neurological and general physical examination, as well as measurement of glucose, serum electrolytes, and liver function tests, electroencephalogram, and CAT scan. If required, further diagnostic studies such as angiography may be performed, with careful attention to the potential risks to the mother and fetus. The emphasis on medical and metabolic evaluation is significant. Hypoxia, hyponatremia, hypocalcemia,[7,58] and hypoglycemia[59] often are seen in conjunction with seizures in a previously asymptomatic patient. A family history of seizure disorders may alert the physician to a patient at increased risk for seizures during pregnancy. Hypocalcemia-induced epilepsy has been associated with lactation, as well as pregnancy.[29] True gestational epilepsy may occur, with seizures absent in the nonpregnant state. About one-third of such patients have recurrent seizures during a given pregnancy, but not necessarily in subsequent pregnancies.[37] Eclampsia must be ruled out, as definitive treatment for eclampsia requires termination of pregnancy. Once the diagnosis of epilepsy is confirmed, management is the same as for preexistent seizures.

When epilepsy antedates pregnancy and drug levels are maintained in the therapeutic range, the incidence of seizures is not increased during pregnancy.[90] However, predictability of seizures is unreliable, and most studies do not correlate plasma drug levels with seizure frequency. There is no uniformity of philosophy, diagnosis, or treatment of the pregnant epileptic.[21] Pregnant patients may take their medication more rigorously, be unable to take it due to nausea and vomiting, or may be taken off all medication due to the pregnancy. Donaldson reviewed five reports of epilepsy in pregnancy since hydantoin became widely used and found epilepsy worsened in 50%, remained unchanged in 42%, and improved in 8% of gravidas. Maternal age, age of onset of seizures, and number of pregnancies were not related.[21,37] The likelihood of increased seizures during pregnancy is related to the control of seizures before pregnancy occurs. Only 25% of patients with one seizure or less during the nine months before pregnancy had an increased incidence of seizures during pregnancy.[56] This is consistent with the observed unpredictability of recurrent seizures in subsequent pregnancies, since interval control of seizures may vary substantially in a given woman.

When the frequency of seizures is increased by pregnancy, the increase often begins in the first half of pregnancy and often is associated with weight gain and fluid retention.[90] An increased dosage of anticonvulsant drug may be needed due to dilutional effects of rising plasma volume, as well as protein binding changes, increased renal blood flow, decreased absorption, and other effects of the altered physiology and hormonal environment of gestation.[38,39,73] Status epilepticus in pregnancy must be treated vigorously, utilizing intravenous phenytoin as the first-line drug and barbiturates or other agents as needed. Metabolic control and careful attention to airway and cardiovascular state are equally important for this life-threatening condition.[73] Healthy infants may be delivered despite status epilepticus.[37,73]

Nevertheless, epilepsy appears to increase the risk of an adverse outcome of pregnancy. A Norwegian study reported a doubled incidence of low-birth-weight babies, an increase in preterm births, hemorrhage, toxemia, and cesarean birth.[7] However, the American collaborative study did not show increased low-birth-weight infants, although the stillbirth rate was higher.[58] Fetal death may occur with seizures, perhaps secondary to altered placental blood flow. Fetal hypoxia and acidosis and fetal heart rate abnormalities may accompany maternal seizures.[63,89-93] Thus, rapid correction of postictal hypoxemia and acidosis is advisable in gravidas.

Management of epilepsy in pregnant women should be based on the least amount of drug therapy needed to control convulsions. The patient should be tapered off her medication before pregnancy if possible. Many patients so treated will be found to require no drugs at all, particularly when very low blood levels have been present all along in the absence of recent seizures. Those who require maintenance drugs should be stabilized at a low level, consistent with minimal to absent seizure activity. At that point, pregnancy may be undertaken. Prepregnancy counseling regarding fetal and neonatal risks, and close weight and sodium control are advisable. Patients should be followed with monthly determinations of the plasma levels of their medications, even when seizure-free, to assure maintenance of a therapeutic level. Some of the commonly used anticonvulsants are associated with folate deficiency, which in itself is associated with congenital abnormalities; therefore, folic acid supplementation is recommended.[6,48,88]

The most commonly used anticonvulsants—diphenylhydantoin, phenobarbital, and carbamazepine—cross the placenta[51,55] and are associated reportedly with an increased incidence of mental retardation, congenital anomalies such as cleft lip and palate, and cardiac defects. It is unclear whether the causative factor is the drug, pregnancy-associated seizures, a genetic trait passed to the fetus associated with the maternal defect, or increasing susceptibility of the fetus to teratogenesis, expressed as seizure disorder in the mother.[9,31,81] Seizures are noted with greater frequency in the offspring of epileptic mothers, so genetic factors cannot be ruled out. Diphenylhydantoin usage is associated, in up to 11% of exposed fetuses, with a syndrome that includes craniofacial anomalies, mental retardation, growth retardaton, and limb defects. The incidence may be higher if diphenylhydantoin is used in conjunction with phenobarbital. Trimethadione is a potent teratogen associated with a syndrome characterized by palatal abnormalities, with associated speech disturbances, low-set ears, growth retardation, cardiac anomalies, and mental retardation, and should be avoided in favor of other anticonvulsants.[23] The frequency of occurrence of these syndromes is greater in treated epileptic mothers than in untreated ones. The patient with a seizure disorder who is taking antiseizure medications at conception should be counseled regarding a threefold increase in risk of congenital malformations and mental retardation in the newborn.[31] Fetuses exposed to diphenylhydantoin are at a risk as high as 11% for major malformations and up to 30% for minor features compatible with the syndrome. Those exposed to trimethadione have a reported 80–85% risk of serious malformations. Phenobarbital has the lowest risk for malformation of the common anticonvulsants.

Postpartum, the patient's medication dosage needs readjustment downward to nonpregnant therapeutic levels. Although most anticonvulsants are transported in breast milk, the dosage to the newborn is low, and breast-feeding is not contraindicated. The neonates must be observed for a coagulation defect resembling vitamin K deficiency, present in 50% of offspring of mothers on anticonvulsants.[57] Neonatal hemorrhage is infrequent but can be fatal. Nevertheless, with careful obstetric management, the prognosis is good for the epileptic mother and her infant.

SPINAL CORD SYNDROMES

Compression of the spinal cord secondary to enlargement of benign hemangiomas during pregnancy has been reported. Under such circumstance, spinal fluid examination suggests subarachnoid block. Hemangiomas usually decrease in size postpartum. Angiomas are the most common spinal cord tumor in pregnancy.[20] Tumors of the cord also may produce a spinal cord transection syndrome.

Relative newcomers to the prenatal high-risk patient population are paraplegics and quadriplegics. Previously, these patients were felt to have potential for serious morbidity and mortality in pregnancy and were discouraged from conceiving. Recent studies have shown that with some precautions pregnancy can be successful, despite spinal cord transection.

Increasing numbers of young women are sustaining and surviving spinal cord injuries.[76] Transient amenorrhea may follow, but ovulatory cycles and fertility usually return within several months in paraplegic women.[16] Pregnancy in this special population poses many problems. The motor innervation of the bladder and ureters in the paraplegic usually is disrupted. This increases the incidence of urinary stasis and infection. In addition, chronic catheterization increases the risk of cystitis and, consequently, chronic pyelonephritis.[62] Often renal calculi are seen. Management in the antepartum period includes monthly urine cultures, evaluation of renal function, and renal ultrasonography when calculi are suspected. In patients with recurrent cystitis, long-term urinary antiseptic therapy is necessary. Agents such as methyl mandelic acid, nalidixic acid, and nitrofurantoin should be utilized to avoid pyelonephritis (Table 37-3).[99]

Anemia frequently is observed in the pregnant paraplegic.[26] Resultant decreased resistance leads to increased susceptibility to infection, as well as to pressure sores in these relatively immobile patients. Oral and parenteral iron therapy and, in refractory cases, blood transfusions should be employed to maintain a near-normal blood count.[26] The risk of hemorrhage at parturition also must be considered. Although oral iron therapy increases constipation, already present in the paralyzed patient, a stool softener alleviates this problem without risk to mother or fetus. Physiotherapy should be continued throughout pregnancy to prevent pressure sores and preserve flexibility.

The intrapartum management of these patients is complex.[16,62,76,99] Labor is usually painless and rapid and usually occurs before 40 weeks. Signs and symptoms of early labor should be discussed with these patients early in

TABLE 37-3. COMPLICATIONS IN THE PREGNANT PARAPLEGIC

Complication	Occurrence
Autonomic hyperreflexia	Pregnancy, labor, postpartum
Urinary infection	Pregnancy, labor, postpartum
Urinary calculi	Pregnancy, labor, postpartum
Anemia	Pregnancy, labor, postpartum
Decubitus ulcers	Pregnancy, labor, postpartum
Muscle spasm	Pregnancy, labor, postpartum
Premature contractions	Pregnancy, labor
Uterine hyperactivity	Pregnancy, labor
Painless cervical dilation	Labor
Fetal stress	Labor
Thrombophlebitis	Postpartum

the third trimester, as they may experience precipitous delivery. Routine pelvic examination after 32 weeks is advisable, but prophylactic hospitalization is unnecessary.

During pregnancy, most women with spinal cord injury develop episodes of autonomic dysreflexia, frequently just before or during labor. The syndrome arises from the dissociation from hypothalamic control of sympathetic spinal reflexes still active below the lesion, usually T6 or higher. Afferent impulses from a distended or contracting hollow viscus, such as the uterus, bowel, or bladder, reach the spinal cord and stimulate a mass reflex response. Due to the spinal cord transection, there is no modulation by the sensory cortex, so that autonomic hyperreflexia develops. The symptoms include severe paroxysmal hypertension, tachycardia, palpitations, anxiety, diaphoresis, headache, facial flushing, piloerection, blockage of nasal air passages, cardiac arrhythmias and bradycardia. In response to the vasoconstriction-induced hypertension, baroreceptors in the aortic and carotid arch stimulate the vagus nerve, with resultant stimulation of the sinoatrial node to slow the heart. Increased secretion of catecholamines is considered to be responsible for the observed symptoms. Increased levels of catecholamines have been found in the urine of such mothers.[76] The syndrome is life-threatening because stroke may result.[50] Episodes of paroxysmal fetal tachycardia parallel to maternal hypertension and tachycardia have been noted. Despite this, the Apgar score is usually good, and cord and tissue pHs are normal.[99] Autonomic dysreflexia also may be seen antepartum when the bladder is overdistended, for example, with a blocked urinary catheter or a stone.

Management of the laboring paraplegic or quadriplegic should include bladder catheterization to prevent distension from precipitating autonomic hyperreflexia, careful monitoring of maternal vital signs, uterine contractions, and fetal heart rate. Some authors recommend only internal monitoring,[91] but external monitoring has been used safely.[99] Fetal monitoring has revealed marked fetal tachycardia and prolonged accelerations of the fetal heart rate during maternal autonomic hyperreflexia, associated with elevated maternal catecholamines.[99]

Although anesthesia for pain relief is not necessary in most patients, regional anesthesia can be used to block the afferent loop of the autonomic reflex arc to reduce or prevent autonomic hyperreflexia (Table 37-4).[87,96] Substantial distortion of the vertebral column may complicate insertion of the epidural catheter. With conduction anesthesia of all kinds, hypotension must be avoided. Hypotension can lead to fetal acidosis[4] or erratic control of blood pressure with possible stroke. Other agents useful in the management of autonomic hyperreflexia in-

TABLE 37-4. SYMPTOMS OF AUTONOMIC HYPERREFLEXIA

Paroxysmal hypertension
Tachycardia
Cardiac arrhythmia
Bradycardia
Headache
Flushes
Diaphoresis
Piloerection
Pupillary dilation
Blocking of nasal passages
Muscle spasms
Anxiety state
Seizures
Loss of consciousness

clude diphenhydramine hydrochloride, promethazine hydrochloride, and diazepam to alleviate symptoms of anxiety, and hydralazine hydrochloride to treat hypertension.[99] Spasm of the muscles of the abdomen, perineum, and extremities occurs in the paraplegic. In labor, abdominal muscle spasm may lead to irregular uterine contractions, and intravenous pitocin may be necessary to regulate uterine contractility. Conversely, prolonged and severe uterine contractions can also occur, accounting for the frequent precipitous labors (Fig. 37-1).[99]

Cesarean section should be performed for obstetric reasons only. Low forceps occasionally may be needed to avoid a prolonged second stage of labor. Postpartum, the quadriplegic is at increased risk for thrombophlebitis and decubitus ulcers, as well as anemia and infection. Therefore, early mobilization and physiotherapy are indicated. The risk of postpartum hemorrhage is not higher among paraplegics,[76] but blood values should be followed closely since these patients are usually chronically anemic. Lactation is normal and breast-feeding is possible.

With careful management of the antepartum course and close maternal and fetal monitoring in labor, the pregnant patient with spinal cord injury can anticipate good outcome. Autonomic hyperreflexia is a life-threatening danger in the paraplegic and must be treated or prevented to ensure a safe pregnancy.

PERIPHERAL NEUROPATHY

The edema of pregnancy predisposes to a variety of nerve compression syndromes. Labor and delivery compound this effect. Patients with nerve compression syndromes usually present with symptoms of clumsiness, paresthesias, numbness, weakness, and, rarely, loss of reflexes.

Bell's Palsy

Bell's palsy is a common syndrome. It results from compression of the facial nerve as it exits through the stylomastoid foramen and within the bony canal. Its incidence may be increased

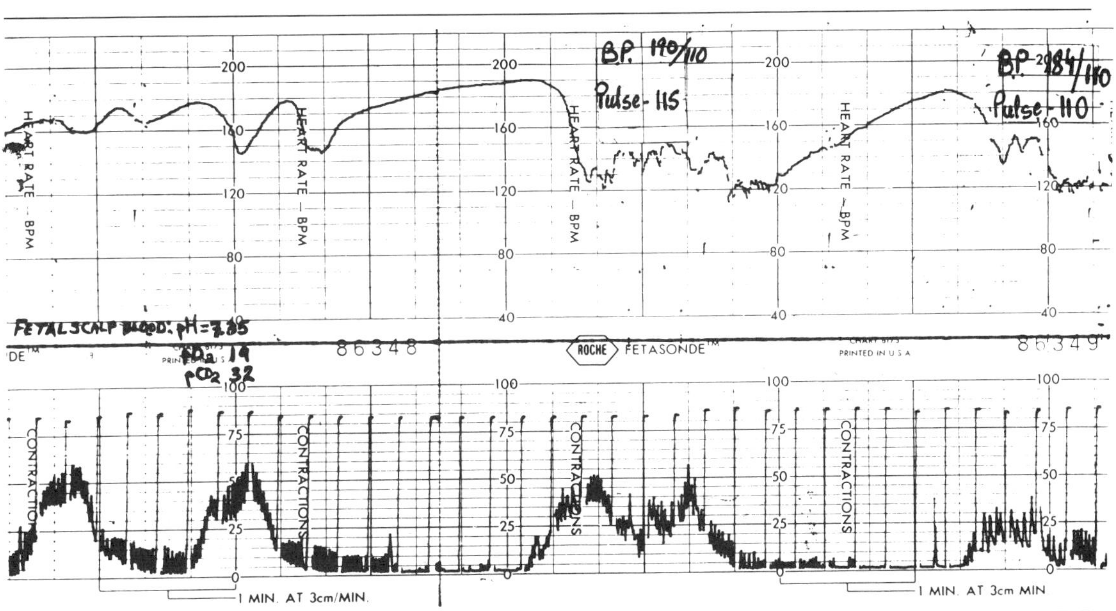

Figure 37-1. Fetal monitoring record showing uterine hyperactivity and intermittent fetal heart rate changes during autonomic hyperreflexia in a paraplegic mother in labor. The neonate was born spontaneously with a normal Apgar score. Continuous tissue pH data shown by the bars on the contraction channel confirm the absence of fetal acidosis, with pH between 7.33 and 7.35 (from Young, B. K., Katz, M., and Klein, S. A.: Pregnancy after spinal cord injury: Altered maternal and fetal response to labor. Obstet. Gynecol. 62:59–63, 1983 with permission.)

in pregnancy, and it may progress to complete paralysis of the face.[2] Recovery is slow, but usually complete, without treatment. Steroid therapy and surgical decompression have been used for paralysis lasting beyond several months postpartum, since about 90% of all lesions have resolved by that time. Steroids also have been advocated for more rapid regression of the paralysis, but the consensus is that specific treatment is unnecessary. Facial massage and ophthalmic solution to prevent corneal abrasion are all that is required until function returns.[47]

Brachial Plexus Syndrome

Brachial plexus syndromes may present with numbness, tingling, and weakness of the hand and arm, most commonly in an ulnar distribution. It may be brachial neuritis, which is often familial and recurrent with subsequent pregnancies, or pressure neuropathy due to breast enlargement and position while sleeping. When severe, there may be pain radiating to the whole arm. Mild anti-inflammatory agents and physical therapy may be helpful.[92]

Carpal Tunnel Syndrome

Carpal tunnel syndrome is the most common peripheral neuropathy seen in pregnancy. It develops from compression of the median nerve at the wrist. Weakness and pain in the pronators of the forearm, long finger flexors, and abductor and opponens muscles of the thumb ensue. Sensory impairment, tingling, and loss of coordination of the hand may be present in varying degrees. When necessary, splinting and local steroid injections may be helpful, but treatment seldom is needed. Symptoms beginning during pregnancy usually abate postpartum. Electrophysiologic studies confirm the diagnosis.

Intercostal Neuralgia

Intercostal neuralgia is another common neuropathy in pregnancy. Typically, the patient complains of severe pain over the lower ribs and upper abdomen. The pain is increased by fetal movements and physical activity and the sitting or lying position.[98] There may be an area of dysesthesia in the same location as the pain. The cause is probably entrapment or torsion of the intercostal nerves or perhaps stretching of the costochondral joints. There is no treatment, but the pain resolves very promptly postpartum.[69]

Lower Extremity Syndromes

Pregnancy predisposes to lower extremity lesions, particularly lumbosacral plexus and peripheral nerve syndromes. Intervertebral disk protrusion, nerve stretching, compression, or injury, especially with anesthesia and difficult delivery, all contribute to the lower extremity neuropathies seen in pregnancy and postpartum.

Lumbosacral plexus syndromes usually are seen as postpartum sensory and motor abnormalities, although they may occur antepartum as well. Depending on the nerves involved, different symptoms appear. Lumbosacral trauma, with pelvic compression of the fibers forming the peroneal nerve, is often due to a snug fit between the fetal vertex and the pelvis associated with midforceps delivery, relative disproportion, and flat posterior pelvis.[97]

With *peroneal nerve trauma*, the patient complains of weakness of the leg, with foot-drop and decreased sensation over the anterolateral aspect of the leg and dorsal foot in severe cases. The peroneal nerve may be compressed at the head of the fibula when the patient is in stirrups in the lithotomy position, as well. Correct positioning at delivery and properly padded stirrups help to avoid this complication.

Meralgia paresthetica presents with numbness, paresthesias, dysesthesias, and pain in the midlateral thigh.[36] It usually results from entrapment of the lateral femoral cutaneous nerve anywhere along its path from the second and third lumbar roots, along the iliac muscles, and under the inguinal ligament to the skin of the thigh. Symptoms usually begin at about 30 weeks of pregnancy, related to the progressive lordosis and weight gain that cause stretching of the nerve.[66,75] The symptoms disappear slowly without treatment, usually by three months postpartum.

Other lower extremity syndromes may result from compression of the nerves subject to stretching or compression during pregnancy or obstetrical procedures. The *obturator nerve* is vulnerable to trauma during delivery, to compression from a hematoma, or to stretching, with adductor weakness and sensory symptoms over the medial thigh. The *genitofemoral nerve* may be traumatized by self-retaining retractors at abdominal surgery, by compression from an adjacent hematoma, and by torsion in pregnancy. The syndrome appears as quadriceps weakness, depressed knee-jerk, and anterior thigh dysesthesia. Both obturator and femoral nerve syndromes are uncommon.

Sciatic nerve compression, which is the most common of the *lumbosacral plexus syndromes*, very frequently appears antepartum. Lordosis and fetal head compression result in low back pain and typical "sciatica" symptoms. A variety of symptoms of weakness, dysesthesias, pain, and diminished reflexes may be present in pregnancy, depending on the site of nerve compression and the degree of radicular stretching. The prognosis for these symptom complexes is excellent, with postpartum recovery the rule. They may be evaluated by electromyography to determine the rate of recovery and eventual prognosis and to rule out underlying disease. Physiotherapy and, rarely, splinting may be helpful, but no treatment is usually necessary.

Lumbosacral Disk Disease

Lumbosacral disk disease may be exacerbated or induced by pregnancy, with development of typical symptoms of neuropathy. Low back pain and sciatic pain due to disk disease appear for the first time in pregnancy or the puerperium in 76% of women with diagnosed disk disease.[60]

The weight gain, lordosis, changes in connective tissue, and loosening of joints associated with pregnancy may predispose to prolapse of lumbosacral disks. Most disk extrusions involve the fifth lumbar or first sacral roots, causing low back pain that radiates down the back of the lower extremity to the foot, the typical sciatic pain. The pain is exacerbated by standing, Lesague's maneuver, prolonged sitting, and Valsalva's maneuver. There may be loss of sensation and decreased or absent knee or ankle reflexes, depending on the nerve roots compressed. Rarely, there is severe extrusion of a disk with loss of bowel or bladder control and bilateral leg weakness or reflex loss. Usually, there is spasm of the back muscles and tenderness over the lumbosacral spine. Electromyography may be useful in differentiating disk disease from peripheral neuropathy. If the symptoms are not severe, further diagnostic tests sch as CAT scan may be deferred until postpartum. Therapy in pregnancy is usually bed rest with a bed board, heat, massage, acetaminophen, an abdominal and back support and avoidance of high-heeled shoes. When labor begins, it should be carried out in the lateral decubitus position with good analgesia, careful moving of the patient, shortening of the second stage with forceps or vacuum extraction, and positioning for delivery wih minimal flexion of the hips. Postpartum, definitive diagnosis and treatment may be carried out.

Traumatic Neuropathy

"Postpartum foot drop" is caused by trauma to the lateral peroneal nerve during delivery with the use of stirrups or following damage to the lumbosacral plexus at L4 and L5 during vaginal birth, for example, with midforceps delivery for transverse arrest. Other traumatic neuropathies also may occur. Obturator nerve injury may follow compression by the fetal head, or the lithotomy position, or pelvic surgery. An abnormal gait and numbness and pain in the medial thigh, hip, and groin may result. The lithotomy position may predispose to femoral neuropathy involving the anterior and medial aspect of the thigh and leg; sciatic neuropathy with sensory loss along the back of the leg and dorsal foot; and saphenous neuropathy, affecting the anterior medial leg below the knee. All these syndromes usually resolve slowly without treatment. Treatment requires physical therapy. Symptoms usually disappear within several months.

NEUROLOGICAL DISORDERS SPECIFIC TO PREGNANCY

The most common complications in the pregnant patient relate to hypertensive disease. Hypertensive disease associated with preeclampsia and eclamptic seizures are discussed in detail in Chapter 32. These pregnancy-specific entities present with neurological symptoms. The neurological symptoms seen with preeclampsia include visual abnormalities such as diplopia, blurred vision, spots or flashes before the eyes, as well as hyprreflexia, clonus, and headache. These indicate severe preeclampsia. Acute grand mal seizures define eclampsia. Treatment of eclampsia requires control of seizures, stabilization of the mother's condition, and prompt delivery.

Besides the clinical diagnosis of eclampsia, many other causes exist for acute onset of seizures in pregnancy. A careful diagnostic evaluation must be made to eliminate the other etiologies, with diligent use of the available means for neurological assessment.

In eclampsia, as in all seizure disorders, the

EEG is acutely abnormal. The abnormalities usually disappear completely by six weeks postpartum but have persisted up to six months in some patients.[82] Computerized tomography and arteriography in eclamptics with transient neurological deficits such as cortical blindness or coma are usually negative for specific lesions. They may be negative for evidence of cerebral edema. However, eclampsia can be associated with cerebral edema, hyperemia, thrombosis, and hemorrhage. Postmortem examinations of fatal cases of eclampsia revealed hemorrhagic lesions in the brain in 78 of 110 patients.[25]

Thus, the syndrome of eclampsia may exist without demonstrable brain lesions or may be associated with a variety of cerebral lesions including edema, hyperemia, thrombosis, and hemorrhage. Unless a specific cause for the seizure is found, the patient is considered to be eclamptic.

FETAL NEUROLOGICAL DISORDERS

The diagnosis of fetal neurological abnormalities has become possible through recent advances in medicine. Significant innovations include the antepartum diagnosis of fetal neural tube defects, the diagnosis and possible in utero treatment of fetal intracranial abnormalities, and the demonstration of fetal brain tumors.

Abnormalities of the nervous system are among the most common congenital malformations. The reported incidence varies from 1 to 8/1000, depending on geographic location. The reported incidence in the United States in an unselected population is 1–2/1000. The risk of recurrence is increased in families with an affected child. [43] Failure of neural plate development in the head is believed to produce anencephaly. Associated defects in the spinal cord are thought to result in spina bifida. The consequences of bearing an anencephalic or spina bifida infant can be devastating for the family. Anencephaly is not compatible with survival. Spina bifida patients exhibit a range of associated abnormalities including paralysis, impaired sensation below the level of the defect, incontinence of bowel and bladder, and communicating hydrocephalus. Some of these patients have diminished intelligence, but most are of normal intelligence. The early prenatal diagnosis of these defects offers parents the option for termination and prepares the neonatal team for management of the affected newborn. Alpha-fetoprotein (AFP) is a stable protein produced by the fetus in large amounts in the early second trimester. Any lesion that allows leakage

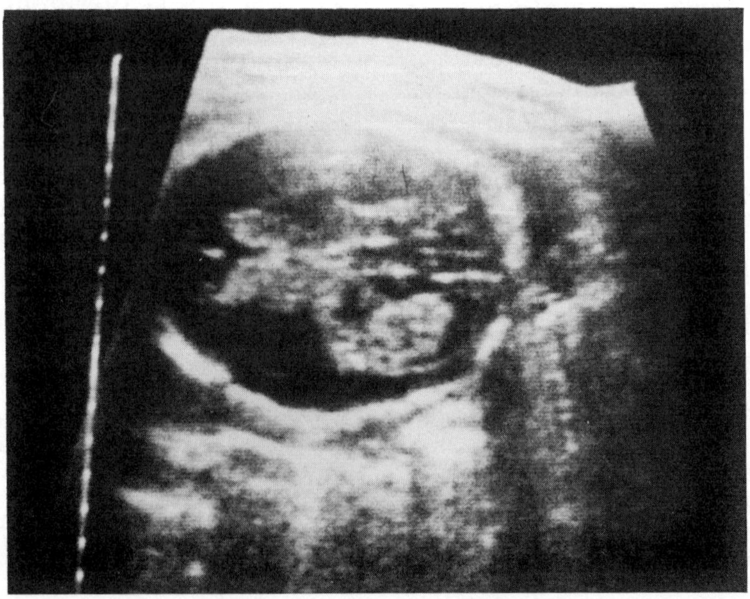

Figure 37-2. Sonogram showing intraventricular hemmorhage in a living intrauterine fetus at 31 weeks' gestation (from Lustig-Gillman, I., Snyder, J. R., Silverman, F., and Young, B. K.: Sonographic anatomy of the fetal cerebral ventricles, with reference to the early diagnosis of hydrocephaly. J. Perinat. Med. 12: 185–191, 1984, with permission.)

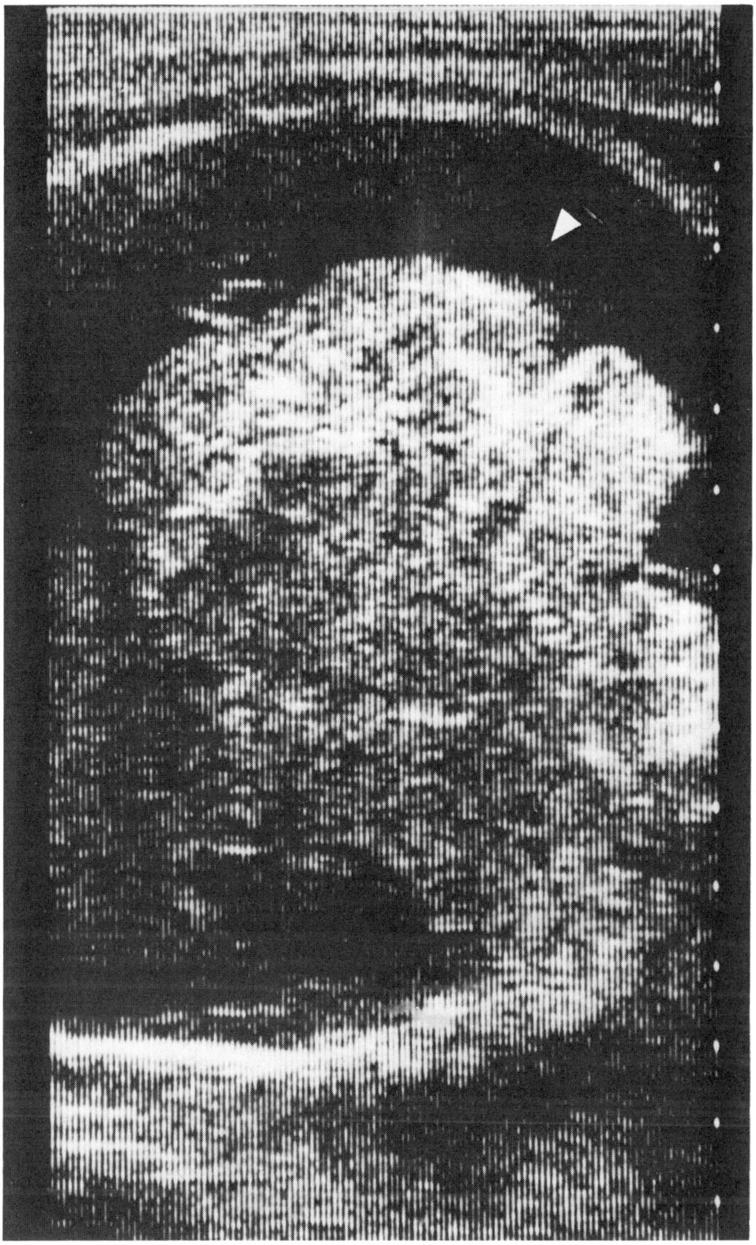

Figure 37-3. Sonogram of fetal head antepartum. Intracranial mass replaces normal anatomical structures. Arrow head shows peripheral fluid around mass (Snyder, J. R., Lustig-Gillman, I., Milio, L., Morris, M., Pardes, J. G., and Young, B. K.: Antenatal ultrasound diagnosis of an intracranial neoplasm—craniopharyngioma. J. Clin. Ultrasound 14: 304–306, 1986, with permission.)

of fetal serum into amniotic fluid increases the intra-amniotic and maternal serum concentrations of alpha-fetoprotein. These lesions include open neural tube defects, encephalocele, imperforate anus, gastroschisis, esophageal atresia, omphalocele, amniotic band syndrome, and congenital nephrosis. Alpha-fetoprotein also is elevated in normal multiple pregnancies.[34]

A protocol for maternal AFP screening has been described and implemented in the United States on Long Island, New York.[44] This protocol involves screening an unselected patient population by measuring maternal serum alpha-fetoprotein levels. An elevation of AFP in two samples drawn at least one week apart places the patient in a high-risk group for neural tube defects. Because values for alpha-fetoprotein are correlated with gestational age, accurate dating of the pregnancy is important, using all criteria available. Patients with elevated AFP in maternal serum then undergo diagnostic ultrasound. Unless multiple pregnancy is diagnosed, amniocentesis is done to obtain amniotic fluid in which to determine alpha-fetoprotein and acetylcholinesterase levels. Six percent of 365 patients undergoing amniocentesis for elevated maternal serum alpha-fetoprotein carried a fetus with open neural tube defects.[43,44]

Because of the time dependency of the initial test and the need for a coordinated approach to diagnosis and intervention, large-scale screening programs in the United States are still under development. Such programs seem likely to be practical in view of their success in Great Britain[8] and in view of recent reports relating low alpha-fetoprotein to chromosomal defects[52] and to intrauterine growth retardation.[46]

Ultrasonography makes possible the diagnosis of fetal neurological disorders including fetal neural tube defects. Development of scanners with improved resolution has permitted early diagnosis of fetal hydrocephalus. It is now

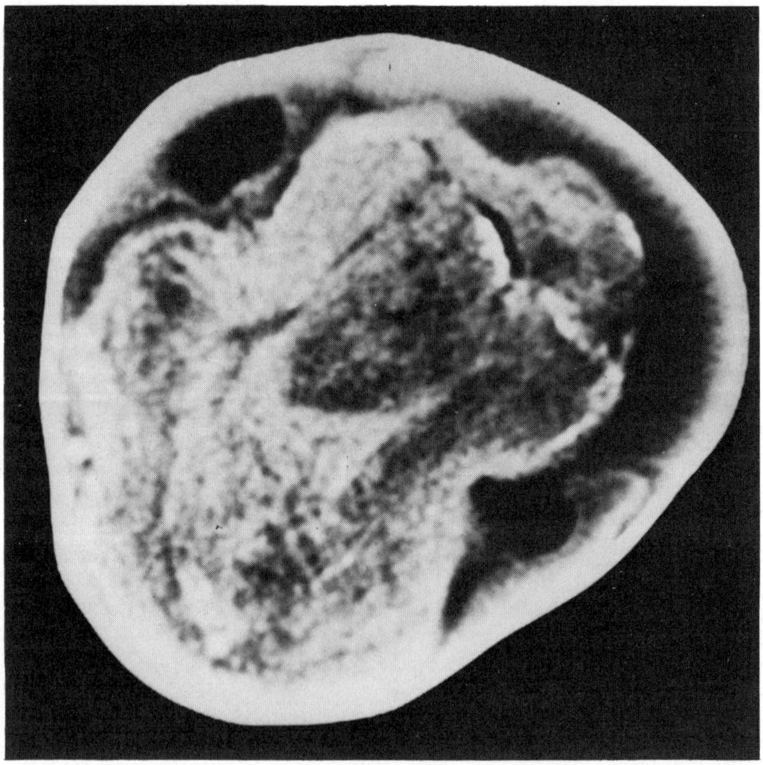

Figure 37-4. CT scan of fetal head postpartum, confirming sonogram with craniopharyngioma obliterating normal anatomy, and peripheral fluid around tumor mass (from Snyder, J. R., Lustig-Gillman, I., Milio, L., Morris, M., Pardes, J. G., and Young, B. K.: Antenatal ultrasound diagnosis of an intracranial neoplasm—craniopharyngioma. J. Clin. Ultrasound 14:304–306, 1986, with permission.)

possible to diagnose hydrocephalus before the circumference of the fetal head is enlarged, by measuring ventricular size and width.[41] The rate of development of the disorder is followed with serial ultrasound examinations. The timing of intervention depends on the rate of fluid accumulation, the persistence of fetal cortex, and the assessment of fetal maturity. Shunting procedures have been performed in utero, but the neonatal outcomes have been dismal.[14] Thus, early delivery and neonatal shunting are performed on fetuses mature enough to withstand surgery. In the event that respiratory distress syndrome and other problems associated with prematurity complicate the neonatal course, repeated lumbar punctures are performed to maintain cerebrospinal fluid pressure at an acceptable level.

Primary hemorrhage of the fetal cerebral ventricles is extremely rare but has been demonstrated in the living intrauterine fetus (Fig. 37-2). Fetal intraventricular hemorrhage is suggested as a possible mechanism for development of hydrocephaly and fetal demise.[42] Further studies are required to elucidate this interesting question. Similarly, hydranencephaly and other types of porencephaly with congenital partial brain agenesis have been ascribed to cerebral artery occlusion in the fetus. Early thrombosis of the anterior or middle cerebral arteries produces destruction of the fetal brain areas they supply.[2]

Finally, antepartum diagnosis of fetal intracranial tumors is possible via sonography. Teratomas[17] and a craniopharyngioma[83] have been described thus far (Figs. 37-3 and 37-4). Such early diagnosis offers hope for neurosurgical treatment of the newborn and raises the possibility of fetal neurosurgery. The fetus is now accessible to neurological diagnosis and may possibly be accessible to therapy in the future.

REFERENCES

1. Adams, R. D. and Victor, M.: Principles of Neurology, 2nd Edition. New York, McGraw-Hill Book Co., 1981.
2. Adorer, K. K. and Wingerd, J.: Idiopathic facial paralysis (Bell's palsy): Factors affecting severity and outcome in 446 patients. *Neurology* **24**:1112–1116, 1974.
3. Allen, J., Eldridge, R., and Koerber, T.: Acoustic neuroma in the last months of pregnancy. , *Am. J. Obstet. Gynecol.* **119**:516–520, 1974.
4. Antoine, C. and Young, B. K.: Fetal lactic acidosis with epidural anesthesia. *Am. J. Obstet. Gynecol.* **142**:55–59, 1982.
5. Bender, A. N., Ringel, S. P., Engel, W. K., Daniels, M. P., and Vogel, Z.: Myasthenia gravis: A serum factor blocking acetylcholamine receptors of the human neuromuscular junction. *Lancet* **1**:607–609, 1975.
6. Biale, Y., Lewentha, H., and Ben-Adereth, N.: Congenital malformations and decreased blood levels of folic acid induced by antiepileptic drugs. *Acta Obstet. Gynecol. Scand.* **55**:187, 1976.
7. Bjerkedal, T. and Bahna, S. L.: The occurrence and outcome of pregnancy in women with epilepsy. *Acta Obstet. Gynecol. Scand.* **52**:245–248, 1973.
8. Brock, D. J. H., Bolton, A. E., and Monaghan, J. M.: Prenatal diagnosis of anencephaly through maternal serum alpha-fetoprotein measurements. *Lancet* **2**:923–924, 1973.
9. Bustamente, S. A. and Stumpff, L. C.: Fetal hydantoin syndrome in triplets. *Am. J. Dis. Child.* **132**:978–979, 1968.
10. Carroll, J. D., Leak, D., and Lee, H. A.: Cerebral thrombophlebitis in pregnancy and the puerperium. *Q. J. Med.* **35**:347–368, 1966.
11. Catanzarite, V. A., McHargue, A. M., Sandberg, E. C., and Dyson, D. C.: Respiratory arrest during therapy for premature labor in a patient with myasthenia gravis. *Obstet. Gynecol.* **64**:819–822, 1984.
12. Cendrowski, W.: Multiple sclerosis in parents and children. *Acta Neurol.* **45**:380–382, 1969.
13. Cendrowski, W.: Multiple sclerosis in twins and other relatives. *Acta Neurol.* **49**:552–556, 1973.
14. Chervenak, F., Berkowitz, R. L., and Romero, R.: The diagnosis of fetal hydrocephalus. *Am. J. Obstet. Gynecol. 147*:703–716, 1983.
15. Cohen, B. A., London, R. S., and Goldstein, P. J.: Myasthenia gravis and pre-eclampsia. *Obstet. Gynecol.* **48**:35S–37S, 1976.
16. Comarr, E.: Observations on menstruation and pregnancy among female spinal cord injury patients. *Paraplegia* **3**:263–271, 1966.
17. Crde, M.: Ultrasonic demonstration in utero of an intracranial teratoma. *JAMA* **247**:1173, 1982.
18. Cross, J. M., Costas, P. O., and Jennett, W. B.: Cerebral strokes associated with pregnancy and the puerperium, *Br. Med. J.* **3**:214–218, 1968.
19. Digre, K. B.; Varner, M. W., and Corbett, J. J.: Pseudotumor cerebri and pregnancy. *Neurology* **34**:721–729, 1984.
20. Divers, S.: A spinal cord neurolemmoma in pregnancy. *Obstet. Gynecol.* **52**:47S–50S, 1978.
21. Donaldson, J. O.: *Neurology of Pregnancy*. Philadelphia, W. B. Saunders Co., 1978.
22. Dublin, A. B. and French, B. N.: Diagnostic image evaluation of hydranencephaly and pictorially similar entities with emphasis on computed tomography. *Radiology* **137**:81–91, 1980.
23. Fedman, G. L., Weaver, D. D., and Lovrien, E. W.:

The fetal trimethadione syndrome. *Am. J. Dis. Child.* **131**:1389–1392, 1977.

24. Gettelfinger, D. M. and Kokmen, E.: Superior sagittal sinus thrombosis. *Arch. Neurol.* **34**:2–6, 1977.
25. Govan, A. D. T.: The pathogenesis of eclamptic lesions. *Pathol. Microbiol. (Basel)* **24**:561–575, 1961.
26. Greenland, V. C. and Young, B. K.: When the mother is a paraplegic. *Contemp. OB/GYN* **24**:201–210, 1984.
27. Gunn, A. and Sanderson, B. W.: Myasthenia gravis complicating pregnancy. *Br. J. Obstet. Gynaecol.* **56**:868–871, 1949.
28. Hanson, J. W. and Buehler, B. A.: Fetal hydantoin syndrome: Current status. *J. Pediatr.* **101**:816–818, 1982.
29. Harrod, R. A. and Kennedy, P. G.: Hypocalcaemia-induced epilepsy during lactation. *Br. Med. J.* **285**:607–608, 1982.
30. Harter, C. A. and Benirschke, K.: Fetal syphilis in the first trimester. *Am. J. Obstet. Gynecol.* **124**:705–711, 1976.
31. Hill, R., Verniaud, W. M., Horning, M. G., McCulley, L. B., and Morgan, N. F.: lnfants exposed in utero to antiepileptic drugs. *Am. J. Dis. Child.* **127**:645–652, 1974.
32. Hokkanen, E.: The aggravating effects of some antibiotics on the neuromuscular blockade in myasthenia gravis. *Acta Neurol. Scand.* **40**:346–352, 1964.
33. Hughes, R. A. C., Newson-Davies, J. M., Perken, G. D., and Pierce, J. M.: Controlled trial of prednisone in acute polyneuropathy. *Lancet* **2**:750–753, 1978.
34. Ishiguro, T.: Alpha fetoprotein in twin pregnancy. *Lancet* **ffl**:1214, 1973.
35. Jones, M. W. and Berry, K.: Chronic relapsing polyneuritis associated with pregnancy. *Ann. Neurol.* **9**:413, 1981.
36. Jones, R. K.: Meralgia paresthetica as a cause of leg discomfort. *Can. Med. Assoc. J.* **111**:541–542, 1974.
37. Knight, A. H. and Rhind, E. G.: Epilepsy and pregnancy: A study of 153 pregnancies in 59 patients. *Epilepsia* **16**:99–110, 1975.
38. Lander, C. M., Edwards, V. E., Eadie, M. J., and Tyrer, J. H.: Plasma anticonvulsant concentrations during pregnancy. *Neurology* **27**:128–131, 1977.
39. Landon, M. J. and Kirkley, M.: Metabolism of diphenylhydantoin (phenytoin) during pregnancy. *Br. J. Obstet. Gynaecol.* **86**:125–132, 1979.
40. Lefyert, A. K. and Osterman, P. O.: Newborn infants to myasthenic mothers: A clinical study and an investigation of acetylcholine receptor antibodies in 17 children. *Neurology* **33**:133–138, 1983.
41. Lustig-Gillman, I., Snyder, J. R., Silverman, F., and Young, B. K.: Sonographic anatomy of the fetal cerebral ventricles, with reference to the early diagnosis of hydrocephaly. *J. Perinat. Med.* **12**:185–191, 194.
42. Lustig-Gillman, I., Young, B. K., Silverman, F., Raghavendra, B. N., Wan, L., Reitz, H. E., Aleksic, S., Greco, A., and Snyder, J. R.: Fetal intraventricular hemorrhage: Sonographic diagnosis and clinical implications. *J. Clin. Ultrasound* **11**:277–280, 1983.
43. Macri, J.: Neural tube defects and alpha fetoprotein. In: *Gynecology and Obstetrics*. J. J. Sciarra (Ed.). Philadelphia, Harper & Row, 1984.
44. Macri, J. N. and Weiss, R. W.: Prenatal serum alpha fetoprotein screening for neural tube defects. *Obstet. Gynecol.* **59**:633–638, 1982.
45. March, C. M., Kletzky, O. A., Davajan, V., Teal, J., Weiss, M., Apuzza, M. L., Mairs, R. P., and Mishell, D. R., Jr.: Longitudinal evaluation of patients with untreated prolactin secreting pituitary adenoma. *Am. J. Obstet. Gynecol.* **139**:835–844, 1981.
46. Mariona, F. G., Hassan, M. M., Synder, F. N., Chik, L. C., and Sokol, R. J.: Maternal serum alpha fetoprotein (MSAFP) and fetal growth. *J. Perinat. Med.* **12**:179–183, 1984.
47. Massey, E. W. and Cefalo, R. C.: Neuropathies of pregnancy. *Obstet. Gynecol. Surv.* **34**:489–492, 1979.
48. Maxwell, J. D., Hunter, J., Stewart, P. A., Ardeman, S., and Williams, R.: Folate deficiency after anticonvulsant drugs: An effect of hepatic enzyme induction. *Br. Med. J.* **1**:297–299, 1972.
49. McAlpine, D.: Some aspects of the natural history: Familial incidence and its significance. In: *Multiple Sclerosis: A Reappraisal*, 2nd edition. D. McAlpine, C. E. Lumsden, and E. D. Achison (Eds.). Edinburgh, Churchill, Livingston, 1972, pp. 42–98.
50. McGregor, J. A. and Meeuwsen, J.: Autonomic hyperreflexia: A mortal danger for spinal cord-damaged women in labor. *Am. J. Obstet. Gynecol.* **151**:330–333, 1985.
51. Melchior, J. C., Svensmark, O., and Troll, D.: Placental transfer of phenobarbitone inepileptic women and elimination in newborns. *Lancet* **2**:860–861, 1967.
52. Merkatz, I. R., Nitowsky, H. M., Macri, J. N., and Johnson, W. E.: An association between low maternal serum alpha fetoprotein and fetal chromosomal abnormalities. *Am. J. Obstet. Gynecol.* **148**:886–894, 1984.
53. Michelsen, J. J. and New, P. F. J.: Brain tumour and pregnancy. *J. Neurol. Neurosurg. Psychiatry* **32**:305–307, 1969.
54. Minielly,R., Yuzpe, A. A., and Drake, C. G.: Subarachnoid hemorrhage secondary to ruptured cerebral aneurysm in pregnancy. *Obstet. Gynecol.* **53**:64–70, 1979.
55. Mirken, B. L.: Diphenylhydantoin in placental transport, fetal localizaton, neonatal metabolism and possible teratogenic effects. *J. Pediatr.* **78**:329–338, 1971.
56. Montouris, G. D., Fenichel, G. M., and McLain, L.

W., Jr.: The pregnant epileptic: A review and recommendations. *Arch. Neurol.* **36**:601-603, 1979.

57. Mountain, K. R., Hirsch, J., and Gallos, A. S.: Neonatal coagulation defect due to anticonvulsant drug treatment in pregnancy. *Lancet* **1**:265-268, 1970.
58. Niswander, K. R. and Gordon, M.: The Collaborative Perinatal Study of the National Institute of Neurological Diseases and Stroke. Dept. of Health, Education, and Welfare Publication No. NIH-73-379, Washington, DC, 1972.
59. Notterman, R. B., Jovanovic, L., Peterson, R., Solomon, G., Druzin, M., and Peterson, C. M.: Spontaneous hypoglycemic seizures in pregnancy. *Arch. Intern. Med.* **144**:189-191, 1984.
60. O'Connell, J. E. A.: Lumbar disc protrusions in pregnancy. *J. Neurol. Neurosurg. Psychiatry* **23**:138-141, 1960.
61. Ohta, M., Matsubara, F., Hayashi, K., Nakao, K., and Nishitani, H.: Acetylcholamine receptor antibodies in infants of mothers with myasthenia gravis. *Neurology* **31**:1019-1022, 1982.
62. Oppenheimer, W. M.: Pregnancy in paraplegic patients: Two case reports. *Am. J. Obstet. Gynecol.* **110**:784-786, 1971.
63. Orringer, C. E., Eustace, J. C., Wunsch, C. D., and Gardner, L. B.: Natural history of lactic acidosis after grand mal seizures. *N. Engl. J. Med.* **297**:796-799, 1977.
64. Osserman, K. E.: *Symposium on Myasthenia Gravis.* New York, Grune & Stratton, 1975.
65. Osserman, K. E., Kornfeld, P., Cohen, E., Genkins, G., Mendelow, H., Goldberg, H., Windsley, H., and Kaplan, L. I.: Studies in myasthenia gravis. *Arch. Intern. Med.* **102**:72-81, 1958.
66. Pearson, M. G.: Meralgia paresthetica: With reference to its occurrence in pregnancy. *J. Obstet. Gynaecol. Br. Emp.* **64**:427-430, 1957.
67. Plauche, W.: Myasthenia gravis in pregnancy. *Am. J. Obstet. Gynecol.* **88**:404-409, 1964.
68. Plauche, W.: Myasthenia gravis in pregnancy: An update. *Am. J. Obstet. Gynecol.* **135**:691-697, 1979.
69. Pleet, A. B. and Massey, E. W.: Intercostal neuralgia of pregnancy. *JAMA* **243**:770, 1980.
70. Poser, S. and Poser, W.: Multiple sclerosis and gestation. *Neurology* **33**:1422-1427, 1983.
71. Poser, S. and Poser, W.: Reply from the authors. *Neurology* **34**:704-705, 1984.
72. Powell, J. L.: Pseudotumor cerebri and pregnancy. *Obstet. Gynecol.* **40**:713-718, 1972.
73. Ramsey, R. E., Strauss, R. G., Wilder, B. J., and Willmore, L. J.: Status epilepticus in pregnancy: Effect of phenytoin malabsorption on seizure control. *Neurology* **28**:85-89, 1978.
74. Reeves, D. L.: Tumors of the brain complicating pregnancy. *West. J. Surg. Obstet. Gynecol.* **60**:211-219, 1952.
75. Rhodes, P.: Meralgia paresthetica in pregnancy. *Lancet* **2**:831, 1957.
76. Robertson, D. N. S. and Guttman, I.: The paraplegic patient in pregnancy and labour. *Proc. R. Soc. Med.* **156**:381-387, 1963.
77. Robinson, J. L., Hall, C. I., and Sedzimir, C. B.: Arteriovenous malformations, aneurysms, and pregnancy. *J. Neurosurg.* **41**:63-70, 1973.
78. Rolbin, S. H., Levinson, G., Shnider, S. M., and Wright, R. G.: Anesthetic considerations for myasthenia gravis and pregnancy. *Anesth. Analg.* **57**:441-447, 1978.
79. Rudolph, J. H., Norris, F. H., Garvey, P. H., and Friederich, M. A.: The Landry Guillain-Barre syndrome in pregnancy: A review. *Obstet. Gynecol.* **26**:265-271, 1965.
80. Scheinhorn, D. J. and Angelillo, V. A.: Antituberculous therapy in pregnancy: Risks to the fetus. *West. J. Med.* **127**:195-198, 1971.
81. Shapiro, S., Hartz, S., Siskind, V., Mitchell, A. A., Slone, D., Rosenberg, L., Monson, R. R., Heinonen, O. P., Idanpaan-Heikkila, J., Saxon, L., and Haro, S.: Anticonvulsants and parental epilepsy in the development of birth defects. *Lancet* **1**:272-275, 1976.
82. Sibai, B., Spinnato, J. A., Watson, D. L., Lewis, J. A., and Anderson, G. D.: Eclampsia IV: Neurologic findings and future outcome. Submtted for publication, 1985.
83. Snyder, J. R., Lustig-Gillman, I., Milio, L., Morris, M., Pardes, J. G., and Young, B. K.: Antenatal ultrasound diagnosis of an intracranial neoplasm—craniopharyngioma. *J. Clin. Ultrasound.* **14**:304-306, 1986.
84. Speroff, L., Glass, R. H., and Kase, N. G.: *Clinical Gynecologic Endocrinology and Infertility*, 3rd Edition. Baltimore, Williams & Wilkins, 1983.
85. Srinivassan, K.: Cerebral venous and arterial thrombosis in pregnancy and the puerperium: Study of 135 patients. *Angiology* **34**:731-746, 1983.
86. Stephanoupoulos, C.: The development of tuberculous meningitis during pregnancy. *Am. Rev. Tuberc.* **76**:1079-1087, 1957.
87. Stirt, J. A., Marco, A., and Conklin, K. A.: Obstetric anesthesia for a quadriplegic patient with autonomic hyperreflexia. *Anesthesiology* **51**:560-562, 1979.
88. Stone, M. L.: Effects on the fetus of folic acid deficiency in pregnancy. *Clin. Obstet. Gynecol.* **11**:1143-1153, 1968.
89. Suidan, J. S. and Young, B. K.: Outcome of fetuses with lactic acidemia. *Am. J. Obstet. Gynecol.* **150**:33-37, 1984.
90. Suter, C. and Klingman, W. O.: Seizure states and pregnancy. *Neurology* **7**:105-118, 1957.
91. Tabsh, K., Brinkman, C. R., II, and Reff, R. A.: Autonomic dysreflexia in pregnancy. *Obstet. Gynecol.* **60**:119-121, 1982.
92. Taylor, R. A.: Heridofamilial mononeuritis multiplex with brachial redilection. *Brain* **83**:113-137, 1960.
93. Teramo, K., Hiilesmaa, V., Bardy, A., and Saari-

kosi, S.: Fetal heart rate during a maternal grand mal epileptic seizure. *J. Perinat. Med.* **7**:3–6, 1979.
94. Toya, S., Shiobara, R., Izumi, J., Shinomiya, Y., Shiga, H., and Kimura, C.: Spontaneous carotid cavernous fistula during pregnancy or in the postpartum stage. *J. Neurosurg.* **54**:252–256, 1981.
95. Turkalj, I., Braun, P., and Krupp, P.: Surveillance of bromocriptine in pregnancy. *JAMA* **247**:-1589–1591, 1982.
96. Watson, D. W. and Downey, G. O.: Epidural anesthesia for labor and delivery of twins of a paraplegic mother. *Anesthesiology* **52**:259–261, 1980.
97. Whittaker, W. G.: Injuries to the sacral plexus in obstetrics. *J. Can. Med. Assoc.* **79**:622–627, 1978.
98. Young, B. K.: Unpublished data.
99. Young, B. K., Katz, M., and Klein, S. A.: Pregnancy after spinal cord injury: Altered maternal and fetal response to labor. *Obstet. Gynecol.* **62**:59–63, 1983.

38

FEVER AND INFECTIONS

Body temperature normally is elevated about 0.5 °F (0.3 °C) in pregnancy, probably as a result of increased progesterone levels. A further rise in temperature is one of the most common signs of infection, but it also may be the result of noninfectious processes such as drug reaction, lymphoma, and collagen disease.

In infections, the febrile response is mediated by endogenous pyrogen, a protein of molecular weight 10,000–20,000, which is elaborated by polymorphonuclear leukocytes and macrophages, probably during phagocytosis.[34] Endogenous pyrogen acts on the temperature center in the anterior hypothalamus to reset the body thermostat. In addition, endotoxin, a lipopolysaccharide present in gram-negative bacteria, is directly pyrogenic even in minute doses. Endotoxin's pyrogenic effect is short-lived because tolerance develops rapidly.

It is debatable whether fever has a beneficial effect in combating infection. Adverse effects of fever are limited to very high fevers in nonpregnant adults. Sustained temperature over 107 °F (42 °C) may lead to brain damage. Fever, even of lower degree, may have other potential adverse effects in pregnancy.

EFFECT OF FEVER PER SE ON THE FETUS

Fever may have three possible effects on the fetus, acidosis–hypoxia, teratogenesis, and premature labor.[22]

Fever as a Cause of Acidosis and Hypoxia

In pregnant baboons, radiant heating to 105–107 °F (41–42 °C) leads to maternal and fetal tachycardia, fetal hypotension, increased uterine activity, and fetal hypoxia and acidosis. However, because the experimental conditions produce profound maternal hypotension, maternal cardiac arrhythmias, and maternal metabolic acidosis, it is difficult to apply this information directly to clinical situations in humans.

Fever as a Teratogen

Patients with hyperthermia during early pregnancy appear to be more likely to deliver newborns with anomalies. Causes of hyperthermia include a variety of infections as well as sauna bathing. Anomalies related to maternal fever in some studies are microphthalmia, anencephaly, midface hypoplasia, and mild impairment of distal limb development. Prospective studies are needed to establish the degree of risk.

Fever as a Cause of Premature Labor

Intrauterine bacterial infection, pyelonephritis pneumonia, and other febrile disorders may lead to premature labor. However, it is not clear whether the labor is a result of the fever, maternal–fetal infection, or maternal cardiovascular deterioration.

Fever usually is recognized as a manifestation of acute infection. While appropriate diagnostic and therapeutic measures are being taken, an important clinical question is whether or not to treat the fever per se with antipyretics to avoid possible fetal effects of maternal fever. Although possible adverse fetal effects of fever are not clearly proven, antipyretics such as acetaminophen appear to have few adverse effects themselves. Accordingly, use of such agents is reasonable as part of the diagnostic and therapeutic plan.

GENITAL SOURCES OF FEVER

Intra-amniotic Infection (Amnionitis, Chorioamnionitis)

Infection of the amniotic cavity is an important cause of perinatal mortality and maternal morbidity. Although a number of terms have been used, we prefer to use intra-amniotic infection (IAI) to distinguish this clinical syndrome from bacterial colonization of amniotic fluid and from histologic inflammation of the cord or placenta.

Incidence. Evident infection occurs in 0.5–2% of pregnancies, most commonly after rupture of the fetal membranes (ROM),[20] but may develop also with intact membranes after labor has begun. On occasion, the infection spreads hematogenously, as with *Listeria monocytogenes*.

Diagnosis of Intra-amniotic Infection. Clinical diagnosis usually is based on a syndrome of maternal fever, maternal or fetal tachycardia, uterine tenderness, foul odor of the amniotic fluid, and leukocytosis.[21] Other causes of fever in parturients include infection of the urinary tract or of other organ systems and possibly dehydration. The differential diagnosis of fetal tachycardia includes prematurity, medications, arrhythmia, and perhaps hypoxia. Possible causes of maternal tachycardia are drugs, hypotension, dehydration, and anxiety. Purulence or foul odor in the fluid coming from the cervix suggests intra-amniotic infection, as does uterine tenderness. Both of these seem to be late, though more specific, signs.

When IAI is suspected, cultures should be obtained from peripheral venous blood and amniotic fluid, if available. It is possible to aspirate amniotic fluid via an intrauterine pressure catheter in about 50% of cases of amnionitis. (In the remainder, flow of fluid cannot be obtained, and a cervical culture should be obtained instead.) Gram staining an uncentrifuged specimen of amniotic fluid also may be helpful (Fig. 38-1). The observation of bacteria on this smear supports the diagnosis, but there may be frequent false positives, especially in patients in labor with ROM. A complete blood count is in order in all patients with suspected infection.

Diagnosis of early neonatal septicemia is difficult because the neonate's response to infection is impaired, and his or her reaction is often nonspecific. The earliest signs are subtle and include changes in color, tone, activity, and feeding, poor temperature control, or an impression that the newborn is not doing well. Other early signs may include abdominal distention, apnea, and jaundice, but these may not appear until late stages and also may be seen in healthy prematures. Late signs may include grunting, dyspnea, cyanosis, arrhythmias, hepatosplenomegaly, petechiae, seizures, bulging fontanelles, and irritability. Focal signs of meningitis or pneumonia may develop.

The cornerstone of the diagnosis of septicemia is a positive blood culture. Multiple cultures spaced over wide intervals are theoretically ideal but usually not practical. Thus, two sets are recommended. Cerebrospinal fluid examination and culture usually are performed because one-third of infants with sepsis also develop meningeal involvement. Either leukopenia (less than 4000/mm^3) or leukocytosis (over 25,000/mm^3) suggests infection in the neonate, but septicemia certainly may occur with intermediate counts. Ominous findings in the CBC in septicemic neonates include extreme leftward shift, more than 50% nonsegmented granulocytes, toxic granulocytes, and less than 80,000 thrombocytes/mm.[3] Inspection of the peripheral smear may show traumatized red blood cells or low platelets, suggesting disseminated intravascular coagulopathy.

Pathogenesis of Intra-amniotic Infection. Intraamniotic infection may be caused by a variety of organisms, often in combination. In a recent study of amniotic fluid, samples were collected via an intrauterine pressure catheter from patients thought on clinical grounds to be infected and from patients apparently uninfected.[19] Seventy percent of the former group IAI showed more than 10^2 colony forming unit flml of high virulence bacteria. Only 8% of the matched control patients had similar findings. In the samples from patients with intra-amniotic infection, the most common pathogenic

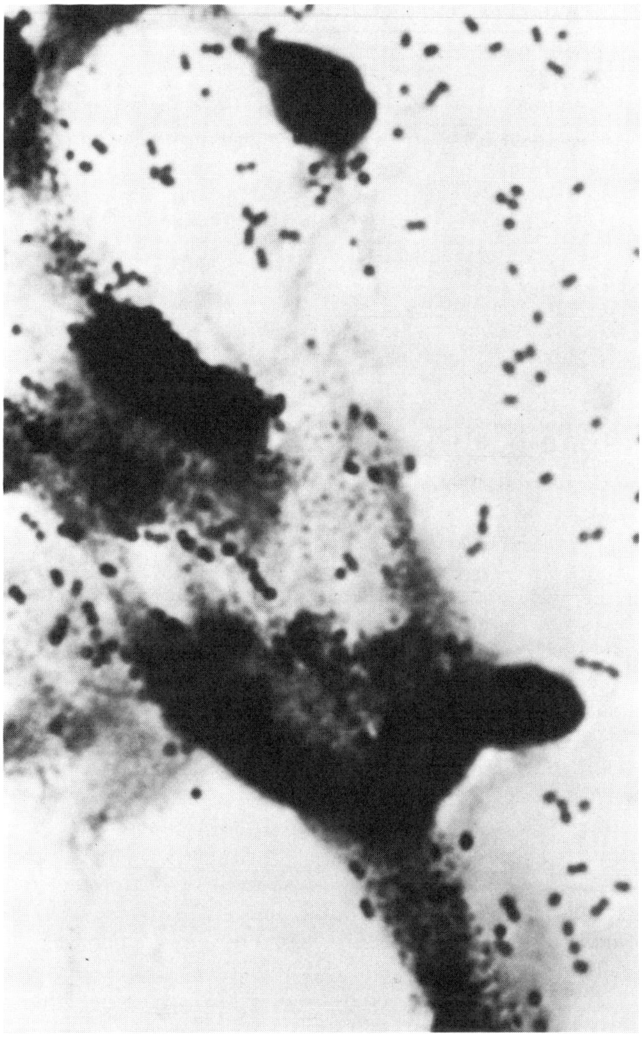

Figure 38-1. Gram stain of uncentrifuged amniotic fluid collected via an intrauterine pressure catheter from patient with clinical intra-amniotic infection. Stain shows numerous polymorphonuclear leukocytes and gram positive cocci, which were group B streptococci.

species were (in decending order) *Bacteroides bivius*, Group B streptococci, and *E. coli*. Other frequently isolated organisms were peptococci and peptostreptococci, *Clostridia* sp., *Bacteroides fragilis* group, *Fusobacteria* sp., *Klebsiella pneumoniae*, alpha streptococci, and enterococci. Other organisms that may cause clinical intra-amniotic infection include *Neisseria gonorrhoeae*, group A streptococci, and *Listeria monocytogenes*. *Mycoplasma hominis* is found significantly more often in amniotic fluid of patients with IAI than in matched controls, but *Ureaplasma urealyticum* is found in 50% of fluids from both groups.[2]

Management. Several studies of management and outcome have been published within the last few years.[20,30,32,47] All have employed similar therapeutic approaches, including use of intrapartum antibiotics (a penicillin usually with an aminoglycoside) and use of cesarean section for standard obstetrical indications. Outcome is summarized in Table 38-1. Bacteremia occurred in 3–10% of mothers and 12% of neonates. The rate of cesarean delivery is higher, but overall maternal outcome is excellent, Cesarean hysterectomy is necessary only infrequently. The outcome is also excellent in term infants, but amnionitis in preterm infants is associated with a greater risk of infection and a higher perinatal mortality; still, the vast majority of infants born from 28 to 34 weeks after amnionitis do well, and few deaths are attributable to infection.[13]

Recent studies have not demonstrated any

TABLE 38-1. STUDIES OF OUTCOME AFTER INTRA-AMNIOTIC INFECTION

Author, Year	Number	Design*	Gestational Age (mean)	Cesarean Delivery	DDI†	Perinatal Mortality
Koh, 1979	140	R	39 weeks	43%	Not given	28/1000
Gibbs, 1980	171	R	36 weeks	34%	5.2 hours	140/1000
Yoder, 1983	67	P	40 weeks	36%	3.1 hours	15/1000
Looff, 1984	104	R	36 weeks	26%	7.2 hours	123/1000

* R = retrospective; P = prospective.
† Diagnosis of intra-amniotic infection to delivery interval (mean).

critical diagnosis-to-delivery time interval. Neither perinatal nor maternal complications are increased with more prolonged intervals. We reserve cesarean section for patients with obstetric indications in addition to chorioamnionitis. With this plan, viable pregnancies usually are delivered within 6–12 hours after diagnosis of chorioamnionitis.

Endometritis

Incidence. Low-grade fever occurs commonly in the postpartum period and often resolves spontaneously.[12] When fever is caused by infection, the genital tract is the most common ste. The overall rate of postpartum infection is 1–8%. Although the absolute risk of death from infection is small among postpartum women, sepsis remains the second most common cause of maternal death in the United States (after toxemia).

Risk Factors. Cesarean section is the major predisposing clinical factor for both frequency and severity of pelvic infection.[14] This observation is particularly important because of increasing cesarean section rates. Patients delivering by cesarean section have a 5- to 30-fold increase in risk of puerperal infection over those who deliver vaginally. Endometritis occurs in 10–50% of patients delivered by cesarean section.

Numerous studies have documented the relationship of labor and rupture of the membranes to postpartum infection. Labor is a more important risk factor than is ROM.[5] Indigent patients have higher puerperal infection rates than do middle-class patients, especially in the presence of other major risk factors such as premature ROM or cesarean section. Possible explanations may include differences in flora, hygiene, nutrition, and amniotic fluid bacterial inhibitor, but indigent patients also may have longer labors and more examinations during labor.

Studies done two decades ago demonstrated that vaginal examination in labor carried no greater infection risk than did rectal examination. However, it is unclear whether or not the number of vaginal examinations is a separate risk from the duration of labor.

Because physicians often use intrauterine fetal monitoring (IFM) in patients with difficult labor, it is not easy to separate the role of IFM from other major predisposing factors, notably cesarean section, ROM, and labor. Most studies conclude that IFM plays little or no direct role in postpartum infection.[1,21,25,35]

Cervical and vaginal traumas increase the likelihood of infection, but only a small percentage of infected women have sustained major trauma at delivery.

Anemia has been associated with puerperal infection, but a causal effect relationship is not established. Likewise, obesity has not been a consistent risk factor for genital infection in patients undergoing cesarean section.

Pathogenesis of Puerperal Infection. Endometritis may be caused by a variety of aerobes and anaerobes, often in combination. Genital mycoplasmas often have been found in blood cultures of women with endometritis.[31] *Chlamydia trachomatis* has been associated with late postpartum endometritis after vaginal delivery but seems to have no role in postcesarean infection.[46]

Diagnosis. The diagnosis of endomyometritis usually is based on symptoms of fever, malaise, abdominal pain, and purulent, foul lochia. However, not all patients demonstrate the complete spectrum. Indeed, many patients with (group A or group B) streptococcal bacteremia have no localizing signs at the onset of fever. In the vast majority of cases, presenting signs and symptoms develop within the first 2–7 days after delivery. Appropriate studies include CBC, venous blood cultures, and a uterine culture. Gram stain of the genital culture may be helpful when hemolytic streptococci or clostridia are suspected.

Treatment. The vast majority of patients improve within a few days with supportive therapy and broad spectrum antibiotics.

Response to antibiotics is poorer among patients with endomyometritis after cesarean than in those with endometritis after vaginal delivery. The cure rate of postcesarean endometritis is about 65–78% after therapy with penicillin plus an aminoglycoside.[8] Patients who do not respond to this regimen require additional antibiotics (notably clindamycin), surgical drainage, or anticoagulants (for septic pelvic thrombophlebitis).

The response rate of endomyometritis after cesarean section is higher when initial therapy consists of clindamycin plus gentamicin. Major infectious complications also may be reduced. This combination has become the benchmark of management. A number of newer cephalosporins and penicillins also yield high cure rates (Fig. 38-2).[4,8,10,16,17,27,41,43,44] Antibiotic failure may be due to a resistant organism, inadequate antibiotic dose, wound infection, pelvic hematoma or abscess, septic pelvic thrombophlebitis, infection of another site, or a noninfectious source.

Septic pelvic thrombophlebitis was first recognized over 35 years ago in autopsies of patients dying of puerperal sepsis.[9] More recently, it has been described as "obscure" or "enigmatic" fever persisting despite multiple antibiotics. These patients characteristically appear nontoxic and are either free of pain or complain only of mild, poorly localized discomfort despite wide swings in temperature. Abdominal and pelvic findings are minimal and vague. Septic pulmonary embolization is a rare complication. In most cases, the diagnosis is presumptive, based on defervescence within 48–72 hours after initiating heparin therapy. This condition has more recently been diagnosed by computerized axial tomography (CAT) scan. Septic pelvic thrombo-phlebitis occurs in approximately 1% of patients with postcesarean endometritis.

Prevention. Perioperative prophylactic antibiotics decrease postcesarean infections to a statistically significant and clinically meaningful degree. Overall, infections are reduced by more than 50%.[42] Thus, in patients at moderate to high risk for postcesarean infection, prophylactic antibiotics should be given in a short course

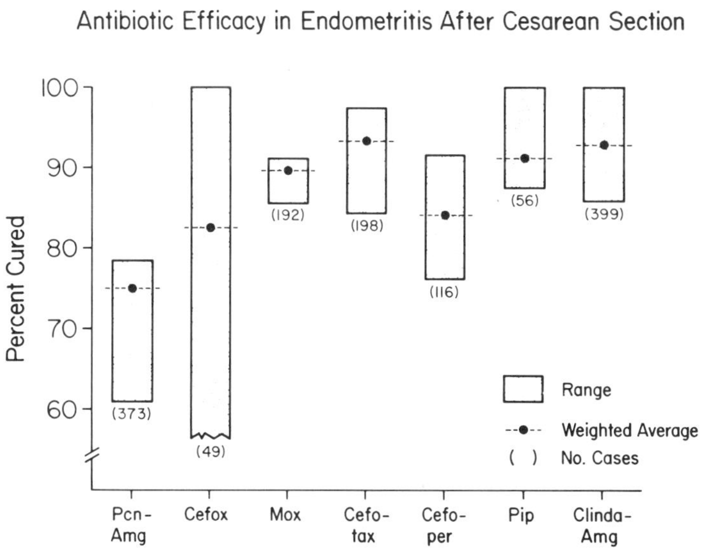

Figure 38-2. Summary of antibiotic efficacy in endometritis after cesarean section.
Legend: Pcn-penicillin; Amg-aminoglycoside; Mox-moxalactam; cefotax-cefotaxime; Cefoper-cefoperazone; Pip-piperacillin; Clinda-clindamycin.

initiated after cord clamping. Excellent results can be expected with ampicillin or a first-generation cephalosporin. Use of newer agents is more expensive and has not led to any greater efficacy.[39] However, prophylactic antibiotics lead to shifts in bacteriology to more resistant species and strains and therefore may have adverse effects. Accordingly, prophylactic antibiotics should not be used in low-risk patients (such as elective sections).

Episiotomy and Other Pelvic Infections

Although episiotomy with repair is performed in most vaginal deliveries, infection is an infrequent complication of this operation.[38] However, on occasion, lethal consequences may develop.

Simple episiotomy infection is a localized infection involving only the skin and subcutaneous tissue (including Camper's fascia of the perineum) adjacent to the episiotomy. Signs are local edema and erythema with exudate. More extensive findings should raise suspicion of a deeper infection. Treatment consists of opening, exploring, and debriding the perineal wound. Drainage alone is usually adequate, but appropriate antibiotics are indicated if there is marked, superficial cellulitis or if group A streptococci are isolated. The episiotomy incision should not be resutured at this time. Most heal by granulation. Those involving the sphincter muscle or rectal mucosa may be repaired when the field is free of infection.

Fascial necrosis is a variant of necrotizing fasciitis. Both layers of the superficial perineal fascia (i.e., Camper's and Colles' fascia) become necrotic, and infection spreads alog the fascial planes to the abdominal wall, thigh, or buttock. Typically, the deep perineal fascia (i.e., inferior fascia of the urogenital diaphragm) is not involved. Skin findings are variable but initially include edema and erythema without clear borders. Later, there is progressive, brawny edema of the skin, and a grayish, watery fluid may be evident. The skin becomes blue or brown, and bullae or frank gangrene may occur. As the infection progresses, there may be loss of sensation or hyperesthesia. Associated findings upon admission include marked hemoconcentration and hypocalcemia (due to saponification of fatty acids). This infection has been associated traditionally with group A streptococci, but anaerobic bacteria also play important roles. Adequate debridement is essential to effective therapy. Indications for surgical exploration are (1) infection extending beyond the labia, (2) unilateral edema, (3) signs of toxicity or deterioration, and (4) failure of the infection to resolve within 24–48 hours. At surgery, necrotizing fasciitis is recognized by separation of the skin from the deep fascia, absence of bleeding along incision lines, and a serosanguinous discharge. Dissection should be carried out until all necrotic tissue is debrided.

Myonecrosis involves the muscles beneath the deep fascia. Often this is caused by myotoxin of *Clostridium perfringens*, but occasionally it may be an extension of necrotizing fasciitis. Onset may be early in the puerperium and is accompanied typically by severe pain. Treatment is extensive debridement and high-dose antibiotics, including penicillin.

Not all puerperal vulvar edema signifies serious perineal infection. Indeed, in most cases, vulvar edema results from less serious causes such as vulvar hematoma, prolonged bearing down in labor, generalized edema from toxemia, allergic reactions, and trauma without serious infection. With these disorders, the edema is usually bilateral, does not extend to the buttock and abdominal wall, and is not accompanied by signs of toxicity.

Within the last few years, a number of cases of *subgluteal or retropsoal infections* have been reported. These severe infections commonly are preceded by paracervical or transvaginal pudendal block. They are characterized by fever and poorly localized hip or pelvic pain. Gas formation in the soft tissues is seen in half the cases. Besides appropriate antibiotic treatment, early debridement is necessary.

PYELONEPHRITIS

Epidemiology

Acute pyelonephritis is one of the most common medical complications of pregnancy, occurring in 1–2.5% of obstetric patients.[23] Recurrence occurs in 10–25% of patients in the same pregnancy. The major predisposing factor for pyelonephritis in pregnancy is asymptomatic bacteriuria. In most populations, asymptomatic bacteriuria is detected in 4–7% of gravidas. Pyelonephritis develops in about 30–40% of these women if untreated. Other predisposing factors are obstructive and neurologic disease of the urinary tract and ureteral or renal calculi. In the preantibiotic era, pyelonephritis was accompanied by premature birth in 20–30% of cases.

Screening for and treatment of asymptomatic bacteriuria lead to dramatic decreases in pyelonephritis in pregnancy.

Diagnosis

The diagnosis of pyelonephritis is based on a history of shaking chills, fever, flank pain, nausea, vomiting, frequency, urgency, and dysuria. Common physical findings are fever, costovertebral angle tenderness (usually in the right), and, at times, lower abdominal tenderness. Confirmation of the diagnosis is based on a urine culture showing 10^5 cfu/ml of a uropathogen.

Microbiology

The organisms causing pyelonephritis are the same that cause asymptomatic bacteriuria and cystitis. The most common isolate is *E. coli*, which accounts for 60–90% of cases. The next most common isolates are *Proteus mirabilis* and *Klebsiella pneumoniae*. *Enterobacter* species, enterococci (*Streptococcus fecalis*), and group B streptococci cause urinary tract infection less frequently in obstetrical patients. Bacteremia develops in approximately 10% of patients with pyelonephritis. On our service, patients with pyelonephritis accounted for 26% of all bacteremias. Of the 29 blood isolates, *E. coli* accounted for 25 (86%).

Treatment

Pyelonephritis is a serious threat to the mother and fetus and requires admission to the hospital. The basis of treatment is close monitoring, supportive therapy, and parenteral antibiotics. Because of nausea, vomiting, and pyexia, dehydration is common. We do not use an indwelling catheter unless the patient is in septic shock. Intravenous fluids with isotonic crystalloid solutions should be administered initially to restore fluid volume. Approximately 20% of patients have transient renal dysfunction with decreased creatinine clearance. This point should be remembered if aminoglycosides are used for therapy.

The initial choice of antimicrobial agents is empiric and is based on knowledge of common pathogeic bacteria. In the past we used i.v. ampicillin, but in view of rising bacterial resistance even in patients with a first episode of pyelonephritis, we now use a first-generation cephalosporin in most patients. For patients with repeated episodes or with septic shock, combination therapy such as ampicillin plus an aminoglycoside should be used. The advantage of using ampicillin (rather than a cephalosporin) in combination with the aminoglycoside is the coverage of enterococci by this combination.

Eighty-five percent of patients become afebrile within 48 hours after initiating intravenous antibiotic therapy. Poor response may be caused by a resistant organism or by obstruction. If cultures do not reveal a resistant organism, a single-shot intravenous pyelogram is in order.

In patients with a good response, intravenous single drug therapy should be continued until the patient has been afebrile for 24–48 hours. Oral therapy should then be continued to complete a 10-day course.

Acute pyelonephritis recurs in 10–18%, and a positive urine culture recurs in another 10–15%. In view of the high likelihood of recurrence, some clinicians favor suppression with antimicrobials throughout pregnancy. Agents used for suppression include nitrofurantoin, ampicillin, or short-acting sulfanomides, each given in small doses once or twice daily. A suitable alternative is regular cultures of the urine (every two to four weeks) with prompt treatment of asymptomatic recurrences. We prefer to employ screening in patients with a single episode and use suppression in patients with one or more recurrent urinary infections (asymptomatic bacteriuria, cystitis, or pyelonephritis).

VIRAL AND PARASITIC INFECTIONS

Rubella

Also known as German measles, rubella is a mild illness causing fever, postauricular or suboccipital lymphadenopathy, arthralgia, and a transient erythematous rash.[3] Rubella in early pregnancy was shown to be teratogenic more than 40 years ago.

Epidemiology. Wild rubella virus is spread by droplets or by direct contact with infected persons or articles contaminated with nasopharyngeal secretions. It is mainly a disease of children, with peak incidence at ages 5–9 years. On rare occasions serious sequelae such as central nervous system involvement or thrombocytopenia develop. By reproductive age, about 75–85% of the population has had rubella, as evidenced by positive titers, although about half of the infections are subclinical. Wild virus infection (even if subclinical) confers life-long immunity.

Before vaccination was available, rubella occurred at six- to nine-year cycles. The last major epidemic was in 1964. Infection during early pregnancy may lead to involvement of the embryo or fetus. The risk of congenital rubella syndrome is about 20% when primary maternal infection occurs in the first trimester of pregnancy. The risk varies from 50% in the first month to 10% by the third month. Cataracts, patent ductus arteriosus, and deafness are the most common abnormalities. When these children are followed for a few years, additional disorders such as diabetes occur more frequently than expected. Congenital rubella syndrome has nearly been eliminated from the United States. In recent years, approximately 2–10 cases are reported to the CDC annually.

Diagnosis. The clinical diagnosis of rubella is often difficult since it resembles a number of other exanthemas. The rubella virus can be isolated from the bloodstream and throat 7–10 days after exposure. Shedding of virus from the throat continues for about a week. The rash, which typically starts in the face, commonly develops 16–18 days after exposure.

Rubella infection stimulates a variety of antibody responses. Hemagglutinating inhibition (HI) antibody, an IgG class antibody, is used most commonly for screening.[33] After wild virus infection, HI titers usually remain positive for life. From 5% to 15% of women with remote rubella infection have stable HI titers equal to or more than 1:256. A titer higher than 1:8 is conclusive evidence of immunity. Because of variations between laboratories and interassay variations within a given laboratory, it is essential that paired serum samples be tested on the same day, in the same laboratory. Complement fixation (CF) antibody, also an IgG class antibody, appears later than HI and may be useful in some diagnostic situations, such as patients with high HI or patients first seen one to five weeks after exposure. This test is not performed routinely.

Rubella specific IgM appears early and lasts for only a few weeks. This test may be helpful in some situations. Although a positive rubella-IgM titer is indicative of recent primary rubella infection, its absence does not necessarily exclude recent infections because IgM may disappear in less than four to five weeks in some patients.

Other serologic responses are detectable by radioimmunoassay, neutralization, or enzyme-linked immunosorbent assay (ELISA). Some of these are more sensitive than HI and probably will replace the HI test for screening.

Even with detailed knowledge of rubella serologic tests, it is not always possible to determine whether there has been acute primary rubella infection.

Counseling and Management. When rubella infection is confirmed in pregnancy, the patient should be advised of the risks and types of congenital anomalies. At present, tests such as culture of amniotic fluid cannot reliably distinguish infected from uninfected fetuses in pregnancies at risk. Counseling should also consider the risks to the mother of pregnancy termination.

Use of immune globulin (IG) after exposure is recommended by some authors. However, the Advisory Committee to the Centers for Disease Control (CDC) notes that IG given after exposure prevents neither infection nor viremia, although it may alter symptoms.[3] Infants with congenital rubella have been born to women who received IG shortly after exposure. Thus, the CDC does not recommend IG for routine postexposure prophylaxis. Yet, CDC suggests that IG might be useful in a susceptible, exposed pregnant woman for whom pregnancy termination is not acceptable. In this situation, IG might offer some protection against fetal infection.

Prevention. All rubella vaccines contain live, attenuated virus. Since January 1979, the rubella vaccine used in the United States is the RA 27/3, which replaced the HPV-77 vaccine. RA 27/3 is administered subcutaneously. After vaccination, approximately 95% of susceptible individuals develop HI antibodies that provide long-term (probably life-long) protection. Among adults who do not show a positive HI titer after vaccinations, nearly all show detectable antibody when a more sensitive test is used. According to the CDC, any detectable rubella antibody or a history of rubella vaccination is presumptive evidence of immunity.

Vaccinees may shed the attenuated virus from the nasopharynx for a few weeks, but there is no evidence that the vaccine virus can be transmitted. Thus, there appears to be no risk to susceptible, pregnant women who contact recently vaccinated children or adults.

Susceptible women of reproductive age are candidates for immunization. Pregnancy should be avoided for 90 days after immunization. The immediate postpartum period is an excellent time for immunization. Vaccinated women may breast-feed without fear of adverse effect to the newborn. Rh-negative women may receive RhD immune globulin, if indicated, as well as the rubella vaccine.

Despite these recommendations, many rubella-susceptible pregnant women have received rubella vaccine within three months of the time of conception. As of 1980, more than 200 of these women had delivered viable infants. After vaccination with the HPV-77 preparation, the virus has been isolated from the products of conception in about 20% of cases. Fewer women who became pregnant within three months of vaccination with the RA 27/3 vaccine have delivered, but this virus appears to be isolated less frequently from the products of conception. Even though the virus may be isolated in the products of conception, none of the 214 infants displayed any anomalies consistent with congenital rubella syndrome. Although the precise risk of teratogenicity from the attenuated vaccine virus is unknown, the risk is considerably less than that of the wild virus and is estimated at 0–3%.

Side effects of the vaccine include arthralgias, but true arthritis occurs in less than 1%. In susceptible adult women, joint symptoms are more frequent and tend to be more severe than in children, but adults usually have not had to disrupt work. Other complaints such as pain or paresthesias are rare.

Contraindications to vaccination are febrile illnesses, immunosuppression, and pregnancy. Precautions are necessary in rare individuals with neomycin allergy.

A recent hospital outbreak of rubella was traced to an obstetrics–gynecology house officer. As a result, it is now advised that hospital workers having contact with pregnant women should be immune to rubella.

Varicella (Chicken Pox)[6]

This common childhood disease usually is marked by typical skin lesions that progress from macules and papules to vesicles and pustules. This highly contagious disorder is acquired by most persons in the United States prior to reproductive age and is generally self-limited. Constitutional and pulmonary symptoms may be more severe in adults who contract the disease. Special problems in obstetrics include possible increase in severity of the disease among pregnant women and effects on the fetus and newborn.

Varicella in the Mother. Varicella is unusual in adults and probably occurs with no greater frequency among pregnant women. Varicella pneumonia probably is no more frequent in pregnant women than in nonpregnant adults, but varicella pneumonia may be more fulminant in pregnancy. When pneumonia develops, pulmonary symptoms begin on the second to sixth day after appearance of the rash, usually initiated by a mild nonproductive cough. If the illness is more severe, there may be additional symptoms of pleuritic chest pain, hemoptysis, dyspnea, and cyanosis. Physical examination reveals fever, rales, and wheezes. Patients should be warned to contact the physician *immediately* if even mild pulmonary symptoms develop. Hospitalization with full respiratory support should be made available.

Varicella in Early Pregnancy. Congenital anomalies due to varicella in early pregnancy were not recognized until the mid-1970s. Maternal varicella infection in the first four months of pregnancy rarely may produce a congenital varicella syndrome, which consists of cutaneous scars, limb hypoplasia, rudimentary digits, and, occasionally, ocular and central nervous system abnormalities.

Although the risk of congenital varicella syndome is small, a number of authorities have recommended administration of varicella immune globulin (also called zoster immune globulin [ZIG]) to pregnant women exposed to varicella who have a negative history for varicella. ZIG should be administered as soon as possible, but within three days of exposure, as this may protect the fetus during the viremia. Once the mother has the rash, there is no reason to administer ZIG, because the viremia already has occurred.

Varicella in the Newborn. Acquisition of maternal antibody usually protects the fetus. However, an infant born after maternal viremia, but before the mother has developed an antibody response, is at high risk for life-threatening, neonatal varicella infection. Those infants whose mothers contract varicella within five days of birth or within the first five days after delivery are at risk. Congenital varicella infection has been reported in 17% of term infants born to mothers with varicella within four to five days of delivery. Nearly one-third of the infants died (4/13). Accordingly, ZIG should be administered to such infants immediately after birth.

Herpes Simplex Virus[24,29]

Herpes simplex virus may infect the adult, the newborn, or, on rare occasions, the fetus. In the adult, typical lesions are vesicular or ulcerative, involving only the skin and mucous membranes. More widespread infection, including the central nervous system, is an unusual complication in adults, most often developing in those with debilitating disease. On the other hand, because of a compromised immune system, the newborn infant is subject to systemic, frequently lethal, disease.

Epidemiology. In adults, the virus commonly causes infection of the mouth and lips and less commonly of the genital tract and skin. Herpes simplex virus, type I, is generally responsible for infection of the mouth and of the skin above the waist, whereas type II virus is mainly responsible for infection of the genitalia and of the skin below the waist. However, approximately 10–15% of genital herpes is now caused by type I.

Herpes virus has been isolated from the genitalia of 0.02–4% of asymptomatic pregnant women. Serologic surveys show that 30–90% of women have antibody to herpes virus, type II, but it may be difficult to differentiate specific serum antibodies of type II from type I. For the mother, the disease does not appear to be more severe or more protracted in pregnancy.

Maternal infection in early pregnancy reportedly has adverse effects on the embryo, including a threefold increase in abortion. Maternal herpes infections occurring after the 20th week allegedly are associated with a higher rate of premature delivery. Both abortion and prematurity are associated more commonly with primary than with recurrent maternal infection.

Transplacental infection of the fetus resulting in congenital infection is a rare sequel to maternal infection. It probably arises from the viremia associated only with primary infections. Only a few cases have been reported.

The major perinatal problem is neonatal herpes infections. Estimates of frequency are subject to error because up to 50% of infants with culture-proved, fatal disease do not have typical lesions of the skin or mucous membranes. In addition, viral laboratories have not been widely available, and recent treatment recommendations (see below) probably have decreased the incidence of neonatal disease. Our best guess is that neonatal herpes occurs in 1 in 2000 vaginal deliveries.

Neonatal herpes is acquired perinatally from an infected, lower maternal genital tract, most commonly during vaginal delivery. Cases have occurred in newborns delivered by cesarean birth performed a number of hours after labor has begun or after the membranes have ruptured. If maternal genital herpes is present at term, the risk of neonatal herpes infection to infants delivering vaginally is probably 40–60%. The risk of death or serious sequelae in infected infants is about 50%. Although the risk of neonatal herpes is probably greater among infants delivered by women with symptomatic herpes, most cases of neonatal disease now occur in infants whose mothers have recurrent, asymptomatic disease. Maternal antibodies thus offer incomplete protection to the neonate.

Diagnosis. The diagnosis of genital herpes is based on observing typical, painful crops of vesicles and ulcers in various stages of progression. Findings in primary infection are regional lymphadenopathy, fever, and other constitutional symptoms. Primary genital herpes usually lasts about two to three weeks. Clinically detectable recurrences are variable, but about 50% of patients will have recurrent disease within six months. Recurrences are milder, with fewer lesions, fewer constitutional symptoms, and a shorter course (usually five to seven days).

Up to two-thirds of women with a positive genital culture for herpes virus do not have typical lesions. Thus, for screening procedures, cytology and cultures are used. Although herpes infection may be suggested by typical changes seen in Papanicolaou smears (intranuclear inclusions and multinucleated giant cells), there are too many false negatives (about 20–50%). The best diagnostic test to rule out herpes infection is the viral culture. Fortunately, this virus grows rapidly. Most positive cultures are identifiable at 48–72 hours. Monoclonal antibody tests may soon be available for examination of clinical specimens. This rapid, inexpensive approach promises to be a major diagnostic advance, provided sensitivity and specificity are high.

Neonatal herpes infection may be limited to the skin or may be systemic, with or without cutaneous involvement. Clinical disease typically begins at the end of the first week of life. Findings depend on the organ system involved and may include skin lesions, cough, cyanosis, tachypnea, dyspnea, jaundice, seizures, or disseminated intravascular coagulopathy. In infants at risk for or suspected of having neonatal herpes, the only reliable diagnostic test is viral culture. One cannot rely on clinical exam or cytologic changes.

A few infants have been recognized with congenital (transplacental) herpes infection. In congenital infection, the typical cutaneous lesions become apparent within 24–48 hours of life. Fetal intrauterine infection presumably occurs a few days before birth. In other cases, there have been less specific clinical signs (microcephaly and spasticity), but serologic evidence of infection has been obtained.

Treatment and Prevention. The main treatment of maternal herpes genital infection in pregnancy is symptomatic—analgesics, hygiene, and topical anesthetics. In nonpregnant women, oral acyclovir shortens the course of primary and recurrent genital herpes and suppresses recurrences in those with frequent recurrences (6–12 per year). There is little experience with acyclovir in pregnancy. Although not teratogenic in laboratory animals, its use in pregnancy cannot be recommended.

Because of the severity of neonatal herpes infection and the lack of satisfactory chemotherapy or immunotherapy, we attempt to prevent neonatal infection by avoiding contact between the fetus and the infected maternal lower genital tract. Accordingly, cesarean section is recommended when there is clinical or culture evidence of active infection at the time of labor, unless the membranes already have been ruptured for a prolonged period. Based on a small number of cases, four to six hours was considered the critical interval between rupture of the membranes and cesarean delivery. Recently, cesarean delivery after more than six hours of membrane rupture has not resulted in neonatal involvement. We now offer cesarean section for up to 12 hours, in women with either primary or recurrent clinical or subclinical infection. Cytologic evidence of herpes infection should not be used to make this important decision. Presence or absence of infection should be proved by cultures.

Cytomegalovirus

Cytomegalovirus[40] (CMV), a DNA virus of the herpes virus group, causes cytomegalic inclusion disease. Characteristic large cells with prominent intranuclear inclusion bodies have been identified in this disease since the early 20th century, but the virus was not isolated until 1956. Initially, CMV was considered rare because only the classic, clinically severe form of the disease was appreciated, but recent studies utilizing viral cultures have identified the frequent presence of "silent" CMV in which no clinical manifestations are present. CMV is the most common cause of intrauterine infection in the United States. Fifty thousand infected infants are born annually. Ten percent of these children have clinically evident disease in the neonatal period. However, absence of detectable infection at birth may not be innocuous. The persistent and progressive nature of these inapparent congenital infections may result in central nervous system (CNS) pathology and neurologic sequelae that may represent the major impact of CMV infection.

The teratogenic potential of CMV is unresolved. Although the virus can cause a reduction in absolute number of cells in various organs, it is unclear whether this is due to a direct effect on the cells or secondary to endothelial and vascular damage. Malformations such as cataracts or congenital heart lesions are seldom seen with CMV. Thus, congenital CMV bears a closer resemblance to congenital toxoplasmosis, in which defects are secondary to destruction of tissue, than to congenital rubella.

Epidemiology. Approximately 50% of females in the United States and Europe are susceptible to CMV when they reach reproductive age. The highest rate of seroconversion occurs between ages 15 and 35 (Table 38-2). CMV infection is more prevalent in lower socioeconomic groups. Although CMV is widespread, it usually produces serious illness only in fetuses, immunodeficient individuals, and patients receiving immunosuppressive therapy. Most adult infections are subclinical, and the remainder (approximately 10%) cause a mononucleosis-like illness.

The virus is excreted persistently. CMV is communicable for long periods of time. Infants infected congenitally excrete CMV for an average of four years. Those who acquire CMV at the time of birth excrete virus for two years. Many seropositive young adults shed CMV intermittently.

Asymptomatic CMV infection and excretion are common during pregnancy. The cervix is involved in 3–18%, breast milk in up to 27%, and

TABLE 38-2. PREVALENCE OF CYTOMEGALOVIRUS INFECTION

	Usual rate
Positive cervical culture for CMV	4%
Previous infection with CMV (seropositivity)	50–60%
Maternal seroconversion in pregnancy to CMV	1–2.5%
Congenital infection (transplacental acquisition by fetus)	0.2–2%
Perinatal infection (acquisition of CMV by neonate from vaginal secretions, milk, etc.)	3%–5% (higher in infants with prolonged nursery stay

the pharynx in 1–2%. The incidence of CMV infection is highest in young, primiparous, unmarried women and in those of low income and low educational status. Asymptomatic infections occur mainly in seropositive women whose antibody status does not change in spite of viral shedding.

In addition to fetuses infected by vertical (i.e., transplacental) transmission from their mothers, an additional 3–5% of liveborn infants acquire CMV peripartum, presumably as a result of exposure to infected cervical secretions, ingestion of infected milk, or mouth-to-mouth contact with the mother. In infants with prolonged hospital stays of more than 30 days, perinatal acquisition of CMV is up to 13%. If maternal genital CMV infection is present at the time of birth, 30–50% of neonates acquire the virus.

Infections transmitted in utero are the major concern, especially as they relate to infant development. Congenital infections may follow either primary or recurrent maternal infection. After maternal seroconversion in pregnancy, approximately 40–50% of infants are infected, but only 10% of them have clinically evident disease. The occurrence of congenital infection in 3.4–6% of infants born to previously immune mothers suggests that recurrent maternal CMV is an important cause of intrauterine transmission of CMV. In fact, the birth of an infant with congenital CMV infection does not ensure that a subsequent fetus will not become infected in utero. Congenital CMV has occurred in consecutive pregnancies, up to three years apart.

It is not clear whether the long-term prognosis for the fetus is different in primary versus recurrent maternal CMV infection. In general, primary maternal infection is considered potentially more dangerous for the fetus, but not all fetuses of mothers with primary CMV infection became infected. The more severely affected infants acquire CMV infection in the first or second trimester of pregnancy. Those born after third trimester maternal infection are normal at birth, but cord sera are positive for CMV IgM antibodies, suggesting "silent" congenital CMV infection.

The prognosis for babies born with clinically apparent disease is poor. CNS and perceptual disabilities usually result in severe mental retardation. The major sites of this chronic morbidity are the brain and perceptual organs with resultant seizures, spastic diplegia, optic atrophy, blindness, and sensorineural deafness. Congenitally infected neonates who appear normal at birth may not develop normally. Significant neurologic sequelae may become apparent with time. Long-term longitudinal follow-up studies have documented progressive sensorineural hearing loss and apparently subtle brain damage resulting in lowered IQ and school-associated behavioral problems.

Diagnosis. More than 90% of maternal CMV infections are asymptomatic. Occasionally, CMV infection presents as a heterophile-negative mononucleosis-like syndrome. Features are leukocytosis with lymphocytosis, abnormal liver function tests, abrupt onset of spiking temperature, and constitutional symptoms such as malaise, myalgias, and chills. The mildness of the pharyngitis, minimal lymphadenopathy, and absence of hepatosplenomegaly and jaundice help to differentiate CMV from infectious mononucleosis.

The spectrum of disease caused by CMV in the fetus and neonate is very broad. Clinically apparent disease ranges from isolated organ involvement to the classic multiorgan disease. In severely infected neonates, clinical features include hepatosplenomegaly, jaundice, thrombocytopenia, purpura, microcephaly, deafness, chorioretinitis, optic atrophy, and cerebral calcifications. The cerebral calcifications of CMV are characteristically periventricular in the subependymal region. A characteristic tetrad of findings has been described in infants who have survived fulminant CMV infection. These are (1) mental retardation, (2) chorioretinitis, (3) cerebral calcifications, and (4) micro- or hydrocephaly.

Several antibody tests are available for detecting CMV infection. The compliment fixation (CF) method is no longer preferred because of considerable cross-reactivity with other herpes viruses. Indirect hemagglutination (IHA), enzyme-linked immunosorbent assay (ELISA), indirect fluorescent antibody, and nutralization tests are available for epidemiologic studies. Since approximately 50% of adults have antibody, a single positive test does not necessarily indicate recent or current infection. Demonstration of seroconversion is the best documentation that primary infection has occurred. If infection has occurred within the previous 30–60 days, IgM-specific antibody may be detected in serum.

The best way to establish the presence of CMV infection is to isolate the virus, but virus isolation does not differentiate primary infection from recurrent. CMV isolation may require two to six weeks.

The small percentage of infections that are clinically apparent in neonates is similar to other congenital infections such as toxoplasmosis, rubella, syphilis, and herpes. The characteristic periventricular calcifications may be helpful in differentiating congenital CMV infection from other infections, but laboratory confirmation is necessary to document CMV infection. Serology can be used as an aid in diagnosis of congenital CMV infection, but virus isolation is more sensitive and direct.

Most neonates with congenital CMV have antibody to CMV when tested with newer methods. Approximately 80% of congenitally infected infants have IgM-specific antibody in their serum during the first few months of life, but this test is available in only a few medical research laboratories. Virus isolation is the best method available for documenting newborn CMV infection. Specimens can be taken from the urine, nasopharynx, conjunctiva, and spinal fluid. Appearance of characteristic cytomegalic inclusions is strongly suggestive of CMV infection. These may be seen in tissues collected at autopsy or by biopsy, for example, of the kidney.

Treatment. There is no known treatment for CMV infection. In mothers with clinical illness, treatment is symptomatic. No satisfactory therapy is available for the treatment of congenital CMV infection. Antiviral agents such as adenosine arabinoside (Ara-A) and cytosine arabinoside (Ara-C) have been used in neonates with severe, clinical infection, but these drugs are quite toxic. Although they temporarily suppress the excretion of CMV, virus shedding resumes when the drugs are stopped. Because of their toxicity, the antiviral agents are not used in asymptomatic CMV infection.

The clinician faces a dilemma when dealing with maternal CMV. The overwhelming majority of maternal infections are undiagnosable and serologic screening programs for maternal CMV infection are very limited. Thus, it is practically impossible to counsel patients about CMV. If a primary CMV infection is documented in the first 20 weeks of pregnancy (e.g., after presentation as a heterophile antigen-negative mononucleosis syndrome), therapeutic termination of pregnancy may be considered. Counseling a mother who already has given birth to an infected infant is even a bigger problem. In such a situation, the incidence of recurrence is unknown, and it is not clear whether subsequent congenital infections have the same prognostic significance as the initial episode.

The development of a CMV vaccine has been suggested as a means of preventing congenital CMV infection, but this approach is unlikely to be successful.

Because large quantities of CMV are excreted by infected infants, it has been suggested that pregnant pediatric health care workers might be at high risk to develop CMV infection. However, annual primary CMV infection rates (as determined by seroconversion) are no higher among pediatric house staff (2.7%) and pediatric nursing staff (3.3%) than among young women in the community (2.5% during pregnancy and 5.5% between pregnancies).[11] The unexpectedly high rate of conversions between pregnancies suggested that exposure to young infants or other social exposures may be the most important factors in horizontal transmission. Thus, standard infection control measures for handling potentially contaminated material in pediatric units seems to provide sufficient protection from CMV infection.

Toxoplasmosis[36]

Toxoplasmosis, a widely distributed illness, is caused by *Toxoplasma gondii*, an intracellular parasite. Knowledge of the disease is necessary to the obstetrician because of potential impact on the fetus.

Epidemiology. Although *T. gondii* is found in many mammalian species, the cat is the only definitive host. The parasite exists in three forms (trophozoite, cyst, or oocyst). Trophozoites are the invasive forms, and cysts are the latent forms. Oocysts are found only in cats. Human infection may be acquired by consuming raw or undercooked meat of infected animals (especially mutton or lamb) or by contact with oocysts from the feces of an infected cat. The oocysts may be spread to humans or to food by handling or by insects. Cats acquire toxoplasmosis by eating infected mice or other animals. Oocysts in cat feces do not become infective for four to five days. Once infected by oocysts from cat feces or by cysts from infected meat, persons may experience a parasitemia during which fetal involvement may occur. Later, *T. gondii* cysts appear in tissues, especially striated muscle and brain, where they persist indefinitely.

Serologic evidence of past infection with *T. gondii* is common in pregnant women. In the United States, the prevalence of *Toxoplasma* antibodies in adults is 20–40%. Seroconversion during pregnancy occurs approximately once in 2000 pregnancies.[28]

When primary toxoplasmosis is acquired during pregnancy, the chance of fetal infection is 30–60%. Sixty-five to 75% of these infections will be subclinical. The rate of fetal infection is higher when maternal infection occurs in the third trimester than when it occurs in the first or second trimester, but the severity of fetal infection is greater when maternal infection occurs in the first trimester. Congenital infection does not affect more than one infant in a particular mother. The role of toxoplasmosis in chronic abortion remains unresolved after 20 years of study.

Diagnosis. Most cases of toxoplasmosis are subclinical. When clinically apparent in an immunocompetent host, the most common manifestation is lymphadenopathy (especially cervical). Fever, fatigue, sore throat, maculopapular rash, and occasionally lymphocytosis or an occasional atypical lymphocyte are seen. Accordingly, this disease is often thought to be "flu" or infectious mononucleosis. Ocular symptoms including haziness of vision, pain, and photophobia occasionally may be the predominant features in adults. Ophthalmologic examination shows clusters of yellow-white patches in the optic fundus, representative of focal necrotizing retinochoroiditis. In healthy adults, clinical toxoplasmosis is mild and self-limited; only in immunosuppressed individuals does it lead to serious pulmonary or central nervous system involvement.

Most infants with congenital toxoplasmosis have only serologic abnormalities. Of those with clinical disease, few have the classic triad of intracerebral calcifications, chorioretinitis, and hydrocephaly. Rather, common contemporary findings in symptomatic infants are chorioretinitis (80%), abnormal spinal fluid (69%), anemia (64%), splenomegaly (56%), jaundice (54%), fever (51%), lymphadenopathy (43%), convulsions (34%), and vomiting (32%). Thus, there is a wide spectrum of disease. Acute, primary toxoplasmosis in pregnancy has been associated also with abortion, prematurity, and growth retardation.

Serologic techniques are used to confirm toxoplasmosis. IgG antibodies are detected by the indirect fluorescent-antibody test, Sabin–Feldman dye test, indirect hemagglutination inhibition test, and complement fixation test. Acute infection is diagnosed by seroconversion. Titers resulting from recent infection nearly always rise to 1:512 or 1:1000 with the indirect fluorescent-antibody and dye tests. These antibodies peak within one to two months of the onset of infection. Low titers persist for years.

IgM antibodies may be detected by an indirect fluorescent-antibody technique. They appear within a week and usually last for a few months.

Histologic techniques may be used in some circumstances (e.g., lymph node biopsy) but in general are not suited to widespread detection.

Prevention. To prevent toxoplasmosis in pregnancy, most authorities advise the following: (1) avoid eating undercooked meat; (2) hand-washing after handling a cat; (3) having someone else change the litter box daily; (4) not permitting indoor cats to go outside, where they may attack an infected mouse; 5) not allowing stray cats in the house; and (6) not feeding raw meat to cats. Based on recent data, routine serologic screening programs are not advisable because of the expense and the low attack rate. Patient education is the recommended alternative.

Treatment. The physician should offer counseling regarding the risk of serious congenital infection and about pregnancy termination to women with confirmed first-trimester toxoplasmosis.

In the United States, the only effective antimicrobial therapy is a combination of sulfadiazine (or triple sulfonamide) with pyrimethamine. Because of bone marrow toxicity of this regimen, folinic acid or baking yeast should be given as well. Spiramycin has been used extensively in Europe but is not available in the United States. Based on studies in Europe, treating of primary toxoplasmosis in pregnancy with spiramycin significantly decreases, but does not eliminate, the risk of congenital infection in the fetus. In the United States, there is no agreement on treatment in pregnancy to control fetal infection. Those who emphasize the lack of efficacy studies and the teratogenicity of pyrimethamine conclude that pregnant women should not be treated except in the rare instance of serious maternal disease. Others avoid pyrimethamine but use sulfadiazine in women with first trimester toxoplasmosis who do not elect abortion.

Symptomatic infants with congenital toxoplasmosis should be treated with sulfadiazine or pyrimethamine (with folinic acid supplementation). Late central nervous system sequelae are possible in infants with asymptomatic toxoplasmosis at birth. Thus, some treat all newborns with toxoplasmosis, and others suggest treatment of newborns with proven toxoplasmosis and abnormal cerebrospinal fluid examination.

MASTITIS

Mastitis appears infrequently after delivery, in both epidemic and endemic form.[7] Epidemic puerperal mastitis occurs among hospitalized women in conjunction with staphylococcal nursery epidemics, whereas endemic puerperal mastitis occurs sporadically among nonhospitalized, nursing women. The latter type often presents as a lobular V-shaped cellulitis of the periglandular connective tissue. Often there is a fissure, crack, or irritation on the nipple. Endemic mastitis is much more common.

With epidemic mastitis, *S. aureus* has been the main culprit. For endemic mastitis, *S. aureus* again is a common pathogen, in either pure or mixed culture, but other common organisms include group A or group B streptococci. In up to 50% of cases, only normal skin flora are cultured from breast milk. Further insight into the relationship of breast symptoms, milk leukocytes, and quantitative breast milk cultures has been provided by recent work in Scandinavia.[45] Asymptomatic women had breast milk that was sterile or contained very low bacterial counts. Milk in these patients showed fewer than 10^6 leukocytes/ml. When bacteria were present in milk from asymptomatic women, the organisms were similar to those normally present on the skin. Most milk specimens revealed mixed cultures. Women with transient, self-resolving breast symptoms had milk with leukocyte counts less than 10^6/ml and cultures similar to those of women without symptoms. This group was said to have "milk stasis."

In symptomatic women with more persistent findings, breast milk showed more than 10^6 leukocytes/ml. Some of these women had negative milk cultures and were said to have "noninfectious inflammation" of the breast. Others had positive cultures and had "true mastitis." Still, approximately half of the cases of "true mastitis" resolved spontaneously without antibiotic therapy, but others developed breast abscesses or toxicity.

Sporadic mastitis most often begins from the second or third postpartum week to a number of months after delivery. Fever, malaise, and localized breast signs are the usual presenting problems. Stasis of milk from weaning is often suggested as the precipitating event for mastitis. However, only a minority of women (perhaps 20%) with mastitis have recently stopped nursing. Leukocyte count and culture of expressed breast milk are appropriate studies.

With early antibiotic treatment, endemic mastitis resolves within 24–48 hours, and abscess formation is unusual (10%). Based on the organisms involved and the well-known resistance of even community-acquired staphylococci to penicillin, the choice of initial antibiotic therapy is a penicillinase-resistant penicillin (such as dicloxacillin) or a cephalosporin. In most cases, antibiotics should be given orally as there is no need for hospitalization. When the milk leukocyte count is low (less than 10^6/ml), spontaneous, prompt resolution can be expected.

In addition to antibiotic therapy, adjunctive measures such as ice packs, breast support, and analgesics have been utilized. In most cases, the mother may continue to nurse from both breasts. If the infected side is too sore, she may pump this breast gently. Regular drainage of the infected breast may be important in preventing abscess. Infants do not seem to suffer any adverse effects from suckling an infected breast, except if an abscess has developed. If abscess develops prompt incision and drainage should be instituted.

WOUND INFECTION AFTER CESAREAN SECTION

Abdominal wound infection following cesarean section complicates approximately 4–10% of cases. A recent case control study has suggested an increased incidence of wound infection in patients with endometritis, chorioamnionitis, and fever or dystocia in labor. Length of labor, interval from ROM to delivery, number of vaginal examinations, operating time, and blood loss are important variables.[18]

Two major factors that determine whether a wound will become infected are the dose of bacterial contamination and the resistance of the patient. Bacterial contamination is either endogenous (from the patient's own microbial flora) or exogenous (from the environment). The source of endogenous bacteria in postcesarean section abdominal wound infections is the vagina and cervix. With labor, rupture of membranes, and repeated examinations, microorganisms from the lower genital tract gain access to the amniotic fluid. At cesarean section, the uterine and abdominal wounds are exposed to the amniotic fluid containing these organisms. The most likely bacteria in these wound infections include group B streptococci, *Escherichia coli, Proteus* species, *Klebsiella* species, and anaerobic bacteria such as Peptococcus, Peptostreptococcus, *Bacteroides fragilis, Bacteroides bivius,* and other *Bacteroides* species. Clostridial organisms also have been noted as part of the normal lower genital tract flora. *S. aureus* also may originate from a genital source. Because the normal flora is composed of aerobic and anaerobic bacteria, endogenous infections are often of mixed aerobic and anaerobic, or polymicrobic, type. The minimal inoculum required to produce an infection is 10^5 bacteria per milliliter or gram.

Factors that increase the rate of infection in clean wounds include razor-shaving the operative site, the use of the electrosurgical knife, the use of drains (especially if brought out through the skin incision), and prolonged preoperative hospitalization. The rate increases with increasing duration of the surgical procedure. Exogenous contamination is less important than the endogenous organisms from the patient's vagina or cervix. However, if general or local host resistance is reduced, a smaller inoculum of bacteria can gain a foothold, and exogenous contamination may become a significant cause of wound infection.

The patient's general resistance is an important determinant of infection. In general, increases in wound infection rate are associated with advancing age, diabetes, malnutrition, obesity, corticosteroid therapy, and immunosuppressive states. The condition of the wound is important in determining local resistance and to a large extent reflects surgical technique. Gentle tissue handling, complete hemostasis, debridement of devitalized tissue, adequate blood supply, obliteration of dead space, and closing of the wound without tension are commonly recognized principles of good surgical technique. The presence of hematomas or foreign bodies in the wound predisposes to the development of infection. Foreign bodies, such as suture material, reduce the minimal inoculum size for infection by a factor of 10,000. Hemoglobin interferes with leukocyte migration and phagocytosis. An inadequate blood supply leads to a lower oxygen tension and acidosis in the wound, with a resultant inability of macrophages to kill bacteria.

Early-Onset Wound Infection. Early-onset wound infection occurs within the first 48 hours after operation. The first signs are elevated temperature and an alteration in appearance of the abdominal wall or the wound. This alteration may be a spreading cellulitis or discoloration of the skin in association with an advancing margin of active infection. Early wound infection is often caused by a single bacterial pathogen, most commonly group A or B streptococci. A gram stain of material aspirated from the active margin of infection is diagnostic. Infection due to group A or B streptococci should be suspected if the patient develops diffuse cellulitis or systematic illness or both. *Clostridium perfringens* may rarely cause early-onset infection. In clostridial infection, cellulitis of the skin and subcutaneous tissue is associated with watery discharge. This is followed by the characteristic bronze appearance of the skin and crepitation in the vicinity of the wound.

The treatment of early wound infection consists of antibiotic therapy and excision of necrotic tissue. Penicillin is the antibiotic of choice for both clostridia and group A or B streptococci; alternatives include ampicillin, cephalosporins, cefoxitin, erythromycin, and chloramphenicol. Extensive debridement and excision of necrotic tissue may be required. It is crucial to remove all nonviable tissue. Failure to treat aggressively an early-onset wound infection exposes the patient to the risk of necrotizing fasciitis, bacteremia, and disseminated intravascular coagulation.

Late-Onset Wound Infection. Late-onset wound infections occur about six to eight days postoperatively. They manifest as fever and a swollen, erythematous, draining wound. In clean cases in which membranes have been ruptured and labor has occurred, the pathogens are the endogenous bacteria from the vagina and cervix (i.e., mixed aerobes and anaerobes), and multiple bacteria are the rule.

The diagnosis is based on the presence of purulent drainage. The treatment of late-onset wound infection is incision and drainage. Antibiotics generally are not required unless there is coexistent extensive cellulitis. Once the wound has been opened and drained and nonviable tissue has been excised, the patient should become afebrile, usually within 12 hours. If response does not occur within this time, broad-spectrum antibiotic therapy aimed at mixed aerobic and anaerobic bacteria should be instituted, and the possibility of a more extensive infection process such as necrotizing fasciitis considered. The diagnosis of this serious complication is based on the presence of edema and necrosis with partial liquefaction of the fascia adjacent to the wound site and the presence of thrombosed microvasculature in the tissue. Necrotizing fasciitis is a polymicrobic infection.

Although necrotizing fasciitis is rare after cesarean section, the necessity for early recognition, extensive surgical debridement, drainage, and antimicrobial therapy is well documented.

LISTERIOSIS[37]

Listeria monocytogenes is a small, non-spore-forming, gram-positive rod that shows alpha or beta hemolysis. In clinical samples, it may be mistaken for the common genital isolate, diphtheroids. *L. monocytogenes* may cause a range of infections in the pregnant woman, the fetus, or the neonate.[26]

L. monocytogenes may be present in genital cultures of asymptomatic pregnant patients, but clinical disease usually is characterized by fever, malaise, and coryza. Because of the resemblance of listeriosis to viral syndromes, any gravida with a febrile illness should have blood and cervical cultures. The laboratory should be informed that *L. monocytogenes* is suspected. Prompt antibiotic treatment is indicated if cultures are positive. On rare occasions, *Listeria* has led to fulminant infection in pregnant women.

When listeriosis occurs in early pregnancy, abortion may result. If maternal infection occurs late, fetal infection may lead to stillbirth or to an acutely ill newborn. In such cases, granulomatous foci of the liver, adrenals, lymph nodes, and other organs have been noted.

Disease also may become evident during the neonatal period. Clinically recognized forms include early-onset and late-onset varieties, reminiscent of group B streptococcal infections.

The antibiotic of choice for *L. monocytogenes* is ampicillin, with erythromycin as an alternative. In serious illness, an aminoglycoside often is recommended in combination with ampicillin.

Because *Listeria monocytogenes* may cause repeated problems, cervical cultures should be performed on pregnant women who have had repeated abortion or previous offspring with *L. monocytogenes* infection. Treatment with oral ampicillin and reculture are appropriate for asymptomatic women with this history and with a positive genital culture for *L. monocytogenes*. High-dose parenteral ampicillin, with or without gentamicin, is in order for a febrile gravida with listeriosis.

REFERENCES

1. Anstey, J. T., Sheldon, G. W., and Blythe, J. G.: Infectious morbidity after primary cesarean sections in a private institution. *Am. J. Obstet. Gynecol.* **136**:205–210, 1980.
2. Blanco, J. D., Gibbs, R. S., Malherbe, H., Strickland-Cholmley, J., St. Clair, P. J., and Castaneda, Y. S.: A controlled study of genital mycoplasmas in amniotic fluid from patients with intra-amniotic infection. *J. Infect. Dis.* **147**:650–653, 1983.
3. Centers for Disease Control. *Morb. Mortal. Wkly. Rpt.* **33**:301–317, 1984.
4. Cunningham, F. G., Hemsell, D. L., DePalma, R. T., Kappus, S., Roark, M., and Nobles, B.: Moxalactam for obstetric and gynecologic infections in vitro and dose-finding studies. *Am. J. Obstet. Gynecol.* **139**:915–921, 1981.
5. D'Angelo, L. J. and Sokol, R. J.: Time-related

peripartum determinants of postpartum morbidity. *Obstet. Gynecol.* **55**:319–323, 1980.

6. DeNicola, L. K. and Hanshaw, J. B.: Congenital and neonatal varicella. (Editorial) *J. Pediatr.* **94**:175–176, 1979.
7. Deveraux, W. P.: Acute puerperal mastitis. *Am. J. Obstet. Gynecol.* **108**:78–81, 197.
8. DiZerega, G., Yonekura, L., Roy, S., Nakamura, R. M., and Ledger, W. J.: A comparison of clindamycin-gentamicin and penicillin-gentamicin in the treatment of post-cesarean section endomyometritis. *Am. J. Obstet. Gynecol.* **134**:238–242, 1979.
9. Duff, P. and Gibbs, R. S.: Pelvic vein thrombophlebitis: Diagnostic dilemma and therapeutic challenge. *Obstet. Gynecol. Surv.* **38**:365–373, 1983.
10. Duff, P. and Keiser, J. F.: A comparative study of two antibiotic regimens for the treatment of operative site infections. *Am. J. Obstet. Gynecol.* **142**:996–1003, 1982.
11. Dworsky, M. E., Welch, K., Cassady, G., and Stagno, S.: Occupational risk for primary cytomegalovirus infection among pediatric health care workers. *N. Eng. J. Med.* **309**:950–953, 1983.
12. Filker, R. and Monif, G. R.: The significance of temperature during the first 24 hours postpartum. *Obstet. Gynecol.* **53**:358–362, 1979.
13. Garite, T. J. and Freeman, R. K.: Chorioamnionitis in the preterm gestation. *Obstet. Gynecol.* **59**:539–545, 1982.
14. Gibbs, R. S.: Clinical risk factors for puerperal infection. *Obstet. Gynecol.* **55**(Suppl):178–184, 1980.
15. Gibbs, R. S.: Diagnosis of intra-amniotic infection. *Semin. Perinatol.* **1**:71–77, 1977.
16. Gibbs, R. S., Blanco, J. D., Castaneda, Y. S., and St. Clair, P. J.: A double-blind, randomized comparison of clindamycin–gentamicin versus cefamandole for treatment of post-cesarean section endomyometritis. *Am. J. Obstet. Gynecol.* **144**:261–267, 1982.
17. Gibbs, R. S., Blanco, J. D., Duff, P., Castaneda, Y. S., and St. Clair, P. J.: A double-blind, randomized comparison of moxalactam versus clindamycin–gentamicin in treatment of endomyometritis after cesarean section delivery. *Am. J. Obstet. Gynecol.* **146**:769–772, 1983.
18. Gibbs, R. S. Blanco, J. D., and St. Clair, P. J.: A case-control study of wound abscess after cesarean delivery. *Obstet. Gynecol.* **62**:498–501, 1983.
19. Gibbs, R. S., Blanco, J. D., St. Clair, P. J., and Castaneda, Y. S.: Quantitative bacteriology of amniotic fluid from women with clinical intra-amniotic infection at term. *J. Infect. Dis.* **145**:1–8, 1982.
20. Gibbs, R. S., Castillo, M. S., and Rodgers, P. J.: Management of acute chorioamnionitis. *Am. J. Obstet. Gynecol.* **136**:709–713, 1980.
21. Gibbs, R. S., Jones, P. M., and Wilder, C. J.: Internal fetal monitoring and maternal infection following cesarean section. A prospective study. *Obstet. Gynecol.* **52**:193–197, 1978.
22. Gibbs, R. S. and Sweet, R. L.: Maternal and fetal infections. In: *Maternal-Fetal Medicine. Principles and Practice.* Philadelphia, W. B. Saunders, 1984, pp. 603–606.
23. Gilstrap, L. C., Cunningham, F. G., and Whalley, P. J.: Acute pyelonephritis in pregnancy: An anterospective study. *Obstet. Gynecol.* **57**:409–413, 1981.
24. Grossman, J. H.: Herpes simplex virus (HSV) infections. *Clin. Obstet. Gynecol.* **25**:555–561, 1982.
25. Hagglund, L., Christensen, K. K., Christensen, P., and Kamme, C.: Risk factors in cesarean section infection. *Obstet. Gynecol.* **62**:145–150, 1983.
26. Halliday, H. L. and Hirata, T.: Perinatal listeriosis: A review of twelve patients. *Am. J. Obstet. Gynecol.* **133**:405–410, 1979.
27. Hemsell, D. L., Cunningham, F. G., DePalma, R. T., Nobles, B. J., Heard, M., and Hemsell, P. G.: Cefotaxime sodium therapy for endomyometritis following cesarean section: Dose-finding and comparative studies. *Obstet. Gynecol.* **52**:489–497, 1983.
28. Hunter, K., Stagno, S., Capps, E., and Smith, R. J.: Prenatal screening of pregnant women for infections caused by cytomegalovirus, Epstein–Barr virus, herpes virus, rubella, and *Toxoplasma gondii. Am. J. Obstet. Gynecol.* **145**:269–273, 1983.
29. Kibrick, S.: Herpes simplex infection at term. What to do with mother, newborn, and nursery personnel. *JAMA* **243**:157–160, 1980.
30. Koh, K. S., Chan, F. H., Monfared, A. H., Ledger, W. J., and Paul, R. S.: The changing perinatal and maternal outcome in chorioamnionitis. *Obstet. Gynecol.* **53**:730–734, 1979.
31. Lamey, J. R., Eschenbach, D. A., Mitchell, S. H., Blumhagen, J. M., Foy, H. M., and Kenney, G. E.: Isolation of mycoplasmas and bacteria from the blood of postpartum women. *Am. J. Obstet. Gynecol.* **143**:104–112, 1982.
32. Looff, J. D. and Hager, W. D.: Management of chorioamnionitis. *Surg. Gynecol. Obstet.* **158**:161–166, 1984.
33. Mann, J. M., Preblud, S. R., and Hoffman, R. E.: Assessing risks of rubella infection. *JAMA* **245**:1647–1652, 1981.
34. Murphy, P. A.: Temperature regulations and the pathogenesis of fever. In: *Principles and Practice of Infectious Diseases*, 2nd Edition. G. L. Mandell, R. G. Douglass, and J. E. Bennett (Eds.). New York, John Wiley & Sons, 1985, pp. 334–339.
35. Rehu, M. and Nilsson, C. G.: Risk factors for febrile morbidity associated with cesarean section. *Obstet. Gynecol.* **56**:269–273, 1980.
36. Remington, J. S. and Desmonts, G.: Toxoplasmosis. In: *Infectious Diseases of the Fetus and Newborn Infant*, 2nd Edition. J. S. Remington, and J. O. Klein (Eds.). Philadelphia, W. B. Saunders, 1983, pp. 144–263.

37. Shackelford, P. G. and Feigen, R. S.: Listeria revisited. *Am. J. Dis. Child.* **131**:391-392, 1977.
38. Shy, K. K. and Eschenbach, D. A.: Fatal perineal cellulitis from an episiotomy site. *Obstet. Gynecol.* **54**:292-298, 1979.
39. Stiver, H. G., Forward, K. R., Livingstone, R. A., Fugure, P., LeMay, M., Verschelden, G., Hunter, J. D. S., Carson, G. D., Beresford, P., and Tyrrell, D. L.: Multicenter comparison of cefoxitin *vs.* cefazolin for prevention of infectious morbidity after non-elective cesarean section. *Am. J. Obstet. Gynecol.* **145**:158-163, 1983.
40. Stagno, S., Pass, R. F., Dworsky, M. E., and Alford, C. A.: Maternal cytomegalovirus infection and perinatal transmission. *Clin. Obstet. Gynecol.* **25**:563-576, 1982.
41. Strausbaugh, L. J. and Llorens, A. S.: Cefoperazone therapy for obstetric and gynecologic infections. *Rev. Infect. Dis.* **5**(Suppl):155-160, 1983.
42. Swartz, W. H. and Grolle, K.: Use of prophylactic antibiotics in cesarean section: Review of literature. *J. Reprod. Med.* **26**:595-609, 1981.
43. Sweet, R. L. and Ledger, W. J.: Cefoxitin: Single-agent treatment of mixed aerobic-anaerobic pelvic infections. *Obstet. Gynecol.* **54**:193-198, 1979.
44. Sweet, R. L., Robbie, M. D., Ohm-Smith, M., and Hadley, W. K.: Comparative study of piperacillin versus cefoxitin in the treatment of obstetric and gynecologic infections. *Am. J. Obstet. Gynecol.* **145**:342-349, 1983.
45. Thomsen, A. C., Espersen, T., and Margaard, S.: Course and treatment of milk stasis, noninfectious inflammation of the breast, and infectious mastitis in nursing women. *Am. J. Obstet. Gynecol.* **149**:492-495, 1983.
46. Wager, G. P., Martin, O. H., Koutsky, L., Eschenbach, D. A., Daling, J. R., Chiang, W. T., Alexander, E. R., and Holmes, K. K.: Puerperal infectious morbidity: Relationship to route of delivery and to antepartum *Chlamydia trachomatis* infection. *Am. J. Obstet. Gynecol.* **135**:1028-1033, 1980.
47. Yoder, P. R., Gibbs, R. S., Blanco, J. D., Castaneda, Y. S., and St. Clair, P. J.: A prospective controlled study of maternal and perinatal outcome after intra-amniotic infection at term. *Am. L. Obstet. Gynecol.* **145**:695-701, 1983.

39

ACUTE RESPIRATORY PROBLEMS

When pregnant women complain of acute respiratory difficulty, a number of conditions must be considered. Historical findings that lead to the correct diagnosis include duration of pregnancy, relationship of the dyspnea to labor, presence of fever or chills, complaint of pleuritic pain, relationship of the dyspnea to anesthetic agents and tocolytic drugs, history of cardiac disease, and past history of similar episodes. Asthmatic patients usually are able to identify a recurrent asthmatic attack and they also can gauge the severity of the attack by comparing it to past episodes.

Physical examination alone is seldom sufficient to make a diagnosis but is quite important. The patient's general appearance should be observed for signs of air hunger, such as use of accessory respiratory muscles, flaring of the nostrils, and tachypnea. These findings all give an indication of the severity of the patient's dyspnea. Cyanosis, if present, confirms the hypoxia. Fever gives a clue to an infectious etiology. The character of the breath sounds audible on auscultation provides an indication of the underlying pathologic process. Rales are indicative of pneumonitis or pulmonary edema. Prolonged expiration with wheezing indicates a bronchospastic process such as asthma. Absence of breath sounds is noted in cases of pulmonary consolidation. A pleural friction rub is sometimes heard in association with pulmonary infarction.

Basic laboratory evaluation includes a complete blood count and a differential count of the leukocytes. Sputum, if present, should be submitted for Gram's stain and culture. Arterial blood gas evaluation should be obtained in all but the mildest cases of respiratory difficulty. Roentgenogram of the chest completes the basic laboratory evaluation. More specific diagnostic tests (arteriograms, pulmonary scans) are reserved for specific indications and are not obtained on all patients.

Based on the initial evaluation of history, physical examination, and laboratory data, a diagnosis can be reached within a short time in most cases of respiratory distress in pregnancy. The causes of dyspnea discussed in this chapter include asthma, pneumonitis, pulmonary edema, aspiration pneumonitis, amniotic fluid embolus, and pulmonary embolus.

Changes in respiratory physiology that occur in pregnancy are discussed in Chapter 3. Pregnancy is basically a state of compensated respiratory alkalosis. Arterial pH remains normal at 7.40–7.47. Arterial blood gas tensions are around 100 mmHg for oxygen (PaO_2) and 25–32 mmHg for carbon dioxide ($PaCO_2$).[15]

ASTHMA

Definition, Incidence, Etiology, and Significance

Asthma is an obstruction of airflow in response to a variety of stimuli. The obstruction is more marked in expiration than in inspiration and results in air trapping in the lungs with resultant hyperinflation. Animal danders, molds, pollens, stress, drugs, steroid withdrawal, and viral upper respiratory infections are among the factors known to provoke asthmatic attacks.[17] The reversible attacks are caused by contraction of bronchiolar smooth muscle accompanied by hypersecretion of mucus and by mucosal edema.

Asthma affects approximately 1% of pregnant women.[15,17] The effect of pregnancy on asthma is variable. Almost half of pregnant asthmatics report no change in the frequency or severity of asthmatic attacks during pregnancy. The other half of pregnant asthmatics is divided almost evenly. Twenty-nine percent report improvement and 22% report worsening of asthma.[15] Asthmatic frequency and severity may differ in different pregnancies in the same woman. Asthmatic attacks may occur at any time in pregnancy.

With good control of asthma during pregnancy, there is no increase in maternal or perinatal mortality.[15] Fetal demise is more likely to occur when there is severe maternal hypoxia (arterial PaO_2 below 60 mmHg). Infants of asthmatic mothers have more than a 50% chance of developing asthma during their lives.

Clinical Findings

The history is of great importance in the diagnosis and treatment of asthma. Almost all patients give a history of similar attacks in the past. Items that should be identified include the duration of the attack, events immediately preceding the attack, current medications, and history of other pulmonary or cardiac disease. History of fever and the presence and character of sputum also should be noted.

Physical examination should be complete. Wheezing and prolonged expiratory phase of respiration are characteristic. In addition to the items listed in the basic physical examination, pulsus paradoxus should be searched for. Pulsus paradoxus is a decrease or even disappearance of the pulse pressure during inspiration. If present during an asthmatic attack, this otherwise nonspecific sign may indicate that the attack is severe.

Basic laboratory investigation includes complete blood count, serum electrolytes, arterial blood gas determination, sputum for Gram's stain, and spirometry. If the patient is febrile or if neutrophils are noted in the sputum, a roentgenogram of the chest should be obtained in search of bronchopneumonia.

The results of the initial investigation allow some determination of the severity of the attack. There are several methods of determining severity. None of them is perfect. One widely used method of determining the need for hospitalization and the possibility of relapse involves the use of seven clinical criteria.[13] This method utilizes simple clinical observations and can be performed by any physician at the bedside. Each of the seven items is given a score of one point if present. If the total score is four or more, the patient should be hospitalized. The seven criteria are:

1. Heart rate—if 120 or more per minute.
2. Respiratory rate—if 30 or more per minute.
3. Pulsus paradoxus—if 18 mmHg or more.
4. Peak expiratory flow rate—if 120 liters per minute or less.
5. Dyspnea—if moderate or severe.
6. Wheezing—if moderate or severe.
7. Use of accessory respiratory muscles—if moderate or severe.

Three of the seven findings are subjective. Not all clinicians have found this index to be as sensitive and specific as first thought.[7,34] Nevertheless, it is widely used to assess the severity of an asthmatic attack.

Other assessment plans for judging the severity of asthmatic attacks, determining the need for hospitalization, and evaluating the response to therapy place more reliance on arterial blood gas determinations. Respiratory alkalosis with an elevated pH and a low $PaCO_2$ (for pregnancy) indicates a mild attack even if the PaO_2 is somewhat low. A combination of depressed PaO_2, normal $PaCO_2$ (for pregnancy), and normal pH indicates possible danger. Respiratory acidosis with a low pH, a low PaO_2, and a $PaCO_2$ elevated for pregnancy indicates a very severe process. A pH below 7.35 or a $PaCO_2$ above 38 mmHg warrants consideration of an intensive care environment.[17] The fetus is in danger from maternal hypoxia when the PaO_2 drops below 60 mmHg.[5,17]

Treatment

The treatment of asthma is altered very little by pregnancy. The goals of therapy are the same, ". . . to prevent death, respiratory failure, status asthmaticus, emergency room visits, and disabling wheezing."[15] Beta adrenergic stimulants, theophylline and its derivative, aminophylline, and glucocorticoids are the mainstays of treatment because they are generally safe for the mother and are not teratogenic.

Epinephrine is still considered the drug of

choice for treating acute asthmatic attacks in pregnancy.[15] It has alpha adrenergic as well as beta adrenergic activity. Some contend that pure beta agonists, such as terbutaline, are preferable to epinephrine. There is no compelling evidence for this conclusion, but terbutaline is certainly a safe alternative. Epinephrine is given subcutaneously as a 1:1000 aqueous solution. The dose is 0.3 ml if the patient weighs less than 60 kg, 0.4 ml if the patient weighs 60–80 kg, and 0.5 ml if she weighs over 80 kg. The dose may be repeated every 20–30 minutes for a total of three doses if there are no adverse effects and if improvement has not occurred. Terbutaline also is administered subcutaneously in a dose of 0.25 mg. It may be repeated once in 15–30 minutes if significant improvement has not occurred. The maximum dose of terbutaline is 0.5 mg every four hours. The maximum effect of terbutaline is reached in 30–60 minutes. It may last as long as four hours. If patients do not respond to either of these adrenergic drugs, other measures should be taken. Patients should NOT be given both epinephrine and terbutaline. Other beta adrenergic agonists may be safe and effective in pregnancy but experience with them is limited.

Beta agonists work by stimulating the beta 2 receptors in bronchial smooth muscle. This results in an increase in cyclic AMP, which causes rapid bronchodilatation and inhibits release of chemical mediators from mast cells.[42]

Theophylline and its derivative, aminophylline, are methylxanthines. They are effective in the treatment of acute asthma because they inhibit the enzyme phosphodiesterase, thus slowing the breakdown of cyclic AMP.[42] Elevated levels of cyclic AMP cause bronchodilatation. Since beta agonists and theophylline increase cyclic AMP via different mechanisms, it has been hypothesized that they should have a synergistic effect. This has not proved to be the case. The combination of epinephrine and aminophylline works no better than epinephrine alone in treating an acute asthmatic attack.[19] Intravenous aminophylline, however, is the drug usually used when beta agonists are ineffective. Some physicians prefer intravenous aminophylline to beta agonists as first-line treatment of an acute asthmatic attack.

The initial intravenous dose of aminophylline is 6–7 mg/kg of body weight[17] mixed in 100 ml of aqueous dextrose solution and infused over 20 minutes. If the patient reports taking oral theophylline prior to the attack, the intravenous loading dose may be reduced to 4 mg/kg or not given at all. However, a history of theophylline ingestion has proved to have little correlation with serum theophylline levels.[19] If serum theophylline levels can be obtained rapidly, this is the best guide to initial therapy. The therapeutic range of theophylline is 10–20 μg/ml of serum.

After the initial loading dose infusion, therapy is maintained at a rate of 0.7 mg/kg/hour for 12 hours and then decreased to 0.5 mg/kg/hour.[21] The serum level of theophylline is used as a guide to therapy.

Additional initial therapy includes the administration of humidified oxygen at a rate of 4–6 liters/minute. Positive-pressure breathing of an aerosol containing a bronchodilator such as isoproterenol is indicated at times. Isoproterenol 1:200 may be added to the nembulizer of the positive-pressure machine; 0.5 ml is added to 2.5 ml of water or saline. This agent should not be used concomitantly with other adrenergic agonists because the combined effects may cause cardiac arrhythmias. Antibiotics such as penicillin or erythromycin are indicated when infection is thought to play a role in the clinical picture. Hydration is important in all but the mildest attacks. An intravenous line should be inserted and fluids given to prevent dehydration.

Corticosteroids are used to treat status asthmaticus, that is, asthma that fails to respond to the usual therapeutic measures. In this situation, corticosteroids are lifesaving. They inhibit chemical mediators and thereby decrease mucosal edema and relieve bronchospasm. They also inhibit inflammatory reaction.[42] The onset of action of corticosteroids requires six hours. This dose may be repeated at intervals of four to eight hours as necessary.[17]

Deaths from asthma are usually from mucus stagnation and impaction which produce asphyxiation. Tension pneumothorax may occur in this setting. Postural drainage, endotracheal intubation, and bronchoscopy are occasionally necessary in the acute treatment of asthma.

Continuing Treatment

The continuing management of bronchial asthma is important to prevent disabling wheezing and recurrent acute attacks. The current *Physician's Desk Reference* lists 58 medications for asthma without mentioning corticosteroids or over-the-counter products. Obviously, there is no single best treatment and this chapter will not deal with them all.

Each drug used in the acute phase of asthma, as well as for outpatient treatment, has its own contraindications and precautions for use. The drugs discussed below are safe for use in pregnancy by women in the absence of specific contraindications to their use. Use of several adrenergic drugs at the same time is to be avoided.

Inhalers are the most commonly used outpatient medication for asthma. Patients can monitor their own therapy and use inhalers as necessary. Commonly used inhalers contain epinephrine, isoproterenol, metaproterenol, or isoetharine—all these have beta adrenergic activity.[42]

Oral preparations are also popular for outpatient therapy. Beta agonists such as oral terbutaline in a dosage of 2.5 mg twice a day to 5.0 mg three times a day may be used, depending on response and side effects. Short- and long-acting theophylline preparations are used in place of, or in addition to, beta agonists. Serum theophylline levels are used to monitor theophylline therapy. The therapeutic range is 10–20 μg/ml. Short-acting preparations are given as 100–200 mg every six hours to achieve this level unless symptoms of toxicity intervene.[17] The development of long-acting theophylline has simplified dosage because it need be taken only twice daily.[44] Ephedrine, though safe, has fallen from favor in the treatment of asthma. Products containing combinations of theophylline, ephedrine, and barbiturates are probably safe but are not recommended in the treatment of pregnant asthmatics.[15]

Women who require corticosteroid treatment for an acute asthmatic attack can occasionally have the drug dosage tapered rapidly and discontinued. More commonly, they require corticosteroids for a longer period of time. In this situation, prednisone 30–50 mg/day is the usual starting dose for oral therapy. The drug is then slowly withdrawn.

If the patient cannot be taken off corticosteroid therapy, several options are available. She can be switched to an alternate day regimen of steroids to decrease side effects. She can be switched to a corticosteroid inhaler such as beclomethasone or triamcinolone. Experience with these inhalers has been good. Most women are able to discontinue oral corticosteroids or to reduce the dose markedly.[1] Systemic effects of the steroid inhalers are much less than those of the oral drugs. The mouth should be rinsed after use of these inhalers to decrease the risk of fungal colonization. A third option is the use of cromolyn sodium inhalers.[17] Cromolyn is an inhaled powder that is ineffective in treating acute asthmatic attacks but is useful in managing steroid-dependent asthmatics. By using this agent, steroid therapy often can be reduced or eliminated. Cromolyn inhibits the degranulation of sensitized mast cells.[42]

PNEUMONIA

Incidence and Significance

Few articles have been written in recent years on pneumonia in pregnancy. In the preantibiotic and early antibiotic eras, most reports on pneumonia in pregnancy noted a high rate of premature delivery and a very high maternal mortality rate. Recently, an article from Southern California placed the incidence of diagnosis of antepartum pneumonia at approximately 1/2300 deliveries.[5] Diagnosis was based on clinical findings of cough, sputum production, fever of 38 °C or higher, and roentgenographic findings compatible with pneumonia. There were no maternal deaths among the 39 patients and preterm delivery was markedly less than that cited in previous reports. The outcome for the mother with antepartum pneumonia and for her fetus has never been better, although the overall perinatal mortality rate was still 40/1000.

Pneumonia is still a potentially serious disease. Twenty-five of the 39 women had arterial blood gas determinations; 12 had a PaO_2 below 70 mmHg and three were in the fetal danger zone below 60 mmHg. Additionally, half of the patients were anemic, as evidenced by a hemoglobin level below 10 g%. Eight of the patients had other significant medical problems.

Sputum and blood cultures were obtained in all patients before antibiotic therapy was started. All blood cultures were negative for pathogens and only 21 of the 39 women had culture-proven bacterial pneumonia. Thirteen women had *Streptococcus pneumoniae* cultured from the sputum. Of the 18 culture-negative pneumonias, two had serologic evidence of mycoplasma as the cause of pneumonia. Sixteen women had no etiologic agent identified.

This report from Southern California is probably not representative of all areas of the nation. Locations with a less favorable climate may well have a higher incidence of pneumonia as well as a poorer outcome.

Etiology, Diagnosis, and Treatment

The most common bacterial cause of pneumonia is *Streptococcus pneumoniae.* It was formerly known as *Diplococcus pneumoniae.* The pneumonia caused by this organism often is termed pneumococcal or diplococcal pneumonia.

Pneumococcal pneumonia usually begins abruptly with rapid appearance of fever, chills, pleuritic chest pain, and a productive cough that is usually purulent and may have a bloody tinge. Dyspnea and tachypnea are present. Auscultation of the lung fields reveals rales, dullness, or bronchial breath sounds. The classic roentgenographic appearance of the lungs is lobar consolidation with air bronchograms, but the infiltrate may appear patchy on occasion.

Gram's stain of the sputum reveals numerous polymorphonuclear leukocytes and Gram positive lancet-shaped diplococci. Culture of the sputum does not always grow the organism, even though it is seen on Gram's stain. Blood cultures are positive for the pneumococcus in approximately 30% of cases.

Pregnant women suspected of having pneumococcal pneumonia should be hospitalized. Laboratory evaluation including cultures and arterial blood gas determinations should be obtained. Treatment with humidified oxygen is usually beneficial. Its continued use is determined by the arterial PaO_2 Fever, if high, should be lowered and antibiotic therapy should be started at once. *S. pneumoniae* is very sensitive to penicillin. Therapy is begun with a total dose of 2.4 million units a day given in divided doses and is continued for three to five days after the patient defervesces. Total duration of therapy is usually seven to ten days. Patients allergic to penicillin should be treated with erythromycin.

Another common cause of pneumonia in pregnancy is *Mycoplasma pneumoniae*. Mycoplasma are the smallest known free living organisms and lack a rigid cell wall. Mycoplasma cause a large percentage of pneumonias in ambulatory patients, so-called "walking pneumonia."

Mycoplasma pneumonia is clinically distinguishable from pneumococcal pneumonia. It typically presents with a gradual onset of sore throat, headache, fever, and nonproductive cough. If sputum is present, it is not purulent and there is usually no leukocytosis. Roentgenogram of the chest reveals patchy infiltrates. Diagnosis usually is based on the serological finding of complement fixing antibodies to mycoplasma. The presence of cold agglutinins in the patient's blood suggests the diagnosis of mycoplasma.

The treatment of choice for *Mycoplasma pneumoniae* in pregnancy is erythromycin. When there is doubt about the causative organism, pneumococcus or mycoplasma, erythromycin is a satisfactory initial choice for antibiotic therapy.

PULMONARY EDEMA

(Pulmonary edema is discussed also in Chapter 49.)

Significance

Pulmonary edema is a true medical emergency caused by fluid leaving the pulmonary vasculature and entering the alveoli. Patients literally can drown in their own edema fluid.

Pathophysiology

Three pathophysiologic mechanisms can act alone or in concert to produce pulmonary edema. Intravascular pressure in the pulmonary vascular bed can rise above the plasma colloidal osmotic pressure. This causes free fluid to leave vessels and enter the interstitial spaces and the alveoli. Alternately, the plasma colloidal osmotic pressure can drop lower than the intravascular pressure with the same result. Finally, increased permeability of the vasculature of the pulmonary circulation will promote transfer of fluid into the interstitial tissue and alveoli despite normal colloidal osmotic and intravascular pressures. The capacity of the pulmonary lymphatics to remove lung fluid is apparently important but its role in the pathophysiology of pulmonary edema is poorly understood.

In clinical practice, intravascular pressure in the pulmonary circulation is measured as the pulmonary capillary wedge pressure (PCWP), which reflects the pressure in the left atrium. Normally, the PCWP is around 10 mmHg. When it rises to levels around 18 mmHg, pulmonary congestion results and, at levels of 25–30 mmHg, pulmonary edema results. The plasma colloidal osmotic pressure (COP) is usually 25 mmHg in healthy adults. Ordinarily, pulmonary edema does not occur as long as the COP is more than 6 mmHg above the PCWP. In pregnancy, and especially at the time of labor, delivery, and the early postpartum period, the COP drops.[10,14] When the COP drops low enough, small rises in PCWP are sufficient to cause pulmonary edema. Increased vessel wall permeability cannot be measured easily but is implied when the other two factors are normal.

Etiologies

There are several causes of pulmonary edema in obstetrics. Maternal cardiac disease is an important cause (see Chapter 31). Mitral stenosis is the classic cardiac lesion causing pulmonary edema. The cardiac output rises in normal pregnancy, labor, and the puerperium. Patients with mitral stenosis often cannot keep up with the physiologic demands because of narrowing of the mitral valve. Pressure in the left atrium rises and is reflected in an increase in the PCWP. Pulmonary edema can result. Failure of the heart as a pump also produces pulmonary edema associated with other conditions.

Abnormal permeability of the pulmonary capillary bed causes progressive respiratory insufficiency from pulmonary edema. Somewhere in the continuum, the patient may develop what has come to be known as adult respiratory distress syndrome (ARDS).[30] Causes of increased pulmonary capillary permeability in obstetric patients include severe preeclampsia, sepsis, shock, aspiration of acid gastric contents, and amniotic fluid embolus.

Excessive hydration can lower COP sufficiently to produce pulmonary edema in otherwise healthy adults. As noted above, obstetric patients tend to have a low COP, which normally drops in labor and after delivery. Excessive hydration may play a role in the genesis of pulmonary edema seen with the use of tocolytic agents to treat premature labor.

Eclampsia and severe preeclampsia cause pulmonary edema by several mechanisms. Studies using balloon flotation catheters have variously identified left ventricular failure, pulmonary capillary leaks, and a combination of low COP and elevated PCWP as the cause of pulmonary edema in patients with severe preeclampsia-eclampsia.[4,40] No single pathophysiological mechanism explains all cases.

Clinical Findings

Patients with pulmonary edema are critically ill. They are apprehensive because of suffocating dyspnea. They are tachypneic, often cyanotic, and produce frothy blood-tinged sputum. Diffuse rales can be heard throughout the chest. Chest roentgenogram shows bilateral perihilar or diffuse infiltrates. Arterial blood gas determinations usually show a respiratory acidosis with a PaO_2 less than 70 mmHg.

Treatment

Conventional treatment is aimed at decreasing blood return to the heart and improving oxygenation. To this end, morphine is often given in small amounts to relieve anxiety. Oxygen may be given by face mask or nasal prongs, but it is better administered by a positive-pressure machine. Positive-pressure respiration helps to retard venous return to the heart and also helps to drive fluid from the alveoli. Phlebotomy and the use of rotating tourniquets are treatments formerly utilized to decrease blood return to the heart. They have largely been abandoned. Rotating tourniquets can be dangerous if not rotated on schedule.

Digitalis preparations have been used in an attempt to increase the strength of cardiac contractions. The use of cardiac glycosides became less important when potent diuretics became available. Furosemide is an important agent in the management of pulmonary edema. The diuretic action of furosemide is well known. It decreases blood volume and venous return. Additionally, furosemide reduces venous tone and promotes pooling of blood in the venous system, further reducing venous return.

Central venous pressure has been shown to be correlated poorly with PCWP in some patients.[4,40] Therefore, balloon flotation catheters should be used to assist in the management of patients with pulmonary edema. Additional means of monitoring the response to therapy include measurement of COP, urinary output, serum electrolytes, and arterial blood gases. Cardiac monitoring is also important.

As discussed in Chapter 49, newer treatments are aimed at reducing the afterload on the heart through the use of vasodilators such as sodium nitroprusside.

Further management of the pregnancy after successful treatment of pulmonary edema depends on the clinical situation. Patients with cardiac disease are usually candidates for continued medical management of the cardiac disease until they go into labor. Patients with excessive hydration usually respond promptly to diuretics; their management can proceed with careful observation of their fluid status. Most preeclamptic patients who develop pulmonary edema do so after delivery,[4] so continued management is not ordinarily a problem. If they are undelivered at the time of pulmonary edema, delivery should be strongly considered once the patient has recovered sufficiently to withstand induction of labor or cesarean delivery. Patients with pulmonary capillary leaks have a tendency to develop the more chronic situation of adult respiratory distress syndrome (ARDS). These women are in greater danger of death and certainly should be placed in an intensive care environment.

ASPIRATION PNEUMONITIS

Definition, Incidence, and Significance

The first anesthetic death to result from aspiration was reported in 1848 by Simpson.[6] Almost 100 years later, Mendelson differentiated aspiration of liquid gastric contents from aspiration of solids. He described aspiration pneumonitis in obstetric patients and in experimental animals.[22] He concluded that aspiration of solid particles caused laryngeal or bronchial obstruction with resultant suffocation. Aspiration of solids was associated with dyspnea, cyanosis, and tachycardia. Atelectasis, consolidation, and mediastinal shift were noted on roentgenograms of the chest.

Aspiration of liquid gastric contents was eight times more common than was aspiration of solids in his series. Aspiration of liquid contents, a condition now called Mendelson's syndrome, was described as "... an apparently hitherto unrecognized asthmatic-like syndrome with distinct clinical, roentgenologic and pathologic features ... due to the irritative action of gastric hydrochloric acid."[22]

Today, 10–15% of maternal mortality is related to anesthetic complications. Aspiration pneumonitis is the leading cause of anesthetic deaths in obstetrics.[9,18,23] The mortality rate of aspiration pneumonitis is more than 50%. In surgical patients, the average hospital stay of survivors is prolonged by three weeks.[39] Aspiration pneumonitis is a significant and expensive problem.

Etiology

Most cases of aspiration occur when patients who have a depressed level of consciousness and consequent loss of protective laryngeal reflexes vomit. This typically occurs with general anesthetics but is also known to occur with sedation from drugs or alcohol. Various neuromuscular disorders can cause aspiration as can iatrogenic mechanisms.

Pregnant women are especially prone to aspiration pneumonitis. The elevated intragastric pressure associated with pregnancy is enhanced by the lithotomy position. The lower esophageal sphincter is less competent during pregnancy, perhaps due to the action of progesterone.[9] The anatomy of the gastroesophageal junction is altered so that reflux of gastric contents meets less resistance. Gastric motility is decreased, especially during labor. This allows for a larger gastric volume that potentially can be aspirated. The onset of labor and the need for emergency cesarean delivery are unpredictable, thus many of the prophylactic measures recommended before elective surgery do not apply in obstetric patients.

Pathophysiology

The pH of aspirated liquid is critical to the development of aspiration pneumonitis. A pH above 2.5 is unlikely to cause the full blown syndrome.[46] The lower the pH, the more severe the syndrome. A pH below 1.8 was associated with 100% mortality in one series.[46] Aspiration of particulate acidic material produces a more prolonged pneumonitis than does aspiration of acidic liquid material only. The volume of aspirated liquid is also important. The critical volume associated with clinical problems seems to be around 0.4 ml/kg—approximately 25 ml in an adult.[31]

The distribution of the aspirated liquid material within the lungs is another factor in determining patient outcome. The aspirate typically localizes in the lower lobes, especially the right lower lobe. When more than one lobe is involved, mortality increases.[6]

The toxic effect of aspirated hydrochloric acid is manifested within 20 seconds.[39] The acid destroys alveolar lining cells, which leads to transudation of fluid, hypovolemia, and shock. It also produces bronchospasm and destroys the surfactant-producing alveolar cells, which leads to atelectasis and shunting within the lungs. All these factors produce hypoxia secondary to a chemical pulmonary edema.[39] Hypotension and decreased pulmonary blood flow also result.

Clinical Presentation

Symptoms typically appear during or just after general anesthetic but also may occur in sedated or obtunded patients. Dyspnea is the most prominent symptom. Signs include cyanosis, tachycardia, shock, and tachypnea. Pulmonary findings are the wheezes associated with bronchospasm and rales and rhonchi secondary to pulmonary edema.

Chest roentgenograms reveal patchy infiltrates that often are localized to the most dependent portion of the lungs at the time of aspiration. The right lower lobe is involved most often. Laboratory findings include leukocytosis and hypoxia.

Resolution of aspiration pneumonitis begins within several days, but several months may be required for complete resolution.

Treatment

When aspiration of gastric contents is noted, the patient should be turned onto her right side in an attempt to lessen the chance of diffuse lung involvement with its associated higher mortality. Endotracheal suction is effective in decreasing the volume of fluid that reaches the alveoli as well as in removing particulate matter.[9] Acidic particles are associated with slower resolution of the process in surviving patients. Tracheobronchial lavage has not proved to be an effective treatment and is not recommended. Bronchoscopy may be helpful in removing large particles that cause airway obstruction.[9]

Perhaps the most critical element in the treatment of aspiration pneumonitis is the early application of oxygen therapy. This is most effective when administered by a positive-pressure apparatus utilizing positive end-expiratory pressure (PEEP).[9,39] PEEP decreases atelectasis, increases the functional residual capacity, and minimizes shunting. Arterial PaO_2 should be maintained above 70 mmHg. Endotracheal intubation or tracheostomy may be required for respiratory care.

Bronchodilators are often effective when there is significant wheezing.[39] Doses of aminophylline similar to those used in the treatment of asthma are employed.

Corticosteroids often are given, although they have never been shown to improve survival in humans.[8,9,39,46] In animal studies, they seem to be of benefit if given within five minutes of aspiration. This time frame is difficult to duplicate in clinical medicine. They are probably of no benefit in the usual clinical situation.

Patients with aspiration pneumonitis often develop hypovolemia and hypotension because of massive fluid loss into the lungs. Intravenous fluid therapy is important, but the optimal fluid to use is still in question. A case can be made for and against both crystalloid and colloid therapy. It is probably appropriate to give 500 ml of colloid solution with every 2500 ml of crystalloid. Furosemide is ineffective in treating the pulmonary edema of aspiration pneumonitis because these patients are hypovolemic.

Antibiotic therapy may become necessary if pulmonary infection develops. Prophylactic use of antibiotics is not appropriate, however.[9,46] Antibiotic use should await documentation of infection.

Patients with aspiration pneumonitis should be in an intensive care environment where they can be monitored properly. Arterial blood gas determinations, balloon flotation catheter monitoring, and monitoring of vital signs and urinary output must all be utilized.

Prevention

Almost all authors writing on aspiration pneumonitis close with a section on prevention. Mendelson stated, "Aspiration of stomach contents into the lungs is preventable."[22] Forty years ago he suggested several items that are still appropriate to decrease the likelihood of aspiration and to treat it quickly if it occurs. They include withholding oral feeding during labor, substitution of local anesthesia for general anesthesia when possible, neutralization of acidic stomach contents prior to general anesthesia, emptying the stomach before general anesthesia, competent administration of general anesthetics, and adequate equipment, including transparent anesthetic masks, tiltable delivery tables, laryngoscopes, suction, and bronchoscopes.

These suggestions are still appropriate, but the way to achieve them has been changed. Patients typically fast after admission to the labor room; ice chips and hard candy sometimes are allowed, but patients generally are encouraged not to eat during labor. General anesthesia rarely is used for vaginal delivery and regional anesthesia has replaced general anesthesia for most cesarean deliveries. Emptying the stomach contents with a nasogastric tube prior to general anesthesia is effective but seldom is employed because of patient discomfort. If a nasogastric tube is used, it should be removed prior to induction of general anesthesia. Metoclopramide accelerates gastric emptying and has been advocated to decrease the volume of gastric contents prior to surgery.[9] Antacids given during labor and prior to general anesthesia are effective at neutralizing the acidic pH of the stomach contents.[31] Colloidal antacids are effective but may cause increased gastric volume.

If aspirated, the colloidal antacids can themselves cause a chemical pneumonitis. Clear antacids (sodium citrate) may be a better choice than colloidal antacids.[9] Cimetadine decreases gastric acidity and volume [18,23] but its onset of action is too slow to be of value in an emergency. The use of endotracheal tubes with large-volume, low-pressure cuffs also decreases the possibility of regurgitated fluid entering the lungs during general anesthesia. Improvements in anesthetic technique, proper equipping of delivery-operating suites, and vigilance by labor and delivery personnel may one day prevent nearly all cases of aspiration pneumonitis.

AMNIOTIC FLUID EMBOLUS

Definition, Incidence, and Significance

Maternal pulmonary embolism by amniotic fluid was described in classic manner in 1941 as a cause of obstetric shock and unexpected death. The condition was described in eight patients and in experimental animals.[38]

As other causes of maternal mortality have decreased in magnitude, amniotic fluid embolus has become increasingly important as a cause of maternal deaths. Currently, up to 10% of maternal deaths in this country are caused by amniotic fluid embolus [11,25] Twelve percent of deaths following legal abortion are attributed to amniotic fluid embolus.[16] The incidence of amniotic fluid embolus is 1/3360 to 1/80,000 deliveries.[11] More than 80% of women who sustain an amniotic fluid embolus die, one-fourth of them within an hour.[25] Amniotic fluid embolus is a rare, but well recognized, deadly condition. The first step to treating it successfully is to recognize that it has occurred.

Etiology

In order for the embolism to occur, amniotic fluid must find an entrance into the maternal circulation. This entry may be via lower uterine segment lacerations, cesarean section incisions, placenta accreta sites, and sites of uterine rupture.[20,26] Conditions associated with amniotic fluid embolus include causes of short, violent labor. In one series, 45% of cases were associated with abruptio placentae, 40% with intrauterine fetal demise, and 35% with meconium-stained amniotic fluid.[26] Amniotic fluid debris can be detected at autopsy in the uterine veins of half of the patients who die of amniotic fluid embolus.[26] Patients are typically of older reproductive age and high parity.[26]

Pathophysiology

Steiner and Lushbaugh noted in 1941 that the syndrome is "composed of several entities."[38] One component is plugging of the pulmonary vasculature with amniotic fluid debris such as vernix, lanugo hair, fetal squames, and meconium. The plugging of the pulmonary vascular bed causes hypoxia, pulmonary vasoconstriction increased pulmonary artery pressure, increased pulmonary vascular resistance, right ventricular failure, and decreased cardiac output which leads to systemic hypotension.[11]

Amniotic fluid has coagulant activity similar to thromboplastin.[45] In animals, intravenous infusion of thromboplastin causes death. In amniotic fluid embolus, the amniotic fluid triggers intravascular coagulation and activates the fibrinolytic system. Fibrin degradation products intensify the consumption of coagulation factors leading to disseminated intravascular coagulation (DIC).[11]

Some patients die quickly from the hypoxia and shock that result from embolization of the pulmonary vasculature. Patients who survive the initial insult then fall victim to the coagulopathy and the accompanying uterine atony. Six of Steiner and Lushbaugh's patients died after delivery; five of them had been treated with an intrauterine pack for postpartum hemorrhage!

Studies in experimental animals have reproduced parts of the syndrome, but none has replicated perfectly the condition seen in humans.[2,28,38] Different species react differently to amniotic fluid infusions. Particulate matter contained in the amniotic fluid seems to be important in producing the initial phase of hypoxia and shock from an embolic effect.

Clinical Presentation

Typically, amniotic fluid embolus is a sudden, unexpected calamity that occurs during labor or shortly after delivery. The prominent presenting symptoms are dyspnea, cyanosis, and shock.[11,24,29,45] Hemorrhage and convulsions are also frequent initial occurrences. Disseminated intravascular coagulation (DIC), pulmonary edema, and, rarely, bronchospasm develop later in the course of the syndrome.[24]

Physical findings include cyanosis, tachycardia, tachypnea, hypotension, rales, and bleeding diathesis.

Laboratory findings include acidosis, hypoxia, thrombocytopenia, low fibrinogen, and prolonged partial thromboplastin time (PTT). Electrocardiogram is consistent with acute cor pulmonale with evidence of right heart strain. Chest roentgenogram reveals bilateral infiltrates and an enlarged pulmonary artery.

Balloon flotation catheter monitoring has been carried out and indicated elevated central venous pressure, elevated pulmonary artery pressure, and elevated pulmonary capillary wedge pressure. These findings were present at the time of diagnosis and persisted for four days.[12]

Diagnosis

When originally described, the diagnosis of amniotic fluid embolus was confirmed only at post mortem examination by finding amniotic fluid debris in the maternal pulmonary vasculature.[26,38] Special stains usually are required to find the debris.

Autopsies of 30 women who died of amniotic fluid infusion revealed that 70% had pulmonary edema at the time of death. All women had mucin in the lungs, and it was the most prominent debris in 24 of them. Twenty-four women demonstrated fetal squames in the maternal lungs and in six of them, squames were the most prominent debris.[26]

Amniotic fluid debris in the maternal pulmonary circulation at autopsy seems to be specific for amniotic fluid embolus. Women who die around the time of delivery without clinical evidence of amniotic fluid embolus almost never have demonstrable amniotic fluid debris in their lungs, even when investigated with special stains.[32,38]

Radioactive chromium-tagged erythrocytes were instilled into the amniotic fluid prior to delivery in an attempt to gain insight into the frequency with which small amniotic fluid infusions occur. In 38 women who delivered by cesarean, or vaginally after spontaneous or induced labor, almost no radioactiity escaped the uterus into the maternal circulation.[37]

All these factors indicate that it is very unusual to find amniotic fluid in the maternal circulation. When such findings occur, they are pathologic. The obstetrician should always alert the pathologist when amniotic fluid embolus is suspected as a cause of maternal death. A recent article notes that microscopic examination of the lungs was omitted in several cases where the suspected cause of death was amniotic fluid embolus.[35]

In the past, when the accurate diagnosis of amniotic fluid embolus had to await autopsy findings, the clinical differential diagnosis was quite important. Depending on the presenting symptom, the differential diagnosis might have included postpartum hemorrhage, pulmonary edema, pulmonary embolism, anesthetic or drug reaction, air embolus, eclampsia, aspiration pneumonitis (the lack of bronchospasm usually rules this out), septic shock, uterine rupture, cerebrovascular accident, or myocardial infarction.[11,24] During that era, if a woman survived a presumed amniotic fluid embolus, the diagnosis was in doubt.[29]

With increased use of hemodynamic monitoring in critically ill obstetric patients, the finding of amniotic fluid debris in blood from the central veins or pulmonary arteries has allowed the diagnosis of amniotic fluid embolus before death or in the absence of death.[12,29,36] Amniotic fluid debris has been found in pulmonary artery blood for as long as three days after an embolic episode.[12] Special stains of the buffy coat of blood from the central veins and pulmonary artery establish the diagnosis. This finding was assumed to be as specific as the autopsy findings, but some doubt has now been cast on that assumption. Two patients without evidence of amniotic fluid embolus were found to have amniotic fluid debris in their pulmonary artery blood.[27] Further investigations may shed light on the development of full-blown amniotic fluid infusion syndrome or perhaps the development of only parts of the syndrome, such as DIC in the absence of pulmonary findings.

Treatment

There is no specific treatment for amniotic fluid embolus. Supportive treatment, however, has improved in recent years.

Hypoxia must be combatted in an intensive care situation that includes oxygen therapy, positive-pressure ventilation, and PEEP. Arterial blood gases should be followed and the PaO kept above 70 mmHg if possible. An arterial line provides access to constant blood pressure monitoring and provides a vehicle for arterial blood sampling. In the rare case with bronchospasm, aminophylline is helpful.[25]

Balloon flotation catheter monitoring is very important to guide fluid administration, and the use of agents such as furosemide, digitalis, and dopamine.[12] All these agents might be used to combat pulmonary edema or shock. Their use will be much more rational when guided by the data provided from the balloon flotation catheter. Use of the catheter also allows establishment of the diagnosis of amniotic fluid embolus with a reasonable degree of certainty.

Uterine atony associated with amniotic fluid embolus has typically been quite resistant to therapy. A recent report documented the successful use of 15-methyl prostaglandin $F_{2\alpha}$ in the treatment of uterine atony from this cause. Several injections were necessary; during the latent period from administration until the prostaglandin analogue began to work, uterine compression was lifesaving (see Chapter 47).[12]

Treatment of the coagulopathy associated with amniotic fluid embolus has been a topic of conjecture. Three decades ago, heparin, fibrinogen, and blood were suggested treatments.[45] Fibrinogen, as such, is no longer on the market and the use of heparin is highly controversial. Blood is definitely indicated and should be used. Amniotic fluid debris in the pulmonary circulation limits the speed with which transfusion is possible. Fresh frozen plasma and cryoprecipitate (Chapter 47), along with platelets, are the agents of choice to combat coagulopathy.

Cryoprecipitate may become the drug of choice to treat amniotic fluid embolus. Cryoprecipitate contains fibronectin, which is a cold-insoluble globulin. Fibronectin is the same as opsonic alpha-2 surface-binding glycoprotein, which helps the reticuloendothelial system to clear cellular debris and particulate matter from the circulation. In one instance, its use in amniotic fluid embolus rapidly and markedly improved pulmonary ventilation and perfusion.[33] Further trials are necessary to establish the utility of fibronectin therapy, but cryoprecipitate is a good source of clotting factors to treat DIC, whether or not fibronectin is effective.

PULMONARY EMBOLUS

Incidence and Significance

Pulmonary embolus is the most common nonobstetric cause of postpartum death (see Chapter 30).

The reported incidence of pulmonary embolus in association with pregnancy varies, but it likely occurs 1/3000 deliveries or 1/2500 cesarean sections. The risk of pulmonary embolus is much higher in pregnancy than in the nonpregnant state. Postpartum pulmonary embolization is three to five times more common than antepartum pulmonary embolization. The lower extremities are the usual sites of origin of venous thrombi that subsequently embolize.

Clinical Findings

The sudden onset of dyspnea, pleuritic chest pain, cough, tachypnea, cyanosis, hemoptysis, and tachycardia are virtually diagnostic of pulmonary embolus. Unfortunately, most patients do not present with such classic findings. The initial symptoms of massive pulmonary embolism can be "deceivingly nonspecific."[43] One study of 90 patients with pulmonary embolus reported clinical findings in decreasing order of frequency as tachypnea (88%), dyspnea (80%), tachycardia (63%), anxiety (61%), loud pulmonic valve closure (60%), rales (50%), hemoptysis (27%), and pleuritic friction rub (17%).[43]

Pulmonary angiography is the most accurate method of diagnosing a large pulmonary embolus. A normal pulmonary angiogram does not exclude the possibility of several small emboli. Because of the complications associated with pulmonary angiography and the reluctance to perform the test during pregnancy, other methods of diagnosis frequently are employed.

The ventilation/perfusion scan (V/Q scan) employs two radioisotopes; one is injected and one is inhaled. It is so important to establish the diagnosis of pulmonary embolus in pregnancy that exposure to the small amount of radiation from the isotopes is justified. Scanning of the lungs in patients with pulmonary embolus characteristically reveals normal ventilation in an area of decreased pulmonary perfusion. Not all authorities agree on the utility of the V/Q scan. It is more accurate than the perfusion scan alone, but it is less accurate than pulmonary angiography.

Patients with pulmonary embolus nearly always have an arterial PaO_2 below 80 mmHg and demonstrate a perfusion defect on lung scan.[41] These findings have led to the belief that a normal arterial PaO_2, above 90 mmHg, or a normal perfusion scan rule out the possibility of pulmonary embolus in a patient with respiratory distress. However, few patients with respiratory distress from any cause have a normal arterial PaO_2 or perfusion lung scan.

Up to 70% of patients with pulmonary emboli have abnormal chest roentgenograms. Abnormal vascular patterns, infiltrates, fluid, and elevated diaphragm are all noted. Abnormal electrocardiographic findings are noted in about 20% of patients. However, if tachycardia is included as an abnormality, the incidence of abnormal electrocardiograms increases greatly.

Treatment

Heparin was established as the treatment of choice for pulmonary embolus in 1960.[3] The goal of heparin therapy is to prevent propagation of the venous thrombus and therefore further embolization. Overt bleeding, severe hypertension, and cerebrovascular hemorrhage are contraindications to heparin therapy.

The initial loading dose for actual or suspected pulmonary embolus is 10,000 units of heparin intravenously. Prior to heparin administration, coagulation studies should be performed to provide a baseline against which to judge the effect of heparin therapy. The preferred method of heparin administration is continuous intravenous infusion. The initial maintenance dose should be 1000–1500 units per hour.

Methods to determine the adequacy of anticoagulant effect include direct measurement of heparin concentration in plasma. The therapeutic range is 0.3–0.4 units/ml. Whole blood clotting time by the Lee–White method seldom is used to monitor heparin therapy because it is time-consuming to perform. If used, therapeutic levels prolong the baseline clotting time by a factor of 2–2.5. Activated partial thromboplastin time (aPTT) should be 1.5–2 times the control value to be in the therapeutic range. Heparin infusion rates are adjusted to achieve the effective range for the chosen test.

Hemorrhage is the most serious complication of heparin therapy. While patients are receiving the drug, their urine and stool should be checked for blood. Hematocrit values should be checked every few days.

Heparin has advantages over other anticoagulants. It essentially does not cross the placenta, so there are no fetal effects. It has a short half-life (one hour) and it can be antagonized readily with protamine sulfate. If rapid reversal of anticoagulant effect is necessary, 1 mg of protamine sulfate neutralizes the effect of 100 units of heparin. In preparing the protamine dose, the half-life of heparin must be taken into consideration. If protamine sulfate is given in excess, it behaves as an anticoagulant.

Oxygen therapy is required because the patients are invariably hypoxic. Mild sedation may be helpful when the patient is extremely anxious.

Surgical therapy may be indicated in treatment of pulmonary embolus. Massive embolization confirmed by pulmonary angiogram and associated with cardiovascular collapse may merit embolectomy. Recurrent embolization while the patient is receiving an adequate dosage of heparin leads to consideration of interruption or blockade of the inferior vena cava and possibly the left ovarian vein to prevent further embolization.

Long-term management of the patient with pulmonary embolus or a history of pulmonary embolus is discussed in Chapter 30.

REFERENCES

1. Abramowicz, M. (Ed.): Corticosteroid aerosols for asthma. *Med. Lett.* **27**:5–6, 1985.
2. Attwood, H. D. and Downing, S. E.: Experimental amniotic fluid and meconium embolism. *Surg. Gynecol. Obstet.* **120**:255–262, 1965.
3. Barritt, D. W. and Jordan, S. C.: Anticoagulant drugs in the treatment of pulmonary embolism: A controlled trial. *Lancet* **1**:1309–1312, 1960.
4. Benedetti, T. J., Kates, R., and Williams, V.: Hemodynamic observations in severe preeclampsia complicated by pulmonary edema. *Am. J. Obstet. Gynecol.* **152**:330–334, 1985.
5. Benedetti, T. J., Valle, R., and Ledger, W. J.: Antepartum pneumonia in pregnancy. *Am. J. Obstet. Gynecol.* **144**:413–417, 1982.
6. Broe, P. J., Toung, T. J. K., and Cameron, J. L.: Aspiration pneumonia. *Surg. Clin. North Am.* **60**:1551–1564, 1980.
7. Centor, R. M., Yarbrough, B., and Wood, J. P.: Inability to predict relapse in acute asthma. *N. Engl. J. Med.* **310**:577–580, 1984.
8. Chapman, R. L., Jr., Downs, J. B., Modell, J. H., and Hood, C. I.: The ineffectiveness of steroid therapy in treating aspiration of hydrochloric acid. *Arch. Surg.* **108**:858–861, 1974.
9. Cohen, S. E.: The aspiration syndrome. *Clin. Obstet. Gynaecol.* **9**:235–254, 1982.
10. Cotton, D. B., Gonik, B., Spillman, T., and Dorfman, K. F.: Intrapartum to postpartum changes in colloid osmotic pressure. *Am. J. Obstet. Gynecol.* **149**:174–177, 1984.
11. Duff, P.: Defusing the dangers of amniotic fluid embolism. *Contemp. OB/GYN* **24**:127–149, 1984.
12. Duff, P., Engelsgjerd, B., Zingery, L. W., Huff, R. W., and Montiel, M.: Hemodynamic observations in a patient with intrapartum amniotic fluid embolism. *Am. J. Obstet. Gynecol.* **146**:112–115, 1983.
13. Fischl, M. A., Pitchenik, A., and Gardner, L. B.: An index predicting relapse and need for hospital-

ization in patients with acute bronchial asthma. *N. Engl. J. Med.* **305**:783–789, 1981.
14. Gonik, B. and Cotton, D. B.: Peripartum colloid osmotic pressure changes: Influence of intravenous hydration. *Am. J. Obstet. Gynecol.* **150**:99–100, 1984.
15. Greenberger, P. A. and Patterson, R.: Management of asthma during pregnancy. *N. Engl. J. Med.* **312**:897–902, 1985.
16. Guidotti, R. J., Grimes, D. A., and Cates, W., Jr.: Fatal amniotic fluid embolism during legally induced abortion, United States, 1972 to 1978. *Am. J. Obstet. Gynecol.* **141**:257–261, 1981.
17. Hernandez, E., Angell, C. S., and Johnson, J. W. C.: Asthma in pregnancy: Current concepts. *Obstet. Gynecol.* **55**:739–743, 1980.
18. Hodgkinson, R., Glassenberg, R., Joyce, T. H., III, Coombs, D. W., Ostheimer, G. W., and Gibbs, C. P.: Comparison of cimetidine (Tagamet® with antacid for safety and effectiveness in reducing gastric acidity before elective cesarean section. *Anesthesiology* **59**:86–90, 1983.
19. Josephson, G. W., MacKenzie, E. J., Leitman, P. S., and Gibson, G.: Emergency treatment of asthma: A comparison of two treatment regimens. *JAMA* **242**:639–643, 1979.
20. Landing, B. H.: The pathogenesis of amniotic fluid embolism. II. Uterine factors. *N. Engl. J. Med.* **243**:590–596, 1950.
21. Marx, C. M. and Fraser, D. G.: Treatment of asthma in pregnancy. (Letter) *Obstet. Gynecol.* **57**:766–767, 1981.
22. Mendelson, C. L.: The aspiration of stomach contents into the lungs during obstetric anesthesia. *Am. J. Obstet. Gynecol.* **52**:191–204, 1946.
23. Moir, D. D.: Cimetidine, antacids, and pulmonary aspiration. *Anesthesiology* **59**:81–83, 1983.
24. Morgan, M.: Amniotic fluid embolism. *Anaesthesia* **34**:20–32, 1979.
25. Mulder, J. I.: Amniotic fluid embolism: An overview and case report. *Am. J. Obstet. Gynecol.* **152**:430–433, 1985.
26. Peterson, E. P. and Taylor, H. B.: Amniotic fluid embolism: An analysis of 40 cases. *Obstet. Gynecol.* **35**:787–793, 1970.
27. Plauche, W. C.: Amnitic fluid embolism. (Letter) *Am. J. Obstet. Gynecol.* **147**:982–983, 1983.
28. Reis, R. L., Pierce, W. S., and Behrendt, D. M.: Hemodynamic effects of amniotic fluid embolism. *Surg. Gynecol. Obstet.* **129**:45–48, 1969.
29. Resnik, R., Swartz, W. H., Plumer, M. H., Benirschke, K., and Stratthaus, M. E.: Amniotic fluid embolism with survival. *Obstet. Gynecol.* **47**:295–298, 1976.
30. Rinaldo, J. E. and Rogers, R. M.: Adult respiratory-distress syndrome: Changing concepts of lung injury and repair. *N. Engl. J. Med.* **306**:900–909, 1982.
31. Roberts, R. B. and Shirley, M. A.: The obstetrician's role in reducing the risk of aspiration pneumonitis: With particular reference to the use of oral antacids. *Am. J. Obstet. Gynecol.* **124**:611–617, 1976.
32. Roche, W. D. and Norris, H. J.: Detection and significance of maternal pulmonary amniotic fluid embolism. *Obstet. Gynecol.* **43**:729–731, 1974.
33. Rodgers, G. P. and Heymach, G. J., III: Cryoprecipitate therapy in amniotic fluid embolization. *Am. J. Med.* **76**:916–920, 1984.
34. Rose, C. C., Murphy, J. G., and Schwartz, J. S.: Performance of an index predicting the response of patients with acute bronchial asthma to intensive emergency department treatment. *N. Engl. J. Med.* **310**:573–577, 1984.
35. Rushton, D. I. and Dawson, I. M. P.: The maternal autopsy. *J. Clin. Pathol.* **35**:909–921, 1982.
36. Schaerf, R. H. M., de Campo, T., and Civetta, J. M.: Hemodynamic alterations and rapid diagnosis in a case of amniotic fluid embolus. *Anesthesiology* **46**:155–157, 1977.
37. Sparr, R. A. and Pritchard, J. A.: Studies to detect the escape of amniotic fluid into the maternal circulation during parturition. *Surg. Gynecol. Obstet.* **107**:560–564, 1958.
38. Steiner, P. E. and Lushbaugh, C. C.: Maternal pulmonary embolism by amniotic fluid as a cause of obstetric shock and unexpected deaths in obstetrics. *JAMA* **117**:1245–1254, 1941.
39. Stewardson, R. H. and Nyhus, L. M.: Pulmonary aspiration: An update. *Arch. Surg.* **112**:1192–1197, 1977.
40. Strauss, R. G., Keefer, J. R., Burke, T., and Civetta, J. M.: Hemodynamic monitoring of cardiogenic pulmonary edema complicating toxemia of pregnancy. *Obstet. Gynecol.* **55**:170–174, 1980.
41. Szucs, M. M., Jr., Brooks, H. L., Grossman, W., Banas, J. S., Jr., Meister, S. G., Dexter, L., and Dalen, J. E.: Diagnostic sensitivity of laboratory findings in acute pulmonary embolism. *Ann. Intern. Med.* **74**:161–166, 1971.
42. Webb-Johnson, D. C. and Andrews, J. L., Jr.: Bronchodilator therapy (First of two parts). *N. Engl. J. Med.* **297**:476–482, 1977.
43. Wegner, N. K., Stein, P. D., and Willis, P. W., III: Massive acute pulmonary embolism: The deceivingly nonspecific manifestations. *JAMA* **220**:843–844, 1972.
44. Weinberger, M. and Hendeles, L.: Slow-release theophylline: Rationale and basis for product selection. *N. Engl. J. Med.* **308**:760–764, 1983.
45. Weiner, A. E. and Reid, D. E.: The pathogenesis of amniotic fluid embolism. III. Coagulant activity in amniotic fluid. *N. Engl. J. Med.* **243**:597–598, 1950.
46. Wynne, J. W. and Modell, J. H.: Respiratory aspiration of stomach contents. *Ann. Intern. Med.* **87**:466–474, 1977.

40

SEPTIC SHOCK

Genital tract infection is one of the most common complications encountered by the obstetrician. Approximately 0.5–1.0% of all pregnant women develop chorioamnionitis.[17] One to 4% of patients who experience vaginal delivery or elective termination of pregnancy develop endomyometritis.[18] The incidence of endomyometritis in women undergoing cesarean section is even higher. It ranges from 15% in middle-class patients undergoing elective abdominal delivery to 85–95% in indigent patients having operative delivery after a period of labor and ruptured membranes.[55] The incidence of bacteremia in women with endomyometritis varies from approximately 5 to 25%.[55]

Serious complications, including pelvic abscess, septic pelvic vein thrombophlebitis, and septic shock, may result from primary intrauterine infection. Approximately 1% of women with puerperal infection develop one of these life-threatening complications.[9] Of these three disorders, septic shock has the most ominous prognosis. In the United States, septic shock is responsible for 20,000–60,000 deaths annually.[43] In certain groups of patients, the mortality due to septic shock is as high as 80%.[16]

The prognosis in septic shock is determined principally by the immunocompetence of the host. The underlying disease is an important determinant of prognosis. Patients with rapidly fatal, ultimately fatal, and nonfatal underlying diseases display progressively lower mortality rates.[16,31,32]

The majority of obstetric patients who develop septic shock fall into the category of nonfatal underlying disease. Mortality is about 18% in such women.[6] Because the obstetric patient's prognosis is so favorable relative to other patients with debilitating medical diseases, she will derive the greatest benefit from prompt, effective treatment of septic shock. Conversely, prognosis is affected adversely if initial medical and surgical therapy is planned poorly. It is essential that the obstetrician thoroughly understand the pathophysiology and therapy of this disorder.

MICROBIOLOGY

Any organism capable of infecting a human host can cause septic shock. Thirty to 50% of cases are caused by *Escherichia coli.* Twenty to 30% are the result of infections caused by *Klebsiella-Enterobacter-Serratia* organisms. Ten percent of cases are caused by *Pseudomonas aeruginosa*, and a similar percentage are due to *Proteus* and *Providencia* species. Among the coliform organisms, no one serotype predominates. The remaining cases of septic shock are due to gram-positive aerobic bacteria, anaerobic gram-negative bacilli, viruses, rickettsiae, and fungi. In approximately 16% of patients, the septicemia is due to multiple organisms.[31,32]

PREDISPOSING FACTORS

Septic shock occurs almost exclusively in hospitalized patients. The microorganisms responsible for sepsis either derive from the patient's endogenous flora or are acquired during hospitalization. The principal pathogens responsible for obstetric septic shock are part of the natural flora of the lower genital tract and are isolated frequently from intrauterine and wound infections.

In obstetric patients, the principal entities that predispose to septic shock are postcesarean endomyometritis, infected abortion, acute pyelonephritis, and, in rare instances, acute chorioamnionitis.[6]

PATHOPHYSIOLOGY

Although still incompletely understood, the pathophysiology of gram-negative shock has been investigated extensively.

Endotoxin is a complex lipopolysaccharide that is present in the cell wall of gram-negative bacteria. The critical component of endotoxin is a substituent termed lipid A,[2] which has a beta 1-6 diglucosamine backbone joined in an ester and amide linkage to long-chain fatty acids. Uninfected individuals have very low titers of antibody against lipid A. Endotoxin is released into the host's circulation at the time of the bacterium's death. Once in the bloodstream, endotoxin initiates the progression of pathophysiologic derangements summarized in Fig. 40-1.

Activation of the Coagulation Cascade

One of the initial effects of endotoxin is direct activation of Hageman Factor (XII), which, in turn, initiates the intrinsic clotting cascade.[11]

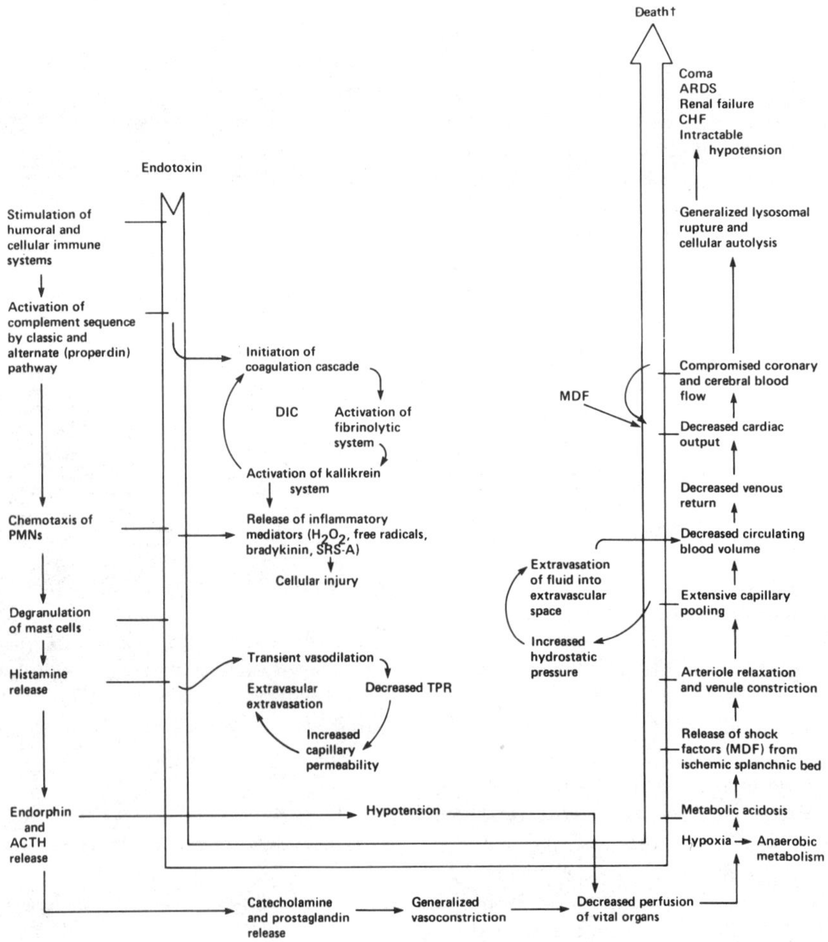

Figure 40-1. Schematic flow diagram summarizes the pathophysiology of septic shock.

Hageman Factor also directly activates Factor VII, thus stimulating the extrinsic coagulation pathway. Activation of the coagulation system leads to concurrent activation of the fibrinolytic system. Plasmin, the active component of the latter system, then acts on Hageman Factor to produce fragments termed prekallikrein activators.[36] These substances activate prekallikrein to form kallikrein. Kallikrein causes conversion of plasminogen to plasmin and also directly activates Hageman Factor. This results in enhanced coagulation and accelerated fibrinolysis and precipitates the phenomenon of disseminated intravascular coagulation. Another major effect of kallikrein activation is the production of a variety of inflammatory mediators such as hydrogen peroxide, free radicals, and bradykinin. These substances cause intense inflammatory injury to vital organs.

Activation of the Complement System

Endotoxin also activates the complement cascade.[12,23,37] Activation of the complement sequence occurs through the classic pathway, the alternate (properdin) pathway, and through direct activation of the first component of complement (Figs. 40-2 and 40-3).

There are three major effects of complement activation. First, C_{5a} and the $C_{5,6,7}$ complex interact to exert a chemotactic effect, promoting migration of leukocytes into injured tissue. Second, leukocytes release a variety of inflammatory mediators termed leukotrienes.[49] (These substances formerly were referred to collectively as "slow reacting substance of anaphylaxis.") They cause vasoconstriction and increased vascular permeability in the postcapillary venules. Leukotrienes also accelerate neutrophil chemotaxis and aggregation, resulting in release of hydrolytic enzymes and superoxides. Progressive vascular injury results in platelet aggregation, release of platelet factor 3, and intensification of the coagulation cascade. Components C_{3a} and C_{5a} interact to cause degranulation of mast cells and release of histamine.

Histamine release induces disruption of endothelial integrity, increase in capillary permeability, decrease in plasma volume, vasodilation, and hypotension.[11] In response to this initial state of hypotension, the host's heart rate and cardiac output increase. Thus, in this early stage of sepsis, the patient appears warm, flushed, and maximally vasodilated. It is for this reason that septic shock often is referred to as "warm shock."

Even in early septic shock, however, when cardiac output is increased, myocardial function is abnormal. Myocardial contractility is impaired and ventricular ejection fractions decrease.[10,29,44,46,57]

Activation of Sympathetic Nervous System

The initial vasodilation and decreased peripheral resistance is usually transient. As sepsis evolves, intense activation of the sympathetic nervous system is manifested by increased catecholamine release from peripheral nerves and the adrenal medulla. This sympathetic discharge causes generalized vasoconstriction in virtually every vascular bed. The vasoconstriction is intensified by the local effects of prosta-

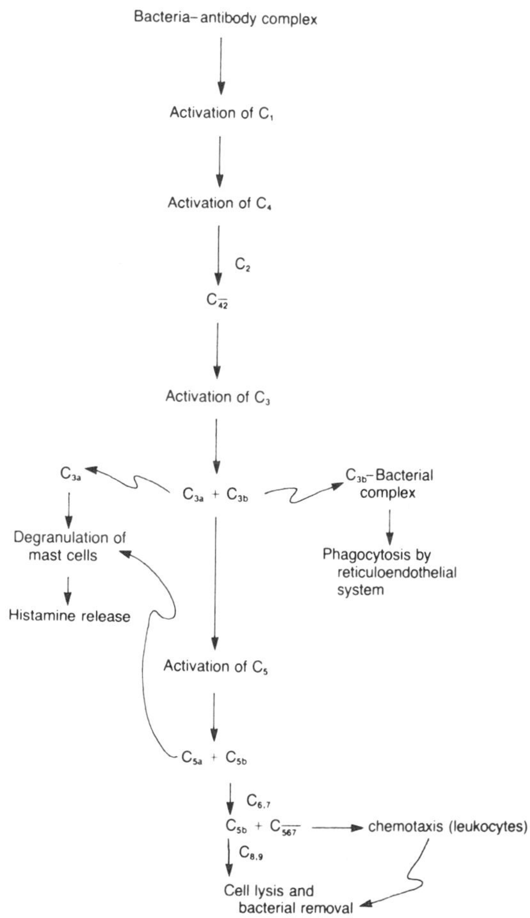

Figure 40-2. Classic pathway of complement activation.

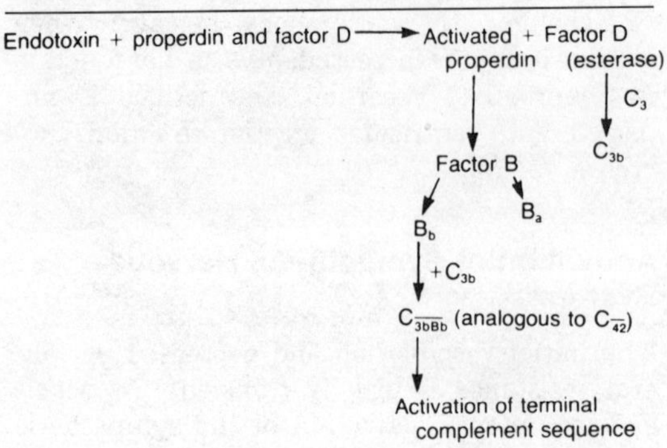

Figure 40-3. Alternate (properdin) pathway of complement activation.

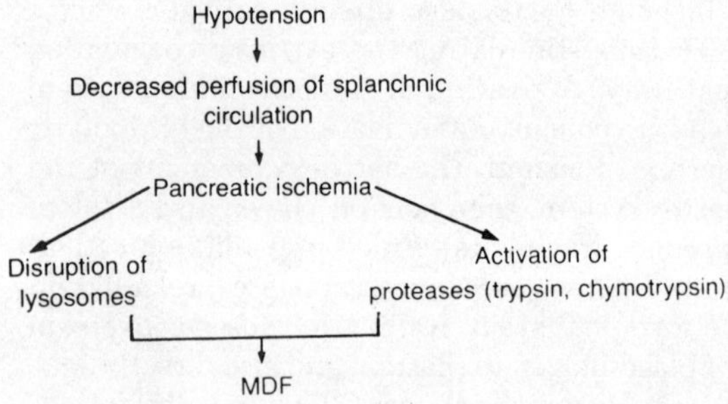

Figure 40-4. Formation of myocardial depressant factor (MDF).

glandins released from injured endothelial tissue.[14]

The most serious effect of generalized vasoconstriction is marked diminution in perfusion of vital organs, resulting in localized tissue hypoxia and acidosis and, ultimately, in systemic metabolic acidosis. As acidosis evolves, there is a marked change in circulatory hemodynamics, characterized by relaxation of smooth muscle in the wall of arterioles and constriction of smooth muscle in the wall of venules. This process leads to extensive pooling in most capillary beds, increased hydrostatic pressure, and transudation of intravascular fluid into the extravascular space.[11,24,41,48] Generalized capillary pooling causes significant decrease in effective circulating blood volume with resultant decrease in venous return to the heart and progressive decrease in cardiac output and systemic blood pressure.

In addition to decreased venous return, at least three other factors contribute to impaired myocardial contractility. First, circulating beta endorphins are increased significantly. These peptides are released from the pituitary gland along with adrenocorticotropin hormone (ACTH) in response to stress. Their principal hemodynamic effects are lowered blood pressure and decreased heart rate.[22,25,39] Second, endotoxin itself has a direct depressant effect on myocardial contractility.

Third, several studies have identified the presence of a specific shock factor, termed myocardial depressant factor (MDF), which apparently is released from the ischemic pancreas during evolution of the shock state (Fig. 40-4). MDF has not been characterized completely, but it appears to be a peptide or glycopeptide with a molecular weight of 500–1000. MDF gradually accumulates in the plasma of shocked animals in direct proportion to the severity of splanchnic ischemia.[34] The most important biologic effect of MDF is depression of myocardial contractility. It also enhances vasoconstriction within splanchnic blood vessels, thus accelerating its own production, and directly depresses the phagocytic capacity of the reticuloendothelial system, resulting in impaired clearance of lysosomal enzymes and MDF from the circulation.

As cardiac output initially begins to fall, local regulatory mechanisms attempt to preserve perfusion of the coronary and cerebral vascular beds. However, if the hemodynamic changes precipitated by septicemia are not corrected, there is progressive diminution in cardiac output and, ultimately, compromise of both coronary and cerebral blood flow. Maintenance of cardiac output correlates directly with ultimate survival.[57]

Respiratory Failure

Endotoxemia also causes profound derangements in the host's respiratory physiology (Fig. 40-5). Endotoxin directly damages the endothelium of the pulmonary vasculature. As disruption of capillaries occurs, platelets adhere to fragments of exposed collagen. Release of platelet factor 3 activates the intrinsic coagulation cascade, resulting in microembolization and stasis of blood flow in the pulmonary microcirculation.[11] Prostaglandins are released from platelets and injured endothelium and cause pulmonary vasoconstriction with subsequent increase in pulmonary vascular resistance. The net effect of these processes is impairment of pulmonary perfusion, ischemia, and progressive

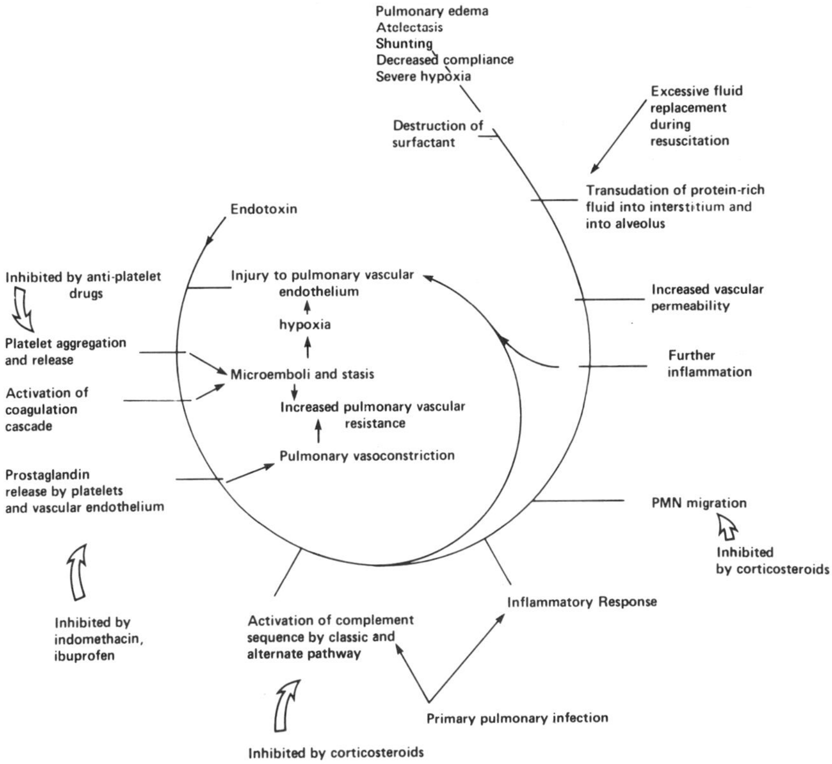

Figure 40-5. Pathophysiology of pulmonary injury in septic shock.

injury to the vascular endothelium. Cerebral ischemia resulting from hypotension intensifies pulmonary vasoconstriction.

Endothelial injury also leads to activation of the complement cascade. Increased serum concentration of C_{5a} is a useful predictor of subsequent development of adult respiratory distress syndrome (ARDS). [23] Complement activation causes damage to the lung by enhancing leukocyte migration into the pulmonary parenchyma. Leukocytes, in turn, release several inflammatory mediators that cause profound injury to lung vasculature and parenchyma. The activity of the proteolytic enzyme, elastase, is increased in bronchoalveolar lavage fluid obtained from patients with ARDS.[33]

Continued inflammation results in increased capillary permeability, transudation of protein-rich fluid into the interstitium and alveolus, and destruction of surfactant.[52] The functional consequences of these events are extensive atelectasis, perfusion–ventilation imbalance, decreased compliance, interstitial and intra-alveolar edema, severe hypoxemia, and, ultimately, respiratory failure (Fig. 40-6).

Other Effects of Endotoxin

Endotoxin adheres to the cell membrane of circulating leukocytes, causing these cells to be removed from the circulation by reticuloendothelial cells in the spleen. Therefore, the early shock state may be distinguished by neutropenia. As cell-mediated immunologic defenses are mobilized, however, rebound leukocytosis usually ensues.[11] This rebound effect, of course, does not occur in immunosuppressed patients, precisely those at greatest risk for developing septic shock.

Endotoxin also exerts a prominent effect on the temperature-regulating center of the hypothalamus. In the early phase of sepsis, the hypothalamic center may be depressed. As a result, hypothermia may be present. As shock evolves, however, the principal effect of endotoxin is activation of the hypothalamic center and eleva-

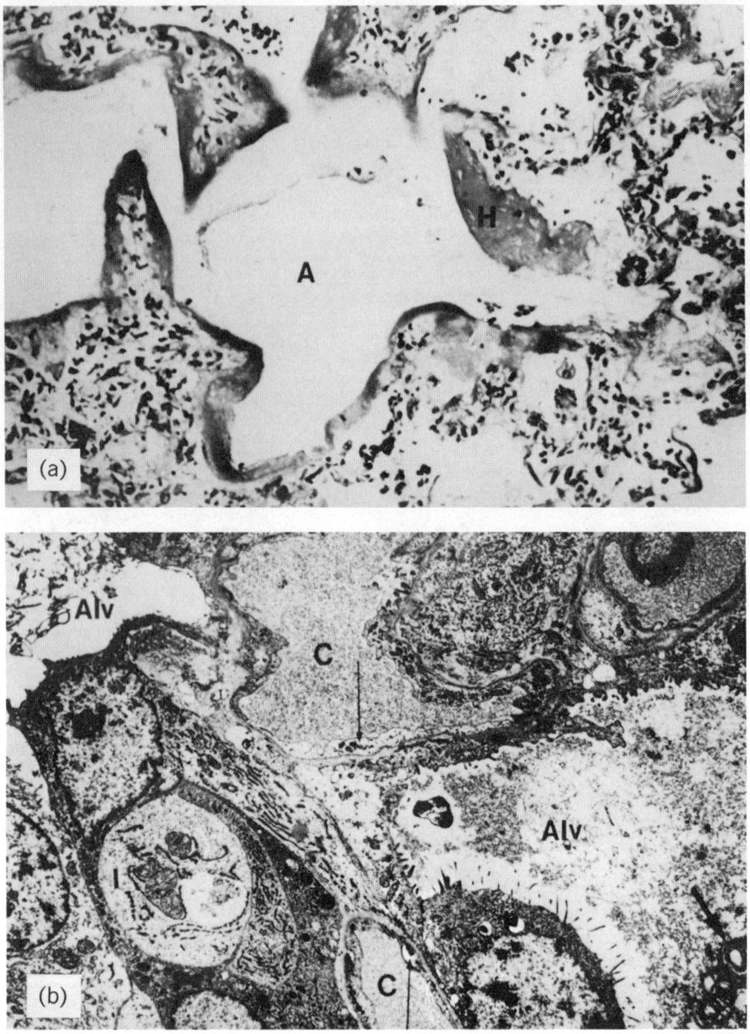

Figure 40-6. Panel A. Photomicrograph of lung tissue from patient with ARDS. Diffuse alveolar damage is characterized by presence of prominent hyaline membranes (H), microatelectasis (arrow) and inflammatory exudate. Air space (A). Hematoxylin and eosin; X 220.
Panel B. Electron micrograph of lung tissue from patient with ARDS secondary to streptococcal septicemia. Proteinaceous debris and cellular fragments (thick arrow) are seen within the alveolar space (Alv). The interstitium (I) is edematous and contains numerous cells, including macrophages and fibroblasts. The endothelium of the capillaries (c) shows focal edema (thin arrows). Uranyl acetate and lead citrate; X 5200.

tion of body temperature, an effect mediated by endogenous pyrogen released from host leukocytes.[2]

The end point of septic shock is a profound hypodynamic state, characterized by intractable hypotension and severe metabolic acidosis. Clinically, this is manifested by coma, complete vasomotor collapse, and multiorgan failure (Figs. 40-7 and 40-8).

CLINICAL MANIFESTATIONS (FIG. 40-9)

Restlessness, anxiety, and disorientation are among the earliest manifestations of septic shock. Another early physical sign is temperature instability. In the initial stages of septic shock, patients frequently are hypothermic. As sepsis progresses, patients typically become hyperthermic.

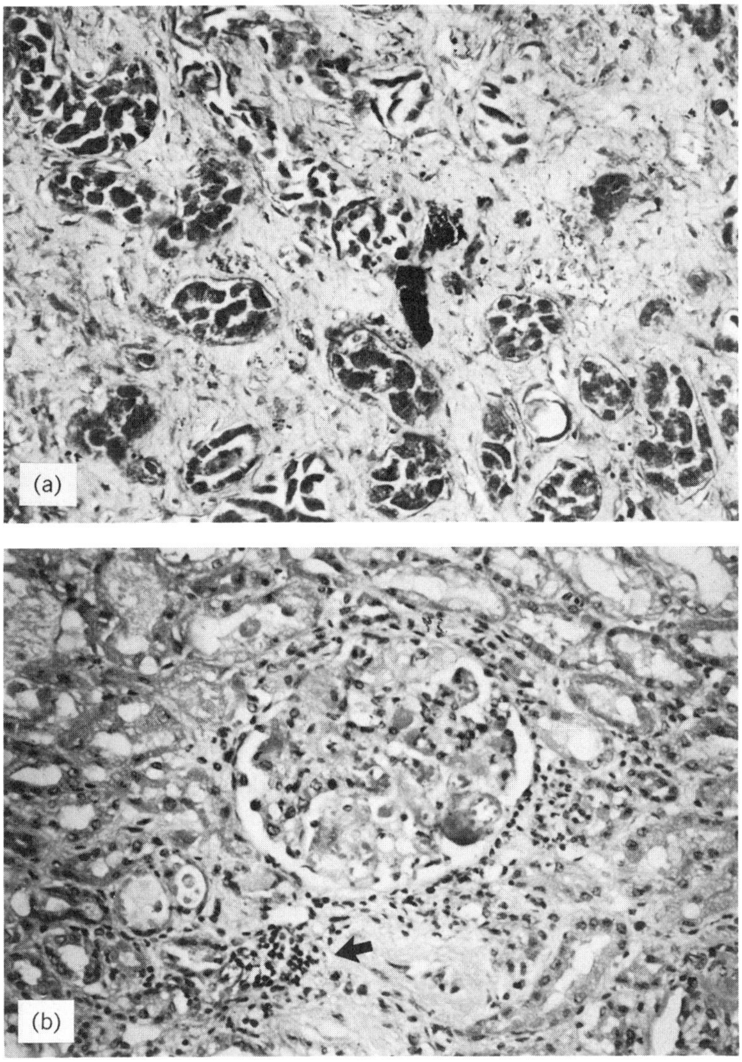

Figure 40-7. Panel A. Photomicrograph of kidney from a patient who died of septic shock demonstrates acute tubular necrosis. Hematoxylin and eosin; X 40.

Panel B. Photomicrograph from same patient shows fibrin deposition within glomerulus and inflammatory infiltrate (arrow). Hematoxylin and eosin; X 40.

The most prominent pathophysiologic changes are those affecting the cardiovascular system.[4,11,41,43,45] In the majority of patients, a hyperdynamic state is present initially. Cardiac output and myocardial oxygen consumption are increased, oxygen consumption by peripheral tissues is increased, and total peripheral resistance is decreased. As the shock state evolves, however, intense, generalized vasoconstriction occurs. Accordingly, there is a transition to a hypodynamic cardiac state characterized by a decrease in cardiac output, systemic blood pressure, and perfusion pressure. Diminished tissue perfusion, in turn, leads to myocardial dysfunction, which is manifested by tachycardia, arrhythmia, myocardial ischemia, and, ultimately, biventricular failure.

Up to 50% of patients with septic shock develop ARDS.[28] The usual clinical signs of this disorder are tachypnea, dyspnea, stridor, and

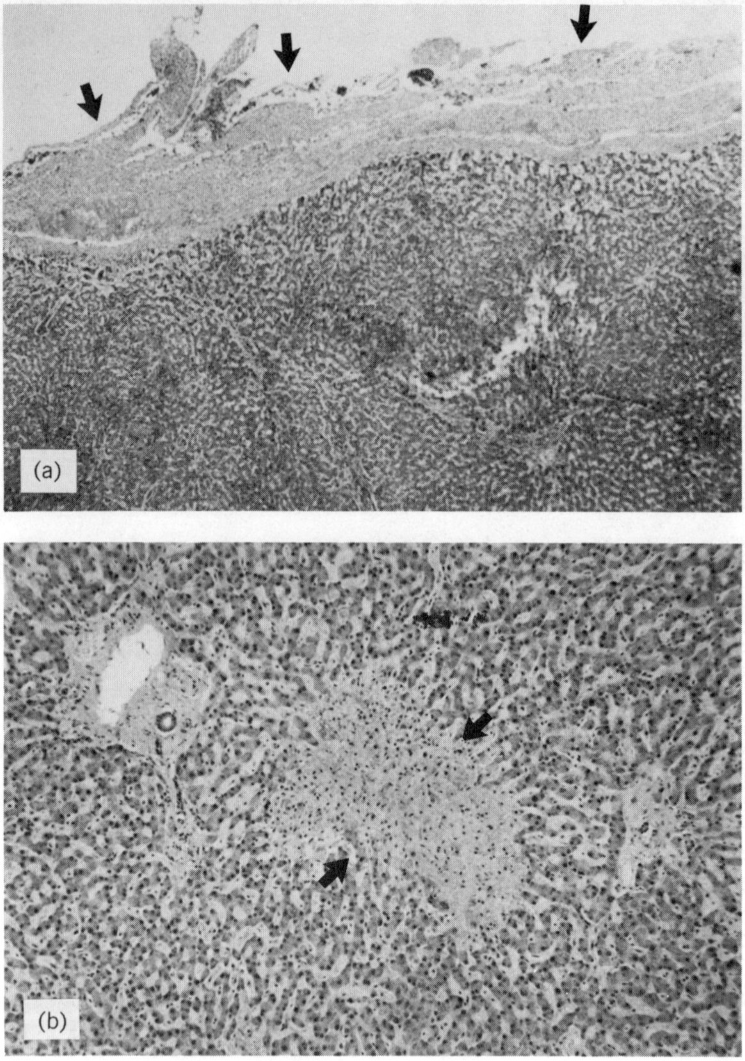

Figure 40-8. Panel A. Photomicrograph of liver from a patient who died of septic shock demonstrates prominent exudate (arrows) on hepatic surface. Hematoxylin and eosin; X 4.
Panel B. Photomicrograph from same patient shows large necrotic area (arrows) within hepatic parenchyma. Hematoxylin and eosin; X 10.

central cyanosis. Examination of the chest demonstrates dullness to percussion, decreased tactile and vocal fremitus, diminished breath sounds, and prominent rales throughout both lung fields.

Examination of the abdomen and pelvis is important in establishing the primary site of infection and in identifying other organ systems compromised by the shock state. Physical examination of the upper abdomen should include a careful search for evidence of hepatobiliary disease such as cholecystitis or ascending cholangitis, renal parenchymal disorders such as acute pyelonephritis or perinephric abscess, and intestinal obstruction. Septicemia also may result from surgical complications such as ureteral injury, wound infection, necrotizing fasciitis, and evisceration.

The finding of generalized peritonitis should direct the physician's attention to problems such as perforated viscus, appendicitis, diverticulitis, or inflammatory bowel disease. Palpation

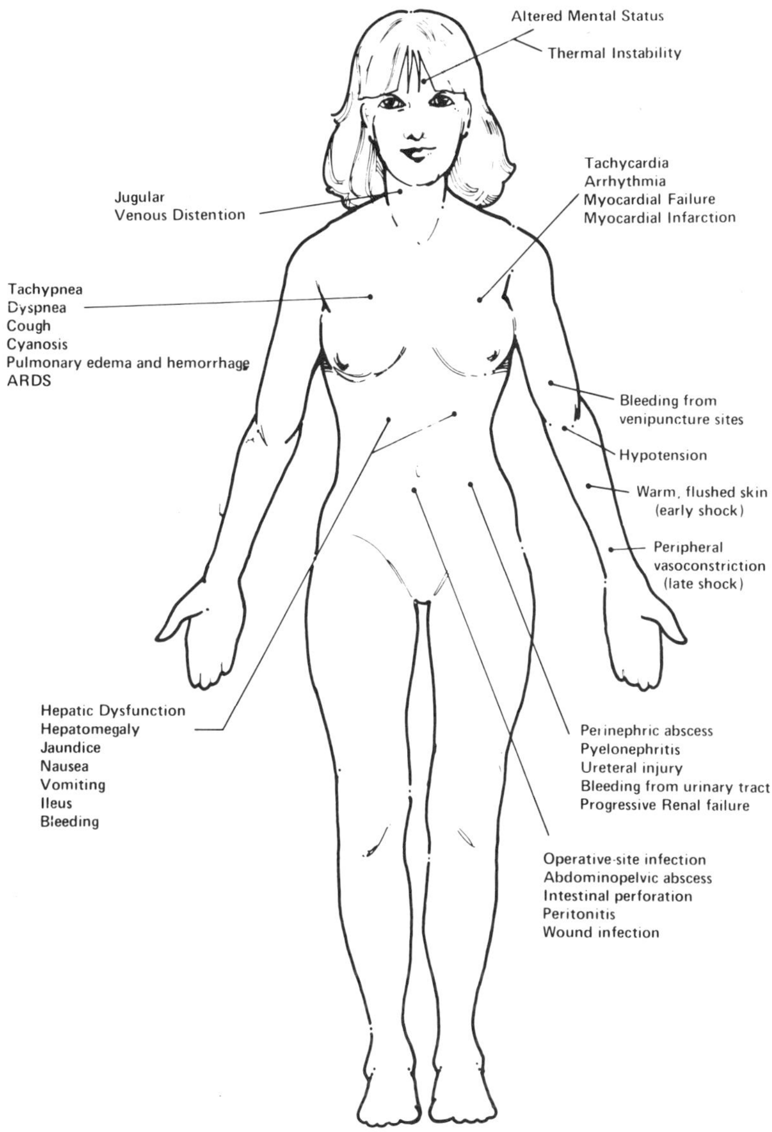

Figure 40-9. Clinical manifestations of septic shock.

of enlarged and/or tender pelvic viscera or a pelvic mass suggests the possibility of disorders such as septic abortion, chorioamnionitis, endomyometritis, ruptured uterus, and pelvic abscess. Depending on the primary site of infection and the severity of the evolving septicemia, other clinical manifestations of septic shock may include hematuria, pyuria, oliguria, jaundice, nausea, and vomiting. Spontaneous hemorrhage from the gastrointestinal or genitourinary tracts or bleeding from venipuncture sites may indicate the presence of a coagulopathy.

DIAGNOSIS

Disorders to be considered in the differential diagnosis of septic shock include cardiogenic and hypovolemic shock, pulmonary embolism, amniotic fluid embolism, cardiac tamponade, aortic dissection, hemorrhagic pancreatitis, and diabetic ketoacidosis. Distinction between septic shock and these entities usually can be made on the basis of history, physical examination, and the selected laboratory tests outlined below.

Hemodynamic monitoring is of critical importance in establishing the diagnosis of septic shock. Electrocardiography should be performed to rule out myocardial infarction or ischemia and to detect arrhythmias. Echocardiography may be of value in detecting valvular dysfunction in patients who have septicemia and endocarditis. Right heart catheterization studies are of particular value in excluding amniotic fluid ebolism, pulmonary embolism, and cardiogenic and hypovolemic shock.

In the initial stages of septic shock, the white blood cell count may be decreased due to sequestration of neutrophils in the spleen. Neutropenia usually is followed by a prominent leukocytosis, however. The hematocrit may be decreased if acute blood loss accompanies sepsis. Alternatively, the hematocrit may be increased as a result of decreased circulating plasma volume.

A variety of coagulation abnormalities may occur in septic shock, including decreased concentration of Factor XII, decreased concentration of antithrombin III, increased concentration of fibrin degradation products (FDP), and thrombocytopenia.[53] Fibrinogen concentrations may be either increased or decreased, reflecting a balance between acute-phase synthesis and consumption of this molecule. Persistence of coagulation abnormalities, particularly thrombocytopenia, is an extremely poor prognostic sign in patients with septic shock.[11,36,53]

Early in the evolution of septic shock, the patient may display respiratory alkalosis as a result of hyperventilation in response to endotoxemia. Respiratory alkalosis typically is followed by a profound metabolic acidosis. Lactate is the major organic acid responsible for the metabolic acidosis. The severity of the patient's circulatory dysfunction and the ultimate prognosis for survival correlate directly with the serum concentration of lactate.[3]

In septic patients with concurrent ARDS, acute respiratory failure also may contribute to the systemic acidosis. This state of mixed metabolic–respiratory acidosis is manifested by decreased arterial pH, decreased serum bicarbonate, and increased arterial $PaCO_2$. Hyperkalemia may develop as intracellular potassium effluxes from the cell in exchange for hydrogen ion.

Renal function may be altered in the patient who has septic shock. As renal blood flow decreases, output diminishes and then ceases. Creatinine and inulin clearance decreases. Serum concentrations of blood urea nitrogen, creatinine, and uric acid then increase.

Abnormalities of liver function also are common in patients with septic shock. These include clinical jaundice and biochemical alterations, such as elevated bilirubin, alkaline phosphatase, and transaminase concentrations.[1]

Serum glucose and insulin concentrations vary with the severity of the shock state. In all patients, glucose uptake by peripheral cells, particularly skeletal muscle cells, is impaired.[8]

Microbiologic cultures are essential to establish the diagnosis of sepsis and to determine the primary site of infection. A sample of urine should be obtained from the indwelling catheter for microscopic examination and culture. Sputum culture and Gram's stain are indicated in patients who have pneumonia. Transbronchial brush biopsy and even open lung biopsy may be necessary to establish the diagnosis of fungal or *Pneumocystis carinii* pneumonia.

Blood cultures should be collected for aerobic and anaerobic bacteria. In patients receiving parenteral hyperalimentation or immunosuppressive drugs, blood specimens also should be cultured for fungal organisms. When appropriate, aerobic and anaerobic cultures of the operative site, wound, or abscess contents should be obtained.

A limited number of radiographic studies are indicated in evaluating the patient with septic shock. Chest x-ray is helpful in detecting the presence of pneumonia, septic pulmonary emboli, pulmonary edema, and ARDS (Fig. 40-10). Immediate recognition of the latter disorder is essential, since it so adversely affects the patient's ultimate prognosis.

Abdominal radiographs are helpful in diagnosing intestinal obstruction or perforated viscus. Intravenous pyelography (IVP) may identify intraparenchymal or perinephric abscess, ureteral fistula, or ureteral injury. Computerized tomography and ultrasonography may aid in delineating a pelvic or abdominal abscess (Figs. 40-11 and 40-12). Of the two tests, CT scan has the greatest sensitivity and predictive value. CT scans correlate well with anatomic findings at exploration or autopsy.[30]

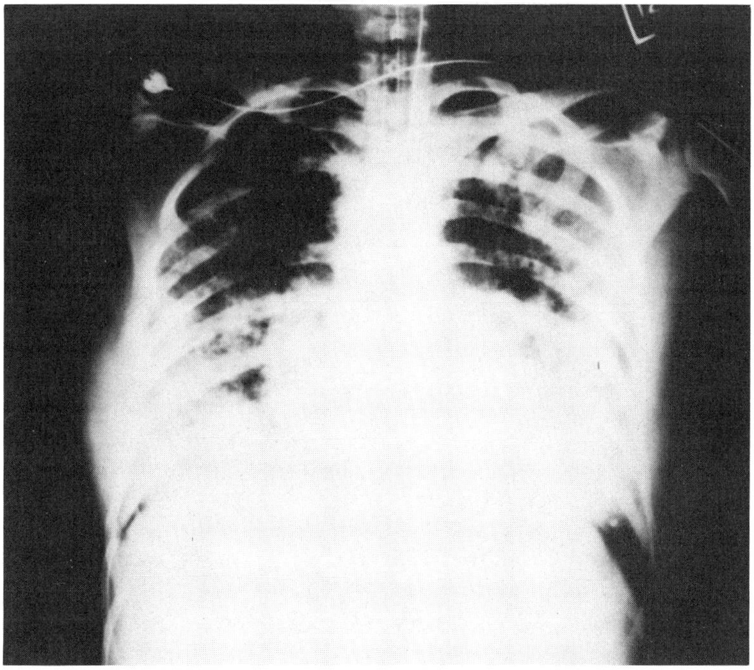

Figure 40-10. Chest X-ray of a 20-year-old woman with ARDS. Note characteristic diffuse bilateral infiltrates reflecting extensive intra-alveolar and interstitial edema.

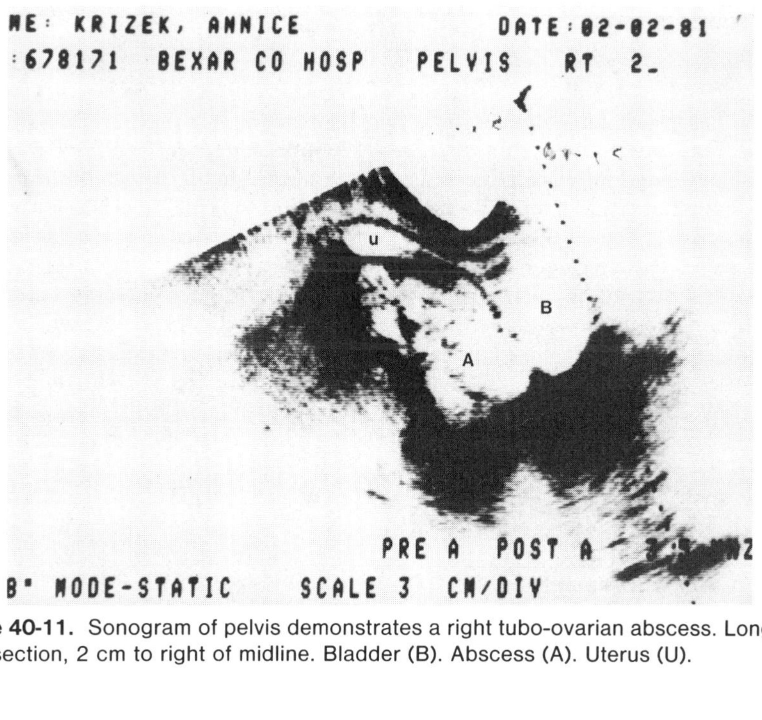

Figure 40-11. Sonogram of pelvis demonstrates a right tubo-ovarian abscess. Longitudinal section, 2 cm to right of midline. Bladder (B). Abscess (A). Uterus (U).

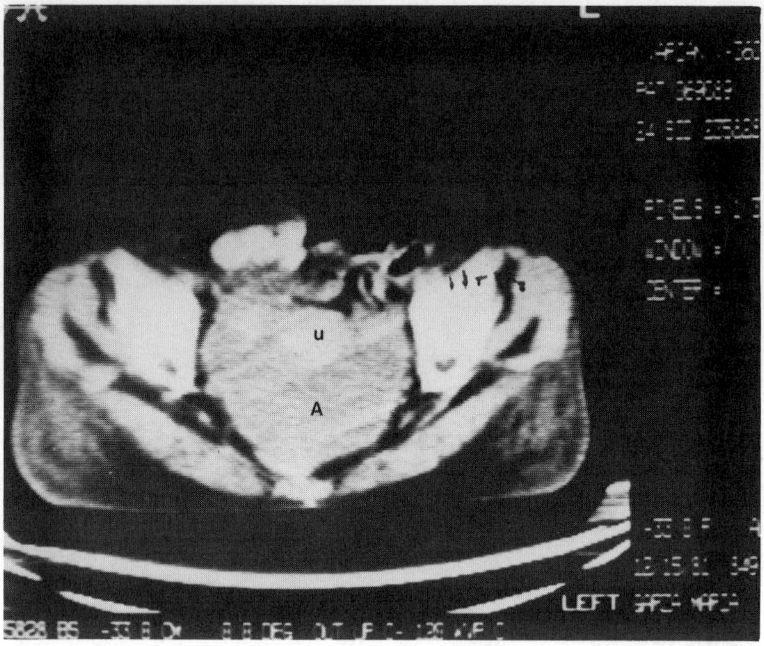

Figure 40-12. CT scan of pelvis demonstrates a normal uterus (U) and large pelvic abscess (A).

MANAGEMENT

Correction of Hemodynamic Derangements

Once the diagnosis of septic shock is established, an arterial catheter and a bladder catheter should be inserted to monitor blood pressure, arterial oxygenation, and urine output. Right heart catheterization should be performed to evaluate cardiac function. Two large-bore intravenous catheters should be inserted to administer fluids and medications.

Fluid resuscitation should be initiated while physiologic monitors are being placed. If the patient has experienced acute blood loss, administration of packed red blood cells may be required. In the absence of blood loss, plasma deficits should be corrected by infusion of isotonic crystalloids such as normal saline or lactated Ringer's solution or colloid solutions such as albumin or Plasmanate. Initial fluid replacement should be in small increments of 150–200 cc infused over 10 minutes. Adjustments in the rate of infusion are made on the basis of evaluation of blood pressure, pulse, jugular venous pressure, and urine output.

Continued restoration of intravascular volume should be guided by direct measurement of pulmonary capillary wedge pressure (PCWP). The optimal PCWP in septic shock is approximately 12 mmHg.[42] Increases in PCWP above this level do not result in corresponding increases in left ventricular stroke work index and cardiac index. PCWP correlates poorly with central venous pressure (CVP) in septic shock, emphasizing the need for right heart catheterization in such critically ill women.

The "7-3 rule" is useful for managing fluid replacement in patients with septic shock. Five to 20 ml/min of fluid are administered for 10 minutes. If PCWP increases more than 7 mmHg above baseline, the infusion should be discontinued temporarily. If PCWP does not increase more than 3 mmHg, the fluid challenge should be repeated and the 7-3 rule applied.

While fluid resuscitation is being initiated, application of a pneumatic antishock garment may result in immediate improvement in cardiac function and tissue perfusion.[56] The antishock garment mobilizes blood that has pooled in the lower portion of the body and returns it to the central circulation. Early use of it may decrease the amount of fluid needed for resuscitation, thereby reducing the risk of iatrogenic pulmonary edema. The unit should be deflated gradually as normal perfusion pressure is reestablished by intravenous fluid administration.

If fluid resuscitation in combination with application of the antishock garment does not restore adequate tissue perfusion, vasopressor therapy is indicated. Dopamine or dobutamine[19,27] are the preferred agents in septic shock. These drugs increase myocardial contractility and heart rate without causing a disproportionate increase in myocardial oxygen consumption. They stimulate dopaminergic receptors in the renal, mesenteric, coronary, and cerebral vasculature to cause vasodilation. Unlike pure beta agonists, they cause vasoconstriction in skeletal muscle. Their net effect is to preserve blood flow to vital organs.[19]

Dopamine is administered by continuous intravenous infusion. Therapy should be initiated at a dose of 2–5 μg/kg/min, and the infusion rate should be increased slowly until the desired hemodynamic response is achieved. In doses exceeding 15–20 μg/kg/min, the principal effect of dopamine is stimulation of alpha receptors. This may lead to transient increase in cardiac output followed by a sustained decrease in tissue perfusion. Other potential adverse effects of dopamine include an increase in venous admixture in the lung.[27]

Dobutamine does not appear to cause these untoward effects and it may be a more effective inotropic agent than dopamine.[27] If these findings are confirmed, dobutamine may supplant dopamine as the initial vasopressor agent in septic shock.

Digitalization is indicated in patients with overt congestive heart failure. This may be accomplished by administering a loading dose of 0.75 mg digoxin in three divided doses, 4–6 hours apart, followed by a daily maintenance dose calculated to provide a therapeutic serum concentration of 0.5–2.5 ng/ml. Usual maintenance doses are 0.125–0.375 mg per day.

In patients who have refractory hypotension despite administration of fluids and vasopressors, infusion of the narcotic antagonist naloxone should be considered. Considerable experimental evidence suggests that endogenous β-endorphins are important in the pathogenesis of septic shock. The principal adverse effects of endorphins are decreased heart rate and systemic blood pressure. The hypotensive and cardiodepressant effects of β-endorphin can be reversed by administration of naloxone.[21,25,47] The principal mechanism of action of naloxone appears to be blockade of opiate receptors in the myocardium and brainstem.[26]

Another experimental modality that appears to be of benefit in correcting certain hemodynamic derangements is administration of prostaglandin inhibitors. Increased prostaglandin concentrations correlate with alterations in cardiac output, mean arterial pressure, heart rate, and pulmonary artery pressure.[35] The principal adverse effect of prostaglandin release in experimental septic shock is pulmonary hypertension.[13] Additional experimental studies using prostaglandin synthetase inhibitors in infected animals appear warranted. To date, however, there is insufficient evidence to establish the efficacy of these drugs in humans.

A final treatment modality that should be considered in patients with refractory hypotension is implementation of intra-aortic balloon counterpulsation. The principal effects of the aortic balloon are increased diastolic blood pressure, increased coronary blood flow, decreased afterload, increased cardiac output, and increased left ventricular stroke work index. Experience with this form of therapy is still too limited to justify its routine use in treatment of septic shock.[15,38]

Treatment of Infection

Antibiotic therapy should be initiated after cultures have been obtained. Although it is not the only acceptable regimen, the antibiotic combination of penicillin (5 million units every 6 hours), tobramycin or gentamicin (3–5 mg/kg/day in divided doses), and clindamycin (900 mg every 8 hours) provides effective coverage for virtually all potential pelvic pathogens. Metronidazole (500 mg every 6 hours) may be substituted for clindamycin.

In certain situations, the obstetrician may need to utilize different antibiotic combinations. Immunosuppressed patients who are neutropenic may require carbenicillin or ticarcillin in conjunction with amikacin to treat infections caused by *Pseudomonas* organisms. Antifungal agents such as amphotericin or miconazole may be necessary for treatment of life-threatening fungal infections. A semisynthetic penicillin should be substituted for penicillin when *Staphylococcus aureus* is suspected or actually isolated. Finally, pentamidine or trimethoprim-sulfamethoxazole may be indicated for treatment of *Pneumocystis carinii* infections in severely immunocompromised patients.

In addition to broad spectrum antibiotics, immunotherapy may be used in selected patients. Passive immunization with antiserum to the lipopolysaccharide core of *E. coli* may reduce mortality in patients with gram-negative bacteremia and gram-negative bacteremia complicated by clinical shock.[58] Such therapy clearly remains experimental at the present time, however.

Elimination of the source of infection may require surgery, for example, to drain an abdominopelvic abscess, to remove infected products of conception, to extirpate grossly contaminated pelvic organs, or to debride devitalized subcutaneous and fascial tissue in the abdominal wall. Surgical intervention, in fact, may be the single most important step in stabilization of the critically ill patient. Definitive surgical therapy should not be delayed simply because the patient's blood pressure and tissue perfusion respond initially to fluid resuscitation.

The management of the gravid patient with septic shock due to chorioamnionitis presents a particularly difficult problem for the obstetrician. The maternal and fetal prognosis in chorioamnionitis has improved remarkably in recent years.[17] This is due to early diagnosis and aggressive treatment with antibiotics highly efficacious against aerobic streptococci and aerobic and anaerobic gram-negative bacilli. The maternal and fetal prognosis may not be so favorable, however, when both chorioamnionitis and septic shock coexist.[40] Prompt delivery of the fetus, by cesarean section if necessary, is indicated if the parturient's cardiovascular dysfunction does not improve with the measures outlined above. If maternal blood pressure, cardiac output, and tissue perfusion do improve, trial of labor is acceptable, provided that the fetus is monitored continuously. Immediate delivery by the most expeditious route is indicated if there is any evidence of deterioration in the condition of the fetus or worsening of maternal cardiovascular performance.

Surgery in the presence of deteriorating maternal cardiovascular function clearly is hazardous. It may be necessary, however, precisely because surgical removal of the focus of infection is the only way to stabilize the critically ill patient. Most investigators recommend endotracheal intubation and general anesthesia for emergency abdominal delivery, particularly in a patient with hemodynamic dysfunction. Regional anesthetics, which often require more time to administer, may aggravate maternal hypotension which, in turn, may result in further decrease in uterine blood flow and progressive fetal hypoxia and acidosis.

The preferred agents for general anesthesia are those that produce the least depressive effect on the cardiovascular system of the mother and fetus. Inhalation gases that result in marked uterine relaxation, such as halothane and enflurane, should be avoided in patients with chorioamnionitis and septic shock, since such patients already are particularly susceptible to uterine atony and postoperative hemorrhage. One acceptable anesthetic regimen for emergency cesarean section is the combination of thiopental (4 mg/kg) for induction, followed by nitrous oxide with oxygen until delivery of the fetus. In the presence of hypotension, ketamine (1.0 mg/kg) may be preferred to thiopental because of the former agent's sympathomimetic properties. Following delivery of the fetus, anesthesia may be deepened by administration of intravenous narcotics and diazepam. Adequate muscle relaxation is pro vided with a continuous infusion of succinylcholine (0.1–0.2%) or with incremental doses of pancuronium.

Administration of Corticosteroids

Many investigators advocate the use of glucocorticoids in treatment of septic shock.[50] Numerous experimental studies, utilizing a variety of animal models, demonstrate improvement in hemodynamic indices and survival in subjects treated with corticosteroids shortly before or after injection of endotoxin. However, clinical studies do not uniformly demonstrate a significant reduction in mortality among patients treated with corticoids compared to patients who received placebo.

There are several reasons for the discordant results reached by different study groups. It is very difficult to separate the effect of corticosteroid administration from the effect of other treatment modalities such as fluid resuscitation, ventilatory support, and timing of surgical intervention. In essence, no two patients will ever be treated exactly the same way, except for the administration of steroids. The dosages of steroids used in different studies often are not comparable, thus making valid conclusions about relative efficacy difficult. Finally, not only the dosage but also the timing of corticosteroid administration appear to be critically important in determining whether the drugs have a beneficial effect on survival. In most of the investigations reporting lack of success with steroid administration, the medication was not given until the shock state was already fully developed.

If corticosteroids are to be of value in the treatment of septic shock, it is clear that they must be given in pharmacologic doses very early in the evolution of the shock state. In medical centers where these agents are used routinely, the most common treatment regimen is methylprednisolone (30 mg/kg) or dexamethasone (3 mg/kg) administered as a single intravenous injection. The infusion should be repeated in 4 hours if there has been no improvement in the patient's clinical status.

When given early in septic shock and in proper dosage, corticosteroids may have several beneficial effects. They exert a positive inotropic effect on the heart and thereby increase cardiac output. They dilate the peripheral vasculature and cerebral vasculature and improve tissue perfusion. They promote gluconeogenesis and thus enhance the availability of glucose to the central nervous system. They suppress the release of myocardial depressant factor from the ischemic pancreas and they decrease the secretion of endogenous opiates. In patients who have an abnormally low hemoglobin saturation (P_{50}) at the onset of sepsis, corticosteroids promote a shift in the oxygen dissociation curve to the right, thereby enhancing release of oxygen to the tissue.[5] Finally, and most importantly, glucocorticoids inhibit the intense inflammatory reaction mediated by initiation of the arachidonic acid and complement cascade and leukocyte aggregation. Accordingly, their net effect on an ultrastructural level is to preserve the integrity of capillary endothelium, thus preventing cellular autolysis and transudation of intravascular fluid into the interstitial spaces. This latter effect of glucocorticoids is particularly important in preventing serious inflammatory injury to the pulmonary vasculature.

Serious side effects occur in approximately 6% of patients receiving pharmacologic doses of corticosteroids for the treatment of septic shock. Complications of steroid therapy include gastrointestinal bleeding, hyperosmolar diabetes, and acute psychosis.[51] Other potential adverse effects include inhibition of neutrophil mobilization and chemotaxis, inhibition of intracellular bacterial killing, and interference with lymphocyte and monocyte function. These effects are difficult to evaluate, but they may be of critical importance in certain patients who survive the initial shock state but then succumb to multiorgan failure resulting from uncontrolled infection.

A recent investigation demonstrated both beneficial and potentially harmful effects of corticosteroids. Early in the course of shock, patients treated with methylprednisolone or dexamethasone were more likely than untreated patients to recover from shock. In the first five days of illness, the mortality was decreased in treated patients. Ultimately, however, no difference in mortality or in the incidence of multiorgan failure was noted in treated patients as compared to controls. Moreover, the incidence of superinfection was increased in patients treated with dexamethasone.[54]

Support of the Respiratory System

The most common cause of death in septic shock is respiratory failure due to ARDS. As noted earlier, 25–50% of patients with septic shock develop ARDS. The mortality rate in septic shock complicated by respiratory failure may be as high as 90%, almost twice that in septic shock without ARDS [7,28]

A major objective in the management of the critically ill patient is *prevention* of respiratory failure. Patients with septicemia and shock are, by definition, hypoxic. Therefore, oxygen should be administered by nasal cannula or face mask. Arterial blood gases should be monitored frequently to detect early onset of respiratory failure. Excessive fluid replacement should be avoided. Most importantly, the patient should be managed with mechanical ventilation at the earliest manifestation of decreased pulmonary compliance, thereby preventing irreversible hypoxic damage to the pulmonary vasculature. Effective ventilatory support, including the application of volume-cycled respirators and positive end-expiratory pressure, is vital in the treatment of the septic patient.

Additional Supportive Measures

It is essential to prevent wide fluctuations in the patient's temperature, since thermal instability may aggravate existing cardiovascular dysfunction. Coagulation abnormalities should be identified promptly and corrected by administration of cryoprecipitate, fresh frozen plasma, fresh whole blood, or platelets. Only in rare circumstances should it be necessary to consider use of heparin for management of a consumption coagulopathy. In immunosuppressed patients, especially those with infections due to *Pseudomonas* organisms, transfusion of compatible white blood cells may be indicated. A study of neutropenic patients with gram-negative bacteremia has documented improved survival in individuals who received white blood cell transfusions in addition to appropriate antimicrobial therapy.[20]

PREVENTIVE MEASURES

Despite immediate, aggressive treatment of septic shock, the mortality associated with this disorder is alarmingly high. Therefore, in providing care to the obstetric patient, the physician should make every effort to eliminate the factors that predispose to septicemia. Asymptomatic bacteriuria should be identified and treated early in the patient's prenatal course. Infected women should remain under continued surveillance in order to detect the recurrence of bladder colonization and development of acute pyelonephritis. Preexisting medical illnesses should be stabilized prior to the onset of labor. Unnecessarily prolonged antepartum hospitalization should be avoided since this increases the patient's risk of becoming colonized with nosocomial bacteria that are resistant to many antibiotics.

In the intrapartum period, the number of vaginal examinations should be restricted, particularly in patients who have ruptured membranes. Examinations should be performed frequently enough, however, to permit prompt identification of labor abnormalities. Such disorders should be corrected promptly to prevent excessively long labors. In women who require operative delivery after an extended period of labor and ruptured membranes, a limited course of prophylactic antibiotics is effective in reducing the incidence of postcesarean endomyometritis,[55] one of the principal obstetric infections that predisposes to septic shock. In such patients, it also is essential to adhere to the established surgical principles of effective hemostasis, obliteration of potential dead space, reduction of operating time, avoidance of excessive intraoperative blood loss, and reduction of tissue necrosis and ischemia.

In the immediate postpartum period, the patient who has a genital tract infection must be identified early in the course of her illness. Once diagnosed, operative-site infections should be treated promptly with antibiotics effective against the major pelvic pathogens, including aerobic and anaerobic streptococci, coliform organisms, and *Bacteroides* species. When therapy is initiated immediately with such antimicrobials, there is a definite decrease in the subsequent incidence of life-threatening complications of pelvic infection, such as pelvic abscess and septic shock.

Nothing substitutes for frequent bedside evaluation of the parturient by her attending physician. Optimal obstetric care requires unrelenting attention on the part of the clinician to every detail of the patient's perioperative care.

REFERENCES

1. Banks, J. G., Foulis, A. K., Ledingham, I. M. A., and Macsween, R. N. M.: Liver function in septic shock. *J. Clin. Pathol.* **35**:1249–1252, 1982.
2. Bernheim, H. A., Block, L. H., and Atkins, E.: Fever: Pathogenesis, pathophysiology, and purpose. *Ann. Intern. Med.* **91**:261–270, 1970.
3. Broder, G. and Weil, M. H.: Excess lactate: An index of reversibility of shock in human patients. *Science* **143**:1457–1459, 1964.
4. Bruni, F. D., Komwatana, P., Soulsby, M. E., and Hess, M. L.: Endotoxin and myocardial failure: Role of the myofibril and venous return. *Am. J. Physiol.* **235**:H150–H156, 1978.
5. Bryan-Brown, C. W.: Effects of methylprednisolone on P[ib]50[ie]. *Crit. Care Med.* **11**;484, 1983.
6. Cavanagh, D., Knuppel, R. A., Shepherd, J. H., Anderson, R., and Rao, P. S.: Septic shock and the obstetrician/gynecologist. *South. Med. J.* **75**:809–813, 1982.
7. Clowes, G. H. A., Jr., Hirsch, E., Williams, L., Kwasnik, E., O'Donnell, T. F., Cuevas, P., Saini, V. K., Moradi, I., Farizan, M., Saravis, C., Stone, M., and Kuffler, J.: Septic lung and shock lung in man. *Ann. Surg.* **181**:681–692, 1975.
8. Clowes, G. H. A., O'Donnell, T. F., Ryan, N. T., and Blackburn, G. L.: Energy metabolism in sepsis: Treatment based on different patterns in shock and high output stage. *Am. Surg.* **79**:684–694, 1974.
9. diZerega, G. S., Yonekura, M. L., Roy, S., Nakamura, R. M., and Ledger, W. J.: A comparison of clindamycin–gentamicin and penicillin–gentamicin in the treatment of post-cesarean section endomyometritis. *Am. J. Obstet. Gynecol.* **134**:238–242, 1979.
10. Ellrodt, G. A., Kimchi, A., Berman, D. S., Riedinger, M., Swan, H. J. C., and Murata, G. H.: Segmental myocardial dysfunction in septic shock: Serial radionuclide observations. (Abstract) *Crit. Care Med.* **11**:229, 1983.
11. Eskridge, R. A.: Septic shock. *Crit. Care. Q.* **2**:55–75, 1980.
12. Fearon, D. T., Ruddy, S., Schur, P. H., and McCabe, W. R.: Activation of the properdin pathway of complement in patients with gram-negative bacteremia. *N. Engl. J. Med.* **292**:937–940, 1975.
13. Fletcher, J. R.: Prostaglandin synthetase inhibi-

tors in endotoxin or septic shock—A review. *Adv. Shock Res.* **10**:9–14, 1983.

14. Fletcher, J. R., Ramwell, P. W., and Herman, C. M.: Prostaglandins and the hemodynamic course of endotoxin shock. *J. Surg. Res.* **20**:589–594, 1976.
15. Foster, E. D., Subramanian, V. A., Vito, L., Hechtman, H. B., and Berger, R. L.: Response to intra-aortic balloon pumping. *Am. J. Surg.* **129**:464–471, 1975.
16. Freid, M. A. and Vosti, K. L.: The importance of underlying disease in patients with gram-negative bacteremia. *Arch. Intern. Med.* **121**:418–423, 1968.
17. Gibbs, R. S., Castillo, M. S., and Rodgers, P. J.: Management of acute chorioamnionitis. *Am. J. Obstet. Gynecol.* **136**:709–713, 1980.
18. Gibbs, R. S., Rodgers, P. J., Castaneda, Y. S., and Ramzy, I.: Endometritis following vaginal delivery. *Obstet. Gynecol.* **56**:555–558, 1980.
19. Goldberg, L. I.: Dopamine—Clinical uses of an endogenous catecholamine. *N. Engl. J. Med.* **291**:707–710, 1974.
20. Graw, R. G., Jr., Herzig, G., Perry, S., and Henderson, E. S.: Normal granulocyte transfusion therapy: Treatment of septicemia due to gram-negative bacteria. *N. Engl. J. Med.* **287**:367–371, 1972.
21. Groeger, J. S., Carlon, G. C., and Howland, W. S.: Naloxone in septic shock. *Crit. Care Med.* **11**:650–654, 1983.
22. Guillemin, R., Vargo, T., Rossier, J., Minick, S., Ling, N., Rivier, C., Vale, W., and Bloom, F.: β-endorphin and adrenocorticotropin are secreted concomitantly by the pituitary gland. *Science* **197**:1367–1369, 1977.
23. Hammerschmidt, D. E., Hudson, L. D., Weaver, L. J., Craddock, P. R., and Jacob, H. S.: Association of complement activation and elevated plasma-C5a with adult respiratory distress syndrome. Pathophysiological relevance and possible prognostic value. *Lancet* **1**:947–949, 1980.
24. Hinshaw, L. B., Emerson, T. E., and Reins, D. A.: Cardiovascular responses of the primate in endotoxin shock. *Am. J. Physiol.* **210**:335–340, 1966.
25. Holaday, J. W. and Faden, A. I.: Naloxone reversal of endotoxin hypotension suggests role of endorphins in shock. *Nature* **275**:450–451, 1978.
26. Janssen, H. F.: Studies on a central site of action for naloxone in endotoxin shock. *Adv. Shock Res.* **10**:73–81, 1983.
27. Jardin, F., Sportiche, M., Bazin, M., Bourokba, A., and Margairaz, A.: Dobutamine: A hemodynamic evaluation in human septic shock. *Crit. Care Med.* **9**:329–332, 1981.
28. Kaplan, R. L., Sahn, S. A., and Petty, T. L.: Incidence and outcome of the respiratory distress syndrome in gram-negative sepsis. *Arch. Intern. Med.* **139**:867–869, 1979.
29. Kimchi, A., Ellrodt, G. A., Berman, D. S., Riedinger, M. S., Swan, H. S. C., and Murata, G. H.: Right ventricular performance in septic shock: Radionuclide and hemodynamic observations. (Abstract) *Crit. Care Med.* **11**:229, 1983.
30. Knochel, J. Q., Koehler, P. R., Lee, T. G., and Welch, D. M.: Diagnosis of abdominal abscesses with computed tomography, ultrasound, and ^{111}In leukocyte scans. *Radiology* **137**:425–432, 1980.
31. Kreger, B. E., Craven, D. E., Carling, P. G., and McCabe, W. R.: Gram-negative bacteremia. III. Reassessment of etiology, epidemiology and ecology in 612 patients. *Am. J. Med.* **68**:332–343, 1980.
32. Kreger, B. E., Craven, D. E., and McCabe, W. R.: Gram-negative bacteremia. IV. Re-evaluation of clinical features and treatment in 612 patients. *Am. J. Med.* **68**:344–355, 1980.
33. Lee, C. T., Fein, A. M., Lippmann, M., Holtzman, H., Kimbel, P., and Weinbaum, G.: Elastolytic activity in pulmonary lavage fluid from patients with adult respiratory distress syndrome. *N. Engl. J. Med.* **304**:192–196, 1981.
34. Lefer, A. M.: Role of a myocardial depressant factor in shock states. *Mod. Concepts Cardiovasc. Dis.* **42**:59–64, 1973.
35. Makabali, G. L., Mandal, A. K., Morris, J. A., Brown, J., Chang, J., and Bankhead, J.: An assessment of the participatory role of prostaglandins and serotonin in the pathophysiology of endotoxic shock. *Am. J. Obstet. Gynecol.* **145**:439–445, 1983.
36. Mason, J. W., Kleeberg, U., Dolan, P., and Colman, R. W.: Plasma kallikrein and Hageman factor in gram-negative bacteremia. *Ann. Itern. Med.* **73**:545–551, 1970.
37. McCabe, W. R.: Serum complement levels in bacteremia due to gram-negative organisms. *N. Engl. J. Med.* **288**:21–23, 1973.
38. Mercer, D., Doris, P., and Salerno, T. A.: Intra-aortic balloon counterpulsation in septic shock. *Can. J. Surg.* **24**:643–645, 1981.
39. Moberg, G. P.: Site of action of endotoxins on hypothalamic-pituitary-adrenal axis. *Am. J. Physiol.* **220**:397–400, 1971.
40. Morishima, H. O., Niemann, W. H., and James, L. S.: Effects of endotoxin on the pregnant baboon and fetus. *Am. J. Obstet. Gynecol.* **131**:899–902, 1978.
41. Motsay, G. J., Dietzman, R. H., Ersek, R. A., and Lillehei, R. C.: Hemodynamic alterations and results of treatment in patients with gram-negative septic shock. *Surgery* **67**:577–583, 1970.
42. Packman, M. I. and Rackow, E. C.: Optimum left heart filling pressure during fluid resuscitation of patients with hypovolemic and septic shock. *Crit. Care Med.* **11**:165–169, 1983.
43. Parker, M. M. and Parrillo, J. E.: Septic shock. Hemodynamics and pathogenesis. *JAMA* **250**:3324–3327, 1983.
44. Pasque, M. K., Murphy, C. E., Van Trigt, Pellom, G. L., Currie, W. D., and Wechsler, A. S.: Myocardial adenosine triphosphate levels during early sepsis. *Arch. Surg.* **118**:1437–1440, 1983.
45. Rackow, E. C. and Weil, M. H.: Recent trends in

diagnosis and management of septic shock. *Curr. Surg.* **40**:181–185, 1983.
46. Raffa, J. and Trunkey, D. D.: Myocardial depression in sepsis. *J. Trauma* **18**:617–621, 1978.
47. Raymond, R. M., Harkema, J. M., Stoffs, W. V., and Emerson, T. E., Jr.: Effects of naloxone therapy on hemodynamics and metabolism following a superlethal dosage of *Escherichia coli* endotoxin in dogs. *Surg. Gynecol. Obstet.* **152**:159–162, 1981.
48. Roberts, J. M. and Laros, R. K.: Hemorrhagic and endotoxic shock: A pathophysiologic approach to diagnosis and management. *Am. J. Obstet. Gynecol.* **110**:1041–1049, 1971.
49. Samuelsson, B.: Leukotrienes: Mediators of immediate hypersensitivity reactions and inflammation. *Science* **220**:568–575, 1983.
50. Schumer, W.: New approaches to shock therapy: Steroids. In: *Molecular and Cellular Aspects of Shock and Trauma.* New York, Alan R. Liss, Inc., 1983, pp. 243–252.
51. Schumer, W.: Steroids in the treatment of clinical septic shock. *Ann. Surg.* **184**:333–339, 1976.
52. Sibbald, W. J., Anderson, R. R., Reid, B., Holliday, R. L., and Driedger, A.A.: Alveolo-capillary permeability in human septic ARDS. Effect of high-dose corticosteroid therapy. *Chest* **79**:33–42, 1981.
53. Smith-Erichsen, N., Aasen, A. O., Gallimore, M. J., and Amundsen, E.: Studies of components of the coagulation systems in normal individuals and septic shock patients. *Circ. Shock.* **9**:491–497, 1982.
54. Sprung, C. L., Caralis, P. V., Marcial, E. H., Pierce, M., Gelbard, M. A., Long, W. M., Duncan, R. C., Tendler, M. D., and Karpf, M.: The effects of high-dose corticosteroids in patients with septic shock. *N. Engl. J. Med.* **311**:1137–1143, 1984.
55. Swartz, W. H. and Grolle, K.: The use of prophylactic antibiotics in cesarean section. *J. Reprod. Med.* **26**:595–609, 1981.
56. Waeckerle, J. F.: Antishock garments. *Crit. Care Q.* **2**:15–26, 1980.
57. Weisel, R. D., Vito, L., Dennis, R. C., Valeri, C. R., and Hechtman, H. B.: Myocardial depression during sepsis. *Am. J. Surg.* **133**:512–520, 1977.
58. Ziegler, E. J., McCutchan, J. A., Fierer, J., Glauser, M.P., Sadoff, J. C., Douglas, H., and Braude, A. I.: Treatment of gram-negative bacteremia and shock with human antiserum to a mutant *Escherichia coli. N. Engl. J. Med.* **307**:1225–1230, 1982.

41

MALIGNANCY

When cancer and pregnancy "collide" in a patient, the obstetrician, the oncologist, and the patient and her family must understand how these two states affect each other. First, they must decide whether the pregnancy should be terminated. The possible effects of available therapeutic options on the mother and fetus and the future reproductive capacities of both must be recognized. In addition, certain compromises in the type or timing of therapy which are rational (in terms of the mother's safety) and which might allow salvage of a healthy infant must be identified.

This clinical situation is made even more complex by the following factors:

1. Good experimental models of the fundamental events in the malignant process, especially etiologic events, are lacking.
2. In vivo studies of therapeutic efficacy in animals are difficult to translate to the human with confidence. For example, in transplant biology, azathioprine, "the aspirin of transplantation," is not particularly effective in animals.[15]
3. In vivo animal studies and in vitro assays of the mutagenicity, carcinogenicity, and teratogenicity of most chemotherapeutic and radiotherapeutic agents and protocols do not correlate well with reported results in pregnant patients with malignancy.
4. Published reports on the utility and risks of antepartum staging techniques and chemo- and radiotherapeutic interventions give only a broad basis for future clinical management. The effects of these treatments, even when performed in a uniform manner, are difficult to predict in any individual patient. Thus, there are as yet no immutable clinical axioms.
5. Patient preference plays a strong role in determining at least the timing of therapy. Some patients will tolerate even the most serious risk to themselves in order to deliver a mature fetus. Individualized plans must balance the patient's wishes with the natural history and stage of the specific disease and the gestational stage at which the malignancy is discovered.
6. Neonatal intensive care units provide effective tertiary care for the premature infant and thus alter the decision-making process. At many institutions the crucial comparison is the difference between outcome for 24-week-old infants (15% survival with significant morbidity) and outcome for 27–28-week-old infants (70–80% survival with acceptable morbidity).[27,80]
7. Timing of delivery may be further refined based on assays used to assess fetal lung maturity antenatally[104] and the potential of parenterally administered steroids to accelerate lung maturity.[28]
8. The coexistence of cancer and pregnancy is not rare. Cancer occurs in about one in 1000 pregnancies.[83] However, because of the plurality of malignant processes observed, few large series involving specific lesions and stages and few prospective series have been reported.

Given the above considerations, we shall review the available data on cancer in pregnancy

TABLE 41-1. MORTALITY IN FEMALES BY AGE GROUP

1–14 Years	15–34 Years	35–54 Years
Accidents	Accidents	Cancer
Cancer	Cancer	Heart disease
Congenital abnormalities	Homicide	Accidents
Homicide	Suicide	Cerebrovascular disease
Heart disease	Heart disease	Cirrhosis

Source: Silverberg, E.: Cancer statistics 1985. *CA* **35**: 19–36, 1985.

and will offer clinical recommendations when appropriate.

EPIDEMIOLOGY

Of the four leading causes of death among women of reproductive age, cancer is the only disease state (Table 41-1). Breast cancer and the hematologic cancers are associated with the highest mortality rates (Table 41-2). The incidence of malignancy in the 25–35-year-old age group is six per 10,000,[85] with essentially the same incidence among pregnant women.[83] In the largest series studying cancer in pregnancy, which involved 700 cases, breast cancer was most common, followed in order of frequency by hematologic malignancies, melanoma, gynecologic cancers, and bone cancer.[5,6] In a large Scandinavian series, cervical cancer was more common than breast cancer, although 50% of the cervical cases were carcinoma in situ; next in frequency were thyroid cancer and melanoma.[83] When hematologic cancer was excluded, malignant lesions of the cervix and breast were the most common cancers found in pregnancy in three other series.[14,73,87] Malignancy can account for up to one-third of maternal deaths.[6]

BREAST CANCER

One in 11 women in the United States develops breast cancer in her lifetime. In 1985, 119,000 new cases of breast cancer are expected to occur in this country,[100] with one of six cases occurring in women under 45 years of age,[56] while 0.7–4.0% of all breast cancers occur in pregnant women. About one in 2500 deliveries is complicated by breast cancer,[105] and about one third of patients with breast cancer in the 30–36-year-old age group are coincidentally pregnant.[78]

Because the incidence of breast cancer is five to 10 times higher in women whose mothers or sisters had the disease, a thorough family history regarding breast disease should be taken at the first prenatal visit. A similar risk exists if the patient's first child was born when the mother was over 30 years of age.[47] Thorough examination of the breasts at the first prenatal visit is crucial because the hypertrophy, increased lymph flow, and increased vascularity occurring later in pregnancy may disguise a subtle dominant lesion, or a dominant lesion may be mistaken for hypertrophy itself.[105] Many attribute the advanced disease and poorer prognosis of gestational breast cancer reported in some series to delays in diagnosis and therapy. The pregnant patient herself finds up to 90% of dominant breast masses,[109] which is greater than the 75% rate of self-discovery in the nonpregnant population.[39]

Cystic masses should be aspirated in the usual fashion, with cytologic study performed on the aspirate. If the mass does not disappear or if cytologic findings are positive, biopsy is mandatory, regardless of mammographic findings.

Mammography is safe in pregnancy if the abdomen is shielded,[109] but the presence of scant radiolucent fat and increased breast tissue in pregnancy makes mammographic images more difficult to interpret.

TABLE 41-2. MORTALITY FROM CANCER IN FEMALES BY AGE AND SITE

1–14 Years	15–34 Years	35–54 Years
Leukemia	Breast	Breast
Central nervous system	Leukemia	Lung
	Uterus	Colon and rectum
Connective tissue	Central nervous system	Uterus
Lymphoma		Ovary
Bone	Skin	

Source: Silverberg, E.: Cancer statistics 1985. *CA* **35**:19–36, 1985.

Bloody discharge from the nipple in pregnancy usually represents a papilloma. Positive cytologic findings are significant, but a negative report does not rule out malignancy, and the duct must be excised.

Rarely, in a lactating patient, the infant refuses to nurse from a particular breast in the absence of an obvious unilateral lesion ("milk rejection sign"). This breast merits closer examination.[105]

Definitive open breast biopsy is relatively safe in pregnancy under local or general anesthesia; with the latter, the rate of miscarriage is less than 1%.[21] One-fifth of both pregnant and nonpregnant patients undergoing breast biopsy have a malignancy.[21] There is no evidence that pregnancy selects for any particular histology. Although inflammatory carcinoma currently is not believed to be more frequent in gravid patients, most oncologists include biopsy to rule out inflammatory carcinoma at the time of incision and drainage of every lactational abscess.[105]

Fifty to 60% of nonpregnant premenopausal women with breast cancer have tumors that are estrogen receptor (ER)-positive.[66] Primary breast cancers that are ER-negative have a higher proliferative index than do the ER-positive lesions, and recurrence is more frequent in the first 20 months after mastectomy.[66] Up to 80% of patients with ER-positive lesions show an objective response to hormonal therapy of recurrence or metastases.

If, on examination of the frozen tissue section, a histologic diagnosis of invasive cancer is returned, retained fresh tissue should be submitted for ER and progesterone receptor (PR) testing. Results of ER studies in pregnant patients demonstrate a high prevalence of ER-negative tumors. These results are consistent with the possibility that high levels of gestational estrogen saturate the receptors and cause translocation of the receptor to the nucleus, thereby depressing the levels of ER in breast cancer cytosols.[105] Given the crucial importance of ER-receptor status in determining whether an early pregnancy should be terminated because of the presence of an ER-positive breast carcinoma, we suggest that ER assays be done, via shipping of frozen tissue, only in laboratories able to perform the special techniques necessary to discern receptor status accurately in the face of the high circulating levels of estrogen of pregnancy.

After initial diagnosis, further evaluation should include shielded chest film and liver function studies (remembering that alkaline phosphatase is elevated in pregnancy). Careful examination, mammography, and even mirror-image biopsy of the opposite breast should be performed, because the incidence of bilaterality may be increased in gestational breast cancer (see below).

Combined results of all recent studies relating stage of disease to presence of bone metastases are presented in Table 41-3. Based on mathematical models, a bone scan results in a radiation dose to the fetus during organogenesis of 99 millirads (rad = a unit of absorbed dose of ionizing radiation equivalent to the absorption of 100 ergs/g of irradiated material).[101,105] To date, there are no data on the short- and long-term fetal effects of this low level of radiation. Therefore, given the low positive yield from bone scans in early disease, bone scanning should be *excluded* from the preoperative metastatic work-up of asymptomatic pregnant patients with clinical Stage I and II disease. (TNM staging of breast cancer is outlined in Table 41-4.) On the other hand, symptomatic patients or those with advanced disease *should* undergo preoperative bone scanning, given the higher probability of disseminated disease, which might alter the initial therapeutic intervention and decisions regarding the pregnancy. Patients with histologically positive axillary nodes should undergo bone scanning postoperatively.

Computerized tomography (CT) of the brain with shielding should be performed only if central nervous system symptoms are present.

Treatment

In the gravida with clinically early breast cancer who is at term, awaiting vaginal delivery for one week is permissible; however, induction should follow promptly if labor does not ensue. Some favor suppression of lactation with bromocrip-

TABLE 41-3. PREVALENCE OF BONE METASTASES BY STAGE OF BREAST CANCER AT PRESENTATION BASED ON BONE SCANS

	Number of Patients	True-Positive Scans
TNM Stage I	533	3%
TNM Stage II	696	7%
TNM Stage III	278	25%

Source: Adapted from Harbert, J. C.: Efficacy of bone and liver scanning in malignant disease. Facts and opinions. In: *Nuclear Medicine Annual 1982.* New York, Raven Press, 1982, pp. 373–401.

TABLE 41-4. TNM STAGING OF BREAST CANCER

Stage I:	T1 a or b, NO or N1a
Stage II:	T3 a or b or N1b
Stage IIIa:	T a or b *or* N2
Stage IIIb:	T4 a, b, or c *or* N3
Stage IV:	Any T, any N with MI

T = Primary tumor

T1	2 cm or less	a. Without fixation of fascia/muscle
T2	2–5 cm	b. With fixation of fascia/muscle
T3	More than 5 cm	

T4 Extension to chest wall/skin
- a. Chest wall
- b. Skin edema/infiltration or ulceration
- c. Both

NO No palpable nodes

N1 Mobile axillary nodes
- a. Not considered metastatic
- b. Considered metastatic

N2 Fixed axillary nodes

N3 Supraclavicular nodes/edema of arm

M Metastases

Source: Modified from Rubin P. (Ed.): *Clinical Oncology*, 6th Edition. New York, American Cancer Society, 1983, p. 125.

tine (Parlodel®) postpartum to reduce hypervascularity and breast size.[1] If the gestation is in the third trimester, amniocentesis (with or without steroid therapy) could be employed to verify fetal lung maturity, after which cesarean section and modified radical mastectomy might be performed under the same anesthetic.

For the gravida who is to be treated while pregnant, the issues of teratogenicity and carcinogenicity of radiation therapy and chemotherapy are prominent. Recent data suggest that disease-free survival rates are equal in patients treated for early breast cancer with lumpectomy and axillary node dissection followed by irradiation of the breast and environs and in those who undergo modified radical mastectomy (mastectomy with sparing of the pectoralis major) and axillary node dissection.[66] Furthermore, adjuvant combination chemotherapy improves survival in premenopausal women in whom axillary lymph nodes contain deposits of breast cancer.[18]

Teratogenicity and Carcinogenicity of Radiation Therapy. During the preimplantation period, the effect of radiation exposure on the embryo is all-or-none—if death does not result, few if any abnormalities will be noted. An overview of radiation effects is presented in Fig. 41-1. During organogenesis, the dose to the fetus is related to leakage of radiation from the radiotherapy unit (reducible by external shielding), the distance of the fetus from the radiation field, and internal scatter radiation from the target tissue (not reducible by external shielding). Using data summarized in Fig. 41-2, one can estimate that radiation to the breast exposes the fetus of up to 12 weeks' gestation to 5000 x 0.2% to 0.3%, or 10–15 rads. At term, parts of the fetus closest to the maternal thorax receive 200 rads, with lesser although still considerable exposure to fetal parts furthest away from the maternal thorax.

The most extensive data on the effects of radiation exposure in utero come from the Hiroshima experience.[77] Microcephaly and mental retardation were observed in almost 20% of infants exposed to 10–20 rads during weeks 6–11 of gestation (Table 41-5). Hydrocephaly, microphthalmia, spina bifida, mongolism, and abnormalities of the extremities and genitalia also were noted. Although in animal models growth stunting alone is observed with radiation after organogenesis, other defects such as microcephaly, mental retardation, chromosomal aberrations, and cataracts have been reported in children heavily irradiated in utero *after* the first trimester.[50] Importantly, some of these stigmata do not evince themselves until 13 months of age.[50]

Existing data on carcinogenesis relative to radiation exposure indicate that exposure up to 100 rads of total-body irradiation causes a 1% incidence of fetal cancers (attributable to radia-

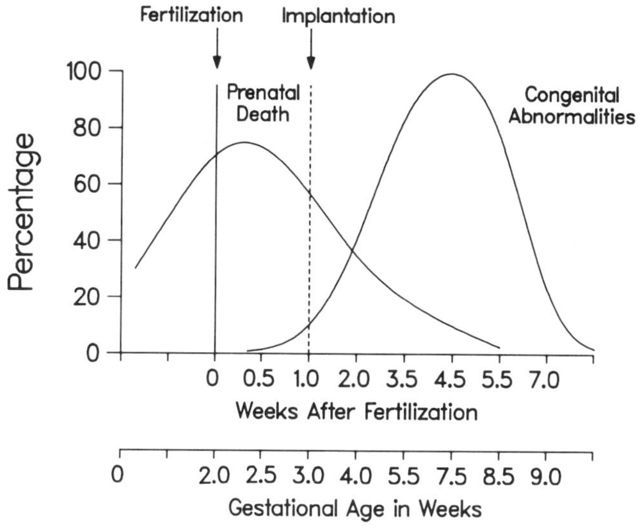

Figure 41-1. Consequences of radiation injury *in utero.* (Modified from Brill, A.B. et al.: Radiation and congenital malformations. Am. J. Obstet. Gynecol. 90:1149–1168, 1964) Reproduced with permission from Orr, J. W., Jr. and Shingleton, H. M.: Cancer in pregnancy, in Hickey, R. C. et al. (eds.): Current Problems In Cancer, Copyright © 1983 by Year Book Medical Publishers, Inc., Chicago.

tion itself) in the populations studied.[86] However, the in utero dose threshold for the induction of subsequent malignancy (often years later) and the differential effect of gestational age at exposure are not known.

The preceding considerations suggest that surgery and not radiation is the initial treatment of choice for the gravida with early breast cancer. Since there are as yet no data on the results of tylectomy and radiotherapy in lactating women with breast cancer, modified radical mastectomy also is recommended for operable patients treated postpartum.

If a woman who has undergone radiation therapy discovers that she is pregnant, some clinicians recommend offering termination to all such patients who have received more than 10 rads to the fetus during organogenesis.[53]

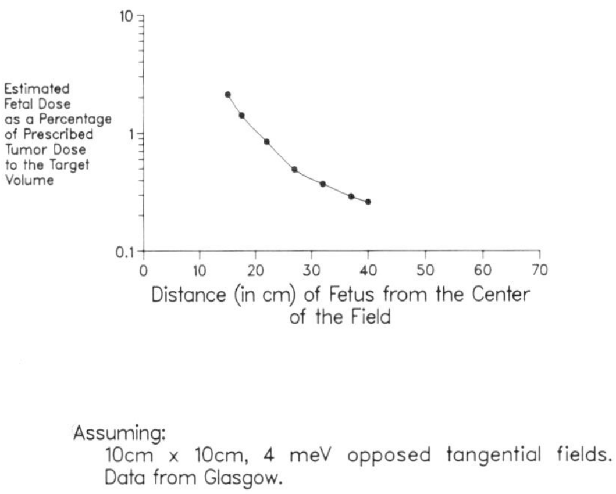

Figure 41-2. Fetal exposure to internal scatter radiation during radiotherapy. Reproduced with permission from Wallack, M. K., Wolf, J. A., Bedwinek, J. Denes, A. E., Glasgow, G. Kumar, B. Meyer, J. S., Rigg, L. A., and Wilson-Krechel, S.: Gestational carcinoma of the female breast, in Hickey, R. C. et al. (eds.): Current Problems In Cancer, Copyright © 1983 by Year Book Medical Publishers, Inc., Chicago.

Chemotherapy. In the gravida with early breast cancer who is a candidate for adjuvant combination chemotherapy (i.e., patients with histologically positive axillary nodes), it is not desirable to delay initiation of chemotherapy

TABLE 41-5. INCIDENCE OF SUBSEQUENT MICROCEPHALY AND MENTAL RETARDATION AFTER IONIZING RADIATION TO THE FETUS DURING WEEKS 6–11 OF GESTATION

Fetal Dose	Incidence
1–9 rads	11%
10–19 rads	17%
20–29 rads	30%
30–39 rads	40%
50–99 rads	70%
100 rads	100%

Source: Modified from Miller, R. and Mulvihill, S.: Small head size after atomic radiation. *Teratology* **14**:355-357, 1976.

for more than a few weeks. Therefore, during the second and third trimester, if delivery of a mature fetus and initiation of chemotherapy postpartum cannot be expected to occur within 3 weeks, chemotherapy should be begun. Chemotherapy in the second and third trimester, even including agents that are severe teratogens in animal studies (e.g., methotrexate), has not resulted in the increased rates of malformations or growth retardation initially predicted. However, methotrexate is prohibitively hepatotoxic when administered preevacuation to patients with high-risk molar pregnancy.[43] This drug is one of the cornerstones of adjuvant chemotherapy for breast cancer (along with cyclophosphamide and 5-fluorouracil). Regimens not including methotrexate for therapy of breast cancer generally include doxorubicin, an agent known to cross the placenta.[65]

The last prenatal dose of chemotherapy should be given 3 weeks prior to the estimated date of confinement or planned delivery to avoid neonatal myelosuppression.

In the first trimester, therapeutic abortion must be discussed prior to adjuvant therapy, and the teratologic risks of the proposed agents based on the available data in humans must be made clear (see below).

Advanced Local Disease. For patients presenting with signs of advanced local disease (edema of the arm, fixation of tumor or nodes, or ulceration), abortion or early delivery is in order because intensive irradiation (exceeding 7000 rads) will be necessary to suppress local and regional disease. This is also true if inflammatory carcinoma is encountered. Chemotherapy can precede or follow radiation; it may be begun first if termination is refused and/or the fetus is viable but the lungs are not yet mature. Radiation therapy and subsequent mastectomy can then be carried out postpartum. Severe focal pain, bleeding, or infection requires immediate irradiation despite the pregnancy.

If recurrent local disease occurs during pregnancy, excision should be performed in order to postpone radiation. If this is not possible, radiation must be undertaken with the fetus in situ unless termination or expeditious delivery is possible.

Disseminated Disease. Metastatic disease (either primary or recurrent) in pregnancy requires chemotherapy or hormonal manipulation, so that knowledge of receptor status is crucial. Termination or delivery and oophorectomy are necessary in ER-positive women if hormonal therapy is elected; fetal risk must be delineated if chemotherapy is to be administered first.

Effect of Pregnancy on Breast Cancer

Pregnant women do not have a higher incidence of breast cancer. Whether pregnancy exerts an adverse effect on the course of the disease and whether termination of pregnancy improves prognosis are controversial issues.

It has been known for two decades that pregnancy enhances both induction and growth of carcinogen-induced, hormone-sensitive mammary tumors in rats.[75] However, varying conclusions have been drawn from many poorly controlled, retrospective studies in humans.

1. The only prospective study that has been carried out is that by Haagensen (Table 41-6).

TABLE 41-6. TEN-YEAR SURVIVAL (%) AFTER RADICAL MASTECTOMY FOR BREAST CANCER ACCORDING TO COLUMBIA CLINICAL CLASSIFICATION*

	Stage A	Stage B	Stage C	Stage D	Total Group
Pregnancy and lactation	60%	27%	13%	0%	33%
All patients	70%	41%	24%	18%	54%

* Patients treated during pregnancy or lactation compared with all patients of all ages in the same series. All patients from Dr. Haagensen's personal series.

Source: Reproduced with permission from Wallack, M. K., Wolf, J. A., Bedwinek, J., Denes, A. E., Glasgow, G., Kumar, B., Meyer, J. S., Rigg, L. A. and Wilson-Krechel, S.: Gestational carcinoma of th› female breast, in Hickey, R.C., et al. (eds): *Curr. Probl. Cancer* **7**(9):1–58, 1983. ›pyright © 1983 by Year Book Medical Publishers, Inc., Chicago.

Staging was based on the Columbia Clinical Classification (Table 41-7). Although the data show a survival disadvantage, stage for stage, at 10 years for gravid and lactating patients, no statistically significant difference evolved.[105] In Haagensen's follow-up report, 10-year survival rates for Stage A and B lesions were 80% and 50%, respectively (versus 70% and 41%, respectively, in the initial report); however, the corresponding figures for pregnancy and lactation in the completed series, involving 935 patients with Stage A and B disease with at least a 10-year follow-up and 591 cases with nearly a 50-year follow-up, are not included.[51]

2. Breast cancer in younger women probably differs from that in the older population. Studies comparing survival in pregnant and lactating patients and nonpregnant younger women are summarized in Table 41-8. No significant overall effect of pregnancy on survival is evident. Maier did observe a survival disadvantage when axillary nodes were positive.[74] In this study, the incidence of positive nodes was similar in the pregnant and nonpregnant groups, whereas the majority of reports suggest a higher incidence of positive nodes in pregnancy—about 65% vs. 35%.[1,66]

TABLE 41-7. COLUMBIA CLINICAL CLASSIFICATION FOR BREAST CANCER

Clinical Stage	Clinical Features
Stage A	No clinically involved axillary nodes No grave signs as in clinical Stage C
Stage B	Clinically involved movable axillary nodes less than 2.5 cm in transverse diameter No grave signs
Stage C	Any one of five grave signs of advanced disease 1. Edema involving less than one-third of the breast 2. Ulceration of skin 3. Solid fixation of tumor to chest wall 4. Axillary nodes 2.5 cm in diameter 5. Fixation of axillary nodes to skin or to deeper structures of overlying axilla
Stage D	1. Two or more of the five grave signs (above) 2. Edema involving more than one-third of the skin over the breast 3. Satellite skin nodules 4. Inflammatory carcinoma 5. Clinically positive supraclavicular nodes 6. Parasternal tumor suggestive of positive internal mammary metastases 7. Arm edema 8. Distant metastases

Source: Haagensen, C. D. and Bodian, C.: A personal experience with Halsted's radical mastectomy. *Ann. Surg.* **199**:143–150, 1984.

3. The careful retrospective analyses of Peters constitute the only large-scale attempt at stratification for age and stage (Table 41-9). Her data show no adverse effect of pregnancy on survival and further suggest that the disease does not present at a more advanced stage in the gravida.

4. The few clinical reports that detail survival in patients who aborted early in pregnancy demonstrate no subsequent advantage gained by that intervention.[35]

5. Few breast cancers in pregnancy have been shown to be ER-positive so far.

6. Estriol, a major component of the increased estrogen produced during pregnancy, is a weak estrogen.

7. Although prolactin can promote carcinogenesis in mouse mammary tumors, its suppression has not proved to be of value clinically.[35]

We conclude that there is no firm evidence that pregnancy per se has an adverse effect on the course of breast cancer. Termination or early delivery should be considered when (1) possible fetal effects of necessary chemotherapy or radiotherapy are of paramount concern, (2) the disease is disseminated, (3) fulminant progression of disease is apparent during pregnancy, or (4) there is clear estrogen-receptor positivity.

Prophylactic oophorectomy in early disease has been evaluated and is of no clinical benefit, whether or not axillary nodes are positive.[82]

Pregnancy after treatment for breast cancer does not appear to shorten the time to recurrence or to increase the incidence of recurrence.[16] Therefore, subsequent pregnancy is allowed, with most clinicians recommending that future childbearing be postponed for up to 3 years, the period during which the rate of recurrence is highest. Because the effects of long-term administration of estrogenic and progestational agents on micrometastases from mammary cancers are not known, oral contraceptives are best withheld. Mechanical barriers, such as intrauterine devices, are preferred. Cases have been reported of patients becoming pregnant during chemotherapy for breast

TABLE 41-8. COMPARISON OF AXILLARY NODAL STATUS AND SURVIVAL BETWEEN PREGNANT AND LACTATING AND NONPREGNANT YOUNGER WOMEN WITH BREAST CANCER

			Negative Nodes				Positive Nodes				Total Survival for Series (%)	
					Survival (%)				Survival (%)			
Reference	Patients Included	Total Patients	Number of Patients	(%)	5 yr	10 yr	Number of Patients	(%)	5 yr	10 yr	5 yr	10 yr
Treves (1958)	<35 yr P, L	51	—	(23)	50	—	—	(77)	20	—	27	(Disease-free)
	<35 yr All patients	367	150	(41)	60	—	217	(59)	21	—	37	(Disease-free)
Horsley (1969)	<35 yr P, L	12	4	(33)	100	100	8	(67)	100	100	100	100
	<35 yr All patients	59	20	(34)	63	56	39	(66)	60	43	61	49
Maier (1978)	<40 yr P,L	79	34	(43)	77	—	37	(47)*	30	—	49	—
	<40 yr Nonpregnant	647	291	(45)	80	—	304	(47)*	48	—	61	—
Rosen (1984)†	≧35 yr P,L	10	—	—	—	—	—	—	—	—	60	—
	<35 yr All patients	166	101	(61)	88	70	63	(39)	61	40	75	60
All series:	Preg, Lac	152									46	—
	Control	1,239									56	—

P, L = Pregnant or up to one year postpartum (maximum) in all studies.

* Not all nodes sampled.

† 14/46 tumors clearly estrogen-receptor positive (30%).

Source: Data from references 74 and 89 and Treves, N. and Holleb, A. I.: *Surg. Gynecol. Obstet.* **107**:271–283, 1958; and Horsley, J. S., Alrich, E. M., and Wright, C. B.: *Ann. Surg.* **169**:839–849, 1969.

TABLE 41-9. FIVE-YEAR SURVIVAL (%) FROM BREAST CANCER ACCORDING TO TNM STAGING*

	Stage I	Stage II	Stage III	Stage IV	Total
Pregnancy and lactation	61%	42%	20%	0%	32%
Control group	73%	27%	24%	4%	34%

* Patients diagnosed during pregnancy and lactation, or up to one year postpartum compared with a control group from the same series, matched for age and stage; distribution of cases among the stages did not differ from that found in the entire population.

Source: Data from Peters, M. V. and Meakin, J. W.: The influence of pregnancy on carcinoma of the breast. *Progr. Clin. Cancer* **1**:471, 1965, adapted from Wallack, M. K., Wolf, J. A., Bedwinek, J., Denes, A. E., Glasgow, G., Kumar, B., Meyer, J. S., Rigg, L. A., and Wilson-Krechel, S.: Gestational carcinoma of the female breast. *Curr. Probl. Cancer* **7**(9):1–58, 1983.

cancer.[60] Contraception should be practiced during adjuvant therapy.

On purely theoretical grounds, breast-feeding is not recommended. Abstention avoids possible viral transmission to the infant, vascular engorgement of the breast, and prolonged prolactin secretion.

No undue symptoms result from the presence of a mammary prosthesis during pregnancy.[47]

Gestational breast cancer may be associated with an increased incidence of bilateral tumors.[105] Simultaneous bilateral invasive breast cancers occur in 2–3% of young women.[89] Furthermore, in the nongravid younger age group, the overall bilateral cancer rate (which includes previous, simultaneous, and subsequent lesions) exceeds 10%.[89] Up to 11% of gravid or lactating patients may present with simultaneous bilateral invasive disease.[93] We recommend careful examination, mammography, and mirror-image biopsy of the opposite breast in patients with gestational breast cancer.

Effect of Breast Cancer on Pregnancy

There are only four well-documented cases of metastases of breast cancer to the placenta, and there was no fetal involvement.[87] Thus, the only effect of breast cancer on pregnancy appears to be the therapeutic dilemma encountered.

HEMATOLOGIC CANCER

Hodgkin's Disease

One in 1000 to 6000 pregnancies is complicated by lymphoma.[84] Hodgkin's disease is by far the most common type observed in gravidas, because 50% of cases occur in women between 20 and 40 years of age.[78] Ninety percent of patients present with peripheral lymphadenopathy affecting, in descending order, the cervical, axillary, and inguinal nodes. Ten percent present with primary mediastinal disease. When present, symptoms include fevers, night sweats, weight loss, malaise, and pruritus. Pain in areas of disease after the ingestion of alcohol is considered pathognomonic.[78]

Definitive diagnosis is by histologic identification of Reed–Sternberg cells after open biopsy, preferably of a cervical node. Needle biopsy is to be avoided. Histologically, the nodular sclerosing subtype is most frequent. Lymphocyte dominance is associated with the best prognosis. Mixed cellular and lymphocyte depletion subtypes are unfavorable and are associated with noncontiguous spread via nearby lymph node chains.

Careful physical examination of lymph nodes, shielded chest radiography, liver function studies, bone marrow biopsy (not simply aspiration), and serum protein electrophoresis can be performed readily in the pregnant patient. A staging laparotomy after the 13th week of pregnancy that involves multiple lymph node biopsies, liver biopsy, and splenectomy can obviate liver/spleen scanning, lymphangiography, and intravenous pyelography and improves the accuracy of staging by 30–40%.[35] Midline surgical oophoropexy at the time of staging laparotomy may be helpful if pelvic radiation therapy is planned. When disease is diagnosed near term, cesarean section often is combined with staging laparotomy. The Ann Arbor staging system is described in Table 41-10.

TABLE 41-10. STAGING OF HODGKIN'S DISEASE—ANN ARBOR CLASSIFICATION

Stage	Description	Substage	
Stage I	Single node region above or below diaphragm, *or*	I	Stages I,II,III do not involve liver or bone marrow; Stages I,II, and IIIA are surgically staged
	Single extralymphatic organ or site alone	IE	
Stage II	Two or more node regions on same side of diaphragm, *or*	II	
	Single node region and localized single extralymphatic organ or site	IIE	
Stage III	Node regions on both sides of diaphragm	III	
	± Localized single extralymphatic organ or site or	IIIE	
	Spleen or	IIIS	
	Both	IIIES	
Stage IV	Diffuse involvement of extralymphatic organs/sites ± node regions (liver, lung, bone marrow, skin)	IV	
All stages further divided	Without weight loss/fever/sweats	A	
	With weight loss/fever/sweats	B	

Source: Modified from Rubin, P. (Ed.): *Clinical Oncology*, 6th Edition. New York, American Cancer Society, 1983.

Treatment. High rates of disease-free survival are now achieved in early disease (up to 85%), and up to 50% disease-free survival has been achieved even in Stages IIIE and IV. Early disease is treated by extended-field radiation therapy alone unless there is contiguous spread to the lung, symptoms are present, there is a large mediastinal mass, or lower abdominal nodes are involved, in which case quadruple chemotherapy with MOPP (mustard, vincristine [Oncovin®] procarbazine, and prednisone) is added subsequent to radiotherapy.[35] Treatment of Stage IIIA depends on histology; nodular sclerosing and lymphocyte dominant subtypes require radiation only, whereas other subtypes require both radiation and chemotherapy. Stages IIIB and IVA and IVB require MOPP as primary therapy with adjunctive radiation.[78]

Only eight cases in which MOPP was used during pregnancy have been reported.[17,22,30,32,62] Of four patients treated during the first trimester, two had abortions; in one of these, the fetus had small malpositioned kidneys. The third patient had a normal-appearing infant, and the fourth had an infant with four toes on each foot and syndactyly. Four patients treated during the second and third trimesters had normal-appearing infants. Most believe that combination chemotherapy is contraindicated during the first trimester,[4] whereas some conclude that forbidding its use completely is premature.[42] The regimen can cause significant leukopenia and thrombocytopenia during pregnancy and lactation.

Although radiation therapy to the mediastinum and subdiaphragmatic areas can be begun during pregnancy if the uterus is shielded,[35] studies suggest that a dose of 3–6 rads is still carried to the pelvis.[110]

Indications for abortion or early delivery include (1) inguinal or abdominal/pelvic disease (which would require direct radiation), (2) disease presenting so early in pregnancy that staging would be delayed several weeks, and (3) desire to be free from the teratogenic risk of quadruple-agent chemotherapy.

Except for the therapeutic issues, Hodgkin's disease has no effect on pregnancy. Miscarriage rates equal those in the general population and there is no proven case of transmission of the disease to a fetus. Pretherapy ovarian biopsies are normal in nonpregnant women.[32] Pregnancy has no effect on the disease, and therapeutic abortion does not increase survival.

Reproductive Performance After Therapy for Hodgkin's Disease. The probability of regular menses after treatment for Hodgkin's disease is shown in Fig. 41-3, and the probability of pregnancy after therapy is shown in Fig. 41-4. In three large recent studies, 56 of 215 women followed gave birth to 55 normal infants;, those followed over the long term showed normal development. There was no increase in the rate of miscarriages in this group.[2,57,106]

In males, prepubertal individuals are most resistant to damage. Pubescent patients are most vulnerable to profound effects on sperm production and endocrine function. Pretherapy sperm cryopreservation can be considered. Effects on libido are variable. Testosterone levels are not affected.[32] In females, hormonal therapy (oral contraceptives) has been utilized to suppress and possibly protect the ovaries during therapy, but results in 15 patients studied to date have been variable.[25,106] Males and females with Hodgkin's disease who are fertile after therapy have good reproductive outcomes.

Non-Hodgkin's Lymphomas

Sixteen cases of non-Hodgkin's lymphoma in pregnancy have been reported. Four gravid patients have been treated with multiple-agent chemotherapy—two beginning in the second trimester, one beginning in the first trimester, and one for 5 months prior to conception and throughout the first and second trimesters. Apparently normal infants were delivered in all four cases [38,71,96]

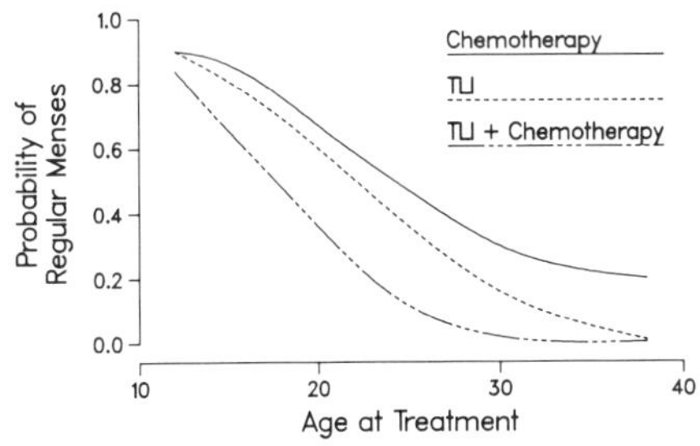

Figure 41-3. Probability of regular menses after chemotherapy, total lymphoid irradiation (TLI), or TLI plus chemotherapy according to age at time of treatment for Hodgkin's disease. (From Horning, S. J., Hoppe, R. T., Kaplan, H. S. and Rosenberg, S. A.: Female reproductive potential after treatment for Hodgkin's disease. N. Engl. J. Med. 304:1377–1382, 1981. Reprinted by permission of the New England Journal of Medicine.)

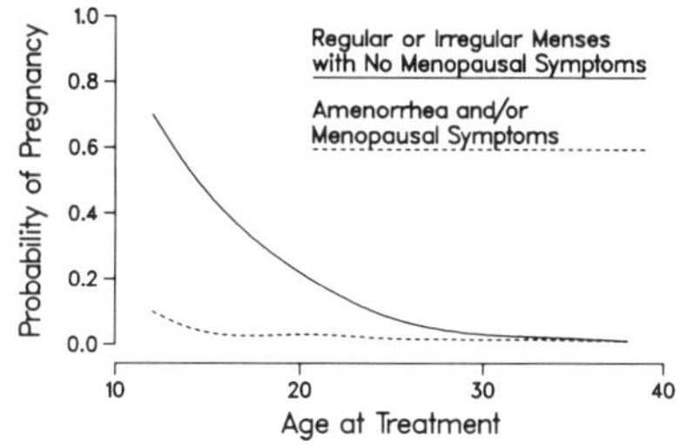

Figure 41-4. Probability of pregnancy after treatment with TLI, chemotherapy, or both for Hodgkin's disease according to menstrual status, menopausal symptoms, and age at treatment. (From Horning, S. J., Hoppe, R. T., Kaplan, H. S. and Rosenberg, S. A.: Female reproductive potential after treatment for Hodgkin's disease. N. Engl. J. Med. 304:1377–1382, 1981. Reprinted by permission of the New England Journal of Medicine.)

If lymphoma that carries a poor prognosis is diagnosed in pregnancy, prompt initiation of chemotherapy regardless of stage of gestation is the only hope for survival.[38] Pregnancy may exert an adverse influence on Burkitt's lymphoma and is not recommended in patients successfully treated for this disease.[84]

Leukemia

Chronic or acute leukemia is diagnosed in one in 40,000 pregnancies.[78] Distribution of cell types is similar in pregnant and nonpregnant women (Table 41-11). The average age at diagnosis of the gravida with acute leukemia is 28 years. [35]

TABLE 41-11. COMPARISON OF LEUKEMIC CELL TYPE IN PREGNANT AND NONPREGNANT WOMEN

	AGL	ALL	CGL	CLL	Other
Pregnant	35.8%	10.8%	45%	1.3%	7.1%
Nonpregnant	35.2%	11.8%	45%	7.8%	0.2%

AGL = acute granulocytic

ALL = acute lymphocytic

CGL = chronic granulocytic

CLL = chronic lymphocytic

Other = blast cell, mist, or AML

Source: Modified from Mitchell, M. S. and Capizzi, R. L.: Neoplastic disease. In: *Medical Complications During Pregnancy,* 2nd Edition. G. N. Burrow and T. F. Ferris (Eds.). Philadelphia, W. B. Saunders, 1982.

Presenting symptoms include anemia, pallor, granulocytopenia, thrombocytopenia, and splenomegaly. Severe infections or bleeding diatheses are not uncommon at the time of diagnosis. Diagnosis is based on peripheral blood smear and bone marrow examination. Unlike acute lymphocytic leukemia (ALL) in children (50% 10-year survival), 50–80% of adults with ALL or acute nonlymphocytic leukemia (ANLL) attain complete remission (CR), but the median duration is only one year. Acute leukemia in adults is a rapidly fatal disease unless aggressive chemotherapy is instituted immediately after diagnosis and stabilization is achieved via administration of blood products and antibiotics.[78]

There have been 31 reported cases of acute leukemia (seven ALL and 24 ANLL) diagnosed and initially treated with multiple-agent chemotherapy during a pregnancy. Cytosine arabinoside (Ara-C), an inhibitor of DNA polymerase and a pyrimidine inhibitor, was the most frequently employed agent. In addition, 10 pregnancies were recorded in nine women on maintenance chemotherapy for ALL (five) or ANLL (four) at the time of conception. Three of these 40 patients undergoing treatment for leukemia died within one month of delivery or abortion (8%). All either had active disease or were in only partial remission at delivery. One had fatal disseminated intravascular coagulation (DIC) secondary to acute promyelocytic leukemia. In a second, delivery occurred during a period of marrow aplasia, and death occurred from pulmonary aspergillosis on the ninth postpartum day. In the third, labor was induced at 38 weeks. The patient was in only partial remission. Death due to urinary sepsis occurred on the seventh postpartum day.

In contrast, maternal outcome in a group of seven women with untreated ANLL at the time of delivery was disastrous. Five of the seven died within one month of delivery (71%). The diagnosis of leukemia was made peripartum in four cases. Postpartum hemorrhage (immediate or delayed) occurred in four of the seven cases. One death occurred in a woman whose labor was induced after diagnosis, but before complete remission was attained.

The 41 pregnancies in patients on chemotherapy for ANLL and ALL yielded 32 viable infants, five therapeutic abortions, two fetal demises (at 24 and 30 weeks), one infant born alive but in "grave condition," and one death one month postpartum (birth weight = 1000 g at 34 weeks). In the seven pregnancies in women with untreated ANLL, two fetuses died in utero secondary to DIC.[24]

Fourteen pregnancies have been observed in 10 women apparently cured of previous childhood ALL. There was one spontaneous abortion; 13 live term infants were delivered. One had calcaneovalgus malformation of the foot, not thought attributable to chemotherapy.[24]

In sum, no major fetal malformations were reported, even though nine patients conceived while on maintenance chemotherapy and six additional patients began intensive chemotherapy during the first trimester. Two infants were born with neutropenia.

It must be noted that fetal outcome with use of first-trimester antileukemic agents is not always so favorable. A woman with ANLL was given Ara-C and 6-thioguanine in the first semester of two separate pregnancies. One infant had absent medial toes and hypoplastic thumbs bilaterally; the other infant appeared completely normal.[95] The following guidelines for acute leukemia in pregnancy can be formulated.

Effect of Pregnancy on Leukemia

1. The incidence of leukemia is not increased in pregnant women, despite the possibility that pregnancy represents a state of decreased immune responsiveness.
2. Evaluation of anemia and fatigue in pregnancy should be done promptly because of the disastrous consequences to mother and infant of a delay in diagnosing acute leukemia.
3. Pregnancy decreases maternal survival in acute leukemia (via the obstetric complications of hemorrhage and infection) in patients with active disease at the time of delivery. Therefore, every effort should be made to delay delivery until complete remission is attained. If therapeutic abortion is elected, termination should be delayed until the acute leukemic phase is under control.
4. Physiologic changes of pregnancy, such as increased blood volume and glomerular filtration rate, may require changes in the dose of chemotherapeutic agents used.

Effect of Leukemia on Pregnancy

1. Two cases have been reported of mothers with ALL who gave birth to infants having the same disease. Both infants died in the first year of life.
2. Intrauterine growth retardation (IUGR) frequently is observed in infants born to mothers with acute leukemia, whether or not chemo-

therapy is given. Possible mechanisms include decreased maternal hemoglobin concentration, aggregation of leukemic cells in the uteroplacental circulation, and DIC secondary to ANLL. If the mother is in complete remission, one should consider early delivery to avoid fetal compromise.

3. Premature labor is common in the gravida with acute leukemia. Tocolytics have been used successfully.[24]

4. The effects of antileukemic chemotherapy on the fetus are uncertain and variable but may be much less than predicted from animal studies.

5. Patients cured of ALL and not on maintenance chemotherapy are not at increased risk for any complications of pregnancy.

Chronic Leukemia

Although chronic granulocytic or lymphocytic leukemia is a more indolent disease than acute leukemia, therapy should not be delayed in the gravida. Chemotherapy and radiation therapy to the spleen with uterine shielding should be provided.[35] The major cytotoxic agents employed are busulfan, hydroxyurea, and cyclophosphamide, all of which pose risks to the fetus.[78]

MELANOMA

The average person has 15 nevi, any of which is capable of becoming a melanoma. This lesion is rare before puberty. Its incidence may be doubling every generation.[84]

After histologic diagnosis, liver function studies, stool guaiac testing (owing to the frequency of GI metastases), and chest radiography are necessary. Computerized tomography and sonography are more sensitive means for detecting liver metastases in melanoma than are liver/spleen scans.[84] The schemas of Clark (level of anatomic invasion of the primary melanoma) and Breslow (actual tumor thickness in millimeters) are related most closely to prognosis. Standard staging criteria are employed also (Table 41-12).

Thin melanomas (less than 0.76 mm) can be treated with local resection alone, with a 2-cm margin. When the primary lesion is 0.76–3.99 mm thick, 50% of patients have regional metastases, and therapy consists of wide local excision and regional lymphadenectomy. Eighty percent of lesions greater than 4 mm in thickness are associated with distant metastases. Dicarbazone (DTIC) or the nitrosureas are associated with a response rate of 20%, although the response is short-lived.[84]

It has been suggested repeatedly that pregnancy exerts an adverse effect on melanoma for the following reasons:

1. The level of melanocyte-stimulating hormone increases in pregnancy after the second month.

2. About one-half of melanomas are estrogen receptor-positive.

3. Animal studies have suggested that the female is a more favorable host for melanoma than is the male.[19]

4. Many earlier case reports describe apparently virulent melanomas found in pregnant women. Cases of spontaneous regression after delivery also have been reported.

5. There are reports on three women whose quiescent disease was possibly exacerbated by pregnancy or oral contraceptives.[78]

Information about melanomas in human pregnancy is limited because of the paucity of data on the thickness or level of invasion of the primary tumor, the varying criteria for including patients under the "melanoma in pregnancy" rubric, and the frequent treatment

TABLE 41-12. STAGING OF MELANOMA

Stage I	Primary melanoma only—no metastases. Includes multiple primary melanomas.
Stage II	Local recurrence or local metastases. All melanotic lesions within 3 cm of primary site (satellitosis).
Stage III	Regional metastases, including intradermal and nodal lesions 3 cm from primary site.
Stage IV	Distant metastases—lung, liver, cutaneous, or nodal.

Source: Adapted by permission from DiSaia, P. H. and Creasman, W. T.: Cancer in pregnancy. In: *Clinical Gynecologic Oncology,* 2nd Edition. St. Louis, C. V. Mosby, 1984, p. 455.

delays when the disease occurs during pregnancy. Nevertheless, some studies have been carried out.

In five human studies[41,58,84,99,102] involving 206 patients with melanoma in pregnancy and 763 nonpregnant female controls with melanoma, survival of subjects with Stage I disease was similar (70–80%), except in one series (31% in the pregnant group). However, fewer than half the patients in this latter group were treated during the pregnancy and all lesions microstaged were Clark's level IV to V.[102] Survival in Stage II disease was also not significantly different (50–60% in both groups), except in a series that included a preponderance of truncal lesions.[99] Indeed, it is of importance that three reports noted a higher incidence of primary lesions in this prognostically much less favorable anatomic location in pregnant women. This distribution may explain the lower survival, stage for stage, seen in pregnancy in earlier studies. Survival is similar in pregnant and nonpregnant women with melanoma when data are stratified for anatomic location.[58]

Transplanted hamster or mouse melanomas do not grow more rapidly or metastasize more readily in pregnant than in nonpregnant females.[19]

In limited trials, administration of antiestrogens or synthetic estrogens has not resulted in consistent clinical responses.[78]

Survival in premenopausal females with melanoma is slightly better than that in males 25–44 years old for all stages of disease.[99]

The following conclusions can be drawn:

1. Therapeutic abortion is not justified once the diagnosis of melanoma is made in pregnancy.

2. Surgical therapy should not be delayed in pregnancy.

3. For reasons that are unclear, pregnancy may predispose to the melanomatous transformation of truncal nevi, which carry a more guarded prognosis.

4. On theoretical grounds, mechanical rather than hormonal birth control is recommended in patients with a history of melanoma.

5. In small groups of patients who were treated for melanoma that was not diagnosed during a pregnancy and who subsequently became pregnant, survival rates have been excellent.[102] Future pregnancy cannot be interdicted in patients with a history of melanoma except on theoretical grounds in those in whom a melanoma was diagnosed during an earlier pregnancy.

6. Although 90% of documented metastases to the fetus are melanoma,[35] the occurrence is sufficiently unusual that it should not be a determinant when one is considering therapeutic abortion or subsequent pregnancy.

GYNECOLOGIC MALIGNANCY

Cervical Intraepithelial Neoplasia (CIN) in Pregnancy

The source of vaginal bleeding during pregnancy, especially in the first trimester, is often the cervix, and examination of this area should not be neglected. Highly suspect cervical lesions should be biopsied even when cytology is normal.

Every pregnant woman should undergo cervical cytologic screening at the first prenatal visit. The Boston Lying-In study of cervical smears in 17,000 pregnant women revealed that the prevalence of dysplasia was 6.5 per 1000 and of carcinoma in situ (CIS) 1.9 per 1000. One in 3300 pregnancies was complicated by invasive cancer of the cervix. [61] Lesions discovered in pregnancy were less likely to regress than those found postpartum or in nonpregnant women, demonstrating that dysplasia in pregnancy is not an interpretative artifact arising from the reserve cell hyperplasia of the exocervix seen in the gravid state.

Subsequent series have reported similar results. [107] The age-corrected prevalence of CIN in pregnant and nonpregnant populations is similar, but a review of gravid patients who presented to a hospital abortion service over a 5-year period revealed nearly a 4% incidence of abnormal Papanicolaou smears (Class III or greater) in this population. The rate of CIS in this group was 1.67 per 1000.[64]

Any gravida with findings suggestive of dysplasia should be examined by an experienced colposcopist, and office biopsies should be performed as needed. Visualization of the entire transformation zone should be possible, especially as pregnancy progresses. No fetal losses were observed after 131 colposcopically directed punch biopsies.[72] The accuracy of such biopsies has been established.[69]

Suggested management of the patient with abnormal cytologic findings in pregnancy is presented in Table 41-13. Biopsy may sometimes be delayed if cytologic findings are consistent with mild dysplasia and an experienced colposcopist sees nothing suggestive of a worse le-

TABLE 41-13. ABNORMAL CYTOLOGY IN PREGNANCY*

BIOPSY RESULT				
Normal	Dysplasia Mild or moderate	Severe dysplasia or CIS	Stage IA, early stromal	R/O adenocarcinoma of cervix
↓	↓	↓	↓	↓
Cytology abnormal	Repeat exam after 4–6 weeks	Repeat colposcopic exam and Pap every month throughout pregnancy	Conization	Conization
↓	↓	↓	↓ (Conization)	↓ (from Conization, Stage IA)
Repeat biopsies	Deliver vaginally at term	Deliver vaginally at term	IA (microinvasion)	IB occult
↓	↓	↓	↓	↓
Conization if multiple successive biopsies fail to explain cytology suggesting severe dysplasia or CIS	Cryosurgery at 6 weeks	Postpartum conization or hysterectomy at 6–8 weeks	Allow progression to term ↓ Postpartum hysterectomy or gravid hysterectomy	Radical management

* Management based on results of colposcopically directed cervical biopsies. No endocervical curettage.

sion.[67] The only absolute indications for performing conization in pregnancy are (1) biopsy results showing microinvasion (early stromal invasion), defined as invasive cancer not penetrating the stroma for more than 3 mm below the basement membrane of the surface epithelium, not manifesting vascular or lymphatic invasion, and free of confluent tongues of tumor; (2) failure to explain cytologic findings of severe dysplasia or CIS in spite of repeated cervical biopsies; and (3) to rule out adenocarcinoma of the cervix.

Patients with CIS or early stromal invasion (with frank invasion ruled out by conization in the latter case) are allowed to deliver vaginally at term. Definitive therapy is deferred until the postpartum period.

Consequences of Conization During Pregnancy. Conization in pregnancy results in transfusion in 10% of patients, fetal wastage in 5%, and stenosis and lacerations complicating labor and delivery in 10%.[3,54] Risk of fetal loss is much higher during the first trimester. Thus, therapeutic conization is never performed during pregnancy. DiSaia recommends placing six hemostatic U-stitches prior to diagnostic conization. The hemostatic sutures also help to evert the squamocolumnar junction and facilitate performance of a shallow conization.[35] Others advocate cerclage placement prior to removing the cone, followed by a Sturmdorf repair.[37]

Diagnostic and therapeutic conization frequently is performed in nongravid females. The subsequent reproductive history of these patients is of much interest. Three recent series, reporting the outcome of 528 pregnancies that followed a total of 860 conizations, reached varying conclusions.[49,70,79] One study showed no increase in fetal wastage, incompetent cervices, premature deliveries, or cesarean sections following conization.[49] A second reported no increased risk except in the 21–25-year-old age group, in which a 30% incidence of premature delivery was not altered by cerclage. However, median gestational age in the premature newborns was 34 weeks and fetal weight averaged 2200 g.[70] In a third series, 15% of patients underwent cerclage in a subsequent pregnancy, and 5% required intrapartum cesarean section for cervical stenosis.[79]

The controversial issue in studies of reproductive performance after conization is in the nature of the controls. However, recent reports taken together suggest that reproductive outcome is quite favorable.

That previous cryosurgery has no effect on

labor and delivery has been documented recently in over 50 patients.[9]

Invasive Cervical Cancer

Invasive cervical cancer occurs in approximately one in 2200 to 3300 pregnancies.[52,61] Pregnancy complicates one in 34 cases of cervical cancer.[52] Histologic diagnosis of frank invasion mandates clinical staging, which includes examination under anesthesia, cystoscopy, sigmoidoscopy, and chest film. Fetal age should be determined accurately.

Definitive therapy should proceed without delay. Survival may decrease 15% for each month that therapy is deferred.[67] The poor prognosis in pregnancy previously noted was probably due to delays in diagnosis and in institution of therapy. For lesions discovered at term, no effect of vaginal delivery on survival has been documented.[84] Normal delivery is allowed unless there is a large and friable or necrotic and infected lesion. Induction should be utilized liberally to avoid delay in instituting therapy.

During the first two trimesters, radical therapy should be carried out as soon as the diagnosis is confirmed and clinical staging is complete. In the third trimester, short delays to gain fetal lung maturity are acceptable prior to cesarean section or induction.

Therapeutic options in Stage IB and IIA lesions include radical hysterectomy with bilateral pelvic lymphadenectomy or radiation therapy. Survival in pregnant patients is similar with either mode of therapy.[67] Sepsis as a serious complication of radiotherapy is much more frequent in pregnancy,[52] whereas blood loss at radical hysterectomy is significantly higher in gravidas. Some favor radical hysterectomy and node dissection in these younger patients because one can preserve the ovaries and because sexual function will not be impaired by vaginal fibrosis. In the first two trimesters, radical hysterectomy can be performed with the fetus in situ or after hysterotomy. In the third trimester, cesarean section can be followed by radical hysterectomy. If radiation is elected in the first trimester, whole-pelvis radiation can be administered, abortion will follow, and brachytherapy can then be given. In second-trimester pregnancy, termination by dilatation, infusion, or hysterotomy is advised prior to radiation, owing to the unpredictable abortifacient properties of radiation at midgestation. In the third trimester, radiation therapy can begin one week after cesarean section or as soon as the wound is healed. Advanced cervical cancer (Stages IIB, III, and IV) is treated with radiation therapy; guidelines by trimester are the same as those given above.

The incidence of lymph node metastases by stage is the same in the pregnant and nonpregnant states.[67] Stage for stage, survival is not significantly different in pregnant and nonpregnant patients (Table 41-14).

One case of adenocarcinoma in situ in pregnancy has been reported. Conization was required to establish the diagnosis. The pregnancy was allowed to go to term. Postpartum hysterectomy revealed no residual disease.[37]

Ovarian Neoplasia in Pregnancy

Ovarian malignancy occurs in one in 18,000 to 25,000 pregnancies,[84] but true ovarian neoplasms are encountered in about one in 1000

TABLE 41-14. FIVE-YEAR SURVIVAL IN PATIENTS WITH CERVICAL CANCER IN PREGNANCY COMPARED WITH ALL CASES, STAGE FOR STAGE

Stage	Pregnancy: Number Treated	Pregnancy: Number Surviving	Pregnancy, % Survival	% Survival, from Annual Report 1954–1963 (All Cases)
IB	474	348	74.5	76.5
II	449	214	47.8	55.0
III/IV	326	53	16.2	27.9
Total	1,249	615	49.2	51.0

Source: Modified from Hacker, N. F., Berek, J. S., Lagasse, L. D., Charles, E. H., Savage, E. W. and Moore, J. G.: Carcinoma of the cervix associated with pregnancy. *Obstet. Gynecol.* **59**:735-747, 1982. Reprinted with permission from The American College of Obstetricians and Gynecologists.

pregnancies.[55] The widespread use of ultrasound in obstetrics may result in more frequent diagnosis of ovarian masses antepartum. In the largest reported series of ovarian neoplasms in pregnancy, one-half were benign cystic teratomas (dermoids); cystadenomas were also common. Malignancy was found in 2.4% of cases, with germ cell tumors seen most often.[20] In other series, the incidence of malignancy ranged from 2.2 to 8.0%.[84] The incidence of malignancy in ovarian masses in nonpregnant women is 15–20%. This difference is probably age-related.[84]

Cysts exceeding 5 cm, 5-cm complex masses, or solid masses persisting into the second trimester require exploratory laparotomy for histologic exclusion of malignancy and to prevent subsequent complications of pregnancy, such as obstructed labor (in up to 15%) or rupture (in up to 35%).[108] Only rupture and hemorrhage, torsion and infarction, or a suspected rapidly growing germ cell tumor represent an indication for laparotomy in the first trimester. By the second trimester, the corpus luteum will have regressed and will no longer masquerade as a neoplasm. The miscarriage rate is 30–35% after first-trimester laparotomy, but only 1–2% after second-trimester procedures.[20] Theoretical concerns about the teratogenicity of administered pharmaceuticals and anesthetics are also lessened after organogenesis. There are two intraoperative concerns: anesthesia and laparotomy.

Anesthesia. Weight gain, increased breast size, and upper airway edema make intubation more difficult, and increased vascularity of the airway mucosa can lead to serious hemorrhage in the event of relatively minor trauma.[33] Decreased functional residual capacity (FRC) results in decreased dilution of inhaled gases and accelerates induction. This outweighs the effect of increased cardiac output in pregnancy.[105]

Even brief periods of airway obstruction or hypoventilation or apnea increase hypoxia secondary to decreased FRC (decreased stored O_2) and increased oxygen consumption in pregnancy. Thus, in addition to ensuring adequate preoxygenation, hypoventilation should strictly be avoided. Hyperventilation is also dangerous, because maternal hypocapnia leads to decreased uterine perfusion and shifts the maternal oxygen-dissociation curve to the left.

Minimum alveolar concentration (MAC) decreases in pregnancy; therefore, more attention must be paid to the clinical depth of anesthesia and to use of the nerve stimulator.[105]

Lower esophageal sphincter tone is decreased and gastric emptying is greatly delayed in pregnancy, with the risk of aspiration significantly increased. Nonparticulate antacids should be given prior to induction of general anesthesia. Given the above considerations, mask anesthesia has no place in pregnancy.

Uterine blood flow is decreased, not only by hypotension and hypovolemia, but also by alpha-adrenergic stimulation secondary to apprehension, vasopressors, or hyperventilation. Patients should be in the left lateral tilt position at all times pre- and intraoperatively to avoid aortocaval compression.[33]

Postoperatively, the additional restrictive defect of abdominal surgery, combined with the already decreased FRC, means that the closing capacity may exceed FRC, resulting in increased atelectasis and hypoxia.[33]

Based on the Ames in vitro assay for mutagenesis, enflurane and isoflurane are not mutagens, unlike halothane and nitrous oxide.[105] However, this assay is rather remote from clinical teratology. On the basis of long-term clinical experience, nitrous oxide in concentrations of 50% or less is acceptable, although it may increase sympathetic tone in the uterine artery in pregnancy.[33] Teratologic data for halogenated hydrocarbons in humans are scant. These agents effectively sustain uterine perfusion. Ketamine directly increass uterine tone and should be avoided.

There is no evidence demonstrating that thiobarbiturates or fentanyl is teratogenic or induces low birth weight when used in single doses. Barbiturates should be used instead of benzodiazepines, based on extrapolation from teratogenicity in animals.[33]

Although regional anesthesia may be preferable in the first trimester to decrease the incidence of spontaneous abortion, spinal anesthesia, with its considerable sympathetic block, can severely decrease blood pressure and cardiac output. Maternal hypotension lasting longer than 2 minutes can produce lasting neurologic changes postpartum, even in term infants.[31] Prehydration with at least 1 liter of crystalloid is mandatory. The prophylactic use of epinephrine is controversial. If epidural anesthesia is employed, the patient should be placed in the left lateral tilt position even for induction of the block.[31] Fluid boluses should not contain dextrose which, when rapidly administered, can result in fetal acidosis and hypoglycemia.

Surgery during pregnancy is associated with premature labor in about 10% of cases. No controlled studies of prophylactic tocolytics have been performed. Fetal monitoring intraoperatively, if possible, and for 36 hours postoperatively is recommended. Postoperatively, external tocodynamic (contraction) monitoring should be added, even in the previable state.

Malignant hyperthermia occurs in one in 52,000 anesthetic administrations and is associated with a 50% mortality. There are three reported cases in pregnancy. Gravidas appear to respond to resuscitative and subsequent prophylactic measures (dantrolene) similarly to nonpregnant women.[29]

Exploratory Laparotomy. A median longitudinal incision is preferred. Cytologic washings and careful perusal of all peritoneal surfaces are necessary, including palpation of the inferior surfaces of both diaphragms. If malignancy is confirmed or if the lesion is grossly suspicious and the frozen section is equivocal, the contralateral ovary must be bisected and biopsied. Pelvic and para-aortic lymph node sampling are performed if nodes are suspicious or if there is potentially a Stage IA lesion with no obvious intraperitoneal spread. Careful documentation of the absence of retroperitoneal tumor is necessary when one is considering conservative therapy or avoidance of adjuvant chemotherapy or radiotherapy, especially in the case of dysgerminomas, which are exquisitely radiosensitive. A part of the greater omentum should be removed for biopsy even in the absence of clinical metastatic disease. Germ cell tumors account for about half of ovarian cancers in pregnancy,[67] with dysgerminoma alone found one-third of the time.[84] Specific criteria must be met to allow the pregnancy to continue and to avoid hysterectomy and bilateral salpingo-oophorectomy:

1. Surgical staging must be complete (see above), even if this requires reoperation during pregnancy.

2. Epithelial tumors must be borderline tumors or low-grade malignancies, Stage IA. The latter must be Stage IA1 (one ovary only, no tumor on the external surface, no rupture, no ascites, no adhesions, and negative peritoneal washings).

3. Stage IA granulosa-thecal cell tumors and Sertoli–Leydig cell tumors.

4. Stage IA germ cell tumors (see below).

Germ Cell Tumors

Dysgerminomas. Proper staging includes at least ipsilateral pelvic and para-aortic node dissections. True Stage IA dysgerminomas have a 10% recurrence rate; radiotherapy is 75% effective in curing recurrence and metastases.[35] Follow-up should include second-look operations and serum alpha-fetoprotein and hCG assays, because a pure dysgerminoma can recur as choriocarcinoma or an endodermal sinus tumor. Tumor markers in ovarian tumors are listed in Table 41-15.

If the primary tumor is greater than 10 cm or presents at a stage more advanced than IA, total abdominal hysterectomy, bilateral salpingo-oophorectomy, omentectomy, and pelvic and para-aortic node dissections are mandatory, followed by postoperative adjuvant abdominal and pelvic radiation therapy. If aortic nodes are positive, the radiation field is extended to include mediastinal and supraclavicular nodes. If the tumor contains areas of endodermal sinus tumor or choriocarcinoma, triple-agent chemotherapy is employed as the adjuvant.

Recurrent dysgerminomas require exploration to excise bulky tumor masses, to define the extent of disease and the histologic type of recurrence (pure dysgerminoma, endodermal sinus tumor, or choriocarcinoma), and to decide on subsequent radiation or chemotherapy, as described above.[35]

Other Malignant Germ Cell Tumors. In true Stage IA lesions (by surgical staging), unilateral

TABLE 41-15. TUMOR MARKERS IN OVARIAN GERM CELL TUMORS AND CHORIOCARCINOMAS

	Human Chorionic Gonadotropin	Alpha-Fetoprotein
Choriocarcinoma	+	−
Embryonal cancers	+	+
Endodermal sinus tumor	−	+
Malignant teratoma	−	−
Pure dysgerminoma	−	−
Benign cystic teratoma (dermoid)	−	−

salpingo-oophorectomy and postoperative triple chemotherapy (beginning within 7 days) improve survival dramatically when compared with more radical surgery and radiation.[35,67,98] In pregnancy, these tumors rapidly become symptomatic (often within one week after discovery). Postoperatively, the patient and her physicians must choose among initiation of chemotherapy during the pregnancy, immediate delivery followed by chemotherapy, or termination of the pregnancy followed by chemotherapy.

Three reports have documented the achievement of four pregnancies in three women previously treated with long-term multiagent chemotherapy, which included cyclophosphamide in each instance. These pregnancies resulted in the birth of three normal infants at term and one ectopic pregnancy located in the stump of the excised tube. No recurrences have been reported, One tumor was found to be ruptured at initial exploration.[59,90,97]

Sex Cord and Stromal Cell Tumors. Thirty-eight cases of granulosa cell and Sertoli–Leydig cell tumors (arrhenoblastomas) in pregnancy have recently been reviewed.[68,108] Two-thirds of the patients had dramatic presentations (e.g., pain, abdominal swelling, hemorrhagic shock, or frank virilization) or obstructed labors; 97% of the tumors were unilateral. All were Stage I. Rupture was common (35%). Treatment was conservative; only four of 36 patients in Scully's series received adjuvant chemotherapy or radiation therapy after initial salpingo-oophorectomy. Only one patient had recurrence and she was successfully treated surgically. In no patient who underwent hysterectomy and contralateral salpingo-oophorectomy was tumor later found in the specimen. All patients with long-term follow-up were disease-free.

Eleven percent of lesions were diagnosed initially as non-neoplastic processes and 35% were classified originally as neoplasms of other types, indicating the need for specialized review of pathologic material in these situations.

Pregnancy luteoma and hyperreaction luteinalis (multiple luteinized follicle cysts), both of which are non-neoplastic lesions, may cause virilization and lead to the erroneous diagnosis of sex cord stromal tumors.

Metastases to Ovary. Endometrial and breast cancer commonly metastasize to the ovary, with gastrointestinal cancers the third most common source of ovarian metastases. Masculinization of a female fetus by a Krukenberg tumor has been reported.[84]

OC 125 Antigen and Ovarian Cancer. Markers are now available for following certain germ cell tumors and trophoblastic neoplasms (Table 41-15). Similar assays for epithelial ovarian tumors have been lacking, but recently a monoclonally derived antibody to an ovarian cancer antigen has been shown to be useful for following the course of ovarian malignancy and may represent an effective screening method for detecting these lesions.[8]

Fallopian Tube Malignancy

Only three cases of tubal adenocarcinoma in pregnancy have been reported. Management was similar to that for ovarian epithelial malignancies.[84] Carcinoma in situ of the fallopian tube found incidentally at postpartum tubal ligation should be treated by hysterectomy and bilateral salpingo-oophorectomy.[35]

Vaginal Cancer: The Diethylstilbestrol (DES) Issue

Clear cell adenocarcinoma of the vagina and cervix has been reported in more than 400 women whose mothers suffered from habitual abortion and were treated while gravid with synthetic estrogens (DES and others) to maintain pregnancy. It is estimated that 6 million persons (including mothers, daughters, and sons) were exposed to these agents.

Benign changes are present in the cervix of nearly every DES-exposed daughter and in the vagina in one-third. Malignancy develops in only about one in 1000 exposed females. All DES cancers have occurred in women under 26 years of age. Benign adenosis does not progress to malignancy. Squamous cell dysplasia is not more common in DES daughters. The incidence of neoplasia in the mothers is not increased significantly.[88]

The most common site of the lesions is the anterior upper one-third of the vagina. The first examination of DES daughters should be performed after menarche or by age 14 if menarche has not occurred. Younger girls should be examined only if they are symptomatic. Palpation is crucial because, on occasion, the cancer lies below the mucosa. Separate cytologic smears of the cervix and vaginal fornices are performed. Application of Schiller's or Lugol's solution is required, but colposcopy generally is not.[88] Initially, very liberal use of biopsies is made. All findings of squamous dysplasia must be verified because immature squamous metaplasia is often difficult to distinguish from dysplasia. If all findings are normal, annual examinations thereafter are sufficient.

Pregnancy Outcome in DES-Exposed Daughters. Results from the four largest studies of reproductive potential in women exposed to DES in utero are presented in Table 41-16. The incidence of spontaneous abortion was nearly twice and preterm delivery three times that seen in nonexposed women. Nevertheless, the majority of patients had surviving infants. Abnormal hysterographic findings are predictive of premature delivery; however, an abnormal hysterosalpingogram by no means precludes normal pregnancy and delivery.

Less sanguine results were reported in a referral population in which all patients had vaginal or cervical lesions. Term delivery was accomplished in only one-third of pregnancies, and in almost one-half of these cerclage was required. Another one-third experienced first-trimester spontaneous abortion and one-sixth suffered second-trimester losses.[10] Frequent evaluation of the cervix and the fetus is necessary during pregnancy in DES-exposed daughters.

Treatment. Eleven squamous carcinomas and three adenocarcinomas of the vagina in pregnancy have been reported. Treatment consists of radical surgery (90% 5-year survival), radioactive implants, or a combination thereof. In Europe, one case of DES-related adenocarcinoma has been managed with needle implants and continuation of the pregnancy with an apparently successful outcome, although the considerable risk of teratogenicity and mutagenicity of irradiation of tissues in such close proximity to the fetus prohibits recommendation of this approach.[84] Another patient with DES-related vaginal adenocarcinoma was followed for 9 weeks during pregnancy without treatment, with no change in size or configuration of the lesion noted.[84] In our opinion, only the insistence of the patient would warrant such delays.

With lesions of the upper half of the vagina, an early pregnancy would be ended and radical surgery, including partial or total radical vaginectomy and radical hysterectomy with simultaneous or delayed creation of a neovagina, would be performed. In late pregnancy, a short wait for fetal lungs to mature is acceptable, followed by induction and definitive surgery postpartum. Treatment of lower vaginal lesions is similar to that of vulvar carcinoma. Multiple biopsies to determine adequate margins of excision are mandatory.

Vulvar Cancer

Any suspicious lesion of the vulva should be biopsied regardless of the stage of pregnancy. If vulvar intraepithelial neoplasia is found during the first trimester, therapy should be deferred until after 12 weeks' gestational age. Wide local excision and multiple additional biopsies can be performed at this time under appropriate anes-

TABLE 41-16. REPRODUCTIVE PERFORMANCE OF WOMEN EXPOSED TO DES IN UTERO AND UNEXPOSED CONTROL WOMEN*

	All Studies Combined	
	Exposed	**Unexposed**
Experienced pregnancy	631	422
Had elective abortion only	157	107
Evaluable women	474	315
Had spontaneous abortions	126 (27%)	51 (16%)
Had ectopic pregnancy	26	3
Had preterm delivery	95 (20%)	23 (7%)
Had term delivery	329 (69%)	292 (93%)
Had surviving infant	316 (79%)†	298 (95%)

*Percentages relate to evaluable women.
† Does not include results in 76 exposed evaluable women.
Source: Adapted from Sandberg, E. C., Riffle, N. I., Higdon, J. V., and Getman, C. E.: Pregnancy outcome in women exposed to diethylstilbestrol in utero. *Am. J. Obstet. Gynecol.* **140**:194–205, 1981.

thesia. Diffuse carcinoma in situ can be treated by simple vulvectomy or skinning vulvectomy with a graft.[67] Paget's disease can be treated with simple vulvectomy, at which time the possibility of an underlying invasive lesion could be ruled out. Some think that treatment of vulvar CIS can be delayed until the postpartum period.[35] All agree that frequent biopsies to rule out invasion cannot be postponed and that vaginal delivery is acceptable.

To date, there have been 20 reported cases of invasive cancer of the vulva in pregnancy. Thirteen were squamous cell carcinomas, three were sarcomas, two were Bartholin's gland adenocarcinomas, one was a melanoma, and one was a yolk sac tumor.[84] There is no indication for therapeutic abortion. Vaginal delivery may be employed after radical vulvectomy and inguinal/femoral node dissection unless there is extensive scarring from a past procedure or the suture lines from a third-trimester procedure are not yet completely healed. Deep pelvic node dissection with the gravid uterus in situ is feasible only up until the early second trimester and must therefore be deferred until after delivery if inguinal or femoral nodes are positive. If the lesion is discovered in late pregnancy and the fetal lungs are mature, labor may be induced and vaginal delivery performed, with radical surgery performed 2 weeks postpartum. Cesarean section should be used if induction is not feasible or if the lesion is extensive or involves the perineum.[67]

Uterine Cancer

There are now nine well-documented cases of adenocarcinoma of the endometrium associated with pregnancy. A review of eight of these shows the following[103]: The last six reported cases were in women under the age of 40 years, the youngest being 21 years old.

In four of the eight cases, the cancer was discovered incidentally in the specimen obtained on dilatation and curettage for spontaneous or therapeutic abortion.

In three cases, the cancer was found after endometrial sampling for menorrhagia. The pregnancy was found incidentally in two cases; in the third, the patient refused therapy and 14 months later delivered a live, term infant.

In one case, biopsy of an extruding polyp at gestational week 28 revealed adenocarcinoma. A live infant was delivered by cesarean section.

Most tumors were well-differentiated adenocarcinomas or adenoacanthomas with minimal invasion, although, in one case, invasion to one-half the myometrium was noted and, in another case, cervical involvement (Stage II) was noted.

All patients with Stage I disease survived; the patient with Stage II succumbed 3 years after surgery and radiation therapy.

The patient who refused therapy had no evidence of disease 10 years after the diagnosis, leading to the speculation that progesterone in the subsequent pregnancy had a salutary effect. However, when all other cases were reviewed, no progesterone-induced histologic changes were noted in the tumors.

TROPHOBLASTIC DISEASE

Considerable strides have been made in the management of molar pregnancy, invasive mole, and choriocarcinoma.[11,13,44,46] Issues of special obstetric interest are choriocarcinoma after term gestation, pregnancy after gestational trophoblastic disease (GTD), and teratologic and carcinogenic effects of chemotherapy for GTD.

Choriocarcinoma After Term Gestation

One-half of choriocarcinomas follow molar pregnancies, one-fourth follow abortion, and one-fourth follow term delivery. Choriocarcinoma should be considered in the diagnosis of pulmonary, intra-abdominal, or vaginal bleeding during pregnancy as well as in pregnant women with lung lesions or brain tumors. In this country, choriocarcinoma occurs once in 13,000 pregnancies or once in 40,000 deliveries; in Asia it occurs once in 250 to 3708 deliveries.[78] Metastatic GTD is usually, but not always, choriocarcinoma; *high-risk* metastatic GTD (see below) is always choriocarcinoma.[44,46]

At the New England Trophoblastic Disease Center (NETDC), 4% of patients with persistent GTD had choriocarcinoma after a term pregnancy.[12] The most common symptoms were vaginal bleeding and hemoptysis. Thirteen percent of patients had previous molar gestations; 87% had metastases at diagnosis, and more than 50% had liver and/or brain metastases.

With combination chemotherapy, complete remission was achieved in all patients with nonmetastatic disease and in 53% of those with metastatic disease. Remission occurred in 87% of patients with an interval from delivery to diagnosis of less than 4 months. Most important, all patients without liver or brain metastases survived, whereas only 28% of those with such involvement lived. The overall survival rate was 67%.

Thus, postpartum patients with choriocarcinoma should have an immediate intensive metastatic work-up. Aggressive combination chemotherapy and adjunctive radiotherapy (e.g., whole-brain) or surgery (e.g., lung resection) should be provided when appropriate.[12]

Fatal pulmonary metastasis of malignant trophoblastic tumors of uncertain origin during an otherwise normal term pregnancy has also been reported.

Management of GTD and Future Conception

The NETDC classification of GTD is presented in Table 41-17. After 6 months of normal hCG titers, patients with Class I or II disease may discontinue oral contraceptives and become pregnant and should be reassured that the risk of repeat molar pregnancy is not high (see below). Nevertheless, placentas from all subsequent pregnancies should be examined histologically to rule out recurrent GTD. Patients with Class III GTD may become pregnant after 12 months of normal hCG titers. Patients with Class IV or V GTD also may become pregnant after 12 months of normal titers;, however, when these patients are not pregnant, hCG titers should be measured every 6 months for 5 years.

Reproductive Performance After GTD

Those who conceive after a molar gestation are at no greater risk for premature delivery or stillbirths, spontaneous abortions, or congenital anomalies than is the general population.[45] At the NETDC, 1.4% of 929 subsequent pregnancies were recurrent moles. One of 150 patients who conceived after a molar pregnancy had a second consecutive molar gestation (10 times the incidence of molar pregnancy in New England). In Chicago, the incidence of consecutive repeat mole is one in 66. Successive moles had more abnormal histologic features and were associated with a higher risk for persistent GTD.[45]

Outcomes of pregnancy after treatment for GTD with chemotherapy (predominantly methotrexate or actinomycin D) are shown in Table 41-18. Reproductive outcome is normal. No chemotherapy-induced ovarian failure is observed and the rate of secondary infertility is only 2%.[45] Data from Charing Cross Hospital in London are similar; however, triple-drug therapy significantly decreased the percentage of women desirous of fertility who had a live birth, but only to 74%. There was no significant increase in congenital malformations.[92]

It also has been shown that, at least at a mean follow-up of about 8 years, the incidence of second tumors in more than 450 women treated for GTD with methotrexate (99%) or methotrexate plus other agents (57%) was not higher than would be expected.[91]

BONE CANCER

Exostoses and endochondromas are benign bony tumors that develop at the pelvic brim and can obstruct the inlet in labor, necessitating cesarean section.

Since the Barber and Brunschwig study, there have been 10 reports of bone sarcomas in pregnancy. The pregnancies did not seem to be affected by the tumor, and there is no documentation of hormonal influence on these lesions, so that termination of pregnancy would not be indicated.[84]

The most frequent primary bone tumors seen in the reproductive age group are Ewing's sarcoma (developing within marrow), osteogenic sarcoma (of the distal femur and proximal humerus), and osteocytoma. Disability from a mass and pain constitutes the usual presentation. In Ewing's sarcoma, the primary tumor is treated with radiation or surgery; survival is currently 60% when aggressive chemotherapy is added. Therapy must be prompt despite the pregnancy. Patients with osteogenic sarcoma also have a 60% survival with surgery and adjuvant combination chemotherapy, and the same admonition applies to this disorder in pregnancy.[34]

Cancers of the breast, uterus, thyroid, and adrenal gland are the most frequent sources of bony metastases in women of reproductive age.

Retroperitoneal sarcomas present obvious anatomic problems in pregnancy; therefore, complete resection of low-grade lesions might be deferred until the fetal lungs have matured and delivery has been accomplished. Management of high-grade lesions must be individualized based on gestational age and patient preference.[35]

One woman with a recurrent knee sarcoma found at 10 weeks' gestation refused therapeutic

TABLE 41-17. THERAPEUTIC CLASSIFICATION OF GESTATIONAL TROPOBLASTIC DISEASE (GTD) UTILIZED AT NEW ENGLAND TROPHOBLASTIC DISEASE CENTER

Class	Characteristics	Therapy
I. Molar pregnancy		
A. Low risk	4% Nonmetastatic complications 0.2% Metastatic complications	Evacuation
B. High risk	19% Nonmetastatic 7% Metastatic complications without prophylaxis hCG >100,000 mIU/ml Uterus >dates Ovaries >6 cm	Evacuation and Act-D prophylactic chemotherapy
II. Low-risk nonmetastatic GTD—endometrial residual after molar evacuation	hCG <5000 mIU/ml Uterine cavity <11 cm Ovaries <6 cm Pathology: Mole only, Grades I to IV	single-agent chemotherapy or TAH plus chemotherapy
III. High-risk nonmetastatic GTD—myometrial residual	hCG >5,000 mIU/ml Uterine cavity >11cm Ovaries >6 cm Pathology: all grades of mole plus choriocarcinoma	Single-agent chemotherapy or TAH plus chemotherapy
IV. Low-risk metastatic GTD	Metastases to lungs, vagina, pelvis, or other organs, excluding liver, brain or bowel hCG <100,000 mIU/ml Duration <4 months from antecedent pregnancy or onset of symptoms Histology: mole or choriocarcinoma	Single-agent chemotherapy; TAH for hemorrhage, sepsis, or large bulky tumor
V. High-risk metastatic GTD	Metastases to liver, brain, or bowel hCG >100,000mIU/ml Duration >4 months from antecedent pregnancy or onset of symptoms All have choriocarcinoma	Triple chemotherapy MTX, Act-D, cyclophosphamide. Whole-brain radiotherapy, hepatic radiotherapy if necessary

Source: Data from Goldstein, D. P. and Berkowitz, R. S.: Preferred management of gestational trophoblastic neoplasms. In: *Reid's Controversy in Obstetrics and Gynecology*, 3rd Edition. F. P. Zuspan and C. D. Christian (Eds.). Philadelphia, W. B. Saunders, 1983, pp. 313–324.

abortion and began undergoing radiation therapy. The estimated fetal dose was 8 centigrays* (cGy) during the first trimester and 7 cGy during the second. (One to 10 cGy is potentially teratogenic.) At 14 months of age the child appears normal.[81]

*One centigray = one rad.

THYROID CANCER

A physiologic moderate diffuse enlargement of the thyroid gland occurs in pregnancy secondary to hyperplasia and increased vascularity. (See Chapter 36.) However, discrete thyroid nodules found on examination must be studied histologically. Use of a radionuclide for diagnosis and therapy is contraindicated in preg-

TABLE 41-18. REPRODUCTIVE OUTCOME IN 91 PATIENTS PREVIOUSLY TREATED FOR GESTATIONAL TROPHOBLASTIC TUMORS WITH CHEMOTHERAPY (INFERTILITY RATE 2/91, OR 2.2% OF WOMEN)

Outcome of pregnancy	Number	(%)
Term delivery	154	(69.1%)
Stillbirth	5	(2.2%)
Premature delivery	10	(4.4%)
Spontaneous abortion		
First trimester	37	(16.5%)
Second trimester	7	(3.1%)
Therapeutic abortion	6	(3.0%)
Ectopic pregnancy	3	(1.3%)
Recurrent mole	1	(0.4%)
Total pregnancies	223	
Problems	**Number/ Deliveries**	**(%)**
Congenital malformations	5/169	(3.0%)
Primary cesarean section*	7/74	(9.5%)

* 1979–1983.

Source: Modified from Goldstein, D. P., Berkowitz, R. S., and Bernstein, M. R.: Reproductive performance after molar pregnancy and gestational trophoblastic tumors. *Clin. Obstet. Gynecol.* **27**:221–227, 1984.

nancy because it can irreparably damage the fetal thyroid, especially *after* the first trimester.[19] Patients with a history of previous thyroid radiation exposure for benign disease are at increased risk for developing thyroid cancer.[86]

Surgical therapy, including node dissection, is the treatment for primary thyroid cancer, with radiation used for metastatic lesions or unresectable primary lesions. Follow-up of 16 women treated for thyroid cancer in pregnancy revealed 100% survival at 6 years.[19] Thyroid cancer is not influenced by pregnancy, and abortion is unnecessary. A history of thyroid cancer is not reason to proscribe future childbearing.

Parathyroid cancer presenting in pregnancy as acute pancreatitis has been reported.[84]

BRAIN TUMORS

Brain tumors are fortunately rare in pregnancy. The most common presenting symptoms are headache (75%) and visual disturbances, with seizures far less common. In 1917, Cushing noted the likelihood of a delay in diagnosis of brain tumors in pregnancy. Nevertheless, the first signs and symptoms occur during pregnancy in 75% of women of reproductive age who develop brain tumors.[26] The cytoplasm of tumor cells of the same histologic type exhibits a more foamy appearance in pregnancy consistent with edema secondary to sodium and water retention. It is believed that this leads to an increase in size of the tumor mass in pregnancy which, in turn, often leads to the onset of symptoms during this period.

Diagnosis is by CT and angiography. If necessary for diagnosis, the latter procedure should not be withheld because of pregnancy. Lumbar puncture is of limited value and should be avoided, especially in the presence of papilledema or other suggestion of increased intracranial pressure.

Gliomas are the most common brain tumor in pregnancy, followed in frequency by meningiomas, acoustic neuromas, and metastases. After metastases, glioblastomas are the most common malignant tumor.[23]

If there is a benign supratentorial lesion with normal intracranial pressure, expectant management is feasible. If ominous signs develop, steroids and mannitol (which crosses the placenta) and sedation are used. Shunts may be required until the postpartum period. Induction with pitocin, no pushing in the second stage, and use of outlet forceps constitute an acceptable approach to delivery. Delivery is followed by resection in the postpartum period.

In cerebral malignancy, therapeutic abortion may be recommended because of the frequent rapid progression of symptoms in pregnancy and the high mortality. Surgery for brain tumors in pregnancy is avoided when possible because of the increased vascularity and the hypotension that usually accompany the operation.[23,26]

GENITOURINARY TUMORS

The rare bladder cancer that occurs during pregnancy is usually of the transitional cell type. Persistent microscopic hematuria or gross hematuria in the pregnant female must be evaluated by cystoscopy (safe in pregnancy) and ultrasound and/or limited IVP as well as urine cytology and cultures for tuberculosis.

Renal cell cancer should be included in the differential diagnosis of any patient with eclampsia in whom symptoms do not respond to delivery. Treatment consists of radical surgery and radiation therapy. Survival is about 35% at 5 years.[84] Brief delays of 2–3 weeks before delivery are acceptable in bladder and renal cancer.

Survival after aggressive therapy for unilateral Wilms' tumor has improved markedly and thus the reproductive future of these patients has become an important consideration. In the Dana–Farber Cancer Institute study of nearly 100 patients treated before puberty with nephrectomy only or with surgery and radiotherapy or with surgery plus radiotherapy and chemotherapy (single-agent), 12% of women had ovarian failure; 5% of males had oligospermia. There were 81 pregnancies in 27 female patients and wives of male patients, with no increased incidence of spontaneous abortion, congenital malformation, or malignancy in the offspring. Premature delivery was more frequent in the radiation and radiation-plus-chemotherapy groups.[48]

Much less reassuring were the outcomes of offspring of treated patients in the Connecticut Tumor Registry. Among 28 Wilms' tumor survivors who were more than 18 years of age, one of two children of one male (treated with nephrectomy and radiation therapy) developed nasopharyngeal rhabdomyosarcoma at age 6. One of four offspring of a female survivor (treated with surgery and radiation) developed Hodgkin's disease at age 15.[63] It is important to note, however, that in the Connecticut study, siblings of the survivors of Wilms' tumor showed a high incidence of non-Wilms' malignant tumors.

Although mutagenesis and subsequent reproductive outcomes in long-term survivors of therapeutic radiation are only beginning to be studied, our knowledge has been advanced by these two reports. At present, there is no reason to suggest that these individuals refrain from childbearing.

GASTROINTESTINAL TUMORS

Colon

Only one of 20 patients with colorectal cancer is under age 40. One in 50,000 pregnancies is complicated by some type of colon cancer. If symptoms warrant, colonoscopy should be performed with caution, since the gravid uterus significantly compresses the large bowel. A diagnostic barium enema will expose the fetus to at least 6 rads of radiation. Fetal exposures during common radiographic procedures are listed in Table 41-19.

In patients with ulcerative colitis, colon cancer develops 10 times more frequently—and at a much younger age—than in other individuals, and such patients bear careful watching during pregnancy. No patient with colon cancer in pregnancy has lived 5 years.[84]

Stomach

In Japan, stomach cancer accounts for one-half of all malignancies, yet only 44 cases of cancer in this organ during pregnancy were reported over the last 60 years. Thus, pregnancy may have a protective effect.[84]

Liver

Although hepatic tumors are rare in pregnant women, one-third present as severe intra-abdominal hemorrhage from liver rupture.[84] A review of over 50 patients with subcapsular hemorrhage (with or without liver rupture) in pregnancy indicated that more than two-thirds of both mothers and fetuses died.[84] Therefore, a suspected hepatic mass in pregnancy should be evaluated with CT and arteriography, if necessary, in addition to ultrasound. Therapeutic abortion may be indicated if pregnancy occurs in a patient with a hepatoma that is only partially resectable.

TABLE 41-19. ESTIMATED FETAL DOSE OF COMMONLY PERFORMED RADIOGRAPHIC PROCEDURES

Isotope or Procedure	Fetal Dose (mrad)
Thyroid scan	15*
Renal scan	03*
Liver/spleen scan	15
Bone scan	100
Chest x-ray	8 (with shielding) per plate
KUB (abdominal film)	300 per plate
Pelvis	40 per plate
Skull	4 per plate
Hip	300 per plate
Spine	275 per plate
Extremity	1 per plate
Cholecystogram	200 total dose
Upper GI	500–2000 (2 rads) total dose
Barium enema	800–6000 (6 rads) total dose
Intravenous pyelogram	400 per plate
Hysterosalpingogram	600 per plate
CT of pelvis	1000 (1 rad) per plate

*Delivers 5000 rads (i.e., 5 x 10^6 mrads) to fetal thyroid.
Source: Data from Orr, J. W., Jr. and Shingleton, H. M.: Cancer in pregnancy. *Curr. Probl. Cancer* **8**(1):1–50, 1983; Barber, H. R. K. and Graber, E. A.: Radiation therapy in pregnancy—Editorial comments. In: *Surgical Disease in Pregnancy*. H. R. K. Barber and E. A. Graber (Eds.). Philadelphia, W. B. Saunders, 1974, pp.736–740; and reference 105.

Hepatocellular cancer in pregnancy is very rare and highly fatal.

Pancreas

The first report of a pancreatic cancer in pregnancy diagnosed antepartum has just appeared, detailing the history of a gravida with twins at 24 weeks' gestation who refused termination and possible resection and chose cholecystostomy and hyperalimentation instead. She delivered healthy twins at 32 weeks and died of advanced disease postpartum.[40] One of 118 women with pancreatic cancer are pregnant.[40] The rarity of this lesion in pregnancy is fortunate, since symptoms so closely mimic the physiologic gastrointestinal effects of pregnancy. We stress that careful physical examination contributed to the timely clinical suspicion and detection in the case just cited.

REFERENCES

1. Anderson, J. M.: Mammary cancers and pregnancy. *Br. Med. J.* **1**:1124–1127, 1979.
2. Andrieu, J. M. and Ochoa-Molina, M. E.: Menstrual cycle, pregnancies and offspring before and after MOPP therapy for Hodgkin's disease. *Cancer* **52**:435–438, 1983.
3. Averette, H. E., Nasser, N., Yankow, S. L., and Little, W. A.: Cervical conization in pregnancy. *Am. J. Obstet. Gynecol.* **106**:543–549, 1970.
4. Barber, H. R. K.: Fetal and neonatal effects of cy totoxic agents. *Obstet. Gynecol.* **58**(Suppl): 41S–47S, 1981.
5. Barber, H. R. K. and Brunschwig, A.: Cancer of the bowel: Radiation and surgical management and pregnancy. *Am. J. Obstet. Gynecol.* **100**: 926–930, 1968.
6. Barber, H. R. K. and Brunschwig, A.: Gynecologic cancer complicating pregnancy. *Am. J. Obstet. Gynecol.* **85**:156–164, 1963.
7. Barber, H. R. K . and Graber, E. A.: *Surgical Disease in Pregnancy*. Philadelphia, W. B. Saunders, 1974, p. 738.
8. Bast, R. C., Jr., Klug, T. L., St. John, E., Jenison, E., Niloff, J., Lazarus, H., Berkowitz, R. S., Leavitt, T., Griffiths, C. T., Parker, L., Zurawski, V. R., Jr., and Knapp, R. C.: A radioimmunoassay using a monoclonal antibody to monitor the course of epithelial ovarian cancer. *N. Engl. J. Med.* **309**:883–887, 1983.
9. Benrubi, G. I., Young, M., and Nuss, R. C.: Intrapartum outcome of term pregnancy after cervical cryotherapy. *J. Reprod. Med.* **29**:251–254, 1984.
10. Berger, M. J. and Goldstein, D. P.: Impaired reproductive performance in DES-exposed women. *Obstet. Gynecol.* **55**:25–27, 1980.
11. Berkowitz, R. S. and Goldstein, D. P.: Pathogenesis of gestational trophoblastic neoplasm. *Pathobiol. Annu.* **11**:391–411, 1981.

12. Berkowitz, R. S., Goldstein, D. P., and Bernstein, M. R.: Choriocarcinoma after term gestation. *Gynecol. Oncol.* **17**:52–57, 1984.
13. Berkowitz, R. S., Goldstein, D. P., and Bernstein, M. R.: Current management of nonmetastatic gestational trophoblastic neoplasms. *Contemp. OB/GYN* **23**(6):139–160, 1984.
14. Betson, J. R. and Golden, M. L.: Cancer and pregnancy. *Am. J. Obstet. Gynecol.* **81**:718–728, 1961.
15. Billingham, R. E.: Contribution of transplantation to modern biology and medicine. *Transplant Proc.* **9**:xxxix–xlvii, 1977.
16. Birks, D. M., Crawford, G. M., Ellison, L. G., and Johnstone, F. R. C.: Cancer of the breast in women 30 years of age or less. *Surg. Gynecol. Obstet.* **137**:21–26, 1973.
17. Blatt, J., Mulvihill, J. J., Ziegler, J. I., Young, R. C., and Poplack, D. G.: Pregnancy outcome following cancer chemotherapy. *Am. J. Med.* **69**:828–832, 1980.
18. Bonadonna, G. and Valagussa, P.: Dose-response effect of adjuvant chemotherapy in breast cancer. *N. Engl. J. Med.* **304**:10–15, 1981.
19. Boronow, R. C.: Extrapelvic malignancy. In: *Surgical Disease in Pregnancy.* H. R. K. Barber and E. A. Graber (Eds.). Philadelphia, W. B. Saunders, 1974, pp. 691–710.
20. Buttery, B. W., Beischer, N. A., Fortune, D. W., and Macaffee, C. A.: Ovarian tumors in pregnancy. *Med. J. Aust.* **1**:345–349, 1973.
21. Byrd, B. F., Bayer, D. S., and Robertson, J. C.: Treatment of breast tumors associated with pregnancy and lactation. *Ann. Surg.* **156**:940–961, 1962.
22. Carcassonne, Y., Dodemant, P., and Favre, R.: Hodgkin's disease in pregnancy. *Acta Haematol.* **66**:67–68, 1981.
23. Carmel, P. W.: Neurologic surgery in pregnancy. In: Surgical Disease in Pregnancy. H. R. K. Barber and E. A. Graber (Eds.). Philadelphia, W. B. Saunders, 1974, pp. 203–221.
24. Catanzarite, V. A. and Ferguson, J. E.: Acute leukemia and pregnancy: A review of management and outcome, 1972-1982. *Obstet. Gynecol. Surv.* **39**:663–678, 1984.
25. Chapman, R. M. and Sutcliffe, S. B.: Protection of ovarian function by oral contraceptives in women receiving chemotherapy for Hodgkin's disease. *Blood* **58**:849–851, 1981.
26. Chaudhuri, P. and Wallenburg, H. C. S.: Brain tumors and pregnancy. *Eur. J. Obstet. Gynecol. Reprod. Biol.* **11**:109–114, 1980.
27. Cloherty, J.: Personal communication.
28. Collaborative Group on Antenatal Steroid Therapy: Effect of antenatal dexamethasone administration on the prevention of respiratory distress syndrome. *Am. J. Obstet. Gynecol.* **141**:276–286, 1981.
29. Cupryn, J. P., Kennedy, A., and Byrick, R. J.: Malignant hyperthermia in pregnancy. *Am. J. Obstet. Gynecol.* **130**:327–328, 1984.
30. Daly, H., McCann, S. R., Hanratty, T. D., and Temperley, I. J.: Successful pregnancy during combination chemotherapy for Hodgkin's disease. *Acta Haematol.* **64**:154–156, 1980.
31. Datta, S.: Avoiding anesthetic complications in cesarean deliveries. *Contemp. OB/GYN* **21**(5): 151–168, 1983.
32. Dein, R. A., Mennuti, M. T., Kovach, P., and Gabbe, S. G.: Reproductive potential of young men and women with Hodgkin's disease. *Obstet. Gynecol. Surv.* **39**:474–482, 1984.
33. Delaney, A. G.: Anesthesia in the pregnant woman. *Clin. Obstet. Gynecol.* **26**:795–800, 1983.
34. DiSaia, P. J.: When extrapelvic malignant disease strikes pregnant women. *Contemp OBflGYN* **21**(5):109–148, 1983.
35. DiSaia, P. J. and Creasman, W. T.: Cancer in pregnancy. In: *Clinical Gynecologic Oncology*, 2nd Edition. P. J. DiSaia and W. T. Creasman (Eds.). St. Louis, Mosby, 1984, pp. 428–464.
36. Donegan, W. L.: Cancer and pregnancy. *Cancer* **33**:194–202, 1983.
37. Drew, N. C.: Adenocarcinoma in situ of the cervix uteri associated with cervical intraepithelial neoplasia in pregnancy. Case report. *Br. J. Obstet. Gynaecol.* **91**:498–502, 1984.
38. Falkson, H. C., Simson, I. W., and Falkson, G.: Non-Hodgkin's lymphoma in pregnancy. *Cancer* **45**:1679–1682, 1980.
39. Feller, W. F.: Evaluating a solitary breast lump. In: Update on General Surgery. *Contemp. OB/GYN* **21**:107–127, 1983.
40. Gambardella, F. R.: Pancreatic cancer in pregnancy. Case report. *Am. J. Obstet. Gynecol.* **149**:15–17, 1984.
41. George, P. A., Fortner, J. G., and Pack, G. T.: Melanoma with pregnancy. *Cancer* **13**:854–859, 1960.
42. Gililland, J. and Weinstein, L.: Effects of cancer chemotherapeutic agents on the developing fetus. *Obstet. Gynecol. Surv.* **38**:6–13, 1983.
43. Goldstein, D. P.: The prevention of gestational trophoblastic disease by the use of actinomycin D in patients with molar pregnancy. *Obstet. Gynecol.* **43**:475, 1974.
44. Goldstein, D. P. and Berkowitz, R. S.: Management of gestational trophoblastic neoplasms. *Curr. Probl. Obstet. Gynecol.* **3**(5):1–42, 1980.
45. Goldstein, D. P., Berkowitz, R. S., and Bernstein, M. F.: Reproductive performance after molar pregnancy and gestational trophoblastic tumors. *Clin. Obstet. Gynecol.* **2**:221–227, 1984.
46. Goldstein, D. P., Berkowitz, R. S., Hammond, C. B., and Suciu, T. N.: Preferred management of gestational trophoblastic neoplasms. In: *Reid's Controversy in Obstetrics and Gynecology*, 3rd Edition. F. P. Zuspan and C. D. Christian (Eds.). Philadelphia, W. B. Saunders, 1983, pp. 313–324.
47. Graber, E. A.: Breast disease in pregnancy. In: *Surgical Disease in Pregnancy.* H. R. K. Barber

and E. A. Graber (Eds.). Philadelphia, W. B. Saunders, 1974, pp. 301–309.

48. Green, D. M., Fine, W. E., and Li, F. P.: Offspring of patients treated for Wilms' tumors in childhood. *Cancer* **49**:2285–2288, 1982.
49. Gronroos, M., Liukko, P., Kilkku, P., and Punnonen, R.: Pregnancy and delivery after conization of the cervix. *Acta Obstet. Gynecol. Scand.* **58**:477–480, 1979.
50. Gustavson, K. H., Jagell, S., Blomquist, H. K., and Nordenson, I.: Microcephaly, mental retardation, and chromosomal aberrations in a girl following radiation therapy during late fetal life. *Acta Radiol. Oncol.* **20**:209–212, 1981.
51. Haagensen, C. D. and Bodian, C.: A personal experience with Halsted's radical mastectomy. *Ann. Surg.* **199**:143–150, 1984.
52. Hacker, N. F., Berek, J. S., Lagasse, L. D., Charles, E. H., Savage, E. W., and Moore, J. G.: Carcinoma of the cervix associated with pregnancy. *Obstet. Gynecol.* **59**:735–747, 1982.
53. Hammer-Jacobsen, E.: Therapeutic abortion on account of x-ray examination during pregnancy. *Dan. Med. Bull.* **6**:113–115, 1959.
54. Hannigan, E. V., Whitehouse, H. H., Atkinson, W. D., and Becker, S. N.: Cone biopsy during pregnancy. *Obstet. Gynecol.* **60**:450–461, 1982.
55. Hill, E. C.: Pregnancy and the surgical patient. In: *Current Surgical Diagnosis and Treatment.* J. E. Dunphy and L. W. Way (Eds.). Los Altos, CA, Lange, 1981, pp. 47–49.
56. Hixenbough, T. J., Jones, L. M., Miller, S. F., and Finley, R. K.: Breast cancer in the pregnant or lactating woman. *Contemp. OB/GYN* **42**(9): 153–158, 1984.
57. Horning, S. J., Hoppe, R. T., Kaplan, H. S., and Rosenberg, S. A.: Female reproductive potential after therapy for Hodgkin's disease. *N. Engl. J. Med.* **304**:1377–1382, 1981.
58. Houghton, A. N., Flannery, J., and Viola, M. V.: Malignant melanoma of the skin occurring during pregnancy. *Cancer* **48**:407–410, 1981.
59. Javaheri, G., Lifchey, A., and Valle, J.: Pregnancy following removal and long term chemotherapy for ovarian malignant teratoma. *Obstet. Gynecol.* **61**(Suppl):8S–9S, 1983.
60. Jochimsen, P. R., Spaight, M. E., and Urdaneta, L. F.: Pregnancy during adjuvant chemotherapy for breast cancer. *JAMA* **245**:1660–1661, 1981.
61. Johnson, L. D., Hertig, A. T., Hinman, C. H., and Easterday, C. L.: Preinvasive cervical lesions in obstetrical patients. *Obstet. Gynecol.* **16**:133–143, 1960.
62. Jones, R. T. and Weinerman, B. H.: MOPP given during pregnancy. *Obstet. Gynecol.* **54**:477–478, 1979.
63. Kantor, A. F., Li, F. P., Frauemeni, J. F., Curren, M. G. M., and Flannery, J. T.: Childhood cancer in offspring of two Wilms' tumor survivors. *Med. Pediatr. Oncol.* **10**:85–89, 1982.
64. Kapnick, S. J., Heyl, P., and Osathanondh, R.: Results of cytologic screening of pregnant patients at high risk for CIN (in preparation).
65. Karp, G. I., von Oeyen, P., Valone, F., Khetarpal, V. K., Israel, M., Mayer, R. J., Frigoletto, F. D., and Garnick, M. B.: Doxorubicin in pregnancy: Possible transplacental passage. *Cancer Treat. Rep.* **67**:773–777, 1983.
66. Keys, H. M., Bakemeier, R. F., and Savlov, E. D.: In: *Clinical Oncology*, 6th Edition. New York, American Cancer Society, 1983, pp. 120–140.
67. Knapp, R. C.: Malignant disease in pregnancy. In: Post-graduate Course in Obstetrics and Gynecology, Harvard Medical School, Brigham and Women's Hospital, 1984.
68. Kristensen, C. B., Baunsgaard, P., and Hesseldahl, H.: Androblastoma associated with pregnancy in two sisters. Case report. *Br. J. Obstet. Gynaecol.* **91**:592–595, 1984.
69. Krumholz, B. A. and Knapp, R. C.: Colposcopic selection of biopsy sites. *Obstet. Gynecol.* **39**:22–26, 1972.
70. Larsson, G., Grundsell, H., Gullber, G. B., and Svennerud, S.: Outcome of pregnancy after conization. *Acta Obstet. Gynecol. Scand.* **61**:461–466, 1982.
71. Lowenthal, R. M., Funnell, C. F., Hope, D. M., Stewart, I. G., and Humphrey, D. C.: Normal infant after combination chemotherapy including teniposide for Burkitt's lymphoma in pregnancy. *Med. Pediatr. Oncol.* **10**:165–169, 1982.
72. Lurain, J. R. and Gallup, D. G.: Management of abnormal Papanicolaou smears in pregnancy. *Obstet. Gynecol.* **53**:484–488, 1979.
73. Lutz, M. H., Underwood, P. B., and Rozier, J. C.: Genital malignancy in pregnancy. *Am. J. Obstet. Gynecol.* **129**:536–542, 1977.
74. Maier, W. P.: Carcinoma of the breast in pregnancy and lactation. *Breast* **4**:12–15, 1978.
75. McCormick, G. M. and Moon, R. C.: Effect of pregnancy and lactation on growth of mammary tumors induced by 7,12-dimethylbenzanthracene (DMBA). *Br. J. Cancer* **19**:160–166, 1965.
76. McGuire, W. L.: Hormone receptors and the hormonal treatment of breast cancer. In: *Principles of Cancer Treatment.* S. K. Carter, E. Glatstein, and R. B. Livingston (Eds.). New York, McGraw-Hill, 1982, pp. 352–357.
77. Miller, R. and Mulvihill S.: Small head size after atomic radiation. *Teratology* **14**:355–357, 1976.
78. Mitchell, M. S. and Capizzi, R. L.: Neoplastic disease. In: *Medical Complications During Pregnancy*, 2nd Edition. G. N. Burrow and T. F. Ferris (Eds.). Philadelphia, W. B. Saunders, 1982, pp. 510–537.
79. Moinian, M. and Andersch, B.: Does cervical conization increase the risk of complications of subsequent pregnancies? *Acta Obstet. Gynecol. Scand.* **61**:101–103, 1982.
80. Molteni, R. A. and Jones, M. D.: Neonatal management. *Clin. Obstet. Gynecol.* **23**:165–179, 1980.
81. Nair, R. P., Nair, T. K. M., and El-Akkad, S.:

Evaluation of fetal dose from megavoltage irradiation of the knee and neonatal followup. *Med. Phys.* **10**:862–865, 1983.

82. Nevinny, H. B., Nevinny, D., and Rosoff, C. B.: Prophylactic oophorectomy in breast cancer therapy. *Am. J. Surg.* **117**:531–536, 1969.
83. Nieminen, N. and Remes, N.: Malignancy during pregnancy. *Acta Obstet. Gynecol. Scand.* **49**:315–324, 1970.
84. Orr, J. W., Jr. and Shingleton, H. M.: Cancer in pregnancy. *Curr. Probl. Cancer* **8**(1):1–50, 1983.
85. Penn, I.: Development of cancer as a complication of clinical transplantation. *Trans. Proc.* **9**:1121–1127, 1977.
86. Pizzarello, D. J., Roses, D. F., Newall, J., and Barish, R. J.: Carcinogenicity of radiation therapy. *Surg. Gynecol. Obstet.* **159**:189–200, 1984.
87. Potter, J. F. and Schoeneman, M.: Metastasis of maternal cancer to the placenta and fetus. *Cancer* **25**:380–384, 1970.
88. Robboy, S. J., Noller, K. L., Kaufman, R. H., Barnes, A. B., Townsend, D., Gundersen, J. H., and Nash, S.: Prenatal DES exposure: Recommendations of the DES-Adnosis (DESAD) project for the identification and management of exposed idividuals. Bethesda, MD, National Cancer Institute, NIH Publ. No. 81-2049, 1981.
89. Rosen, P. P., Lesser, M. L., Kinne, D. W., and Beattie, E. J.: Breast carcinoma in women 35 years of age or younger. *Ann. Surg.* **199**:133–142, 1984.
90. Rosenheim, N. B., Grumbine, F. C., Woodruff, J. D., and Ettinger, D. S.: Pregnancy following chemotherapy for an ovarian immature embryonal teratoma. *Gynecol. Oncol.* **8**:234–239, 1979.
91. Rustin, G. J. S., Rustin, F., Dent, J., Booth, M., Salt, S., and Bagshawe, K. D.: No increase in second tumors after cytotoxic chemotherapy for gestational trophoblastic tumors. *N. Engl. J. Med.* **308**:473–476, 1983.
92. Rustin, G. J. S., Booth, M., Dent, J., Salt, S., Rustin, F., and Bagshawe, K. D.: Pregnancy after cytotoxic chemotherapy for gestational trophoblastic tumors. *Br. Med. J.* **288**:103–106, 1984.
93. Sahni, K., Sanyal, B., Agrawal, M. S., Pant, G. C., Khanna, N. S., and Khanna, S.: Carcinoma of the breast associated with pregnancy and lactation. *J. Surg. Oncol.* **16**:167–173, 1981.
94. Sandberg, E. C., Riffle, N. L., Higdan, J. V., and Getman, C. E.: Pregnancy outcome in women exposed to DES in utero. *Am. J. Obstet. Gynecol.* **140**:194–205, 1981.
95. Schafer, A. I.: Teratogenic effects of antileukemic chemotherapy. *Arch. Intern. Med.* **141**:514–515, 1981.
96. Schapira, D. V. and Chudley, A. E.: Successful pregnancy following continuous treatment with combination chemotherapy before conception and throughout pregnancy. *Cancer* **54**:800–803, 1984.
97. Schwartz, P. E. and Vidone, R. A.: Pregnancy following combination chemotherapy for mixed germ cell tumor of the ovary. *Gynecol. Oncol.* **12**:373–378, 1981.
98. Schwartz, R. P., Chatwani, A. J., Strimel, W., and Putong, P. B.: Endodermal sinus tumor in pregnancy: Report of a case and review of the literature. *Gynecol. Oncol.* **15**:434–439, 1983.
99. Shiu, M. H., Schottenfeld, D., and Maclean, B.: Adverse effect of pregnancy on melanoma. *Cancer* **37**:181–187, 1976.
100. Silverberg, E.: Cancer statistics. *CA* **35**:19–36, 1985.
101. Smith, E. M. and Warner, G. G.: Estimation of radiation dose to the embryo from nuclear medicine procedures. *J. Nucl. Med.* **17**:836–840, 1976.
102. Sutherland, C. M., Loutfi, A., Mather, F. J., Carter, R. D., and Krementz, E. T.: Effect of pregnancy upon malignant melanoma. *Surg. Gynecol. Obstet.* **157**:443–446, 1983.
103. Suzuki, A., Konish, I., Okamura, H., and Nakashima, N.: Adenocarcinoma of the endometrium associated with intra-uterine pregnancy. *Gynecol. Oncol.* **18**:261–269, 1984.
104. Torday, J., Carson, L., and Lawson, E. E.: Saturated phosphatidylcholine in amniotic fluid and prediction of respiratory distress syndrome. *N. Engl. J. Med.* **301**:1013–1018, 1979.
105. Wallak, M. K., Wolf, J. A., Bedwinek, J., Denes, A. E., Glasgow, G., Kumar, B., Meyer, J. S., Rigg, L. A., and Wilson-Krechel, S.: Gestational carcinoma of the female breast. *Curr. Probl. Cancer* **7**(9):1–58, 1983.
106. Whitehead, E., Shalet, S. M., Blackledge, G., Todd, I., Crowther, D., and Beardwell, C. G.: Effect of combination chemotherapy on ovarian function in women treated for Hodgkin's disease. *Cancer* **52**:988–993, 1983.
107. Yoonessi, M., Wieckowska, W., Mariniello, D., and Antkowiak, J.: Cervical intraepithelial neoplasia in pregnancy. *Int. J. Gynaecol. Obstet.* **20**:111–118, 1982.
108. Young, R. H., Dudley, A. G., and Scully, R. E.: Granulosa cell, Sertoli-Leydig cell, and unclassified sex-cord-stromal tumors associated with pregnancy: A clinicopathologic analysis of thirty-six cases. *Gynecol. Oncol.* **18**:181–205, 1984.
109. Zinn, J. S.: The association of pregnancy and breastcancer. *J. Reprod. Med.* **22**:297–302, 1979.
110. Zucali, R., Marchesini, R., and DePalo, G.: Abdominal dosimetry for supradiaphragmatic radiation of Hodgkin's disease in pregnancy. *Tumori* **67**:203–208, 1981.

42

PREGNANCY-RELATED PSYCHIATRIC SYNDROMES

This chapter reviews the relationship of some of the major psychiatric illnesses to pregnancy. In addition, some nonpathologic emotional reactions of pregnancy will be discussed and compared to more serious psychiatric syndromes. When possible, diagnostic terms will utilize the nomenclature published by the American Psychiatric Association.[1] Hopefully, this will make terminology clear and diagnosis easier. The psychotropic agents commonly prescribed for these syndromes and their implications to mother and fetus also are discussed.

The numerous physiologic changes that occur during pregnancy as well as the startling changes in body size and shape add stress to the emotional impact that a healthy pregnancy can have on a woman and her family. The added burden of interacting with a complex health care system makes this task enormously challenging, even for those physically fit and mentally healthy. For patients unfortunate enough to have either a coexisting medical complication of pregnancy, such as pregnancy-induced hypertension, multiple gestation, herpes simplex, or diabetes, the ordinarily healthy expectations of pregnancy may be eroded by fear and concern. For patients who have a history of serious mental illness such as a Major Affective Disorder, concern for their own well-being is compounded by apprehension about the health of the fetus. Of course, this is also true of a woman who has any serious chronic illness and is facing a pregnancy. However, patients with psychiatric disorders are confronted with the stigma of mental illness. For these reasons, the care of the pregnant woman with a psychiatric illness requires that the obstetrician have basic information about the illness and the treatment of the illness.

POSTPARTUM DEPRESSION

Historical Background

Although descriptions of postpartum mood disorders date back to Hippocrates, who described "puerperal fever" as early as 460 B.C., there has been a lack of diagnostic clarity from the beginning. This confusion was the result of an absence of diagnostic criteria as well as poorly constructed studies. For many decades, diagnostic clarity was not so important because treatment options were limited. However, with the advent of modern psychopharmacology, excellent treatment options exist. Clinicians caring for the pregnant woman now have the opportunity to relieve the pain and turmoil associated with postpartum depression.

The postpartum depression is a relatively common disorder with great potential for suicide, disruption of family or marriage, interruption of maternal participation in infant bonding, and economic loss as a result of afflicted mothers being unable to return to their roles as breadwinners, homemakers, or both. The experience of postpartum depression can lead to recurrent anxiety about future pregnancy and possible recurrence. It also can scar its victims' psyches with guilt and the stigma of mental illness. Prompt recognition and treatment have the potential to spare the afflicted woman the prolonged pain of depression as well as the need for hospitalization. Untreated, the patient with this severe illness may, in desperation, turn to suicide, depriving herself and her family of the opportunity to experience the joy that accompanies a newborn child.

Although the French obstetrician, Louis V. Marce, wrote a treatise on madness after childbirth in 1858, little attention is directed toward this problem in today's obstetric literature.[3,12]

Careful attention to symptoms and historical risk factors will allow the contemporary obstetrician to identify the significant postpartum mood disorders early, to treat them effectively, and to prevent the tragic sequellae that can emerge if this syndrome goes unrecognized and untreated.

DIAGNOSIS OF POSTPARTUM DEPRESSION AND POSTPARTUM BLUES

The changes in psychiatric diagnosis that came with the publication of the Diagnostic and Statistical Manual of the American Psychiatric Association (DSM)[1] represent a great advance in the recognition of mood or affective disorders. It is now reasonably well accepted that depressive symptoms in the postpartum period are similar, in terms of symptoms, to the depressive syndromes seen at other periods of life. For this reason, there is no specific nomenclature in the DSM that separates depression during the postpartum period from that recognized at other times in life. The diagnosis of postpartum depression, then, really entails the diagnosis of what the psychiatric literature refers to as Major Depression. In order to make this diagnosis, the patient must fulfill the following criteria:

A. A mood or affect of dysphoria, irritability or depression must be prominent, but not necessarily the dominant symptom.
B. Four of the following symptoms must be present nearly every day for at least two weeks: (1) an appetite change with either a significant increase or decrease in appetite or weight; (2) insomnia or hypersomnia; (3) psychomotor retardation or agitation; (4) loss of interest or pleasure in usual activities; (5) loss of energy or fatigue; (6) feelings of worthlessness or self-reproach or excessive or inappropriate guilt; (7) diminished ability to think or concentrate or slowed thinking or indecisiveness; and (8) recurrent thought of suicide, death, or morbid ideation.

These criteria allow for the possibility of hallucinations, as long as they are mood congruent. They exclude the diagnoses of schizophrenia or organic mental disorders such as those seen in association with myxedema or uremia.

The terms "Postpartum Blues," "Maternity Blues," or "Baby Blues" often are confused with true postpartum depression. The latter is a pathologic, longer-lasting syndrome. Many women experience a limited kind of transient depression with vegetative symptoms after childbirth that lasts for three to ten days. This shorter, "mini" depression may be considered as an Atypical Depression.[1] It occurs after approximately 50% of deliveries and resolves within two weeks of delivery without requiring intervention beyond support.[5,7]

INCIDENCE OF POSTPARTUM AFFECTIVE SYNDROMES

Affective disorders affect 15–30% of people sometime during their lives. Women are afflicted twice as frequently as men. Postpartum depressive episodes appear to occur following 3–15% of pregnancies, whereas only 4% have similar symptoms during pregnancy.[5,7,15] On the other hand, as noted earlier, the incidence of some type of transient depressive symptomatology is quite common.

ETIOLOGY OF POSTPARTUM AFFECTIVE SYNDROMES

Postpartum mood disorders may rest on both psychological and biological foundations. Understanding of pregnancy-related mood disorders is confused by additional variables, both psychological and neuroendocrine, introduced by the pregnant state. It is now clear that monoamines play a role in the regulation of mood.[8] The notion that biological factors influence mood is not new to postpartum syndromes. Hippocrates speculated that suppressed lochial discharge was carried to the head, resulting in psychiatric symptoms. Biological factors implicated in postpartum depression include hormonal interactions with monoamines. Some investigators believe that the estrogen changes in the postpartum period may lead to changes in the density of brain serotonin receptors as they do in animals, linking hormonal change associated with parturition to mood alteration.[7] Further understanding of the neuroendocrine basis of mood disorders may provide a beacon that also will illuminate the postpartum syndromes.

There are no apparent significant differences in precipitating environmental factors between groups of patients with and without postpartum depression.[7] However, problematic life events and/or long-standing difficult circumstances may play an important etiological role in episodes of postpartum depression.[15]

TREATMENT OF POSTPARTUM DEPRESSION

The utilization of psychopharmacologic agents in the treatment of affective disorders represents a major advance in medicine. The art and science of psychoactive drug use has been refined considerably since the 1930s when the amphetamines were introduced into medical practice for the treatment of depression. The advances in this field point toward genetic and neuroendocrine interaction that makes certain individuals more vulnerable to mood-related syndromes at childbirth or at any time. The treatment of postpartum depression is the same as the treatment of major depression at other times, with the exception of concerns related to the passage of the antidepressant medication into the breast milk and on to the infant. When patients are appropriately selected for drug treatment and carefully managed, the response rates are good. Response rates of 70% have been reported in patients with unipolar depressive syndromes.[2]

However, a variety of factors complicate therapy. For one thing, depressive syndromes are not all alike. Some depressed patients experience hypersomnic depression, whereas others develop insomnia. These variations in symptom clusters probably represent neuroendocrine differences among subtypes of illness. Therefore, the selection of the antidepressant agent ideally should be fitted to the individual. For example, the antidepressant, amitriptyline (a potent serotonin re-uptake inhibitor) is very sedating and would be more suitable for a patient with insomnia than for one who was lethargic with hypersomnia. Unfortunately, biologic profiles of patients are not yet available to assist the clinician in drug selection. At present, an awareness of the side effects of the various agents and their match with patient symptoms must suffice. In addition to matching the subtype of illness with the individual drugs, it is also important to obtain the desired symptom relief without causing impairment from the side effects. The following facts influence the success of drug treatment of postpartum depression: (1) The antidepressants do not act immediately but require 7–21 days to yield good clinical response. (2) Serum levels of antidepressant need to be followed in patients who are experiencing poor response or who are having side effects. Individuals metabolize these drugs very differently, and a therapeutic serum level range is necessary for response. (3) Side effects are often more prominent initially and become more tolerable over time. (4) The same drugs that have the potential to be lifesaving can be lethal when taken in overdosage. Patients should be evaluated for suicidal potential and prescriptions limited in amount to reflect this concern. (5) Patients treated medically still require patience and support. Personal concerns must not be overlooked. It is worthwhile to talk with other family members as well.

Most episodes of depression are limited to 3–12 months. For others, recurrent depressive episodes may be a way of life, and maintenance treatment may be helpful. In any case, careful attention to target symptoms in the postpartum period will allow prompt recognition of patients with this syndrome. Patients with previous episodes of depression or postpartum depression are more likely to have subsequent episodes.

Patients who are experiencing the briefer "mini" depression or postpartum "blues" are likely to benefit from the knowledge that their experience is common and will probably be shortlived. If symptoms persist more than two weeks, the more serious diagnosis, Major Depression, should be entertained and appropriate treatment should be instituted.

Selection of an antidepressant may be facilitated by combining the patient's sleep pattern with knowledge of the particular antidepressant's side effects. The following algorithm is useful (Fig. 42-1).[14]

While using antidepressant drugs, the clinician must not overlook the despair common in depressed patients. The potential for suicide should be evaluated carefully at each visit. Depressed patients deserve the same emergency access to the physician as does the hemorrhag-

Insomnia	Hypersomnia
Select amitriptyline or doxepin	Select imipramine or desipramine

Dosage may be increased as tolerated up to 150 mg, gradually over 7–10 days. (May be taken at h.s.) Reevaluate in 7 days.

Progress	No Progress
Continue at 150 mg daily dosage and follow vegetative symptoms	Consider increase in dosage up to 250 mg in next 7–10 days if tolerated or until vegetative symptoms improve

Reevaluate

Progress	No Progress
Maintain present dosage and follow as is appropriate	Psychiatric consultation/measure serum level

Figure 42-1. Patients with major depression.

ing patient. Because the antidepressants have a therapeutic lag time of 7–21 days, emotional support is especially vital early on. Improper drug selection and/or inadequate blood levels are common causes of treatment failure. The antidepressant drugs may be lethal when taken in overdoses and must be prescribed and supervised carefully, with prompt referral to a psychiatrist when any question of need for hospitalization or concern about suicide arises. Depression is one of the two afflictions that account for the majority of suicides in this country.[9] Early treatment with support and medication may prevent the tragedy of suicide in the postpartum depressed woman.

HYPEREMESIS GRAVIDARUM

Hyperemesis gravidarum is a condition characterized by persistent vomiting. It usually occurs in the first trimester of pregnancy and at times leads to severe dehydration, electrolyte imbalance, and desperation on the part of the patient, spouse, physician, and nursing staff. Fortunately, the condition is uncommon, occurring in about 3.5 per 1000 deliveries (see Chapter 35). The challenge of maintaining the nutrition of the mother and fetus is significant. There are a large number of psychological theories concerning this syndrome; however, they lack validation. For this reason, the syndrome rarely is discussed in the psychiatric literature. The relative paucity of information concerning this syndrome may be related to a lack of special attention to it because of its somewhat distasteful features.

Patients with hyperemesis gravidarum are approached best with a combination of nutritional support (including the appropriate use of parenteral fluids), psychological support, and attention to obstetrical problems that may develop, such as careful establishment of dates to document fetal growth. It is important to offer treatment with intravenous fluids in a positive manner, and not as a punishment. When extended hospitalization is necessary, involvement of specialists in dietetics and occupational therapy may be worthwhile. Psychiatric consultation may be helpful, if it is presented to the patient and her family as a positive opportunity to explore the emotional factors that may lead to stress and persistent vomiting. At the same time, it is important to clarify to the patient and her family that we do not understand the nature of this syndrome and that psychiatric care is merely one of several ways to approach treatment. Physicians and nurses commonly avoid these patients, perhaps to allow the patient to get ample rest or perhaps to protect themselves from futile attempts to treat this poorly understood disorder of pregnancy.

ANOREXIA NERVOSA AND PREGNANCY

Women suffering from active Anorexia Nervosa are seen infrequently during pregnancy. This disorder is seen more commonly by the infertility specialist, because the patient is seeking assistance with conception.[6] This syndrome is diagnosed when the following criteria[1] are fulfilled: (1) An intense fear of obesity, undiminished by weight loss. (2) Body image disturbance, leading the patient to "feel" fat when emaciated. (3) Weight loss of at least 25% of original body weight. (4) Refusal to maintain weight over a minimal normal weight determined for age and height. (5) No known "physical illness" that would account for the weight loss.

The syndrome of Anorexia Nervosa may also have a neuroendocrine etiology. Some evidence suggests that these patients have a variant of an affective disorder and may benefit from combined treatment with antidepressant medication and behavioral therapies. The Anorexia Nervosa patient, if pregnant, may be vulnerable to severe nutritional deficiency, leading to intrauterine growth retardation (IUGR) or even maternal demise, if untreated. Psychiatric consultation is advisable when Anorexia Nervosa and pregnancy coexist.

PREGNANCY LOSS

Obstetricians ordinarily are fortunate to participate in the happy experience of healthy childbirth. When pregnancy loss occurs, early or late, or when the outcome of a pregnancy is unhappy, as with severe congenital malformations, the environment becomes troubled for the patient, for her family, and for the physician. Each individual circumstance presents different challenges to the physician. Even in these unhappy circumstances, the physician has the opportunity to offer assistance that usually will be appreciated by the saddened woman and her family. Most physicians have the ability to participate in the rituals of a healthy birth. The exceptional ones are also able to function in the less comfortable situations and, with skill and empathy, attend the needs of the family in this very stressful situation. Guidelines for effective intervention in such clinical experiences are: (1) When a situation of unmet expectations arises, as in the case of a stillborn, the role of the physician is one of facilitation of the grieving process and not one of denial. People need permission to emote, often in the form of crying or vocalization of despair. Efforts to suppress this will fail and lead to anger that may be directed toward the physician. People cannot be talked out of grief. Their grieving will not be shortened by pointing out the positive aspects of the experience, even though this advice is well intended. (2) Although it is easy to assume a defensive posture in the current medical–legal climate, defensiveness may be more destructive than beneficial. No one likes to assume blame for a loss. Defensive responses from the physician may leave the patient with additional guilt about her responsibility for the loss or with anger directed toward the physician. (3) Following hospital discharge, the family will appreciate an offer for a follow-up visit to discuss their feelings, as well as to review information regarding the loss that they may be unable to assimilate at the time it occurs. (4) When the family seems to be unable to move ahead with their grief, referral to a mental health professional or support group may be worthwhile. (5) Recommendations as to the timing of subsequent pregnancies should be individualized, as couples process their feelings of loss at different rates.

It is unfortunate that our own feelings often interfere with the opportunity that we have to offer the treatment that can be so genuinely helpful to our patients. If we take time to examine our own reactions to the loss before we initiate a response, we may be more effective and find our efforts accepted with respect and appreciation.

PSYCHOTROPIC DRUGS, PREGNANCY, AND LACTATION

The commonly prescribed antidepressant drugs include the tricyclic antidepressants, the monoamine oxidase inhibitors, and more recently introduced agents, including the tetracyclics. Although it would be preferable to avoid these agents during pregnancy because of concerns about teratogenicity and possible later behavioral effects in offspring, for some patients there is little choice. Some women would find it impossible to cope with the pregnancy or even to carry out their routine daily functions without medical intervention.

When treatment of depression during pregnancy is necessary, it is worthwhile to maintain the lowest possible serum concentration necessary for response. If it is possible, avoid drug treatment for the first trimester or for the entire pregnancy, as might be desirable in some patients who have limited episodes of affective illness. In circumstances where antidepressants are necessary, use of the well established tricyclic antidepressants is wise. These agents include amitriptyline, imipramine, desipramine, nortriptyline, and protriptyline. Monoamine oxidase inhibitors are seldom necessary. Although the tricyclic agents have allegedly been shown to increase the risk of teratogenicity, large studies are lacking. Rodents exposed to imipramine have shown morphologic and behavioral abnormalities.[4] There are unanswered questions about the passage of the tricyclic antidepressants into breast milk. It would seem wise for mothers on tricyclic antidepressants to avoid breast-feeding their infants.

Lithium carbonate is used for the treatment of bipolar mood disorders and has also been used for the treatment of recurrent depressive syndromes. The impact of this drug on psychiatric treatment has been most remarkable. Lithium carbonate has transformed the lives of patients with bipolar mood disorders (Manic–Depressive Illness) from lives of chaotic disruption and recurrent hospitalization to normalcy. For this reason, patients desiring pregnancy who are under treatment with lithium carbonate face a dilemma. Cessation of drug treatment may lead to exacerbation of manic or depressive episodes and possibly to the need for hospitalization, but continued treatment with lithium during pregnancy has the potential to cause congenital malformations and other problems.

Lithium carbonate has been linked to a rare cardiac anomaly (Ebstein's Anomaly) when exposure occurs in the first trimester of pregnancy.[4] Other infant-associated problems include goiter, nephrogenic diabetes insipidus, and hypotonia. Lithium also passes into breast milk. Infants of breast-feeding mothers who are taking lithium may have serum levels similar to those of their mother. These infants may develop hypotonia or lethargy and may feed poorly. Because of the significant concerns related to lithium use in pregnancy, bipolar patients require careful psychiatric scrutiny during pregnancy. In the event that depressive symptoms develop during pregnancy, tricyclic antidepressants may be a safer alternative to lithium carbonate.

Neuroleptic agents (antipsychotic) such as the phenothiazines are not well documented as teratogens. The neuroleptics are secreted into breast milk.[10] This is not a serious problem, because breast-feeding can be foregone in favor of needed drug treatment.

Antianxiety drugs rarely are needed during pregnancy. Diazepam and its active metabolite have been found in the breast milk and infant's blood, but it is seldom necessary to consider the use of benzodiazepines in lactating women. The benzodiazepines, such as chlordiazepoxide and diazepam, are not thought to be significant teratogens, although there are conflicting reports about the association between diazepam and oral clefts. At this writing, it is not clear that the risk of oral clefts is increased in infants exposed to diazepam in the first trimester of pregnancy.[13]

Anxiety about pregnancy is best managed by support and acknowledgment that apprehension is an acceptable emotion, as opposed to statements suggesting that "there is nothing to worry about." When patients experience panic attacks or agoraphobic behavior during pregnancy, the possibility of an affective illness should be explored because of the common occurrence of these anxiety-related problems in depression.[11]

SUMMARY

Pregnancy challenges the expectant mother, her family, and the physician. The multiple psychologic factors, physiologic changes, and the potential for superimposed complications require the obstetrician's undivided and well-informed attention. Awareness of major psychiatric syndromes and their treatment during pregnancy and the puerperium allows the obstetrician to deal with syndromes that may jeopardize the expectant mother, the unborn fetus, or the newborn child. Conditions in pregnant women once thought to be purely emotional reactions may actually be as biologic in their genesis as is pregnancy itself.

REFERENCES

1. American Psychiatric Association: *Diagnostic and Statistical Manual of Mental Disorders*, 3rd Edition. Washington, DC, 1980.
2. Amsterdam, J., Brunswick, D., and Mendels, J.: The clinical application of tricyclic antidepressant pharmacokinetics and plasma levels. *Am. J. Psychiatry* **137**:653–662, 180.
3. Burrows, G. N. and Ferris, T. F.: *Medical Complications of Pregnancy*. Philadelphia, W. B. Saunders, 1982.
4. Committee on Drugs, American Academy of Pediatrics: Psychotropic drugs in pregnancy and lactation. *Pediatrics* **69**:241–244, 1982.
5. Cox, J. L., Connor, Y., and Kendell, R. E.: Prospective study of the psychiatric disorders of childbirth. *Br. J. Psychiatry* **140**:111–117, 1982.
6. Eisenberg, E.: Toward an understanding of reproductive function in anorexia nervosa. *Fertil. Steril.* **36**:543–550, 1981.
7. Garvey, M. J. and Tollefson, G. D.: Postpartum depression. *J. Reprod. Med.* **29**:113–116, 1984.
8. Green, A. R. and Costain, D. W.: The biochemistry of depression. In: *Psychopharmacology of Affective Disorders*. E. S. Paykel and A. Coppen (Eds.), New York, Oxford University Press, 1979, pp. 14–40.
9. Hudgens, R. W.: Preventing suicide. *N. Engl. J. Med.* **308**:897–898, 1983.
10. Oyewmi, L. K.: Neuroleptics under high risk conditions. *Can. J. Psychiatry* **28**:398–403, 1983.

11. Pariser, S. F., Jones, B. J., Pinta, E. P., et al.: Panic attacks: Diagnostic evaluations of 17 patients. *Am. J. Psychiatry* **136**:105–106, 1979.
12. Pritchard, J. A., MacDonald, P. C., and Gant, N. F.: *Williams' Obstetrics*. Norwalk, CT, Appleton-Century-Crofts, 1984.
13. Rosenberg, L., Mitchell, A. A., Parsells, M. S., Pashyan, H., Louik, C., and Shapiro, S.: Lack of relation of oral clefts to diazepam use during pregnancy. *N. Engl. J. Med.* **309**:1282–1285, 1983.
14. Votolano, N. A. and Pariser, S. F.: Psychoactive drugs. In: *Drug Therapy in Obstetrics and Gynecology*. W. F. Rayburn and F. P. Zuspan (Eds.), Norwalk, CT, Appleton-Century-Crofts, 1982, pp. 359–374.
15. Watson, J. P., Elliot, S. A., and Brough, D. I.: Psychiatric disorder in pregnancy and the first postnatal year. *Br. J. Psychiatry* **144**:453–462, 1984.

PART III

Operative Obstetrics

43

EPISIOTOMY

Episiotomy, which was first introduced into obstetrics in 1742,[7] is a very popular adjunct to delivery. In the United States, and in most industrialized nations where deliveries are done in the hospital setting, incision of the perineal body at the time of vaginal delivery has become nearly routine. Eighty to 90% of patients undergo episiotomy in many hospitals.[5,7] However, both advocates and opponents of episiotomy voice strong opinions based on rather minimal evidence. This chapter reviews perineal anatomy, the operative technique of episiotomy and repair, and the risks and benefits of the procedure.

PERINEAL ANATOMY

As the fetal head approaches the vaginal outlet in the late second stage of labor, the resistance of the pelvic floor is encountered. In the midline, the pelvic floor is composed of interdigitating fibers of the levator ani muscles and fascial coverings. The medial portion of the levator ani muscle group is the pubococcygeus complex comprised of the pubourethralis, pubovaginalis (bulbocavernosus) and the puborectalis muscles. Coursing medially from the ischiopubic rami to join the pubococcygeus group are the superficial and deep transverse perinei separated by the inferior fascia of the urogenital diaphragm (see Chapter 7, Fig. 7-1, for illustration).[4]

The portion of the medial pelvic floor that lies posterior to the vaginal introitus and anterior to the anus is commonly designated the perineal body and is the usual site of episiotomy.

Delivery of the fetus through the musculofascial support of the pelvic floor requires significant stretching of these structures and their attachments, often with resultant trauma. The intended purpose of episiotomy is to substitute a surgical incision limited to a reparable portion of the perineum.

EPISIOTOMY AND REPAIR

Optimal use of episiotomy is predicated upon: satisfactory anesthesia; allowing the fetal head to distend the perineal body sufficiently to decrease blood loss and extension of the incision; and an incision that extends twice as far toward the vaginal apex as down the perineum posteriorly. Plans for perineal anesthesia for delivery should be discussed with the patient and decided on in late pregnancy or early labor (see Chapter 7). Vaginal delivery may be complicated by twins, breech presentation, or the necessity for a midforceps operation. Under these circumstances, episiotomy may be necessary prior to distention of the perineal body. In most vertex vaginal deliveries, however, it is desirable to allow distention of the perineum prior to episiotomy incision. As the head crowns, the operator's index and second fingers are placed inside the introitus to expose the mucosa, posterior fourchette, and perineal body (Fig. 43-1). Mayo scissors are placed in the midline at the fourchette, and a 3 cm incision is made either directly posteriorly (midline) or posteriorlaterally at a 45° angle to the midline (mediolateral). Under visualization, the incision is extended approximately 6 cm into the vaginal mucosa. The anatomic structures incised during midline episiotomy include the posterior vaginal fourchette, the vaginal mucosa and submucosa, the interdigitating fibers of the superficial and deep transverse perinei and pubococcygeus muscle group, and the inferior fascia of the urogenital diaphragm. During mediolateral episiotomy, in addition to the above, the medial portions of the bulbocavernosus and pubococcygeus muscles also may be incised. The advantages and disadvantages of midline and mediolateral episiotomies are outlined in Table 43-1. Most obstetricians in the United States have abandoned the routine use of mediolateral episiotomy. The disadvantages of this mediolateral incision include increased blood loss from incision of bulbocavernosus and pubococcygeus muscle bellies, an incidence of rectal sphincter injury as high as 9% despite lateral approach, and severe postpartum discomfort. Despite the increased risk of sphincter injury with midline episiotomy, satisfactory repair and healing can be expected in nearly all cases.

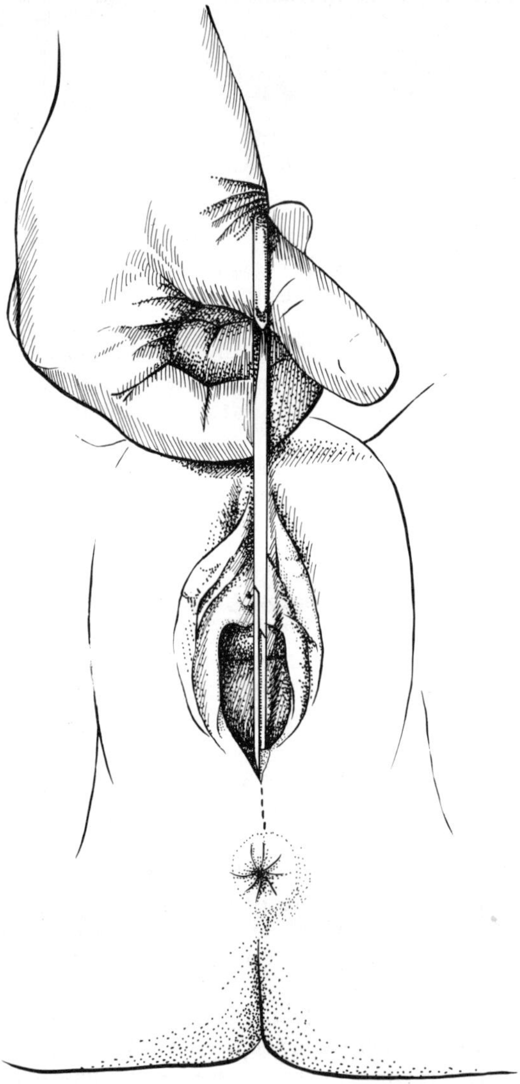

Figure 43-1. To perform a median episiotomy, the scissors are placed in the midline. The incision is extended into the vaginal mucosa and perineal body.

Extensions or lacerations complicating midline episiotomies are classified as first degree (involving only vaginal mucosa), second degree (involving vaginal mucosa and perineal body without sphincter injury), third degree (rectal sphincter injury), and fourth degree (injury to rectal mucosa).

Repair of the midline episiotomy begins with a careful survey of the region to rule out rectal mucosa or rectal sphincter injury. Suture repair proceeds by reapproximation of tissues in layers. Repair of an uncomplicated episiotomy begins with suturing of the vaginal mucosa with a continuous suture of 2-0 or 3-0 chromic catgut (Figs. 43-2–43-5). When the level of the hymenal ring is reached, the bulbocavernosus muscles are reapproximated at the midline ("crown stitch"). The needle is then passed through the vaginal tissues, to exit on the perineal side of the episiotomy incision. The continuous suture is held at that point, and interrupted sutures of 2-0 chromic catgut are used to approximate the muscles and fascia of the perineal body. The remainder of the continuous suture is then used to close the subcutaneous layer of muscle and fascia. When the inferior margin of the incision has been reached, the suture is carried upward as a subcutaneous suture to close the skin.

Third and fourth degree extensions of median episiotomies are common. Prompt recognition and careful repair usually yield excellent outcome. Repair of a midline episiotomy with injury to the rectal mucosa and sphincter is demonstrated in Fig. 43-6. The margins of the lacerations to the vaginal mucosa and submu-

TABLE 43-1. COMPARISON OF MIDLINE AND MEDIOLATERAL EPISIOTOMIES

	Midline	Mediolateral
Blood loss	Minimal	May be excessive
Extension to sphincter	3.6%	0.6%
Repair	Easy	More difficult
Pain	Minimal	85% of patients
Healing	Good	10% esthetically poor

cosa, perineal body, and rectal sphincter and mucosa are identified. While maintaining exposure, a continuous suture of 4-0 chromic catgut is begun at the apex of the rectal mucosal laceration and carried to the anus, approximating submucosa to submucosa, thus inverting the mucosal edges. Interrupted sutures are used to reapproximate more lateral submucosal tissue, further imbricating the rectal mucosa. The fascial sheath of the rectal sphincter is then reapproximated end-to-end with interrupted 3-0 chromic catgut (or polyglycolic acid) figure-eight sutures placed circumferentially (Fig. 43-7). Once the rectal mucosa and sphincter are reapproximated, the repair proceeds as if the laceration were second degree. The apex of the vaginal incision is identified and, beginning at this point, the mucosa and submucosa are reapproximated with a continuous interlocking suture. Deep to the hymenal ring, the suture is directed under the posterior fourchette and into the anterior portion of the perineal body and laid aside untied. Reapproximation of the superficial transverse perinei is a critical step in the repair of the midline episiotomy. Interrupted deep horizontal sutures are placed, reapproximating the perineal muscle and fascia from

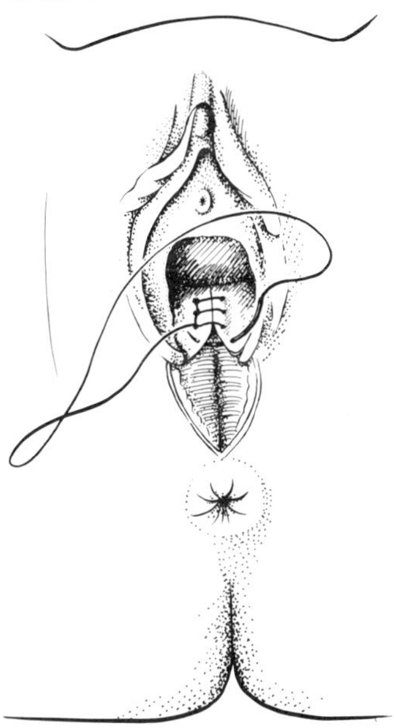

Figure 43-2. Repair of an uncomplicated episiotomy begins with suturing the vaginal mucosa utilizing a continuous technique, usually with 00 or 000 chromic catgut.

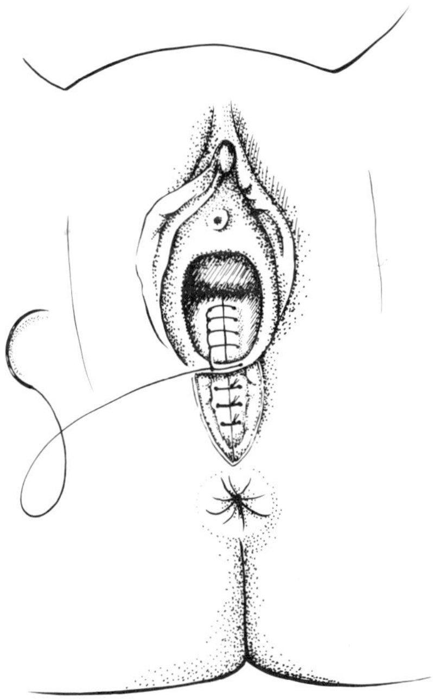

Figure 43-3. The repair is carried to the level of the introitus, and the bulbocavernosus muscle is reapproximated. The needle is then passed through to the perineal side and held for later use. Interrupted sutures are then placed in the perineal muscles and fascia.

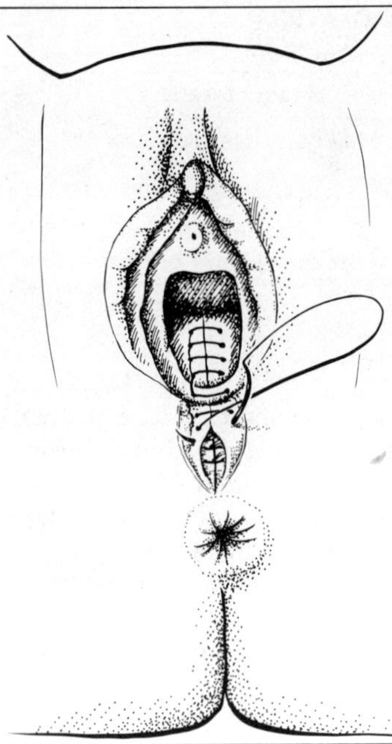

Figure 43-4. The continuous suture is now utilized to approximate the superficial subcutaneous structures.

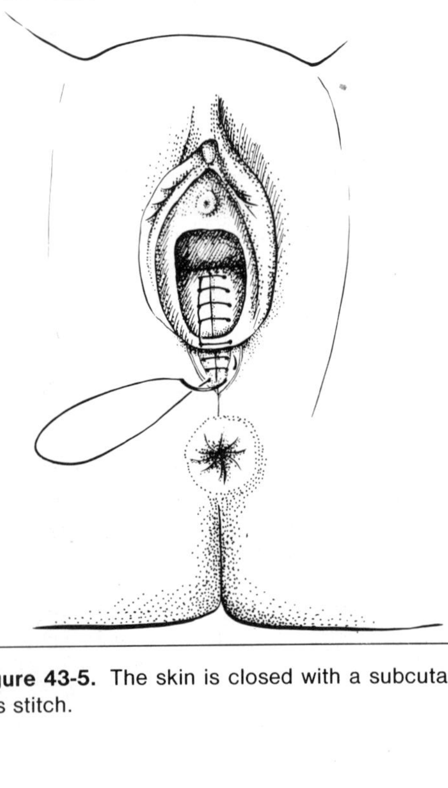

Figure 43-5. The skin is closed with a subcutaneous stitch.

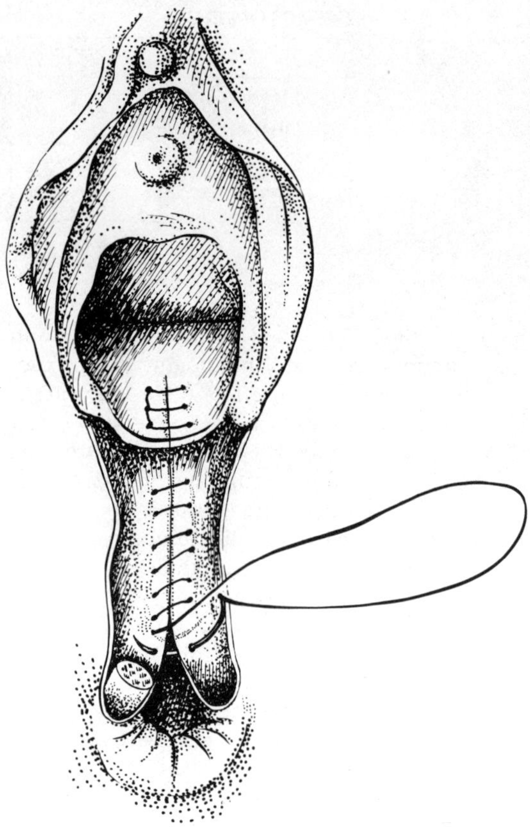

Figure 43-6. The tear in the rectal mucosa is closed with a continuous suture of 4-0 chromic catgut. The suture line starts above the apex of the laceration and is carried to the anus. The suture line is then reinforced with interrupted sutures, used to bring lateral tissues to imbricate the suture line.

the subvaginal vestibule posteriorly to the rectal sphincter. After thus reconstructing the perineal body, the continuous vaginal mucosal suture is continued posteriorly, to reapproximate the subcutaneous tissue overlying the perineal body. The suture is brought out subcuticularly at the posterior apex of the cutaneous incision. It is then used to reapproximate the skin as a subcuticular continuous suture. Upon arrival at the posterior fourchette, the suture is again directed beneath the fourchette and hymenal ring and tied inside the vaginal introitus, thus burying or "interiorizing" all knots.

Reabsorbable sutures should be used in episiotomy repair. The synthetic sutures are reabsorbed by hydrolysis rather than by polymorphonuclear phagocytosis and are associated with

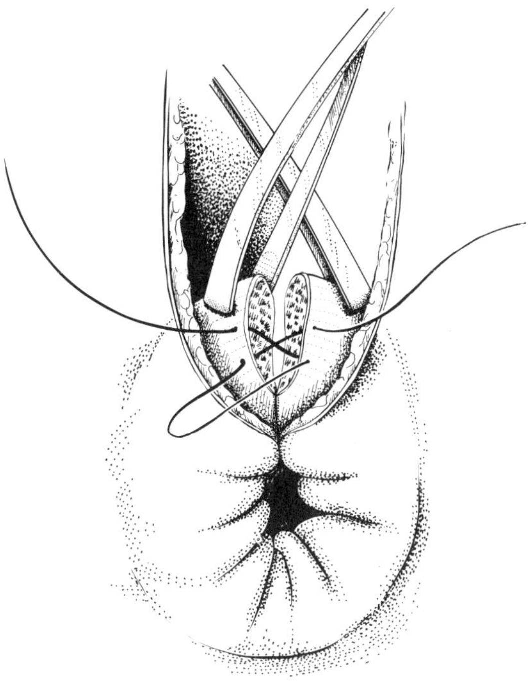

Figure 43-7. The retracted ends of the anal sphincter are grasped with Allis forceps, and held in approximation. Four figure-eight sutures are placed circumferentially through the fascia of the anal sphincter.

less postpartum discomfort. However, they are not well absorbed from mucosal surfaces. Patients may complain of retained suture material or of dyspareunia for 4–6 weeks.[1,8]

BENEFITS AND RISKS OF EPISIOTOMY

The benefits and risks of episiotomy have not been studied in prospective randomized trials. Although most obstetricians agree that episiotomy is useful in relaxing the vaginal introitus in cases of midforceps deliveries, delivery of breech or twins, and in the management of shoulder dystocia, considerable controversy exists regarding other alleged benefits.

It is commonly stated that episiotomy is indicated because it shortens the second stage of labor, thereby decreasing trauma to the fetal head and the musculofascial support of the pelvic floor. No studies to date have demonstrated that the routine use of episiotomy prevents fetal intracranial trauma in term vertex deliveries.[2] The liberal use of episiotomy is believed by some to be responsible for the decrease in pelvic relaxation and vesicovaginal fistulas noted in recent years. However, the same era has brought with it other marked changes such as improved maternal nutrition and lower parity that must be considered confounding variables. No long-term randomized studies have examined the effects of episiotomy on the supports of the pelvic floor.

Another alleged benefit of episiotomy is substitution of an incision in a reparable location for the uncontrolled and unpredictable trauma of vaginal delivery without episiotomy. Randomized comparative studies of "liberal" versus "restricted" use of episiotomy demonstrate that approximately 20%–25% of patients are able to maintain intact perinei during vaginal delivery.[5] The incidence of lacerations that require suturing is similar in the groups with and without episiotomy. It is clear, therefore, that some patients are able to deliver without episiotomy. Assuming that the patient is agreeable to episiotomy, whether or not to perform an episiotomy must be left to the discretion of the attendant delivering the infant.

As with most surgical procedures, episiotomy carries risks of anesthesia, bleeding, and infection. Additional risks include extension of the incision with rectal and anal sphincter involvement and postpartum pain and dyspareunia. Anesthesia commonly is provided for relief of the pain associated with childbirth. Episiotomy is performed without additional anesthesia. Alternatively, infiltration of the perineal body with a local anesthetic or a pudendal nerve block may be used for episiotomy. Measures to avoid intravascular injection minimize risks. Routine vaginal delivery is associated with a 500–600 cc blood loss. Exact quantitation of blood loss is difficult, therefore obfuscating the results of comparative studies of patients with and without episiotomy. Although third-degree extension of median episiotomy occurs in approximately 3.6% of cases, repair is successful and without sequelae 99% of the time.[6] Postpartum discomfort and dyspareunia associated with episiotomy may be minimized by use of fine gauge absorbable suture material and by avoidance of knots near the hymenal ring or on the perineal skin. Necrotizing fasciitis of a perineal laceration is an uncommon complication. There is no evidence to suggest that necrotizing fasciitis is more common in patients with episiotomy than in those with sutured spontaneous lacerations.[3]

Episiotomy is useful in three situations: (1) to facilitate delivery; (2) to create more room when it is needed, such as in breech presentations and shoulder dystocia; and (3) to prevent perineal lacerations when it appears likely that the perineum will tear in the absence of episiotomy. ln practice, this means that episiotomy will be offered to most primigravidas and to many multiparas. The procedure should be used for indication, rather than as a routine. Careful attention should be given to the operation and to ensuring anatomical repair.

REFERENCES

1. Anscombe, A. R., Hira, N., and Hunt, B.: The use of new absorbable suture material (polyglycolic acid) in general surgery. *Br. J. Surg.* **57**:917–920, 1970.
2. Bowe, N. L.: lntact perineum: A slow delivery of the head does not adversely affect the outcome of the newborn. *J. Nurse-Midwifery* **26**:5–11, 1981.
3. Ewing, T. L., Smale, L. E., and Elliott, F. A.: Maternal deaths associated with postpartum vulvar edema. *Am. J. Obstet. Gynecol.* **134**:173–179, 1979.
4. Huff, R. W. and Pauerstein, C. J. (Eds.): Developmental and anatomic correlates of reproduction. In: *Human Reproduction: Physiology and Pathophysiology*. New York, John Wiley & Sons, 1979, pp. 16–18.
5. Sleep, J., Grant, A., Garcia, J., Elbourne, D., Spencer, J., and Chalmers, I.: West Berkshire perineal management trial. *Br. Med. J.* **289**:587–590, 1984.
6. Thacker, S. B. and Banta, H. D.: Benefits and risks of episiotomy. *Women Health* **7**:161–177, 1982.
7. Thacker, S. B. and Banta, H. D.: Benefits and risks of episiotomy: An interpretative review of the English language literature, 1860–1980. *Obstet. Gynecol. Surv.* **38**:322–338, 1983.
8. Wallace, W. R., Maxwel, G. R., and Cavalares, C. J.: Comparison of polyglycolic acid suture to black silk, chromic, and plain catgut in human oral tissues. *J. Oral Surg.* **28**:739–746, 1970.

44

FORCEPS AND VACUUM EXTRACTOR

FORCEPS

The past 25 years brought an explosion of knowledge to medicine. In obstetrics and gynecology, there has been an expansion of the understanding of basic physiology and pathophysiology, unequaled in the history of the specialty.

As our comprehension of reproductive science has increased, previously accepted modalities have undergone a critical appraisal. Evaluation of the use of obstetric forceps turned many away from their use, a decision reinforced by the liberalization of indications for cesarean section.

We are now taking another look at some of the changes that have occurred in the practice of obstetrics. There has been growing concern over the increasing number of cesarean sections performed. Not only is the use of obstetric forceps being reappraised, but vacuum extraction also is growing in popularity.

A recent survey conducted among 144 members of the Association of Professors of Gynecology and Obstetrics from the United States and Canada revealed some enlightening information concerning the use of obstetrics forceps.[23] Although this survey is difficult to validate, it demonstrated that forceps are still actively used in obstetrics training programs and have not been discarded from the everyday clinical practice of obstetrics.

To understand the proper use of obstetric forceps and the vacuum extractor, it is imperative to be knowledgeable about the history of these instruments, their construction, design, function, and the indications for their proper use.

The ancient Japanese attempted to extract a fetus with fillets of whale bone placed over the fetal head. Hindu writings long before the birth of Christ refer to a knife and a hook for perforation and extraction. The utilization of destructive procedures persisted for centuries and was described by Hippocrates in 400 B.C. and by Soranus in the early second century A.D.

Only one of the great physicians of antiquity, Avicenna, alluded to the possibility of an instrument that would extract the infant alive. He wrote that unsuccessful manual extraction should be followed by the use of the fillet. He added that, if the fillet is unsuccessful, "let the forceps be applied, and let it be delivered by them," Avicenna concluded with the statement that, should the forceps be unsuccessful, the infant must be withdrawn by incision "as in the case of a dead fetus."[12]

The era of modern operative obstetrics began more than 300 years ago with the introduction of the Chamberlen forceps. The Chamberlens were a family of physicians who for four generations, between 1600 and 1728, practiced midwifery in England. Which member of the family invented the forceps is not known, but all achieved fame as accoucheurs. Sharing of new medical discoveries was seldom practiced in those times. They kept their forceps a family secret for more than 100 years.

The Chamberlen forceps was a simple but effective instrument (Fig. 44-1). Each branch was about 12 inches long and had a fenestrated blade with a cephalic curve. The success of the instrument was based on the fact that the branches were separable and could be inserted individually. Once applied, they were rejoined with either a rivet or a thong. The forceps then functioned as a first-class lever (like a scissors), and the infant could be extracted alive.[12]

During the next 200 years, more than 800 varieties of forceps appeared. Most were minor modifications in design or material; many were elaborate but nonfunctional mechanical innovations. A very few represent significant contributions to the function of obstetric forceps. This is all the more intriguing when one realizes that there are only four basic principles of forceps design.

The two major innovations that contributed to the ultimate design of the most popular forceps employed today were the movable locking mechanism, introduced by Dusée, and the pelvic curve, introduced independently by Pugh, Levret, and Smellie.

Another major contribution came over 100 years later, when there was better understanding of the function of obstetric forceps. During the years 1877–1881, Tarnier developed and refined an axis-traction forceps. His principles are still employed today, not only in technique, but also in axis-traction handles and in the perineal curve that has been added to many of the new instruments.

Two specially designed instruments appeared a little over 50 years ago. These are the Kielland and Barton forceps; the former still enjoys great popularity for the management of occiput transverse and posterior positions.

Recently, there has been a resurgence of interest in divergent forceps. These instruments function as third-class rather than first-class levers, reducing the amount of compression applied to the fetal head as compared with crossed forceps.

Construction and Design

Forceps are best categorized into four groups determined by the relationship of their branches. The branches either cross in the shape of an X, diverge in the shape of a V, are parallel, or converge toward the toes of the blades (Fig. 44-2). Converging forceps are no longer employed. Examples of parallel forceps are the spatulas of Thierry and the Shute forceps.

The majority of obstetric forceps in use today are patterned after the Chamberlen instrument. They are the crossed type, with the fulcrum near the middle of the X. There are two major subdivisions of the crossed forceps, depending on the blade length and shank relation-

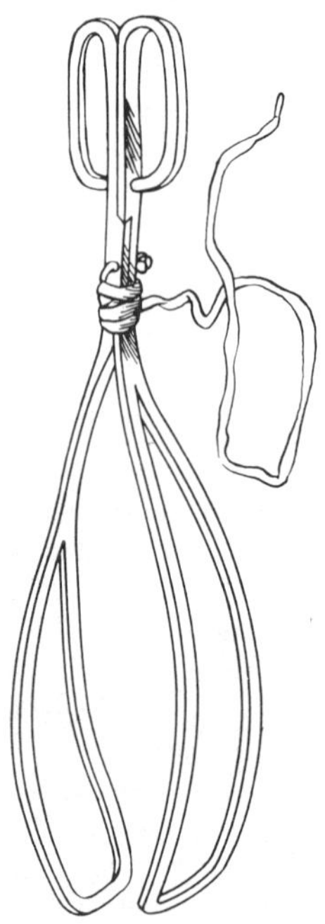

Figure 44-1. Chamberlen forceps. (Reprinted from Laufe, L. E.: *Obstetric Forceps*, New York, Hoeber Medical Division, Harper & Row, 1968, by permission of the publisher.)

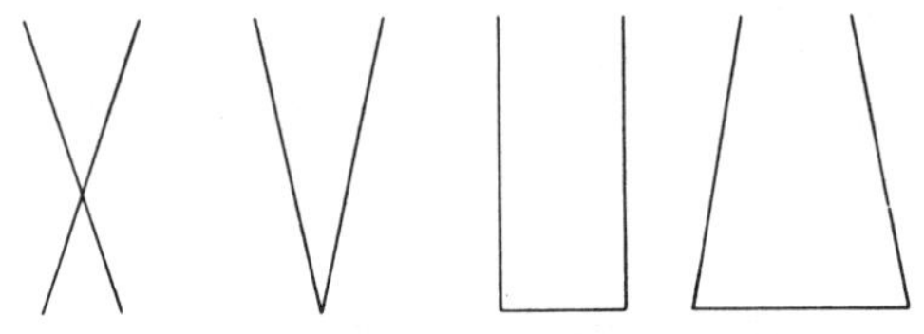

Figure 44-2. Types of forceps (Reprinted from Laufe, L. E.: *Obstetric Forceps*, New York, Hoeber Medical Division, Harper & Row, 1968, by permission of the publisher.)

ship. Forceps with overlapping shanks and 15-cm blades are modifications of the Elliot forceps. Instruments with parallel shanks and 18-cm blades are designed after the Simpson forceps (Fig. 44-3).

Divergent forceps first were introduced by Thenance in 1781. Thenance's forceps were long and unwieldy, and the principle never gained popularity. This is unfortunate, because divergent forceps act as third-class levers and reduce the compression force applied to the fetal head (Fig. 44-4).

Modern divergent outlet forceps were introduced in 1968[27] (Fig. 44-5). During the past 15 years these forceps have achieved a considerable degree of international popularity. In some institutions they are used in more than 50% of forceps deliveries.[11,21]

Irrespective of their design principle, all obstetric forceps have the same component parts.

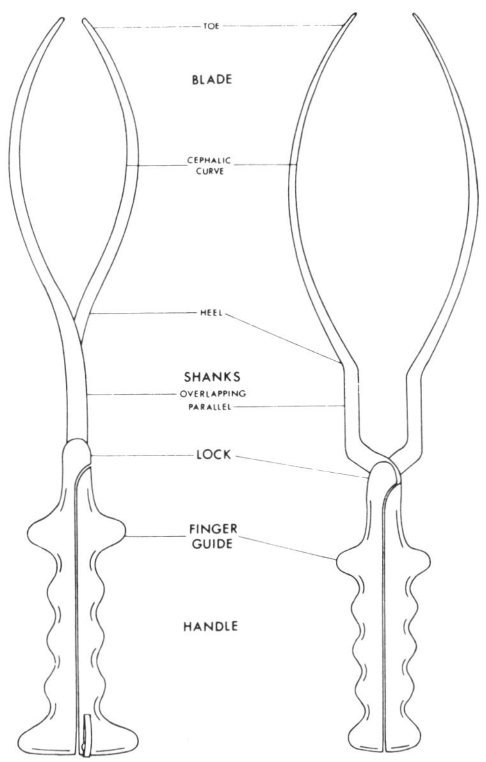

Figure 44-3. Anatomy of Elliott (left) and Simpson (right) obstetric forceps (superior view). (Reprinted from Laufe, L. E.: *Obstetric Forceps*, New York, Hoeber Medical Division, Harper & Row, 1968, by permission of the publisher.)

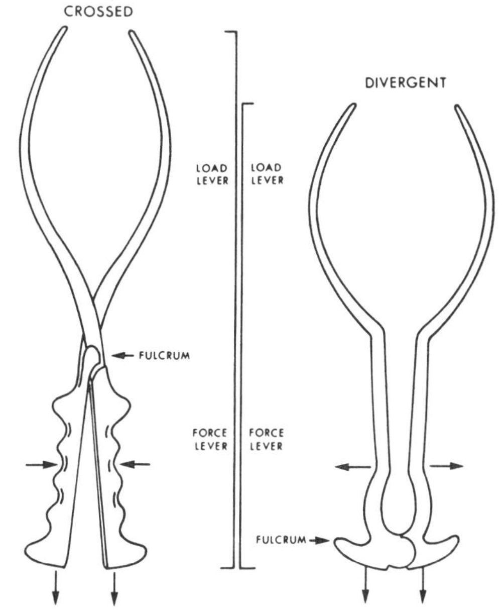

Figure 44-4. Mechanics of crossed and divergent obstetric forceps. (Courtesy of Medical Research Engineering)

Each has two branches, or vecti, designated right or left by their orientation to the pelvic walls. Each branch consists of three major parts: the blade, which fits the fetal head and maternal pelvis; the handle, with which the operator manipulates the instrument; and the shank, which is the portion between the blade and handle. Each branch articulates with its mate by a locking mechanism, usually located at or near the junction of the shanks and handles.

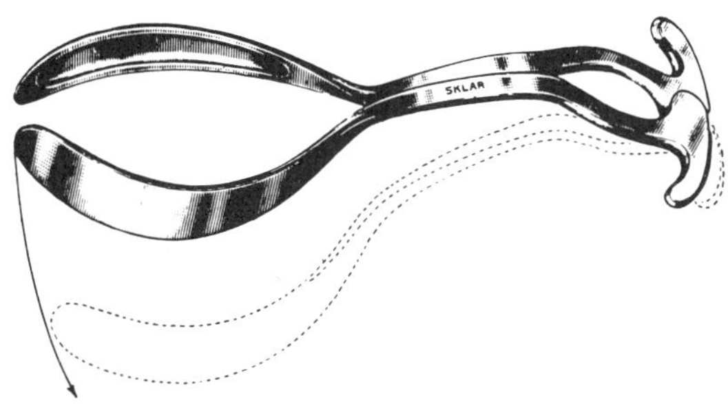

Figure 44-5. Divergent outlet forceps (Courtesy of Misdom Frank and Sklar Instrument Company)

The blades have two curves, pelvic and cephalic, are usually 15 or 18 cm in length, depending on their degree of taper, and may be solid, fenestrated, or pseudofenestrated (Luikart's modification). The shanks of the instruments also vary in length, design, and contour. Their lengths range from 4 cm in the short Elliot forceps to 15 cm in the Piper forceps. The shanks may be parallel or overlapping. They may be straight or designed with a perineal curve to augment axis traction.

A variety of locking mechanisms have evolved. Traditionally, they are classified by the country of origin—English, French, or German. The sliding lock is relatively new and was introduced by Kielland and Barton. The pivot lock owes its ultimate development to Boerma. It is a basic component to the development of the outlet divergent forceps (Fig. 44-6).

The handles of most forceps are similar. They are hollow and many have lateral indentations to enhance grip. Kielland forceps handles are solid, quite narrow, and separated. The divergent forceps terminate in finger grips rather than traditional handles. Perhaps the most significant change in handle design was the development of the axis-traction bar. The concept originated with Tarnier, but the most popular refinement is the detachable traction handle of Bill, which can be used with almost any conventional forceps (Fig. 44-7).[13]

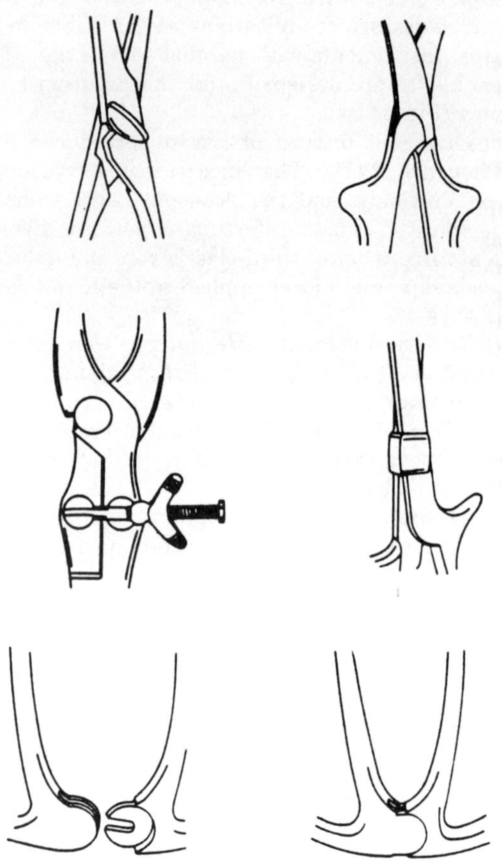

Figure 44-6. Locks of obstetric forceps. *Top, left.* French lock. *Top, right.* English lock. *Middle, left.* German lock. *Middle, right.* Sliding lock. *Bottom.* Pivot lock. (Reprinted from Laufe, L. E.: *Obstetric Forceps,* New York, Hoeber Medical Division, Harper & Row, 1968, by permission of the publisher.)

Function

Obstetrics forceps perform two functions: traction and rotation. To accomplish these, however, a third action, compression, simultaneously occurs. This factor is undesirable and spurs continued efforts to improve forceps design.

Over 100 years ago, Kristeller introduced a metric forceps that measured the force of traction. Unfortunately, this unique effort failed to stimulate interest and concern about the forces generated by the use of forceps. During the past two decades, however, interest in the forces of traction and compression has been rekindled.[20,37,43] The forces of crossed and divergent forceps have been studied. For outlet forceps deliveries of primigravidas utilizing crossed forceps, the peak force of traction averages about 40 lb and the peak force of compression about 5 lb.

Measurement of the forces of traction and compression lends insight into how forceps function. For crossed forceps, the ratio is almost constant. Total compression is 25% of total traction irrespective of parity. This results because all crossed forceps are first-class levers and function on the scissors principle (Fig. 44-4). For divergent forceps, the C/T ratio is reduced significantly relative to crossed forceps, and the C/T ratio decreases with increasing parity (Table 44-1).

The first use of the obstetric forceps as a rotator was recorded in 1752. It was not until 1881, however, that the principles of rotation were clarified. To accomplish rotation about an axis it is necessary for the handles to describe a wide arc. With this maneuver, the toes of the blades

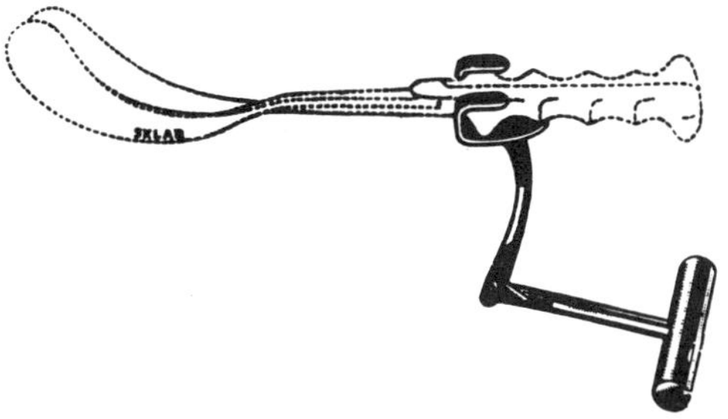

Figure 44-7. Bill axis-traction handle. (Courtesy of Misdom Frank and Sklar Instrument Company)

become the central point of rotation (Fig. 44-8). Relatively little is known about the forces generated in rotation. Instrumentation is available that should provide the missing data.

Many factors contribute to the forces generated by the use of obstetric forceps: size of the fetal head, pelvic contour, station, position, and soft tissue resistance. Other obstetric factors include the patient's age and parity. A variety of physical factors, including the laws of acceleration and friction, also contribute to the forces of traction, compression, and rotation.

The timing of episiotomy is also critical. If episiotomy is performed prior to traction, a significant reduction in peak and total tractive forces is achieved.[29]

Although theoretic knowledge regarding the forces generated by obstetric forceps is meager, sufficient clinical data govern their use. The obstetrician must fully appreciate each phase of the delivery, the instrument, the object, the resistance, and the force applied.

Status of Forceps Deliveries

There has been a radical change in the practice of operative obstetrics during the past 15 years. Although outlet forceps still enjoy popularity, operative forceps deliveries have decreased significantly as the rate of cesarean section has increased. The recognition of the vulnerability of some breech presentations to vaginal delivery and the compromised intrauterine environment of high-risk mothers are justifiable indications for the liberalization of cesarean sections. The introduction, acceptance, and widespread dissemination of fetal monitoring equipment also have increased the tendency to surgical intervention. Another factor influencing obstetric practice is physician and institutional liability. Collectively, these factors make physicians broaden their indications for cesarean section, which is perceived as a quick and safe solution for almost any problem and should therefore lower perinatal mortality. However, when the experience at the National Maternity Hospital in Dublin is compared with a similar 15-year experience in the United States, efficacy of cesarean section is not demonstrated.[28] With a cesarean section rate that remained unchanged at slightly less than 5%, the perinatal mortality rates at the National Maternity Hospital have

TABLE 44-1. TOTAL FORCES: CROSSED VERSUS DIVERGENT FORCEPS

Parity	Compression/Traction Ratio X	Compression/Traction Ratio V	% Reduction
0	0.236	0.170	28
1	0.228	0.153	33
2–3	0.236	0.140	41

X = crossed forceps; V = divergent forceps.

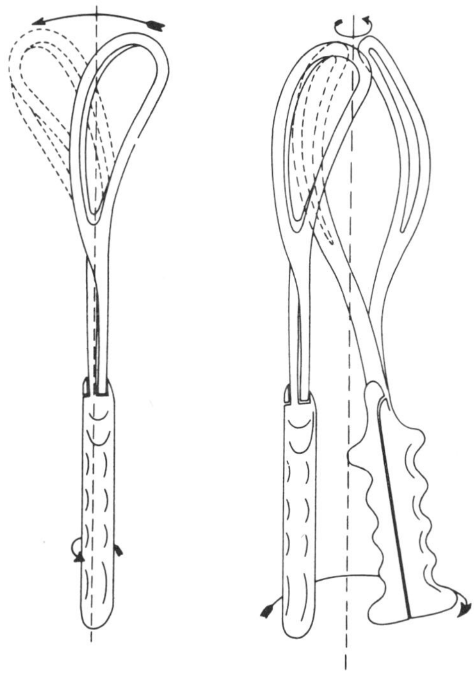

Figure 44-8. Rotation of forceps. (Reprinted from Laufe, L. E.: *Obstetric Forceps*, New York, Hoeber Medical Division, Harper & Row, 1968, by permission of the publisher.)

improved similarly to those in the United States. Although no information is given regarding morbidity and the use of other means of intervention (forceps or VE), the National Maternity Hospital has demonstrated that vaginal delivery after cesarean section and the active but judicious use of oxytocin in first labors can significantly reduce the cesarean section rate.

The benefits of routine fetal monitoring and the increased utilization of cesarean section must be evaluated in relation to maternal morbidity and mortality as well as to fetal outcome. We must appraise the costs of routine fetal monitoring against the benefits received.

Cesarean section has become the tenth most common operation in the United States. This prompted a task force inquiry sponsored by the National Institute of Child Health and Human Development.[9] The Task Force report stated that low priority and emphasis were given to forceps delivery in some obstetric training programs and emphasized the diminishing opportunity for residents to develop skills and knowledge in the techniques of midforceps delivery.

Indications and Prerequisites for Use

Indications for the use of obstetric forceps may be maternal or fetal. The primary maternal indication is the need to shorten the second stage of labor when the mother's physical reserve is limited or exhaustion is impending. Fetal indications include arrest of rotation, fetal distress, certain abnormal positions, and the aftercoming head in breech presentation.

Outlet forceps deliveries can be categorized as "prophylactic." This concept advocates interference to spare the fetal head from prolonged pounding against the perineum and to avoid maternal exhaustion during the second stage and overstretching of the pelvic tissues. With increased interest in vaginal delivery of selected breeches, the aftercoming head forceps assumes renewed importance.

The primary maternal prerequisite for successful forceps delivery is adequate pelvic capacity for that particular infant. Soft tissue factors may be involved in addition to the bony pelvis. The bladder and rectum should be empty. The membranes must be ruptured. The cervix must be fully dilated and retracted over the fetal head. The tension and thickness of the perineal tissues must be evaluated, so that episiotomy can be performed prior to overstretching of the soft tissues. Early episiotomy can reduce peak traction force by as much as 25%.[29]

The fetal head must be well engaged in the pelvis and its position and attitude accurately determined. Well-molded and large fetal heads dictate the use of forceps with long tapered blades, whereas average-sized heads are better fitted by blades with an increased cephalic curve. Higher pelvic stations of the fetal head may dictate the choice of an instrument that accentuates axis traction.[6]

Types of Obstetric Forceps

Obstetric forceps can be categorized as conventional or special. The former are used primarily for the conduct of outlet and basic midforceps deliveries. The latter are employed in management of deliveries requiring rotational procedures, increased traction, or management of the aftercoming head.

Conventional. Most conventional forceps are offspring of two classic prototypes, the Simpson and the Elliot. The classic Simpson forceps is 35 cm long and has parallel shanks with an English lock. The blades are 18 cm long, fenestrated, and gradually tapered to provide a shallow cephalic curve (Fig. 44-3). This forceps is suited for well-molded and large fetal heads. The DeLee forceps, both short and long models, are modifications of the Simpson instrument.

The short Elliot forceps is characterized by its overlapping shanks and 15-cm fenestrated blades with their accentuated cephalic curve (Fig. 44-3). They are most suitable for the average-sized fetal head. There is a "long" version of the Elliot forceps that has 18-cm blades but partially retains the accentuated cephalic curve. The most popular modification of the Elliot instrument is the Tucker–McLane forceps with either solid or semisolid (pseudofenestrated or Luikart) blades (Fig. 44-9).

The basic principle of divergent outlet forceps is placement of the fulcrum at the rear and conversion of the instrument to a third-class lever. The forceps contains Elliot-type blades with Luikart modification, parallel shanks with a perineal curve, a pivot lock to allow the branches to diverge, and finger grips rather than traditional handles (Fig. 44-5). When crossed and divergent forceps are compared, the divergent instrument reduces total compression force to the fetal head by 33% (Table 44-1).

The data regarding forces generated by ob-

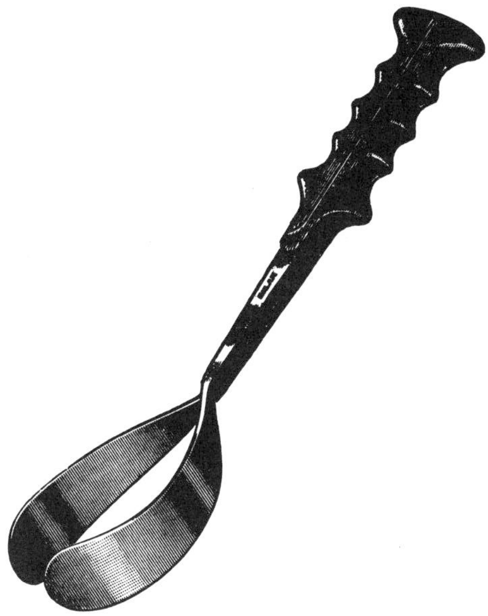

Figure 44-9. Tucker-McLane forceps. (Courtesy of Misdom Frank and Sklar Instrument Company)

stetric forceps represent only a small bit of information about the forces acting on the fetus. We do not know the compressive forces generated against the fetal head in spontaneous labor. More important, we do not know the forces generated in augmented labors or in the gamut of forceps operations that are employed. Until we know what these forces are, we cannot correlate them to fetal outcome.

Special. Special obstetric forceps have been designed to facilitate instrumental rotation, allow for increased traction, and manage the aftercoming head in breech delivery.

The two forceps most commonly used to accomplish rotation and extraction of the fetal head from an occiput transverse or posterior position are the Kielland and Barton forceps. Although they were designed contemporaneously, they are based on different principles.

Christian Kielland introduced his forceps in 1916.[25] It is a long (40 cm), well-designed and engineered instrument intended to accomplish a biparietal forceps application to the fetal head in the transverse diameter. The forceps is characterized by its bayonet appearance, offset pelvic curve, wide fenestrated 15-cm blades, overlapping shanks, sliding lock, directional markers on the finger grips, and solid separated handles. (See Figure 44-19.)

The unique features of the Barton forceps are its hinged anterior blade, sliding lock, and the 500 offset angulation of the shanks with the blades. (See Figure 44-18.) The forceps was designed by Lyman G. Barton and introduced in 1925. Barton's intent was to apply traction to the transverse fetal head without prior rotation. To accomplish this, the cephalic and pelvic curves of the blades are parallel and allow for the instrument's unique function.[4]

Instruments that were designed to augment traction, such as the Dewey forceps, although popular for a while, rarely are employed today. The device most frequently employed to augment traction is the Bill axis-traction handle which may be applied to any conventional forceps. The Bill handle allows for traction to be applied in the proper plane and axis of the pelvis (Fig. 44-7).

The Piper forceps introduced in 1924 was designed to manage the aftercoming head. The instrument is characterized by light construction. The forceps has an overall length of 44.5 cm, tapered fenestrated blades, parallel shanks with a perineal curve, and hollow handles (Fig. 44-10).

The classic Piper forceps has been modified to a short outlet instrument. The essential alteration, replacing the handles with finger grips and a pivot lock, converted the forceps to a third-class lever similar to the divergent outlet forceps (Fig 44-11).[26]

Classification of Forceps Operations

The following classification of forceps operations has been proposed by the American College of Obstetrics and Gynecology[3]:

1. Outlet Forceps. The application of forceps when the scalp is or has been visible at the introitus without separating the labia, the skull has reached the pelvic floor, and the sagittal suture is in the anteroposterior diameter of the pelvis.
2. Midforceps. The application of forceps when the head is engaged but the conditions for outlet forceps have not been met. In the context of this term, any forceps delivery requiring artificial rotation, regardless of the station from which extraction is begun, shall be designated a *midforceps* delivery. The term *low midforceps* is disapproved. A record shall be made of the position and the station of the head when

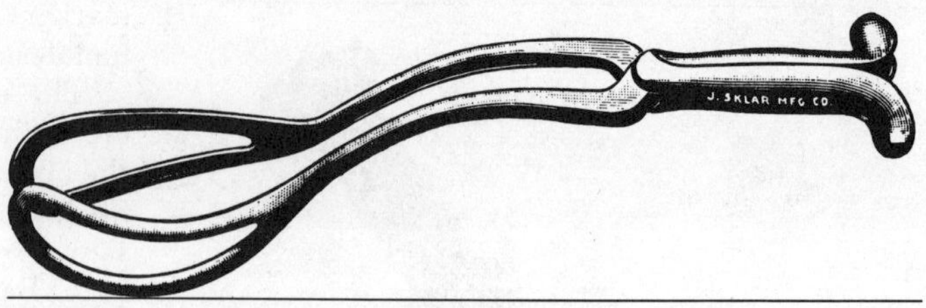

Figure 44-10. Piper forceps. (Courtesy of Misdom Frank and Sklar Instrument Company)

the delivery is begun. In addition, a description of the various maneuvers and of any difficulties encountered in the application of the forceps and in the extraction of the infant shall be recorded.

3. High Forceps. The application of forceps at any time prior to full engagement of the head. High forceps delivery is never justifiable.

This system of classification does not employ the terms *low forceps* and *low midforceps.* The latter category had become extremely popular with increased utilization of conduction anesthesia. The designation low midforceps becomes an inviting category in which to conceal true midforceps rotations and extractions. Therefore, forceps operations can usefully be categorized into outlet forceps deliveries, basic midforceps deliveries, and special midforceps procedures. No matter which procedure is undertaken, all prerequisites for a forceps operation must be fulfilled. The clinician must be familiar with the forceps of his choice and must know its limitations as well as his own. A forceps delivery is a surgical procedure involving a vulnerable subject, not a contest of strength.

Outlet Forceps Techniques. Outlet forceps procedures constitute the majority of forceps operations. For vertex presentations, the fetal head must reach the pelvic floor, the scalp must be visible at the introitus, and the sagittal suture must be in the anteroposterior diameter of the pelvis for the operation to be a true "outlet forceps."

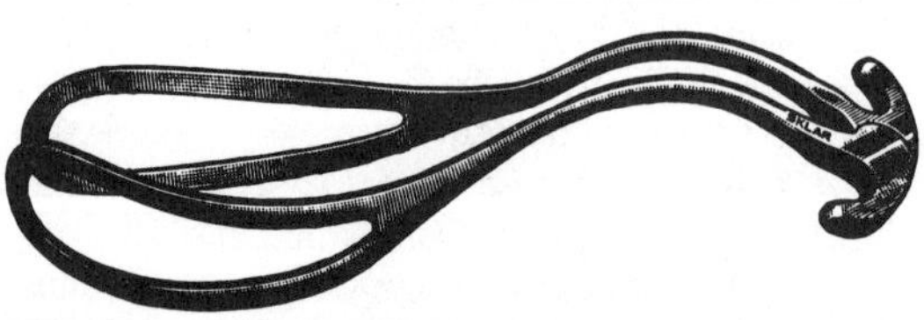

Figure 44-11. Short Piper forceps. (Courtesy of Misdom Frank and Sklar Instrument Company)

If there has been extensive molding or if the infant is large, an instrument with long tapered blades is indicated. The Elliot forceps and its modifications are best suited for average-sized and well-rounded fetal heads. For routine outlet forceps deliveries when extensive molding has not taken place, divergent forceps are preferred because the compressive force applied to the head is reduced significantly.

The essential steps for performance of an outlet forceps delivery are (1) insertion of the branches, (2) application to the fetal head, (3) adjustment if necessary, and (4) articulation and locking of the handles.

In application of conventional forceps, the left branch is inserted first to facilitate articulation, since the lock usually is on the left side. The forceps should be moistened or lubricated prior to use. The operator should insert the middle and index fingers of the right hand into the vagina along the left side of the fetal head. The left branch is now held upright with the left hand and the right thumb placed at the heel of the blade. The handle is lowered in a sweeping arc which begins toward the operator's left and ends at the midline when the handle reaches the horizontal. The rate of descent and insertion are controlled by the right thumb while the middle and index fingers guide the toe of the blade and protect the vaginal tissue.

The right branch is now inserted in similar manner. If one of the blades has to be adjusted, this is best performed by placing the index finger beneath the shank at the heel of the blade and controlling the handle with the opposite hand (Fig. 44-12). This must be done prior to articulation.

Once both blades have been inserted and applied to the fetal head, the branches are articulated and the lock engaged. The position of the blade and that of the fetal head must be re-

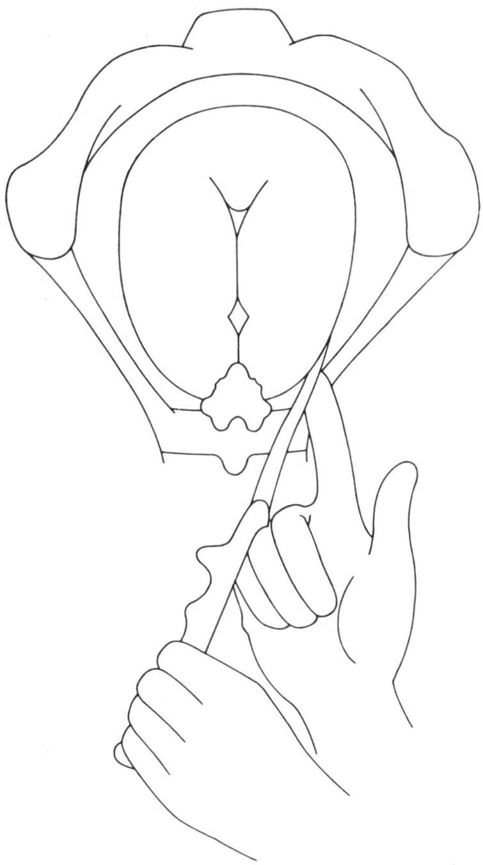

Figure 44-12. Adjustment of left forceps branch. (Reprinted from Laufe, L. E.: *Obstetric Forceps*, New York, Hoeber Medical Division, Harper & Row, 1968, by permission of the publisher.)

checked and appropriate adjustments made if resistance is met during any part of the application procedure. To minimize compression, the operator should always avoid squeezing the handles.

There are three cardinal rules for assuring proper forceps application:

1. The sagittal suture must be equidistant between the branches. If the shanks are parallel, the sagittal suture should be midway between them; if overlapping, directly in line with them.
2. The posterior fontanelle should be one finger-width above the shanks.
3. If the blades are fenestrated, they should admit one finger between the heel of the blade and the fetal head.

Once the application has been checked, traction (the only function of outlet forceps) may be instituted. This is best accomplished from a sitting position. The forceps is grasped from below; all the force applied is derived from the forearm. The plane of traction must be continuous with the curve of the pelvis (Fig. 44-13). This is best accomplished by the Saxtorph–Pajot maneuver (Fig. 44-14).

The first effort should be *trial traction*. This will indicate how much resistance will be encountered and how much effort must be expended and provides another opportunity to check the accuracy of forceps application. There is no predetermined number of traction efforts. The operator must remember that the desired result is to mimic the forces of labor. Early episiotomy reduces the total number of traction pulls as well as the peak traction force.

After the occiput passes beneath the pubic bone, the direction of the forceps is altered upward to produce extension of the fetal head. When the biparietal diameter of the head has passed the vulvar ring, the forceps may be removed. The branches are unlocked and removed in reverse order to their application. The operator must avoid excessive force and desist if descent does not occur easily.

When divergent forceps are employed, either branch may be inserted first because of the pivot lock. Because of the perineal curve, traction is accomplished in a continuous line with the shanks (Fig. 44-15). Because the instrument

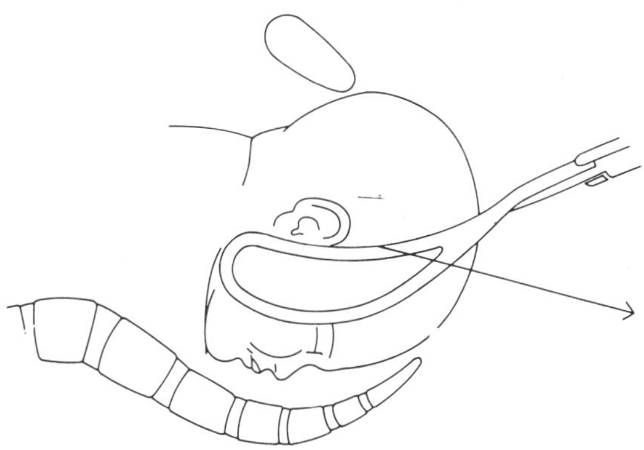

Figure 44-13. Traction in the axis of the pelvis, outlet forceps. (Reprinted from Laufe, L. E.: *Obstetric Forceps*, New York, Hoeber Medical Division, Harper & Row, 1968, by permission of the publisher.)

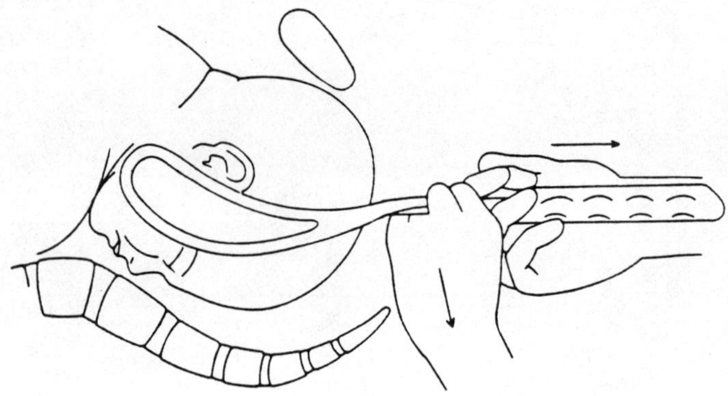

Figure 44-14. Saxtorph-Pajot maneuver. (Reprinted from Laufe, L. E.: *Obstetric Forceps,* New York, Hoeber Medical Division, Harper & Row, 1968, by permission of the publisher.)

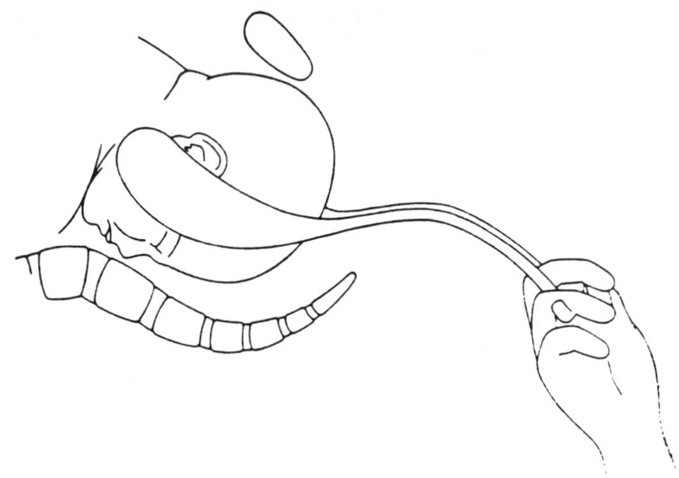

Figure 44-15. Divergent forceps: application and traction. (Reprinted from Laufe, L. E.: *Obstetric Forceps,* New York, Hoeber Medical Division, Harper & Row, 1968, by permission of the publisher.)

diverges and reduces compression, removal of the forceps can be deferred until the head has been delivered.

For occiput posterior outlet forceps, certain relationships change. The widest diameter of the fetal head (biparietal) is now in the posterior pelvic segment and will produce increased perineal distension. The toes of the blades curve away from, rather than toward, the ears. For this reason, a long tapered blade is best. The posterior fontanelle will be one finger-width *beneath* the shanks and the head will deliver by *flexion* rather than extension.

Delivery of the aftercoming head in breech presentation may also be considered a prophylactic forceps delivery. Deep application of forceps to assist the aftercoming head is fraught with danger to both mother and child. When vaginal breech delivery is indicated (see Chapter 24), the use of forceps to the aftercoming head avoids the sudden explosive delivery of the fetal head through the introitus.

There are three cardinal principles in applying forceps to the aftercoming head:

1. The forceps is inserted and applied from below upward.
2. The application is pelvic rather than purely cephalic.
3. The mechanism of extraction is flexion of the fetal head, accomplished by elevating the handles of the forceps.

The short Piper forceps is less unwieldly and functions as a third-class lever. It also affords the attendant better control of the instrument and of the fetal body.

Basic Midforceps Techniques. Basic midforceps operations are those that require increased axis traction or rotation of the fetal head less than 90°. Any forceps rotation of 90° or greater is classified as a major midforceps operation. Basic midforceps procedures from either a left occipitoanterior (LOA) or right occipitoanterior (ROA) position are quite frequent because of the increased use of conduction anesthesia. Formerly, these procedures were called low forceps or low midforceps.

The basic technique for insertion and application of the forceps for LOA or ROA is similar to that described for a direct occiput anterior. The posterior blade must be inserted first (Fig. 44-16A). The insertion of the anterior blade requires the handle to describe a wider arc so the blade will be directed toward the anterior segment of the pelvis (Fig. 44-16B). This procedure decreases the amount of wandering of the blade necessary to achieve proper biparietal application.

Once applied and locked, the forceps must be checked for adequacy of insertion, symmetry of application, and blade–cephalic relationship. Rotation is now performed to align the sagittal suture with the anteroposterior diameter of the pelvis. This is accomplished by slightly elevating the handles through an arc in the desired direction (Fig. 44-16C).

Traction for midforceps deliveries is performed as for outlet forceps, but adjustment is made to the station (Fig. 44-17).

Instrumental axis traction is a valuable adjunct to the management of large infants, late failure of the powers of labor, or midpelvis arrests because of conduction anesthesia. Axis traction is best achieved by the addition of the Bill traction handle to the forceps of choice. It should be restricted to average-sized infants whose vertex is at midpelvis. Proper traction is accomplished by following the lateral markers on the handle. The attendant must remember that augmented axis traction means increased traction force with resultant increased compression of the fetal head. The operation must be performed slowly and the traction handle and forceps loosened between pulls to avoid sustained force. For large or well-molded heads, an axis-traction instrument with long tapered blades is desirable.

It is not so long since the merits of "trial forceps" were debated in the literature.[15] In current obstetric practice, a "trial forceps" operation is rarely valid.

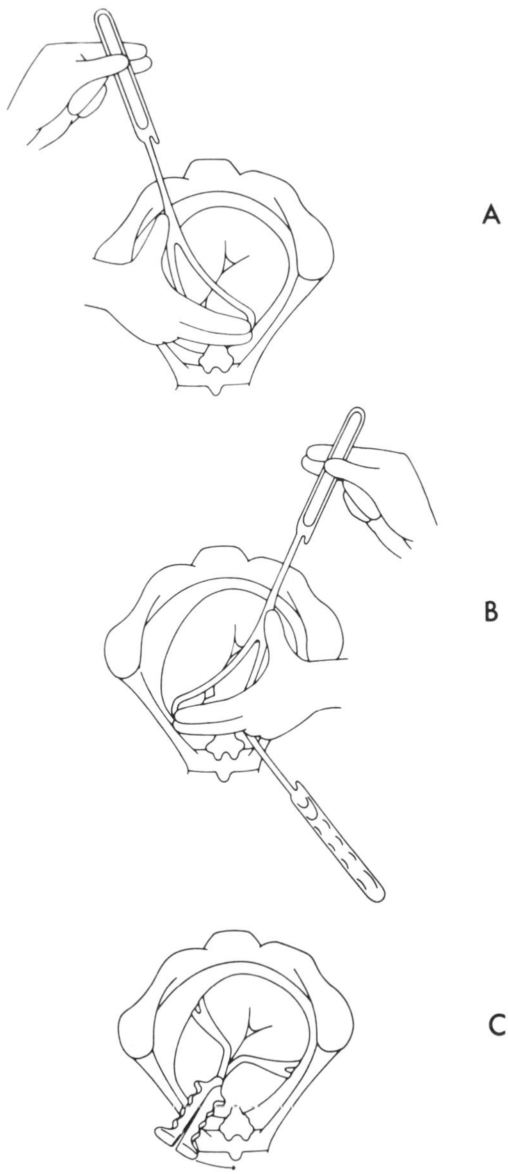

Figure 44-16. Insertion, application, and rotation of basic midforceps, LOA. (Reprinted from Laufe, L. E.: *Obstetric Forceps*, New York, Hoeber Medical Division, Harper & Row, 1968, by permission of the publisher.)

Special Midforceps Techniques. Special midforceps operations deal with transverse arrest, occiput posterior positions, and face presentations. These problems have always attracted the attention of obstetricians. No manipulative

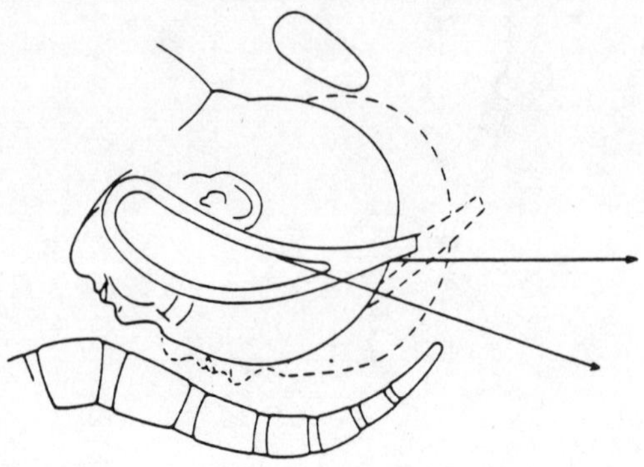

Figure 44-17. Traction in the axis of the pelvis depending on station. (Reprinted from Laufe, L. E.: *Obstetric Forceps*, New York, Hoeber Medical Division, Harper & Row, 1968, by permission of the publisher.)

procedure for these complications should be undertaken if the safety of the fetus or mother will be jeopardized. Delivery room gymnastics with forceps do not equate with quality obstetric care.

Transverse Arrests. Transverse arrests are classified as "high" or "low." In the former, the arrest has occurred above the midpelvis and cesarean section is the procedure of choice. Low arrests are those in which the vertex has failed to progress beyond station plus 2 following an adequate trial of second-stage labor. There are a variety of causes. A prominent sacrum or ischial spines may inhibit internal rotation; late failure of the powers can prevent internal rotation; increasing size of successive infants can produce relative as well as real disproportions; and, not uncommonly, premature use of conduction anesthesia predisposes to incomplete rotation. Finally, a transverse position of the vertex can be a normal mechanism of delivery in a flat pelvis.

Once the etiology of a transverse arrest has been determined, the attendant can choose from a variety of instrumental procedures. Instrumental procedures in transverse arrest are probably the most difficult of all forceps operations. Two cardinal rules are fundamental: the anterior branch must be applied first, since the anterior pelvic segment is limited, and asynclitism must be accounted for. All transverse arrests have a deflexed attitude that must be corrected prior to rotation.

The special forceps designed to manage transverse arrests are the Barton (Fig. 44-18) and the Kielland (Fig. 44-19).[17] Each employs a sliding lock, which is mandatory when asynclitism exists.

The Barton forceps is the choice for dealing with a transverse arrest in a flat pelvis. It is the only forceps designed to apply traction in the transverse diameter of the pelvis. The classic technique for using the Barton forceps for transverse arrest is illustrated in Fig. 44-20. Rotation of the hinged or anterior blade is usually over the occiput but can be performed over the face if resistance is met. When there is marked anterior asynclitism, the hinged blade can be directly applied to the anterior parietal bone.

The Kielland forceps is the choice for managing a transverse arrest by rotation followed by traction. The *classic* or *inversion* technique of inserting, applying, rotating, and extracting with the Kielland is illustrated in Fig. 44-21. This is the only forceps operation that utilizes intrauterine insertion of a blade. The forceps was designed to take advantage of the triangular space between the side of the head, the anterior shoulder, and the lower uterine segment.

Many who favor the Kielland forceps have abandoned the *classic* technique because of the potential danger of trauma to the fetus and maternal tissues. These individuals employ a *wandering* technique of insertion and application as utilized with other forceps. As is true of the Barton forceps, a *direct* anterior blade application can be made when there is marked anterior asynclitism. Rotation corrects any asynclitism, and no special adjustment of the blades is necessary.

The most important concept in the management of transverse arrests from below is individualization. The operator must be willing to abandon any instrument if he or she suspects it is leading to use of undue force. Those who rely exclusively on a given instrument or procedure do not comprehend the various etiologies of transverse arrests and the obstetric forceps designed to manage them.

Occiput Posterior Positions. Occiput posterior positions are amenable to forceps delivery. Occiput posterior positions are a normal mechanism of labor in the anthropoid pelvis. Many deliver spontaneously or with outlet forceps.

Occiput posterior arrests can occur in any pelvis with a reduced transverse diameter, a reduced capacity, or converging lateral pelvic walls. Contributing factors include deflexion of

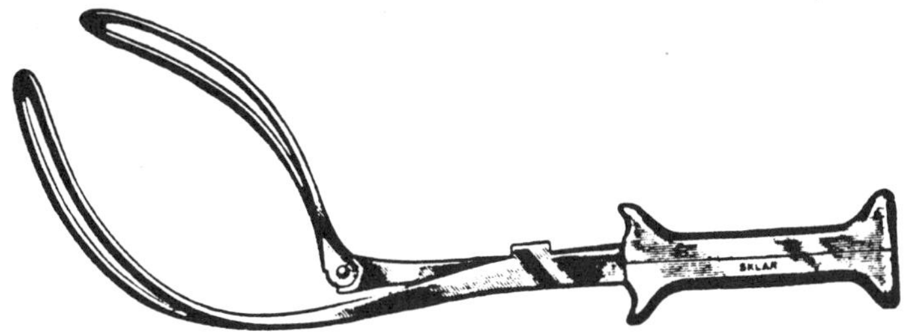

Figure 44-18. Barton forceps. (Reprinted from Laufe, L. E.: *Obstetric Forceps*, New York, Hoeber Medical Division, Harper & Row, 1968, by permission of the publisher.)

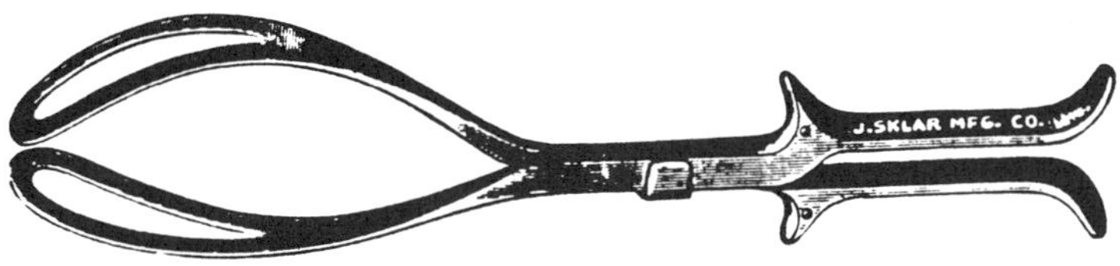

Figure 44-19. Kielland forceps. (Reprinted from Laufe, L. E.: *Obstetric Forceps*, New York, Hoeber Medical Division, Harper & Row, 1968, by permission of the publisher.)

the fetal head, late uterine inertia, and premature use of conduction anesthesia. A variety of instrumental procedures are available for the management of the problem.

Before attempting any of the rotational procedures available for management of posterior arrest, each case should be evaluated. No disproportion must exist, an adequate trial of labor must be given, and the attendant must be familiar with the limitations of the instrument chosen.

The best-known rotary maneuver is the Scanzoni maneuver. As originally described, the forceps is applied as if to an occiput anterior head. The head is rotated until the sagittal suture reaches the transverse plane. A second forceps application is made to achieve a true cephalic application in the occiput transverse position and rotation is completed to the OA position, followed by extraction.

The Scanzoni maneuver has been modified repeatedly and includes primary rotation all the way to an OA position, retention of one blade in the pelvis as a "splint" to prevent the head from rotating back to its original position, and the inverted Scanzoni maneuver. The latter technique has achieved some popularity and simplifies the procedure to a single forceps application, illustrated in Fig. 44-22. These procedures rarely are performed now.

No matter which instrument is used, the operator must correct deflexion of the fetal head prior to rotation. When the Barton forceps is used, the hinged blade is inserted first. The rigid blade is then applied and the branches are articulated. Rotation is performed in the appropriate direction, sweeping the handles through a wide arc (Fig. 44-23). If the Barton forceps is to be used for traction in the OA position, it is wise to add the special traction handle to counteract the effects of the now offset shanks and handles.

The Kielland forceps functions extremely well as a rotator because of the negated pelvic curve. The blades are applied to an occiput posterior with the directional markers oriented to the posterior fontanelle (Fig. 44-24). Once applied and articulated, the handles are elevated in the plane of the sagittal suture to correct the deflexion, and rotation is then performed as if one were turning a key in a lock. If the Kielland is used for extraction, a wide episiotomy is indicated because of the spaciousness of the posterior segment of the blades. Traction is performed with the handles 45° below the hori-

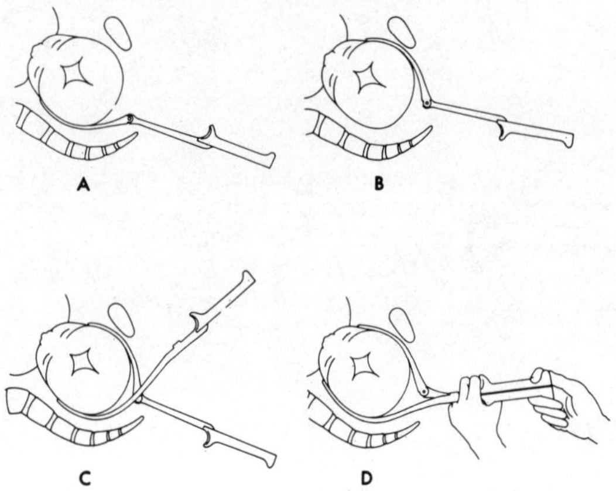

Figure 44-20. Insertion, application, and traction of Barton forceps, LOT. (Reprinted from Laufe, L. E.: *Obstetric Forceps*, New York, Hoeber Medical Division, Harper & Row, 1968, by permission of the publisher.)

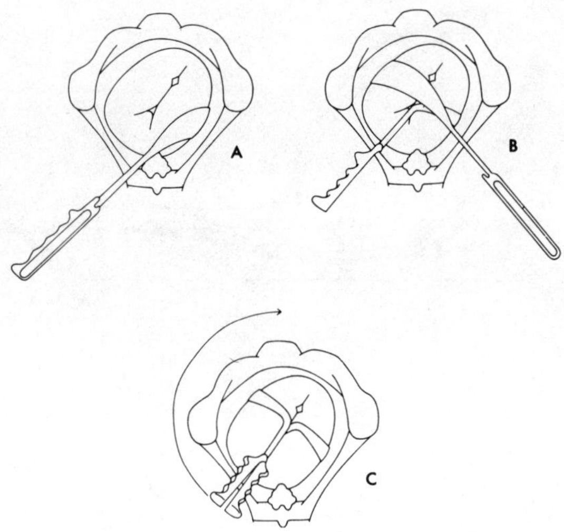

Figure 44-22. Inverted Scanzoni maneuver, Tucker-McLane forceps, insertion and rotation, ROP. (Reprinted from Laufe, L. E.: *Obstetric Forceps*, New York, Hoeber Medical Division, Harper & Row, 1968, by permission of the publisher.)

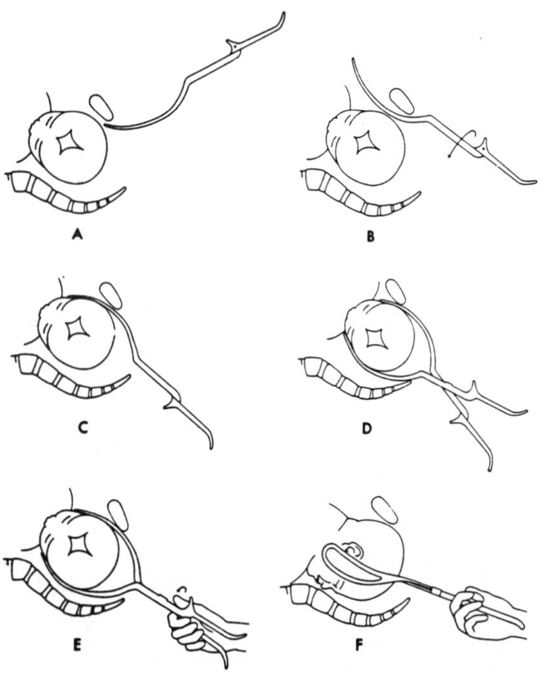

Figure 44-21. Inversion technique of insertion, application, articulation, rotation, and traction using Kielland forceps. LOT. (Reprinted from Laufe, L. E.: *Obstetric Forceps*, New York, Hoeber Medical Division, Harper & Row, 1968, by permission of the publisher.)

zontal to compensate for the offset pelvic curve of the blades (Fig. 44-21). If the handles are elevated, the toes of the blades may cause vaginal lacerations.

If the operator prefers, a forceps with a conventional pelvic curve for traction can be employed after either the Barton or Kielland forceps is used for rotation. When performing a forceps rotation, the operator should place one hand on the lower abdomen and, as the shoulder of the fetus rotates, the external hand can assist by applying gentle pressure in the proper direction.

Brow and Face Presentations. Current concepts for managing brow and face presentations stress the liberalization of indications for cesarean section (see Chapter 25).

Most brow presentations are transitional and convert to a face or an occiput. When a persistent brow is diagnosed, ultraconservatism is the keynote of management.

Because of their distinctive feel on vaginal examination, face presentations are usually diagnosed earlier than brow presentations. They may be allowed a trial of labor as long as progress is being made and the fetus is not compromised. Forceps procedures are restricted to mentum anteriors. The Kielland forceps is the instrument of choice (Fig. 44-24), although the

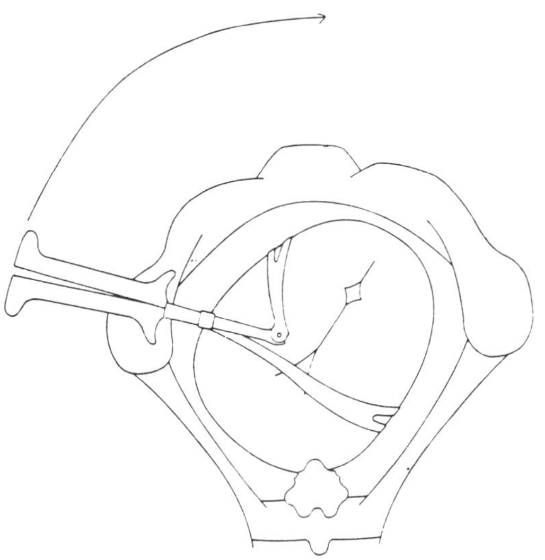

Figure 44-23. Barton forceps: application and arc of rotation, ROP. (Reprinted from Laufe, L. E.: *Obstetric Forceps,* New York, Hoeber Medical Division, Harper & Row, 1968, by permission of the publisher.)

Simpson forceps is acceptable and is preferred by many.

The indications for the use of obstetric forceps have been reduced significantly during the past 15 years. Increased use of fetal monitoring and better identification of the high-risk fetus have resulted in increased use of cesarean section. This is more appropriate than is subjecting mother and fetus to a difficult forceps operation that could inflict long-term trauma to both.

Not enough is known about the safe parameters of a forceps delivery to define completely the role of forceps in obstetric care. Clinicians must be knowledgeable about what can and cannot be done safely with obstetric forceps.

VACUUM EXTRACTOR

The use of vacuum-cup deliveries to facilitate vaginal delivery dates back to the 18th century. James Yonge mentions, in his 1706 paper on benign cystic teratomas, that he could not "draw it (an infant's head) out by a cupping-glass fixed to the scalp with an airpump."[47] This is perhaps the first mention of a vacuum type extractor. The first description of a true vacuum extractor was by John Simpson who, in 1849, described an instrument consisting of a slender, short brass syringe worked by a double-valve piston, attached to an inner metal cup, covered by an outer, more flexible cup made of "vulcanized caoutchouc," (a type of rubber). The inner cup was covered by a diaphragm of sponge-covered brass mesh, "with a view of preventing any injury to the scalp."[42] This early attempt at vacuum extraction (VE) was with a pliable cup. Simpson went on to state that:

> The air-tractor seemed to possess various advantages over the forceps. It was far less dangerous to the mother, as it was attached only to the exposed part of the scalp of the infant; the forceps were required to be passed high up between the head and maternal passages, and in incautious and inexperienced hands were apt to injure one or both. The materials of the air-tractor were safer to the mother and child than the material of the forceps (steel). The forceps always took up a certain amount of space between the head and passages; the air-tractor did not. The air-tractor was greatly less in size, and subsequently, far more portable. It could be applied with sufficient firmness and power to enable us to rotate the head, or change its position; as from, for example, an occipito-posterior to an occipital- anterior position (the form of rotation most frequently required in practice). . . . If found perfectly easily of application, it may enable

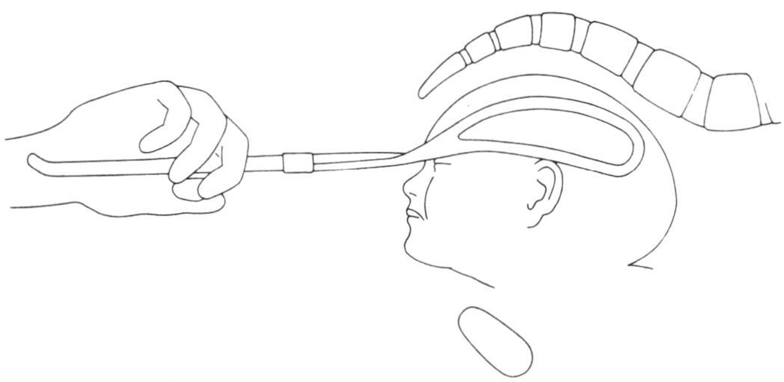

Figure 44-24. Kielland forceps application, mentum anterior. (Reprinted from Laufe, L. E.: *Obstetric Forceps,* New York, Hoeber Medical Division, Harper & Row, 1968, by permission of the publisher.)

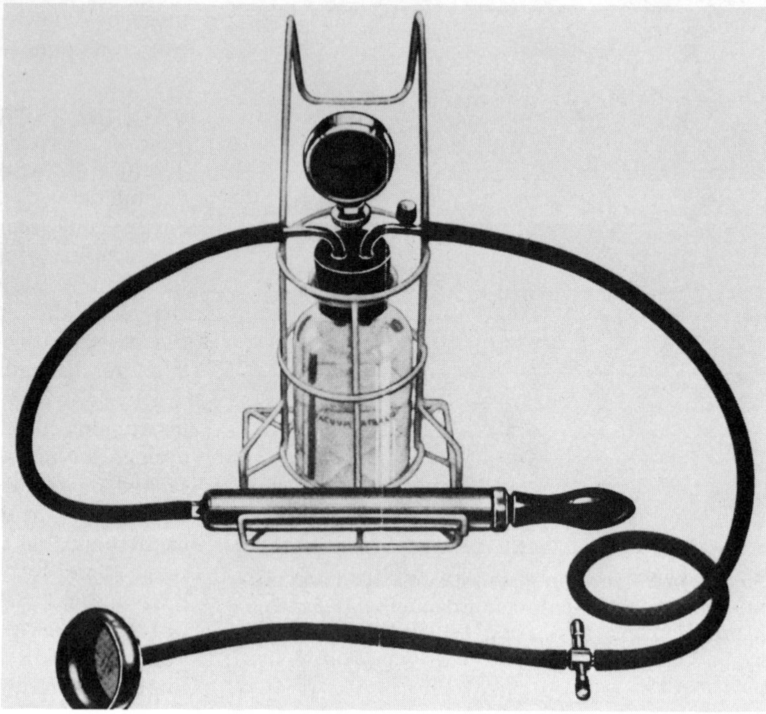

Figure 44-25. The Malmström Vacuum Extractor.

> the accoucheur, by adding a few pounds to the strength of each pain, to bring to a safe and speedier termination cases that would otherwise go on tediously, hour after hour, in what we would still not choose to use so formidable an instrument as the forceps.[44]

Thus, even the inventor of a forceps was in favor of a smaller, more flexible instrument and proclaimed its virtues. However, it was not until Malmström introduced his metal vacuum extractor (VE) in 1952 that the instrument came into general use (Fig. 44-25).

The VE has nearly replaced forceps in Europe[16] due to the influence of Malmström, Chamberlain, and Bergman.[5,10,31] Subsequently, considerable literature evaluating the Malmström VE and its maternal and fetal sequelae has been published. [2,3,7,10,40,44] These papers report reduced maternal trauma[7,10,16,22,35,44,46] but some scalp injuries to the fetus. A few series have reported serious fetal cranial injury and death.[1,2,34,39] These injuries probably resulted from the constant suction force on the caput succedaneum created with the metal cup.

There has been a general reluctance to use the VE in the United States because of the scalp effects.[34,39] The more severe injuries appear to be caused by the use of the VE at a high station or when the cervix is not completely dilated.[45] In 1973, Kobayashi introduced a pliable plastic VE. This instrument offers the advantage of less scalp trauma because it can shape to the baby's head and has no rigid metal edge. Serious cranial hemorrhage might be avoided by restricting its use to the second stage of labor. To date there are few reports available to substantiate these considerations.[24,32,38] Recent research[6] has indicated that this instrument is superior to the metal cup and is certainly as safe and effective as forceps for vaginal delivery. Because of the increased safety and convenience of the pliable cup, this device has nearly replaced the Malmström instrument for use in VE deliveries in this country.

Pliable Vacuum Extractor

Design. The Kobayashi cup VE (Fig. 44-26) consists of a single-unit pliable cup and a stainless steel valve. The cup measures 65 mm in diameter, easily fitting into the vagina but precluding application through an incompletely dilated cervix. The valve is a simple sliding piston with a small relief hole that allows a drop in pressure from 0.8 kg per square centimeter to 0.2 kg per square centimeter or 700 mmHg to 200 mmHg when depressed. This allows for re-

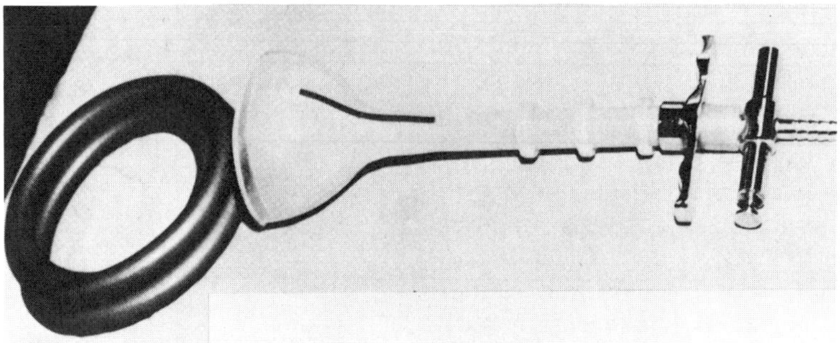

Figure 44-26. The Kobayashi vacuum extractor.

lief of a significant amount of the suction force to the infant's scalp between contractions without loss of application of the cup to the vertex. A blue line is marked on the cup for orientation when applied to the scalp.

Several types of vacuum systems exist. They consist of an electric vacuum pump with a manometer to monitor negative pressure. The maximum pressures are regulated not to exceed 0.7–0.8 kg per square centimeter as recommended by earlier studies.[5] The pumps can compensate for leakage to maintain constant pressure, a definite advantage over hand pump models that require continual monitoring by nursing staff. Timers limit the total suction time and a foot pedal release facilitates removal after the head is delivered.

Indications for VE

Indications for VE are essentially the same as those for forceps delivery. This covers obstetrical problems from prolapsed cord to delivery of the fetal head at cesarean section. Most applications are for problems in the second stage of labor with prolonged second stage predominant. The generally accepted indications for VE in the second stage of labor for low and midforceps applications are:

1. Obstetrical complications, such as dystocia, prolonged second stage, malpresentation.
2. Maternal complications such as toxemia, abruption, and exhaustion, cardiovascular disease.
3. Fetal distress.
4. Elective outlet application.

Malpresentation presents some special considerations. In the deflexed or malpresent position, especially occiput-posterior, the pliable cup VE is more likely to fail than with occiput-anterior presentation. However, if the cup can be maneuvered over the occiput, flexion can be enhanced. Rotation usually occurs spontaneously when traction is maintained in synchrony with contractions. Rotation can be assisted by putting torque on the shaft during traction. Brow or face presentations are contraindications to VE delivery.

VE use for fetal distress varied from 2.5% to 44.5% in early studies but has decreased with the increase in abdominal delivery, especially for this indication. In our experience, 31% of vacuum-extracted deliveries were associated with abnormal fetal heart tracings.[6] Because of the need for formation of the caput, which takes 6–10 minutes, the Malmström instrument has not been commonly used, because outlet forceps delivery could be performed more rapidly. The pliable VE obviates this time restraint because full suction can be obtained within a few seconds.

Caution must be interjected. Intercerebral bleeding occurs in babies who are asphyxiated, whether there is trauma or not, especially in term babies who are normally much more resistant to intracranial hemorrhage than are premature infants.[33] Instrumental delivery, whether by VE or forceps, may increase this risk because of compressive forces and increases the medical–legal risk over that of cesarean section in this setting.

Contraindications

The following are contraindications to VE:

A. Absolute Contraindications
   1. Nonvertex presentation or uncertain presentation and orientation
   2. Suspected fetal macrosomia ($\geqq$4000 g)
   3. Suspected cephalopelvic disproportion
B. Relative Contraindications
   1. Suspected fetal anomaly
   2. Less than 35 weeks' gestation
   3. Previous scalp sampling

4. High station
5. Incompletely dilated cervix
6. Fetal demise

Since cephalopelvic disproportion is not always possible to diagnose, every VE should be considered to be a trial and should be abandoned when unsuccessful. Our studies support the use of VE in this way. Failed VE adds no significant morbidity to subsequent immediate cesarean section. However, combined VE and forceps delivery increases superficial injury to the infant scalp even when successful.

Experience involving the delivery of premature infants with the VE contributed to many of the reports of serious fetal injury and death.[1,2,40] Reports studying the VE in term deliveries yield much more encouraging results. With the pliable cup, there is no significant increased morbidity over that of forceps deliveries.[6,22,45] Restricting the use of the VE to term deliveries should eliminate most, if not all, of the serious complications of VE deliveries.

There is one report of exsanguination of an infant subsequent to a VE delivery. This occurred after scalp sampling and was secondary to bleeding from the sampling site.[35] This is the only such report; however, it would be advisable to refrain from using the VE after scalp sampling. The nearly transparent pliable cup allows for monitoring of bleeding, but such an application requires extreme caution and should be abandoned if any significant blood is seen under the cup or in the suction tubing.

Technique of Vacuum Extraction

Anesthesia. In general, anesthetic requirements for vacuum extractor are less than for forceps.[22] The degree of pelvic relaxation required is reduced because the instrument is smaller and works with the normal second-stage pushing of the mother. Pudendal block or local infiltration are used more often than are saddle block or epidural, although these are also suitable methods. The anesthetic requirements generally are for the insertion and application of the suction cup and for episiotomy, not for pelvic relaxation.

Application of the Cup. The instrument should be used for vertex presentation only when the contraindications mentioned above are not present. It should be sterilized. Proper functioning of the pump should be confirmed. It is important to ascertain the attitude and position of the vertex and to determine any malrotation that may be present. The pliable cup is collapsed into the smallest possible diameter and inserted carefully, keeping pressure toward the posterior vagina. Once the cup is manipulated inside the vagina, there is generally no difficulty in applying it to the scalp. Simple rotation unfolds the cup edge. The border of the cup should then be traced to avoid inclusion of the cervix, vagina or bladder in the application. At this point low-level suction, a vacuum of approximately 200 mmHg, should be initiated and the application rechecked. The extractor should be applied with the blue line oriented toward the occiput.

At the beginning of a contraction, the vacuum setting is increased to 600–700 mmHg and traction applied along the pelvic axis. Between tractions, the vacuum is released to 200 mmHg by use of the trumpet-valve that is part of the stainless steel handle of the instrument. No settings need to be changed on the pump.

There is no significant waiting time because formation of the caput succedaneum is not required for traction. If the cup slips when traction is applied, it should be reapplied and delivery attempted again. Should this occur more than once, the situation should be reevaluated. If the vertex does not descend with a satisfactory application and use of adequate force, there is no reason to persist until the cup dislodges. This is a built-in safety factor of the pliable cup. Excessive force cannot be applied to deliver the infant in the face of cephalopelvic disproportion.

As the vertex is delivered, the cup should assume a 90° orientation as the head is flexed. The suction is then released using the foot pedal, and delivery is accomplished with the usual maneuvers.

Traction should be synchronized with labor pains, with one hand pulling on the stainless steel handle and the other hand maintaining contact between the cup and the fetal head. In this way the fetal head movements can be monitored and the direction of traction can be adjusted accordingly. Usually, three to five tractions, synchronized with labor pains, are sufficient to obtain delivery. The total extraction time should not exceed 15 minutes of maximum suction as this has been correlated with increased scalp injuries and cephalohematomas.[18] Using the pliable cup with release of suction between each contraction, 15 minutes represents approximately 15 contractions, much in excess of what a normal low or midpelvic delivery should require. In most cases it is advisable to perform an episiotomy to avoid vaginal tears and dislodging of the cup at the introitus, although if the patient is able to increase her intra-abdominal pressure adequately, the head can be delivered spontaneously, sometimes avoiding the need for episiotomy.

One of the difficulties with the metal versions is that the different parts have to be assembled for use after they are sterilized. The pliable VE is a single unit with a plastic hose and only requires attachment to the suction bottle by the nurse. Thus, it is quickly assembled and ready for use in emergency situations. The scalp electrode can be left in place, because adequate suction usually can be obtained around the scalp electrode wire. Thus, the infant can be monitored continually throughout the delivery process.

Complications. Injury to the mother is reduced significantly with the VE over forceps, but neonatal scalp injuries have negated this benefit in the past. Since the VE is applied inside the biparietal diameter as opposed to the cradling effects of forceps, one could expect that injury to the maternal birth canal would be less frequent. Studies have shown reduced maternal lacerations and blood loss with the use of the VE as compared to forceps.[10,22,35,45,47]

Present studies using the pliable instrument also have reported promising results and have noted no significant increase in morbidity over that associated with spontaneous vaginal delivery.[6] In addition, superficial skin injuries were not greater than those occurring with forceps used under similar circumstances.

Neonatal Morbidity. American obstetricians generally have not accepted the VE because of scalp injuries. The very pronounced caput succedaneum generated with the metal cup seems to be the primary source for these injuries. The Kobayashi cup molds to the scalp, creating much less caput and hence less injury.

Although scalp abrasions and lacerations with the Malmström cup are reported more frequently than are forceps marks, we found no such increase with the pliable instrument.[6] Cosmetic injuries are an important consideration in both VE and forceps delivery. Parents must be informed that transient caput or forceps marks may occur and that they will resolve over the first few days of life. After such preparation, the reactions of parents, relatives, and nursery personnel are accepting. In general, the caput is preferred to facial abrasions.

Cephalohematomas. These lesions are caused by bleeding under the periosteum of the cranial bones. They are restricted to a single bone plate, absorb over 4–6 weeks, may calcify, and frequently cause anemia and jaundice as the blood pigment is broken down. Plauche, in his review of the literature, found an incidence of cephalohematomas of 1–16% for the Malmström VE.[39] Others have reported up to 40%.

Although the incidence of cephalohematoma with the plastic VE was increased over that of forceps and spontaneous birth it was well below the incidence for the metal cup, probably because of the small caput generated and release of vacuum pressure between contractions. These lesions could be confirmed with ultrasound on 3 of our 12 cases of clinical cephalohematomas. Unlike classic cephalohematomas, the soft-cup VE lesions resolve within 1–2 weeks and do not calcify. None of the infants required transfusion.

Subgaleal Hematomas. These lesions are caused by trauma to the diploic vessels in the loose subaponeurotic tissue of the scalp. Because there is no periosteal membrane to contain the bleeding, massive hemorrhage can occur, sometimes leading to fatalities. In most cases, these lesions are associated with asphyxia and difficult deliveries involving application at high stations or in the first stage of labor. No subgaleal hemorrhage has been reported with the soft cup.

Retinal Hemorrhage. The incidence of retinal hemorrhage is increased significantly in Malmström vacuum extractor deliveries. The incidence of retinal hemorrhage is about 20% in spontaneous vaginal deliveries, 30% in forceps deliveries, and 60% following use of the Malmström vacuum extractor.[18,41] Although neither long-term visual loss nor intracranial hemorrhage are associated with these lesions, some types of hemorrhage may cause permanent damage, especially when the macular region of the eye is involved. There is an association between retinal hemorrhage, the degree of delivery trauma, and the difficulty of application of the instrument. Our studies did not show an increase in retinal hemorrhage with the pliable VE device as compared to forceps or spontaneous vaginal delivery.

Intracerebral Hemorrhage (ICH). Although ICH has been reported in up to 40% of premature births,[14] the incidence is probably less than 1% in term infants. The occurrence of ICH associated with VE varies from 0% to 0.35%[39] but is increased markedly in preterm deliveries or when asphyxia is present. Selecting term infants and avoiding prolonged applications, we were unable to identify any instance of ICH, except in one instance of clotting abnormalities combined with severe asphyxia. This infant manifested subarachnoid hemorrhage only.

ICH occurs so rarely in term infants that it is reasonable to assume that anatomic or developmental abnormalities are predisposing factors. A-V malformations or persistent germinal matrix may be more important etiologies than method of delivery.

Long-term follow-up studies of term infants delivered by VE have shown no increase in mental retardation or cerebral palsy.[8] When children entering school were examined, developmental problems or minor neurological symptoms were found in 5.9% of the spontaneous vaginal delivery group and in 5.3% of the VE group.[7]

Trial of VE

There is little published information about the soft vacuum cup and none about failure rates with this instrument. Our research indicates that failure is marginally higher than with the Malmström cup. The reported failure rate for the Malmström VE is from 1.1% to 27%. Nearly all the failures require cesarean section for delivery.[19,22] Of 129 pliable VE deliveries studied prospectively, 84 were completed with VE alone, 36 with mid or low forceps, and 9 required cesarean section.[6] The group that required forceps completion consisted of 78% midpelvic VE applications, of which all but one were converted to outlet forceps deliveries.

The pliability and lack of "chignon" generated with the pliable instrument convey improved safety and cosmetic outcome to newborn and mother but cause the instrument not to hold onto the scalp as firmly as the Malmström cup, increasing the need for forceps as an adjuvant procedure. Even when unsuccessful, the VE reduced a potentially difficult midforceps to an outlet procedure in 93% of the cases. There was no increase in serious neonatal morbidity secondary to a trial of VE. Thus, a trial of VE is safe. The minimal cost of an unsuccessful application is balanced by the maternal benefits when difficult midforceps delivery or cesarean section can be avoided. With the current decreased exposure to midforceps in residency training, the tendency is to solve most dystocia problems by utilizing abdominal delivery. VE is an easy instrument to master and teach and may resolve many midpelvic arrests.

Conclusion

The VE is an effective and safe method of delivery. It requires less skill than do forceps and causes less injury to the mother and infant, especially for midcavity applications.

With the new pliable cup VE and electric pump, technical problems have become infrequent. Scalp injury and caput have been reduced markedly. With appropriate counseling and selection of patients, it may well be "time the obstetricians in the United States take a careful look at the European experience [and our own], and give the VE a fair trial."[35]

REFERENCES

1. Aguero, O. and Alvarez, H.: Fetal injury due to the vacuum extractor. *Obstet. Gynecol.* **19**:212–217, 1962.
2. Ahuja, G. L., Willoughby, M. L. N., Kerr, M. M., and Hutchison, J. H.: Massive subaponeurotic hemorrhage in infants born by vacuum extractor. *Br. Med. J.* **3**:743–745, 1969.
3. American College of Obstetricians and Gynecologists: *Manual of Standards in Obstetric-Gynecologic Practice*, 2nd Edition. Chicago, 1965.
4. Barton, H. G. and Dossert, F. C.: *The Barton Forceps*. New York, Chazy Free Press, 1949.
5. Bergman, P. and Malmstrœm m, T.: Natal and postnatal foetal mortality in association with vacuum extraction and forceps delivery. *Gynaecologia* **154**:65–72, 1962.
6. Berkus, M. D., Ramamurthy, R. S., O'Connor, P. S., Brown, K., and Hayashi, R. H.: A cohort study of Silastic Obstetrical Vacuum Cup deliveries: Safety of the instrument. *Obstet. Gynecol.*, **66**:503–509, 1965.
7. Bjerre, I. and Dahlin, K.: The long-term development of childrendelivered by vacuum extraction. *Dev. Med. Child. Neurol.* **15**:378–381, 1974.
8. Blennow, G., Svenningsen, N. W., Gustafson, B., Sunden, B., and Cronquist, S.: Neonatal and prospective follow-up study of infants delivered by vacuum extraction (VE). *Acta Obstet. Gynecol. Scand.* **56**:189–194, 1977.
9. Cesarean childbirth: Report of a Consensus Development Conference sponsored by the National Institute of Child Health and Human Development in conjunction with the National Center for Health Care Technology and assisted by the Office for Medical Applications of Research. (NIH) 82-2067, National Institutes of Health, Bethesda, MD: U.S. Dept. of Health and Human Services, Public Health Service, National Institutes of Health, 1981, 537 pp.
10. Chamberlain, G.: Forceps and vacuum extraction. *Clin. Obstet. Gynaecol.* **7**:511–527, 1980.

11. Cutter, B.: Laufe's divergent forceps: The Canberra experience. *Aust. N.Z. J. Obstet. Gynaecol.* **15**:215–218, 1975.
12. Das, K. N.: *Obstetric Forceps: Its History and Evolution*. St. Louis, Mosby, 1929.
13. Dennen, E. H.: *Forceps Deliveries*, 2nd Edition. Philadelphia, Davis, 1964.
14. Donat, J. F., Okazaki, H., Kleinberg, F., and Reagan, T. J.: Intraventricular hemorrhages in full-term and premature infants. *Mayo Clin. Proc.* **53**:437–441, 1978.
15. Dyer, I.: Trial and failed forceps. *Clin. Obstet. Gynecol.* **8**:914–918, 1965.
16. Earn, A. A.: An appraisal of Malmström's vacuum-tractor (vacuum extractor). Obstetric and pediatric results. *Am. J. Obstet. Gynecol.* **99**:732–743, 1967.
17. Eastman, N. J. and Hellman L. M.: *Williams Obstetrics*, 13th Edition. New York, Appleton-Century-Crofts, 1966.
18. Ehlers, N., Jensen, I. K., and Hansen, K. B.: Retinal haemorrhages in the newborn. Comparison of delivery by forceps and by vacuum extractor. *Acta Ophthalmol. (Kbh)* **52**:73–82, 1974.
19. Fahmy, K.: Failed trial vacuum extraction followed by cesarean section. *Int. Surg.* **49**:262–269, 1968.
20. Fleming, A. R., Brandeberry, K. R., and Pearse, W. H.: Introduction of a metric forceps, *Am. J. Obstet. Gynecol.* **78**:125–133, 1959.
21. Forster, F. M. C.: On modern forceps delivery and Laufe's divergent forceps. *Aust. N.Z. J. Obstet. Gynaecol.* **15**:209–214, 1975.
22. Greis, J. B., Bieniarz, J., and Scommegna, A.: Comparison of maternal and fetal effects of vacuum extraction with forceps or cesarean deliveries. *Obstet. Gynecol.* **57**:571–577, 1981.
23. Healy, D. L. and Laufe, L. E.: Survey of obstetric forceps training in North America in 1981. *Am. J. Obstet. Gynecol.* **151**:54–58, 1985.
24. Kappy, K. A.: Vacuum extractor. *Clin. Perinatol.* **8**:79–86, 1981.
25. Kielland, C.: The application of forceps in transverse presentation. *Monatsschr. Geburtsh. Gynak.* **43**:48–78, 1916.
26. Laufe, L. E.: An improved Piper forceps. *Obstet. Gynecol.* **29**:284–286, 1967.
27. Laufe, L. E.: A new divergent outlet forceps. *Am. J. Obstet. Gynecol.* **101**:509–512, 1968.
28. Laufe, L. E.: Obstetric forceps. In: *Gynecology and Obstetrics*. J. W. Sciarra (Ed.). Philadelphia, Harper & Row, 1985, pp. 1–20.
29. Laufe L. E. and Leslie D. C.: The timing of episiotomy. *Am. J. Obstet. Gynecol.* **114**:773–774, 1972.
30. Luikart, R.: A modification of the Kielland, Simpson and Tucker-McLean forceps to simplify their use and improve function and safety. *Am. J. Obstet. Gynecol.* **34**:686–687, 1937.
31. Malmström, T.: The vacuum extractor. I. Indications and results. *Acta Obstet. Gynecol. Scand.* **43**:5–52, 1961.
32. Maryniak, G. M. and Frank, J. B.: Clinical assessment of the Kobayashi vacuum extractor. *Obstet. Gynecol.* **64**:431–435, 1984.
33. Mitchell, W. and O'Tuama, L.: Cerebral intraventricular hemorrhages in infants: A widening age spectrum. *Pediatrics* **65**:35–39, 1980.
34. Munsat, T. L., Neerhout, R., and Nyirjesy, I.: A comparative clinical study of the vacuum extractor and forceps. Part II. Evaluation of the newborn. *Am. J. Obstet. Gynecol.* **85**:1083–1090, 1963.
35. Ott, W. J.: Vacuum extraction. *Obstet. Gynecol. Surv.* **30**:643–649, 1975.
36. Palma, P. A., Miner, M. E., Morriss, F. H., Jr., Adcock, E. W., III, and Denson, S. E.: Intraventricular hemorrhage in the neonate born at term. *Am. J. Dis. Child.* **133**:941–944, 1979.
37. Pearse, W. H.: Electronic recording of forceps delivery. *Am. J. Obstet. Gynecol.* **86**:43–51, 1963.
38. Pelosi, M. A. and Apuzzio, J.: Use of the soft, silicone obstetric vacuum cup for delivery of the fetal head at cesarean section. *J. Reprod. Med.* **9**:289–292, 1984.
39. Plauche, W. C.: Fetal cranial injuries related to delivery with the Malmstroom m vacuum extractor. *Obstet. Gynecol.* **53**:750–757, 1979.
40. Rosemann, G. W. E.: Vacuum extraction of premature infants. *S. Afr. J. Obstet. Gynaecol.* **7**:10–12, 1969.
41. Schenker, J. B. and Gombos, G..: Retinal hemorrhage in the newborn. *Obstet. Gynecol.* **27**:521–524, 1966.
42. Simpson, J. V.: On a suction-tractor or new mechanical power as a substitute for forceps in tedious labours. *Edinburgh Monthly J. Med. Sci.* **32**:556–559, 618–620, 1848/1849.
43. Ullery, J. C., Teteris, N. J., Botschner, A. W., and McDaniels, B.: Traction and compression forces exerted by obstetric forcps and their effect on fetal heart rate. *Am. J. Obstet. Gynecol.* **85**:1066–1070, 1963.
44. Vacca, A., Grant, A., Wyatt, G., and Chalmers, I.: Portsmouth operative delivery trial: A comparison vacuum extraction and forceps delivery. *Br. J. Obstet. Gynaecol.* **90**:1107–1112, 1983.
45. von Barsewisch, B.: *Perinatal Retina Haemorrhages: Morphology, Aetiology, and Significance*. New York, Springer-Verlag, 1979.
46. Wider, J. A., Erez, S., and Steer, C. M.: An evaluation of the vacuum extractor in series of 201 cases. *Am. J. Obstet. Gynecol.* **98**:24–31, 1967.
47. Yonge, J.: An account of the balls of hair taken from the uterus and ovaria of several women. *Philosophical Transactions* **25**:2387, 1706–7.

45

SHOULDER DYSTOCIA

The greatest battles in obstetrics have too often been fought with the outward icily calm, but inward extremely harassed, obstetrician attempting to disguise how hard he is really pulling on the fetal head, while up on the table, kneeling, heedless of the proprieties, and of the picture she must present to the anesthetist, the nurse pushes, stiff-armed and with all her might on the fundus. Meanwhile, the plum-colored, excessively fat and cherubic face of the baby gazes reproachfully at the world.[14]

As the fetus descends through the birth canal during normal labor, the shoulders usually rotate from the direct AP plane of the maternal pelvis to an oblique plane. The anterior shoulder usually comes to rest under the ramus of the pubis and subsequently emerges from the maternal vaginal introitus after expulsion of the head. On occasion the anterior shoulder fails to rotate under the symphysis pubis, but rather becomes lodged behind it. Arrest of delivery after expulsion of the fetal head is termed *shoulder dystocia*. The usual problem is impaction of the anterior shoulder with the posterior shoulder occupying the hollow of the sacrum. On occasion the posterior shoulder is also lodged against the sacrum, resulting in more severe impaction.

The first sign of this disorder is recoil of the fetal head into the maternal perineum, described by some as the "turtle sign." Shoulder dystocia is one of the most catastrophic events that occurs during the birth process. It has the potential to cause death or lifelong injuries to the fetus and occasionally to the mother. Predelivery recognition of patients at risk for this complication and appropriate treatment of this circumstance in the delivery suite are the subject of some debate.

Shoulder dystocia is usually the result of fetal macrosomia. When the size of the fetus exceeds 4000 g, there is a statistically significant disproportionate increase in the size of the fetal trunk relative to the size of the fetal head (Table 45-1).[16] In macrosomic infants who experience shoulder dystocia, this difference is even more exaggerated and probably represents the primary etiology of the disorder (Table 45-2).

Several factors influence the reported incidences of shoulder dystocia. These factors include the incidence of macrosomic fetuses (4000 g), the primary cesarean section rate, and the inclusion or exclusion in the calculations of patients not at risk for shoulder dystocia (e.g., cesarean section, low-birth-weight infants). The expected incidence of shoulder dystocia in the general population is 2–4/1000 deliveries (Table 45-3). This incidence of shoulder dystocia increases if low-birth-weight infants and patients undergoing cesarean section are excluded. It is not possible to determine from the available data what effect the increased use of cesarean section has had on the incidence of shoulder dystocia in the United Sates. If more babies at risk for shoulder dystocia are delivered by cesarean section, the incidence of shoulder dystocia obviously would decrease.

TABLE 45-1. COMPARISON OF ANTHROPOMETRIC MEASUREMENTS IN NEWBORN INFANTS WITH BIRTH WEIGHTS GREATER THAN AND LESS THAN 4000 g, EXCLUDING LOW BIRTH WEIGHTS (<2500 g) AND INFANTS OF DIABETIC MOTHERS

Anthropometric Measurements*	Birth Weights >4000 g (*n* = 202)	Birth Weights >4000 g (*n* = 100)	*P*
Birth weight (g)	4247 ± 471	3399 ± 363	NS†
Gestational age (wk)	40.7 ± 1.3	39.6 ± 3.9	<0.001
Length (cm)	54.6 ± 2.8	51.7 ± 2.6	<0.001
Head circumference (cm)	36.3 ± 1.2	34.6 ± 1.3	<0.001
Chest circumference (cm)	36.2 ± 2.8	33.6 ± 1.8	<0.001
Chest–head (cm)	0.06 ± 1.6	−1.1 ± 1.5	<0.001

* Mean ± 1 SD.
† NS = Not significant.
Source: Adapted from Modalnou et al.[16]

TABLE 45-2. COMPARISON OF ANTHROPOMETRIC MEASUREMENTS IN NEWBORN INFANTS WITH BIRTH WEIGHTS >4000 g DELIVERED VAGINALLY WITH SHOULDER DYSTOCIA VERSUS THOSE WITHOUT SHOULDER DYSTOCIA

Anthropometric Measurements*	Shoulder Dystocia (*n* = 10)	No Shoulder Dystocia (*n* = 130)	*P*
Birth weight (g)	4416 ± 294	4254 ± 323	NS†
Gestational age (wk)	41.2 ± 1.6	40.4 ± 3.6	NS
Length (cm)	54.5 ± 1.9	54.8 ± 2.3	NS
Head circumference (cm)	36.1 ± 1.6	36.2 ± 1.1	NS
Chest circumference (cm)	37.7 ± 1.5	36.0 ± 3.3	NS
Chest–head (cm)	1.6 ± 2.2	0.2 ± 1.8	<0.025

* Mean ± 1 SD.
† NS = Not significant.
Source: Adapted from Modanlou et al.[16]

TABLE 45-3. INCIDENCE OF SHOULDER DYSTOCIA

Author	Incidence	Total Number Shoulder Dystocia/ Total Number Deliveries	Year
Benedetti and Gabbe[5]	3.4/1000	34/9864	1978
Parks and Zeil[17]	19/1000	127/6680	1978
Seigworth[21]	3.8/1000	51/13491	1966
Schwartz and McClelland[20]	1.5/1000	31/20599	1960
Johnstone[12]	2.1/1000	47/22663	1976

Several clinical circumstances increase the chance that shoulder dystocia will occur during vaginal delivery. All agree that fetal macrosomia increases the incidence of shoulder dystocia. If one evaluates the risk of brachial plexus injury due to shoulder dystocia on the basis of birth weight only, a statistically significant increase is noted at birth weights in excess of 4 kg. However, the relative risk increases from 2.6 for infants weighing between 4 and 4.5 kg to 21.6 for infants weighing in excess of 4.5 kg.[15] Unfortunately, accurate prediction of fetal macrosomia, whether defined as weighing more than 4000 g or weighing more than 4500 g, still eludes clinical detection.

In the absence of accurate clinical prediction

of fetal weight, investigators have turned to other factors that might be associated with increased risk of fetal macrosomia. Prepregnant maternal weight of over either 180 or 200 lb,[17,20,21] a history of prior infants weighing in excess of 4000 g,[19-22] and gestation prolonged beyond 42 weeks,[12,17] all increase the risk of shoulder dystocia, undoubtedly because of the increased incidence of fetal macrosomia associated with each of these conditions. However, none of the factors, considered alone or in combination, yields a high predictive value for shoulder dystocia.

A more useful approach to prediction of shoulder dystocia is consideration of labor and delivery factors. Abnormalities of the first and second stages of labor have been associated with shoulder dystocia.[5,9,12,13,19] Midforceps deliveries also are associated with a high incidence of shoulder dystocia, but in many studies associated labor abnormalities are not identified.[5,11,21] Few studies consider multiple factors in a way that is clinically meaningful for the practicing obstetrician.

The incidence of shoulder dystocia following second-stage labor abnormalities, considering fetal weight and method of delivery, is illustrated in Table 45-4.[5] In the presence of a normal second stage of labor, midpelvic delivery even of a macrosomic fetus results in only a 1.2% incidence of shoulder dystocia. However, when a macrosomic fetus is delivered from the midpelvis after a prolonged second stage of labor, the incidence of shoulder dystocia is 23%.

Clinically, a combination of the historical and labor high-risk factors outlined above should alert the obstetrician to the patient at increased risk for shoulder dystocia. However, accurate identification of the macrosomic fetus has continued to elude the obstetrician. Recently, the use of ultrasound has provided some hope in this area. Based on anthropometric observations in macrosomic neonates which showed differences from those in normal neonates, some investigators have attempted to reproduce these measurements on intrauterine fetuses, using real-time ultrasound.

Standard measurement of fetal biparietal diameter combined with measurement of the fetal abdominal diameter just below the level of the heart has been used in these studies. The abdominal diameter is an average of the transverse diameter and the anterior posterior measurement $\frac{TV + AP}{2}$. In diabetic patients, fetal macrosomia correlates positively with a difference between chest and biparietal diameter of greater than 1.4 cm.[6] This method has been used to study a group of 29 patients judged to be at high risk for shoulder dystocia using three criteria (Class A diabetes, estimated fetal weight greater than 4 kg, fundal height over 42 cm). All eight patients who subsequently suffered shoulder dystocia were predicted correctly using the AD-BPD diameter of more than 1.4 cm.[25]

This new method may aid in detection of patients at risk for shoulder dystocia. However, further clinical trials involving all patients at risk for shoulder dystocia rather than a selected sample are necessary before this technique can be advocated as a standard method of identification. Furthermore, the method requires identification prior to labor or in early labor. Difficulty in obtaining these measurements after labor has advanced into the second stage may preclude its use in many patients not identified prior to this time.

DELIVERY ROOM MANAGEMENT OF SHOULDER DYSTOCIA

Nearly 70–80% of shoulder dystocias follow spontaneous deliveries and occur without prior warning. Although the Woods maneuver[26] commonly is advocated to relieve shoulder dystocia, there are no data published regarding the out-

TABLE 45-4. RELATIONSHIP BETWEEN SHOULDER DYSTOCIA, WEIGHT, AND METHOD OF DELIVERY[5]

Method of Delivery	Weight (g)	Incidence	Percent	P
*PSS and midpelvic delivery	<4000	6/360	1.6	<0.01
	>4000	13/56	23	
All other vertex vaginal deliveries	<4000	6/7836	0.07	<0.01
	>4000	8/638	1.2	

* Prolonged second stage of labor

come of this method. The maneuver requires the obstetrician to apply fundal pressure with one hand while using two fingers to rotate the posterior shoulder in a clockwise direction. Most obstetricians recognize that, although intellectually attractive, this method of relieving shoulder dystocia is rarely successful. The same can be said of the procedure decribed by Hibbard,[10] which depends on appropriately timed fundal pressure to accomplish delivery. Fundal pressure is an inappropriate way to relieve shoulder dystocia for two reasons: (1) it often results in further impaction of the shoulder against the symphysis, and (2) it can result in catastrophic uterine rupture.

The successful management of shoulder dystocia requires some critical judgments on the part of the obstetrician. The first one is recognition of the problem before excessive lateral traction which may result in brachial plexus injury applied to the fetal neck. If the usual delivery maneuvers fail to dislodge the shoulder from behind the symphysis, lateral traction should be abandoned until further preparations are made. These preparations include summoning anesthesia assistance and informing the patient and the nurses present that there is a problem in delivering the baby. Careful, clear, and calm directions must be given to each participant in the delivery process in order to maximize the possibility of favorable outcome.

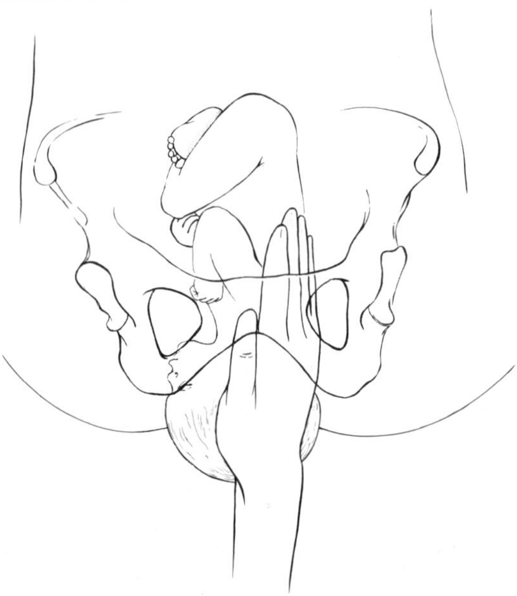

Figure 45-1. The attendant's hand is inserted along the back of the fetus and pressure is applied against the scapula in an attempt to rotate the shoulder from behind the symphysis.

The next step should be to try to slip one's hand along the fetal back underneath the symphysis to try to rotate the shoulders (Fig. 45-1). At the same time ask the nurse to exert suprapubic pressure in an oblique direction (Fig. 45-2). The purpose of these actions is to rotate the shoulder internally so that it slips from behind the symphysis to a position under the pubic ramus. In cases of mild shoulder impaction, these maneuvers will dislodge the shoulders and no further actions are necessary.

In the event that these initial maneuvers fail to relieve the impacted shoulders, the McRoberts maneuver[8] should be tried. The parturient should be instructed to grasp her posterior thighs and to flex them against her abdomen and chest. If the patient is anesthetized, the assistants present in the delivery room should aid the patient in asuming this position. This maneuver results in anterior rotation of the symphysis and a flattening of the angle of inclination of the symphysis that frequently dislodges the impacted shoulder (Figs. 45-3 and 45-4).

If this maneuver fails to relieve the shoulder dystocia, preparation should be made to extract the posterior arm. A proctoepisiotomy should be made with the incision extending approximately 4 cm into the rectum. The delivery attendant's hand should be inserted posteriorly and the humerus located. The humeral shaft should be traced until the antecubital fossa is located. The forearm should be flexed, the hand grasped and the arm swept across the chest and out the vaginal introitus. This will disimpact the obstructed wedge created by the fetal shoulders. Efforts should be redirected toward delivery of the anterior shoulder after delivery of the posterior shoulder. If gentle traction still fails to effect delivery of the anterior shoulder, the obstetrician should rotate the posterior shoulder in a clockwise direction 180 degrees to effect delivery of the anterior shoulder. These maneuvers are illustrated in Figs. 45-5–45-10.[2-4]

Rarely, the posterior shoulder also is found to be impacted against the sacrum or the posterior arm is found to be trapped along the dorsal (back) surface of the fetus (Fig. 45-11). In this instance, the obstetrician has no choice but to fracture the fetal humerus and "green stick" the arm into the ventral aspect of the fetus and out the introitus. This injury to the fetus will infre-

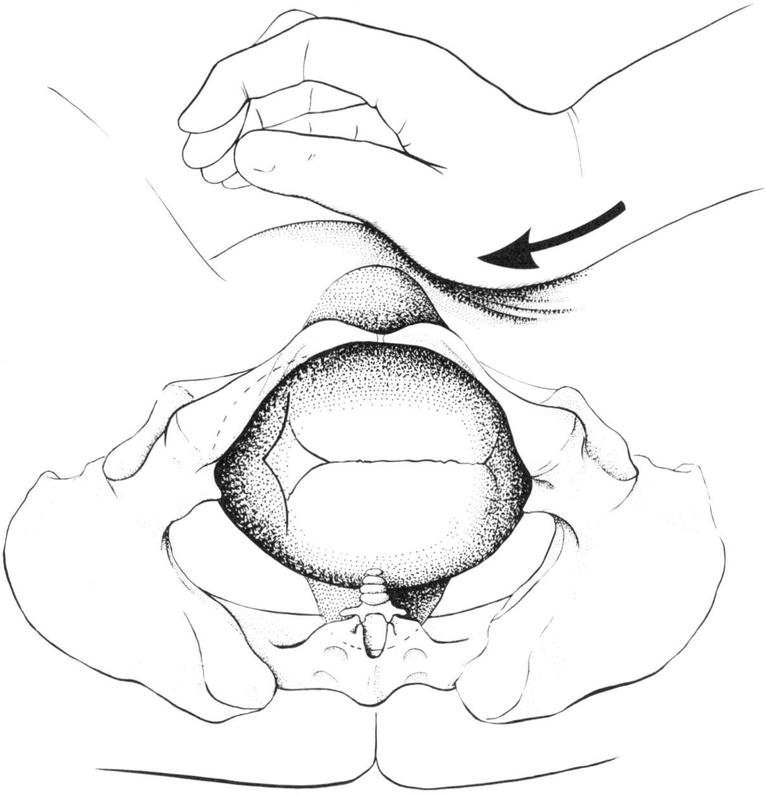

Figure 45-2. Suprapubic pressure is applied in an oblique direction to aid in the rotation of the fetal shoulder from behind the symphysis.

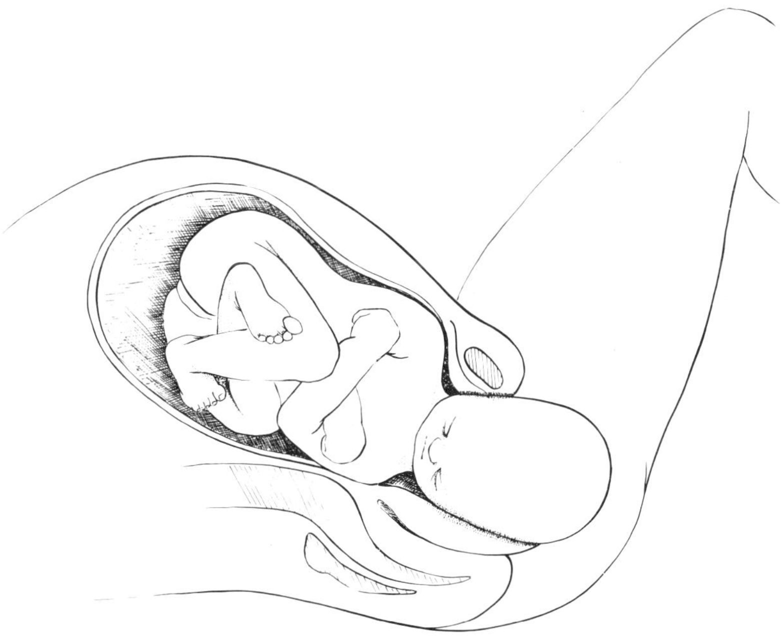

Figure 45-3. Impacted shoulder while mother is in the dorsal lithotomy position.

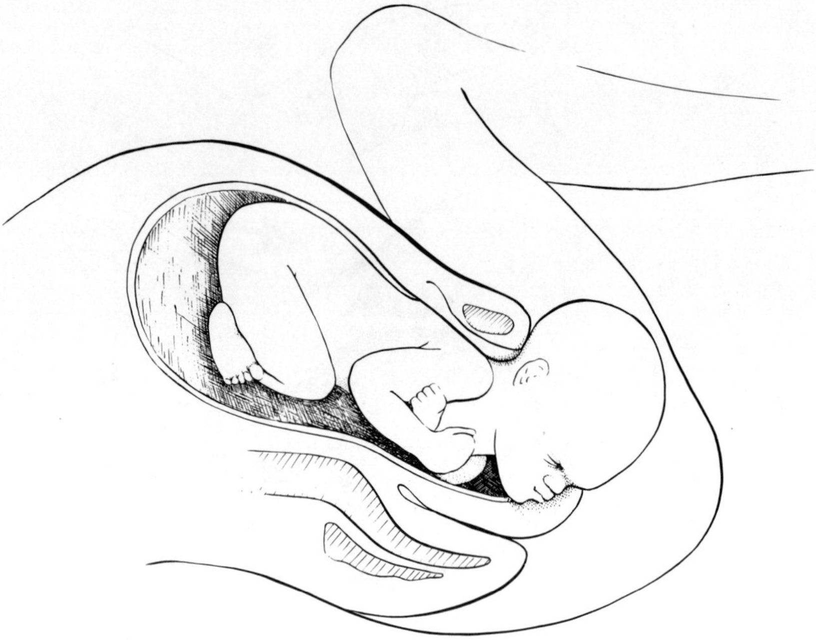

Figure 45-4. Dorsiflexion of the hips results in the cephalad rotation of the symphysis and concomitant flattening of the angle of inclination of the symphysis. This often allows release of the impacted shoulder.

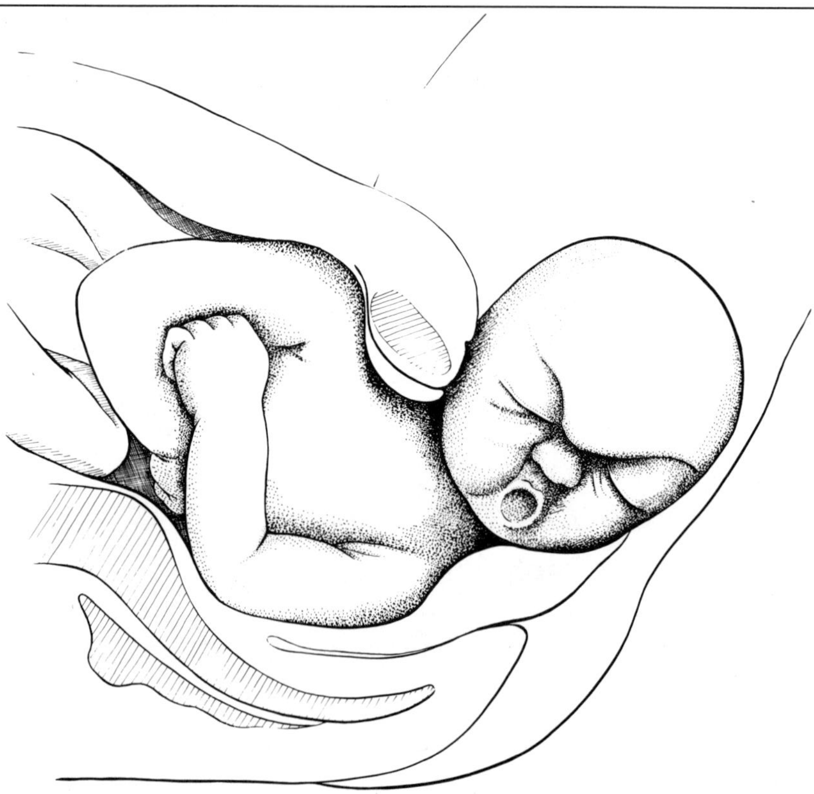

Figure 45-5. Impaction of the anterior shoulder.

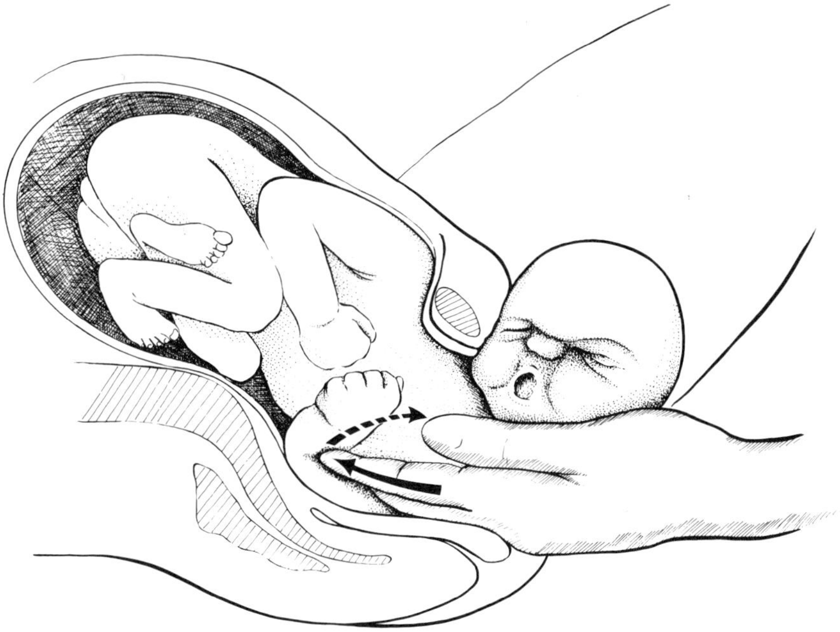

Figure 45-6. To bring the wrist within reach, exert pressure with the index finger at the bend of the fetal elbow. This maneuver is similar to the Pinard maneuver during breech delivery.

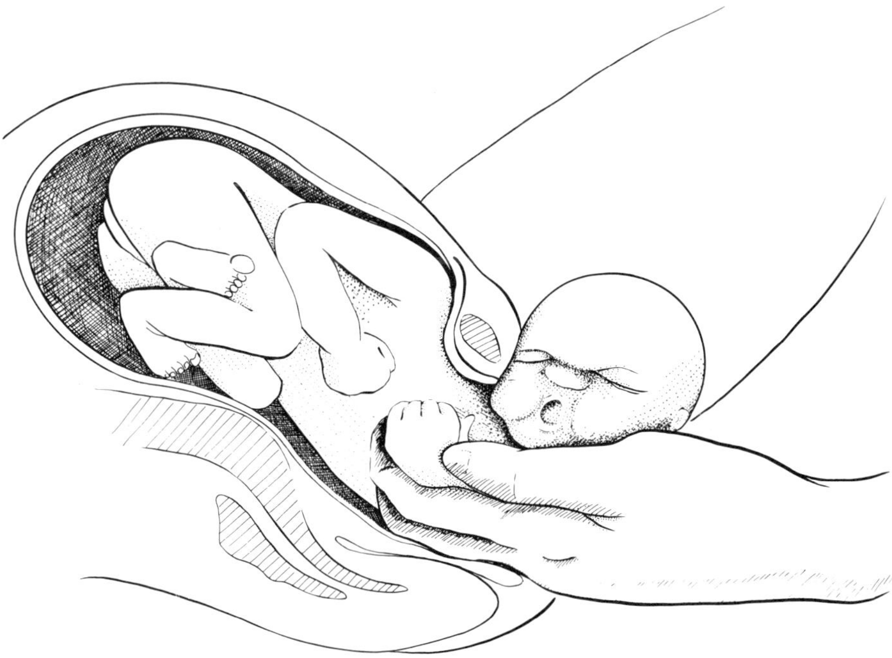

Figure 45-7. Sweep the fetal forearm down across the front of the fetal chest.

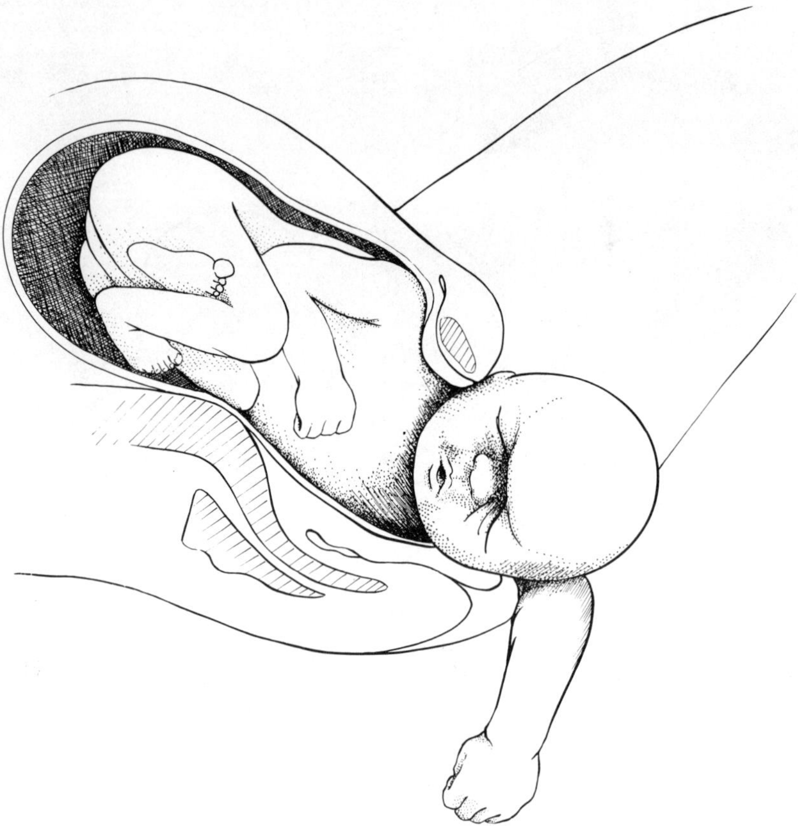

Figure 45-8. Deliver the posterior arm through the introitus.

quently result in permanent injury and is certainly preferable to a brachial plexus injury or a prolonged period of hypoxemia.

I am aware of three instances of shoulder dystocia where all efforts failed to result in delivery of the fetus. In each instance, the obstetrician forced the fetal head back into the vagina and performed a cesarean section. Two of these instances resulted in a liveborn, undamaged fetus. In the third instance, the fetus was known to be dead prior to delivery but was so massive that it could not be delivered vaginally. Rather than attempt a destructive procedure, the obstetrician elected to reposit the head and perform cesarean section.

It is not always possible to deliver an undamaged infant after shoulder dystocia. The most serious injuries are to the brachial plexus. It is preferable to fracture the humerus rather than to risk injury to the brachial plexus from excessive lateral traction on the fetal head. However, even when this emergency is managed optimally, brachial plexus injuries occur. I believe that some injuries to the brachial plexus are associated with the process of impaction at the symphysis or during arrested descent into the pelvis. A number of cases of brachial plexus injury in vertex infants delivered by cesarean section tend to support this hypothesis.[1,7,15] In such instances, injury to the brachial plexus seems unavoidable.

It is essential that there be clear documentation in the chart of the exact events that have taken place during delivery of an infant after shoulder dystocia. If the infant is unfortunate enough to suffer permanent brachial plexus injury, there is a high likelihood of malpractice litigation. The best defense can be mounted if there is a clearly documented description of the efforts made to deliver the fetus.

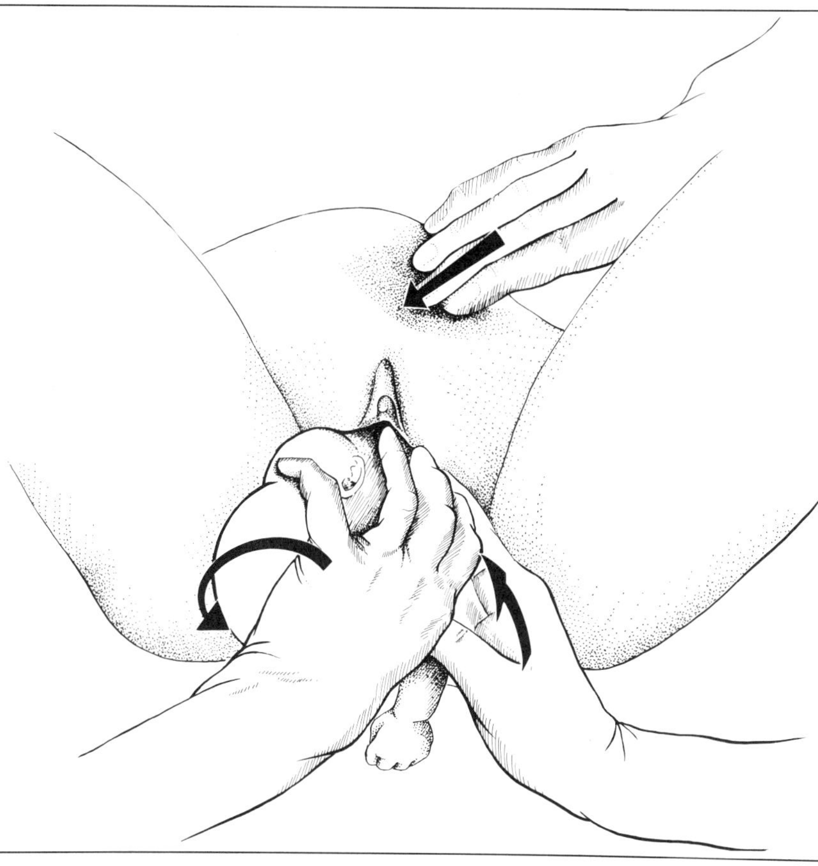

Figure 45-9. If unable to deliver the fetus with downward traction after releasing the posterior arm, grasp the occiput with one hand and the posterior shoulder with the other hand. Have an assistant apply suprapubic pressure.

BRACHIAL PLEXUS INJURY

In a recent study analyzing more than 210,000 births in the state of Washington, brachial plexus injury was reported on the birth certificates in 104 instances.[15] Assuming that the incidence of shoulder dystocia was 3/1000 among the population of vertex vaginal deliveries, the incidence of brachial plexus injuries after shoulder dystocia is one in six.

Brachial plexus palsies have been classified according to the pattern of nerve root involvement. The majority of infants have upper root (C5, C6) damage, which is Erb's palsy. Clinically, the shoulder girdle muscles are most affected, whereas the hand is relatively normal. The next most frequent injury is the complete lesion in which there is some damage to the entire brachial plexus (C5–T1). In the third type of injury, Klumpke's paralysis, the C8–T1 nerve roots are the site of damage, resulting in poor hand function with good shoulder function. In most brachial plexus injuries, sensory changes are minimal because of the dermatomal overlap from functioning root levels.

The risk of permanent brachial plexus injury has been reported to be from 22–44% (Table 44-5).[7,9,18,23,24] This figure varies depending on the severity of residual injury and the length of follow-up after the injury. The lowest figures are quoted from follow-up studies on infants with brachial plexus injuries recognized at birth. The higher figures tend to be reported by neurologists who first see the infant a few days to months after birth. The longer the palsy persists, the poorer is the prognosis for complete recovery.

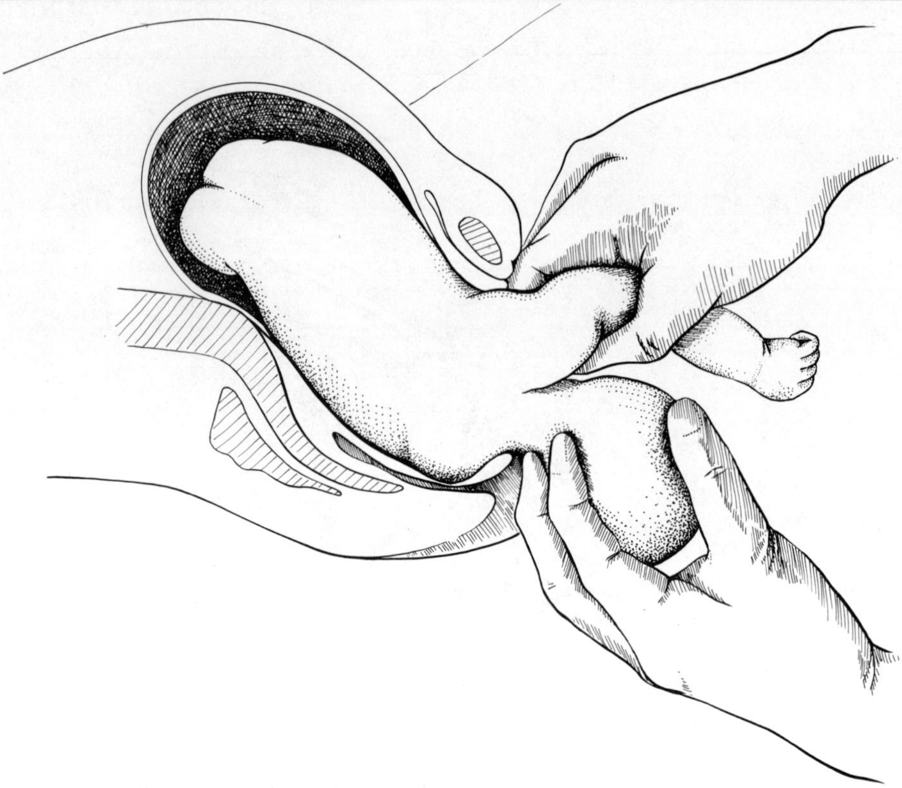

Figure 45-10. Completion of the rotation of the fetus usually results in the complete release of the impaction.

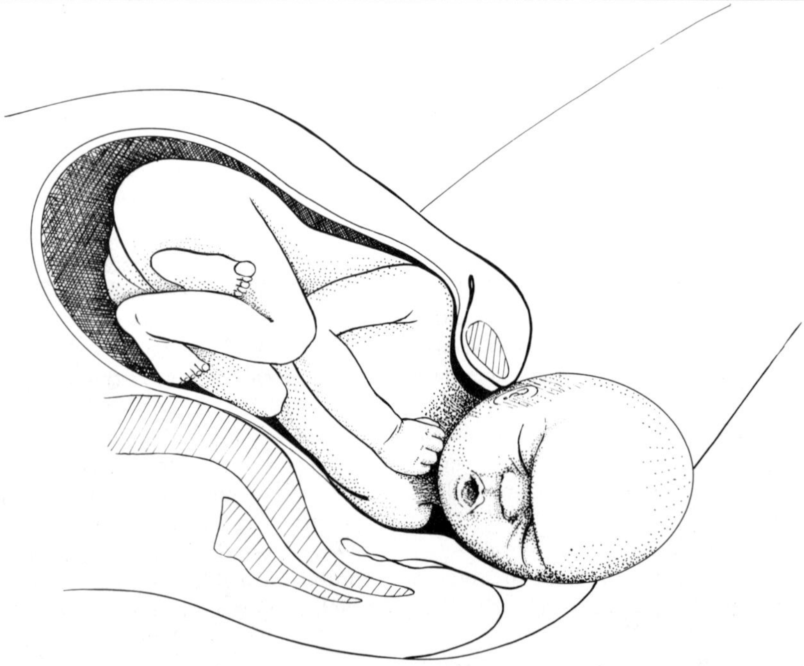

Figure 45-11. In the uncommon event that the posterior arm is trapped behind the fetus, the humerus may be purposefully fractured by inserting the attendant's finger at mid-shaft in the humerus and flexing the attendant's finger. The posterior arm may then be delivered after grasping the forearm of the fetus and delivering the arm as illustrated in figures 45-6–45-8.

TABLE 45-5. NEONATAL FOLLOW-UP OF INFANTS WITH BRACHIAL PLEXUS INJURY

Author	Number of Infants	Lost to Follow-up	Length of Follow-up	Permanent Injury
Gordon et al.[9]	60	8	48 months	7%
Tan[23]	57	22	9 months	34%
Rubin[18]	18	?	?	22%
Eng et al.[7]	135	16	>24 months	30%
Wickstrom[24]	75	0	24 months	44%

SUMMARY

Shoulder dystocia can have devastating long-term consequences for the infant. Avoidance of shoulder dystocia involves being constantly aware of patients at risk for development of this obstetric emergency. Risk factors include maternal obesity, previous macrosomic infant, maternal diabetes, prolonged pregnancy, and arrest disorders of the first and second stage of labor. Methods of accurate estimation of fetal weight are still under development. The obstetrician should clinically estimate fetal weight when faced with high-risk factors. A fetal weight judged to be more than 4000 g in combination with arrest disorders of labor and high-risk historical factors warrants strong consideration of cesarean section. Suspicion of fetal weight in excess of 4500 g should be considered an indication for cesarean section. In these instances, attempted midpelvic delivery is a poor choice. Avoidance of midpelvic delivery in the patient at high risk for shoulder dystocia is the best way to prevent the 25–30% of shoulder dystocias that are potentially avoidable.

At present, most shoulder dystocias are not preventable and occur sporadically and without warning. The obstetrician must be forearmed with a logical plan for management of these emergencies that focuses on the avoidance of brachial plexus injury to the fetus.

REFERENCES

1. Adler, J. B. and Patterson, R. L. J.: Erb's palsy long term results of treatment in 88 cases. *J. Bone Joint Surg.* **49A**:1052–1064, 1967.
2. Barnum, C. G.: Dystocia due to the shoulders. *Am. J. Obstet. Gynecol.* **50**:452, 1945.
3. Benedetti T. J.: Managing shoulder dystocia. *Contemp. OB/GYN* **14**:33–40, 1979.
4. Benedetti, T. J. and Chez, R. A.: How to manage a shoulder dystocia during delivery. *Contemp. OB/GYN* **19**:203–209, 1982.
5. Benedetti, T. J. and Gabbe, S. C.: Shoulder dystocia: A complication of fetal macrosomia and prolonged second stage of labor with midpelvic delivery. *Obstet. Gynecol.* **52**:526–529, 1978.
6. Elliott, J. P., Garite, T. H., Freeman, R. K., McQuown, D. S., and Patel, J. M.: Ultrasonic prediction of fetal macrosomia in diabetic patients. *Journal.* **60**:159–162, 1982.
7. Eng, G. D., Hoch, B., and Smokvina, M. D.: Brachial plexus palsy in neonates and children. *Arch. Phys. Med. Rehabil.* **59**:458–464, 1978.
8. Gonik, B., Stringer, C. A., and Held, B.: An alternate maneuver for management of shoulder dystocia. *Am. J. Obstet. Gynecol.* **145**:882–885, 1983.
9. Gordon, M., Rich, H., Deutschberger, J. and Green, M.: The immediate and long-term outcome of obstetric birth trauma: Brachial plexus. *Am. J. Obstet. Gynecol.* **117**:51–56, 1973.
10. Hibbard, I. T.: Shoulder dystocia. *Obstet. Gynecol.* **34**:424–429, 1969.
11. Hughey, M.: Midforceps delivery. *J. Reprod. Med.* **20**:253–260, 1978.
12. Johnstone, N. R.: Shoulder girdle dystocia: A study of 47 cases. *Aust. N.Z. J. Obstet. Gynaecol.* **19**:28–31, 1979.
13. Khatree, M. D. H., Gamsu, H. R., Rudd, P., and Studd, J. W.: Features predictive of brachial plexus injury during labor. *S. Afr. Med. J.* **61**:232–233, 1982.
14. Kinch, R. A.: Shoulder girdle dystocia. *Clin. Obstet. Gynecol.* **5**:1031–1043, 1962.
15. McFarland, L. V., Raskin, M., Benedetti, T. J., and Daling, J. R.: Erb-Duchenne palsy: A consequence of macrosomia and method of delivery, *Obstet. Gynecol.* (submitted).
16. Modanlou, H. D., Komatsu, G., Dorchester, W., Freeman, R. K., and Bosu, S. K.: Large for gestational age neonates. Anthropometric reasons for shoulder dystocia. *Obstet. Gynecol.* **60**:417–423, 1982.
17. Parks, G. D., and Zeil, H. K.: Macrosomia: A proposed indication for primary cesarean section. *Obstet. Gynecol.* **52**:407–409, 1978.
18. Rubin, A.: Birth injuries: Incidence, mechanisms, and end results. *Obstet. Gynecol.* **23**:219–221, 1964.
19. Sack, R. A.: The large infant. *Am. J. Obstet. Gynecol.* **104**:195–204, 1969.

20. Schwartz, B. C. and McClelland, D. D.: Shoulder dystocia. *Obstet. Gynecol.* **11**:468–471, 1958.
21. Seigworth, G. R.: Shoulder dystocia: Review of five years experience. *Obstet. Gynecol.* **28**:764–767, 966.
22. Swartz, D. P.: Shoulder girdle dystocia in vertex delivery: Clinical study and review. *Obstet. Gynecol.* **15**:194–205, 1960.
23. Tan, K. L.: Brachial palsy. *J. Obstet. Gynaecol. Br. Commonw.* **80**:60–62, 1973.
24. Wickstrom, J.: Birth injuries of the brachial plexus. *Clin. Orthop.* **23**:187–196, 1962.
25. Williams, J., III, Kirz, D. S., Worthen, N. J., and Oakes, G. K.: Ultrasound prediction of shoulder dystocia. Presented at the Fifth Annual Meeting of the Society of Perinatal Obstetricians, Las Vegas, NV, 1985, p. 27 (Abstract 11).
26. Woods, C. E.: The principle of physics as applicable to shoulder delivery. *Am. J. Obstet. Gynecol.* **45**:796–802, 1943.

46

CESAREAN DELIVERY AND CESAREAN HYSTERECTOMY

CESAREAN DELIVERY

History

Major landmarks in the evolution of cesarean childbirth (Table 46-1) are discussed briefly in succeeding paragraphs. A recent monograph offers a detailed review of the history of cesarean section.[68]

In the eighth century B.C., the Roman ruler Numa Pompilius established a law requiring that postmortem abdominal delivery be performed whenever a woman died late in pregnancy. The purpose of the statute was twofold: to attempt to save the life of the fetus and to permit separate entombment of mother and fetus. This law, originally termed *lex regia*, was continued under the rule of the Roman emperors and became known as *lex caesarea*.

Although isolated references to cesarean delivery appear in early scientific writings, the details of the operations are poorly documented. It was not until 1500 that cesarean delivery was allegedly performed on a living patient.[68] In that year, Jacob Neufer, a German farmer, reportedly performed the operation on his wife. The woman survived and subsequently delivered two other children vaginally. This remarkable achievement was not described in the literature until 1591, and several historians question the authenticity of the report.

In 1668, the French obstetrician Francois Mauriceau reviewed the European obstetric experience with cesarean delivery and concluded that the procedure almost invariably resulted in maternal death and therefore should be performed only in rare and desperate situations.[68]

In 1822, Francis and Beck[23] reported the first self-performed cesarean delivery in the United States. The patient was a 14-year-old servant girl who was pregnant with twins.

> While the family was at dinner, she went a distance of perhaps fifty rods from the house, and placed herself on a snowdrift, near a fence, where she was first discovered by her master in the act of covering something with snow, which afterwards proved to be a naked child. As soon as she perceived that she was observed, she immediately ran to the house, with the second child hanging out at the wound, together with a considerable portion of her intestines; laid by her razor and large needle, which were the instruments she had previously prepared for the operation, and shortly began to complain.[23]

In 1830, John Lambert Richmond became the first American physician to successfully perform a cesarean delivery.[38] The patient had been in labor for over 30 hours, but her cervix remained minimally dilated. She was experiencing recurrent eclamptic convulsions when he took over her care from two midwives. Alarmed by the deterioration in the woman's condition, Richmond, "feeling a deep and solemn sense of my responsibility, with only a case of common pocket instruments, about one o'clock at night..." performed a cesarean section. Despite making a classical uterine incision, Richmond was unable to extract the fetus.

> . . . As soon as the gush of blood partially subsided, I commenced my efforts to remove the child, but it was

TABLE 46-1. MAJOR DEVELOPMENTS IN THE HISTORY OF CESAREAN DELIVERY

8th century B.C.	Roman leader Numa Pompilius established the *Lex regia* requiring postmortem cesarean delivery.
2nd–6th century A.D.	Poorly documented references to cesarean delivery included in the Talmud.
1500	First cesarean delivery in a living patient. Report not published until 1591.
1822	First self-performed cesarean section in the United States.
1830	Richmond is first American physician to perform cesarean section.
1876	Porro performed first cesarean hysterectomy in which both mother and infant survived.
1882	Sanger described closure of uterine wall with wire sutures.
1907	Frank described the extraperitoneal approach for cesarean delivery.
1909	Latzko reported major modification of Frank's technique, ensuring that the operation was entirely extraperitoneal.
1912	Krönig described vertical incision in lower uterine segment.
1919–1922	Beck and DeLee popularized the vertical lower-segment incision in the United States.
1926	Kerr described the transverse lower-segment incision.
1950–present	Improvements in anesthetic techniques, blood-banking technology, and supportive medical care.
1965–present	Increased understanding of the pathophysiology, treatment, and prevention of postcesarean infection.

uncommonly large. . . . Thinking the danger to the mother very great and believing . . . the child was dead from detachment of the placenta, and considering at all events that a childless mother was better than a motherless child, I determined to do all I could for the preservation of the mother. Accordingly I made a transverse incision across the back of the foetus . . . by which means I was enabled easily to extract it. . . .[38]

The patient ultimately survived, despite developing a pelvic abscess. "She commenced work in twenty-four days from the operation, and in the fifth week walked a mile and back the same day."

Until the early twentieth century, a high maternal mortality was associated with cesarean section. In 1865, the maternal mortality from cesarean delivery was 85% in Great Britain and Ireland. For the 90 years ending 1876, French obstetricians were unable to report a single patient who survived the operation. The vast majority of deaths were the result of either exsanguination or overwhelming septicemia.[61]

In the late nineteenth century, two major innovations greatly improved the safety of abdominal delivery. In 1876, Porro[56] performed the first cesarean hysterectomy in which both mother and child survived. Hysterectomy was recommended as a means of preventing the serious intra-abdominal sepsis that resulted when an infected uterus was left in place. In 1882, Sanger described a technique for closure of the uterine wall with wire sutures.[21] Sanger had used this technique in only one operation and based his recommendation primarily on reports of 16 operations performed by American frontier surgeons.

Frank Polin (1852) was the first American physician credited with use of sutures to close the uterus after cesarean delivery. He used silver wire sutures, as J. Marion Sims had recently recommended for closure of vesicovaginal fistulae. Although his patient survived, Polin did not publish a report of his success. Sixteen years later, in 1868, Brickell published the first American report describing use of sutures for uterine closure.[21] Maternal mortality in these early American reports was "only" 50%, and Sanger acknowledged that the new technique was a major deterrent to exsanguinating hemorrhage.

The next major development in cesarean delivery was Frank's description in 1907 of extraperitoneal cesarean section.[24] Frank opened the peritoneal cavity just above the pubis and then sutured the parietal peritoneum to the visceral peritoneum at the point of the vesicouterine reflection. This sealed off the peritoneal cavity before opening the uterus through a vertical incision. Two years later, Latzko[40] reported a major modification of the procedure, which avoided entry into the peritoneal cavity. The extraperitoneal operation was designed to prevent the peritoneal contamination that occurred once the uterus was opened.

In 1912, Krönig used a transperitoneal approach, dissected the bladder away from the lower uterine segment, and entered the uterus through a short vertical incision.[61] In the early 1920s, Beck[7] and DeLee and Cornell[12] popularized the vertical lower segment operation in the United States. In 1926, Munro Kerr[37] of Glasgow modified Krönig's technique and performed a transverse incision in the lower uterine segment. It was not until 1949, however, at the Twelfth British Congress of Obstetricians and Gynecologists, that Kerr finally noted general acceptance of his procedure. Raising his arms over his head, he proclaimed, "Allelujah! The strife is o'er, the battle done."[49] The Kerr procedure now is the most popular type of cesarean section.

Several developments during the past 30 years have enhanced further the safety of cesarean delivery. Improvements in anesthetic techniques, blood-banking technology, and supportive medical care, particularly intravenous fluid therapy, have benefited all surgical patients. Obstetric patients have particularly benefited from improved understanding of the pathophysiology and microbiology of postcesarean infection.

Indications for Cesarean Delivery

The past 30 years have seen a marked increase in the number of cesarean deliveries performed in the United States. The average incidence of cesarean delivery rose from approximately 4% in 1950 to almost 15% in 1980[47] (Fig. 46-1). Some medical centers report cesarean delivery rates that exceed 20%. The increased incidence of operative deliveries has coincided with changes in obstetric practice, most notably: (1) widespread application of ultrasound and electronic fetal monitoring, (2) intensified multidisciplinary approach to management of pregnant women with major medical illnesses, and (3) enhanced safety of the operation. The increase has coincided with an equally marked decrease in the perinatal mortality rate. This latter is due primarily to other changes in obstetric practice and only in part to the increased incidence of operative delivery.

Four indications account for most of the increase in the cesarean delivery rate: dystocia, repeat cesarean section, breech presentation, and fetal distress[47] (Fig. 46-2). It is our opinion that the incidence of cesarean delivery can (and should) be reduced without adversely affecting

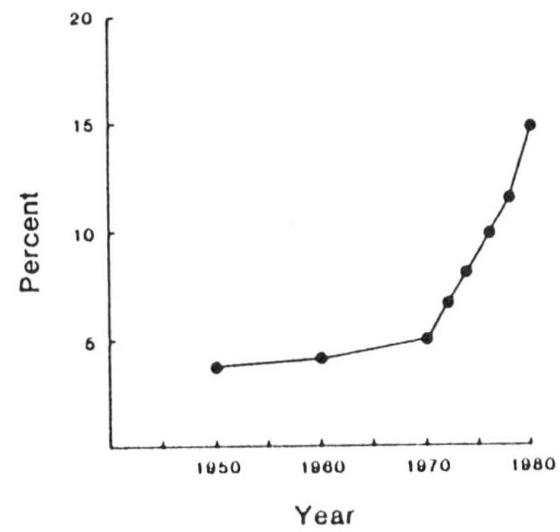

Figure 46-1. Incidence of cesarean delivery in the United States, 1950 to 1980.

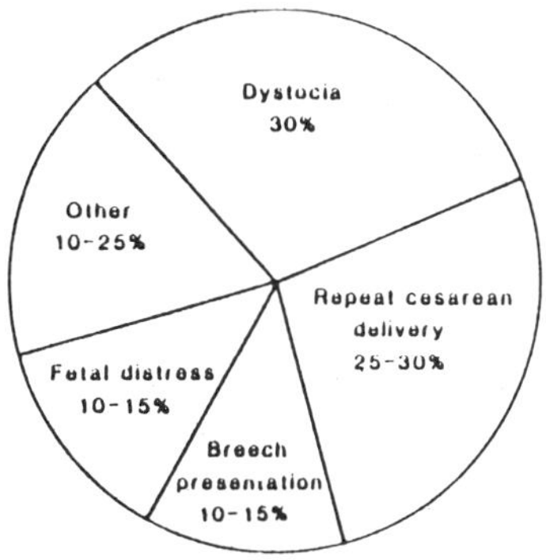

Figure 46-2. Principal indications responsible for the increased incidence of cesarean delivery in the United States.

either perinatal or maternal outcome. The clinical entities that warrant additional attention are active management of abnormal labor, trial of labor after previous cesarean delivery, and breech presentation.[47]

Table 46-2 lists clinical situations in which cesarean delivery may be indicated. Each of these indications is discussed in detail in other chapters of this book. The leading indication is dystocia or dysfunctional labor, which accounts for approximately 50 to 60% of cesarean sections. Breech presentation is responsible for an additional 15–25%, fetal distress for 3–15%, and abruptio placentae and placenta previa together account for 6–11% of primary cesarean sections. In aggregate, these entities are the indications for 80–90% of primary abdominal deliveries.

TABLE 46-2. SELECTED INDICATIONS FOR CESAREAN DELIVERY

Arrest of progress in labor (dystocia)
- Failed induction
- Inadequate uterine contractility despite administration of oxytocin
- Arrest of dilation in the active phase of labor
- Arrest of descent in the second stage of labor

Abnormal presentation
- Preterm breech (estimated fetal weight <2000 g)
- Term breech
  - Incomplete breech
  - Hyperextended breech head
- Shoulder
- Compound
- Face—persistent mentum posterior
- Brow

Fetal distress
- Persistent abnormal fetal heart rate tracing
- Declining scalp pH or single scalp pH <7.20

Third-trimester bleeding
- Abruptio placentae
- Placenta previa

Repeat cesarean delivery in patients who are not candidates for trial of labor
- Prior classical cesarean section
- Recurrent indication for abdominal delivery

Fetal anomalies
- Hydrocephalus
- Abdominal wall defect—gastroschisis, omphalocele
- Sacrococcygeal teratoma

Prior uterine surgery that weakened myometrial integrity
- Cornual resection
- Resection of intramural leiomyoma

Medical or obstetric indication for delivery and cervix unfavorable for induction of labor
- Hypertensive disorder
- Diabetes
- Rh disease
- Intrauterine growth retardation
- Abnormal antepartum surveillance test

Perioperative Complications

Maternal Mortality. In the twentieth century, maternal mortality secondary to operative delivery has declined sharply.[47] For example, in 1970, maternal mortality for cesarean delivery was 113.8 per 100,000 operations. By 1978, mortality had decreased to 40.9 per 100,000. A recent report documented no maternal deaths in 10,231 cesarean deliveries performed during the 11-year period 1968–1978.[25]

The leading causes of maternal death associated with cesarean section are infection, hemorrhage, pulmonary embolism, and complications of anesthesia. Foremost among the latter are aspiration pneumonitis and cardiopulmonary arrest.[47] In reviewing maternal mortality data, it is not always possible to determine precisely whether death was due to the operation itself or to the condition that created the requirement for abdominal delivery. However, despite major improvements in anesthetic and surgical techniques, cesarean delivery still is associated with at least a two- to fourfold increased risk of maternal death compared to vaginal delivery.[47]

Urinary Tract Injury. The incidence of bladder injuries at cesarean section is about 0.3%. The incidence of bladder injury associated with primary and repeat cesarean section is 0.19% and 0.60%, respectively. Injury typically occurs in patients who have had prior cesarean deliveries and have extensive adhesions between the bladder and lower uterine segment or between the bladder and under surface of the anterior abdominal wall. The most common site of injury is the lower posterior wall of the bladder. Primary intraoperative repair of the bladder defect usually results in healing without subsequent development of a vesicovaginal fistula.[22]

The incidence of ureteral injuries is about 0.09%. Most ureteral injuries occur when the ureter is ligated accidentally during efforts to control hemorrhage from the major uterine vessels. Ureteral injuries identified intraoperatively can be repaired primarily. When the ureter has been ligated, removal of the ligature is the only treatment necessary. If the ureter is crushed by a clamp or actually severed, resection of the damaged tissue followed by ureteroureteral anastomosis or ureteroneocystostomy is necessary.

Infection. Infection is the most common complication of cesarean delivery. Figure 46-3 summarizes the range and mean incidence of specific postcesarean infections reported in selected studies published in the American obstetric literature since 1970.[17] All patients underwent surgery without antibiotic prophylaxis.

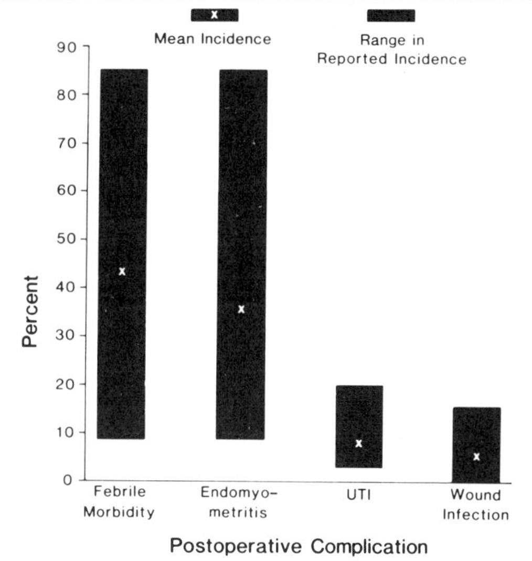

Figure 46-3. Incidence of infection after cesarean section.

Principal risk factors for postcesarean infection are young age, low socioeconomic status, multiple vaginal examinations, and extended duration of both labor and ruptured membranes. Variables such as type of anesthesia, duration of internal fetal monitoring, preoperative hematocrit, and level of experience of the surgeon bear an inconsistent relationship to incidence of infection. The lowest incidence of infection occurs in middle-class, private patients undergoing scheduled abdominal delivery. The highest incidence of infection occurs in indigent patients undergoing cesarean delivery after long labors with ruptured membranes. In certain patient populations, the incidence of infection is even higher. For example, as many as 85% of indigent women who have ruptured membranes for more than 6 hours and who subsequently require cesarean delivery for cephalopelvic disproportion may develop endometritis.[13]

Endometritis is the most common postcesarean infection. Approximately 10% of women with endometritis have associated bacteremia.[17] Fortunately, the vast majority of infected patients, including those with bacteremia, are cured readily with broad spectrum antibiotic therapy. Less than 2% of patients with endometritis develop life-threatening complications such as septic shock, pelvic abscess, and septic pelvic thrombophlebitis.[17]

Hemorrhage. The average blood loss during cesarean delivery is 1000–1100 cc. Placenta previa, abruptio placentae, preeclampsia, and multiple gestation predispose to excessive blood loss at cesarean section.

Surgical technique itself may influence intraoperative blood loss. A classical uterine incision usually causes more blood loss than a low transverse or low vertical incision. When the lower uterine segment is poorly developed, as in preterm gestation, lateral extension of the incision into the major uterine vessels may occur. Vertical extensions of the lower segment incision into the vagina or the uterine fundus also may result in excessive intraoperative blood loss. Tubal ligation or incidental appendectomy generally do not increase the incidence of intraoperative hemorrhage.

The need for perioperative transfusion depends on several variables, the most important of which are the original indication for surgery, the socioeconomic status of the patient, the patient's preoperative hematocrit, and the surgical skill of the obstetrician. Less than 10% of middle-class patients undergoing elective repeat cesarean section or primary cesarean section for arrest of progress in labor require transfusion. The requirement for transfusion may be higher in indigent, anemic women undergoing emergency cesarean delivery.[47]

Operative Technique

Skin Incision. The peritoneal cavity may be entered through either a vertical or transverse skin incision (Figs. 46-4 and 46-5). The vertical incision usually is made in the midline, extending from a point approximately 2 cm above the pubic symphysis to just below the umbilicus. The principal advantages of the vertical incision are that it permits more rapid entry into the abdominal cavity, facilitates operative exposure, and results in less blood loss than does the transverse incision. The major disadvantage is the greater susceptibility to dehiscence.

The vertical skin incision is extended downward through the subcutaneous tissue to the level of the anterior fascial sheath of the *rectus abdominis* muscle. The fascia is incised in the midline with the scalpel. This incision then is extended vertically in either direction utilizing scalpel or Mayo scissors. Once the anterior rectus sheath has been incised, the *rectus abdominis* muscle is separated in the midline by sharp or blunt dissection (Fig. 46-6). Once the muscles have been separated, the transversalis fascia and parietal peritoneum are visible.

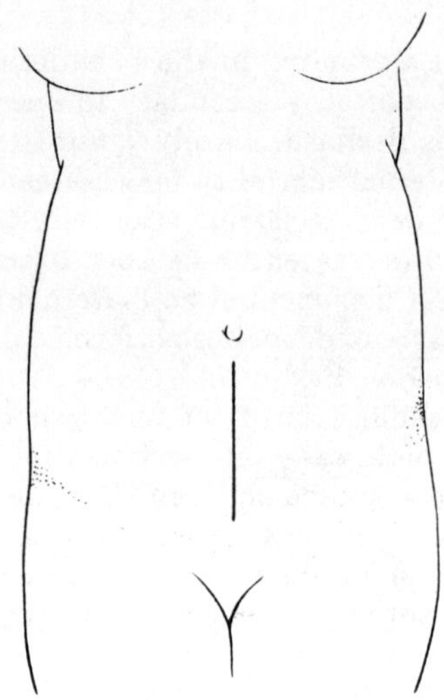

Figure 46-4. Midline skin incision for cesarean delivery.

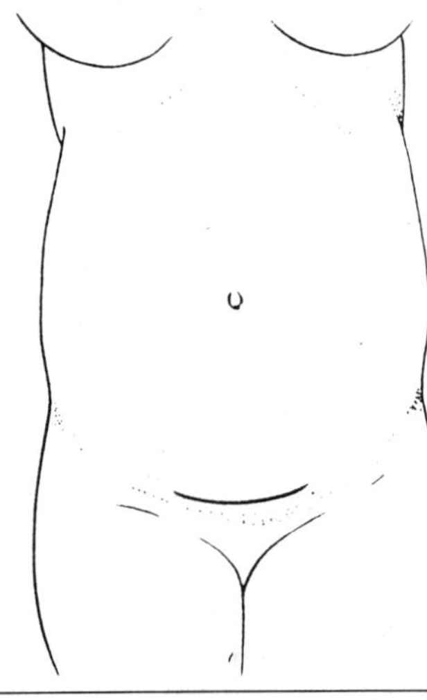

Figure 46-5. Transverse (Pfannenstiel) incision for cesarean delivery.

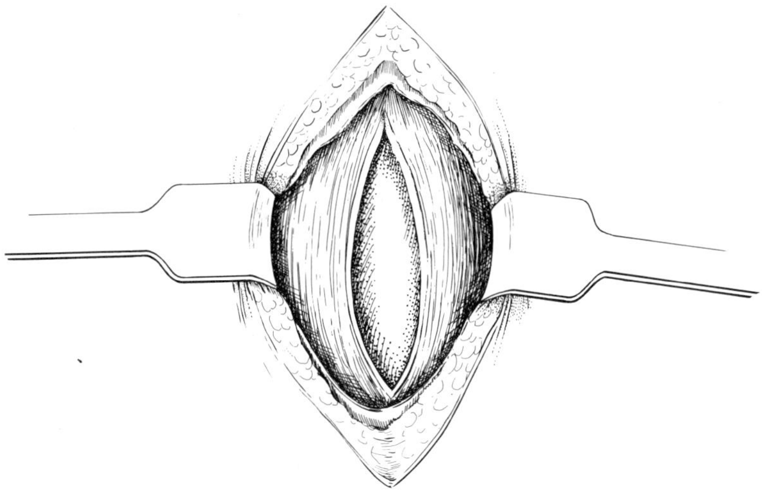

Figure 46-6. Separation of rectus muscles in the midline.

These layers are then elevated (Fig. 46-7a) and incised throughout the entire length of the incision (Fig. 46-7b). Care must be taken to be certain that bowel is not adherent to the undersurface of the peritoneal membrane. At this point, the operative field is exposed and preparations can be made for the uterine incision.

The transverse or Pfannenstiel incision extends transversely for approximately 6 cm on either side of the midline at a point 2 cm above the pubic symphysis. The principal advantage of this incision is that it is less likely to result in dehiscence than is the vertical incision. In addition, it affords a better posthealing cosmetic appearance. Disadvantages of the transverse incision include slower entry into the peritoneal cavity, greater blood loss, decreased operative exposure, and a slightly increased risk of wound infection.

The transverse skin incision is extended downward through the subcutaneous tissue to the level of the anterior rectus sheath. The fascia is incised in the midline, and the incision is extended curvilinearly on either side for approximately 6–8 cm (Fig. 46-8). At this point, the fascia is grasped at its superior margin on either side of the midline. The fascia is then separated from the underlying muscle by sharp and blunt dissection (Fig. 46-9). The same maneuvers are repeated at the inferior fascial margin.

The rectus muscles are then separated in the midline. The posterior fascial sheath and parietal peritoneum then should be grasped and incised as above. The initial incision in the parietal peritoneum should be as far cephalad as possible to avoid injuring the bladder.

Low Transverse Uterine Incision. The low transverse, or Kerr, incision[37] is the procedure most frequently performed for cesarean delivery. It generally is associated with less intraoperative blood loss than is either the low vertical or classical incision. Its principal advantage is that it heals more securely than the vertical incisions and is less likely to disrupt during subsequent pregnancies.[12,37] Improved healing is a consequence of the fact that the lower segment incision is made at a point in the uterus where there are relatively few myometrial fibers. Therefore, during the process of uterine involution, the incision is not subjected to contractile forces that would tend to disturb the integrity of the wound.

The operative technique is illustrated in Figs. 46-10–46-19. After the peritoneal cavity is entered, the visceral peritoneum is identified. The vesicouterine fold of the visceral peritoneum is incised in the midline at a point just above the reflection of the bladder onto the lower uterine segment (Fig. 46-10). The incision is then extended by sharp dissection for approximately 6 cm on either side of the midline (Fig. 46-11). The inferior margin of the peritoneal reflection is then grasped in the midline and the posterior wall of the bladder is separated from

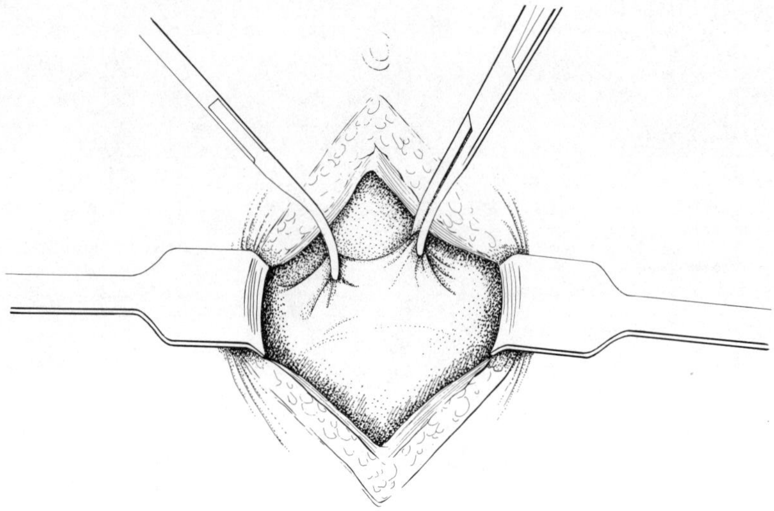

(a)

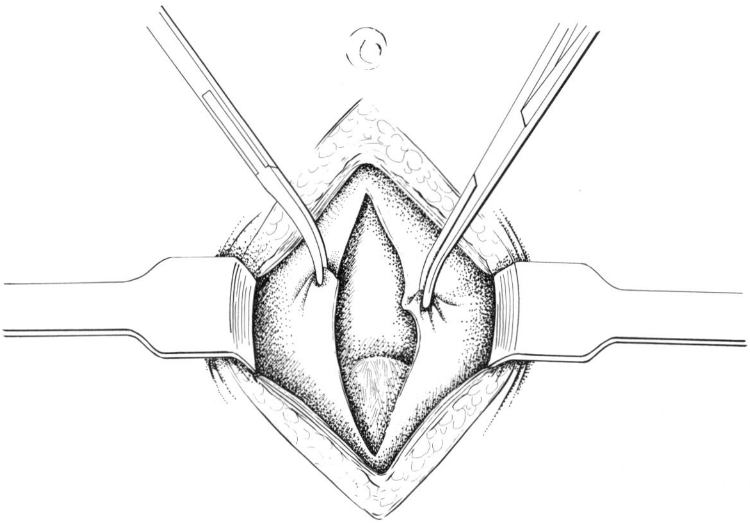

(b)

Figure 46-7. Panel A. Elevation of transversalis fascia and parietal peritoneum. Panel B. Extension of peritoneal incision.

the lower uterine segment. In a primary cesarean delivery, this separation is best accomplished by blunt dissection (Fig. 46-12). If there are adhesions between the posterior bladder wall and uterus, sharp dissection should be utilized to avoid blunt trauma to the bladder.

After the plane between the bladder and the lower uterine segment has been developed, the bladder is retracted inferiorly, and a horizontal incision is made in the lower uterine segment at a point just below the bladder reflection (Fig. 46-13). This incision should be extended upward and laterally for approximately 6 cm on either side of the midline. This can be accomplished by sharp or blunt dissection (Fig. 46-14). It is essential that the incision be curvilinear in order to avoid lateral extension into the uterine artery and vein.

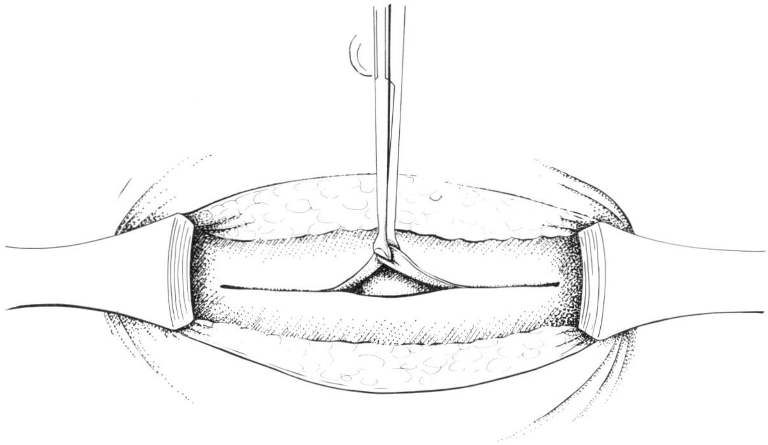

Figure 46-8. Fascial incision is extended laterally for approximately 6 cm from the midline.

Once the uterus has been opened, the membranes should be ruptured if they remain intact. The operator places his hand below the fetal head so that the occiput is in the palm of the hand. The head then should be flexed gently and elevated into the incision (Fig. 46-15). (Should the head be arrested at a deep pelvic station, it is useful to have an assistant place a gloved hand under the drapes and into the vagina to displace the head upward. This greatly facilitates delivery and helps to avoid extension of the uterine incision.) At this point, extraction of the fetus is facilitated by having the assistant exert downward pressure on the uterine fundus. The naso- and oropharynx of the fetus are suctioned and the umbilical cord doubly clamped and ligated (Fig. 46-16).

After the fetus is delivered, umbilical cord blood should be obtained for fetal hematocrit, blood type, and antibody screen. Umbilical artery and vein blood gases should be evaluated if any significant fetal heart rate abnormality has been noted.

The placenta is then removed by manual extraction. Following removal of the placenta, a dilute infusion of oxytocin should be administered to prevent excessive blood loss due to uterine atony. At this point, although it is not absolutely necessary to do so, the uterus can be elevated out of the abdominal incision. The margins of the uterine incision should be grasped with instruments such as Pennington or DuVal clamps (Fig. 46-17). This gains temporary hemostasis. The operator then inspects the incision carefully to be certain that the incision has not extended inferiorly into the vagina, superiorly into the contractile portion of the myometrium, or laterally into the uterine vessels and broad ligament. Inferior extension is particularly likely to occur when the fetal head has been impacted at a deep station.

After ensuring that no extension of the incision has occurred, the operator removes all fragments of membranes and placenta from the endometrial cavity. The hysterotomy incision is then reapproximated in two layers, with either continuous sutures or interrupted sutures. Uterine closure utilizing a continuous suture is illustrated in Fig. 46-18. The important principles in closing the uterine incision are to achieve hemostasis, to coapt the margins of the incision evenly, and to minimize the amount of tissue incorporated into the closure.

After the uterine incision is closed, the margins of visceral peritoneum should be reapproximated (Fig. 46-19). The rationale for this step of the operation is to provide at least a partial "seal" over the uterine incision, thereby minimizing continual seeding of the peritoneal cavity by bacteria that gained access to the lower uterine segment during labor.[7,12,37] This rationale for peritoneal closure is theoretical. No rigorously designed investigation has proved conclusively that peritoneal closure is necessary.

After approximation of the visceral peritoneum, the tubes and ovaries are inspected. The abdominal wall is then elevated with a retractor and the uterus is reposited into the peritoneal

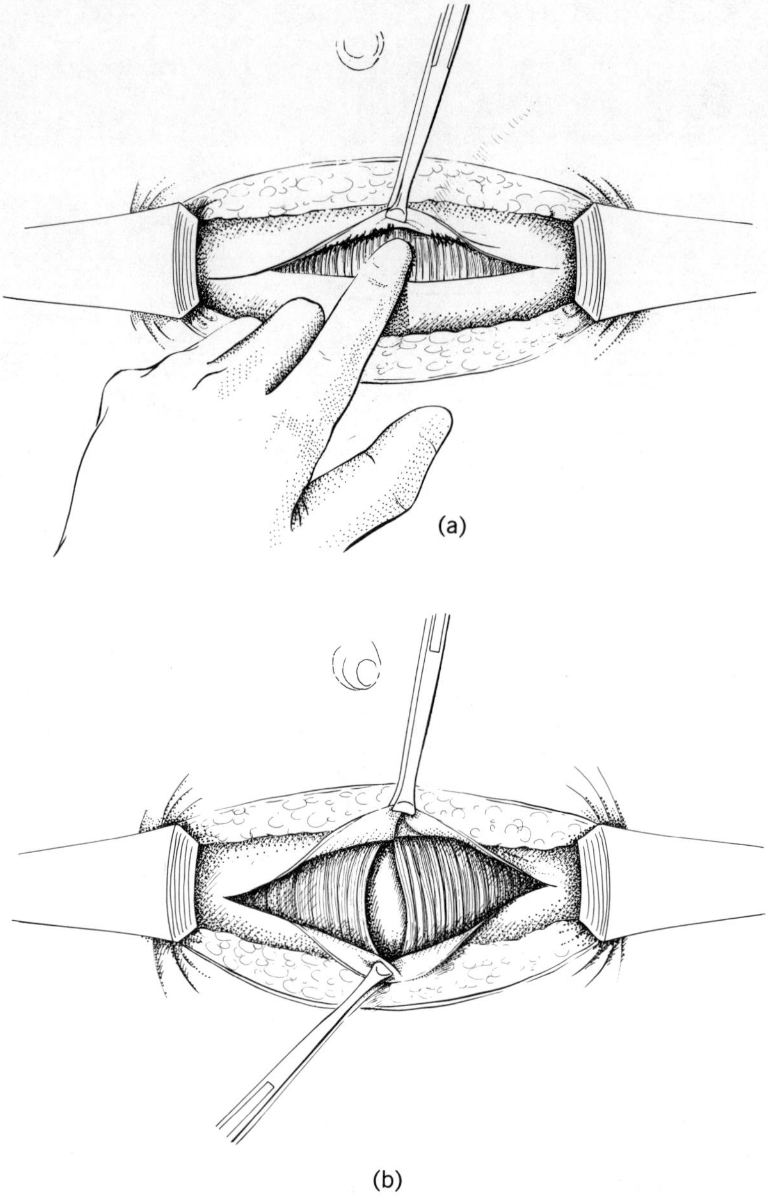

Figure 46-9. Panel A. Superior margin of fascia is grasped with clamps, and the fascia is separated from the underlying muscle by blunt dissection.
Panel B. Separation of fascia and muscle is completed by sharp dissection.

cavity. Blood clots and amniotic fluid debris should be removed from the pelvic cavity before closing the anterior abdominal wall.

Low Vertical Uterine Incision. There are two principal indications for the low vertical or Krönig incision. It is used preferentially for delivery of the very small preterm fetus, especially the fetus in breech presentation, when the lower uterine segment is poorly developed. In this circumstance, a transverse incision may result in exposure inadequate for atraumatic delivery of

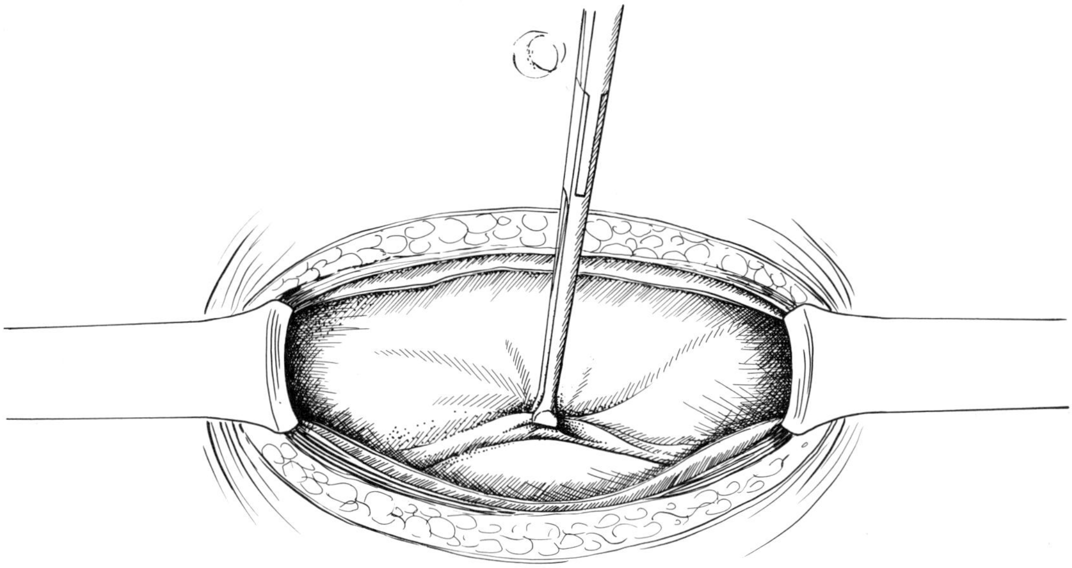

Figure 46-10. Vesicouterine peritoneal reflection is identified and elevated.

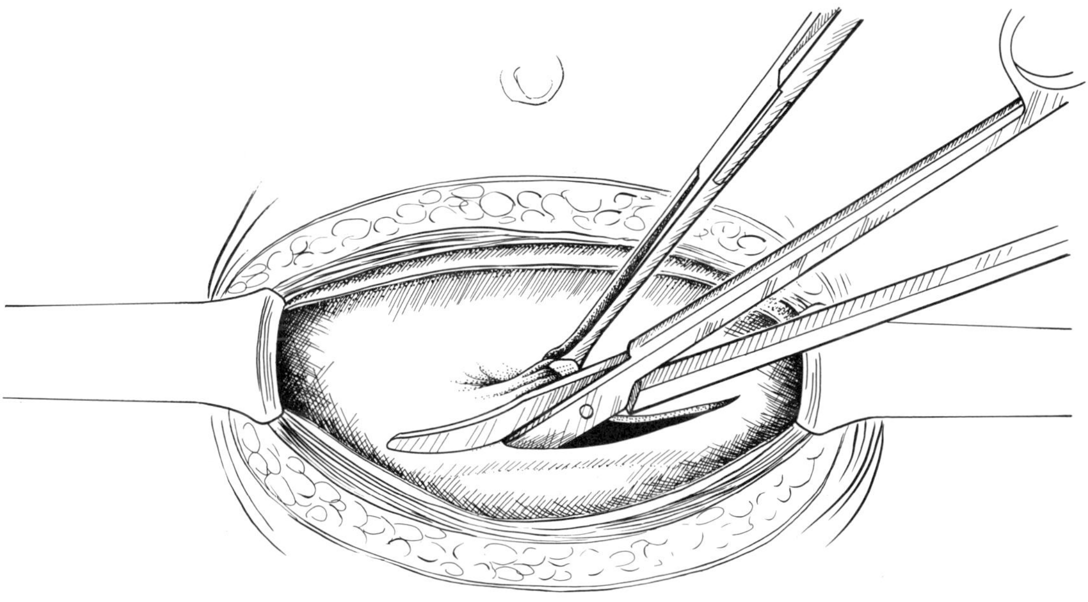

Figure 46-11. Visceral peritoneum is incised.

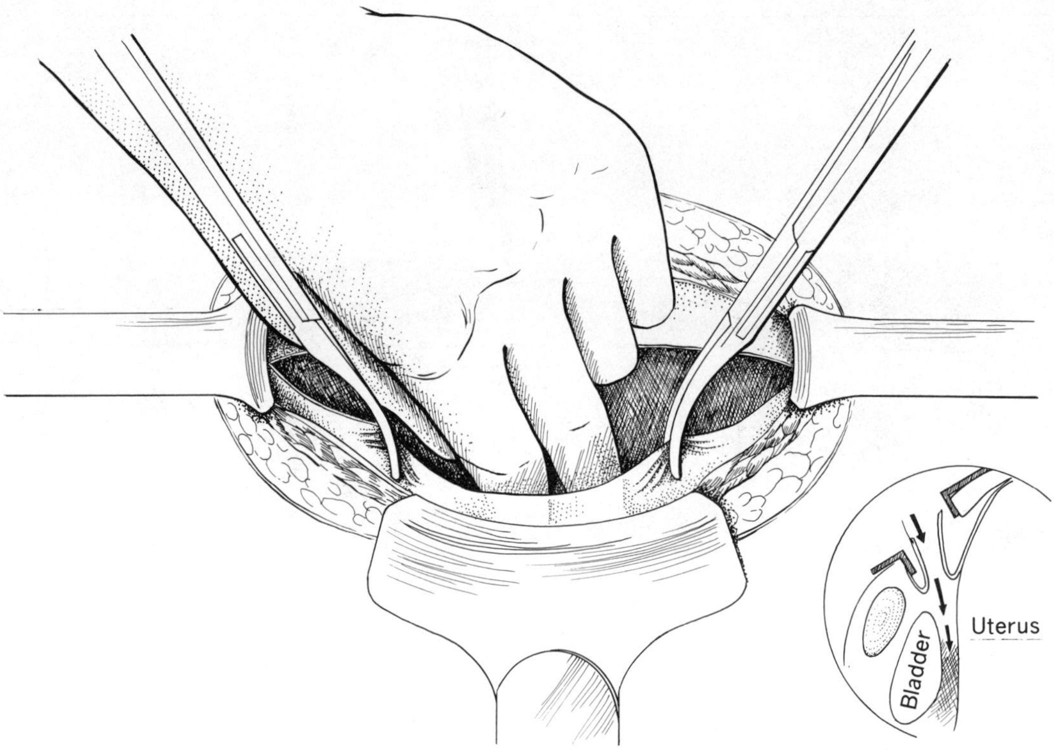

Figure 46-12. Space between posterior bladder wall and lower uterine segment is developed by blunt dissection.

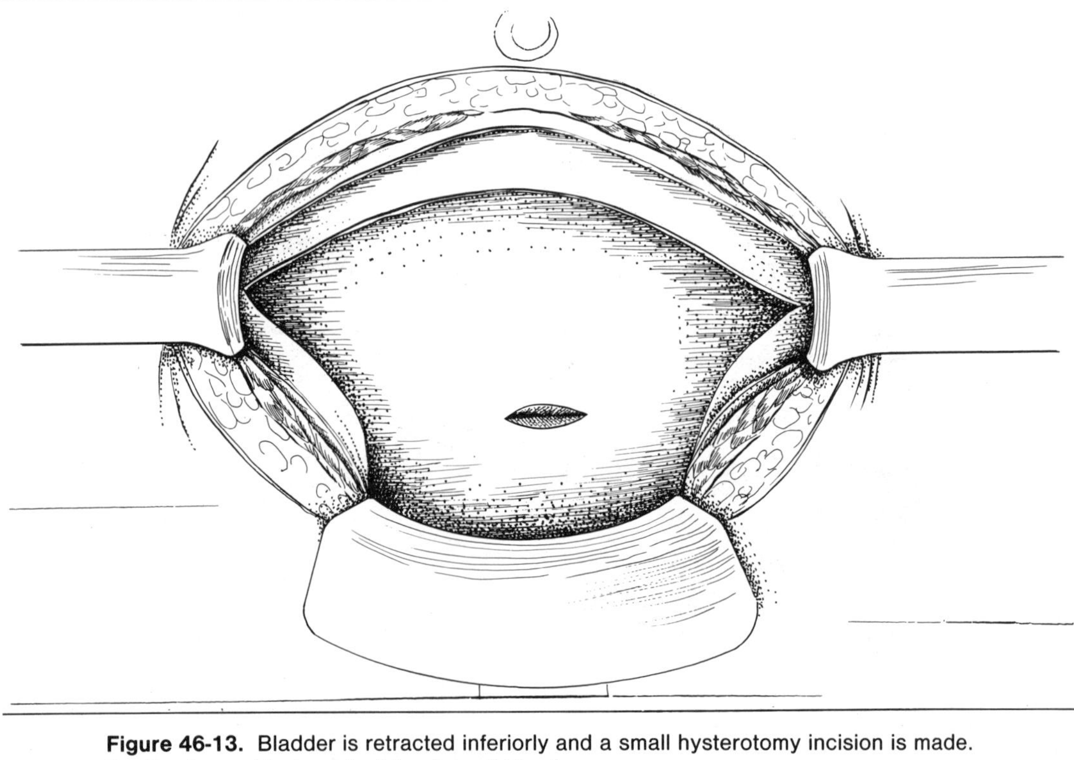

Figure 46-13. Bladder is retracted inferiorly and a small hysterotomy incision is made. Suction is used to keep incision free of blood.

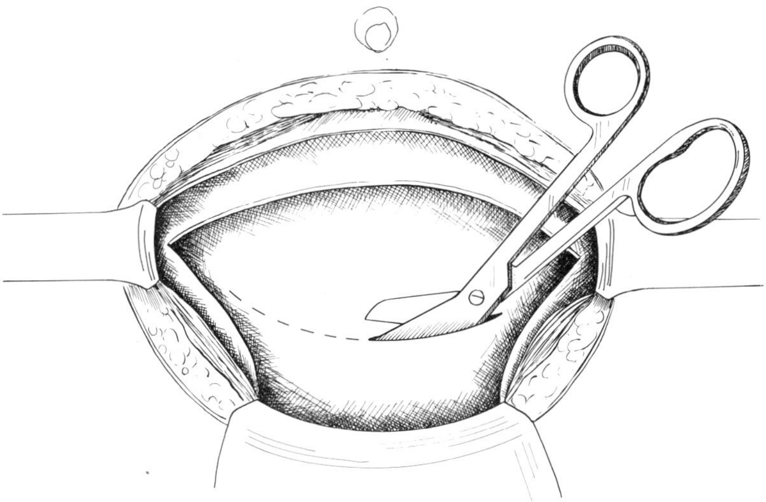

(a)

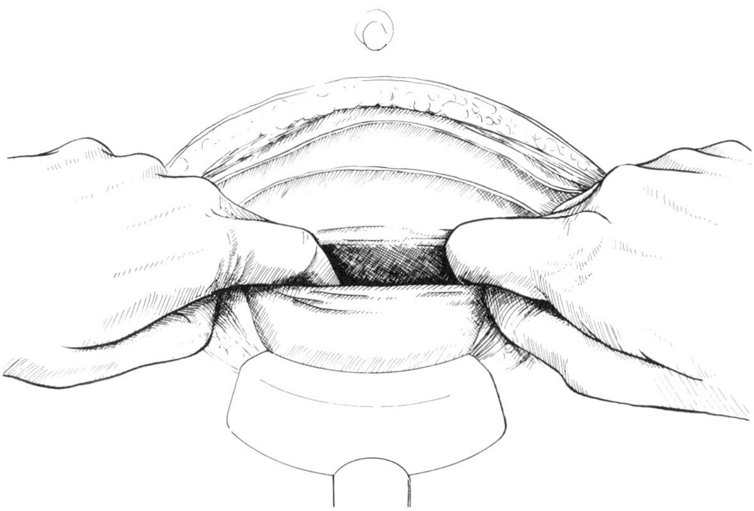

(b)

Figure 46-14. The incision may be enlarged in a curvilinear arc by utilizing scissors (panel A) or the incision may be extended curvilinearly by lateral traction with the index fingers (panel B) to expose the chorioamnionitic membranes.

the fetus. It also may result in lateral extension of the incision and laceration of the uterine artery and vein.

The low vertical incision is also useful when cesarean hysterectomy is planned. In this instance, the vertical incision avoids the risk of laceration of the major uterine vessels prior to performance of the more extensive surgical procedure.

The initial steps of the low vertical procedure are the same as described above for the low transverse incision. After the plane between bladder and lower uterine segment has been developed, the bladder is retracted inferiorly. A vertical hysterotomy incision is made starting at the lowermost boundary of the lower uterine segment and extending upward for approximately 8 cm (Fig. 46-20). At its upper limits, this

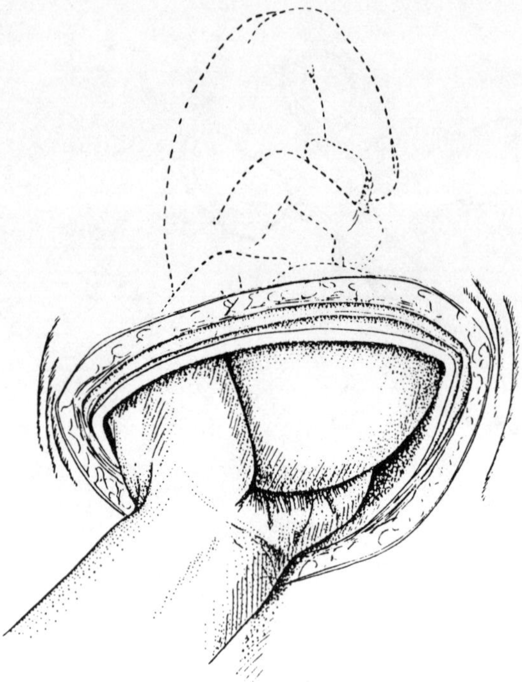

Figure 46-15. The fetal head is rotated so that the occiput rests in the palm of the surgeon's hand. Gentle fundal pressure is then applied to elevate the fetal head into the uterine incision.

incision usually extends, at least partially, into the upper uterine segment.

After delivery of the fetus and placenta, the margins of the incision should be grasped with instruments in order to control bleeding. The endometrium and myometrium are then reapproximated in two layers, using either continuous or interrupted sutures. After the uterine incision has been closed, the visceral peritoneum is reapproximated.

Classical Uterine Incision. The classical uterine incision is indicated rarely in modern obstetric practice. Its principal disadvantage is that it is much more likely than the low transverse incision to disrupt in a subsequent pregnancy.[47,49] Disruption may occur before the onset of labor. In addition, it usually results in increased intraoperative blood loss, compared to either the low transverse or low vertical incision.

The major advantage of the classical incision is that it provides complete access to the endometrial cavity. In selected clinical situations, such access may be necessary to accomplish safe delivery of the fetus (Table 46-3).

The classical incision should extend vertically from a point just above the bladder reflection to the superior portion of the uterine fundus (Fig. 46-21). It is not necessary to separate the bladder from the lower uterine segment. Once the fetus and placenta are delivered, the margins of the incision are grasped with clamps to minimize blood loss. The myometrium is then closed in at least two, and sometimes three, layers. Sutures may be placed in either a continuous or an interrupted manner.

Extraperitoneal Cesarean Section. The extraperitoneal procedure was developed to decrease the risk of peritoneal contamination in patients who already had chorioamnionitis or

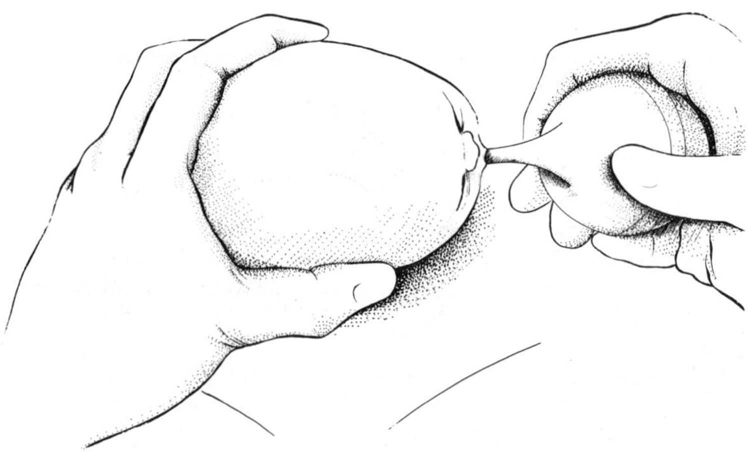

Figure 46-16. The oro- and nasopharynx of the fetus are suctioned with a bulb syringe.

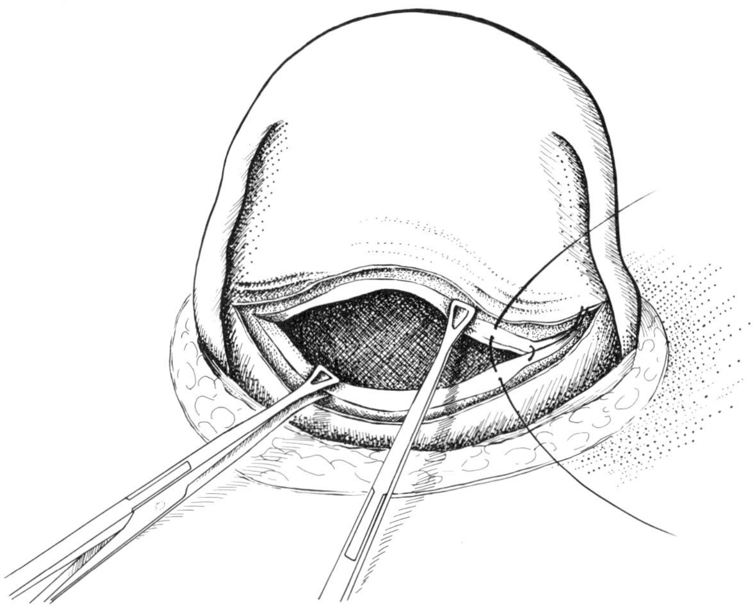

Figure 46-17. Bleeding from uterine incision is controlled by grasping the margins of the incision with clamps.

who were at high risk for postoperative infection because of prolonged rupture of membranes.[24,40] Waters[70] stated that:

> (t)he indication for a true extraperitoneal operation is therefore the probable or actual existence of intrauterine infection. If properly done, it should largely remove peritonitis as a cause of postoperative morbidity, and at the same time it conserves the uterus.

In the preantibiotic era, the rationale for extraperitoneal cesarean delivery was unquestionable. Maternal mortality rates were dramatically higher than at present, and sepsis was one of the two major causes of maternal death. With the advent of broad spectrum antibiotics, the theoretical and practical advantages of the extraperitoneal procedure are questionable.

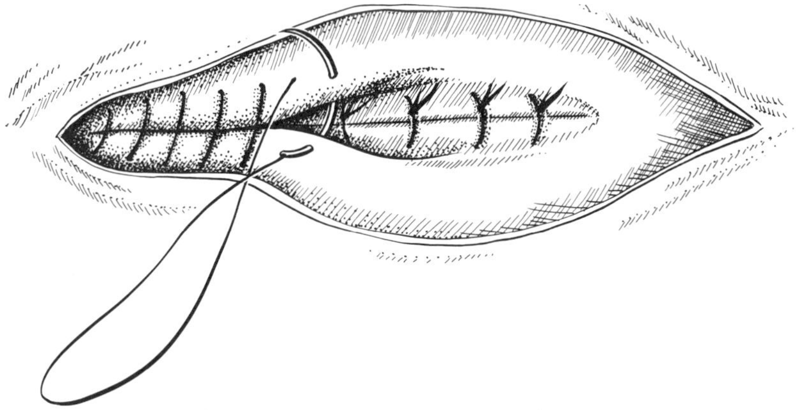

Figure 46-18. The myometrium is reapproximated with two layers of continuous sutures.

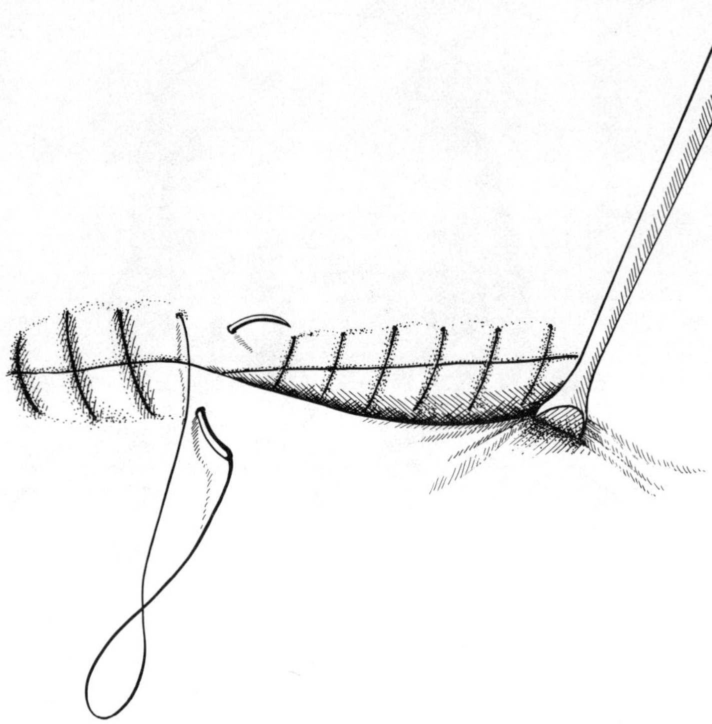

Figure 46-19. Reapproximation of visceral peritoneum with a simple continuous suture.

Several authors[30] continue to recommend extraperitoneal operative delivery in patients at high risk of infection and have demonstrated that the operation can be performed as quickly and safely as the transperitoneal procedure.

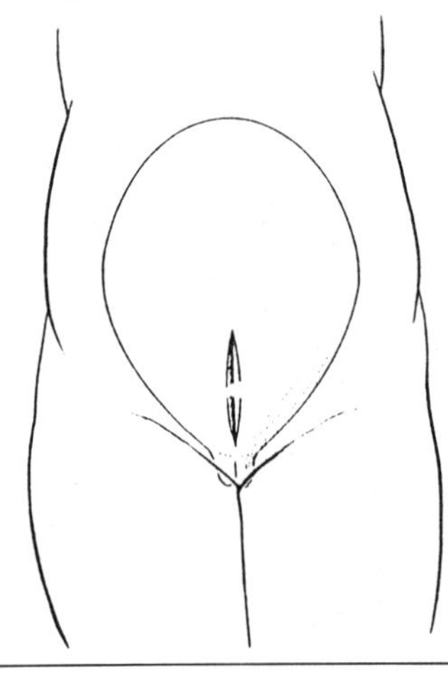

Figure 46-20. Low vertical uterine incision.

However, flaws in these studies weaken conclusions concerning the efficacy of the procedure. Only one recent investigation[69] specifically compared extraperitoneal cesarean section to other techniques for preventing postoperative infection. The authors concluded that extraperitoneal cesarean section was not an effective means of reducing the incidence of postoperative endometritis.

In most clinical situations, extraperitoneal cesarean section, although not harmful, does not display any significant advantage over the transperitoneal procedure. There are instances, however, where the extraperitoneal approach to the uterus clearly should not be utilized. It is contraindicated whenever there is a need for concurrent adnexal surgery or cesarean hysterectomy. It cannot be utilized if a classical uterine incision is necessary. In addition, it may be extremely difficult to perform whenever there are anatomic alterations in the lower uterine segment, a low-lying anterior placenta or placenta previa, or extensive vesicouterine adhesions.

The extraperitoneal procedure can be performed through either a vertical or transverse

TABLE 46-3. INDICATIONS FOR CLASSICAL UTERINE INCISION

Transverse lie with fetal back down
Fetal anomaly • Severe hydrocephalus • Large abdominal wall defect • Large sacrococcygeal teratoma
Premature twin gestation
Multiple fetuses (>2)
Extensive adhesions between bladder and lower uterine segment
Placenta previa combined with prominent varicosities of the lower uterine segment
Large leiomyoma obstructing access to the lower uterine segment

skin incision. The initial part of the operation is the same as that described for transperitoneal cesarean delivery. The technique differs once the rectus abdominis muscles are separated and the underlying transversalis fascia and parietal peritoneum are exposed. At this point, as illustrated in Figs. 46-22–46-24, the thin layer of transversalis fascia overlying the bladder is incised. Prior to this step, the bladder should be distended with a solution of methylene blue in saline. Once the transversalis fascia has been dissected free of the bladder, the left lateral vesicle margin should be identified. The thin fascial layer that is posterior to the bladder and overlying the lower uterine segment is then incised, and the bladder is retracted to the patient's right. The vesicouterine peritoneal reflection is then inspected to be certain that it is intact. A transverse incision is made in the lower uterine segment and the fetus extracted. Uterine closure is accomplished as outlined previously for the transperitoneal procedure. Drainage of the retrovesical and supravesical space is recommended.

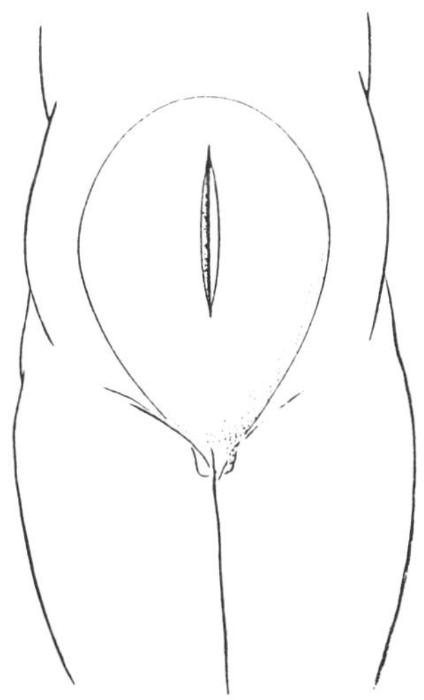

Figure 46-21. Classical uterine incision.

Selection of Suture for Uterine Closure

Although there are differences of opinion with respect to the selection of suture for uterine closure, the synthetic resorbable fibers such as polyglycolic acid and polyglactin appear to be the best choices. Compared to chromic suture, these materials have increased tensile strength and cause less inflammation. Improved manufacturing techniques, especially coating of the suture with polyglycolic or polyglactin polymer, have made these materials comparable to chromic suture in terms of ease of handling. Knot slippage is a possibility with the new synthetic materials, but this can be minimized by tying a minimum of four square knots.

Abdominal Wall Closure. It is not necessary to reapproximate the parietal peritoneum. Peritoneal closure neither improves the ultimate tensile strength of the wound nor prevents the formation of adhesions between the bowel and under surface of the anterior abdominal wall.

The fascial edges may be reapproximated with either a continuous suture or interrupted sutures (Fig. 46-25). The latter sutures may be placed as single loops or as double loops. The latter technique is especially useful in patients who have a vertical incision and who have associated disorders that place them at risk for wound dehiscence. Such risk factors include obesity, diabetes, chronic pulmonary disease, and use of immunosuppressive or cytotoxic drugs.

The selection of suture material for closure of the abdominal wall is, in large part, a matter of personal preference. The current trend is toward synthetic resorbable sutures rather than chromic sutures. In patients at increased risk for wound dehiscence, a strong, nonreactive, mono-

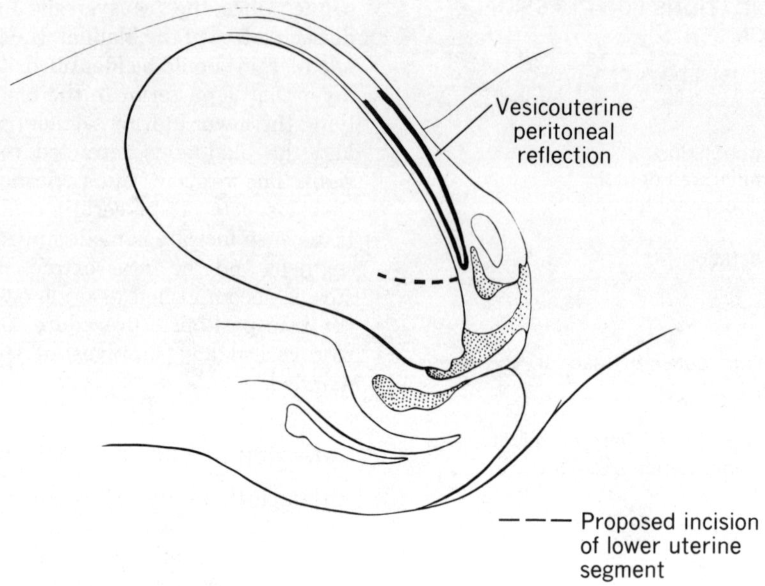

Figure 46-22. Schematic representation of operative approach in extraperitoneal cesarean section. The point of access to lower uterine segment is inferior to the vesicouterine peritoneal reflection.

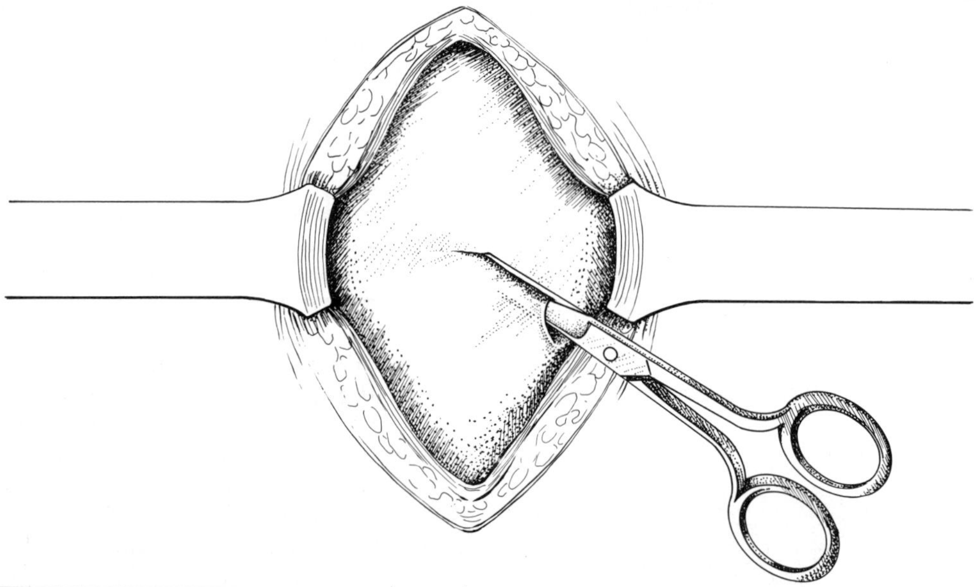

Figure 46-23. Incision of transversalis fascia which overlies the bladder.

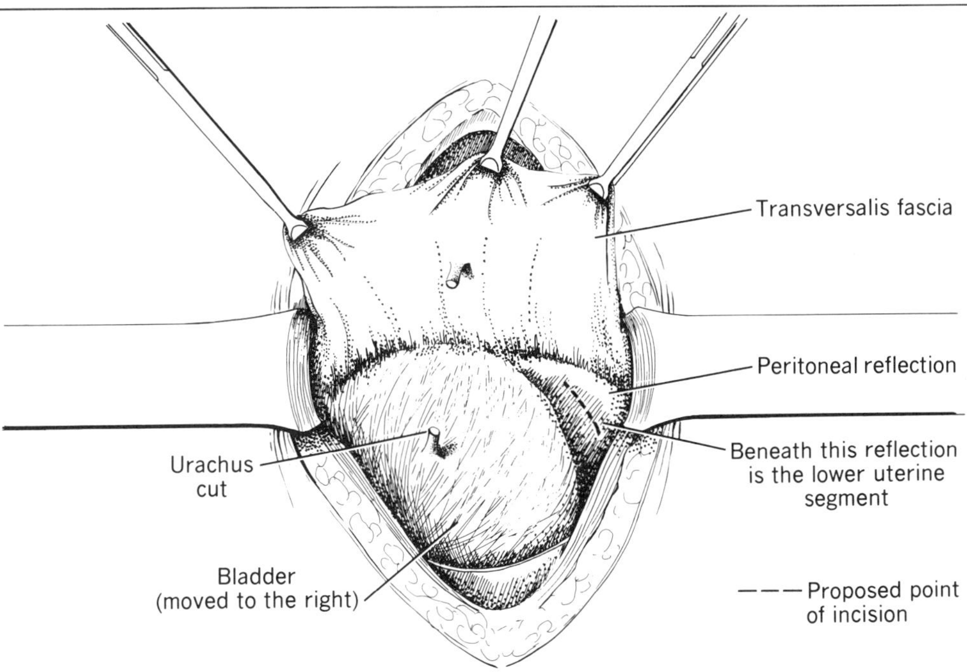

Figure 46-24. Bladder is retracted to the patient's right, exposing the lower uterine segment.

filamented suture such as nylon or stainless steel wire should be used to close the fascia.

It is not necessary to reapproximate the subcutaneous tissue. The skin edges may be closed utilizing stainless steel staples, clips, or sutures (Fig. 46-26).

Anesthesia for Cesarean Delivery

Cesarean delivery can be performed under local anesthesia. This technique, however, does not provide optimal anesthesia and may require use of near-toxic doses of the local anesthetic agent. Therefore, in virtually all circumstances, regional or general anesthesia should be utilized for abdominal delivery. In the United States, general anesthesia is used in 32–55% of cesarean deliveries. Spinal anesthesia is used in 24–39% of cesareans, and epidural anesthesia is used in 3–32% of cesarean sections.[47]

The most frequent complications of spinal anesthesia are maternal hypotension and postspinal headache. Epidural or caudal anesthesia is more difficult to perform than subarachnoid block and, therefore, more frequently results in technical failure. Peridural anesthesia is less likely, however, than subarachnoid block to cause maternal hypotension because it produces more gradual blockade of sympathetic vasomotor fibers. With either technique, systemic absorption of the local anesthetic agent may occur and lead to toxic manifestations, including seizures and cardiac arrest. Similarly, with either technique, unexpectedly high levels of blockade may occur, resulting in paralysis of the accessory muscles of respiration. Infection or prolonged neurologic injury are exceedingly rare complications of regional anesthesia.[47]

In those situations in which general anesthesia is indicated for cesarean delivery, the patient must be intubated to minimize the risk of aspiration pneumonitis. Induction of general anesthesia usually is accomplished by administering thiopental intravenously (2–4 mg/kg). In the presence of hypotension, ketamine (1.0 mg/kg) may be preferred to thiopental because of its sympathomimetic properties. Succinylcholine (0.1–0.2%) usually is administered intravenously during the induction sequence to prevent laryngospasm during intubation. Nitrous oxide (50–75%) with oxygen then is given by inhalation to maintain a light plane of anesthesia until the fetus is delivered. After delivery of the infant, the plane of anesthesia can be deepened by

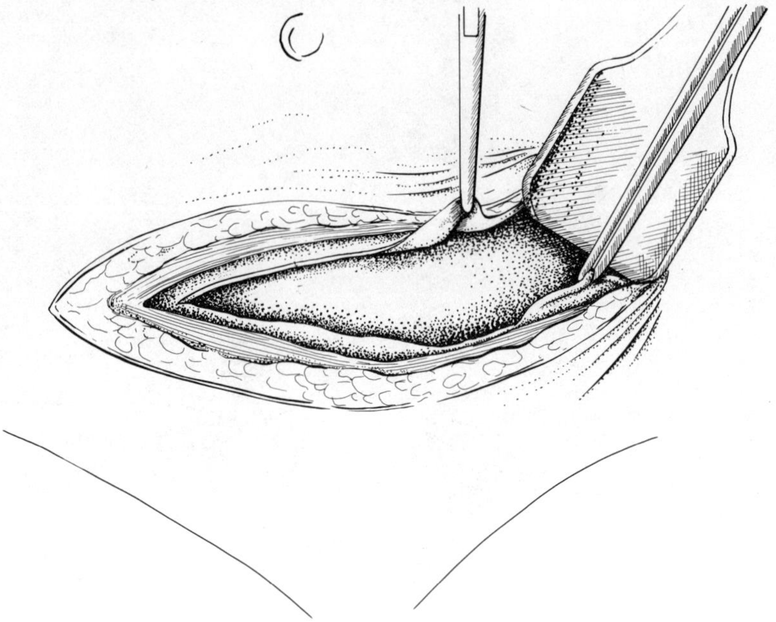

(a)

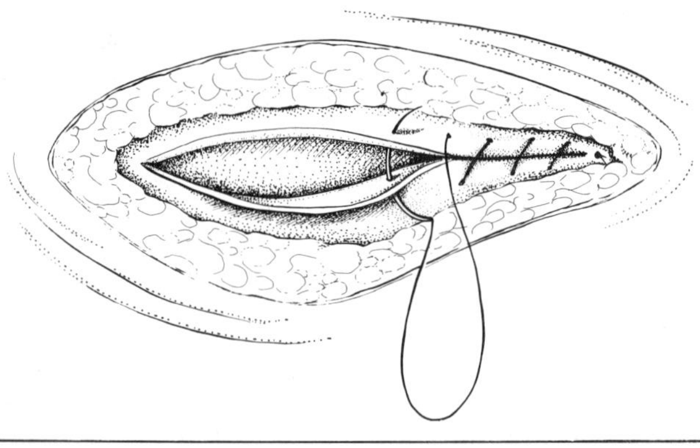

Figure 46-25. Panel A. Lateral margin of incision is exposed, and the apex of fascial incision is identified.
Panel B. Fascial edges are reapproximated with a continuous suture. Needle is inserted approximately 1.5 to 2.0 cm from the fascial edge. Fascial edges are coapted evenly, and the sutures are tied without excessive tension.

administering intravenous narcotics and diazepam. If uterine relaxation is required, this can be achieved by administering one of the nonflammable agents such as halothane, enflurane, or isoflurane. Adequate muscle relaxation can be maintained during delivery by administering a continuous intravenous infusion of succinylcholine or incremental doses of pancuronium.

Postmortem Cesarean Section

Postmortem cesarean delivery rarely is performed except in unusual and tragic circumstances. In the small series of postmortem cesarean sections reported in the literature, neonatal survival has ranged from 0% to 40%.

Postmortem cesarean section can be consid-

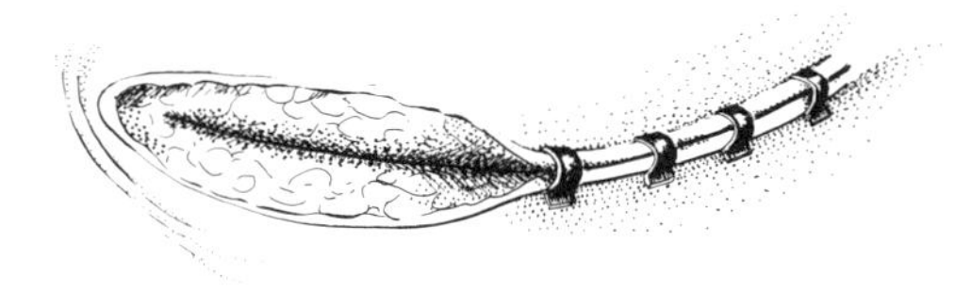

(b)

Figure 46-26. Reapproximation of skin edges with clips.

ered whenever maternal death is imminent and pregnancy has progressed to the point of fetal viability. In exceptional situations, it may even be appropriate to prolong maternal life for a short period of time after brain function has ceased in order to enhance the chances for neonatal survival.[4]

In considering the possibility of postmortem cesarean delivery, the attending physician must be aware of the strict definition of brain death. All of the following criteria must be fulfilled before a patient is declared to be "brain dead":

- There is no response to painful stimuli.
- There is no muscular movement and no spontaneous breathing for one hour (or three minutes off of the respirator).
- There are no reflexes, ocular movements, or blinking.
- The pupils are fixed and dilated.
- The electroencephalogram is flat and isoelectric during two separate recordings obtained 24 hours apart.
- The observations above must not have occurred as a result of barbiturate intoxication or hypothermia.

In ideal circumstances, the physician should discuss the procedure in advance with the patient's nearest relative. In the case of sudden maternal death, however, lack of prior approval does not mandate that the operation not be done. If this intervention is planned, a surgical instrument set should be kept at the bedside of critically ill obstetric patients, so that delivery can be completed as soon as possible after the declaration of maternal death. Cardiopulmonary support must be maintained in the interval between maternal death and delivery of the fetus.

Ancillary Surgical Procedures at the Time of Cesarean Delivery

Tubal Ligation. Sterilization may be performed at the time of cesarean section by one of several methods. These techniques are discussed in detail in Chapter 9. In general, tubal ligation does not increase the morbidity associated with cesarean section. Counseling for permanent sterilization should be conducted well in advance of delivery. The operative permit for tubal ligation should be completed before the final weeks of pregnancy. Prior to performing tubal ligation at the time of cesarean section, the surgeon should ascertain that the initial neonatal evaluation is normal.

Appendectomy. The principal rationale for removal of the appendix at the time of cesarean section is that it prevents future cases of appendicitis that may be associated with increased risk of mortality in older patients. It also eliminates appendicitis as a diagnostic consideration should patients subsequently experience acute abdominal pain. In addition, in a small percentage of cases, histologic abnormalities may be present in an apparently normal appendix.

The major argument against performance of incidental appendectomy is that it may result in prolonged ileus and serious infection, including abdominal or pelvic abscess. Although such complications have been reported, they are rare. Moreover, it is not always possible to determine whether the ileus or the infection was the direct result of the appendectomy or whether it was due to the primary operation.

There is little doubt that incidental appendectomy can be performed safely at the time of cesarean delivery. When considering performance of elective appendectomy at the time of cesarean section, the surgeon should observe the following guidelines:

- The procedure should be explained to the patient prior to cesarean delivery.
- The primary operation should be performed under nonemergency conditions.
- The appendix should be easily accessible through the incision selected for cesarean section.
- The surgeon should be skilled in performance of appendectomy.

Trial of Labor After Previous Cesarean Delivery

In 1916, Edwin Cragin[10] presented a paper before the Eastern Medical Society of the City of New York in which he directed his associates' attention to the dangers associated with cesarean delivery, particularly the danger of maternal death due to overwhelming infection.

Let me say, that it pays to be charitable toward any careful man who is unfortunate enough to have in his practice a case of puerperal infection. To criticize is easy, but alas! the tables may soon be turned and we may be the next unfortunate to spend anxious days and sleepless nights over a case of puerperal infection which came we know not how.

Cragin noted that most instances of severe infection occurred in situations where cesarean delivery followed a long period of labor and an extended duration of ruptured membranes.

If the woman has been a long time in labor with membranes ruptured many hours, the mortality of two to three percent rises to a mortality of ten to fifteen percent, and the operation ceases to be a conservative procedure and becomes one of considerable hazard. This emphasizes the importance of an early diagnosis in all cases with a positive indication for Caesarean Section so that the operation can be performed either just before or in the early stages of labor.

He cautioned, however, that cesarean delivery should be performed only in exceptional circumstances:

(o)ne thing must always be borne in mind, viz., that no matter how carefully a uterine incision is sutured, we can never be certain that the cicatrized uterine wall will stand a subsequent pregnancy and labor without rupture. This means that the usual rule is, *once a Caesarean always a Caesarean*.... I believe that the extension of Caesarean section to conditions other than dystocia from contracted pelvis or tumors should be exceptional and infrequent.

Cragin's paper was presented at a time when cesarean delivery was not safe and when the vast majority of operations were performed through classical uterine incisions. For over 50 years, however, his dictum, "once a Caesarean always a Caesarean" was accepted without reservation by most American obstetricians. In spite of contrary rationale,[52] as late as 1984 more than 95% of women who previously had had cesarean deliveries were delivered by repeat cesarean section.[28]

In recent years, more than 30 papers describing trials of labor in patients with previous cesarean section have been published. The reader is referred to three recent review articles[36,41,49] for detailed information concerning these investigations. The findings of these studies may be summarized as follows.

- During a subsequent pregnancy, the classical incision is much more likely to disrupt than the low-segment transverse incision. The incidence of disruption of the classical incision is approximately 5% compared to 0.5–1.5% for the transverse incision. The incidence of rupture of the low vertical incision has not been defined precisely but appears to be intermediate between the low transverse and classical incisions.
- Disruption of the classical incision usually is a true rupture of the uterus. It may occur prior to the onset of labor and typically is associated with potentially life-threatening maternal hemorrhage. Maternal mortality may be as high as 5%. Fetal mortality has ranged from 40% to almost 75%. The usual clinical manifestations are fetal distress, pain, shock, and cessation of labor.
- Disruption of the low transverse incision typically takes the form of a small dehiscence of the scar. It usually does not become apparent prior to the onset of labor, nor is it associated with major maternal blood loss. Only in rare circumstances does fetal mortality occur. Dehiscence of the lower uterine segment scar usually is asymptomatic but may present with fetal distress, mild to moderate abdominal pain, and loss of coordinated uterine activity.
- The low transverse incision heals more rapidly and securely than the vertical incision because the former incision is not subjected to the same disruptive contractile forces as the latter.
- The majority of women who have had a prior cesarean delivery are acceptable candidates for subsequent trial of labor. The principal contraindications to trial of labor are prior classical incision, prior low transverse incision complicated by vertical extension into the thickened myometrium, and present indication for abdominal delivery such as placenta previa, abruptio placentae, malpresentation, or marked fetopelvic disproportion.
- Overall, the maternal morbidity and mortality associated with a management protocol that allows trial of labor for selected patients is significantly less than that associated with a policy that dictates elective repeat cesarean section for all patients.
- More than one prior low transverse incision does not contraindicate trial of labor. Patients with more than one prior low transverse cesarean section do not appear to have a disproportionately increased risk of uterine scar dehiscence.[55]

- On the average, 60–75% of women who are allowed trial of labor will deliver vaginally. In selected series, 80–90% of patients have had successful trials of labor.
- Unless markedly decreased pelvic capacity has been demonstrated conclusively, a prior diagnosis of cephalopelvic disproportion is not a contraindication to trial of labor. Among women with a previous cesarean delivery for failure to progress or for cephalopelvic disproportion, approximately 50–60% will have a successful trial of labor. Of those delivering vaginally, 20–30% will have a larger infant than during the first delivery.[60]
- In women who have an unsuccessful trial of labor, the incidence of postcesarean infection is significantly higher than that in patients who undergo elective repeat cesarean section.[44]
- There is no contraindication to use of regional anesthesia in women undergoing trial of labor. Regional anesthesia will not mask clinical manifestations of overt scar dehiscence.
- There is no contraindication to administration of oxytocin for induction or augmentation of labor in patients undergoing trial of labor, *provided that uterine hyperstimulation is avoided.*[48]
- In women delivering vaginally, small scar defects that are not bleeding do not need to be repaired. If such defects are noted during repeat cesarean section, they should be repaired as the uterine incision is closed. Only in exceptional circumstances will hysterectomy be necessary because of disruption of a transverse lower-segment scar.

The recent obstetric literature clearly supports a change in approach. Repeat cesarean sections now account for almost one-third of all operative deliveries. Up to three-fourths of these procedures could be avoided without increasing significantly the risk for either mother or fetus. Table 46-4 outlines the criteria that should be fulfilled before an obstetric service implements such a policy.

TABLE 46-4. CRITERIA FOR TRIAL OF LABOR AFTER PREVIOUS CESAREAN DELIVERY

- Prior operations were low transverse procedures and there were no vertical extensions of the incision into the uterine fundus.
- Prior operative report has been reviewed by the attending physician.
- Patient has been informed of expected risks and benefits of trial of labor.
- Recurrent indication for abdominal delivery is not present. Cephalopelvic disproportion, unless conclusively documented, is not a contraindication to trial of labor.
- Continuous internal electronic fetal monitoring is utilized.
- Availability of pediatric, anesthesia, and blood-banking services makes it possible to perform cesarean delivery within 20 to 30 minutes should complications of trial of labor develop.

Scheduling of Repeat Cesarean Delivery

In patients who have had previous cesarean delivery and who are not candidates for trial of labor, the timing of repeat cesarean section is important to optimal maternal and neonatal outcome. Inadvertent delivery of a preterm infant, usually due to failure of the attending physician to satisfy rigid criteria for establishment of gestational age, is a major complication of repeat cesarean section.

One way to avoid miscalculation of gestational age is to perform amniocentesis to document a mature surfactant profile prior to elective delivery. However, amniocentesis increases costs, and third-trimester amniocentesis may be associated with serious complications, including fetal and placental bleeding, rupture of membranes, infection, and initiation of labor. Although the usual incidence of such complications is less than 3%, the incidence of complications in patients undergoing amniocentesis for assessment of fetal lung maturity may be as high as 11%.[32]

Another method for avoiding elective prematurity is to delay repeat cesarean until the patient is in labor. One disadvantage of the policy of awaiting onset of labor is that patients with prior classical uterine incisions may experience disruption of their scar prior to labor. Disruption of a classical incision may be associated with severe maternal hemorrhage and a high incidence of fetal mortality. Therefore, at least in this select group of patients, delivery should be performed on a scheduled basis prior to onset of labor. Other disadvantages are: (1) the patient may go into labor during the night or weekend hours, when the surgical team is not immediately available and (2) the patient may go into labor soon after eating a meal.

If strict criteria are observed for documenting gestational age, elective repeat cesarean delivery can be performed without antecedent amniocentesis. Ideally, all the following criteria should be fulfilled before scheduling an elective delivery.

- Known last menstrual period
- History of regular menses
- Early serial physical examinations before 20 weeks' gestation that are consistent with menstrual dates
- Documentation of fetal heart tones by doptone at 12 weeks' gestation
- Documentation of fetal heart tones with fetoscope at 18–20 weeks' gestation
- Second-trimester sonogram that is consistent with menstrual dates
- Second sonogram immediately prior to delivery that demonstrates biparietal diameter $\geqq$ 9.2 cm
- Gestational age > 38 weeks

In patients who do not have a reliable menstrual history and/or clinical evaluation, elective delivery still may be scheduled safely if two sequential sonograms, obtained prior to 30 weeks' gestation, support a gestational age of 38 weeks. Documentation of a fetal biparietal diameter $\geqq$ 9.2 cm in such patients offers additional confirmation that the fetus is mature.[32] If these minimal criteria are not fulfilled, or if the patient has any medical complication that might influence fetal maturation, amniocentesis should be performed prior to elective delivery. Repeat cesarean section should then be delayed until a mature surfactant profile is documented.

Prophylactic Antibiotics for Cesarean Section

Pathogenesis of Postcesarean Infection . Postoperative endometritis is a polymicrobial infection caused by bacteria normally present in the host's lower genital tract. The major microorganisms responsible for endometritis are aerobic gram-negative bacilli, principally *E. coli*; anaerobic gram-negative bacilli, principally *Bacteroides* species and *Gardnerella vaginalis;* aerobic gram-positive cocci, primarily Group B and Group D streptococci; and anaerobic gram-positive cocci, specifically *Peptococcus* species and *Peptostreptococcus* species.[17]

The development of clinical infection is dependent on a complex balance between host defense mechanisms and bacterial virulence factors. Cesarean delivery alters this balance so as to predispose the patient to infection. During labor and abdominal delivery, the endometrium and peritoneal cavity invariably are contaminated with large numbers of highly pathogenic aerobic and anaerobic bacteria. The serosanguineous fluid that collects in the abdomen after surgery and the injured uterine tissue at the site of the hysterotomy incision provide excellent culture media for microbial growth. The bacterial inoculum is particularly large when cesarean section is performed after multiple vaginal examinations and extended duration of labor and ruptured membranes.

Rationale for Prophylaxis. Antibiotic prophylaxis is intended to reduce the size of the bacterial inoculum and to change the characteristics of the culture medium at the operative site during the brief time that host defenses are impaired by the trauma of surgery.

Three clinical criteria should be fulfilled to justify perioperative use of prophylactic antibiotics.[43] First, the surgical procedure, by necessity, must be performed through a contaminated operative field. Second, there must be a high incidence of postoperative infection in the absence of prophylaxis. Finally, sequelae that may result from the primary infection must be significant.

Most cesarean deliveries fulfill these criteria. The major objective in using prophylactic antibiotics is to reduce the incidence of postcesarean endometritis. This disorder causes the patient considerable discomfort and results in increased duration of hospitalization. In addition, it is the usual precursor for serious complications such as pelvic abscess, septic shock, and septic pelvic thrombophlebitis. A second objective of prophylaxis is to reduce the incidence of these life-threatening complications.

The third objective of prophylaxis is to reduce the incidence of major wound infections. Such disorders usually require a second surgical procedure to open and debride the incision and may lead to dehiscence and evisceration. Wound infection is even more likely than endometritis to result in marked prolongation of the patient's hospitalization.

Results of Clinical Trials. Since 1970, more than 20 reports of prophylactic antibiotics in cesarean section have been published in the American obstetric literature (Figs. 46-27 and 46-28).[17] The studies summarized in the figures are restricted to prospective, randomized, placebo-controlled investigations in which antibi-

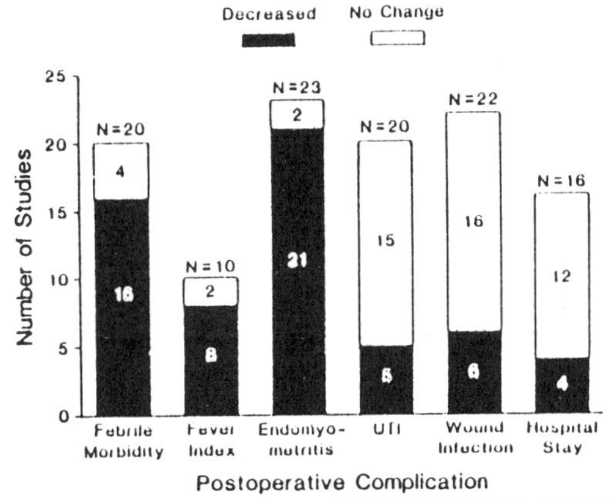

Figure 46-27. Effects of systemic antibiotic prophylaxis in patients undergoing cesarean section.

otic use was limited to a maximum of 24 hours immediately after surgery.

The drugs most commonly utilized for systemic prophylaxis have been ampicillin and the first-generation cephalosporins. Only one study directly compared a first-generation cephalosporin to an extended spectrum cephalosporin. In that study, cefoxitin and cefazolin were equally effective in reducing the incidence of febrile morbidity, endometritis, and wound infection and in decreasing the fever index.[63]

In the majority of investigations, the principal benefit of prophylaxis has accrued to women undergoing abdominal delivery after extended

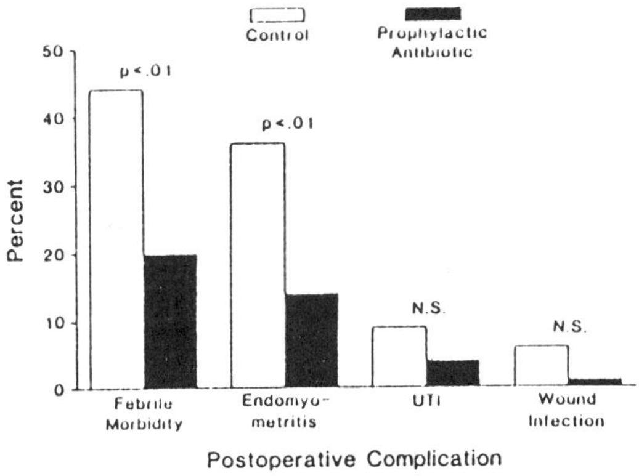

Figure 46-28. Mean incidence of postcesarean infection in control patients and patients receiving prophylactic antibiotics.

duration of labor and ruptured membranes. Most studies do not show a statistically significant decrease in the incidence of wound infection or endometritis in women who receive prophylaxis at the time of elective cesarean section.

Most clinicians utilize a three-dose regimen for prophylaxis. However, a single injection of systemic antibiotics may provide a degree of prophylaxis that is comparable to two-, three-, and four-dose regimens.

There is little reason to believe that a course of antibiotics extended over 3–5 days is any more effective in decreasing the incidence of postcesarean complications than is perioperative prophylaxis limited to 3 or 4 doses of antibiotic.

Delay in administration of antibiotics until after clamping of the cord or delivery of the fetus does not diminish the effectiveness of prophylaxis.

Finally, most investigations do not demonstrate that antibiotic prophylaxis decreases the incidence of abdominal wound infection. However, the failure to demonstrate statistically significant reductions in wound infection may be due to low incidences of infection in the control groups.

Alternatives to Systemic Antibiotics

Intraoperative Irrigation. Some clinicians advocate irrigation of the uterine and peritoneal cavity with an antibiotic solution as an alternative to systemic antibiotic prophylaxis. Intraoperative antibiotic irrigation appears to exert its primary effect by delivering a high concentration of antibiotic directly to the site of injured tissue and the site of maximum bacterial contamination. Systemic absorption of antibiotic does occur with topical irrigation, especially when both intrauterine and intraperitoneal irrigation are performed. However, the concentration of antibiotic in endometrial tissue is much higher than that achieved by systemic administration of the same dose of drug.

Additional investigation of antibiotic irrigation is indicated. The optimal agent for prophylaxis has not yet been determined. Reported differences in treatment with various antibiotics appear to relate more to pharmacokinetic properties of the drugs than to differences in spectrum of activity. In addition, it is not clear that topical irrigation is an appropriate alternative to systemic prophylaxis in all women undergoing cesarean delivery.

Early Treatment of Established Infection

In patient populations where the risk of postcesarean endometritis and wound infection is very low, early treatment of overt infection with antibiotics highly effective against anaerobes, aerobic streptococci, and aerobic gram-negative bacilli is an acceptable alternative to routine administration of prophylactic antibiotics. Broad spectrum single agents such as the third-generation cephalosporins and the new semisynthetic penicillins or the combination regimens of clindamycin plus an aminoglycoside cure 90–95% of patients who have operative site infections.[66] In isolated patients who fail to respond to one of these antibiotic regimens, cure usually can be effected by modifying antibiotic therapy. It is rare for such patients to develop complications such as septic shock, pelvic abscess, or septic pelvic thrombophlebitis.

Complications of Antibiotic Prophylaxis

Maternal Side Effects. To date, no serious maternal side effects related to use of antimicrobial prophylaxis for cesarean section have occurred. There are reports, however, of deaths from anaphylaxis in patients who received intraoperative injections of cephalothin during orthopedic procedures.[62] The anesthetized state masks the early warning symptoms of an anaphylactic reaction. The possibility of untoward side effects must always be considered when a decision is made to utilize prophylactic antibiotics. Even intraoperative antibiotic irrigation yields sufficient systemic absorption of the antibiotic to elicit an allergic reaction.

Neonatal Side Effects. Until recently, prophylactic antibiotic regimens provided for administration of the first dose of drug just prior to surgery. As a result, the fetus was exposed to at least minimal concentrations of a broad spectrum antibiotic. Most of the early investigations of prophylaxis did not examine specifically the incidence of infection-related complications in neonates exposed prenatally to antibiotics. Investigations that did ask this question did not demonstrate an increased incidence of neonatal infection in such infants.

Excellent evidence now demonstrates that delay in administration of antibiotics until after the umbilical cord is clamped does not reduce the success of prophylaxis. Therefore, there is no reason to expose the fetus to broad spectrum antibiotics prior to birth in order to provide prophylaxis for the mother.

Selection of Resistant Microorganisms. When antibiotic prophylaxis fails and patients develop endometritis, the organisms cultured are less likely to be aerobic and anaerobic cocci and *Bacteroides* species and more likely to be *E. coli* and enterococci.[27] The clinical significance of these changes in the flora of the lower genital tract is not clear. The incidence of serious complications is not increased in women who become infected despite administration of prophylactic antibiotics. The increased isolation of enterococci in women receiving prophylactic antibiotics is of concern, however. Many antibiotics used singly or in combination for treatment of postcesarean infection do not provide effective coverage against Group D streptococci, particularly enterococci. If prophylactic antibiotics are to be used routinely on an obstetric service, careful surveillance must be maintained to detect unusual changes in antimicrobial susceptibilities.

Conclusions Regarding Prophylactic Antibiotics

- The principal rationale for use of prophylactic antibiotics is reduction in the incidence of postcesarean endometritis. In selected patient populations, prophylaxis also has been effective in decreasing the incidence of major wound infection and decreasing the duration of hospitalization.
- In patients undergoing abdominal delivery after extended duration of labor and ruptured membranes, prophylactic antibiotics are indicated. The definition of "extended duration" will vary, depending on the characteristics of the patient population.
- In populations with a low risk of infection, prophylactic antibiotics are of only marginal benefit in women scheduled for elective repeat cesarean delivery.
- Administration of prophylaxis should be deferred until after delivery of the fetus. Prophylaxis should be limited to no more than 3 perioperative doses.
- In some patient populations, intraoperative irrigation of the endometrium and peri-

toneal cavity with an antibiotic solution appears to provide prophylaxis as effective as systemic administration of the same drug.

- The antibiotic selected for prophylaxis should provide reasonable, but not necessarily complete, coverage against the major pathogens responsible for postcesarean endometritis. The drug should be inexpensive, easy to administer, and should possess minimal toxicity. It should not be a drug ordinarily used for therapy of an established infection.
- If prophylactic antibiotics are used routinely on an obstetric service, physicians must maintain careful surveillance to detect untoward effects such as superinfection and alterations in microbial antibiotic susceptibility patterns.

CESAREAN HYSTERECTOMY

Historical Evolution of Cesarean Hysterectomy* (Table 46-5)

In 1768, Joseph Cavallini described experimental cesarean hysterectomy in laboratory animals and suggested that there might be instances in which such a procedure would be necessary as a lifesaving measure for the gravid patient.

> All things having been duly weighed, I do not doubt that the uterus is not at all necessary to life, but whether it may be plucked out with impunity from the human body we cannot be certain without a further series of experiments of this kind which, perhaps, a more fortunate generation may obtain.[58]
>
> In speculative moments, I have sometimes felt inclined to persuade myself that the dangers of the Caesarean operation might be considerably diminished by removal of the uterus. Perhaps this method of operating may prove an eminent and valuable improvement.[74]

Forty years later, Feser and Georg Rein published additional investigations in laboratory animals.

Cavallini's investigations stimulated other scientists to investigate cesarean hysterectomy. In 1823, James Blundell published his study of cesarean hysterectomy in the rabbit model.

In 1869, Horatio Storer[64] performed the first subtotal hysterectomy in a living patient. Abdominal delivery was necessary because the patient's birth canal was obstructed by a large pelvic tumor. Removal of the uterus was performed because of life-threatening hemorrhage. Although the infant survived, the patient died on the third day after surgery.

In 1876, Eduardo Porro[56] described the first cesarean hysterectomy in which both infant and mother survived. By a strange coincidence of fate, Porro's patient was also named Cavallini. Julia Cavallini was a 25-year-old dwarf. She was 4 feet 9 inches tall, and her pelvis was markedly distorted by rickets. After delivery of the infant, Porro performed a subtotal hysterectomy and unilateral salpingo-oophorectomy utilizing a snare called "Cintrat's constrictor."

Despite the lack of blood products, intravenous fluids, and antibiotics, Julia Cavallini survived a turbulent 40-day hospitalization. The successful outcome in this case was due to Porro's adherence to surgical principles that are well recognized today, but which certainly were not firmly established in 1876. He achieved hemostasis by use of the occluding snare. He irrigated the peritoneal cavity with carbolized sponges, drained the operative bed, and exteriorized the cervical stump in an effort to prevent infection. He closed the abdominal wound with wire to reduce the risk of dehiscence. Porro personally attended the patient during the first 24 hours after surgery, feeding her "champagne and laudanum."

Porro's paper, "Della Amputazione Utero-ovarica come Complemento de Tiaglo Cesereo," stimulated a flurry of interest in cesarean hysterectomy. Within months of his report, Inzana and Previtali in Italy and Hegar in Germany presented single-case reports of cesarean hysterectomy. Although two of the three infants survived, all three mothers died in the immediate postoperative period. These fatalities are not surprising, in view of the fact that one patient had osteosarcoma affecting the bones of the pelvis, one had eclampsia, and one had chorioamnionitis.

Two years after publication of Porro's paper, Muller of Switzerland described a modification of Porro's technique. His patient had been in labor for three days. Chorioamnionitis had developed, resulting in fetal death. Muller's innovation was to remove the uterus from the peritoneal cavity and elevate it onto the abdominal wall before making the hysterotomy incision.

> The object in removing the uterus from the abdomen before evacuating its contents was to control the hem-

* Unless otherwise specified, much of this historical information has been gleaned from References 19, 58, and 74.

TABLE 46-5. MAJOR EVENTS IN THE EVOLUTION OF CESAREAN HYSTERECTOMY

Year	Event
1768	Cavallini performed cesarean hysterectomy in laboratory animals.
1869	Storer performed first subtotal cesarean hysterectomy.
1876	Porro performed first cesarean hysterectomy in which both mother and infant survived.
1878	Muller described technique for exteriorizing uterus prior to hysterotomy incision.
1880	Harris reported first series of patients undergoing cesarean hysterectomy.
1881	Richardson performed first successful cesarean hysterectomy in United States.
1882	Wells performed first total cesarean hysterectomy.
1884	Godson described use of low transverse uterine incision.
1892	Von Waerz recommended retention of cervical stump in pelvic cavity and reapproximation of visceral peritoneum.

orrhage more early and lessen the risk of its putrid contents escaping into the peritoneal cavity. . . .

In 1880, Robert P. Harris[31] of the United States reviewed the world literature and collected 50 cases of cesarean hysterectomy, reported from seven countries. The cumulative maternal mortality was 58%; fetal survival was 86%.

The first report of cesarean hysterectomy in the United States was included in Harris' investigation. The operation was performed in 1880 by Isaac Taylor of New York, who used a uterine ligature technique similar to Porro's. Taylor's patient died of pulmonary embolism on the 26th postoperative day.

The first successful cesarean hysterectomy in the United States was performed by Richardson in 1881. His patient, like Porro's, was a young dwarf, 3 feet, 10 inches tall. Richardson utilized Muller's technique of exteriorizing the uterus. Once the uterus was positioned on the abdominal wall, a wire snare was placed around the cervix at the level of the internal os and tightened to secure hemostasis. After delivery of the fetus, the uterus was amputated, and the cervical stump was cauterized with carbolic acid and placed back into the pelvis. Both mother and infant survived.

One year later, the first cesarean hysterectomy was performed in Great Britain by Croom, Hart, and Caird. In that same year, Wells,[73] also of Great Britain, completed the first total cesarean hysterectomy; all previous operations had been supracervical procedures. The indication for surgery in Wells' patient was invasive cervical carcinoma. The first two British patients died in the immediate postoperative period.

In 1884, Godson[29] performed the first cesarean hysterectomy in Great Britain that resulted in maternal survival. He also was first to use a low transverse uterine incision. Additional modifications in Porro's operative technique were made by Tait,[67] Von Waerz, and Weiss. Each of these investigators directed special attention to management of the cervical stump after supracervical hysterectomy. Tait recommended exteriorization of the uterus, excision of the corpus, and suture of the cervical stump to the abdominal wall. Von Waerz and Weiss advocated leaving the cervical remnant within the pelvis and reapproximating the visceral peritoneum over the stump. Another modification in technique was suggested by several authors, including Reymond and Cazalis in 1911, LeCoq in 1917, and Solieri and Rogers in 1922. These investigators described performance of hysterectomy *before* cesarean delivery and reported survivals in both mother and infant.

Figure 46-29 illustrates the operative technique most commonly employed at the turn of the century.

Changing Indications for Cesarean Hysterectomy

Cesarean Hysterectomy for Sterilization. From its development in the mid-1800s until 1900, cesarean hysterectomy was performed exclusively as a lifesaving measure for the mother. In 1900, Reed outlined the following indications

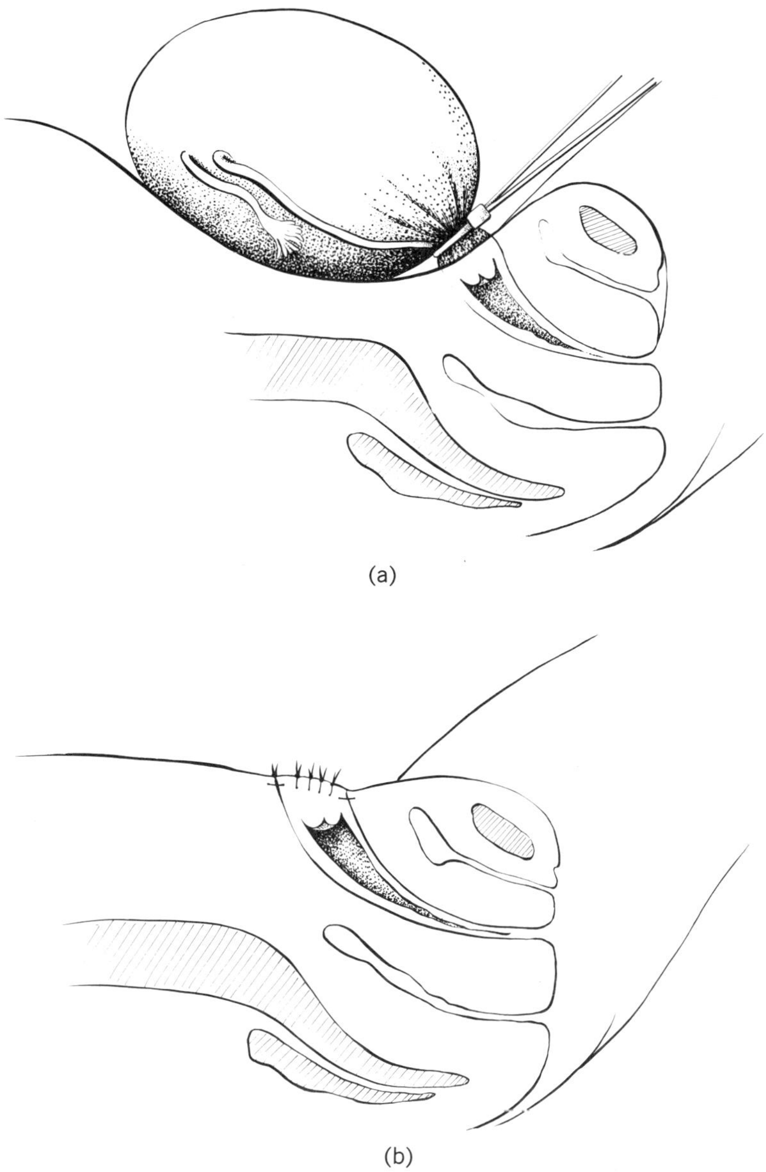

Figure 46-29. Panel A. Operative techniques for subtotal cesarean hysterectomy at beginning of the 20th century. Note the use of a constricting device to amputate the uterine fundus and to provide hemostasis.
Panel B. The cervical stump then is exteriorized and sutured to the anterior abdominal wall.

for the Porro procedure: (1) intrauterine fetal demise in association with chorioamnionitis; (2) cervical cancer; (3) hemorrhage due to uterine atony; (4) uncontrolled hemorrhage due to placenta previa, placenta accreta, or abruptio placentae; (5) ruptured uterus.

In the early 1900s, some clinicians began to extend the indications for cesarean hysterectomy. Duncan and Targett[18] of Great Britain were among the first to suggest that subtotal hysterectomy be performed for sterilization at the time of indicated cesarean delivery. In 1922,

J. W. Harris of Johns Hopkins reported 64 subtotal cesarean hysterectomies, of which 18 were performed for sterilization. Harris justified these elective procedures by citing an improved maternal mortality of 4.68% compared to the 58% incidence reported earlier by Robert P. Harris.

In 1935, Lash and Cummings listed the following indications for cesarean hysterectomy: intrauterine infection, acute blood loss, chronic renal disease, tuberculosis, and any case in which sterilization is indicated. Two years later, Wilson reported that 8.7% of all cesarean sections at the University of Rochester were accompanied by hysterectomy. He cited uterine leiomyoma, uncontrolled hemorrhage, intrauterine infection, and sterilization as acceptable indications for the procedure.

In 1951, M. E. Davis[11] of the Chicago Lying-In Hospital advocated the extreme view that sterilization by cesarean hysterectomy was justified "... in women near the end of their reproductive period, in whom the uterus no longer serves a useful function ..." and that "when reproduction is no longer desirable the uterus can be dispensed with, for, although it contributes little or nothing, the aging organ is subject to degeneration and serious disease." Addressing his contemporaries' concern with the psychological aspects of elective hysterectomy, Davis dismissed their fears by noting that "the complete removal of the uterus at delivery does not interfere with normal sex life, it actually improves it.... The roomy, plastic vagina, combined with the freedom from fear of conception results in ideal marital life."

Davis reported a series of 140 patients who underwent cesarean hysterectomy. Fifty-six percent of these procedures appear to have been performed solely for sterilization. Davis documented surprisingly low perioperative morbidity and an absence of maternal mortality.

Proponents of cesarean hysterectomy base some of their argument on the observation that a significant percentage of all women who undergo cesarean section subsequently require hysterectomy for treatment of a gynecologic disorder. In a well-publicized investigation by Weed, the average interval between cesarean section and hysterectomy was 6 years.[72]

The Present Controversy. The appropriate role of cesarean hysterectomy in modern obstetric practice is unsettled.[54] One extreme view argues that the overall results with cesarean hysterectomy justify the use of hysterectomy as a preferred method of sterilization in elective cases.[9,71]

At the other extreme are clinicians who believe that hysterectomy should not be used solely to effect sterilization at the time of cesarean section because the physical and emotional morbidity outweigh the benefits. Other clinicians perform elective cesarean hysterectomies in selected situations.

Emergency Versus Nonemergency Procedures. Table 46-6 summarizes selected publications on this subject. The incidence of cesarean hysterectomy in the studies listed ranges from 0.16% to 1.80% with a mean of 0.59%. The following conclusions concerning acceptable indications for surgery are based on the reports listed in Table 46-6.

Early investigators usually classified procedures as either elective or indicated. Elective procedures were those done for the sole purpose of effecting sterilization. Indicated procedures included operations performed because of obstetric emergencies and those done because of coexisting gynecologic disorders. This method of classification makes it difficult to separate morbidity associated with the operation itself from the morbidity associated with the underlying disorder. Therefore, it is more useful to classify indications for cesarean hysterectomy as emergency or nonemergency.[54] The latter category can be subdivided into procedures done to treat a coexisting gynecologic disorder and those done purely to accomplish sterilization.

Table 46-7 summarizes the most common indications for emergency cesarean hysterectomy. However, the disorders listed do not invariably require cesarean hysterectomy. For example, improved blood-banking services now make it possible to manage many coagulopathies medically. A well-planned revision of a uterine scar may obviate the need for hysterectomy. Excessive bleeding from an atonic uterus, unresponsive to oxytocin and ergot alkaloids, may be managed successfully with prostaglandin preparations.[33] Selective embolization of the pelvic vessels and hypogastric artery ligation also may be effective in controlling obstetric hemorrhage.[50]

It is rarely necessary to perform cesarean hysterectomy for treatment of chorioamnionitis. Early diagnosis and treatment of infection with broad spectrum antibiotics have greatly improved the prognosis for the patient with chorioamnionitis.[26]

TABLE 46-6. SUMMARY OF REPORTS OF CESAREAN HYSTERECTOMY

Authors	Institution	Year of Study	Number of Patients
Alford et al.[1]	Charity Hospital, New Orleans, LA	1949–1959	272
Amirikia and Evans[2]	Wayne State University	1965–1974	56
Barclay[5]	Tulane University	1938–1959	1000
Barclay[6]	University of Arkansas	1970–1974	242
Brenner et al.[8]	New York Medical College	1958–1968	198
Britton[9]	Tuomey Hospital, Sumter, SC	1968–1977	112
Davis[11]	Chicago Lying-In Hospital	1947–1951	140
Easterday[20]	Boston Lying-In Hospital	1933–1968	113
Haynes and Martin[34]	University of Louisville	1953–1977	149
Hofmeister[35]	Lutheran Hospital, Milwaukee, WI	1963–1967	32
Langer et al.[39]	New Jersey College of Medicine	1968–1973	150
Mickal et al.[45]	Louisiana State University	1959–1963	384
Morton[46]	Loma Linda University	1941–1961	250
Patterson[51]	University of Tennessee	1954–1967	327
Plauche et al.[53]	Howard Memorial Hospital, Biloxi, MS	1967–1977	108
Pletsch and Sandberg[54]	Stanford University	1949–1961	169
Prevedourakis[57]	University of Athens, Greece	1955–1968	79
Schneider and Tyrone[59]	Ochsner Foundation Hospital, New Orleans, LA	1946–1969	249
Webb and Gibbs[71]	University of Tennessee	1954–1966	72
	TOTAL		4102

Selected obstetric emergencies still may require cesarean hysterectomy, however. Uterine rupture that cannot be repaired securely should be managed by removal of the uterus. Hemorrhage unresponsive to medical management and lesser surgical maneuvers must be controlled by hysterectomy. Hemorrhage due to placenta accreta, increta, and percreta is particularly likely to mandate cesarean hysterectomy. Finally, fulminant intrauterine infection that precipitates septic shock and fails to respond promptly to medical management may require cesarean hysterectomy as a lifesaving measure.

Nonemergency cesarean hysterectomies include procedures performed for treatment of a coexisting gynecologic disorder and operations performed for sterilization. Gynecologic indications for hysterectomy include, but are not limited to, symptomatic leiomyomata, endometriosis, severe dysmenorrhea or dysfunctional uterine bleeding that is unresponsive to medical management, and Grade III cervical intraepithelial neoplasia in patients who desire sterilization.

TABLE 46-7. INDICATIONS FOR EMERGENCY CESAREAN HYSTERECTOMY

1. Uncontrolled hemorrhage
    a. Uterine atony
    b. Abruptio placentae complicated by coagulopathy
    c. Placenta accreta, increta, or percreta
    d. Uterine artery laceration
    e. Cervical laceration
2. Overwhelming infection
3. Uterine rupture not amenable to surgical repair

In nonindigent patients, the overall incidence of perioperative complications associated with cesarean hysterectomy appears to be similar to the incidence associated with cesarean section and interval hysterectomy. In this setting, the combined procedure may be justified provided that both acceptable obstetric and gynecologic indications for surgery exist. In some public hospitals where indigent patients are treated by physicians-in- training, the incidence of major complications associated with cesarean hysterectomy may be high enough to mandate that cesarean section and interval hysterectomy be done in preference. In either setting, use of the operation solely to effect sterilization is probably not justified because it exposes the patient to an unacceptably high risk of morbidity and mortality.

Special mention should be made of the fact that cesarean hysterectomy does have an established role in treatment of the pregnant patient who has an invasive cervical malignancy. Radical hysterectomy can be accomplished safely at the time of cesarean section. Radical cesarean hysterectomy is accepted treatment for Stage IA and IB cervical cancer that is identified during pregnancy. (See also Chapter 40.)

Complications Associated with Cesarean Hysterectomy

Figure 46-30, based on the reports listed in Table 46-6, summarizes the complications described most frequently in patients undergoing cesarean hysterectomy. Serious complications are most likely to occur during performance of an emergency cesarean hysterectomy but may occur with surprisingly high frequency during a nonemergency procedure. Major perioperative complications may be grouped into the following categories: (1) operative mortality, (2) perioperative hemorrhage, (3) infection-related complications, and (4) urinary tract injury.

Operative Mortality. The operative mortality in patients undergoing cesarean hysterectomy ranges from 0% to 10.1%, with a mean of 0.9% (Table 46-8). In contrast, the operative mortality in patients undergoing cesarean section ranges from 0.07% to 0.11%, with a mean of 0.09%.[3] In patients undergoing abdominal hysterectomy, operative mortality ranges from 0.10% to 0.24%, with a mean of 0.17%.[14]

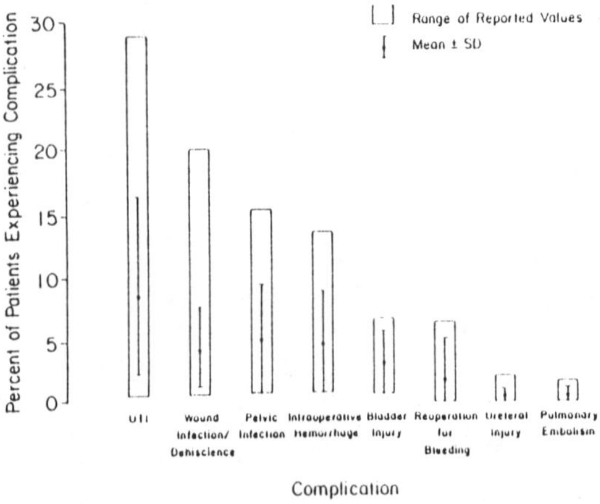

Figure 46-30. Incidence of perioperative complications associated with cesarean hysterectomy. Percentages are based upon the reports listed in Table 46–6.

Most deaths related to cesarean hysterectomy occur in indigent patients undergoing emergency operations. Acute hemorrhagic shock and pulmonary embolism are the leading causes of perioperative death. Most of the reported deaths occurred before the development of modern blood-banking procedures and anesthetic techniques and before the introduction of broad-spectrum antibiotics. Recent series from both public and private hospitals document several hundred elective and emergency procedures without a fatality. Nevertheless, when large series are considered cumulatively, the operative mortality associated with cesarean hysterectomy is five to eight times that associated with abdominal hysterectomy or cesarean section.

Perioperative Hemorrhage. Many cesarean hysterectomies are performed because of life-threatening hemorrhage due to obstetric disorders such as placenta previa, placenta accreta, and abruptio placentae. It is not surprising, then, that 56–100% (mean—75%) of patients undergoing emergency cesarean hysterectomy receive multiple blood transfusions. The average blood replacement during emergency surgery is 2.8 units of whole blood.

Excessive blood loss also may occur during elective cesarean hysterectomy. Twelve to 66% of patients (mean—39.6%) having elective operations receive transfusions. The average replacement is 1.3 units of whole blood. Even in this group of patients, the percentage of individuals requiring transfusions is approximately eight times that of patients having cesarean section[3] and three to four times that of women having abdominal hysterectomy.[14]

Perioperative hemorrhage is not always the result of an underlying obstetric disorder but often is due to technical difficulty with the surgical procedure itself. One to 13% of patients undergoing cesarean hysterectomy experience such extensive intraoperative blood loss that an unplanned surgical procedure such as adnexectomy, hypogastric artery ligation, or supracervical hysterectomy (rather than total hysterectomy) must be performed to control hemorrhage. Approximately 2% (range 0–6.3%) of patients require reexploration for control of postoperative hemorrhage. In these instances, bleeding usually has occurred from either the infundibulopelvic ligament or the uterine vascular pedicle. The incidence of reoperation for

TABLE 46-8. CAUSES OF MATERNAL DEATH IN PATIENTS UNDERGOING CESAREAN HYSTERECTOMY

Authors	Number of Patients	Number of Deaths	Percent	Etiology
Alford et al.[1]	272	1	0.4	Pulmonary embolism
Amirikia and Evans[2]	56	1	1.8	Pulmonary embolism
Barclay[5]	1000	9	0.9	Infection—2 Hemorrhage—2 CVA—2 Transfusion reaction—2 Renal failure—1
Haynes and Martin[34]	149	1	0.7	Pulmonary embolism
Morton[46]	250	3	1.2	Infection—2 Hemorrhage—1
Patterson[51]	327	1	0.3	Amniotic fluid embolism
Prevedourakis[57]	79	8	10.1	Hemorrhage—8

CVA = Cerebrovascular accident.

bleeding is well in excess of that reported in patients undergoing cesarean section[81] or abdominal hysterectomy.[42]

Infection-Related Complications. Postoperative soft-tissue pelvic infection, abdominal wound infection and disruption, and urinary tract infection constitute the second most common group of complications associated with cesarean hysterectomy. It is difficult to evaluate the reported incidence of perioperative infection for several reasons. Some authors use standard febrile morbidity to define infection. Standard morbidity does not accurately reflect the true incidence of overt clinical infection. The sporadic uncontrolled use of "prophylactic antibiotics" probably affects the reported incidence of infection-related complications. Finally, varying criteria are used for the diagnosis of pelvic infection. Many studies of cesarean hysterectomy were published before the pathophysiology of operative-site infection was well understood. Accordingly, many patients who were treated with antibiotics for "fever of unexplained etiology" may have had pelvic cellulitis. Therefore the true incidence of this disorder has likely been underreported.

With these caveats in mind, several general conclusions appear to be warranted. The most common perioperative infection is lower urinary tract infection (UTI), which occurs, on the average, in 9% of patients. Paradoxically, incidence of UTI after cesarean hysterectomy is apparently lower than that associated with abdominal hysterectomy. In patients undergoing the latter operation, the reported incidence of UTI ranges from 2% to 57% with a mean of 20%.[15,16] The incidence of UTI after cesarean section is approximately 13% in patients who do not receive prophylactic antibiotics.[65]

Pelvic cellulitis is the second most common infection, occurring in 0.7–15% of patients with a mean incidence of 6.1%. In contrast, pelvic cellulitis occurs in 2–33% (mean—13%) of patients undergoing abdominal hysterectomy. Endometritis occurs in 30–40% of patients delivered by cesarean section without antibiotic prophylaxis.

The highest reported incidence of pelvic abscess in patients having cesarean hysterectomy is 3.8% of a series of 1000 indigent patients.[5] Most investigators describe an incidence of abscess of less than 0.5%. By comparison, the reported incidence of pelvic abscess following abdominal hysterectomy or cesarean section ranges from less than 1% to 4%.[14-16,42,65]

Wound infection is the third most frequent infection and occurs, on the average, in 4–5% of patients. Comparable figures for patients undergoing abdominal hysterectomy and cesarean section are 15%[15,16] and 5–7%,[65] respectively.

Figure 46-31 summarizes the incidence of infection in patients undergoing cesarean hysterectomy, abdominal hysterectomy, and cesarean section. The lowest incidence of each of these infections is associated with cesarean hysterectomy.

Urinary Tract Injury. Inadvertent injury to the urinary bladder occurs in 0.9–6.7% (mean—3.5%) of patients undergoing cesarean hysterectomy. Most injuries occur in patients who have a history of prior cesarean section and who have extensive adhesions between the bladder and lower uterine segment. Approximately 15% of

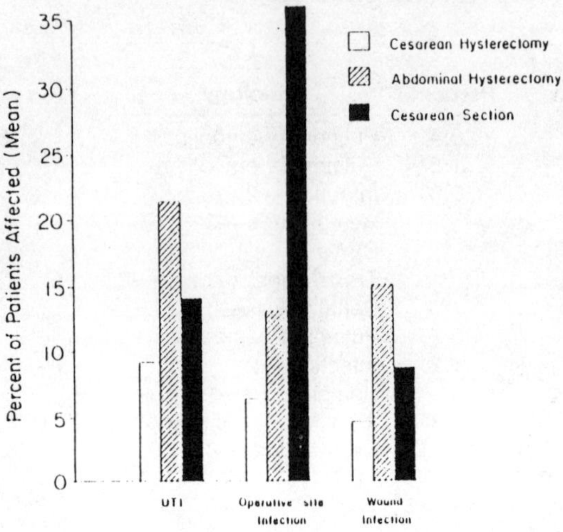

Figure 46-31. Comparison of incidence of infection in patients undergoing cesarean hysterectomy, abdominal hysterectomy, and cesarean section.

bladder injuries result in vesicovaginal fistulas. Virtually every reported case of fistula developed because the original bladder injury was not recognized and repaired primarily.

The reported incidence of ureteral injury varies from 0% to 1.8% with a mean of 0.6%. Ureteral injury most commonly occurs at three anatomic sites. The ureter may be incorporated into the pedicle containing the infundibulopelvic ligament when adnexectomy is performed. It may be ligated or transected as the uterine vessels are clamped and incised. It also may be injured as it courses through the paracervical tissue and enters the bladder. Although ureteral injury is relatively rare, 33–40% of patients who sustain such injuries develop ureterovaginal fistulas. If recognized promptly, most ureteral injuries may be managed by either reanastomosis or ureteroneocystostomy.

Urinary tract injury is 5 to 10 times less likely to occur during abdominal hysterectomy and cesarean section than during cesarean hysterectomy.[2,22]

Operative Technique

The reported operating time required for cesarean hysterectomy ranges from 65 to 132 minutes with a mean of 100 minutes. The operative technique for cesarean hysterectomy is illustrated in Figs. 46-32–46-36.

Skin Incision. When cesarean hysterectomy is performed for treatment of invasive cervical malignancy, the surgeon must have sufficient operative exposure to allow thorough exploration of the abdominal viscera and upper periaortic lymph nodes. Most oncologists prefer a vertical incision for this purpose.

When surgery is performed because of an obstetric emergency, a vertical incision should be utilized, since it permits the most rapid abdominal entry and assures maximal surgical exposure. When cesarean hysterectomy is performed for nonemergency indications, either a transverse incision or a vertical incision is acceptable. Operative exposure may be limited with the former incision, however, particularly when surgery is done under conduction anesthesia.

Dissection of the Bladder. In order to reduce the risk of bladder injury, sharp dissection of individual adhesions should be employed if necessary to free the bladder from the underlying uterus (Fig. 46-32). In the presence of adhesions, efforts to separate the bladder by blunt dissection may result in trauma to the posterior bladder wall. The surgeon should be particularly careful to avoid extension of the dissection laterally into the highly vascular bladder pillars. The dissection initially should be extended in-

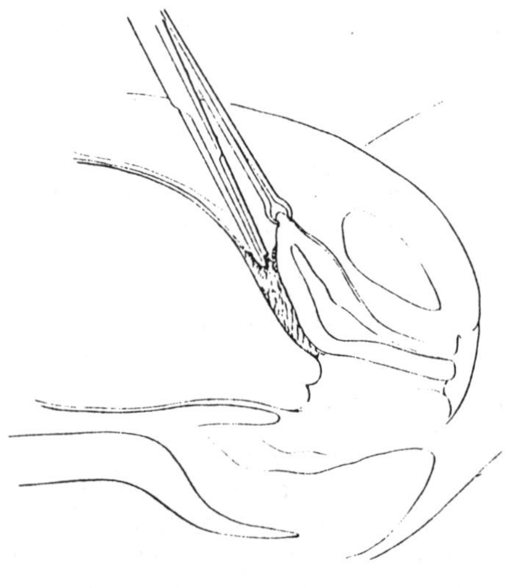

Figure 46-32. The bladder should be separated from the lower uterine segment by sharp dissection to prevent injury to the posterior bladder wall. Elevation of the bladder with an atraumatic clamp facilitates identification and lysis of individual adhesions.

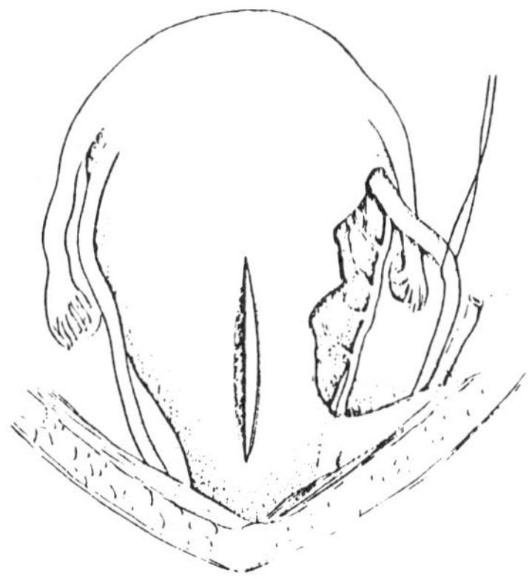

Figure 46-33. The low vertical (Krönig) hysterotomy incision minimizes the risk of lateral extension of the incision into the uterine vessels and broad ligament.

feriorly only so far as is necessary to permit safe ligation of the uterine vascular pedicle.

Bladder injuries must be recognized and repaired immediately in order to prevent formation of a vesicovaginal fistula. When bladder dissection has been difficult, bladder competency should be evaluated at the conclusion of the procedure by instilling marker media (such as sterile evaporated milk) through the urinary catheter.

Uterine Incision. A classical uterine incision should be performed for selected obstetric indications such as transverse lie with the fetal back down, compound presentation, premature breech presentation, and placenta previa associated with multiple varicosities of the lower uterine segment. In other clinical situations, a low transverse or low vertical incision is acceptable.

The most serious complication associated with a transverse incision is extension of the incision into the uterine vessels and broad ligament, resulting in severe intraoperative hemorrhage. Lateral extension is particularly likely to occur in patients in whom the lower uterine segment is poorly developed. In contrast, a low vertical incision provides excellent access for delivery of the fetus and minimizes the risk of lateral extension of the incision into the broad ligament. It also facilitates exposure of the cervix and separation of cervix from vagina during removal of the uterus (Figs. 46-33 and 46-34).

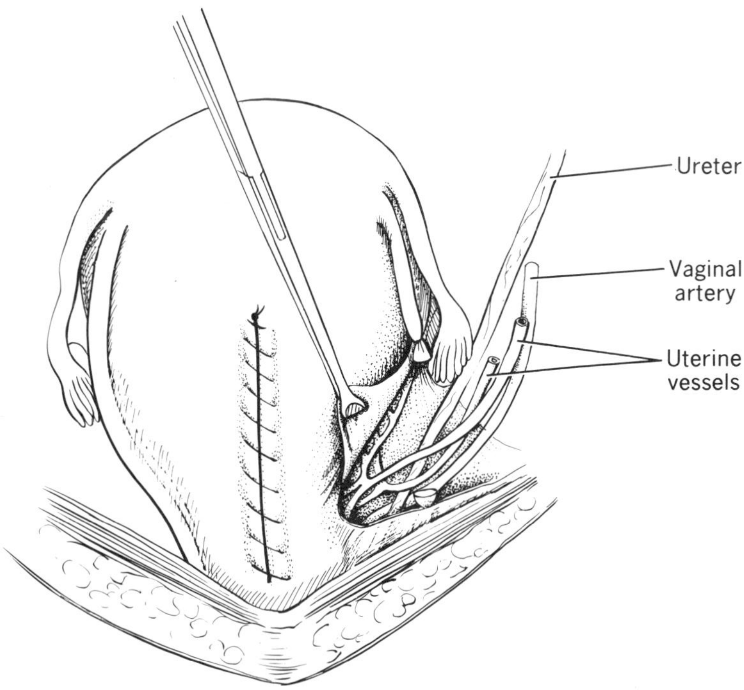

Figure 46-34. The low vertical incision is reapproximated with through-and-through sutures or with towel clips. The round ligament then is ligated and incised, and the visceral peritoneum is opened to expose the ureter. Note that the ureter courses along the medial leaf of the broad ligament and beneath the uterine artery and vein.

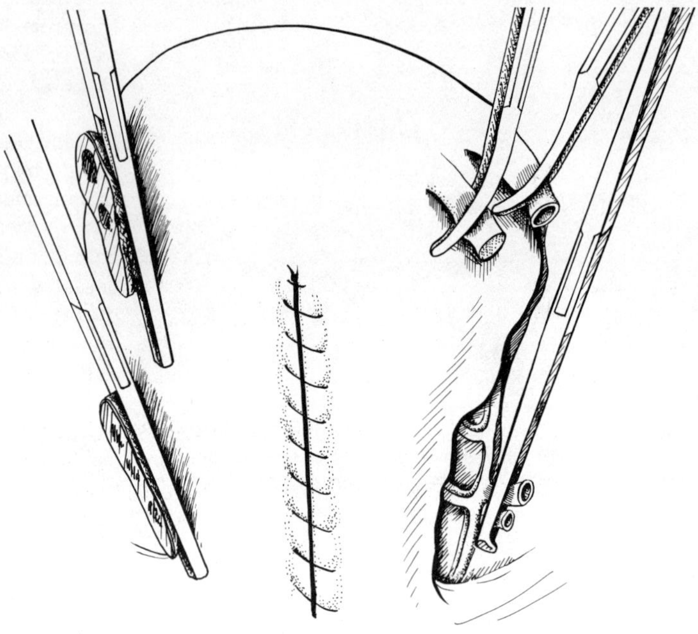

Figure 46-35. Pedicles along the lateral margin of the uterus are isolated and ligated. Clamps may be applied to the proximal side of the pedicles to prevent retrograde bleeding.

Identification of the Ureter. Ureteral injuries are largely preventable by employing meticulous surgical technique. Even when adnexectomy is not contemplated, the visceral peritoneum should be opened and the ureter should be identified as it courses along the medial leaf of the broad ligament (Fig. 46-34). Dissection of the ureter is continued to the point where it passes below the uterine artery and vein so that the uterine vascular pedicle may be isolated without risk of injury to the adjacent ureter. Careful separation of the bladder from the lower uterine segment also ensures that the ureters are displaced laterally away from the uterine vascular structures.

If radical cesarean hysterectomy is to be per-

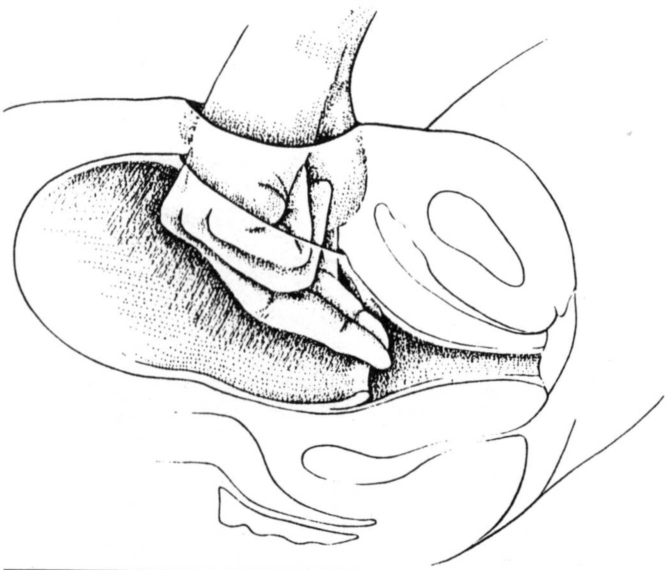

Figure 46-36. Surgeon places finger through the cervix into vaginal fornices to identify cervicovaginal junction and to ensure that entire cervix is excised.

formed, the ureter must be dissected free from the paracervical tissue, and the point of insertion of the ureter into the bladder must be identified. In simple cesarean hysterectomy, this additional dissection is not necessary. It is prudent, however, to palpate the ureter in the distal third of its course to ensure that it is lateral to the point where clamps and ligatures are applied to the cardinal ligaments, uterosacral ligaments, and upper vagina (Figs. 46-35 and 46-36).

Isolation and Ligation of Vascular Pedicles. One to 13% (mean—5.6%) of patients undergoing cesarean hysterectomy experience severe intraoperative hemorrhage because of uncontrolled bleeding from either the ovarian or uterine vascular pedicle. Unilateral or bilateral adnexectomy may be necessary to manage this complication.

During pregnancy, the ovarian and uterine vessels are dilated to 10 times their normal caliber and blood flow is increased many times above that of the nonpregnant state. All vascular pedicles must be clearly identified, isolated, and securely clamped and ligated. The amount of tissue included in each pedicle should be minimized, and both leaves of the broad ligament should be incorporated into the pedicle to prevent retraction of vessels and bleeding from denuded peritoneal surfaces. Retrograde bleeding from the uterine side of pedicles may be prevented by clamping or ligating the proximal side of each pedicle (Fig. 46-35).

Prevention of Perioperative Infection. There are no prospective, randomized, controlled investigations of the use of prophylactic antibiotics in patients undergoing cesarean hysterectomy. Therefore, conclusions about their value must be extrapolated from data reported for cesarean delivery or abdominal hysterectomy.

Prophylactic antibiotics decrease the incidence of lower urinary tract infection after abdominal hysterectomy and cesarean section. However, prevention of cystitis is not an acceptable rationale for the use of prophylactic antibiotics. Infections of the lower urinary tract rarely cause serious morbidity in obstetric patients. In most instances, such infections can be treated successfully with oral antibiotics without prolonging the patient's hospital stay.

Although prophylactic antibiotics are effective in decreasing the incidence of endometritis after cesarean section, they are not of proven value in decreasing the occurrence of posthysterectomy pelvic cellulitis. Since the incidence of pelvic cellulitis after cesarean hysterectomy appears to be lower than that associated with abdominal hysterectomy, prophylactic antibiotics are unlikely to be of value in decreasing significantly the incidence of pelvic infection after the former procedure.

Prophylactic antibiotics are of value in decreasing the incidence of incisional infections in selected patients undergoing cesarean section and abdominal hysterectomy. In patient populations displaying a high incidence of wound infection, use of perioperative antibiotics as prophylaxis for wound infection is justified since wound infections may cause serious morbidity (dehiscence, evisceration, necrotizing fasciitis) and prolonged hospitalization.

If prophylactic antibiotics are given to patients undergoing cesarean hysterectomy, administration should be delayed until after the infant has been delivered and should be restricted to no more than 3 doses in the perioperative period. Antibiotics used in prophylaxis should have minimal toxicity and a broad spectrum of activity against recognized pelvic pathogens. They should not be drugs that are commonly used as initial therapy for established infections.

Anesthesia for Cesarean Hysterectomy. Nonemergency, scheduled cesarean hysterectomies may be performed under either regional or general anesthesia. Most clinicians recommend endotracheal intubation and general anesthesia for emergency cesarean hysterectomy. Regional anesthetics usually require more time to administer and may exacerbate maternal hemodynamic dysfunction in the setting of such an obstetric emergency.

The preferred agents for general anesthesia are those that produce the least depressive effect on the cardiovascular system of the mother and fetus. Inhalation gases that result in marked uterine relaxation, such as halothane and enflurane, should be avoided in patients with severe hemorrhage. The anesthetic regimen most commonly used for emergency cesarean hysterectomy is the same as the one outlined previously for emergency cesarean delivery.

REFERENCES

1. Alford, C. D., Miller, A. C., and Simpson, J. W.: Cesarean section hysterectomy: A 10 year review. *Am. J. Obstet. Gynecol.* **82**:664–668, 1961.

2. Amirikia, H. and Evans, T. N.: Ten year review of hysterectomies: Trends, indications, and risks. *Am. J. Obstet. Gynecol.* **134**:431–437, 1979.
3. Amirikia, H., Zarewych, B., and Evans, T. N.: Cesarean section: A 15-year review of changing incidence, indications, and risks. *Am. J. Obstet. Gynecol.* **140**:81–90, 1981.
4. Arthur, R. K.: Postmortem cesarean section. *Am. J. Obstet. Gynecol.* **132**:175–177, 1978.
5. Barclay, D. L.: Cesarean hysterectomy at the Charity Hospital in New Orleans—1000 consecutive operations. *Clin. Obstet. Gynecol.* **12**:635–651, 1969.
6. Barclay, D. L., Hawks, B. L., Frueh, D. M., Power, J. D., and Struble, R. H.: Elective cesarean hysterectomy: A 5 year comparison with cesarean section. *Am. J. Obstet. Gynecol.* **124**:900–910, 1976.
7. Beck, A. G.: The advantages and disadvantages of the two flap low incision cesarean section, with a report of eighty-three cases done by fifteen operators. *Am. J. Obstet. Gynecol.* **1**:586–594, 1921.
8. Brenner, P., Sall, S., and Sonnenblick, B.: Evaluation of cesarean section hysterectomy as a sterilization procedure. *Am. J. Obstet. Gynecol.* **108**:335–339, 1970.
9. Britton, J. J.: Sterilization by cesarean hysterectomy. *Am. J. Obstet. Gynecol.* **137**:837–842, 1980.
10. Cragin, E. B.: Conservatism in obstetrics. *N.Y. Med. J.* **104**:1–3, 1916.
11. Davis, M. E.: Complete cesarean hysterectomy. A logical advance in modern obstetric surgery. *Am. J. Obstet. Gynecol.* **62**:838–850, 1951.
12. DeLee, J. B. and Cornell, E. L.: Low cervical cesarean section (laparotrachelotomy). *JAMA* **79**:109–112, 1922.
13. De Palma, R. T., Cunningham, F. G., Leveno, K. G., and Roark, M. L.: Continuing investigation of women at high risk for infection following cesarean delivery. *Obstet. Gynecol.* **60**:53–59, 1982.
14. Dicker, R. C., Greenspan, J. R., Strauss, L.T., Cowart, M. R., Scally, M. J., Peterson, H. B., De Stefano, F., Rubin, G. L., and Ory, H. W.: Complications of abdominal and vaginal hysterectomy among women of reproductive age in the United States. The collaborative review of sterilization. *Am. J. Obstet. Gynecol.* **144**:841–848, 1982.
15. Duff, P.: Antibiotic prophylaxis for abdominal hysterectomy. *Obstet. Gynecol.* **60**:25–29, 1982.
16. Duff, P.: Antibiotic prophylaxis for abdominal hysterectomy: A review. *Infect. Dis. Ltr. Obstet. Gynecol.* **5**:49–54, 1983.
17. Duff, P.: Antibiotic prophylaxis for cesarean section: A review of the American literature since 1970. *Sex. Med. Today,* **9**:18, 1985.
18. Duncan, W. and Targett, J. H.: Porro-Cesarean hysterectomy with retro-peritoneal treatment of the stump in a case of fibroids obstructing labour; with remarks upon the relative advantage of the modern Porro operation over the Sanger Cesarean in most other cases requiring abdominal section. *Trans. Obstet. Soc. Lond.* **42**:244, 1900.
19. Durfee, R. B.: Evolution of cesarean hysterectomy. *Clin. Obstet. Gynecol.* **12**:575–589, 1969.
20. Easterday, C. L.: Cesarean hysterectomy at the Boston Hospital for women. *Clin. Obstet. Gynecol.* **12**:652–659, 1969.
21. Eastman, N. J.: The role of frontier America in the development of cesarean section. *Am. J. Obstet. Gynecol.* **24**:919–920, 1932.
22. Eisenkop, S. M., Richman, R., Platt, L. D., and Paul, R. H.: Urinary tract injury during cesarean section. *Obstet. Gynecol.* **60**:591–596, 1982.
23. Francis, J. W. and Beck, J. B.: Case of self-performed caesarean section. *N.Y. Med. Phys. J.* **2**:40–44, 1823.
24. Frank, F.: Suprasymphysial delivery and its relation to other operations in the presence of contracted pelvis. *Arch. Gynaekol.* **81**:46, 1907.
25. Frigoletto, F. D., Jr., Ryan, K. J., and Phillippe, M.: Maternal mortality rate associated with cesarean section: An appraisal. *Am. J. Obstet. Gynecol.* **136**:969–970, 1980.
26. Gibbs, R. S., Castillo, M. S., and Rodgers, P. J.: Management of acute chorioamnionitis. *Am. J. Obstet. Gynecol.* **136**:709–713, 1980.
27. Gibbs, R. S., St. Clair, P. J., Castillo, M. S., and Castaneda, Y. S.: Bacteriologic effects of antibiotic prophylaxis in high-risk cesarean section. *Obstet. Gynecol.* **57**:277–282, 1981.
28. Gleicher, N.: Cesarean section rates in the United States. The short-term failure of the National Consensus Development Conference in 1980. *JAMA* **252**:3273–3276, 1984.
29. Godson, C.: Porro's operation. *Br. Med. J.* **1**:142–154, 1884.
30. Hanson, H. B.: Current use of the extraperitoneal cesarean section: A decade of experience. *Am. J. Obstet. Gynecol.* **149**:31–34, 1984.
31. Harris, R. P.: Results of the first fifty cases of "cesarean ovarohysterectomy," 1869–1880. *Am. J. Med. Sci.* **80**:129–134, 1880.
32. Hayashi, R. H., Berry, J. L., and Castillo, M. S.: Use of ultrasound biparietal diameter in timing of repeat cesarean section. *Obstet. Gynecol.* **57**:325–329, 1981.
33. Hayashi, R. H., Castillo, M. S., and Noah, M. L.: Management of severe postpartum hemorrhage due to uterine atony using an analogue of prostaglandin $F_{2\alpha}$. *Obstet. Gynecol.* **58**:426–429, 1981.
34. Haynes, D. M. and Martin, B. J.: Cesarean hysterectomy: A twenty-five year review. *Am. J. Obstet. Gynecol.* **134**:393–398, 1979.
35. Hofmeister, F. J.: Tubal ligation versus cesarean hysterectomy. *Clin. Obstet. Gynecol.* **12**:676–687, 1969.
36. Horowitz, B. J., Edelstein, S. W., and Lippman, L.: Once a cesarean...always a cesarean. *Obstet. Gynecol. Surv.* **36**:592–598, 1981.
37. Kerr, J. M. M.: The technic of cesarean section, with special reference to the lower uterine segment incision. *Am. J. Obstet. Gynecol.* **12**:729–734, 1926.

38. King, A. G.: America's first cesarean section. *Obstet. Gynecol.* **37**:797-802, 1971.
39. Langer, R., Pelosi, M., Hung, C. T., Devanesan, R., Caterini, H., Harrigan, J. T., and Sama, J.: Comparison of sterilization by tubal ligation and hysterectomy. *Surg. Gynecol. Obstet.* **140**:235-238, 1975.
40. Latzko, W.: Der extraperitoneale Kaiserschnitt, seine Geschichte, seine Technik and seine Indikationen. *Wien. Klin. Wochenschr.* **22**:477-482, 1909.
41. Lavin, J. P., Stephens, R. J., Miodovnik, M., and Barden, T. P.: Vaginal delivery in patients with a prior cesarean section. *Obstet. Gynecol.* **59**:135-147, 1982.
42. Ledger, W. J. and Child, M. A.: The hospital care of patients undergoing hysterectomy: An analysis of 12,026 patients from the Professional Activity Study. *Am. J. Obstet. Gynecol.* **117**:423-433, 1973.
43. Ledger, W. J., Gee, C., and Lewis, W. P.: Guidelines for antibiotic prophylaxis in gynecology. *Am. J. Obstet. Gynecol.* **121**:1038-1044, 1975.
44. Merrill, B. S. and Gibbs, C. E.: Planned vaginal delivery following cesarean section. *Obstet. Gynecol.* **52**:50-52, 1978.
45. Mickal, A., Begneaud, W. P., and Hawes, T. P.: Pitfalls and complications of cesarean section hysterectomy. *Clin. Obstet. Gynecol.* **12**:660-675, 1969.
46. Morton, J. H.: Cesarean hysterectomy. *Am. J. Obstet. Gynecol.* **83**:1422-1430, 1962.
47. National Institute of Child Health and Human Development: Report of a Consensus Development Conference on Cesarean Childbirth. National Institutes of Health Publication No. 82-2067, 1981.
48. O'Connor, R. M.: How safe is induction of labour following a previous cesarean section? *J. Obstet. Gynaecol.* **44**:86-87, 1983.
49. O'Sullivan, M. J., Fumia, F., Holsinger, K., and McLeod, A.G.W.: Vaginal delivery after cesarean section. *Clin. Perinatol.* **8**:131-143, 1981.
50. Pais, S. O., Glickman, M., Schwartz, P., Pingoud, E., and Berkowitz, R.: Embolization of pelvic arteries for control of postpartum hemorrhage. *Obstet. Gynecol.* **55**:754-758, 1980.
51. Patterson, S. P.: Cesarean hysterectomy. *Am. J. Obstet. Gynecol.* **107**:729-734, 1970.
52. Pauerstein, C. J.: Once a section, always a trial of labor. *Obstet. Gynecol.* **28**:273-276, 1966.
53. Plauche, W. C., Gruich, F. G., and Bourgeois, M. O.: Hysterectomy at the time of cesarean section: Analysis of 108 cases. *Obstet. Gynecol.* **58**:459-464, 1981.
54. Pletsch, T. D. and Sandberg, E. C.: Cesarean hysterectomy for sterilization. *Am. J. Obstet. Gynecol.* **85**:254-259, 1963.
55. Porreco, R. P. and Meier, P. R.: Trial of labor in patients with multiple previous cesarean sections. *J. Reprod. Med.* **28**:770-772, 1983.
56. Porro, E.: Dell'amputazione utero-ovarica come complemento de taglio cesareo—Milan, frat Rechiedei, 1876.
57. Prevedourakis, C. N.: Emergency cesarean hysterectomy. *Int. Surg.* **59**:33-34, 1974.
58. Riva, H. L.: Indications and techniques for cesarean hysterectomy. *Clin. Obstet. Gynecol.* **12**:618-634, 1969.
59. Schneider, G. T. and Tyrone, C. H.: Cesarean hysterectomy. *Surg. Gynecol. Obstet.* **130**:501-504, 1970.
60. Seitchik, J. and Rao, V. R.: Cesarean delivery in nulliparous women for failed oxytocin-augmented labor: Route of delivery in subsequent pregnancy. *Am. J. Obstet. Gynecol.* **143**:393-397, 1982.
61. Speert, H.: *Obstetrics and Gynecology in America: A History.* Baltimore, MD, Waverly Press, 1980.
62. Spruill, F. G., Minette, L. G., and Sturner, W. Q.: Two surgical deaths associated with cephalothin. *JAMA* **229**:440-441, 1974.
63. Stiver, H. G., Forward, K. R., Livingstone, R. A., Fugeéere, P., Lemay, M., Verschelden, G., Hunter, J. D. W., Carson, G. D., Beresford, P., and Tyrrell, D. L.: Multicenter comparison of cefoxitin versus cefazolin for prevention of infectious morbidity after nonelective cesarean section. *Am. J. Obstet. Gynecol.* **145**:158-163, 1983.
64. Storer, H. R.: Successful removal of the uterus and both ovaries by abdominal section; the tumor, fibrocystic, weighing thirty-seven pounds. *Am. J. Med. Sci.* **51**:110-139, 1866.
65. Swartz, W. H. and Grolle, K.: The use of prophylactic antibiotics in cesarean section: A review of the literature. *J. Reprod. Med.* **26**:595-609, 1981.
66. Sweet, R. L., Yonekura, M. L., Hill, G., Gibbs, R. S., and Eschenbach, D. A : Appropriate use of antibiotics in serious obstetric and gynecologic infections. *Am. J. Obstet. Gynecol.* **146**:719-739, 1983.
67. Tait, L.: Address on the surgical aspect of impacted labour. *Br. Med. J.* **1**:657-661, 1890.
68. Trolle, D.: *The History of Cesarean Section.* Copenhagen, Denmark, University Library, CA, Reitzel Booksellers, 1982.
69. Wallace, R. L., Eglinton, G. S., and Yonekura, M. L.: Extraperitoneal cesarean section: A surgical form of infection prophylaxis? *Am. J. Obstet. Gynecol.* **148**:172-179, 1984.
70. Waters, E. G.: Supravesical extraperitoneal cesarean section. *Am. J. Obstet. Gynecol.* **39**:423-432, 1940.
71. Webb, C. F. and Gibbs, J. V.: Preplanned toal cesarean hysterectomies. *Am. J. Obstet. Gynecol.* **101**:23-27, 1968.
72. Weed, J. C.: The fate of the postcesarean uterus. *Obstet. Gynecol.* **14**:780-785, 1959.
73. Wells, T. S.: Observations on recent improvements in the mode of removing uterine tumors. *Br. Med. J.* **1**:909-910, 1881.
74. Young, J. H.: *The History of Cesarean Section.* Lewis, London, 1944.

47

POSTPARTUM HEMORRHAGE

DEFINITION, INCIDENCE, AND IMPORTANCE

Postpartum hemorrhage is defined as the loss of 500 ml or more of blood from the reproductive tract after the third stage of labor. Bleeding also may be classified as early or late postpartum hemorrhage, depending on whether or not it occurs in the first 24 hours after delivery.[3] The definition needs revision. Several investigators using different methods of measuring usual blood loss after delivery obtained similar estimates of blood loss that often far exceeded 500 ml. The usually quoted incidence of postpartum hemorrhage is 4–5%. With accurate measurement of blood loss, almost 40% of women lose 500 ml of blood after normal vaginal delivery. Thus, the current definition rests on consistent underestimation of normal blood loss after delivery. An appeal to express blood loss at delivery as a percentage of the woman's estimated blood volume and to define postpartum hemorrhage as blood loss greater than 15% of the estimated blood volume[39] has received little acceptance.

An analysis of 2000 deliveries in Canada in 1941 defined postpartum hemorrhage as the loss of more than 1% of the patient's body weight. The average blood loss for nulliparas was 388 ml. Twenty-one percent of nulliparas had a blood loss in excess of 600 ml. In 1200 multiparas, the average blood loss was 323 ml. Twelve percent of these women lost more than 600 ml of blood. Overall, 16% of the 2000 women lost more than 600 ml of blood. Factors associated with increased blood loss included multiple gestation, large infants, maternal obesity, increasing length of labor, use of forceps, perineal incisions or lacerations, and long duration of the third stage of labor.[13]

Studies on the effects of the routine use of oxytocics to decrease postpartum bleeding found the least blood loss in women of parity between 1 and 4. Women of higher or lower parity lost more blood. The authors used the acid–hematin spectrophotometric method of measuring blood loss. Correcting for 10% error and for maternal blood lost with the placenta, the mean blood loss at delivery and in the first hour after delivery was calculated to be 577 ml. They thought their method 90% accurate in estimating blood loss. When comparing their results to clinical estimates of blood loss, they found a 46% error in the clinical estimate. Specifically, when the clinical estimate was 500 ml, the measured loss was 750 ml, and the total loss, including blood in the drapes, clots, and blood in the placenta, was approximately 950 ml![40,41]

Blood volume changes in the puerperium were investigated using chromium-tagged erythrocytes. After vaginal delivery, 75 women investigated lost an average of 505 ml of blood. Thirty-two percent of the women lost between 500 and 1000 ml of blood and 7% of women lost more than 1000 ml. The average loss was 9% of the woman's blood volume. Elective cesarean delivery without labor was associated with an average loss of 930 ml and elective cesarean hysterectomy without labor had an average blood loss of 1435 ml—30% of the total blood volume. The standard deviations in all these averages were quite large; nevertheless, spontaneous and operative deliveries are often associated with substantial blood loss that usually is underestimated by the physician.[50]

Hemorrhage continues to be among the leading causes of maternal mortality. Postpartum hemorrhage is one of the leading causes of obstetric hemorrhage. When pregnancies not associated with abortive outcomes are considered, obstetric hemorrhage is the third most common cause of maternal mortality in the United States.[33] In the most recent analysis of maternal deaths in England and Wales,[15] hemorrhage—excluding abortion, ectopic pregnancy, and ruptured uterus—was also the third leading cause of maternal death. Postpartum hemorrhage accounted for 74% of hemorrhage deaths. This is little changed from 1941, when postpartum hemorrhage accounted for 30% of all maternal deaths in Alberta, Canada.[13] A review of 501 consecutive maternal deaths in Texas from 1969 to 1973 also demonstrated that postpartum hemorrhage was one of the leading causes of maternal death.[19] This was not because of inadequate facilities or difficulty in transporation, but rather because the excessive bleeding was not anticipated or because it was not recognized promptly. This is very similar to the situation reported from England and Wales where women died of postpartum hemorrhage because the blood loss was underestimated, was not reported early enough, and was not properly investigated, diagnosed, or managed.

ETIOLOGY

Uterine Atony

Uterine atony is the most common cause of postpartum hemorrhage. Factors that predispose to uterine atony usually can be anticipated prior to delivery. Overdistention of the uterus from polyhydramnios, multiple gestation, or a macrosomic infant is associated with atony. Prolonged labor, oxytocin use in labor, and precipitous labor are associated with uterine atony. Some drugs, especially the anesthetic agents halothane and ethyl ether, cause uterine relaxation. This action is beneficial when uterine relaxation is desired, but the relaxation induced by halothane is not readily reversible with oxytocics. Magnesium sulfate infusion during labor has been associated with postpartum uterine atony. Multiparity, past history of uterine atony, amniotic fluid embolus, and intra-amniotic infection have all been associated with uterine atony.

At term, approximately 600 ml of blood per minute pass through the spiral arteries of the uterus to enter the intervillous space. With separation of the placenta from the uterus in the third stage of labor, the parturient is in danger of bleeding to death unless hemostasis at the placental site is achieved promptly. Normal clotting mechanisms do not act rapidly enough to obtain hemostasis. Rather, uterine muscle contractions produce a tourniquet-like effect on the vasculature. This provides initial hemostasis until clotting mechanisms effect a permanent hemostasis. Uterine atony and consequent loss of the tourniquet effect cause most postpartum hemorrhages. Almost all cases of postpartum hemorrhage due to uterine atony occur in the first hour or two following delivery. Consequently, it is very important that the woman who has just delivered be very closely observed for excessive bleeding in the early puerperium. Some clinicians refer to the first hour after delivery of the placenta as the fourth stage of labor. This designation emphasizes the importance of close observation during this time.

The diagnosis of postpartum hemorrhage due to uterine atony is not difficult. It rests on the identification of an atonic, boggy uterus in the absence of any other cause of postpartum hemorrhage. The management of uterine atony is discussed later in the chapter.

Lacerations

Lacerations of the genital tract can occur in the uterine fundus and lower uterine segment where they are more properly considered uterine ruptures. More commonly, lacerations involve the cervix, vagina, and perineum. Perineal lacerations are usually easy to see and to repair. The cervix and vagina must be searched for lacerations. Good exposure and adequate lighting are essential to find and to repair lacerations. Too often, therapy for postpartum hemorrhage is directed at treatment of uterine atony when, in fact, the cause of bleeding is a laceration. Lacerations can coexist with uterine atony and with other causes of postpartum hemorrhage. Cervical and vaginal lacerations may occur spontaneously during labor and delivery. If an operative delivery is performed, however, the operator usually is credited with causing the laceration, whether or not it is true. (See Chapter 48 for a detailed discussion of lacerations.)

Retained Placental Fragments

Retention of fragments of the placenta within the uterus after the third stage of labor is another main cause of postpartum hemorrhage. The condition is suspected by examination of the placenta. When missing pieces are noted, manual exploration of the uterus should be performed to find them. Occasionally, the presence of vessels in the membranes suggests that an accessory lobe of placenta has remained in the uterus.

Retained placental fragments produce postpartum hemorrhage by interfering with uterine contractions in the area of placental attachment. This implies that the mechanism is a localized uterine atony. The diagnosis of retained fragments is not difficult. Manual exploration of the uterus is easy to perform immediately postpartum. Some physicians advocate exploration of the uterus routinely after every delivery. Arguments against this practice are based on the possibility of introducing infection and producing discomfort to the patient unless she has received an anesthetic or an analgesic for the procedure. Everyone agrees that if the placenta appears fragmented or if the woman is bleeding excessively, the uterus should be explored. A clean, sterile glove should be placed on the exploring hand, which is then introduced through the cervix into the uterus. The opposite hand is placed on the abdomen to control the uterus. A systematic palpation of the uterus follows in order to detect placental pieces and membranes as well as uterine ruptures. If fragments are encountered, they usually can be removed by the hand. If more abrasive action is required, a gauze pad can be wrapped around the fingers. Occasionally curettage is necessary to remove the fragments. When curettage is performed, a large curette (25–30 mm diameter) should be used to lessen the chance of perforation of the soft postpartum uterus.

Uterine atony, lacerations, and retained placental fragments account for over 90% of cases of postpartum hemorrhage. Less common causes of postpartum hemorrhage are discussed below.

Placenta Accreta

Placenta accreta is defined as "an abnormal adherence, either in whole or in part, of the afterbirth to the underlying uterine wall." The pathologic basis for the condition was described in a classic paper in 1937.[29] Complete or partial absence of the decidua basalis allows the placenta to attach directly to the myometrium. More severe degrees of the same process produce placenta increta or placenta percreta: conditions in which the placenta invades the myometrium or penetrates through it. The true incidence of placenta accreta is unknown, but it probably occurs about once in 2500 deliveries.

Although the pathologic anatomy of placenta accreta is known, the pathogenesis is still uncertain. Placenta previa and previous cesarean delivery are two of the most important predisposing factors.[18] The finding of a placenta previa in a woman who has had a previous cesarean delivery should certainly make the physician consider the possibility of a placenta accreta. In our clinic, placenta accreta is present 20% of the time in this circumstance. The risk of placenta accreta complicating placenta previa rises with the number of cesarean deliveries a woman has had. After two or more cesarean sections, the risk of placenta accreta complicating placenta previa approaches 50%.[11] Placenta accreta is quite uncommon in primigravidas and is seen most commonly in elderly multigravidas. Many women wih placenta accreta have a history of uterine curettage or of manual removal of the placenta in a previous pregnancy (possibly from a partial accreta then). In cases where there is a placenta previa accreta, antepartum bleeding is common. Uterine rupture can occur in any stage of pregnancy. In one series of 622 cases, rupture of the uterus occurred 13.8% of the time.[18]

Because the decidua basalis is defective and the placenta implants directly on the myometrium, there is no plane of cleavage for separation of the placenta. Postpartum hemorrhage is common in this situation and it can be catastrophic. It was noted almost 50 years ago that hysterectomy produced excellent results in placenta accreta. Nineteen women were treated by hysterectomy with no attempt to remove the placenta and all survived, whereas 20 of 30 women treated by manual extraction of the placenta died.[29] More recently, the overall maternal mortality associated with placenta accreta is 9.5%. Patients treated by immediate hysterectomy had the lowest mortality (6.1%). Conservative management in an attempt to preserve the uterus yielded the highest mortality (25.6%) and conservative management followed by hysterectomy was accompanied by an intermediate mortality of 14.8%.[18] Twenty-two cases of placenta accreta were reported in 1980 from a single institution. Fourteen of the women had placenta previa and six of this group had a previous cesarean delivery. There was one maternal death in the series, a woman with placenta percreta who received 20,000 ml of blood before she died. Fourteen of the women were treated by hysterectomy. Manual removal of the placenta, curettage, sharp dissection, suture of the implantation site, and uterine artery ligation were used in various combinations to treat the eight women who did not undergo hysterectomy. The average amount of blood transfused was 7.9 units. Five women required 10 or more units of blood.[51]

When the placenta is retained in the uterus after delivery and attempts at manual removal reveal no cleavage plane, the presence of placenta accreta is likely. Blood should be crossmatched promptly. There should be no prolonged effort at manual extraction. Women still die from placenta accreta, but hysterectomy is an effective lifesaving therapy. If hysterectomy is not chosen, there should be a good reason. Whenever a woman with a placenta previa and a previous cesarean delivery is to undergo a repeat cesarean section, blood should be ready. If an accreta is found, hysterectomy should be performed promptly. If this is unacceptable to the patient, some of the conservative measures mentioned above may be tried. The patient's condition should not be allowed to deteriorate before performing hysterectomy.

Inverted Uterus

Inversion of the puerperal uterus is an unusual complication that is estimated to occur in 1 in 2000 to 1 in 20,000 deliveries. The condition was associated with a maternal mortality as high as 10% in the recent past.[62] Death usually occurs from hemorrhage and shock. One alleged cause of uterine inversion is improper management of the third stage of labor with traction on the umbilical cord and downward pressure on the uterus (Credé's maneuver). However, it is dubious whether such maneuvers actually cause uterine inversion. Other etiologic factors include increased intra-abdominal pressure, uterine hypotonia, fundal implantation of the placenta, and primigravidity.

Uterine inversion is classified in several ways. One method is by the extent of the inversion. An incomplete inversion is simply a dimple in the uterine fundus. With complete inversion, the fundus is through the cervix. With prolapse, the entire uterus is inverted and the fundus is out of the introitus. A classification by the time of inversion with respect to delivery is also used. Acute inversion occurs immediately after delivery and the placenta often is still attached to the fundus. Subacute and chronic inversions also occur but are not seen in the context of postpartum hemorrhage. Uterine inversions also may be recurrent.

Inversion of the uterus is diagnosed when the placenta appears at the introitus still attached to the inverted uterine fundus. If the placenta has been delivered before the uterine inversion occurs, the sudden presence of the uterine fundus at the introitus can give the physician quite a surprise. Undiagnosed second twin or submucous myoma is often the first thought.[21] The patient suffers pain, hemorrhage, and shock in varying degrees. Hemorrhagic shock occurred in approximately 30% of a recent series of patients suffering acute uterine inversions.[49]

Once a diagnosis of uterine inversion has been made, prompt action is necessary. If attached, the placenta should be removed. Following this, upward pressure should be directed against the uterine fundus to replace it into the abdominal cavity. If this is done promptly, before a contraction ring of cervix traps the inverted fundus, approximately half the patients can be treated successfully without general anesthesia. It is critical to be sure that the uterus is fully repositioned. Generally, the operator's hand has to reach so high that the elbow of that arm is at the patient's introitus. Should a cervical contraction ring be present, uterine relaxation with a general anesthetic such as halothane or with a beta-sympathomimetic such as terbutaline sulfate can relax the ring sufficiently to allow repositioning of the uterus.[34] Several methods have been described for repositing the uterus; one method is based on indenting the fundus first and elevating the uterus, another method elevates around the sulcus first and allows the fundus to follow this restoration.[21,31] These two techniques are not necessarily exclusive. One can be tried and, if it does not work, the other may be tried.

If attempts at transvaginal replacement of the uterus are unsuccessful, a laparotomy should be performed. At surgery, the inverted uterus resembles a funnel with the round ligaments and oviducts disappearing into it. Traction on the round ligaments and uterine tissue with Allis clamps often successfully repositions the uterus, especially if an assistant is pressing upward on the inverted fundus from below.[21] If this procedure is unsuccessful, a longitudinal incision in the back of the uterus allows repositioning of the fundus in virtually all cases.

After the uterus has been replaced, a hand should be kept in the uterine cavity until the myometrium contracts firmly. This is to avoid recurrent inversions. In one woman who had several recurrent uterine inversions within 24 hours of delivery, packing the uterus with gauze and administering 15-methyl prostaglandin $F_{2\alpha}$ to stimulate uterine contractions stopped the recurrent inversions and avoided hysterectomy.[28]

Uterine inversion is an obstetric emergency. Fortunately, if it is recognized and treated promptly, good results are the rule.

Ruptured Uterus

The first description of rupture of the pregnant uterus is credited to Smellie. Since that description, hundreds of articles have been written on the topic. Rupture of the uterus continues to be an important cause of maternal mortality. In England and Wales, the combination of postpartum hemorrhage, ectopic pregnancy, and uterine rupture constitutes the largest cause of maternal mortality.[15] The reported incidence of uterine rupture varies. In the United States, uterine rupture occurs in from 1 in 1000 to 1 in 1500 deliveries.

Etiologic factors associated with uterine rupture are well known. The most common factor is the presence of a uterine scar, especially from a cesarean delivery.[56] High parity and the use of oxytocin are each associated with uterine rupture. When these two factors occur together, the risk of uterine rupture is as high as 2%.[6] Placental problems such as placenta percreta and gestational trophoblastic disease are associated with rupture of the uterus. Trauma, whether from obstetric procedures such as forceps delivery or internal version and breech extraction or from external trauma such as automobile accident can rupture the pregnant uterus. Obstructed labor, which might occur with transverse lie, brow presentation, or with an undiagnosed hydrocephalic fetus, can proceed to uterine rupture. Women with type IV Ehlers–Danlos syndrome are at a 25% risk of death from pregnancy complications such as rupture of the uterus, aorta, vena cava, or bowel, as well as from vaginal laceration and other forms of postpartum hemorrhage.[55] Cornual pregnancy can cause uterine rupture as can uterine anomalies. Previous uterine curettage and previous manual removal of the placenta have a positive association with uterine rupture. Hypertonic uterine contractions associated with spontaneous labor, abruptio placentae, or ecbolic agents can rupture the uterus in labor. Although rupture of the uterus occurs as early as the first trimester, almost all ruptures occur in the third trimester. Rupture of the uterus of the primigravida from any cause is rare.

Spontaneous rupture after previous uterine surgery is the largest cause of uterine tears. Although reports of uterine rupture after myomectomy, cervical cerclage procedures, tubal implantations, uterine perforations, and uterine unification procedures exist, the majority of cases follow a previous cesarean section. The rate of rupture is much higher after a classical scar (3–4%), than after a lower uterine segment scar (0.25%). Healing differences between a scar in the upper segment (mainly muscle) and in the lower segment (mainly collagen) partially explain the variation in rates of rupture. The difference in the rare of rupture after low-segment cesarean section is important because of the increasing number of cesareans performed in the United States and the advocacy by many of vaginal delivery after a low cervical transverse cesarean section. Patients with classical scars should not be allowed a trial of labor because of the higher rate of uterine rupture and of the often more serious outcome when such a scar ruptures.

Classification of ruptured uterus is confusing because no two authors use the same system. One simple classification considers only rupture of a scarred uterus and rupture of an unscarred uterus. Most classifications are more complicated. Rupture associated with oxytocin use is considered spontaneous in one classification, traumatic in another, and in a separate category in a third classification scheme.

The maternal mortality report from England and Wales classifies ruptures in three categories.[15]

1. Rupture associated with a scar
2. Traumatic rupture
3. Spontaneous rupture
   a. With oxytocin
   b. Without oxytocin

The system seems to be as useful as any other system of classification.

Some authorities do not consider dehiscence of a uterine scar to be a true rupture so they do not include this condition in their data; others include dehiscence. Uterine dehiscence is a gradual, painless separation of the uterus in the area of an old scar, producing a window-like defect. Typically, the membranes are intact, there is no bleeding, and the fetus is not extruded into the abdominal cavity. Dehiscences are limited to the area of an old scar—usually a low cervical transverse scar. There is usually no hemorrhage, no shock, and no maternal or fetal mortality. True ruptures, on the other hand, are characteristically sudden and explosive in onset and associated with pain, hemorrhage, shock, rupture of the membranes, extrusion of the fetus into the peritoneal cavity, and high fetal and maternal mortality.[56] Scars in the corpus usually rupture rather than separate and, in so doing, they often extend into unscarred areas of myometrium.

If rupture of an unscarred uterus occurs during labor, the site of rupture is usually the lower uterine segment. Rupture of the unscarred uterus prior to labor is likely to occur in the corpus. Ruptures are classified as complete or incomplete. A complete rupture has communication between the uterine cavity and the peritoneal cavity. An incomplete rupture is variously defined as extending through the serosa and myometrium but not through the endometrium, or as rupture into the broad ligament.

The signs and symptoms of uterine rupture vary from mild, vague pain that can be confused with early labor; through continuous or intermittent pain that is thought to be due to placental abruption; to an acute, general collapse with shock. The clinical presentation depends on the location of the rupture, whether or not it is complete, the cause of the rupture, the amount of peritoneal spill, and the type of anesthesia that the patient has received. The classic presentation includes abdominal pain, a tearing sensation, tenderness, vaginal bleeding, shock, cessation of labor, elevation of or change in the presenting part, and easily palpable fetal parts. Loss of fetal heart tones and loss of intrauterine pressure reading via an intrauterine pressure catheter may be noted. This presentation commonly is experienced by women who rupture a classical cesarean scar in labor; it usually indicates complete rupture of the uterus in the corpus. The dehiscence of a low cervical transverse scar usually produces no symptoms; it is most often noted after delivery when the interior of the uterus is explored.

The pregnant uterus can rupture spontaneously prior to the onset of labor. In fact, half of the ruptures of classical cesarean scars occur prior to the onset of labor. Rupture of the uterus prior to labor is usually in the corpus and can be difficult to diagnose because the symptoms can be so vague. Maternal mortality is highest in patients with uterine rupture prior to labor. Abdominal pain and tenderness in the absence of fetal heart tones usually suggest a placental abruption. Peritoneal irritation may suggest a bowel problem. A completely asymptomatic uterine rupture diagnosed only at the time of puerperal tubal sterilization three days after delivery has been reported.[4]

The diagnosis of uterine rupture is made after delivery by manually exploring the uterus and detecting the rent. Postpartum hemorrhage, especially in the presence of a contracted uterus, suggests the possibility of genital tract damage and should lead to exploration of the uterus, cervix, and vagina. Failure to examine the uterine cavity and delay in surgical treatment are the two leading causes of maternal mortality from uterine rupture.[15]

The treatment of uterine rupture is surgical. Two-thirds of patients with uterine rupture develop shock. Although transfusion therapy is necessary, the presence of shock does not contraindicate surgical therapy. The choice of operation is influenced to some extent by the patient's condition, her wishes, and by the findings at operation. Hysterectomy is usually the treatment of choice for ruptures. Prior to laparotomy, a careful vaginal examination should be done to discover and repair any vaginal lacerations.

During surgery, manual compression of the aorta helps to prevent excessive bleeding. Hypogastric artery ligation may be necessary, especially if there is hematoma formation in the broad ligaments. Total or subtotal hysterectomy usually is performed. If the woman strongly desires to preserve her childbearing capacity, simple repair of the rupture may be performed. Results of such surgery have been disappointing. Two of a group of seven women who had a rupture repaired had another rupture in a subsequent pregnancy. One of them died.[56] Uterine dehiscence generally does not require hysterectomy. Trimming back the thinned margins of the defect to good tissue and suturing the defect suffice as treatment.

Coagulopathy

Failure of maternal blood to clot is an important, though uncommon, cause of postpartum hemorrhage. As noted earlier, hemostasis immediately after delivery is most dependent on myometrial contractility. Women with a coagulopathy may not bleed immediately after delivery if the uterus is well contracted. Lacerations and surgical incisions bleed excessively if there is a coagulopathy.

For practical purposes, three entities account for most cases of coagulopathy in obstetrics. Consumptive coagulopathy from disseminated intravascular coagulation is associated with abruptio placentae and with amniotic fluid embolus. Inherited coagulopathies are almost always due to von Willebrand's disease. Circulating clotting factor inhibitors are usually to Factor VIII and they produce a condition that appears similar to von Willebrand's disease (see Chapter 30).

The coagulopathy associated with abruptio placentae is discussed in Chapter 15 and the syndromes associated with amniotic fluid embolus are discussed in Chapter 39. Delayed postpartum hemorrhage 7–12 days after delivery occurs in up to 25% of women with von Willebrand's disease. Women who do not have a rise in Factor VIII levels to normal levels during pregnancy should be treated with cryoprecipitate during labor and for several days postpartum. Cryoprecipitate is the agent of choice to treat the disorder; it comes from single units of plasma so the risk of transmitted disease is lower than with multidonor products and it produces an "overresponse" in the patient's Factor VIII level. Eight to 10 units of Factor VIII should be given patients deficient in the factor prior to cesarean delivery. After delivery, Factor VIII levels should be checked daily and cryoprecipitate given to keep the level above 25%.[36,43]

Rarely, acquired Factor VIII inhibitors appear around the time of delivery to produce a von Willebrand's type syndrome. These inhibitors are antibodies against Factor VIII and they can lead to life-threatening hemorrhage. Therapy with blood transfusions, cryoprecipitate, fresh frozen plasma, and Factor VIII concentrate has been used with some success. Treatment with Autoplex, a product made from pooled plasma and containing precursors and activated clotting factors, has been successful at controlling the hemorrhagic diathesis associated with this condition. It does not eliminate the inhibitor.[52]

TREATMENT

Management of the Third Stage of Labor

It is better to avoid postpartum hemorrhage than to have to treat it. Prophylaxis against postpartum hemorrhage begins with proper management of the third stage of labor.[7] In 1933, Brandt described a technique that is now accepted as the best method of managing the third stage of labor. Some authors have referred to the Brandt maneuver as cord traction, but this is not the way Brandt described it. In his description, Brand stated that the placenta separates from the uterus within 8–10 minutes after delivery of the infant. Following separation, the placenta is in the cervix or upper vagina. To test for this, the cord is clamped close to the vulva and the clamp is held with one hand. The operator's other hand is then placed on the woman's abdomen. The thumb of the abdominal hand is placed parallel to the patient's symphysis and the palm and fingers are against the uterus. As the cord is held taut, the abdominal hand gently pushes upward against the uterus. If the placenta has not separated, tension develops in the cord; if this occurs, nothing further is done for several minutes. The process is then repeated. If the placenta has separated and is in the cervix or upper vagina, there will be only slight tension as the uterus is elevated. When the uterus is high in the abdomen, the placenta should be in the upper vagina; it is then expressed by pressing downward with the abdominal hand just above the symphysis. Traction, as such, is not applied to the cord and the uterus is not massaged or squeezed. Downward pressure is not applied to the uterine fundus. Brandt reported this management in 800 cases. The average duration of the third stage of labor was eight minutes. Of the 800 women, there were only 10 instances of excessive bleeding after delivery. The average blood loss was approximately 210 ml.

The routine use of oxytocics after delivery to promote uterine contractions and thereby to avoid postpartum hemorrhage is practiced widely. Scientific evidence for such action is lacking. The average blood loss of patients receiving oxytocics is not statistically different from that of women not given oxytocic prophylaxis.[41] Support for the routine use of ecbolic agents, however, derives from the same study because there were fewer instances of excessive bleeding among women given oxytocics than among controls. Prompt treatment of postpartum hemorrhage kept the average blood loss the same in both groups.

Advocates of puerperal administration of oxytocic agents utilize various regimens. In some clinics, oxytocin alone is given by continuous intravenous drip. Others give ergonovine (0.2 mg, i.m. or i.v.), methylergonovine (0.2 mg i.m.), or oxytocin (10 units, i.m.) with delivery of the anterior shoulder. Clinicians employing the latter regimen must be certain that a second infant is not in utero and must be willing to accept the possibility of occasionally trapping the placenta. Another popular regimen is the intramuscular administration of 10 units of oxytocin after the birth of the infant, followed by injection of ergonovine or methylergonovine (0.2 mg) after delivery of the placenta.

Ergot alkaloids cause undesirable systemic manifestations such as hypertension, tachycardia, headache, nausea, and vomiting. Although some deny that methylergonovine causes such side effects when administered during the third stage of labor, others have noted all these systemic effects in similar patients. These agents can be particularly dangerous in women with previous hypertension.

Oxytocin and other ecbolic agents probably should be reserved for patients who are at increased risk for immediate postpartum hemorrhage. Patients who fall into this category are those with an overdistended uterus (large baby, multiple pregnancy, polyhydramnios), high parity, history of previous puerperal hemorrhage, or prolonged labor. Similarly, women who are delivered under general anesthesia and those who are delivered operatively display an increased frequency of postpartum hemorrhage and merit ecbolic prophylaxis.

Some authorities claim that ergot derivatives are superior to oxytocin for puerperal use, whereas others state that continuous intravenous infusion of oxytocin is without peer in the puerperium. No clinical data demonstrating clear superiority for any single regimen are existent. We prefer to use oxytocin. When oxytocin is given intravenously, response begins within one minute. However, if given as a single injection, the uterine response begins to subside within 10 minutes. For these reasons, we prefer to administer oxytocin by intravenous drip. Utilizing 20 units of oxytocin in 500 ml of fluid produces a concentration of 40 mU/ml. We start this infusion immediately after delivery of the placenta.

Management of Postpartum Hemorrhage

Medical. When postpartum hemorrhage is diagnosed, the physician should immediately go through a mental checklist of causes and rule them in or out by examination. One hand should be placed inside the uterus immediately. This hand checks for retained placental fragments, uterine inversion, and uterine rupture; it also evaluates uterine tone. If uterine atony is the only problem detected, the hand is withdrawn from the uterus into the vagina and fashioned into a fist. The physician's other hand is then placed on the abdomen and the flaccid uterus is compressed between the abdominal hand and the fist in the vagina. Uterine compression is quite effective in controlling hemorrhage from uterine atony. During uterine compression intravenous lines can be placed, blood crossmatched, and ecbolic agents given to promote uterine contractions. Uterine compression is a life-saving temporary treatment. After uterine tone has been restored, continued bleeding suggests genital tract trauma; if this has not been found previously, another search should be conducted. Coagulopathy is suspected when the blood lost does not clot.

Oxytocin and methylergonovine are the mainstays of medical treatment of postpartum uterine atony, but improper use of them causes profound effects on the cardiovascular system. Intramuscular or subcutaneous injection of 10 units of oxytocin produces no cardiovascular effect. Dilute intravenous infusion produces little cardiovascular effect, but intravenous injection of a bolus of 5 units of oxytocin produces a rapid, precipitous fall in blood pressure that begins within 20 seconds and is accompanied by tachycardia. The hypotensive response to bolus oxytocin is the same in males and also occurs if the patient is already in shock. The hypotensive effect dissipates rapidly. Blood pressure is back to normal in 10 minutes. The magnitude of the fall in blood pressure and the time to return to normal are proportional to the amount of oxytocin injected.[25] Ergonovine and methylergonovine maleate produce hypertension, especially after intravenous injection. Three minutes is required for hypertension to develop. The cardiovascular effects of ergots is slower to resolve than is the cardiovascular effect of oxytocin. To be safe, ergot preparations should be given intramuscularly.

Uterine atony unresponsive to oxytocin and methylergonovine maleate can be treated successfully with prostaglandins. Prostaglandin E_2 vaginal suppositories[26] and intramyometrial injections of prostaglandin $F_{2\alpha}$[30] have been utilized to treat uterine atony in the immediate puerperium as well as delayed postpartum hemorrhage resistant to conventional treatment.[5]

Clinical trials of an analogue of prostaglandin $F_{2\alpha}$, [Prostin/15 M® (carboprost tromethamine)] in treatment of severe postpartum hemorrhage have been reported recently.[23,24,61] The analogue was administered after conventional therapy with intravenous oxytocin solutions, intramuscular methylergonovine, and uterine compression had failed to correct postpartum uterine atony. The drug was given in a 0.25 mg dose intramuscularly. Up to five repeat doses were used at intervals of 1.5 hours (shorter intervals were occasionally necessary). The drug was tolerated well and atony was managed successfully in 44 of 51 women (86%).[24] Uterine tone increased approximately 45 minutes after the first injection. Thirty women responded to the first injection and nine women responded to a second injection. Uterine atony associated with intra-amniotic infection responded poorly to the prostaglandin analogue; four of eight with atony on the basis of infection were treatment failures and required surgical therapy. Other causes of uterine atony, including amniotic fluid embolus, responded well to treatment with 15-methyl prostaglandin $F_{2\alpha}$. Antepartum intrauterine infection was associated with the only treatment failure in 16 cases of severe postpartum hemorrhage treated with the same analogue by investigators in Egypt.[61] The role of intra-amniotic infection in the production of postpartum hemorrhage due to uterine atony awaits further investigation.

Medical management of postpartum hemorrhage from uterine atony is based on the use of oxytocin and ergot preparations. Should these agents fail to produce uterine contractions, 15-methyl prostaglandin $F_{2\alpha}$ can be used to promote contractions and to avoid surgical treatment.

Packing. The most controversial therapy for postpartum hemorrhage involves the use of an intrauterine and intravaginal pack. Use of the gauze pack has fallen into disfavor. Some authorities have termed uterine tamponade useless, archaic, and dangerous. Critics of intrauterine packing contend that the procedure merely hides blood loss and gives the physician a false sense of security.[63] It also is said that a flaccid uterus cannot be packed for it merely distends more, whereas a contracted uterus does not need packing. The author has never packed a uterus but includes this section on use of the intrauterine pack because advocates of uterine packing make a good case for its effectiveness and report excellent results in the treatment of postpartum hemorrhage [16,27,35,59]

Use of an intrauterine pack should be part of a careful management plan for treatment of postpartum hemorrhage. Before resorting to a pack, the patient's vulva, vagina, and cervix should be inspected for lacerations. The uterus should be evaluated for inversion, rupture, perforation, and retained placental fragments. Ecbolic agents and manual compression should be used while the clotting status of the patient is evaluated and while fluids and blood are given and the patient is monitored.[16] Improper use of a poorly placed pack probably has contributed to the lowly esteem of this form of therapy.

Authors differ in the manner of placing an intrauterine pack. Dry gauze 20 feet in length and 36 inches wide is used by one author. The gauze is folded lengthwise four times to produce a pack of 16 plies that is 2 inches wide. The pack is placed through a Holmes packing instrument into the uterus.[35] Sponge forceps are satisfactory for use in packing with dry gauze. The pack may be placed successfully by hand if the operator does not have access to a mechanical packer. Gauze moistened with saline is said to be easier to pack manually than is dry gauze.[35]

All authors agree that correct technique is of the utmost importance in the use of a pack. Failure of a pack to control hemorrhage is attributed most often to poor technique in placing the pack. Anesthesia may be of great value. An indwelling catheter should be placed in the urinary bladder. Sterile technique should be practiced. While an assistant holds the fundus and an oxytocin solution is running, the pack is inserted. Starting in the fundus, the pack is placed from one side of the uterus to the other. Particular attention is paid to filling the lower uterine segment completely. The packing is continued, filling the vagina to the introitus. Prophylactic antibiotics are used by some clinicians, but infection does not seem to be a prominent complication of packing. If successful, the pack is removed in 24-36 hours. Some authors recommend removal in a delivery room or operating room. If the patient's condition deteriorates after the pack is placed, surgical therapy should be undertaken without delay.

Surgical. When medical management fails to control postpartum hemorrhage, surgical therapy is indicated. Hysterectomy is the definitive treatment for hemorrhage from uterine atony. In a series of 70 emergency hysterectomies for obstetric hemorrhage, uterine atony was the most common indication (43%), followed by placenta accreta (30%) and uterine rupture (13%).[12]

Frequently, however, hysterectomy can be avoided by choosing other procedures such as arterial ligations or arterial embolization.

Internal iliac (hypogastric) artery ligation is well known for its ability to control pelvic hemorrhage. Reich and Nechtow popularized the operation in 1961.[53] They described it as "... a life-saving procedure for uncontrollable gynecologic and obstetric hemorrhage." The technique they popularized is basically the technique still in use; it will be described below.

In the 1960s, Burchell investigated the physiology and hemodynamics of internal iliac artery ligation.[8-10] After ligation of one internal iliac artery, blood still flows through its uterine artery branch. However, pulse pressure decreases by 77%; when both internal iliacs are ligated, pulse pressure in the uterine artery decreases by 85%. Blood flow through the uterine artery is halved whether one or both internal iliac arteries are ligated. Burchell noted, "With the trip-hammer effect of arterial pulsation virtually eliminated, clotting developed and persisted so that pressure alone could control bleeding from the severed uterine artery."[8] The source of collateral circulation to the pelvis was elucidated by arteriographic studies immediately or several years after internal iliac artery ligation. Collateral circulation is established immediately after ligation. Ligation reverses flow in some vessels, but all pelvic arteries receive blood. The three principal systems of collateral circulation are:. lumbar–iliolumbar, middle sacral–lateral sacral, and superior hemorrhoidal–middle hemorrhoidal. The three pairs of vessels involved in the anastomoses have small diameters; this results in the fundamental change noted after ligation, dampening of pulse pressure.[10] The adequacy of blood supply following internal iliac artery ligation is attested to by successful pregnancies following the procedure, even when combined with ovarian artery ligation.[38] Prophylactic internal artery ligation at the time of elective cesarean hysterectomy does not decrease operative blood loss.[48]

The operative technique for internal iliac artery ligation is diagrammed in Fig. 47-1. A transperitoneal approach is used. The common iliac artery bifurcates into internal and external iliac branches at the level of the sacral promontory. The ureter crosses the common iliac at the level of the bifurcation. An 8–10 cm incision is made parallel with and lateral to the ureter. The flap of peritoneum is then retracted medially with the ureter still attached. The bifurcation of the common iliac should be identified clearly and the internal iliac artery bluntly dissected free for approximately 5 cm. This is to avoid ligation above the posterior branch of the internal iliac. Ligation above the posterior branch can compromise the success of the procedure by allowing more anastomoses; it also may compromise blood supply to the buttocks. Once the anterior branch of the internal iliac artery is identified, a delicate longitudinal incision is made into the adventitia, which is stripped away from the artery. The vessel then bulges forward and away from the internal iliac vein which lies posteromedially to the artery. A right angle clamp may now be carried beneath the artery with less chance of injuring the internal iliac vein. Two silk sutures are used to ligate the internal iliac artery. Number 1 or 0 silk suture is acceptable for this purpose. The ties are placed 1 cm apart; there is no need to divide the artery between the ties.

Complications of internal iliac artery ligation include the following: injury to the vein, which is very difficult to repair; ligation of the external iliac artery, which may not be diagnosed until the abdomen is closed; ischemic damage to the pelvic organs; and failure of the procedure to yield the desired effect. In a recent series of postpartum hypogastric ligations, 8 of 14 women required subsequent hysterectomy.[17] However, only two cases were done for uterine atony and the procedure was successful in both instances. The procedure was much less effective in treating hemorrhage from placenta accreta or uterine lacerations.

Since the operation simply reduces blood flow and pulse pressure through the vessels below the ligation, hemostasis depends on an intact clotting mechanism. If a coagulopathy coexists with an atony, internal iliac artery ligation may be unsuccessful in controlling hemorrhage. In this circumstance, immediate hysterectomy may be more prudent.

Ovarian artery ligation often is performed as an adjunct to internal iliac artery ligation in the control of postpartum hemorrhage. If the infundibulopelvic ligaments are ligated bilaterally, both the ovarian artery and vein are occluded. Should the internal iliac artery ligation be unsuccessful, hysterectomy with bilateral salpingo-oophorectomy becomes necessary. A technique for ovarian artery ligation that avoids infundibulopelvic ligament ligation is shown in Fig. 47-2. With this technique, the ovarian artery is ligated in the mesovarium near its anastomosis with the uterine artery. Blood flow to the ovary is not compromised and the ovaries

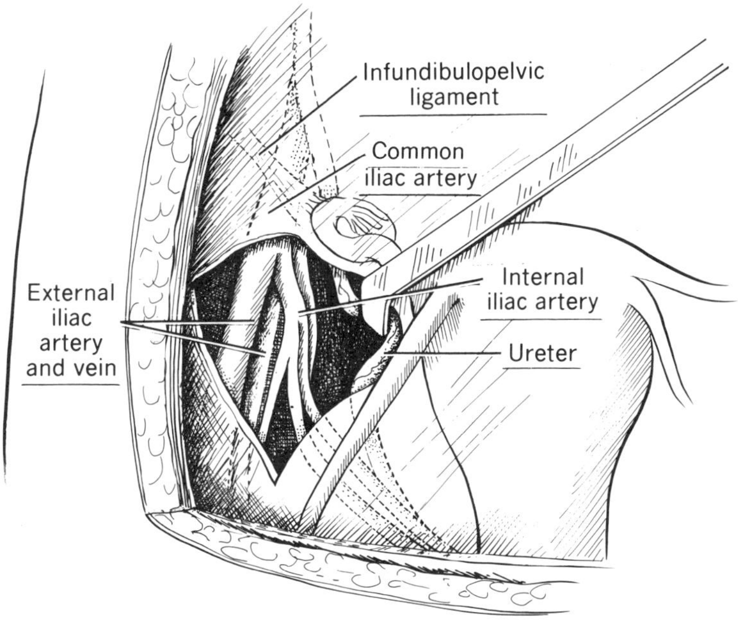

(a)

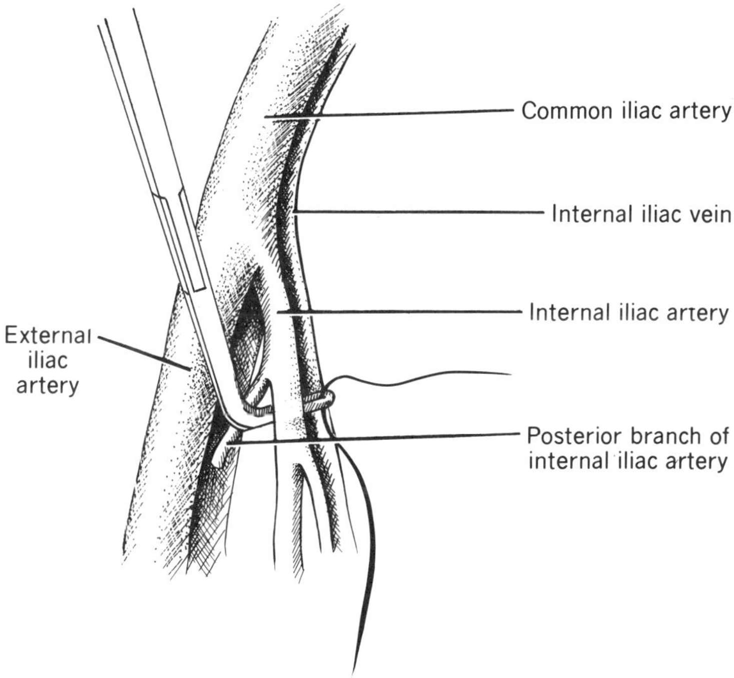

(b)

Figure 47-1. Operative technique of internal iliac artery ligation

Panel A. The retroperitoneal space over the right internal and external iliac vessels has been opened and the ureter retracted medially.

Panel B. A right angle clamp is passed between the iliac artery and vein to receive a ligature of number 0 silk. The vessel should be doubly ligated as described in the text.

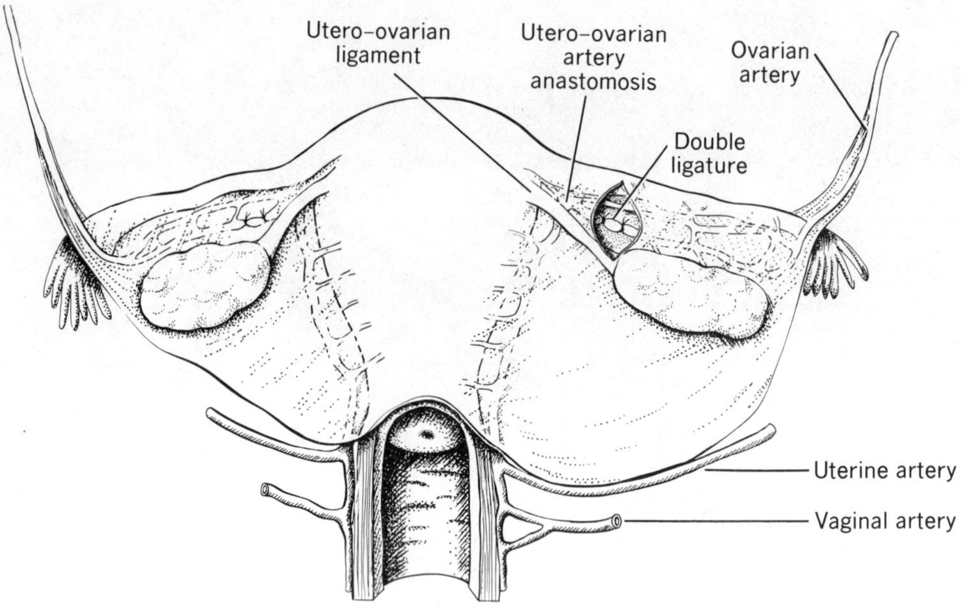

Figure 47-2. Area for ovarian artery ligation 14
Two free ties of 2-0 silk suture are used to ligate the ovarian artery bilaterally near its anastomosis with the uterine artery. An avascular area of mesovarium near the junction of the utero-ovarian ligament with the ovary is the site chosen.

may be retained even if hysterectomy becomes necessary.[14]

Uterine artery ligation to manage postpartum hemorrhage was described in very colorful language in 1952 by Walters. He wrote, ". . . the uterine artery ligation will not surmount basic ignorance and carelessness. It is not offered to eliminate hysterectomy . . . nor as a panacea for bad obstetrics. It will overcome uterine atony without sacrificing the uterus."[63]

The procedure is based on ligation of the ascending branch of the uterine artery to control postpartum bleeding from uterine atony and from other causes. During pregnancy, 90% of the uterine blood flow passes through the uterine arteries. Ligation of these vessels is said to be easier, faster, and more effective at controlling uterine hemorrhage than is internal iliac artery ligation.[44] In a series of 66 cases of uterine artery ligation done for hemorrhage, there were six failures of the procedure. Placenta previa placenta accreta and atony with intrauterine infection were associated with the failures. All 30 cases of uterine atony were successfully treated.[45]

Uterine artery ligation is performed by mobilizing the bladder inferiorly as if for a transverse low-segment cesarean section (Fig. 47-3). While an assistant elevates the uterus and exposes the broad ligament, the surgeon passes a large atraumatic Mayo needle with No. 1 chromic catgut through the avascular space of the broad ligament and through the myometrium. The suture should include 2–3 cm of myometrium. A single suture is tied on either side to occlude each uterine artery. The uterine vein is also ligated by this procedure. If the procedure is done after a low transverse cesarean section, the ligature should be placed below the incision in the uterus. The procedure is said to have the same hemostatic effect as a supracervical hysterectomy. This accounts for failure of the procedure in cases of placenta previa and placenta accreta.[45]

Arterial infusion of vasopressin and embolization of gelatin sponge (Gelfoam®) or coils have been successful in the treatment of pelvic hemorrhage postpartum, postabortal, and postoperatively. The procedure can be performed in less than two hours by a skilled angiographer.[22,37,46,54]

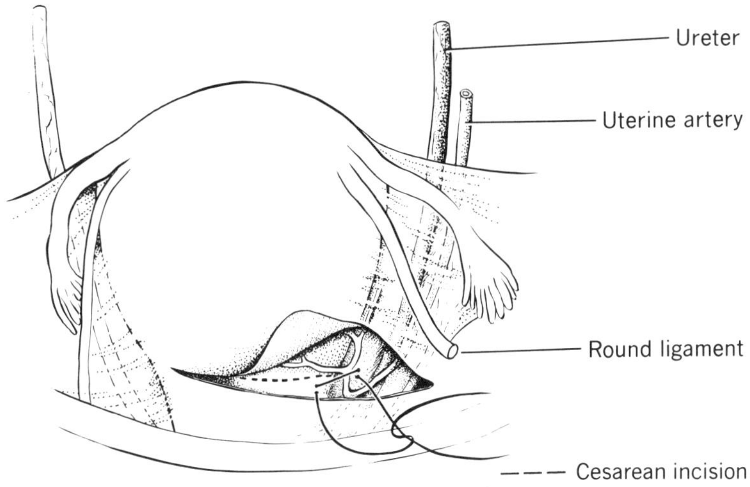

Figure 47-3. Operative technique for uterine artery ligation 45
The vesico-uterine fold of visceral peritoneum has been incised transversely and the bladder mobilized inferiorly. A number 1 chromic catgut suture on a large smooth needle has been placed through the avascular space of the broad ligament and through the uterus. The suture includes the uterine vessels and several centimeters of myometrium.

Transfusion Therapy

The etiology and treatment of postpartum hemorrhage have been discussed above. Transfusion therapy is an integral part of the prevention or management of hemorrhagic shock, which complicates blood loss from any cause. For the woman of average size with a normally expanded blood volume in pregnancy, consideration of transfusion therapy should begin when estimated blood loss reaches a liter. The onset of hemorrhagic shock or an estimated acute blood loss of 1500 ml almost always requires transfusion therapy.

Common wisdom suggests that the loss of blood be replaced with blood. Fresh whole blood, however, is seldom available for transfusions in an emergency situation. Since the 1970s, the emphasis in most blood banks has been to separate freshly donated whole blood into several products or components. These products are then given to patients as required to treat specific problems. From a 500 ml unit of whole blood, the following products are obtained.[1]

Packed Red Blood Cells. After centrifugation, the red blood cells are compressed into a volume of 200 ml. This product has a useful "shelf life" of 35 days when stored at 1–6 °C. One unit of packed red blood cells raises a patient's hematocrit approximately 3–5%. Because of the high viscosity of this component, it cannot be given rapidly unless diluted with normal saline immediately before infusion; 200 ml of diluent is sufficient. When there is a possibility of cardiovascular overload, the packed cells should not be diluted. Normal saline is the recommended diluent for packed red blood cells. Glucose solutions may cause hemolysis and balanced salt solutions may cause clot formation because of their calcium content.

Packed red blood cells may be washed and frozen for prolonged periods of time. When frozen cells are required for therapy, time must be allowed for thawing and washing the cells; they must be used within 24 hours of thawing.

Fresh Frozen Plasma. The fluid portion of one unit of blood which is separated from the cellular portion within six hours of donation and is then frozen solid at −18 °C or colder is called fresh frozen plasma. This product contains coagulation factors, labile as well as stable. It also contains plasma proteins, immunoglobulins, fats, carbohydrates, and other constituents of plasma. Fresh frozen plasma must be thawed before use and must be used promptly after thawing.

A tenfold increase in the use of fresh frozen

plasma within a decade led to a National Institutes of Health Consensus Development Conference on the indications and risks of fresh frozen plasma in 1984.[42] The group concluded that there was no indication to use the component as a volume expander or as a nutrition source. It is indicated for the treatment of isolated clotting factor deficiencies when specific component therapy is not available (Factors II, V, VII, IX, X, and XI). Fresh frozen plasma also reverses the anticoagulant effect of warfarin on the vitamin K-dependent coagulation factors. One of the most common uses for fresh frozen plasma is in the treatment of coagulation disorders that occur after massive blood transfusions with packed red blood cells, a product that contains no clotting factors. Although the consensus group gave this indication lukewarm endorsement, other authorities recommend the administration of 1 unit of fresh frozen plasma for every 4 units of packed red blood cells given.[1] Another possible use of fresh frozen plasma not addressed by the N.I.H. Conference is in treatment of consumption coagulopathy from disseminated intravascular coagulation. Other indications for use of fresh frozen plasma which the Consensus Conference mentioned include treatment of immunodeficiencies in infants with protein-losing enteropathy, treatment of thrombotic thrombocytopenic purpura, and as a source of antithrombin III for patients deficient in this inhibitor who are receiving heparin to treat thrombosis or who are undergoing surgery.

Cryoprecipitate and Single Donor Plasma. Cryoprecipitate may be removed from donated blood. When this is done, fresh frozen plasma cannot be prepared because cryoprecipitate contains coagulation Factors I, V, VIII, and XIII. Instead of fresh frozen plasma, single donor plasma is left. Single donor plasma contains the stable coagulation factors and is effective in the management of patients who require reversal of warfarin treatment. It contains coagulation Factors II, VII, IX, and X. Single donor plasma shares other indications with fresh frozen plasma, including treatment of antithrombin III deficiency and deficiency of immune globulins.

Each unit of cryoprecipitate is 40 ml in volume. It is indicated to treat disseminated intravascular coagulation, von Willebrand's disease, and hemophilia A. Each unit of cryoprecipitate administered increases the patient's fibrinogen concentration by 10 mg/dl.

Platelet Concentrate. Each unit of donated blood yields a unit of platelets that is contained in 50 ml of relatively fresh plasma along with some red blood cells. Platelet transfusions are used most often in patients with thrombocytopenia; however, they may be indicated in the management of coagulopathy associated with massive transfusion therapy. Patients with platelet counts below 100,000 per microliter who are to have surgery should be considered for platelet transfusion. Each unit of platelets given raises the platelet count by approximately 7500 per microliter. The "shelf life" of platelet concentrate is only three days.

In addition to the components derived from a single unit of donated whole blood, specific coagulation factors are available from pooled plasma sources. These include Factors VIII, IX, and XIII.

Risks of transfusion therapy are not insignificant and include allergic reactions that range from urticaria to pulmonary edema, alloimmunization, volume overload, and transmission of diseases such as hepatitis and acquired immunodeficiency syndrome. The decision to use transfusion therapy should not be a casual one.[1]

Treatment of Hemorrhagic Shock

Shock is caused by inadequate cardiac output; this leads to decreased tissue perfusion with the subsequent development of hypoxia, anaerobic metabolism, acidosis, and tissue damage. Types of shock based on etiologic factors are traditionally arranged into three broad categories: hypovolemic shock from hemorrhage or fluid loss, vasogenic shock from an abnormally expanded vascular space with decreased venous return to the heart, and cardiogenic shock which results from failure of the heart to pump. This section deals with hypovolemic shock due to blood loss.

The general appearance of patients in shock is one of pallor; cyanosis or diaphoresis may be present. Mental status often is altered and the patient may exhibit anxiety, confusion, or coma. Alterations in vital signs typically include hypotension, tachycardia, and tachypnea; the pulse is weak and thready. Anemia and oliguria are common. In women with postpartum hemorrhage, the blood loss is usually apparent rather than concealed, so the physicians and nursing staff caring for the patient can anticipate development of shock. When blood loss is excessive, treatment should begin before the woman develops hypotension and tachycardia. Early treatment of shock leads to prompt reversal of the pathophysiology. In longstanding shock, progressive acidosis and tissue damage may render the pathophysiology irreversible.

In hemorrhagic shock, loss of blood volume is so large that vasoconstriction cannot compensate. Venous return to the heart drops and, consequently, cardiac output drops. The initial steps in treating hypovolemic shock are aimed at restoring the circulating blood volume. One or more large intravenous lines should be placed. Agents used to treat blood loss include crystalloid solutions, colloid solutions, and red blood cells. Generally, crystalloid solutions are used first. They are readily available, inexpensive, and safe to use. Crystalloid solutions consist of water and electrolytes with or without glucose. Normal saline with glucose replenishes intravascular volume as well as any other preparation. Different authors prefer different solutions. Lactated Ringer's solution is mentioned often as the crystalloid of choice for initial expansion of blood volume.

Crystalloids alone are not sufficient treatment for most cases of hemorrhagic shock. Colloid solutions and/or blood are also needed. Plasma colloids may be replaced with 5% albumin solution or plasma protein fraction. Neither of these products carries a risk of hepatitis and both provide 11–12 grams of albumin in 250 ml of volume. Colloid fluids tend to remain in the vascular compartment and maintain colloidal osmotic pressure, thus preventing edema formation. Excessive fluid replacement with electrolyte solutions can lead to the development of pulmonary edema.[58] Colloids and crystalloids are both important in treatment of hemorrhagic shock. Colloids may also be given as whole blood or fresh frozen plasma, but, as mentioned above, whole blood may not be available and the use of fresh frozen plasma for whole blood or this purpose is controversial.

Red blood cell transfusion is necessary to restore oxygen carrying capacity. When many units of blood are transfused it is prudent to be prepared to replace components such as platelets and other coagulation factors through the use of fresh frozen plasma. The generally accepted goal of transfusion therapy is to keep the patient's hematocrit above 30%. Oxygen therapy is of value in increasing oxygen supply to the tissues.

While placing intravenous lines, blood can be drawn for laboratory studies. A minimum evaluation includes blood type and crossmatch, hematocrit, and a tube for observation of clotting time. Depending on the circumstances, a complete clotting profile and a serum chemistry analysis can be ordered. Arterial blood gas determinations are helpful in all but early cases of mild shock.

Methods of evaluating the adequacy of treatment should be instituted. This may be as simple as frequent hematocrit determinations and hourly quantitation of urinary output. A useful rule of thumb is to keep the hematocrit above 30% and the urine output above 30 ml/hour. Invasive monitoring with a central venous pressure line or, preferably, with a balloon flotation catheter (Swan–Ganz) is desirable for patients with more critical problems. Use of the balloon flotation catheter is discussed in Chapter 49. These methods of monitoring allow the physician to replace the patient's fluids vigorously while minimizing the chances for overhydration and pulmonary edema.[2]

A useful approach to fluid replacement for patients in shock is based on the response of central venous pressure or pulmonary capillary wedge pressure to a fluid challenge.[57] This approach is based on a normal central venous pressure of 5–15 cm of water or a normal pulmonary capillary wedge pressure of 6–18 Torr. The fluid challenge test is summarized in Table 47-1.

Under ordinary circumstances, definitive treatment of the source of hemorrhage awaits the emergency management of the hypovolemic shock. Exceptions to this statement abound, however. Medical management of uterine atony can proceed while the patient is being transfused. Occasionally, surgical treatment must be undertaken even though the shock has not been fully reversed. Reasons for such management include refusal of blood, unavailability of blood, and inability to keep up with blood loss without surgical intervention.

Goals in management of hypovolemic shock include restoration of blood volume and oxygen carrying capacity, stabilization of vital signs, and definitive teatment of the source of bleeding. The physician should be alert to detect and treat complications of shock such as coagulopathy, transfusion reactions, acidosis, adult respiratory distress syndrome, and acute tubular necrosis. More unusual complications such as cerebrovascular accident, myocardial infarction, pituitary necrosis, and renal cortical necrosis may occur.

Treatment of hemorrhagic shock requires prompt implementation of a plan of action. Rapid replacement of fluid and components, monitoring their replacement, stopping the

TABLE 47-1. FLUID INFUSION TEST AFTER SHUBIN AND WEIL[57]

Initial Central Venous Pressure	Initial Pulmonary Capillary Wedge Pressure	Infuse in 10 Minutes
<10 cm H_2O	<12 Torr	200 ml
10–15 cm H_2O	12–20 Torr	100 ml
>15 cm H_2O	>20 Torr	50 ml
Interpretation of Infusion Test		
Central Venous Pressure Rise	**Wedge Pressure Rise**	**Action**
>5 cm H_2O	>7 Torr	Stop infusion
2–5 cm H_2O	3–7 Torr	Wait 10 minutes and reevaluate
<2 cm H_2O	<3 Torr	Repeat infusion

hemorrhage, and detecting and managing complications of shock should be parts of the plan.

Supportive Measures

Development of a red blood cell substitute has been a research goal for a number of years. Compounds in the perfluorocarbon family are capable of dissolving 40 volume % of oxygen. Studies in experimental animals led to the use of the milky emulsion Fluosol-DA 20% in women who refuse blood transfusions. Early research trials in the treatment of such patients have been encouraging.[32]

Circumferential pneumatic compression is not widely used in the treatment of intra-abdominal hemorrhage despite reports of its effectiveness.[20,47] Authors cannot even agree on the name of the treatment. It has been called G suit, gravity suit, military or medical antishock trousers (MAST), pneumatic pressure, circumferential pressure, and external counterpressure.

Treatment involves placement of pneumatic trousers on the lower extremities and a pneumatic bladder around the abdomen from the pubis to the xiphoid. Pressure is then raised in the pneumatic bladders. There have been virtually no guidelines for use and no controlled clinical trials have been conducted. Generally, pressure of 20–25 Torr is used. The circumferential pressure produces an "autotransfusion" of 250–1000 ml of blood from the lower extremities and abdomen. Associated with this is an increase in blood pressure and a decrease in heart rate. The right atrial pressure, stroke volume, and pulmonary capillary wedge pressure increase and the vital capacity decreases by approximately 20%. Cardiac output is variably influenced but is usually unchanged.[47] Hemostasis is achieved by keeping disrupted vessel walls together.

Pneumatic pressure usually is maintained from 12 to 36 hours. Deflation of the device should take place over 30 minutes. If there is a fall in blood pressure during the deflation process, deflation should be stopped and fluids given to raise the blood pressure. Slow deflation is then resumed. Coagulopathy is a contraindication to deflation of the bladders.

Indications for pneumatic compression in obstetrics include postpartum hemorrhage due to uterine atony, bleeding into the space of Retzius, postcesarean section or hysterectomy bleeding, bleeding after cesarean section for placenta previa, and oozing after virtually any surgical procedure.[20]

Complications of pneumatic compression in experimental animals include severe metabolic acidosis and decreased renal function when pressures above 40 Torr have been use. Neither of these problems have been reported in humans. Some decrease in pulmonary function has been noted. Contraindications to pneumatic compression are not well studied but are assumed to include pregnancy, cerebral edema, pulmonary edema, congestive heart failure, and bleeding above the diaphragm.[20]

LATE POSTPARTUM HEMORRHAGE

Delayed postpartum hemorrhage is defined as excessive bleeding between 24 hours and six weeks after delivery.[3] In a report on delayed postpartum hemorrhage from the Mayo Clinic,[60] the incidence was reported as 1 in 107 deliveries. Of 148 patients reported, 35% were treated successfully with oxytocin infusion alone. Ninety-four women required surgical treatment: 87 had one curettage, 3 had two curettages, 3 required hysterectomy, and 1 was treated with myomectomy. Over three-fourths of the patients treated with curettage had retained placental fragments removed; two of four women with delayed postpartum hemorrhage after cesarean delivery had retained fragments. Other authors mention abnormal involution of the placental site as a cause of late postpartum hemorrhage and report a much lower incidence of the disorder.

In the Mayo Clinic series, age and parity were not associated with late postpartum hemorrhage and there were no patients with genital malignancies or blood dyscrasias. There was an association with multiple gestation, precipitate labor, succenturiate lobe of the placenta, and circumvallate placenta. The peak time of onset of late postpartum hemorrhage was 8 days after delivery. One-third of cases occurred by day 6 and more than 75% of cases occurred by day 18.

A trial of medical management has been recommended before resorting to uterine curettage. The reason for this recommendation is that some women hemorrhage more profusely during curettage and may require hysterectomy. The recommendation seems sound but has not been tested.

REFERENCES

1. A.C.O.G. Technical Bulletin: Blood component therapy. No. 78, July 1984.
2. A.C.O.G. Technical Bulletin: Hemorrhagic shock. No. 82, December 1984.
3. A.C.O.G. Committee on Terminology: *Obstetric-Gynecologic Terminology*. E. C. Hughes (Ed.). Philadelphia, F. A. Davis Company, 1972, p. 417.
4. Alper, M.M. and Dudley, D.K.: Asymptomatic rupture of the uterus: A case report. *Can. Med. Assoc. J.* **130**:153–155, 1984.
5. Andrinopoulos, G. C. and Mendenhall, H. W.: Prostaglandin $F_{2\alpha}$ in the management of delayed postpartum hemorrhage. *Am. J. Obstet. Gynecol.* **146**:217–218, 1983.
6. Awais, G. M. and Lebherz, T. B.: Ruptured uterus, a complication of oxytocin induction and high parity. *Obstet. Gynecol.* **36**:465–468, 1970.
7. Brandt, M. L.: The mechanism and management of the third stage of labor. *Am. J. Obstet. Gynecol.* **25**:662–667, 1933.
8. Burchell, R. C.: Internal iliac artery ligation: Hemodynamics. *Obstet. Gynecol.* **24**:737–739, 1964.
9. Burchell, R. C.: Physiology of internal iliac artery ligation. *J. Obstet. Gynaecol. Br. Commonw.* **75**:642–651, 1968.
10. Burcell, R. C. and Olson, G.: Internal iliac artery ligation: Aortograms. *Am. J. Obstet. Gynecol.* **94**:117–124, 1966.
11. Clark, S. L., Koonings, P. P., and Phelan, J. P.: Placenta previa/accreta and prior cesarean section. *Obstet. Gynecol.* **66**:89–92, 1985.
12. Clark, S. L., Yeh, S. Y., Phelan, J. P., Bruce, S., and Paul, R. H.: Emergency hysterectomy for obstetric hemorrhage. *Obstet. Gynecol.* **64**:376–380, 1984.
13. Conn, L. C., Vant, J. R., and Cantor, M. M.: A critical analysis of blood loss in 2,000 obstetric cases. *Am. J. Obstet. Gynecol.* **42**:768–785, 1941.
14. Cruickshank, S. H. and Stoelk, E. M.: Surgical control of pelvic hemorrhage: Method of bilateral ovarian artery ligation. *Am. J. Obstet. Gynecol.* **147**:724–725, 1983.
15. Department of Health and Social Security: *Report on Confidential Enquiries into Maternal Deaths in England and Wales 1976-1978.* J. Tomkinson (Ed.). London, Her Majesty's Stationery Office, 1982.
16. Drucker, M. and Wallach, R. C.: Uterine packing: A reappraisal. *Mt. Sinai J. Med.* **46**:191–194, 1979.
17. Evans, S. and McShane, P.: The efficacy of internal iliac artery ligation in obstetric hemorrhage. *Surg. Gynecol. Obstet.* **160**:250–253, 1985.
18. Fox, H.: Placenta accreta, 1945–1969. *Obstet. Gynecol. Surv.* **27**:475–490, 1972.
19. Gibbs, C. E. and Locke, W. E.: Maternal deaths in Texas, 1969 to 1973. *Am. J. Obstet. Gynecol.* **126**:687–692, 1976.
20. Gunning, J. E.: For controlling intractable hemorrhage: The gravity suit. *Contemp. OB/GYN* **22**:23–32, 1983.
21. Harris, B. A.: Acute puerperal inversion of the uterus. *Clin. Obstet. Gynecol.* **27**:134–138, 1984.
22. Haseltine, F. P., Glickman, M. G., Marchesi, S., Spitz, R., Dlugi, A., and DeCherney, A. A.: Uterine embolization in a patient with postabortal hemorrhage. *Obstet. Gynecol.* **63**:78S–80S, 1984.
23. Hayashi, R. H., Castillo, M. S., and Noah, M. L.: Management of severe postpartum hemorrhage due to uterine atony using an analogue of prostaglandin $F_{2\alpha}$. *Obstet. Gynecol.* **58**:426–429, 1981.
24. Hayashi, R. H., Castillo, M. S., and Noah, M. L.: Management of severe postpartum hemorrhage with a prostaglandin $F_{2\alpha}$ analogue. *Obstet. Gynecol.* **63**:806–808, 1984.
25. Hendricks, C. H. and Brenner, W. E.: Cardiovascular effects of oxytoxic drugs used postpartum. *Am. J. Obstet. Gynecol.* **108**:751–760, 1970.
26. Hertz, R. H., Sokol, R. J., and Dierker, L. J.: Treatment of postpartum uterine atony with prostaglandin E_2 vaginal suppositories. *Obstet. Gynecol.* **56**:129–130, 1980.
27. Hester, J. D.: Postpartum hemorrhage and re-

evaluation of uterine packing. *Obstet. Gynecol.* **45**:501–504, 1975.

28. Heyl, P. S., Stubblefield, P. G., and Phillippe, M.: Recurrent inversion of the puerperal uterus managed with 15(S)-15-methyl prostaglandin $F_{2\alpha}$ and uterine packing. *Obstet. Gynecol.* **63**:263–264, 1984.
29. Irving, F. C. and Hertig, A. T.: A study of placenta accreta. *Surg. Gynecol. Obstet.* **64**:178–200, 1937.
30. Jacobs, M. M. and Arias, F.: Intramyometrial prostaglandin $F_{2\alpha}$ in the treatment of severe postpartum hemorrhage. *Obstet. Gynecol.* **55**:665–666, 1980.
31. Johnson, A. B.: A new concept in the replacement of the inverted uterus and a report of nine cases. *Am. J. Obstet. Gynecol.* **57**:557–562, 1949.
32. Karn, K. E., Ogburn, P. L., Jr., Julian, T., Cerra, F. B., Hammerschmidt, D. E., and Vercellotti, G.: Use of a whole blood substitute, Fluosol-DA 20%, after massive postpartum hemorrhage. *Obstet. Gynecol.* **65**:127–130, 1985.
33. Kaunitz, A. M., Hughes, J. M., Grimes, D. A., Smith, J. C., Rochat, R. W., and Kafrissen, M. E.: Causes of maternal mortality in the United States. *Obstet. Gynecol.* **65**:605–612, 1985.
34. Kovacs, B. W. and De Vore, G. R.: Management of acute and subacute puerperal uterine inversion with terbutaline sulfate. *Am. J. Obstet. Gynecol.* **150**:784–786, 1984.
35. Lester, W. M., Bartholomew, R. A., Colvin, E. D., Grimes, W. H., Fish, J. S., and Galloway, W. H.: Reconsideration of the uterine pack in postpartum hemorrhage. *Am. J. Obstet. Gynecol.* **93**:321–329, 1965.
36. Lipton, R. A., Ayromlooi J., and Coller, B. S.: Severe von Willebrand's disease during labor and delivery. *JAMA* **248**:1355–1357, 1982.
37. Magrina, J. F., Moffat, R. E., Masterson, B. J., and Krantz, K. E.: Selective arterial infusion of Pitressin for the control of puerperal hemorrhage after hypogastric artery ligation. *Obstet. Gynecol.* **58**:646–648, 1981.
38. Mengert, W. F., Burchell, R. C., Blumstein, R. W., and Daskal, J. L.: Pregnancy after bilateral ligation of the internal iliac and ovarian arteries. *Obstet. Gynecol.* **34**:664–666, 1969.
39. Nelson, G. H.: Consideration of blood loss at delivery as percentage of estimated blood volume. *Am. J. Obstet. Gynecol.* **138**:1117–1119, 1980.
40. Newton, M.: Postpartum hemorrhage. *Am. J. Obstet. Gynecol.* **94**:711–714, 1966.
41. Newton, M., Mosey, L. M., Egli, G. E., Gifford, W. B., and Hull, C. T.: Blood loss during and immediately after delivery. *Obstet. Gynecol.* **17**:9–18, 1961.
42. N.I.H. Consensus Development Conference: Fresh frozen plasma: Indications and risks. Vol. 5, No. 5, 1984.
43. Noller, K. L., Bowie, E. J. W., Kempers, R. D., and Owen, C. A.: von Willebrand's disease in pregnancy. *Obstet. Gynecol.* **41**:865–872, 1973.
44. O'Leary, J. L. and O'Leary, J. A.: Uterine artery ligation in the control of intractable postpartum hemorrhage. *Am. J. Obstet. Gynecol.* **94**:920–924, 1966.
45. O'Leary, J. L. and O'Leary, J. A.: Uterine artery ligation for the control of postcesarean section hemorrhage. *Obstet. Gynecol.* **43**:849–853, 1974.
46. Pais, S. O., Glickman, M., Schwartz, P., Pingoud, E., and Berkowitz, R.: Embolization of pelvic arteries for control of postpartum hemorrhage. *Obstet. Gynecol.* **55**:754–758, 1980.
47. Pelligra, R. and Sandberg, E. C.: Control of intractable abdominal bleeding by external counterpressure. *JAMA* **241**:708–713, 1979.
48. Pelosi, M., Langer, A., and Hung, C.: Prophylactic internal iliac artery ligation at cesarean hysterectomy. *Am. J. Obstet. Gynecol.* **121**:394–398, 1975.
49. Platt, L. D. and Druzin, M. L.: Acute puerperal inversion of the uterus. *Am. J. Obstet. Gynecol.* **141**:187–190, 1981.
50. Pritchard, J. A., Baldwin, R. M., Dickey, J. C., and Wiggins, K. M.: Blood volume changes in pregnancy and the puerperium. *Am. J. Obstet. Gynecol.* **84**:1271–1281, 1962.
51. Read, J. A., Cotton, D. B., and Miller, F. C.: Placenta accreta: Changing clinical aspects and outcome. *Obstet. Gynecol.* **56**:31–34, 1980.
52. Reece, E. A., Fox, H. E., and Rapoport, F.: Factor VIII inhibitor: A cause of severe postpartum hemorrhage. *Am. J. Obstet. Gynecol.* **144**:985–987, 1982.
53. Reich, W. J. and Nechtow, M. J.: Ligation of the internal iliac (hypogastric) arteries: A life-saving procedure for uncontrollable gynecologic and obstetric hemorrhage. *J. Int. Coll. Surg.* **36**:157–168, 1961.
54. Rosenthal, D. M. and Colapinto, R.: Angiographic arterial embolization in the management of postoperative vaginal hemorrhage. *Am. J. Obstet. Gynecol.* **151**:227–231, 1985.
55. Rudd, N. L., Nimrod, C., Holbrook, K. A., and Byers, P. H.: Pregnancy complications in type IV Ehlers-Danlos syndrome. *Lancet* **1**:50–53, 1983.
56. Schrinsky, D. C. and Benson, R. C.: Rupture of the pregnant uterus: A review. *Obstet. Gynecol. Surv.* **33**:217–232, 1978.
57. Shubin, H. and Weil, M. H.: Bacterial shock. *JAMA* **235**:421–424, 1976.
58. Stein, L., Beraud, J. J., Cavanilles, J., daLuz, P., Weil, M. H., and Shubin, H.: Pulmonary edema during fluid infusion in the absence of heart failure. *JAMA* **229**:65–68, 1974.
59. Taylor, E. S.: Intrapartum and postpartum hemorrhage. *Clin. Obstet. Gynecol.* **3**:646–665, 1960.
60. Thorstein, V. T. and Kempers, R. D.: Delayed postpartum bleeding. *Am. J. Obstet. Gynecol.* **107**:565–571, 1970.
61. Toppozada, M., El-Bossaty, M., El-Rahman, H. A., and Shams El-Din, A. H.: Control of intractable atonic postpartum hemorrhage by 15-methyl

prostaglandin $F_{2\alpha}$. *Obstet. Gynecol.* **58**:327–330, 1981.

62. van Vugt, P. J. H., Baudoin, P., Blom, V. M., and van Deursen, C. Th. B. M: Inversio uteri puerperalis. *Acta Obstet. Gynecol.* **60**:353–362, 1981.

63. Walters, E. G.: Surgical management of postpartum hemorrhage with particular reference to ligation of uterine arteries. *Am. J. Obstet. Gynecol.* **64**:1143–1148, 1952.

48

POSTPARTUM LACERATIONS AND HEMATOMAS

Maternal injury may occur at any time during the birth process and at any site along the genital tract. Vaginal, vulvar, and perineal tears usually occur during delivery. Cervical lacerations occur during cervical dilatation or at delivery, whereas uterine rupture occurs prior to and during active labor. Similar to lacerations, genital hematomas also happen at various times during labor and delivery and may occur in the upper or lower genital tract. Hematomas may result from a vessel lacerated by a transmucosal tear or from deep trauma that does not break the mucosal or skin surface. Each complication has different clinical presentations, predisposing factors, management schemes, and eventual prognosis.

UTERINE RUPTURE

An unusual, but often catastropic event, uterine rupture may result in fetal and/or maternal death. This entity is discussed in Chapter 47.

CERVICAL LACERATIONS

Cervical lacerations can result from several causes, including precipitous labor; the patient pushing before complete cervical dilation; instrumental deliveries; and previous scars, incisions, or lacerations of the cervix. Deliberate incision of the cervix in order to effect vaginal delivery is rarely performed except in the unusual instance of vaginal breech delivery with entrapment of the fetal head by an incompletely dilated cervix.

The diagnosis of cervical laceration is often first suspected during the first stage of labor when rapid cervical dilation occurs accompanied by vaginal bleeding. It is not unusual to find small cervical abrasions or lacerations that are of no consequence and require no intervention after vaginal deliveries. Some lacerations, however, demand intervention to stop bleeding and to restore anatomical relationships. The cervix should be inspected in all patients after vaginal delivery. The softness of the tissues renders manual palpation unsatisfactory. Good lighting is important. Visual inspection is assisted by the use of sponge forceps to retract the vaginal walls or to grasp the cervix itself. Several sponge sticks may be used to grasp the cervical margin and manipulate it so that the entire circumference of the cervix is visualized. Some causes of cervical tears are forceps delivery, delivery before full dilatation, attempts at manual dilatation of the cervix, rapid labor and delivery, macrosomia, and prior cervical scarring or strictures. With prolonged labor, portions of the cervix may become edematous. If compressed sufficiently, portions of the cervix may necrose and separate.

Lacerations that are actively bleeding should be repaired, as should all lacerations over 1.5 cm in length, whether or not they are bleeding. Most cervical lacerations occur at 3 and 9 o'clock, and they may extend superiorly high enough to involve the descending branch of the uterine artery and vein or to involve the parametrium. Therefore, it is important to visualize the upper margin of the laceration. With superior extension into the parametrium, a transvaginal approach is inadequate. Laparotomy is needed for repair of lacerations that extend into the lower uterine segment or the broad ligament. Most lacerations, however, can be repaired transvaginally.

Exposure to identify the apex of the defect is imperative to the repair of a cervical laceration. This often requires the help of an assistant to hold the ring forceps while the operator finds the apex of the laceration. Vaginal retractors allow visualization of the cervix, and sponge forceps are used to grasp the torn edges of the cervix. The defect is repaired with interrupted or "running-lock" stitches of 2-0 or 3-0 chromic catgut on an atraumatic round needle. The first suture is placed several millimeters above the apex of the laceration to prevent bleeding above the tear from torn vessels that may have retracted.

Visual inspection of the cervix prevents the complications of an unrepaired cervical laceration—vaginal bleeding and cervical incompetence.

VAGINAL AND VULVAR LACERATIONS

Lacerations of the upper vagina are similar in etiology and method of repair to cervical lacerations. Postdelivery genital inspection should include visualization of the vaginal fornices. A common cause of upper vaginal lacerations in the region of the ischial spines is trauma due to forceps. Lacerations also may result from extension of an episiotomy or congenital anomalies such as a septum. Vaginal fornix lacerations may be unilateral or bilateral and are usually superficial. The most common are longitudinal and lateral. Rarely, these tears extend into the peritoneal cavity along the cul-de-sac of Douglas. Vaginal side-wall lacerations and sulcus tears can bleed profusely; it has been estimated that the average blood loss from such a laceration is close to a liter. With vaginal lacerations there is often no discrete arterial bleeding source that can be ligated. More often, there is a generalized venous oozing from the base of the laceration. Exposure, assistance, and good lighting are essential for repair. Small lacerations can be repaired with a running, locking suture of absorbable material; the repair should begin above the apex for the same reasons cited above. Repair of longer, deeper lacerations is more difficult. Simply approximating the vaginal mucosa is not adequate treatment because the patient may then develop a hematoma beneath the suture line. The apex of the tear must be seen and a suture applied above. Interrupted sutures in the depths of the laceration may achieve hemostasis after which the vaginal mucosa can be closed with a running, locking suture. If good hemostasis cannot be achieved with suture material, consideration should be given to packing and counterpacking. With this technique a retention catheter is placed in the urinary bladder. Next, the depths of the laceration are packed with gauze. After the laceration has been packed, the vagina is counterpacked tightly. This provides sufficient pressure to stop troublesome oozing. The packs are removed in 24–36 hours. Prophylactic antibiotics are not necessary. If blood appears after the pack is in place, the source of bleeding must be investigated promptly. Damage to adjacent structures such as rectum, bladder, or ureter should be sought, and care should be exercised not to include these structures in the sutures.

Lacerations of the lower vagina and vulva usually result from episiotomy extension or from delayed performance of episiotomy. Posterior lacerations are repaired with a technique similar to episiotomy suture (see Chapter 43). Anterior lacerations are usually superficial and involve only the vaginal mucosa. These shallow lacerations require sutures only if bleeding persists and is not controlled after a brief period of pressure. With anterior lacerations, damage to the urethra and bladder should be excluded.

Anterior lacerations that are deep or continue to bleed should be repaired with 3-0 or 4-0 chromic. An indwelling catheter may be inserted for drainage and to avoid damage to the urethra during suturing. Proper anatomical approximation is important to prevent distortion of the urethra and bladder-neck which may result in voiding difficulties.

URINARY FISTULA

Urinary fistula, a rare event, can occur after delivery. Common causes of vesicovaginal fistulas are prolonged labor, misuse of forceps, and improper technique at cesarean section. The rate of fistula formation at two institutions from 1946 to 1955 varied from 0.01 per 1000 to 0.05 per 1000 deliveries.[3] Two types of fistula are encountered—immediate and late. An immediate fistula is due to trauma and laceration at the time of delivery, usually due to instrumentation, such as incorrectly applied forceps. Diagnosis is prompt because urine leaks from the laceration. Bleeding from the laceration often results in immediate repair. Adequate bladder drainage with an indwelling catheter is useful to prevent further injury during repair. Prolonged drainage aids healing.

Patients with a late urinary fistula experience urine loss 3–7 days after delivery. Necrosis and tissue damage from prolonged compression of the bladder, urethra, and anterior vaginal wall between the fetal head and pubic arch result in sloughing of these tissues with urine loss. The fistula can be quite small and urinary incontinence must be excluded. Injection of methylene-blue into the bladder to observe the point of leakage is useful. With leaks high in the vagina, dye in the bladder and a tampon in the vagina may assist in localization. Drainage of the bladder is critical in the initial treatment, and many fistulas will close spontaneously. Even with a persistent fistula, drainage is important so that the tissues are revitalized prior to the attempted surgical repair.

SYMPHYSIOLYSIS

Separation of the symphysis pubis rarely occurs. In an African population known to have "generally contracted pelvices," 18 of 4500 (0.4%) deliveries resulted in spontaneous symphisiolysis.[2] Surprisingly 15 of the 18 followed uninstrumented vaginal deliveries and only 3 were after forceps deliveries. Reported incidences in other populations range from 1 in 521 to 1 in 30,000.[1] This wide diversity in prevalence may result from the many asymptomatic patients in whom radiography must be performed to arrive at a diagnosis.

Symptomatic patients often complain of exquisite pain and tenderness at the symphysis pubis, inability to walk, or a waddling gait, and urinary retention. Treatment consists of bed rest, a pelvic binder, and time. Most patients are able to walk and do well after 10–14 days. Occasionally, prolonged urinary drainage is required.

HEMATOMAS

Peripartal hematomas may develop at any site along the genital tract. The extent of spread is determined by the muscular and fascial planes surrounding the bleeding. The anatomic classification of Pieri is useful to understand the extent of spread and to plan optimal treatment (Table 48-1).[4]

The rate of genital hematomas varies from 1 in 500 to 1 in 1000 deliveries.[4] Trauma is the major cause. Hematomas may occur after spontaneous vaginal delivery because of damage to a submucosal vessel. More commonly, hematomas follow delivery with forceps or the use of needles for anesthesia. Excessive uterine manipulation or massage may result in hematomas, as may inadequate hemostasis in an episiotomy.

VULVAR HEMATOMAS

It is unusual to see vulvar hematomas develop rapidly enough to be diagnosed at the delivery table. Commonly, the first symptom of a vulvar hematoma is the complaint of severe pain in the pelvis. Visual inspection of the genitalia also identifies many hematomas. A tensely swollen, edematous, and often ecchymotic labium majorus and perineum commonly are noted with vulvar hematomas. These hematomas are superficial and do not extend into the vaginal canal. The fascial and muscular planes of the pelvis limit the spread of the vulvar hematoma to the area below the levator ani muscles. Even though the hematoma may distort the episiotomy, the source is not necessarily a bleeding vessel from the episiotomy.

Unless the hematoma is very small, not increasing in size, and physical exam reveals no extension, the hematoma should be evacuated. A linear incision over the area of maximal distension or, if involved, at the hymenal ring, is performed. The blood clot is thoroughly evac-

TABLE 48-1. ANATOMIC CLASSIFICATION OF PELVIC HEMATOMAS

I. VULVAR—Below the pelvic diaphragm

II. VAGINAL
   A. Above the pelvic diaphragm
   B. Below the cardinal ligaments

III. SUBPERITONEAL—Above the cardinal ligaments

Source: Reprinted with permission from the American College of Obstetricians and Gynecologists. Modified from Pieri, R. J.: Pelvic hematomas associated with pregnancy. *Obstet. Gynecol.* **12**:249–258, 1958.

uated and bleeding vessels are sought. Most often, the cavity oozes diffusely and no single bleeding site is noted. With a small cavity, 2-0 or 3-0 chromic sutures easily obliterate the cavity. Large cavities should be packed with gauze after evacuation. A vaginal pack should be utilized to compress the walls of the cavity and prevent bleeding. If packing of the vagina is properly done, a catheter is required for adequate urinary drainage. After 12–24 hours, the packing can be withdrawn progressively.

Vulvar hematomas may contain large amounts of blood. The patient may require fluid and blood replacement, and administration of fresh-frozen plasma, cryoprecipitate, or fresh blood to reverse disseminated intravascular coagulation.

VAGINAL HEMATOMAS

Vaginal hematomas are less common than vulvar hematomas and are harder to diagnose. Pelvic pain is often the only complaint, although blood loss may be sufficient to result in hypovolemia, shock, and cardiovascular collapse. Bimanual examination reveals a mass distorting the vaginal canal. The anatomic planes of the pelvis limit the extent of vaginal hematomas to the area from the levator ani to below the vaginal fornix, but the depth, and therefore size, is impossible to ascertain. Because of inability to gauge the extent and spread of the hematoma, vaginal hematomas should be evacuated. A longitudinal incision of the vaginal mucosa at the point of maximal distension is performed and drainage effected. Because of the many surrounding structures that may be injured by random sutures to close the defect, these patients should be treated with a vaginal pack to apply pressure to the hematoma site. Ligation of any bleeding vessels that are identified is useful. Bladder drainage with a catheter is necessary.

SUBPERITONEAL HEMATOMA

The rarest of all the pelvic hematomas, a subperitoneal hematoma, may be the most catastrophic. Many of these patients are asymptomatic until they develop marked hypotension from hypovolemia. Others may present with evidence of intra-abdominal bleeding. Pelvic exam may reveal the hematoma if it extends between the leaves of the broad ligament, but retroperitoneal spread may not be easy to detect on bimanual exam. Treatment requires aggressive blood and fluid replacement and early surgical intervention. Since the extent and location of the hematoma may vary, the procedure to be performed at laparotomy depends on the findings at surgery. Hypogastric artery ligation is often useful in controlling bleeding and therefore the spread of the hematoma. Incision of the hematoma and hysterectomy also may be necessary.

REFERENCES

1. Cibils, L. A.: Rupture of the symphysis pubis: A case report. *Obstet. Gynecol.* **38**:409–410, 1971.
2. Hyslop, C. M.: Separation of the symphysis pubis in East African parturients. *J. Obstet. Gynaecol. Br. Commonw.* **71**:284–286, 1964.
3. McCausland, A. M., Caillouette, J. C., Bennallack, D. A., and Holmes, F.: A comparative study of vesicovaginal fistulas following delivery. *Am. J. Obstet. Gynecol.* **79**:1110–1113, 1960.
4. Pieri, R. J.: Pelvic hematomas associated with pregnancy. *Obstet. Gynecol.* **12**:249–258, 1958.

49

HEMODYNAMIC MONITORING IN OBSTETRICS

Use of the pulmonary artery catheter in obstetrics has been limited. This device optimizes the care of women with severe preeclampsia. Although routine use of invasive hemodynamic monitoring is not indicated, Swan–Ganz catheterization may aid in the management of patients who develop pulmonary edema or oliguria or who require massive fluid and blood product replacement.

THE PULMONARY ARTERY CATHETER

The clinical utilization of flow-directed pulmonary artery catheterization was popularized in the early 1970s. The initial catheter introduced by Swan and Ganz had two lumina.[74] The device has since been modified. The catheter now most widely used contains three lumina, one for control of the inflation of a balloon located at the catheter tip, and the others terminating either proximal to or at the catheter tip (Fig. 49-1). These portals allow recording of pressure and sampling of blood from various positions in the right heart and pulmonary circuits. More sophisticated devices that allow for cardiac pacing and recording of electrocardiograms from the bundle of His are available.

A thermistor is located at the catheter tip. Injection of 5% dextrose at 0 °C into the proximal port allows calculation of cardiac output by thermodilution principles. In clinical practice a bedside computer is employed to perform the calculations.

Intermittent balloon inflation allows measurement of pulmonary capillary wedge pressure (PCWP). As the balloon is inflated, it is carried by pulmonary artery blood flow into a more peripheral and smaller vessel. The balloon becomes wedged in the smaller vessel. Pressure readings from the catheter tip in this position reflect hydrostatic pressure in the pulmonary capillary circuit. In the absence of mitral valvular disease, PCWP closely approximates left ventricular end-diastolic pressure (LVEDP).[50,73]

In addition to determination of cardiac output and PCWP, the pulmonary artery catheter allows measurement of right atrial (central venous) and pulmonary artery pressures and collection of central venous blood samples. With these and other readily measured parameters (blood pressures, arterial blood gases, hemoglobin, height, and weight), systemic and pulmonary vascular resistances, oxygen delivery and utilization, and indices of ventricular performance may be calculated. Serial determinations allow construction of left ventricular function curves and assessment of the impact of therapy on the patient's hemodynamic status.[14,26,27]

The Swan–Ganz catheter is passed into the vena cava from any of the larger peripheral or central veins. After insertion and balloon inflation, the catheter is drawn into and through the right side of the heart by venous and pulmonary arterial blood flow. The progress of the catheter is monitored by recording pressure at the catheter tip and by observing the characteristic pressure waveforms in the vena cava, right atrium, right ventricle, and pulmonary artery (Fig. 49-2). Generally, fluoroscopy is not re-

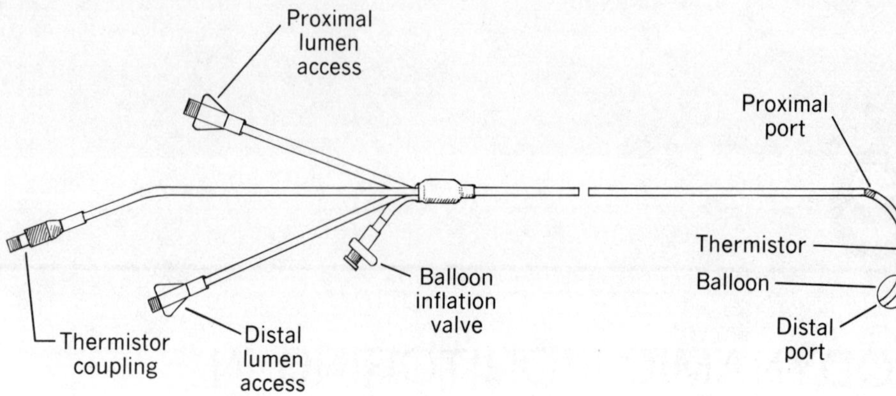

Figure 49-1. Diagram of pulmonary artery catheter (see text).

quired but may be useful in difficult catheterizations.

Complications that may occur with insertion of the pulmonary artery catheter include hematoma formation, laceration of adjacent arteries or nerves, and pneumothorax and air embolism. The incidence of these complications appears to be related to operator training.[65] In experienced hands, the rate of complications is low.

Cardiac arrhythmias occur in 30–78% of cases and have been attributed to balloon or catheter trauma to the right atrium or ventricle.[23,65] Transient ectopy is fairly common, but sustained or life-threatening arrhythmias are

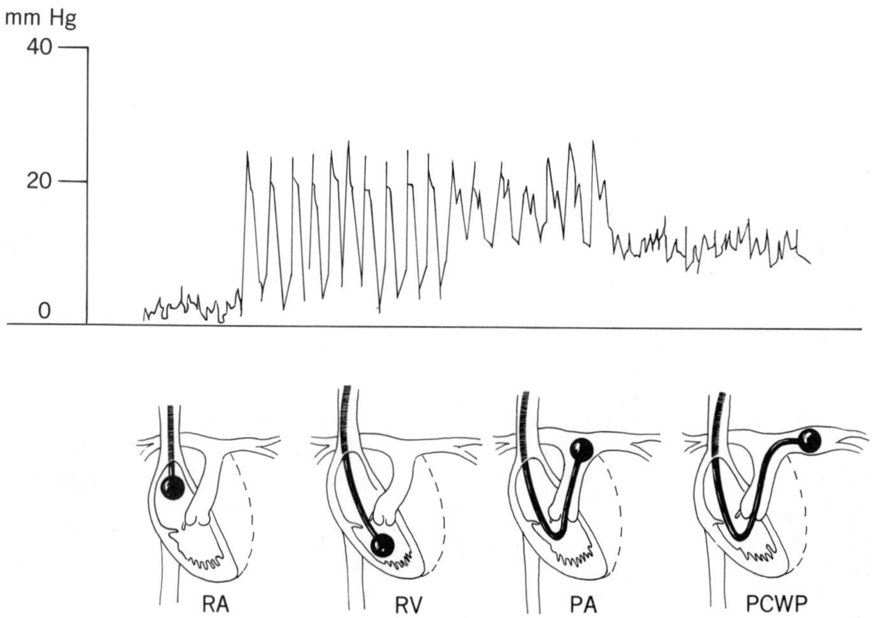

Figure 49-2. Catheter progress is assessed by monitoring waveforms in right atrium (RA), right ventricle (RV), and pulmonary artery (PA). Wedging of catheter balloon in a branch of the pulmonary artery results in pulmonary capillary wedge pressure (PCWP) measurement.

rare.[68] The occurrence of arrhythmias also is related to operator experience. The underlying disease state of the patient also appears to be a significant factor.[68]

Infectious complications occur in about 3% of patients.[23,65] Though adherence to strict aseptic technique minimizes this occurrence, bacterial colonization of the catheter is related to the underlying disease and to the duration of catheter usage.[2,23]

Pulmonary damage, including pulmonary infarction and pulmonary artery rupture, may occur. Avoidance of prolonged balloon inflation and protracted catheter use and prevention of peripheral migration of the catheter tip limit these occurrences.[25,46] Hemoptysis is an early sign of pulmonary damage and should be investigated diligently.[5,56]

Mechanical difficulties such as balloon rupture and catheter knotting are infrequent. The former appears related to excessive catheterization time and trauma to the balloon during insertion. Knotting may be prevented by ensuring that the balloon is fully inflated at the time of catheter advancement and by avoiding introduction of an excessive length of the catheter.[24]

DETERMINANTS OF PULMONARY EDEMA FORMATION

The relationship of factors involved in the transfer of fluid across a capillary wall is expressed in the Starling equation:

$$J = k[(P_c - P_t) - \Theta\ (\pi c - \pi t)]$$

where J = net volume of fluid filtered; k = the capillary permeability coefficient; P_c, P_t = capillary and tissue hydrostatic pressures; Θ = the Staverman reflection coefficient; and πc, πt = plasma and tissue colloid osmotic pressures.

In the lung the physical forces that determine transfer of fluid include the hydrostatic and oncotic pressures in the capillary and interstitial spaces, and the surface tension within the alveolus (Table 49-1). Although the exact magnitude of interstitial pressures is unknown, it appears that in the normal state a net transfer of fluid from the capillary to the interstitium and into the lymphatics occurs constantly.[55] Physical forces also favor the transfer of fluid from alveolar surfaces into the lymphatics.[47] Lymphatic capacity is crucial in the control of fluid balance within the lung.[69] When lymphatic capacity is exceeded, interstitial congestion and ultimately alveolar edema ensue.

The Starling equation predicts that transfer of fluid from the capillary to the interstitium increases with increased vessel wall permeability, lowered plasma oncotic pressure, or elevated capillary hydrostatic pressure. In the intact patient, measurement of all parameters of the Starling equation is not possible. Plasma colloid oncotic pressure (COP), however, is determined easily and capillary hydrostatic pressure is approximated closely by the PCWP. Although this method of procedure has been criticized by some,[16] simplification of the Starling relationships by utilizing the COP-PCWP gradient appears to be a clinically useful tool.[78]

PCWP is normally about 10 mmHg. Levels above 18 mmHg are associated with pulmonary congestion and levels above 25–30 mmHg are associated with pulmonary edema.[14] The COP is usually about 25 mmHg in healthy subjects. Thus, a COP-PCWP gradient of approximately 15 mmHg usually prevents excessive fluid transfer from the capillary to the interstitium.

Colloid oncotic pressure may be unusually low in critically ill patients and in postoperative patients for a variety of reasons. In seriously ill patients, if the COP-PCWP gradient is less than 0 mmHg, pulmonary edema uniformly develops.[78] On the other hand, if the gradient is greater than 6 mmHg, pulmonary edema rarely occurs. However, it is important to be aware that pulmonary edema can occur despite nor-

TABLE 49-1. FORCES ACTIVE IN THE DETERMINATION OF NET FLUID MOVEMENT WITHIN THE LUNG

Location	Force	Activity
Capillary	Hydrostatic pressure	Favors fluid movement to interstitial space
	Oncotic pressure	Retards fluid movement from capillary to interstitium
Interstitium	Hydrostatic pressure	Favors fluid movement from capillary and alveolus
	Oncotic pressure	Favors fluid movement from capillary and alveolus
Alveolus	Surface tension	Favors fluid movement into alveolus
Lymphatic	Hydrostatic pressure	Favors fluid movement from interstitium
	Oncotic pressure	?

mal PCWPs and normal left ventricular function.[70]

Central venous pressure measurement commonly is used to estimate volume status and cardiac filling pressures in the management of postoperative and critically ill patients. In a variety of disease states, including preeclampsia, central venous pressure may not accurately reflect left ventricular end-diastolic pressure.[21,75] This is particularly true where the function of one ventricle is impaired more severely than is that of the other. In such situations reliable estimation of left ventricular filling pressures and left ventricular performance can be obtained only through direct measurement of LVEDP or by determination of PCWP.[75]

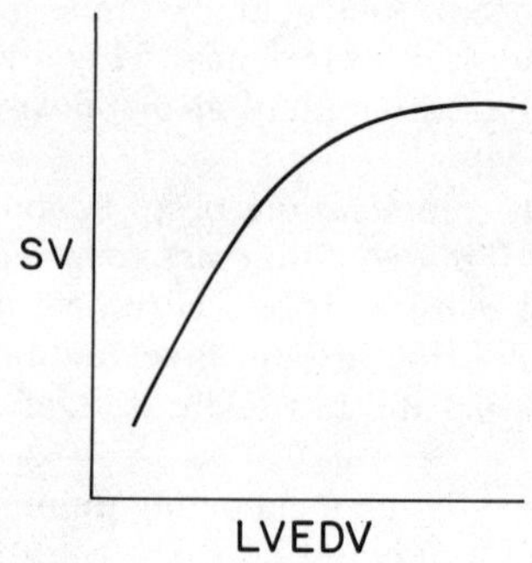

Figure 49-3. Ventricular function curve demonstrating relationship between stroke volume (SV) and left ventricular end-diastolic volume.

CARDIOVASCULAR HEMODYNAMICS

Cardiac function is determined by the interaction of several variables. These include preload (ventricular wall tension at end-diastole), afterload (the tension exerted on the ventricular wall after ejection onset), and the intrinsic inotropic state of the heart.[12,67] These factors are interrelated. Isolation of the effect of alteration of one factor is difficult in the clinical setting. Data derived from experimental preparations, in which reflex adjustments can be controlled, provide insights into the relationship of each factor to overall cardiac performance. These observations provide the basis for hemodynamic monitoring. At any given inotropic level, if heart rate and systemic vascular resistance are held constant, then (within certain limits) left ventricular stroke volume varies directly with left ventricular end-diastolic volume (preload). This relationship forms the basis of Starling's law of the heart and is represented graphically by the familiar Frank–Starling curve (Fig. 49-3). Depending on loading characteristics and level of inotropy, ventricular function may be represented by a series of Frank–Starling curves. The absolute level and shape of any given curve are determined by both the inotropic state and the degree of afterload.[58]

Stroke volume is inversely related to afterload.[44] If all other factors are controlled for, as afterload increases a greater proportion of ventricular work is expended in the generation of greater wall tension. Myocardial fiber shortening is lessened, and stroke volume is reduced (Fig. 49-4).

Cardiac response to altered loading depends on the intrinsic inotropic level of the heart and the adequacy of preload reserve mechanisms.[57] In the resting state, the point defining cardiac function is located on the ascending portion of a given Frank–Starling curve (point A, Fig. 49-5). An acute increase in preload results in increased myocardial length at end-diastole and an increase in stroke volume (point B, Fig. 49-5). If inotropic level, heart rate, and afterload are held constant, cardiac output increases progressively with progressive increases in preload. However, the magnitude of each progressive rise is proportionately smaller (point C, Fig. 49-5). Eventually, further elevation of preload results in no increase in cardiac output (point D, Fig. 49-5). At this point, preload reserve mechanisms are exhausted and preload and afterload are mismatched. Further elevation of cardiac output is achieved only by diminishing afterload or by raising the inotropic state (shift to a higher Frank–Starling curve).

Similarly, cardiac reflex adjustments to af-

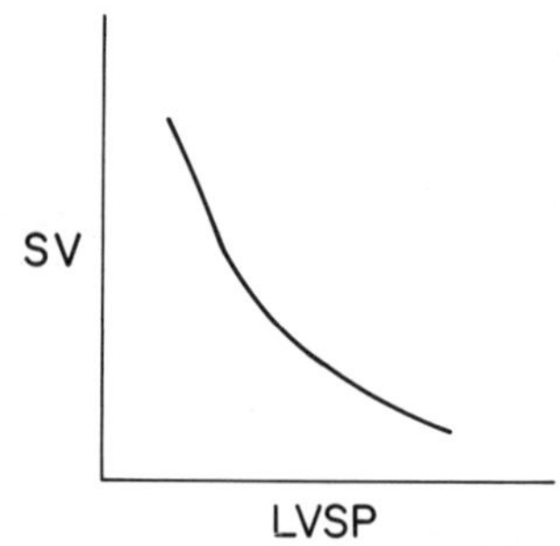

Figure 49-4. The influence of increasing afterload upon ventricular function. SV (stroke volume), LVSP (left ventricular systolic pressure).

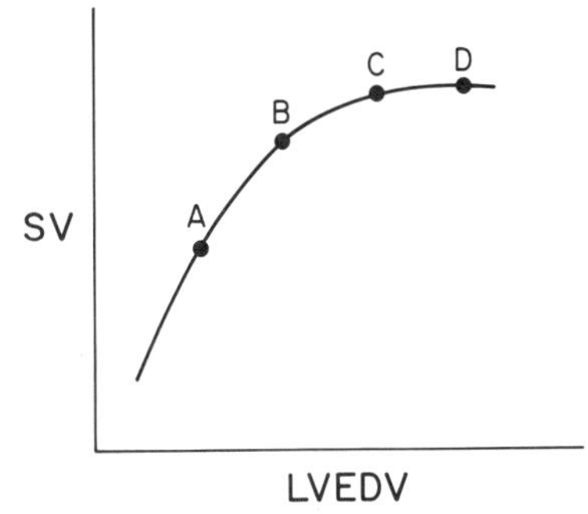

Figure 49-5. Effect of increasing preload on ventricular stroke volume. Stroke volume (SV) is augmented after an increase in left ventricular end-diastolic volume (LVEDV) from resting Level (A to B). Augmentation of stroke volume is smaller at higher initial preload level (B to C). With preload reserve exhausted, a further increase in LVEDV is not accompanied by an increase in stroke volume (C to D).

terload elevation involve Frank–Starling mechanisms.[57] Acute afterload elevation results in a fall in stroke volume and cardiac output (Fig. 49-6). At a higher level of afterload, cardiac function is described by a lower Frank–Starling curve. Decreased stroke volume, however, results in an increased end-diastolic volume (preload). If adequate reserves are present, preload elevation reflexly increases stroke volume, and cardiac output is returned toward normal (point B, Fig. 49-6). In this reflex adjustment, however, a portion of preload reserve is lost, since stroke volume is normalized by an increase in preload. If afterload is further increased, ventricular performance is shifted to still lower Frank–Starling curves, and end-diastolic volumes rise progressively. Reflex adjustments designed to return output toward normal fail, as preload reserve is taxed. Eventually, the reserve is exhausted and end-diastolic volume rises without concomitant reflex augmentation of stroke volume (point D, Fig. 49-6). Furthermore, as ventricular end-diastolic volume increases, ventricular compliance diminishes. Thus, successive increases in end-diastolic volume result in disproportionately greater increases in end-diastolic pressure.[45]

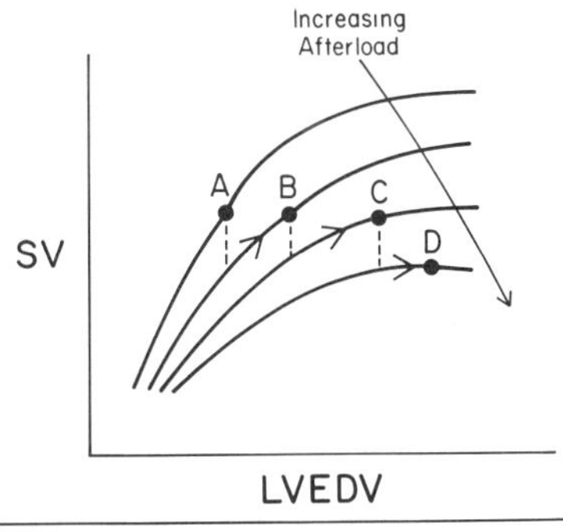

Figure 49-6. Afterload elevation results in a downward shift of ventricular function curve. Frank-Starling mechanisms (———→———) serve to restore stroke volume (SV) toward normal levels (A,B,C). As preload reserve is exhausted, no further increase in SV occurs despite elevation of left ventricular end-diastolic volume (LVEDV) (D).

The effects of afterload elevation on ventricular performance have important clinical consequences. The level of the systemic blood pressure generally is assumed to represent the degree of afterload to which the ventricle is subjected. In patients with markedly elevated systemic vascular resistance, this assumption may not be valid. Blood pressure (BP) is determined by both systemic vascular resistance (SVR) and cardiac output (CO). The relationship of these factors is represented by the equation: BP = CO x SVR. Since CO and SVR are inversely related and extreme elevations of SVR depress cardiac output, an elevated SVR may not be reflected in an elevated BP. Thus, varying levels of cardiac output and systemic vascular resistance may yield similar blood pressures. Furthermore, SVR may be elevated significantly in a normotensive person.[18]

Hypertensive cardiac dysfunction frequently is seen in a certain subset of patients after myocardial infarction. These patients may respond dramatically to therapeutic maneuvers that lower systemic vascular resistance (vasodilator therapy).[19] Hypertensive cardiac dysfunction may develop in certain patients with otherwise normal hearts who suffer from disease processes associated with marked elevations of systemic vascular assistance. These include patients with malignant hypertension and some patients with preeclampsia[72] (see below).

VENTRICULAR ADAPTATION TO CHRONIC LOADING CHANGES

Cardiac hypertrophy occurs in the presence of chronic overload states. The nature of the hypertrophy depends on the type of overload to which the ventricle is subjected. Ventricular hypertrophy is apparently an adaptation that attempts to normalize ventricular wall stress.[33]

The determinants of ventricular wall stress may be represented by a simplification of the LaPlace relationship[37]: wall stress $= \frac{P \times r}{2h}$ where P = intraventricular pressure, r = ventricular radius and h = the ventricular wall thickness. Because ventricular wall stress is a major determinant of myocardial oxygen consumption, limitation of wall stress has adaptive advantages.

As noted above, the ventricle responds to an elevated preload by increasing end-diastolic dimensions and by augmenting ventricular output by Frank–Starling mechanisms. Increased end-diastolic volume, however, necessarily results in increased ventricular wall stress. Ventricular adaptation to chronic preload elevation (chronic volume overload) includes an increase in myocardial cell mass and wall thickness, as well as an increase in ventricular end-diastolic and stroke volumes. This type of hypertrophy, termed eccentric, results in a larger ventricle with a thicker wall. The ventricular radius to wall thickness ratio is close to normal, and wall stress is minimized.[33]

Ventricular hypertrophy in response to chronic afterload elevation (hypertension) also serves to limit wall stress. In this situation, however, the ventricular alteration results in an increase in myocardial wall thickness and is termed concentric.[33] The resulting chamber is only modestly enlarged but has a much thicker wall. Radius-to-wall thickness ratio is reduced and wall stress is minimized. In the absence of dysfunction, ejection fraction and stroke volume remain normal.[64]

CARDIOVASCULAR ALTERATIONS IN NORMAL PREGNANCY

Circulating volume increases 40–50% during normal pregnancy.[15,59,60] In response to this natural overload state, eccentric cardiac hypertropy develops. Left ventricular end-diastolic volume increases 15–20%[38] and stroke volume is augmented by 10–20%.[62] Concomitantly, heart rate rises 10–15% over nonpregnant levels[48] (see Chapters 3 and 31). When studies are performed in the left lateral position, these alterations appear to be progressive throughout pregnancy, though near maximal values are attained early in the third trimester.

Systemic vascular resistance declines during normal gestation reaching a low of approximately 900 dyne • sec • cm^{-5} at 20–28 weeks, before returning to nonpregnant levels at term (1200 dyne • sec • cm^{-5}). [61] Blood pressure changes reflect the changes in SVR. Mean arterial blood pressure (MAP) parallels the changes in SVR. These alterations limit the afterload placed on a volume overloaded ventricle and thus limit wall stress.

The net effect of these changes is a 30–40% increase in cardiac output.[48] The functional state of the myocardium is probably little altered during pregnancy,[43] although myocardial contractility may be enhanced.[63] Most studies suggest that ventricular ejection fraction and mean velocity of circumferential shortening (mVcf) are maintained within normal limits.[41,77] Similarly, despite elevated end-diastolic volumes, LVEDP and PCWP remain normal during normal pregnancy.[4]

CARDIOVASCULAR ADJUSTMENTS IN PREECLAMPSIA

Preeclampsia is a vasospastic disease. In preeclampsia, vascular reactivity to pressor agents is augmented.[29] Refractoriness to the pressor effect of angiotensin II, which characterizes normal gestation, is lost in preeclampsia. Elevated anteriolar resistance is either directly or indirectly responsible for many of the signs and symptoms of the disease (Chapter 32). Preeclampsia is a chronic process. Abnormal vascular reactivity antedates the onset of clinical signs of hypertension, proteinuria, and edema by several weeks.[29] The well-documented contraction (or lack of expansion) of circulating blood volume precedes the onset of clinical signs [11,28,35]

In the majority of women with preeclampsia, left ventricular function is maintained within normal pregnancy ranges.[7,34,52,53] Echocardiographic studies demonstrate that, despite elevated ventricular afterload (increased MAP), left ventricular ejection fraction and mVcf are maintained within normal limits. The preservation of normal function is accomplished apparently by a major alteration of the geometry of the left ventricle.[41,77]

Concentric cardiac hypertrophy occurs in pregnancies complicated by preeclampsia.[42] This type of hypertrophy, resulting in a thicker-walled myocardium, appears to provide the preeclamptic gravida the ability to cope more efficiently with an acute elevation in afterload.

Ventricular response to acute elevations in afterload involves Starling mechanisms. Stroke volume is maintained by an increase in LVEDV. Such an adjustment in the normal gravida with an eccentrically hypertrophic heart results in a rapid increase in ventricular wall stress. It is possible that the preeclamptic is adapted to handle acute elevations of afterload.[77] With a concentrically hypertrophic heart, ventricular wall stress is minimized as end-diastolic volume increases.

Left ventricular end-diastolic and stroke volumes are increased in the majority of preeclamptic patients as compared to nonpregnant women, but lower than those observed in normal pregnant women.[41] These alterations appear to be the consequence of diminished circulating plasma volume in preeclampsia. Such observations suggest that cardiovascular performance suffers because of diminished volume. Thus, plasma volume expansion has been advocated as a therapeutic means to correct a suspected volume deficit. However, although the plasma volume of the preeclamptic is smaller than that of the normal gravida, the condition reflects a chronically contracted vascular space.[3,15,66] Response to maneuvers designed to test orthostasis lends further evidence for the absence of a volume deficit.[49]

Hemodynamic data demonstrate that efficient cardiac adaptation to the preeclamptic state is the rule.[7,8,53] The majority of patients with preeclampsia exhibit cardiac function that is in a hyperdynamic zone in terms of Frank–Starling relationships. Thus, despite diminished intravascular volume and presumed lower preload, the level of preload present is sufficient to maintain excellent function.

Ventricular function is load-dependent, and response to altered loading conditions depends on the adequacy of preload reserves. Most preeclamptics respond to hydration with increased cardiac output reflecting efficient adaptation to a condition of chronic afterload elevation. Despite increased afterload, most still function on the ascending portion of their ventricular function curves and have adequate preload reserves. It is apparent, however, that this may not be true of all patients. Hydration causes pulmonary edema in certain preeclamptic patients.[8]

PULMONARY EDEMA IN PREECLAMPSIA

The etiology of pulmonary edema, as a complication of severe preeclampsia, has been variously ascribed to altered hydrostatic/oncotic pressure relationships, left ventricular hypertensive dysfunction, or alteration in the permeability of pulmonary capillaries. In any given patient, a combination of factors may be operative.

Hydrostatic/Oncotic Pressure Alterations

During normal human pregnancy there is a progressive decrease in plasma colloid osmotic pressure (COP).[54] Intrapartum plasma COP in normal pregnant women is significantly lower than that observed in nonpregnant controls (mean 21.0 ± 2.1 mmHg vs. 28 mmHg). COP is reduced significantly (to a mean level of 15.4 ± 2.1 mmHg) in the postpartum period.[22] Plasma COP is significantly lower in preeclamptic than in normal pregnant controls, both intra- (17.9 vs. 22.0 mmHg) and postpartum (13.7 vs. 17.2 mmHg). The drop in COP postpartum presumably is due to a combination of intrapartum fluid therapy and mobilization of peripheral edema associated with the recumbent position.[6]

Postpartum plasma COPs are maximally depressed by 6 hours postpartum.[31] The maximal depression, thus is coincident with the peaks in cardiac output and PCWP that occur in the immediate postpartum period as initial uterine involution takes place.[32,34,76] Simultaneous alterations of two factors important in the rate of edema formation within the lung account for the fact that the majority of cases of pulmonary edema complicating preeclampsia occur in the immediate puerperium.[36]

Altered hydrostatic/oncotic pressure relationships were said to be etiologic in more than half the women in a recently reported series of cases of pulmonary edema complicating preeclampsia.[8] In this subgroup, pulmonary capillary wedge pressures were modestly elevated (14–22 mmHg) and COPs moderately depressed (10.4–18.8 mmHg). COP-PCWP gradients were all 1 mmHg or less. Of note was that CO was normal or elevated (7.5–12.5 liters/min). Infusion of large volumes of fluid was thought to contribute to the occurrence of pulmonary edema in these patients.

Left Ventricular Dysfunction

Although normal left ventricular function generally is maintained in preeclampsia, occasional patients manifest hypertensive cardiac dysfunction. Cardiac performance in patients with severe preeclampsia seems to follow a continuum from low output to hyperdynamic, depending on the level of systemic vascular resistance.[52] In patients with very elevated SVR, CO may be depressed as the ventricular contractile apparatus fails to adjust to the elevated afterload.[72] As LVEDP rises in an effort to augment CO by Frank–Starling mechanisms, capillary hydrostatic pressure in the lung increases and pulmonary edema may eventuate.

Ventricular contractility probably rapidly returns to normal once blood pressure is normalized in patients with hypertensive left ventricular dysfunction.[77] In this setting, ventricular dysfunction likely results from mechanical overload of a previously normal heart and does not represent the unmasking of latent dysfunction in an abnormal ventricle. Rapid response to vasodilator therapy in similar patients supports this contention.[72]

Increased Pulmonary Capillary Permeability

Adult respiratory distress syndrome (ARDS) is a disorder of progressive respiratory insufficiency that is relatively refractory to simple oxygen therapy. The basic defect present in patients with ARDS is abnormal permeability of the pulmonary capillary.[13] Left ventricular function and pulmonary capillary wedge pressure are normal. The pulmonary edema that develops is thus "noncardiogenic." Transudation of plasma proteins and red blood cells into the pulmonary interstitium and alveolar spaces results in alveolar flooding. Hypoxemia develops due to significant intrapulmonary shunting. Lung compliance is reduced. Diffuse infiltrates are present on chest radiographs. Severe preeclampsia is a recognized cause of ARDS,[10,39] though the syndrome is more likely to occur in obstetrical patients with sepsis, shock, amniotic fluid embolism, or after aspiration of gastric contents.[1]

The precise mechanism of altered pulmonary capillary permeability in patients with preeclampsia is unclear. Apparently, it is not due to vasospastic endothelial damage, since the pulmonary vasculature is not involved in the vasospastic process of preeclampsia.[7,53] Whatever the mechanism, transudation of protein-rich fluid into the alveolar spaces occurs. Altered capillary permeability is the second leading cause of pulmonary edema complicating preeclampsia.[8]

Indications For and Use of Pulmonary Artery Catheterization

Routine placement of the Swan–Ganz catheter in all patients with severe preeclampsia is difficult to justify, but placement in selected instances can help to optimize care. Pulmonary artery catheterization is useful in patients who require large volumes of fluid or blood products, in those with oliguria, and in those with pulmonary edema.[9,20]

Placement of the pulmonary artery catheter should be performed by a physician with demonstrated proficiency. If this expertise is present in members of the obstetrical team, placement and management may be carried out solely by the obstetrical service.[17] If infrequent catheterizations are performed on a particular service, then placement and management is best performed in the unit with the most experience in the technique. In this situation, close cooperation between intensive care staff and perinatal staff is vital, because each is proficient in different aspects of patient management. Attention also should be paid to nursing personnel. If the obstetrical nursing staff is familiar with central monitoring, then management in the Labor and Delivery area is acceptable. If experience with these techniques is lacking, then the patient will benefit from nursing care in a special care unit or by movement of special care nurses to the Labor and Delivery area.

Fluid and Blood Product Therapy

Most preeclamptic patients, even those with severe disease, may be maintained adequately with a balanced salt solution infused at rates of 75–100 cc/hour. Circumstances surrounding the administration of anesthesia, regional or general, the occurrence of postpartum hemorrhage, disseminated intravascular coagulation, or placental abruption may dictate fluid or blood product administration in excess of this rate. In these circumstances pulmonary artery catheterization is of particular value.

In situations where the right and left heart are subject to different loading characteristics, central venous pressure monitoring may be inadequate for optimal care. This situation holds in a significant portion of patients with severe preeclampsia who demonstrate poor correlation between CVP and PCWP.[21]

In this setting, Swan–Ganz catheterization provides an accurate measure of left ventricular filling pressures. Fluid and blood product administration should be administered at a rate sufficient to keep the PCWP in the 6–8 mmHg range. Concomitant plasma colloid oncotic pressure determination may be beneficial, because a significantly low COP is associated with the occurrence of pulmonary edema in spite of "normal" cardiac filing pressures. Should plasma COP fall below 15 mmHg, consideration should be given to the use of loop diuretics, if PCWP is elevated, or to the infusion of colloids if PCWP is low. This scheme maximizes cardiac performance and the risk of pulmonary edema is lessened.

Oliguria

Oliguria is not uncommon in patients with severe preeclampsia. Oliguria is usually secondary to hypovolemia and thus responds to hydration.[17] However, occasional patients develop oliguria because of peripheral vasospasm and diminished cardiac output secondary to elevated afterload. These conditions are indistinguishable from each other utilizing clinical and laboratory criteria. The underlying etiology may be discovered only by the use of pulmonary artery catheterization. In situations of hypovolemia, low PCWP and hyperdynamic left ventricular function are apparent. In the case of oliguria due to peripheral vasospasm, a normal or elevated PCWP will be found in the presence of marked elevation of systemic vascular resistance and low cardiac output.

If oliguria persists after a bolus of 300–600 cc of normal saline is administered, Swan-Ganz catheterization is recommended. If low PCWP and normal SVR are encountered, cautious hydration therapy may proceed. If CO is diminished and systemic vascular resistance is high, vasodilator therapy as outlined below is indicated. As with other situations of low urinary output, measurement of urinary specific gravity, calculation of fractional sodium excretion and BUN/creatinine ratio are helpful in assessing the cause of oliguria. Acute renal failure rarely complicates preeclampsia in the absence of hemorrhagic complications. Acute tubular necrosis or, more uncommonly, bilateral renal cortical necrosis may occur. In these situations pulmonary artery catheterization may be of benefit in the initial stabilization of the patient.

Pulmonary Edema

The occurrence of pulmonary edema in a severe preeclamptic is a medical emergency. Supportive measures, including oxygen therapy, rotating tourniquets, and morphine should be provided immediately. Furosemide administered intravenously in a bolus of 40–80 mg is recommended, both for its diuretic activity and for its immediate venodilatory effect. Intake and output in the preceding hours should be reviewed. In most cases excess fluid administration is evident, and a provisional diagnosis of overload can be made. Pulmonary artery catheterization should be utilized for diagnostic and therapeutic reasons.

After placing the pulmonary artery catheter COP, PCWP, and COP-PCWP gradients may be determined. This information, in concert with determination of cardiac output, systemic vascular resistance, and left ventricular stroke volume, should help to determine the etiology of the pulmonary edema. Arterial line placement is useful, because frequent blood gas determination and other blood samples generally are needed. Should vasodilator therapy be necessary, it is mandatory.

Pulmonary edema due to fluid overload can be recognized by a low colloid oncotic pressure (generally less than 16 mmHg) and high normal or moderately elevated pulmonary capillary wedge pressure (12–18 mmHg), in the presence of normal cardiac output. Diuretic therapy and fluid restriction are usually adequate to restore physiology. Because of the propensity to elevate preload further and the possibility of concomitant pulmonary capillary permeability changes, colloid containing solutions are not recommended.

Adult respiratory distress syndrome and/or rapidly progressive hypoxemia in preeclampsia are diagnosed as outlined above. Rapidly progressive hypoxemia must be treated aggressively. Diuretic therapy is useful in lowering PCWP to the 2–6 mmHg range to eliminate the possibility of elevated hydrostatic pressure contributing to further edema formation. The mainstay of treatment for ARDS is ventilator therapy with concomitant application of positive end-expiratory pressure (PEEP).[30] PEEP levels of 15–20 mmHg, or even higher, are occasionally necessary to provide adequate oxygenation. At these levels, cardiac output may fall due to impairment of venous return to the heart. Pulmonary artery catheterization provides immediate documentation of any adverse effect of ventilation therapy on cardiac function. Furthermore, it helps to guide fluid therapy to assure that the preload is sufficient.

Occasionally, pulmonary edema occurs secondary to hypertensive cardiac dysfunction. As noted above, most instances represent mechanical overload of a previously normal ventricle by extremely elevated afterload. Pulmonary artery catheter parameters reveal low cardiac output, high levels of SVR (usually greater than 2000–2200 dyne • sec • cm^{-5}) and elevated PCWP.[72] It is emphasized that the level of vasospasm present may not be reflected by an elevation of blood pressure in this setting. Elevated afterload may depress ventricular function so severely that patients are normotensive or even hypotensive. Vasodilator therapy is the key to management of hypertensive cardiac dysfunction. Rapid digitalization is recommended by most authorities, but it is likely that the benefit from inotropic agents is not great. Vasodilators, by decreasing ventricular afterload, shift the cardiac function curve upward and to the left.[18,19] The normal, but overloaded, left ventricle responds rapidly to removal of the overload.[71]

Hydralazine, used either in intermittent boluses or by continuous intravenous infusion, has been used successfully as a vasodilator in obstetrics for many years. It acts directly on arteriolar smooth muscle to increase blood flow in the coronary, cerebral, splanchnic, and renal beds to a greater extent than it increases flow to skeletal muscle and skin.[40] Hydralazine exerts minimal effect on venous capacitance vessels. Uterine perfusion, in the absence of hypotension, is either unaffected or increased by hydralazine.

The use of sodium nitroprusside in obstetrics has been limited, mainly due to uncertainty regarding potential fetal toxicities of its metabolites, cyanide and thiocyanate.[71] For this reason, it is recommended that antepartum use be limited to the stabilization of patients with life-threatening emergencies due to severe arteriolar vasospasm, prior to operative delivery.

Advantages of nitroprusside therapy include rapid onset of action (2–3 min), rapid loss of activity with cessation of infusion (generally within 5 minutes), and the fact that both arteriolar and venous capacitance vessels are affected. Therapy is begun at a rate of 0.5 μg/kg/min and titrated upward as necessary to a maximal rate of 10 μg/kg/min. Adequate therapeutic response generally is attained at levels of 3–4 μg/kg/min.[51] Cyanide toxicity is a potential complication of nitroprusside therapy. Circulating cyanide is metabolized in the liver to thiocyanate by hepatic rhodanase. Hepatic dysfunction in severe preeclampsia theoretically may lower the therapeutic margin of safety. Cyanide intoxication is accompanied by mental status changes, muscular spasms, and a rapidly progressive metabolic acidosis. Therapy for cyanide intoxication involves the use of nitrates that induce the formation of methemoglobin to which the cyanide ion is tightly bound.

Pulmonary artery catheterization and continuous arterial blood pressure monitoring are mandatory for the effective use of nitroprusside therapy. The initial response of the dysfunctional ventricle to the vasodilating agent may be signaled by a paradoxic rise in arterial blood pressure.

REFERENCES

1. Anderson, H. F., Lynch, J. P., and Johnson, T. R. B.: Adult respiratory distress syndrome in obstetrics and gynecology. *Obstet. Gynecol.* **55**:291–295, 1980.
2. Applefield, J. J., Caruthers, T. E., Reno, D. J., and Civetta, J. M.: Assessment of the sterility of long-term cardiac catheterization using the thermodilution Swan–Ganz catheter. *Chest* **74**:377–380, 1978.
3. Assali, N. S. and Vaughn, D. L.: Blood volume in pre-eclampsia: Fantasy and reality. *Am. J. Obstet. Gynecol.* **129**:355–359, 1977.
4. Bader, R. A., Bader, M. E., Rose, D. J., and Braunwald, E.: Hemodynamics at rest and during exercise in normal pregnancy as studied by cardiac catheterization. *J. Clin. Invest.* **34**:1524–1536, 1955.
5. Barash, P. G., Nardi, D., Hammond, G., Walker-Smith, G., Capuano, D., Laks, H., Kopriva, C. J., Baue, A. E., and Geha, A. S.: Catheter induced pulmonary artery perforation: Mechanisms, management and modifications. *J. Thorac. Cardiovasc. Surg.* **82**:5–12, 1981.
6. Benedetti, T. J. and Carlson, R. W.: Studies of colloid osmotic pressure in pregnancy-induced hypertension. *Am. J. Obstet. Gynecol.* **135**:308–311, 1979.
7. Benedetti, T. J., Cotton, D. B., Read, J. C., and Miller, F. C.: Hemodynamic observations in severe pre-eclampsia with a flow-directed pulmonary artery catheter. *Am. J. Obstet. Gynecol.* **136**:465–470, 1980.
8. Benedetti, T. J., Kates, R., and Williams, V.: Hemodynamic observations in severe preeclampsia complicated by pulmonary edema. *Am. J. Obstet. Gynecol.* **152**:330–334, 1985.
9. Berkowitz, R. L. and Rafferty, T. D.: Invasive hemodynamic monitoring in critically ill pregnant patients: Role of Swan–Ganz catheterization. *Am. J. Obstet. Gynecol.* **137**:127–134, 1980.
10. Berkowitz, R. L. and Rafferty, T. D.: Pulmonary

artery flow-directed catheter use in the obstetric patient. *Obstet. Gynecol.* **55**:507–510, 1980.
11. Blekta, M., Hlavaty, V., Trnkova, M., Bendl, J., Bendova, L., and Chytil, M.: Volume of whole blood and absolute amount of serum proteins in the early stage of late toxemia of pregnancy. *Am. J. Obstet. Gynecol.* **106**:10–13, 1970.
12. Braunwald, E.: Determinants and assessment of cardiac function. *N. Engl. J. Med.* **296**:86–89, 1977.
13. Brigham, K. L.: Mechanisms of lung injury. *Clin. Chest Med.* **3**:9–24, 1982.
14. Buchbinder, N. and Ganz, W.: Hemodynamic monitoring: Invasive techniques. *Anesthesiology* **45**:146–155, 1976.
15. Chesley, L. C.: Plasma and red cell volumes during pregnancy. *Am. J. Obstet. Gynecol.* **112**:440–450, 1972.
16. Civetta, J. M.: A new look at the Starling equation. *Crit. Care Med.* **7**:84–91, 1979.
17. Clark, S. L., Horenstein, J. M., Phelan, J. P., Montag, T. W., and Paul, R. H.: Experience with the pulmonary artery catheter in obstetrics and gynecology. *Am. J. Obstet. Gynecol.* **152**:374–378, 1985.
18. Cohn, J. N. and Franciosa J. A.: Vasodilator therapy of cardiac failure (first of two parts). *N. Engl. J. Med.* **297**:27–31, 1977.
19. Cohn, J. N. and Franciosa, J. A.: Vasodilator therapy of cardiac failure. (second of two parts) *N. Engl. J. Med.* **297**:254–258, 1977.
20. Cotton, D. B. and Benedetti, T. J.: Use of the Swan–Ganz catheter in obstetrics and gynecology. *Obstet. Gynecol.* **56**:641–645, 1980.
21. Cotton, D. B., Gonik, B., Dorman, K., and Harrist, R.: Cardiovascular alterations in severe pregnancy-induced hypertension: Relationship of central venous pressure to pulmonary capillary wedge pressure. *Am. J. Obstet. Gynecol.* **151**:762–764, 1985.
22. Cotton, D. B., Gonik, B., Spillman, T., and Dorman, K. F.: Intrapartum to postpartum changes in colloid osmotic pressure. *Am. J. Obstet. Gynecol.* **149**:174–177, 1984.
23. Elliott, C. G., Zimmerman, G. A., and Clemmer, T. P.: Complications of pulmonary artery catheterization in the care of critically ill patients: A prospective study. *Chest* **76**:647–652, 1979.
24. Fibuch E. E. and Tuohy, G. F.: Intracardiac knotting of a flowdirected balloon-tipped catheter. *Anesth. Analg.* **59**:217–219, 1980.
25. Foote, G. A., Schabel, S. I., and Hodges, M.: Pulmonary complications of the flow-directed balloon-tipped catheter. *N. Engl. J. Med.* **290**:927–931, 1974.
26. Forrester, J. S., Diamond, G., Chatterjee, K., and Swan, H. J. C.: Medical therapy of acute myocardial infarction by application of hemodynamic subsets. *N. Engl. J. Med.* **295**:1356–1362, 1976.
27. Forrester, J. S., Diamond, G., Chatterjee, K., and Swan, H. J. C.: Medical therapy of acute myocardial infarction by application of hemodynamic subsets. *N. Engl. J. Med.* **295**:1404–1413, 1976.
28. Gallery, E. D. M., Hunyor, S. N., and Gyory, A. Z.: Plasma volume contraction: A significant factor in both pregnancy-associated hypertension (preeclampsia) and chronic hypertension in pregnancy. *Q. J. Med.* **192**:593–602, 1979.
29. Gant, N. F., Daley, G. L., Chand, S., Whalley, P. J., and MacDonald, P. C.: A study of angiotensin II pressor response throughout primigravid pregnancy. *J. Clin. Invest.* **52**:2682–2689, 1973.
30. Gong, H.: Positive-pressure ventilation in the adult respiratory distress syndrome. *Clin. Chest Med.* **3**:69–85, 1982.
31. Gonik, B., Cotton, D., Spillman, T., Abouleish, E., and Zavisca, F.: Peripartum colloid osmotic pressure changes: Effects of controlled fluid management. *Am. J. Obstet. Gynecol.* **151**:812–815, 1985.
32. Goodlin, R., Kurpershoek, C., and Hesslein H.: Colloid osmotic pressure changes during hypertensive pregnancy. *Clin. Exp. Hyper. (B)* **1**:49–56, 1982.
33. Grossman, W., Jones, D., and McLaurin, L. P.: Wall stress and patterns of hypertrophy in the human left ventricle. *J. Clin. Invest.* **56**:56–64, 1975.
34. Hankins, G. D., Wendel, G. D., Cunningham, F. G., and Leveno, K. J.: Longitudinal evaluation of hemodynamic changes in eclampsia. *Am. J. Obstet. Gynecol.* **150**:506–512, 1984.
35. Hays, P. M., Cruikshank, D. P., and Dunn, L. J.: Plasma volume determination in normal and preeclamptic pregnancies. *Am. J. Obstet. Gynecol.* **151**:958–966, 1985.
36. Henderson, D. W., Vilos, G. A., Milne, K. J., and Nichol, P. M.: The role of Swan–Ganz catheterization in severe pregnancy-induced hypertension. *Am. J. Obstet. Gynecol.* **148**:570–574, 1984.
37. Hood, W. P., Rackley, C. E., and Rolett, E. L.: Wall stress in the normal and hypertrophied human left ventricle. *Am. J. Cardiol.* **22**:550–558, 1968.
38. Katz, R., Karliner, J. S., and Resnik, R.: Effects of a natural volume overload state (pregnancy) on left ventricular performance in normal human subjects. *Circulation* **58**:434–441, 1978.
39. Keefer, J. R., Strauss, R. G., Civetta, J. M., and Burke, T.: Noncardiogenic pulmonary edema and invasive cardiovascular monitoring. *Obstet. Gynecol.* **58**:46–51, 1981.
40. Koch-Weser, J.: Hydralazine. *N. Engl. J. Med.* **295**:320–323, 1976.
41. Kuzniar, J., Peila, A., and Skret, A.: Left ventricular function in preeclamptic patients: An echocardiographic study. *Am. J. Obstet. Gynecol.* **146**:400–405, 1983.
42. Larkin, H., Gallery, E. D. M., Hunyor, S. N., Gyory, A. Z., and Boyce, E. S.: Cardiac and hemodynamic measurements in hypertensive pregnancy. *Clin. Sci.* **59**:357s–360s, 1980.

43. Lim, Y. L. and Walters, W. A. W.: Systolic time intervals in normotensive and hypertensive human pregnancy. *Am. J. Obstet. Gynecol.* **126**:26–32, 1976.
44. MacGregon, D. C., Covell, J. W., Mahler, F., Dilley, R. B. and Ross, J.: Relations between afterload, stroke volume, and descending limb of Starling's curve. *Am. J. Physiol.* **227**:884–890, 1974.
45. McCullagh, W. H., Covell, J. W., and Ross, J.: Left ventricular dilatation and diastolic compliance changes during chronic volume overloading. *Circulation* **45**:943–951, 1972.
46. McDaniel, D. D., Stone, J. G., Faltas, A. N., Khambatta, H. J., Thys, D. M., Antunes, A. M., and Bregman, D.: Catheter induced pulmonary artery hemorrhage: Diagnosis and management in cardiac operations. *J. Thorac. Cardiovasc. Surg.* **82**:1–4, 1981.
47. Mellins, R. B., Levine, O. R., Skalak, R., and Fishman, A. P.: Interstitial pressure of the lung. *Circ. Res.* **24**:197–212, 1969.
48. Metcalfe, J. and Ueland, K.: Maternal cardiovascular adjustments to pregnancy. *Prog. Cardiovasc. Dis.* **16**:363–374, 1974.
49. Nisell, H., Hjendahl, P., Linde, B., and Lunell, N.: Sympathoadrenal and cardiovascular reactivity in pregnancy-induced hypertension. *Am. J. Obstet. Gynecol.* **152**:554–560, 1985.
50. Pace, N. L.: A critique of flow-directed pulmonary arterial catheterization. *Anesthesiology* **47**:455–465, 1977.
51. Palmer, R. F. and Lasseter, K. C.: Sodium nitroprusside. *N. Engl. J. Med.* **292**:294–297, 1975.
52. Phelan, J. P. and Yurth, D. A.: Severe preeclampsia. I. Peripartum hemodynamic observations. *Am. J. Obstet. Gynecol.* **144**:17–22, 1982.
53. Rafferty, T. D. and Berkowitz, R. L.: Hemodynamics in patients with severe toxemia during labor and delivery. *Am. J. Obstet. Gynecol.* **138**:263–270, 1980.
54. Robertson, E. G. and Cheyne, G. A.: Plasma biochemistry in relation to oedema of pregnancy. *J. Obstet. Gynaecol. Br. Commonw.* **79**:769–776, 1972.
55. Robin, E. D., Cross, C. E., and Zelis, R.: Pulmonary edema. *N. Engl. J. Med.* **288**:239–246, 1973.
56. Rosenbaum, L., Rosenbaum, S. H., Askanazi, J., and Hyman, A. I.: Small amounts of hemoptysis as an early warning sign of pulmonary artery rupture by a pulmonary artery catheter. *Crit. Care Med.* **9**:319–320, 1981.
57. Ross, J.: Afterload mismatch and preload reserve: A conceptual framework for the analysis of ventricular function. *Prog. Cardiovasc. Dis.* **18**:255–264, 1976.
58. Ross, J. and Braunwald, E.: The study of left ventricular function in man by increasing resistance to ventricular ejection with angiotensin. *Circulation* **29**:739–748, 1964.
59. Rovinsky, J. J. and Jaffin, H.: Cardiovascular hemodynamics in pregnancy. I. Blood and plasma volumes in multiple pregnancy. *Am. J. Obstet. Gynecol.* **93**:1–13, 1965.
60. Rovinsky, J. J. and Jaffin, H.: Cardiovascular hemodynamics in pregnancy II: Cardiac output and left ventricular work in multiple pregnancy. *Am. J. Obstet. Gynecol.* **95**:781–786, 1966.
61. Rovinsky, J. J. and Jaffin, H.: Cardiovascular hemodynamics in pregnancy. III. Cardiac rate, stroke volume, total peripheral resistance, and central blood volume in multiple pregnancy. Synthesis of results. *Am. J. Obstet. Gynecol.* **95**:787–794, 1966.
62. Roy, S. B., Malkani, P. K., Virik, R., and Bhatia, M. L.: Circulatory effects of pregnancy. *Am. J. Obstet. Gynecol.* **96**:221–225, 1966.
63. Rubler, S., Damani, P. M., and Pinto, E. R.: Cardiac size and performance during pregnancy estimated with echocardiography. *Am. J. Cardiol.* **40**:534–540, 1977.
64. Sasayama, S., Ross, J., Franklin, D., Bloor, C. M., Bishop, S., and Dilley, R. B.: Adaptations of the left ventricle to chronic pressure overload. *Circ. Res.* **38**:172–178, 1976.
65. Sise, M. J., Hollingsworth, P., Brimm, J. E., Peters, R. M., Virgilio, R. W., and Shackford, S. R.: Complications of the flow-directed pulmonary-artery catheter: A prospective analysis in 219 patients. *Crit. Care Med.* **9**:315–318, 1981.
66. Soffronoff, E. C., Kaufman, B. M., and Connaughton, J. F.: Intravascular volume determinations and fetal outcome in hypertensive diseases of pregnancy. *Am. J. Obstet. Gynecol.* **127**:4–9, 1977.
67. Sonnenblick, E. H. and Strobeck, J. E.: Derived indexes of ventricular and myocardial function. *N. Engl. J. Med.* **296**:978–982, 1977.
68. Sprung, C. L., Jacobs, L. J., Caralis, P. V., and Karpf, M.: Ventricular arrhythmias during Swan-Ganz catheterization of the critically ill. *Chest* **79**:413–415, 1981.
69. Staub, N. C.: The pathophysiology of pulmonary edea. *Hum. Physiol.* **1**:419–432, 1970.
70. Stein, L., Beraud, J., Morissette, M., DaLuz, P., Weil, M. H., and Shubin, H.: Pulmonary edema during volume infusion. *Circulation* **52**:483–489, 1975.
71. Stempel, J. E., O'Grady, J. P., Morton, M. J., and Johnson, K. A.: Use of sodium nitroprusside in complications of gestational hypertension. *Obstet. Gynecol.* **60**:533–538, 1982.
72. Strauss, R. G., Keefer, J., Burke, T., and Civetta, J. M.: Hemodynamic monitoring of cardiogenic pulmonary edema complicating toxemia of pregnancy. *Obstet. Gynecol.* **55**:170–174, 1980.
73. Swan, H. J. C.: The role of hemodynamic monitoring in the management of the critically ill. *Crit. Care Med.* **3**:83–89, 1975.
74. Swan, H. J. C., Ganz, W., Forrester, J., Marcus, H., Diamond, G., and Chonette, D.: Catheterization of the heart in man with use of a flow-

directed balloon-tipped catheter. *N. Engl. J. Med.* **283**:447–451, 1970.

75. Toussaint, G. P. M., Burgess, J. H., and Hampson, L. G.: Central venous pressure and pulmonary wedge pressure in critical surgical illness. *Arch. Surg.* **109**:265–268, 1974.
76. Ueland, K. and Hansen., J. M.: Maternal cardiovascular dynamics. III. Labor and delivery under local and caudal analgesia. *Am. J. Obstet. Gynecol.* **103**:8–18, 1969.
77. Veille, J. C., Hosenpud, J. D., Morton, M. J., and Welch, J. E.: Cardiac size and function in pregnancy-induced hypertension. *Am. J. Obstet. Gynecol.* **150**:443–449, 1984.
78. Weil, M. H., Henning, R. J., and Puri, V. K.: Colloid oncotic pressure: Clinical significance. *Crit. Care Med.* **7**:113–116, 1979.

PART IV

Medical–Legal Considerations

50

MEDICAL–LEGAL CONSIDERATIONS IN CLINICAL OBSTETRICS

In America today, a medical malpractice lawsuit is one of the greatest threats to a physician's career. If a doctor produces results that deviate even slightly from the patient's expectations, a liability action against the doctor becomes a distinct possibility. Never before have society's expectations been so high and malpractice actions so numerous. In Cook County, Illinois, in 1984 alone, 2047 medical malpractice actions were initiated.[9]

Since the 1930s, claims against the medical profession have proliferated—a development that parallels the expansion of modern medicine and the growth of sophisticated technology. Along with these new, complex medical and technical advancements came an expansive list of new risks of injury to the patient. Ironically, this progress also caused society to expect perfection in the medical field—hence the burgeoning of medical malpractice claims.

Apace with the multiplying malpractice suits was a drastic increase in the amount of money damages being awarded to the injured party. Today, million-dollar payouts are not uncommon. Consequently, physicians' costs for professional liability insurance have risen to prohibitive levels. Moreover, insurers are discovering that it is no longer profitable to provide medical malpractice insurance, and many are therefore withdrawing from that marketplace.

The decrease in the availability of medical liability insurance caused the profession to suffer its first "crisis" in 1974. An outgrowth of this crisis was doctor or hospital-sponsored insurance companies, which now comprise 60% of the malpractice market.[17] Although these new companies facilitated efforts to obtain coverage, they could do little to tame the high premiums. As a result, the medical profession currently is experiencing a new crisis of even more threatening proportions.

Obstetricians are among the doctors hardest hit by the recent crisis. In 1984, the national midpoint verdict award for injuries to newborns was $1,452,000.[8] Statistics such as this have forced some obstetricians to pay premiums totaling $55,000 for one year of coverage.[7] An additional shocking fact is that, nationally, "the incidence of malpractice suits rose in 1983 to 16 suits for every 100 obstetricians, up from five suits in 1975."[7] In light of these statistics, it is not surprising that fewer and fewer medical students are entering the field of obstetrics, while those already in the field are deserting it en masse. Florida, for example, has recently lost one-fourth of its obstetricians.[8]

The purpose of this chapter is to inform the obstetrician of:

1. the basic concepts of medical malpractice litigation,
2. malpractice considerations particular to the obstetrician;
3. ways in which obstetrical malpractice claims can be avoided; and
4. how to anticipate and respond to malpractice lawsuits.

BASIC CONCEPTS OF MEDICAL MALPRACTICE LITIGATION

Every physician must seriously consider the possibility of being implicated in a medical malpractice case. This section focuses on some basic legal concepts that should be studied by the doctor in order to better understand the nature of malpractice litigation.

Medical malpractice is a deviation from accepted standards. The issue to be resolved in a malpractice case is: What would a reasonable health care provider have done under similar circumstances? The particular standard by which this question may be answered is established by "expert" testimony, authoritative textual materials such as package inserts, articles, by-laws, rules and regulations, or by the testimony of the defendant-doctor. The injured party's or plaintiff's burden in a malpractice action is to prove by a "preponderance of the evidence" (more likely true than not—as opposed to more stringent standards such as "beyond a reasonable doubt" as required in most criminal cases) the existence of the following elements:

1. the standard of care;
2. a deviation therefrom;
3. injury; and
4. proximate cause.

The Doctrine of *Res Ipsa Loquitor*

Under the doctrine of *Res Ipsa Loquitor* (the thing speaks for itself), the plaintiff is excused from carrying the burden of proof in a malpractice case. This doctrine is an evidentiary exception that allows the drawing of logical conclusions from circumstantial facts. Its use is permitted only when it is clear that the plaintiff did nothing wrong, the injury would not have existed normally absent negligence on the part of the defendant, and information about the occurrence and control over the situation were exclusively with the defendant. In essence, this doctrine shifts the burden of proof to the defendant. General examples of *Res Ipsa* cases include laparotomy sponge or instrument left in the patient following surgery and surgery performed on the wrong leg.

Although *Res Ipsa* often is alleged in a complaint, rarely will a plaintiff rely solely on this doctrine. The reason for this lack of faith is that courts are aware that medicine is an inexact science. Thus, a physician normally should not be held responsible for even the most serious of complications resulting from his/her medical procedures without some proof of negligence. If *Res Ipsa* were applied using a more flexible standard, the effect would be virtually to deem physicians insurers of perfect health.[6]

Expert Testimony

In negligence actions the plaintiff and defendant usually must prove their case through expert testimony. Experts are necessary in malpractice cases, particularly due to the complex nature of the medical practices involved. If the facts and circumstances are within the common knowledge of the laypersons who compose the jury, expert testimony can be omitted. The issue of whether experts are required in a case is one for the judge to decide.

The general purpose of an expert is to explain to the jury why medical negligence did or did not occur. In theory, the expert should be qualified in the particular medical field which he or she is to testify about. An expert is qualified based on knowledge, skill, experience, and education in the specific area. For example, a licensed and experienced obstetrician should be qualified to testify as to another obstetrician's alleged negligent performance of a cesarean section. In practice, however, courts often permit doctors to testify as experts about medical specialities in which they have little or no training or experience. When confronted with this situation, the opposing attorney should immediately challenge the competency of the expert by motion. Should the expert be permitted to testify anyway, the opposing attorney should then highlight the expert's lack of credentials before the jury, so that the jurors may determine the weight or credence to be given to the testimony accordingly.

Respondeat Superior: Captain of the Ship

Physicians can be held liable for the actions of other health care providers under a general legal theory known as vicarious liability. In order to impose vicarious liability, the existence of an agency or master–servant relationship must be demonstrated. Once such a relationship is established, the legal doctrine of *respondeat superior* (let the master speak) comes into play. Under this doctrine, the physician can be held vicariously liable for negligent acts of employees committed within the scope of their employment.

The doctrine of *respondeat superior* also extends to the operating or delivery room settings through the "borrowed servant" or "captain of the ship" doctrine. This doctrine holds the physician responsible if he instructs or supervises other doctors, nurses, or hospital personnel during the particular medical treatment. Note that the hospital under some circumstances may share liability with the physician under *respondeat superior* principles.

The Statute of Limitations

All physicians should know that laws exist in every state that prevent a malpractice claim from being pursued after the expiration of a certain time period. The laws enacted that work to bar these cases are statutes of limitation. The purpose of these statutes is to prevent the bringing of stale claims. Specifically, public policy mandates that one who incurs liability not be forever vulnerable to suit for the same offense. Rather, claims must be brought while the proofs are still fresh.

In some states the statute of limitations for medical liability begins to run from the date the injury is incurred, whereas in other states the discovery of the injury commences the statute. In a third group of states, which includes Illinois, only after the plaintiff has discovered the injury *and* knows that it was wrongfully caused will the limitations statute begin running.[19] Because injuries caused by doctors may not discovered for years, physicians often are sued long after their last contact with the plaintiff, a result that appears to defeat the purpose behind the statute of limitations. Many states have reacted to this criticism by placing an absolute maximum time period within which the malpractice suit may be brought. For example, in Illinois, a suit based on medical negligence may not be brought more than four years after treatment was rendered.[16] However, exceptions to these remedial statutes often exist when foreign objects are left in the body, or when the doctor has fraudulently concealed the injury from the patient.[16]

Most state statutes of limitations allow special privileges in the case of a minor plaintiff. When a minor is the victim of medical malpractice,the statute ceases (is tolled) until the child reaches majority. Due to the fact that this exception can cause the physician to defend himself as long as 18 years after treatment, states such as Alabama and Iowa have modified their statutes to begin operating at some point before the child reaches majority.

MALPRACTICE AGAINST THE OBSTETRICIAN

The preceding statements focused on general concepts applicable to all medical malpractice actions. Yet obstetrical malpractice is unique from a legal standpoint in many respects. This section will educate the obstetrician about those unique features associated with obstetrical malpractice.

Potential Complaints

The legal duty of an obstetrician extends beyond the patient to the fetus and spouse. Consequently, the obstetrician is exposed to malpractice liability through as many as three potential claimants: the mother, the father, and the child. These claimants often join together in one suit against the physician, each one asserting his/her own independent theories of recovery.

Length of Treatment

The length of treatment is unique to the practice of obstetrics. Care of a pregnant woman typically lasts as long as 40 weeks. This period of treatment can be subdivided into various stages, each of which carries separate and distinct risks. These subdivisions include antepartum care, intrapartum care, postpartum care, and possibly preconceptual care. These stages of treatment and some of the hazards associated with them are discussed below.

Theories of Liability

Negligence. Negligence in the care and treatment of the mother and fetus is the most common theory on which plaintiffs base their complaints against obstetricians. In order to prove a case of negligence, the plaintiff must show:

1. the existence of a legal duty owed to the plaintiff;
2. that this duty was in fact breached by some act or omission which falls below the standard of care;
3. an injury; and

4. that the breach of the duty was the proximate cause of the injury suffered by the plaintiff.[16]

Negligence in the practice of obstetrics can occur at any of the stages of treatment mentioned above. For example, during the antepartum stage, an obstetrician may negligently administer drugs suspected or known to be teratogens to the pregnant mother. Such drugs include phenytoin sodium, thalidomides, doxylamine/ pyridoxine (Bendectin®), and antithyroid drugs.[10] (See Chapter 14.) As a result, the infant may be born defective. Malpractice also may stem from the careless performance or interpretation of amniocentesis during the antepartum period.

Injury to the infant due to faulty obstetrical procedures also may occur intrapartum or postpartum. Negligent induction of labor through oxytocin, improper fetal monitoring, breech deliveries, or cesarean sections are common instances of alleged malpractice during delivery. The failure to order Rho-gam to desensitize the mother's blood after delivery also may form the basis of a malpractice suit. The obstetrician is never really free of risk when caring for the mother and fetus.

The damages that can be considered in a negligence action are:

1. Nature, extent, and duration of the injury.
2. The aggravation of any preexisting ailment or condition.
3. The disability and disfigurement resulting from the injury.
4. The reasonable expense of necessary medical care, treatment, and services received and the present cash value of the reasonable expenses of medical care, treatment, and services reasonably certain to be received in the future.
5. The value of time, earnings, profits, salaries lost and the present cash value of the time, earnings, profits, salaries reasonably certain to be lost in the future.
6. The present cash value of earnings reasonably certain to be lost in the future after the plaintiff has reached the age of (male 21) (female 18).
7. The reasonable expense of necessary help in his home, which has been received as a result of his injury and the present cash value of such expense reasonably certain to be required in the future.[13]

Willful and Wanton Misconduct. Willful and wanton misconduct is a course of action that shows actual or deliberate intention to harm or that, if not intentional shows an utter indifference to or conscious disregard for a person's own safety and the safety of others.[14] Rarely can a plaintiff succeed in proving that a doctor displayed such gross misconduct. However, if the plaintiff is able to prove willful and wanton behavior against the obstetrician, exemplary or punitive damages may be awarded. The purpose of punitive damages is to punish the defendant while simultaneously deterring others from committing a similar offense.

Wrongful Death. Wrongful death actions are based on the premise that a life has been ended which should not have ended. This cause of action is brought by a personal representative of the deceased for the benefit of next of kin (or a widow) for their pecuniary injury.[15] For example, if an infant is born alive but dies in the delivery room as a result of negligence in the cutting of the umbilical cord, a wrongful death action against the obstetrician may be brought by a legal representative of the child's estate (usually a parent).

A more interesting case develops when a wrongful death action is brought on behalf of an unborn fetus. The courts are split as to whether negligence by a physician that causes the death of an unborn fetus is legally compensable. Most courts, however, have recognized this cause of action if the fetus was viable (able to sustain life separate and independent from the mother) at the time of death.[21]

Wrongful Birth. Wrongful birth suits are brought against the physician by the parents of unwanted children. These suits allege that the physician's negligence is the proximate cause of their child's birth. Against obstetricians in particular, the claim is premised on the negligent failure to inform the parents of the possibility of their bearing a severely defective child. The parents further argue that had they been so informed, they would have obtained an abortion.

The case of *Goldberg* v. *Ruskin* is a prime example of a successful wrongful birth suit. Here the physician failed to inform the parents of the risk of Tay-Sachs disease and that testing procedures were available that could detect the disease. The court held that a cause of action did in fact exist.[11] The Goldberg case, along with other successful wrongful birth cases, magnifies the importance of performing proper prenatal testing and maintaining good obstetrician–patient communications.

Wrongful Life. A relatively new cause of action that has yet to be fully recognized in more than two states across the country is wrongful life. A wrongful life suit involves a minor's claim that, had the physician properly informed the parents of the possibility of their bearing a severely defective child, the minor would never have been born.

Wrongful life is "the child's equivalent of the parents' wrongful birth action."[12] Yet, although wrongful birth has received nationwide acceptance, wrongful life actions have been widely rejected.[12]

California became the first state to recognize the right of a child born with a hereditary affliction to bring a cause of action against the physician who negligently advised the parents regarding the possibility of the hereditary condition, thereby depriving them of the right to abort the child.[20] Because of the difficulty in comparing the value of impaired life to nonlife, general damages were not awarded in either the wrongful life cause of action or the wrongful birth cause of action. However, the court did award the child and his parents recovery of the extraordinary expenses to be incurred during the child's lifetime, with the condition that both the parents and the child could not recover for the same expenses. A short time after this case, the Supreme Court of Washington upheld a cause of action for wrongful life.[12]

Such widespread rejection of this theory is based primarily on two grounds. First, it is impossible to decide whether the child has suffered an injury in being born impaired, rather than not being born. Second, it is difficult to determine a measure of damages. How can a court measure the difference in value "between life in an impaired condition and nonexistence?"[11]

Malpractice Liability at the Preconception Stage

The area of preconceptional liability differs from the typical prenatal case in that the former involves a plaintiff who was not in existence at the time of the wrongful conduct. The Illinois Supreme Court in 1977 upheld such an action in the case of *Renslow* v. *Mennonite Hospital.*[18] In this case, the plaintiff mother alleged that back in 1965 when she was 13 years old, the physician negligently gave her an Rh-positive blood transfusion, thereby sensitizing her Rh-negative blood. She further alleged that this act caused her child (born in 1974) to suffer permanent damage to his brain and nervous system. The court held that there was a right to be born "free from prenatal injuries forseeably caused by a breach of duty to the child's mother."

The effect of the *Renslow* decision on the practice of obstetrics is significant in that it adds to the already expansive list one more way an obstetrician can be brought into court. It also has the effect of avoiding the statute of limitations for certain acts or omissions. Thus, a failure to give the mother Rho-gam after the birth of her first child may lead to a malpractice action against the obstetrician 10 years later by a second child who suffers from physical abnormalities as a result of isoimmunization.

CAUTIONARY MEASURES THAT CAN BE FOLLOWED IN ORDER TO AVOID MALPRACTICE

Although a malpractice claim poses a significant threat to any medical practice today, certain precautions that may help avoid liability can be incorporated into a practice. This section sets forth some of those cautionary measures.

Maintain Good Communication and Good Rapport with the Patient

With the increasing sophistication of modern medicine and the advent of impersonal mechanisms such as HMOs, preferred providers, and diagnosis-related groups, the relationship with the patient has suffered. Therefore, improving and maintaining effective and constant communication and a healthy rapport with the pregnant woman, her spouse (if one exists), and other involved family members (if any) are of primary importance in an attempt to avoid a malpractice claim.

The obstetrician can achieve good doctor–patient rapport by displaying the appropriate attitude toward his or her patient. Amiability and understanding should be expressed. Never ignore questions the mother may have or any pains she may be experiencing. It is much more difficult to sue a doctor who has projected genuine respect and caring for the patient and her family.

Informed Consent. Good communication with the patient and family has traditionally included providing them with the relevant information pertaining to the condition of the mother and fetus (or baby), any treatments they might undergo, and the risks associated with the treatments. Consistent with this tradition, the law has developed a doctrine referred to as informed consent, that actually imposes a duty on the physician to disclose certain information. Generally, this doctrine requires that the physician inform patients of their condition, possible alternative treatments available, the monetary costs of each treatment, the risks associated with each treatment, and projected results. The physician must make sure that all involved fully comprehend the nature of the condition. Any misconceptions must be corrected immediately. It is very important that all communications be recorded in the medical record.

Once the above information is imparted, the patient can then make an educated decision as to which treatment she desires. A written consent form should be signed by the patient, doctor, and one witness, and dated, after a decision has been reached. Note that the best evidence that informed consent was obtained is the recordings in the medical records and not the form itself. Only then have the duties required by the doctrine been satisfied. Failure to communicate relevant information prior to obtaining the patient's consent may be actionable medical negligence.

Maintain Up-to-Date and Detailed Records for Each Patient

There is no better evidence that quality care was received by a patient than the medical record. Similarly, a poorly maintained record is strong ammunition for the plaintiff in proving that the care she received was well below the accepted standards. Thus, the medical record is of paramount importance in physician care.

The purpose of medical documentation is twofold:

1. It is the primary method of communication among treating physicians and other members of the health care team.
2. It preserves a written record of treatment rendered, the procedures used, the problems confronted, all findings, the overall management plan, and the patient's reactions, attitudes, and complaints.

According to the American College of Obstetricians and Gynecologists a "good" record should display the following six characteristics:

1. *Accuracy.* This includes using clear and consistent terminology and abbreviations, as well as noting all treatment rendered, with dates, times, and the physician's signature.
2. *Objectivity.* This requires that notations be limited to clinical facts and judgments.
3. *Legibility.*
4. *Timeliness.* Do not procrastinate in making notations, as other medical providers depend on the record in adjusting their own treatment of the patient.
5. *Comprehensiveness.* A good record will contain the following:
   a. Notes concerning the history of the patient and all physical examinations
   b. Progress notes
   c. Consent forms
   d. Laboratory tests and results
   e. A record of all pertinent correspondence and communications with other medical personnel and with the patient and her family
6. *Unaltered.* Never erase an entry (a simple line through the mistake, followed by the date and the physician's initials will do) and do not attempt to change or destroy the record. Such action would only serve to undermine the credibility of the doctor in the minds of the judge and/or jury.[3]

Communicate on a Frequent Basis with Other Medical Personnel Contributing to the Care of the Patient

It is essential that all members of a health care team communicate with one another on a consistent and frequent basis. The most efficient method of ensuring that vital information passes among them is through the medical record (discussed above). Documentation of all orders, instructions, and clinical facts and judgments will prevent inconsistent or incorrect care from being given to the patient. However, reliance on the medical record as the primary method of communicating naturally requires that all personnel always consult the record prior to rendering any type of treatment to the patient. Note that one of the largest verdicts in

Illinois medical malpractice history featured a physician who testified at his deposition that he never bothered to read nursing notes or medicine orders.[4]

Use the Prenatal Period to Identify Potential Complications

The prenatal period allows the obstetrician to discover potential problems that may arise during the intrapartum or postpartum periods. Often these complications may be detected simply by obtaining a complete medical history of the parents, performing proper physical examinations of the mother and fetus throughout pregnancy, and maintaining effective doctor–patient communication. Certain information received may indicate that the patient is predisposed to a specific problem. If the obstetrician is lucky enough to discover this at an early state, the proper monitoring and course of treatment can begin immediately. Such early detection and close monitoring can alleviate many of the pressures associated with later discovery that are experienced by the patient as well as the physician. Moreover, early detection of future complications provides the obstetrician with ample time to assure that his care and treatment are consistent with the standard of care.

Prenatal testing is also important in discovering possible complications. All test results must be *read* and *interpreted* by qualified medical personnel. Failure to assess properly the conditions of the mother and fetus during the period of obstetrical care provides strong grounds for a successful malpractice suit against the obstetrician.

Remain Up-to-Date with All Medical Advances

All physicians should educate themselves on a frequent basis concerning all new medical procedures and technologies. Failure to keep up with the state of the art may be cause for a malpractice action. Many state medical associations and other medical groups offer seminars designed to keep the doctor well informed.

ANTICIPATING AND RESPONDING TO MALPRACTICE LAWSUIT

In today's litigious society, an obstetrician can expect to be named as a defendant in a malpractice lawsuit at least once during his or her career. Whether or not the plaintiff's claim is meritorious, the physician should know how to respond. An inappropriate reaction at any stage after receiving the summons could have a negative impact on the outcome of the case.

In anticipation of being involved in a malpractice suit, all physicians should obtain adequate medical liability insurance as soon as possible after entering the profession. Professional liability insurance protects against "legal liability due to negligence for failure to use due care and the degree of skill expected of a person in that profession."[1]

The physician should definitely shop around for the best insurance policy. In determining which policy is best suited to his or her needs, cost, along with the following factors, should be considered:

1. Insurer's obligations include payment for injury (or damages) subject to policy limits plus defense costs.
2. The written consent of the insured before settling claims.
3. Coverage for acts or omissions committed by any person for whom the insured is legally responsible.
4. A provision to pay for medical expenses incurred by a patient without any admission of fault on the part of the insured (this may be referred to by some insurers as an emergency medical fund, which provides payment without admission of guilt up to a maximum of $10,000).
5. Office or office-related coverage.[1]

A doctor should also be cognizant of the difference between Claims-Made policies and Occurrence policies. A Claims-Made agreement provides coverage only for claims reported to the insured during the policy year. Occurrence policies differ in that the date the claim is filed or reported is irrelevant. Rather, the significant event is the date of the alleged malpractice. Therefore, if the incident complained of occurred during the policy period, the physician should be covered whenever suit is filed or claim is made (unless, of course, there is some other unsatisfied condition that prevents coverage).

A further precautionary measure that can be taken by the physician is the purchase of excess insurance. The purpose of excess coverage is to guard against the possibility of being liable for monetary damages that exceed the primary insurer's liability limits. Only when a doctor is liable for a sum greater than the amount stipulated in the original insurance policy does excess insurance apply. This added coverage is simply more assurance that the physician will not be forced to satisfy a large money judgment from his or her own pocket. Because courts today do not hesitate to assess damages against an obstetrician of more than one million dollars, excess insurance should be given serious consideration.

Once a summons is received, the physician is thereafter on notice that he or she is being sued. The remainder of this chapter suggests steps that should be taken in preparation for the trial and during the trial.

Preparing for Trial

Notify the Insurance Carrier. Immediately upon receiving the summons, the physician's insurance carrier should be notified in writing of the claim. A photocopy of the records and a copy of the relevant hospital charts, if available, shuld be furnished to the carrier. If the carrier requests any information, the doctor must cooperate and comply. Most insurance policies contain a provision requiring the insured's full cooperation. The physician should not compound problems by failing to do what is requested.

If the physician has excess insurance, the same notice and level of cooperation should be extended to the second carrier.

Open a File. The physician should maintain a file containing all documents, records, and correspondence relating to the case. These documents may be needed for reference during the case or for insurance purposes.

Get to Know the Attorney. A cooperative and trusting working relationship with the attorney is crucial to a physician's case.

Take an Active Role in the Case. Being a defendant should never be a passive experience. The physician should make sure that the attorney knows all the relevant facts in the case. If the physician should suddenly discover new details the attorney should be notified immediately. Furthermore, the defendant physician should attend the pretrial questioning sessions or depositions of the plaintiff and the plaintiff's expert. Not only will this aid in the doctor's understanding of the nature of his or her alleged offense, but it will allow the attorney and physician to work together in anticipating future obstacles. After hearing the opposing expert's deposition, the physician can also undertake a search for literature, authoritative treatises or other doctors that either will provide additional support for the defense or will refute the plaintiff's position.

Prepare to Give a Deposition. The physician and his or her attorney should discuss the types of question to expect when questioned by the plaintiff's attorney. Demeanor during the session also should be discussed. The case file, medical records, and pertinent medical research or literature should be reviewed prior to attending the deposition.

The Trial

If the case eventually goes to trial, it is important that the physician prepare according to the attorney's instructions. As a defendant, the doctor should be especially concerned with his or her demeanor in the courtroom. Displays of arrogance, disdain, or hostility often will cause the jurors to look on the defendant with disfavor. Rather, a cooperative and professional attitude should be expressed. In addition, a physician should make sure to review all previous statements he or she has given. An inconsistency between trial testimony and a previous statement could seriously harm the defense.

If the physician is going to take the witness stand, the American College of Obstetricians and Gynecologists suggests that the following steps be followed:

1. Walk carefully and calmly to the spot from which you will testify. Speak clearly and audibly; listen carefully to all questions and other statements made. Sit comfortably, but upright, and do not fidget, frown, or grin. Keep all your body movements composed. Answer all questions concisely and accurately, without embellishment. During cross-examination, answer promptly, but allow a moment for your attorney to object if he so wishes. Do not recite your testimony as if it were memorized.
2. As you speak, listen to yourself to assure that your voice is calm and your statements correct. Do not bring to the witness stand notes, records, or documents unless you do not mind their being introduced as evidence in their entirety.

3. Always be completely honest. Do not make self-deprecating jokes or confessions. Try to avoid being tense or defensive during cross-examination. If the plaintiff's lawyer provokes you or makes outrageous remarks, remain calm and dignified and he will appear the ill-mannered individual that he hoped you would be.
4. If you are the defendant, never belittle the plaintiff's injury or pain, even if you think there is none. If you are an expert witness, you will likely be asked about your fee for testimony; answer that you are being reimbursed for your expertise, training, experience, and time.
5. Never attempt to outsmart or manipulate a lawyer. They make their living doing that. You make yours healing people. When your testimony is complete, leave the stand quietly, carefully, and with composure. When back at your seat, do not wince, remark, or respond physically to others' testimony.
6. Finally, always take some time with your attorney to prepare for any conversation, deposition, or trial appearance where you will confront your former patient or her attorney.[2]

CONCLUSION

In the mid-1980s, alleged torts relating to obstetrical care are clearly among the hottest areas for legal scrutiny. The number of cases filed alleging obstetrical negligence is increasing dramatically.

Well-qualified obstetricians have shown a disturbing willingness, nay enthusiasm, to criticize their colleagues in even the most equivocal cases.

Heavily publicized verdicts or settlements of obstetrical care cases guarantee that the high level of legal attention will continue. The huge monetary damages that a newborn can generate over a projected life expectancy of 70-plus years make these cases among the most dangerous in all of our civil justice system.

Obstetricians must be advertent to the increasingly hostile legal atmosphere in which they will work. They also must be sensitive to the legal pitfalls outlined in this chapter.

The specialty of obstetrics has made invaluable contributions to the improvement of maternal and newborn survival. We hope that the concerns shared in this chapter will serve to allow the continuance of the specialty's contributions.

REFERENCES

1. American College of Obstetricians and Gynecologists: The Assistant: Information for Improved Risk Management: Insurance Principles and Policies. Chicago, IL, September 1983.
2. American College of Obstetricians and Gynecologists: The Assistant: Information for Improved Risk Management: Responding to Claims and Lawsuits: The Lawyer, The Deposition, The Trial. Chicago, IL, September 1983.
3. American College of Obstetricians and Gynecologists: The Assistant: Information for Improved Risk Management: Six Elements of Improved Recordkeeping. Chicago, IL, September 1983.
4. *Batteaste* v. *St. Bernard Hospital* et al.: No. 77 L 12460 (tried in the Circuit Court of Cook County, Illinois, May 7, 1984 through June 29, 1984—appeal pending).
5. *Black's Law Dictionary*, 5th Edition. St. Paul, Minnesota, West Publishing Company, 1979, p. 1103.
6. *Carpenter* v. *Campbell*: 149 Ind. App. 189, 271 N.E.2d, 163 (Ind. ct. App. 1971).
7. *Chicago Daily Law Bulletin*, February 14, 1985, p. 3, Col. 1.
8. *Chicago Sun Times*, March 5, 1985, p. 33, Col. 2.
9. *Cook County Jury Verdict*, 1984.
10. Forfar, J.: Epidemiology of drug-induced malformations. *Biochem. Soc. Trans.* **2**:690–695, 1974.
11. *Goldberg* v. *Ruskin*, 128 Ill. App. 3d, 1029, 471 N.E.2d, 530 (First Dist. 1984).
12. *Harbeson* v. *Parke-Davis, Inc.*, 98 Wash. 2d, 460, 656 P.2d 483, 494, 1983.
13. Illinois Pattern Jury Instructions—Civil, 20.00–30.09, 1971.
14. Illinois Pattern Jury Instructions—Civil, 1401, 1971.
15. Illinois Pattern Jury Instructions—Civil, 31.00, 1971.
16. Illinois Revised Statutes, ch. 110, Par. 13-212, 1983.
17. *New York Times*, February 24, 1985, F4, Col. 3.
18. *Renslow* v. *Mennonite Hospital*, 67 111. 2d 348, 367 N.E. 2d, 1250, 1977.
19. *Tabor* v. *Riordan*, 83 Ill. App.3d 900, 403 N.E.2d, 1349 (Second Dist., 1980).
20. *Turpin* v. *Sortini*, 31 Cal. 3d 220, 643 P.2d, 954, 1982.
21. *Wallace* v. *Wallace*, 421 A. 2d 134, 1980.

INDEX